ASTNA
PATIENT TRANSPORT
PRINCIPLES AND PRACTICE

ASTNA
PATIENT TRANSPORT
PRINCIPLES AND PRACTICE

Fourth Edition

Air and Surface Transport Nurses Association

Edited by
Reneé Semonin Holleran, RN, PhD, CEN, CCRN, CFRN, CTRN, FAEN
Former Chief Flight Nurse
University Air Care
Cincinnati, Ohio
Former Manager
Adult Transport Services
Intermountain Life Flight
Salt Lake City, Utah

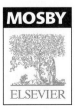

MOSBY

ELSEVIER

3251 Riverport Lane
St. Louis, Missouri 63043

ASTNA Patient Transport: Principles and Practice   ISBN: 978-0-323-05749-3

Notice

Neither the Publisher nor the Editors assume any responsibility for any loss or injury and/or
damage to persons or property arising out of or related to any use of the material contained in
this book. It is the responsibility of the treating practitioner, relying on independent expertise
and knowledge of the patient, to determine the best treatment and method of application for
the patient.

The Publisher

Library of Congress Cataloging-in-Publication Data

ASTNA patient transport : principles and practice / Air and Surface Transport Nurses Association ;
edited by Reneé Semonin Holleran. – 4th ed.
p. ; cm.
Rev. ed. of: Air and surface patient transport / edited by Reneé Semonin Holleran. 3rd ed. c2003.
    Includes bibliographical references and index.
    ISBN 978-0-323-05749-3 (hardcover : alk. paper) 1. Aviation nursing. 2. Transport of sick and
    wounded. 3. Airplane ambulances. I. Holleran, Reneé Semonin. II. Air & Surface Transport
    Nurses Association (U.S.) III. Air and surface patient transport.
    [DNLM: 1. Air Ambulances. 2. Emergency Nursing. 3. Aerospace Medicine. 4. Emergency
    Medical Services. 5. Transportation of Patients. WY 154 A855 2010]
    RC1097.F55 2010
    362.18'8—dc22   2009025489

Managing Editor: Maureen Iannuzzi
Developmental Editor: Laurie Sparks
Publishing Services Manager: Anne Altepeter
Project Manager: Cindy Thoms
Designer: Kim Denando

Printed in United States of America
Last digit is the print number: 9 8 7 6 5 4 3 2

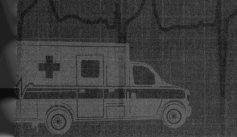

Teri Campbell, RN, BSN, CEN, CFRN
Flight Nurse
University of Chicago Aeromedical Network
University of Chicago
Chicago, Illinois

Wesley Chasteen, NREMT-P, CCEMT-P, FP-C
Flight Paramedic
Education Coordinator
PHI Air Medical of Kentucky
Lexington, Kentucky

Cheryl Erler, MSN, RN
Clinical Assistant Professor
Environments for Health
Indiana University
Indianapolis, Indiana

Michael Frakes, APRN, MS, CCNS, CFRN, CCRN, EMTP
Clinical Nurse Specialist
Boston MedFlight
Boston, Massachusetts

Eileen Frazer, RN, CMTE
Executive Director
Commission on Accreditation of Medical Transport Systems
Anderson, South Carolina

Jonathan D. Gryniuk, FP-C, CCEMT-P, NREMT-P, RRT, CMTE
CAMTS Representative and Past President – International
    Association of Flight Paramedics
Business Manager – Life Net of New York/Guthrie Air
Community Based Services Division
AirMethods Corporation
Albany, New York

Catherine Janson Hesse, RN, MSN, NP
Manager
Emergency Services
Kaiser Permanente
Vallejo, California

Kevin High, RN, MPH, EMT, CFRN
Trauma Program Manager
Department of Emergency Medicine
Vanderbilt Medical Center
Nashville, Tennessee

Sally Houliston, RN, BN, MN
Certified NZ Flight Nurse
Hastings, New Zealand

Timothy L. Hudson, RN, PhD, FACHE
Chief
Hospital Education Division
Martin Army Community Hospital
Fort Benning, Georgia
Lieutenant Colonel
Army Nurse Corps
United States Army

Jill Johnson, RN, MSN, FNP-BC, CCRN, CEN, CFRN
Emergency Department
St. Joseph Hospital
Education/Consultant
Nurse Nerd, Inc.
Lexington, Kentucky

Rose Linsler, RN, BSN, CCRN
Intermountain Healthcare
Life Flight
Salt Lake City, Utah

Katherine Logee, RN, MSN, CPNP, CNE
Flight Nurse
REACH Air Medical Services
Santa Rosa, California
Registered Nurse
CHW Health System
Sacramento, California

Russell D. MacDonald, MD, MPH, FCFP, FRCPC
Medical Director
Research and Development
Ornge Transport Medicine
Attending Staff, Emergency Services
Sunnybrook Health Sciences Centre
Assistant Director and Co-Director, Fellowship Programs
Division of Emergency Medicine
Faculty of Medicine, University of Toronto
Toronto, Ontario, Canada

Kyle Madigan, RN, CFRN, CTRN, CCRN, CEN
Chief Flight Nurse
Dartmouth Hitchcock Advanced Response Team
Dartmouth Hitchcock Medical Center
Lebanon, New Hampshire
President Elect
Air & Surface Transport Nurses Association

Christopher Manacci, MSN, ACNPC, CCRN
Director, ACNP Flight Nursing Program
Frances Payne Bolton School of Nursing
Case Western Reserve University
Lead Nurse Practitioner
Critical Care Transport
Cleveland Clinic
Cleveland, Ohio

Debbie K. Martin, RN, MSN, CCRN, CMTE
Flight Nurse
Spirit Medical Transportation Services
St. Joseph's Hospital – Ministry Health Care
Marshfield, Wisconsin

Heather McLellan, RN, BN, MDE
Emergency Department
Foothills Hospital
Coordinator/Instructor – ACCN Emergency Nursing Program
Advanced Specialty Health Studies
Mount Royal
Calgary, Alberta, Canada

Debra A. Milliner, MSN, MBA/HCM, CEN, CFRN, NREMT-P
Flight Nurse
Care Flight
REMSA
Reno, Nevada

Steven W. Neher, RN, MSN, CEN, CFRN, NREMT-P
Professional Practice Specialist
Division of Transport Medicine
Children's National Medical Center
Washington, DC

Christopher T. Paige, MSN, FNP, BC, CFRN, CEN, NREMT-P
Major
Nurse Corps
Air University – Maxwell Air Force Base
United States Air Force

Carol Rhoades, RN, BSN, CFRN
Nurse Manager
Life Flight
Intermountain Healthcare
Salt Lake City, Utah

Michael Rouse, CRNA, MSN
Visiting Assistant Professor of Clinical Nursing
Department of Adult Health, College of Nursing
University of Cincinnati
CRNA
UAA Anesthesia Department
University Hospital
Cincinnati, Ohio

Scott R. Singel, RN, MSN, ACNP
Flight Nurse
Pegasus Flight Operations
University of Virginia
Charlottesville, Virginia

Stephanie L. Steiner, MSN, ACNP-C, CFRN
Acute Care Nurse Practitioner
Critical Care Transport Services
Cleveland Clinic
Lecturer
Bolton School of Nursing – National Flight Nurse Academy
Case Western Reserve University
Cleveland, Ohio

Leslie C. Sweet, RN, BSN
Mechanical Circulatory Support Device Coordinator
Cardiac Surgery
Washington Hospital Center
Washington, DC

Frank Thomas, MD, MBA
Intermountain Life Flight
Salt Lake City, Utah

Christine Tijerina, RN, MHSc, EMT-B
Clinical Coordinator
Transport Department
Driscoll Children's Hospital
Corpus Christi, Texas

Denise M. Treadwell, MSN, CRNP, CEN, CFRN, CMTE
Executive Vice President
AirMed International, LLC
Birmingham, Alabama
AirMed Asia Company Limited
Hong Kong
AirMed Hawaii, LLC
Honolulu, Hawaii

Allen C. Wolfe, Jr., RN, MSN, CFRN, CCRN
Critical Care Clinical Specialist/Chief Flight Nurse
MedSTAR Transport
Washington Hospital Center
Washington, DC

Gordon H. Worley, RN, CEN, CFRN
Flight Nurse/Clinical Safety Advisor
REACH Air Medical Services
Santa Rosa, California

REVIEWERS

Rebecca D. Baute, RN, BSN, MBA, CMTE
Cincinnati Children's Hospital Medical Center
Cincinnati, Ohio

George J. Brand II, RN, BSN
Lieutenant, United States Navy
Ship's Nurse
USS George Washington, CVN-73

Tony Bright, BS
Air Care & Mobile Care University Hospital
Cincinnati, Ohio

Judi Carpenter, BSN, MSN, APRN
Nursing
Intermountain Healthcare
Life Flight
Salt Lake City, Utah

Lori Carpenter, AAS, RRT
Respiratory Therapist
Intermountain Medical Center
Salt Lake City, Utah

Brian R. Carriere, RN, NREMTP, CFRN, CEN, BA, MDE
Education Team Leader
Alberta Shock Trauma Air Rescue Society
Grande Prairie, Alberta, Canada

Mike Clumpner, BS, MBA, NREMT-P, CCEMT-P, PNCCT, EMT-T, FP-C
Clinical Faculty
Emergency Health Sciences
University of Maryland at Baltimore County
Baltimore, Maryland
Flight Paramedic
Regional One Helicopter
Spartanburg Regional Medical Center
Spartanburg, South Carolina
Fire Captain/Paramedic
Charlotte Fire Department
Charlotte, North Carolina

Topper Cramer, RN, BS, CCRN, CFRN, CTRN, CMTE, NREMT-P
Clinical Nurse Educator
Lifeline Air and Ground Transport Services
The Johns Hopkins Hospital
Baltimore, Maryland

Laura M. Criddle, PhD, RN, CEN, CPEN, CFRN, CCRN, FAEN
Affiliate Faculty
Nursing
Oregon Health & Science University
Portland, Oregon
Clinical Nurse Specialist
The Laurelwood Group
Scappoose, Oregon

Jack B. Davidoff, MD, BCEM, BCDM, EMT-P
Chief Medical Director
Mercy Flight Central, Inc.
Canandaigua, New York

Scott DeBoer, RN, MSN, CEN, CCRN, CPEN, CFRN
Flight Nurse
UCAN
University of Chicago Hospitals
Chicago, Illinois
Transport Nurse
Superior Ambulance Service
Elmhurst, Illinois
Founder
Peds-R-Us Medical Education
Dyer, Indiana

John Delgado, RN, CEN, BSRN, PADI
Virginia Mason Medical Center
Airlift Northwest
University of Washington Medical Center
Seattle, Washington

Bryan S. Dunlop, RN, BSN
Omniflight Helicopters, Inc./Native Air
Mesa, Arizona

Teresa Duquette-Frame, RN, BSN, MBA, CCRN
Lieutenant Colonel, United States Army
Critical Care Flight Nurse
Army Medical Department Center & School
Fort Sam Houston, Texas

Jessica Strohm Farber, MSN, RN, CCRN, CFRN, CMTE
Transport Nurse
Division of Transport Medicine
Children's National Medical Center
Washington, DC

Kathleen Flarity, ARNP, PhD, CFRN, FAEN
Nurse Practitioner
Walk-in Clinic
Wenatchee Valley Medical Center
Wenatchee, Washington
Commander, Lieutenant Colonel, USAFR
34th Aeromedical Evacuation Squadron
Peterson Air Force Base
Colorado Springs, Colorado

Joyce Foresman-Capuzzi, RN, BSN, CEN, CTRN, CCRN, CPN, EMT-P
Clinical Nurse Educator, Emergency Department
The Lankenau Hospital, Main Line Health System
Wynnewood, Pennsylvania

Michael Frakes, APRN, MS, CCNS, CFRN, CCRN, EMTP
Clinical Nurse Specialist
Boston MedFlight
Boston, Massachusetts

Steven D. Glow, MSN, NP, RN, EMT-P, CEN, CFRN
Associate Clinical Professor
College of Nursing
Montana State University
Missoula, Montana

Linda F. Greenberg, RN, BSN, MS, CCRN, CEN, EMT-P
Critical Care Transport Nurse
Boston MedFlight
Bedford, Massachusetts

Colin K. Grissom, MD
Associate Clinical Professor
Pulmonary and Critical Care Division
Department of Internal Medicine
University of Utah
Salt Lake City, Utah
Attending Physician
Critical Care Medicine, Shock Trauma ICU
Assistant Medical Director
Life Flight
Intermountain Medical Center
Murray, Utah

Cindy Hayes, ACS, CFC, OPS Control
LifeFlight
Intermountain Healthcare
Salt Lake City, Utah
NAACS President 2006-2008
National Association of Air Medical Transport Specialists
Nashville, Tennessee

Evelyn Hickman, RN, BSN, CTRN, CEN, NREMT-P
Clinical Supervisor, Children's Transport Team
Children's Health Care of Atlanta
Atlanta, Georgia

Robert L. Howe
Clinical Engineering Supervisor
Intermountain Medical Center
Salt Lake City, Utah

Lori Hutchinson, RN
Grade XVI Survival, Life Flight
Intermountain Healthcare
Salt Lake City, Utah

Jill Johnson, RN, MSN, FNP-BC, CCRN, CEN, CFRN
Emergency Department
St. Joseph Hospital
Education/Consultant
Nurse Nerd, Inc.
Lexington, Kentucky

Kent Johnson, ATP, BS
Chief Pilot
Intermountain Life Flight
Salt Lake City, Utah

David Brian Jones, MSN, ACNP-BC, EMT-P
Acute Care Nurse Practitioner
Cardiothoracic Surgery
Hospital of the University of Pennsylvania
Flight Nurse
PennSTAR Flight
Hospital of the University of Pennsylvania
Philadelphia, Pennsylvania

Kristine A. Karlsen, PhD, NNP-BC
Founder/Author
National Program Director
The S.T.A.B.L.E. Program
Park City, Utah

Patricia M. Kenney, MN, APRN, RNC, FNP-BC
Palmetto Health Richland
Columbia, South Carolina

Sandra Koopman-Bryant, RN, JD, CCRN
Airlift Northwest
Seattle, Washington

Major Debra T. Krupa, RN, MS
Medical Administrative Officer/Deputy Commander
147 Medical Group
147 Reconnaissance Wing
Ellington Field Joint Reserve Base
Texas Air National Guard
Houston, Texas

Gitte Y. Larsen, MD, MPH
Associate Professor
Pediatric Critical Care
University of Utah
Attending Physician, Pediatric Intensive Care Unit
Medical Director of Life Flight Children's
    Transport Services
Co-Chair – Medication Safety, Primary Children's
    Medical Center
Chair – Pediatric Quality Team, Intermountain Health Care
Pediatric Critical Care
Primary Children's Medical Center
Salt Lake City, Utah

Ken Lawson-Williams, CD, BHSc, RN, REMT-P, FP-C
Transport Nurse
Children's Transport Team
Legacy Emanuel Children's Hospital
Portland, Oregon
Critical Care Flight Paramedic
Medflight Air Ambulance
Yellowknife, Northwest Territories

Rose Linsler, RN, BSN, CCRN
Intermountain Healthcare
Life Flight
Salt Lake City, Utah

Katherine Logee, RN, MSN, CPNP, CNE
Flight Nurse
REACH Air Medical Services
Santa Rosa, California
Registered Nurse
CHW Health System
Sacramento, California

Kyle Madigan, RN, CFRN, CTRN, CCRN, CEN
Chief Flight Nurse
Dartmouth Hitchcock Advanced Response Team (DHART)
Dartmouth Hitchcock Medical Center
Lebanon, New Hampshire
President Elect
Air & Surface Transport Nurses Association

Dawn McKevitt, RN, LLB
Clinical Resource Nurse
Alberta Children's Hospital
Calgary, Alberta, Canada

Debra A. Milliner, MSN, MBA/HCM, CEN, CFRN, NREMT-P
Flight Nurse
Care Flight
REMSA
Reno, Nevada

Paris M. Napoli, FP-C, NREMT-P
Paramedic Team Lead
Intermountain Life Flight
Salt Lake City, Utah

Robyn Neely, RN, BS/BSN, EMT-P, CMTE
Assistant Director of Clinical Services/Chief Flight Nurse
MedCenter Air – Carolinas HealthCare System
Charlotte, North Carolina

Christopher A. O'Connell, RN, BSN, CFRN, EMT-B
Colonel, USA Nurse Corps
Dartmouth Hitchcock Advanced Response Team
    (DHART) Program
Dartmouth Hitchcock Medical Center
Lebanon, New Hampshire

Pamela Peterson, RN, MSN, CCRN, CFRN, CEN
Trauma Program Manager/Clinical Nurse Manager
Emergency Services
Providence St. Peter Hospital
Olympia, Washington

Rebecca Pusateri, RN, MSN
AeroCare Medical Transport Systems, Inc.
Sugar Grove, Illinois, and Scottsdale, Arizona

Mark A Randall, RN, BSN, CEN, CCRN, CFRN
Flight Nurse
AirCare
University of Mississippi Health Care
Jackson, Mississippi

Jacqueline C. Stocking, RN, MSN, MBA, CMTE, CEN, CFRN, FP-C, NREMT-P
Air Methods
Englewood, Colorado

Charlotte Thomas, RN, MSN, EMP-P
Outreach Coordinator and New Business Development
MedCenter Air
Carolinas HealthCare System
Charlotte, North Carolina

Renata J. Wheeler, RN, MSN, CEN, CCRN, CFRN, NREMT-P
Clinical Educator
Dartmouth Hitchcock Advanced Response Team
    (DHART) Program
Dartmouth-Hitchcock Medical Center
Lebanon, New Hampshire

Kyle Williams, EMT-P, CCEMT-P, RN, CFRN, CEN
Flight Nurse and Paramedic
Air Methods-Kentucky
Hazard, Kentucky

Bryan Woodford, MSN, MBA, RN, NREMT-P, CMTE
Flight Nurse/Director of Materials Management
The Center for Emergency Medicine (affliated with
  The University of Pittsburgh Medical Center)
  Pittsburgh, Pennsylvania
STAT MedEvac
West Mifflin, Pennsylvania
Career Firefighter/Paramedic
Cumberland Trail Fire District #4
St. Clairsville, Ohio

Jared Worthington, FP-C, NREMT-P
Flight Paramedic
AirMed
University of Utah
HRT Firefighter Paramedic
Salt Lake City Fire Department
Salt Lake City, Utah

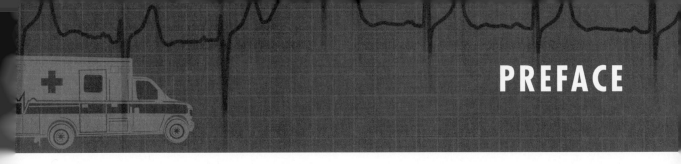

PREFACE

The Air and Surface Transport Nurses Association recognized the need for a comprehensive textbook that provided a foundation for the art and science of transport nursing more than 20 years ago. The first edition of this book was published in 1991 and edited by Genell Lee. Believe it or not, this is the fourth edition of this book and the third one edited by me.

In this edition, we have continued the collaborative focus of the transport process. The care and transport of patients involves multiple persons—nurses, paramedics, physicians, respiratory therapists, communication specialists, pilots, vehicle operators, mechanics, and the communities that support them.

The fourth edition not only contains updates to previous chapters but also the addition of several new chapters. These chapters were added after extensive reviews from experts in the transport field and have been written and reviewed by experienced transport personnel. The new chapters include:

- Airway
- Mechanical Ventilation
- Use of Technology in Transport
- Mechanical Circulatory Support Devices in Transport
- Military Transport

All of the chapters were reviewed by multiple transport specialists representing all of the disciplines that participate in patient transport. Included in many of the chapters are competencies and case studies, just as in previous editions. Some of the case studies are new; others are classic teaching tools and remain the same.

Patient transport cannot be done in a vacuum. It is a collaborative process, one which has recently come under intense scrutiny from many sources, including regulatory, medical, and consumer groups. These are important entities and we must learn to work closely with them to provide the safest and most competent care.

"You must be the change you want to see in the world" (Mahatma Gandhi). The broader-focused we are, the better prepared we are, and the more open to change we are, the better care we can provide to those we serve.

Reneé Semonin Holleran
RN, PhD, CEN, CCRN,
CFRN, CTRN, FAEN

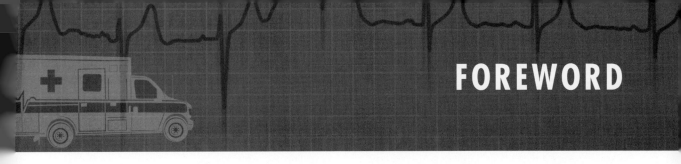

This marks the fourth edition of a textbook originally intended to serve the needs of the National Flight Nurses Association (NFNA) and a small cadre of other professionals interested in the care of patients during transport. Just as the NFNA has grown to be the Air and Surface Transport Nurses Association (ASTNA) in an effort to include and address issues for all nurses involved in patient transport, so also has Principles and Practice grown.

In this edition, the original themes have been expanded to meet the educational and resource needs of all healthcare providers dedicated to expert care delivery in transport.

ASTNA is so appreciative for the unending dedication Reneé Semonin Holleran has given to this effort. Truly, without her passion and expertise, this text would not be a reality.

The ASTNA Board of Directors is thankful for the commitment of those members who have authored chapters—we thank you for your time and expertise. Nurses are the integral key in critical care transport. The work of the authors, reviewers, and contributors demonstrates a dedication to high quality and excellence. We are also grateful to authors from all other medical disciplines for their contributions to this work.

In closing, a wish for all involved in the care of the sick and injured in transport: pursue excellence daily, add value to your team, and be engaged in your personal safety, the patient's safety, and the safety of your team members.

Kevin High, RN, MPH, CFRN, CEN
President
Air and Surface Transport Nurses Association

ACKNOWLEDGMENTS

The fourth edition of this book would not have been possible without the work of those visionary nurses who wrote and edited the first edition of *Flight Nursing: Principle and Practice.* I thank those from other disciplines who are key in patient transport and willing to devote their time and energies to make this fourth edition possible. If we do not continue to take pleasure in what makes us the same, we will never become what our patients need.

I also acknowledge and thank Maureen, Laurie, and Jackie for all they did to make this book possible once again!

CONTENTS

xx **Contents**

UNIT I

History and the Current Role of Ground and Air Transport Nurses

CHAPTER 1

HISTORY OF PATIENT TRANSPORT

Jill Johnson, Reneé Semonin Holleran

PATIENT TRANSPORT BY AMBULANCE

The history of patient transport begins before the invention of the wheel, when patients were carried or dragged to care. Ambulance systems were first established in the 1400s for the transportation of war casualties. These ambulances assumed many forms, from horse-pulled stretchers to wagons developed specifically for patient transport.

During the Civil War, the United States Army developed an organized ambulance system for transport of the wounded. Plans also were developed for effective evacuation and treatment of casualties from the battlefield. At this time, trains and steamboats were used in addition to conventional ambulance transport.[4,6,11,38]

An intense interest in resuscitation began in the 18th century. The first organized effort was started in 1767 in Amsterdam by a group of wealthy men known as the Society for the Recovery of Drowned Persons. One of the group's suggestions was that persons who needed resuscitation should be taken to receiving houses (hospitals) where trained individuals could resuscitate them.[5] Identification of a method of civilian-based transport thus became an important issue.

In 1865, the first hospital-based ambulance service in the United States was started at Cincinnati Commercial Hospital (Figure 1-1).

The first electric ambulance was used in 1899 at the Michael Reese Hospital in Chicago. In 1905, a bulletproof ambulance was introduced for military use on the battlefield. During World War I, buses were converted into mobile surgical units for treatment of the wounded. The Model T Ford was also placed into action during World War I for transport of patients. As ground and air transport of the ill and injured progressed, the care needed before and during transport also advanced. Not until the 20th century were reliable methods of resuscitation developed, studied, and used consistently outside the hospital. In the 1960s, the work of Safar and Elam, mouth-to-mouth-resuscitation or the "kiss of life," was combined with that of Kouwenhoven, who demonstrated the benefits of cardiac massage.

1

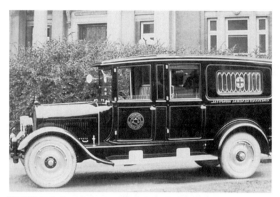

FIGURE 1-1   **Early ambulance dispatched from Cincinnati Hospital to transport patients.**

A Mobile Coronary Care Unit, staffed with both nurses and physicians, was started in Belfast in 1966. In 1968, similar units went into service in Great Britain, the United States, and Australia. In the United States, cardiopulmonary resuscitation then was taken from within the walls of the hospital to the field through the pioneering work of emergency medical systems in Los Angeles, Miami, and Warren, Ohio, in the late 1960s and 1970s.[5-7]

The initial equipment used in hospital resuscitation was large and not transportable; it operated only on AC power. The advent of battery-operated portable monitors and defibrillators greatly improved the care of the critically ill or injured patient during transport. The safety of equipment was improved so that it could be used in any type of transport vehicle without interference with vehicle operations. Today, the monitors used during transport offer multiple functions, such as continuous multilead rhythm monitoring, 12-lead analysis, waveform capnography, invasive monitoring, noninvasive blood pressure (NIBP) monitoring, pulse oximetry (SpO_2) monitoring, defibrillation, and external pacing.[8] The value of trained personnel who provide critical care outside the hospital continues to grow into the systems that exist throughout the world today.[5]

PATIENT TRANSPORT BY AIRPLANE

Despite an old claim that balloons once were used to transport the injured from the battlefield, patient air medical transport was not used until 1915.[10] The French successfully used planes to evacuate patients during World War I, which led to their development of ambulance aircraft.

During World War I, the United States successfully completed air ambulance transports with old JN-4 aircraft that were converted into air ambulances. The JN-4 aircraft were large, old, and costly to maintain. As the aircraft started to break down, the military decided against investing in their maintenance. The military was interested in a smaller, less costly aircraft for patient transport. A military air ambulance service was used to evacuate wounded from the Spanish Civil War in 1936 for treatment in Nazi Germany.[15,16]

The first fixed-wing civilian air ambulance service in the world was established in 1928 in the Australian outback. This organization became the Royal Flying Doctor Service, which is still in operation today, with more than 35,000 evacuations annually.[17,18]

The first civil air service in the United Kingdom was sponsored by the Department of Health for Scotland through local authorities who continued development and gradual expansion over the decades. It continues to this day as the Scottish Ambulance Service (Air Wing).[19]

The first civilian air ambulance service in Africa was established in Morocco in 1934 by the legendary French nurse and pilot Marie Marvingt.[20-22] That same year, Austin Airways started operations in Northern Canada with two Waco cabin biplanes, one of which had a new feature: a removable panel on the port side behind the cabin that facilitated the loading of a stretcher. This aircraft became North America's first private air ambulance.[23]

The first government-funded civilian fixed-wing air ambulance in North America was established by the Saskatchewan government in 1946 and is still in operation today.[24,25] Schaefer Air Service became the first commercial civilian air ambulance service in the United States in 1947; it was also the first Federal Aviation Administration (FAA)–certified air ambulance service in the United States.[26]

African Medical and Research Foundation (AMREF) in Kenya was established in 1957 by three surgeons; since then, the Flying Doctors have been involved in many healthcare projects in East Africa, including the Air Ambulance Services.[27]

Today, fixed-wing transport continues to play a major role in patient transport, particularly in rural, underdeveloped parts of the world.

PATIENT TRANSPORT BY HELICOPTER

The French pioneer Paul Cornu lifted an untethered twin-rotored helicopter into the air entirely without assistance from the ground for a few seconds on November 1907. By 1936, many problems that had prevented the helicopter from becoming a useful aircraft had solutions. With the introduction of the Focke-Wulf Fw 61 for the German military, the practical helicopter was a reality.[28] The first useful helicopter was the Focke-Achgelis Fa 223 Drache, which first flew in October 1940.[29] It could reach speeds of up to 109 mph and heights up to 23,294 ft. The Dragon, as the aircraft came to be known, could transport loads up to 2200 lbs.[30]

Igor Sirkorsky is considered to be the "father" of modern helicopters; he invented the first commercially successful helicopters on which further designs were based. The military subsequently became interested in the potential of helicopters. The US Army commissioned Sirkorsky to produce several helicopters for general military use. They found that the helicopter was successful at getting into small areas, and thus, the military used it to drop off special units in remote areas.[31]

The first helicopter patient evacuation took place in April 1944. A US Army Sikorsky YR-4B helicopter was used to rescue a wounded British soldier from more than 100 miles behind Japanese lines, 15 miles west of Mawlu, Burma.[32] This rescue was the beginning of patient transport by helicopter in the military.

Two weeks after arrival in Korea, Marine Corp pilots of the HMR-161 made the first of 20,000 medical evacuations by helicopter. Seventy-four casualties were flown a distance of 7 miles in a Sikorsky HRS-1 cargo helicopter.[33] A special helicopter unit soon was formed; it used the smaller Bell 47 and was attached to the Mobile Army Surgical Hospital (MASH; Figure 1-2).

Swiss Air-Rescue (REGA) was established in April 1952.[33] REGA is still the only air service that provides emergency air medical assistance in Switzerland. REGA brings citizens by fixed-wing or helicopter

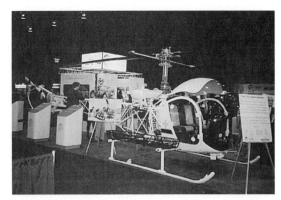

FIGURE 1-2 **Helicopter used to transport patients during Korean War.**

from anywhere in the world. REGA is believed to be the first civilian-based helicopter in the world to routinely use a hoist for rescue. REGA also is believed to be the first civilian-based program that is solely funded by donations and volunteer service groups.[34-36]

During the Vietnam War, the care and transport of the ill and injured continued to mature. Approximately 200,000 injured were transported by helicopter during this conflict. Medics were placed on ships to provide triage and care from the battlefield to the field hospital.[3]

Two programs were implemented by the US government in 1969 to assess the impact of medical helicopters on mortality and morbidity rates in the civilian area. Project CARESOM was established in Mississippi. Three helicopters were purchased through a federal grant and located strategically in the northern, central, and southern areas of the state. On completion of the project, which was considered a success, each area was afforded the opportunity to keep the aircraft; only the one located in Hattiesburg chose to keep the helicopter. This program became the first civilian-based helicopter program in the United States.[37]

The second program, the Military Assistance to Safety and Traffic (MAST) system, was established at Fort Sam Houston in San Antonio, Texas, in 1969. This program was an experiment (established in several areas of the United States) by the Department of Transportation to study the feasibility of military helicopter use to augment existing civilian emergency medical services.[39]

The first permanent civilian ambulance helicopter in Germany, Christoph 1, entered service at the Hospital of Harlaching, Munich, in 1970. The program's success led to a quick expansion of the concept of helicopter transport throughout Germany. As of 2007, 77 helicopters in Germany were named after St Christopher and performed more than 90,000 flights a year.[39,41]

In May 1972, Loma Linda Medical Center in California started the first American hospital-based helicopter program; this was followed by St Anthony's Hospital in Denver in October 1972 (Figure 1-3). Loma Linda closed after 6 months of operations because of a lack of funding and reopened the program the following year. Flight for Life Colorado began with a single Aloutte III helicopter, based at St Anthony Central Hospital in Denver, in October 1972 and continues today, making St Anthony's Hospital the longest running hospital-based program in the United States.[14,40]

During the 1980s, hospital-based programs opened at an amazing pace. By 1987, 150 programs existed. Special operations were added to the Helicopter Emergency Medical Services (HEMS) role in the 1990s when STAR Flight in Austin, Texas, became the first American HEMS program to offer

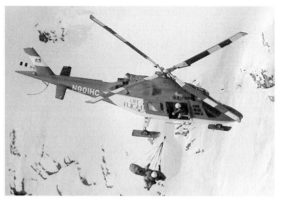

FIGURE 1-4   **Intermountain Life Flight Hoist Rescue Operation.** (Courtesy Intermountain Life Flight.)

long-line helicopter rescue in 1993.[43] Intermountain Life Flight in Salt Lake City became the first FAA-approved civilian helicopter hoisting program in the United States in 2001 (Figure 1-4). By the start of the second millennium, more than 400 air medical transport programs existed worldwide.[42]

THE HISTORY OF NURSING IN CRITICAL CARE TRANSPORT

The word *nursing* is derived from the Latin word *nutrire,* to nourish.[1] Florence Nightingale is considered the founder of modern nursing practice and was one of the original nurses to practice in the "field."[1] In 1854, Florence Nightingale was put in charge of the Female Nursing Establishment of the English General Hospitals in Turkey during the Crimean War. Within 6 months, the death rate in the military hospitals went from 47% to 2.2% under her leadership. She went to the front lines where she visited and cared for the ill and injured until she became ill with Crimean fever and was sent back to England. Her work during the Crimean War laid the foundation for prehospital nursing practice.

In the United States, the history of transport nursing began with the Civil War, which furnished nurses with an opportunity to demonstrate their skills and administer care to ill and injured soldiers. Nurses served in volunteer corps and offered care to both the Union and Confederate Armies.

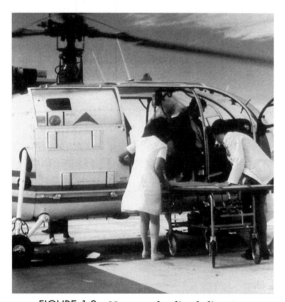

FIGURE 1-3   **Nurses unloading helicopter.**

Clara Barton emerged as the symbol of nursing's philosophy to meet the health needs of all humans, regardless of race, creed, or color. She was an outspoken opponent of slavery, and she gave care on the battlefield to Northerners, Southerners, blacks, and whites.[4] She went on to establish the American Red Cross in 1882. Many transport nurses today are Mobile Assist Teams (MAT) nurses who play an integral role in the delivering of care to victims of disasters.

In the 20th century, nurses were active participants in World War I, World War II, the Korean and Vietnam Wars, and more recently, the Gulf War. Nurses, physicians, and corpsmen, working only miles from the battlefront, have staffed hospitals known as MASH and Medical Unit Self-contained Transportable (MUST). The war experiences of the 20th century have shown that field stabilization and rapid transport can decrease mortality and morbidity rates. Nurses have played a significant role in the delivery of this care in the field, particularly through flight nursing.

The first recorded flight nurse and probably the true founder of flight nursing was Marie Marvingt (1875-1963). She was the most decorated woman in the history of France. She was also a surgical nurse and a pioneering aviator. In 1910, she designed the first air ambulance capable of carrying a stretcher (Figure 1-5). Between the two World Wars, she worked as a medical officer with French Forces in North Africa. While in

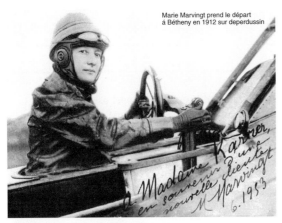

Marie Marvingt prend le départ
á Bétheny en 1912 sur deperdussin

FIGURE 1-5   **Marie Marvingt, Reims, 1912.** (From Hargrave L: *The pioneers: aviation and aeromodeling – interdependent evoluations and histories,* available at www.ctie.monash.edu.au/hargrave/marvingt.html, retrieved June 1, 2008.)

Morocco, she invented metal skis and suggested their use on air planes that landed in sand.

Marvingt devoted the remainder of her life after World War I to the concept of air medical evacuation and gave more than 3000 conferences and seminars related to air medical transport all over the world. She was one of the organizers of the first International Congress on Medical Aviation in 1929. In 1931, she created the Captain Echeman Challenge, which gave a prize for the best air ambulance performance.

In 1934, she established the first civil air ambulance service in Morocco and subsequently was awarded the Medal of Peace of Morocco. In that same year, she developed training courses for Nurses of the Air and in 1935, became the first person in the world licensed to practice aviation paramedicine.

In 1934 and 1935, she wrote, directed, and appeared in two documentary films that described the history and development of air ambulances: *Wings which Save* and *Saved by a Dove.* In 1935, she was made a Chevalier of the Legion of Honor.

During World War II, she served as a surgical nurse and invented a new type of surgical suture. In 1955, at the age of 80 years, she earned her helicopter license with turbine rating and piloted a US Air Force supersonic fighter jet.[20-22]

The origin of American flight nursing can be traced to Laureate M. Schimmoler, who formed the Emergency Flight Corps in 1933. Ms Schimmoler influenced the military to open its first flight nurse training program in 1942 at the 349th Air Evacuation Group, Bowman Field, Louisville, Kentucky. The training program lasted 6 weeks and included flight physiology. The "Bees" was the insignia for these nurses (Figure 1-6; a description of its meaning is included in the figure).

To become a flight nurse, a nurse had to send an application to the Army Nurse Corps and work 6 months at an Army Air Force Hospital. After completion of flight school, one could submit a request to the Commanding General of the Army Air Force for the designation Flight Nurse. Many nurses desired to enter the program because flight nursing represented the elite of the corps (Box 1-1).

On February 18, 1943, the first class of flight nurses graduated from the specialized course of

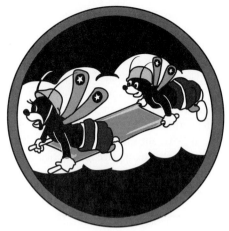

FIGURE 1-6   **Bees insignia.** Insignia of US Army Air Force's School of Air Evacuation was dark blue disc with two honeybees, whose bodies were or (gold) and sable (black) with argent (white) wings bearing stars, carrying a brown litter, all in front of an argent cloud. Blue and gold are the Air Corps colors. The honeybees, helmeted and wearing red cross armbands, are indicative of the industry displayed by the personnel of the organization. The litter is symbolic of evacuation of the sick and wounded, the cloud indicative of the area in which the mission is carried out. The insignia was designed by Mrs Don Rider of Buechel, Kentucky, who was greatly impressed by the work of the air evacuation personnel during the flood in Louisville in 1942.

medical training at Bowman Field in Louisville. General David Grant, one of the driving forces behind this new field of military nursing, officiated at the ceremony. When he realized that no one had thought of an insignia for this new group of nurses,

---

BOX 1-1 **"The Song of the Army Nurse Corps"**

We march along with faith undaunted beside our
    gallant fighting men;
Whenever they are sick or wounded, we nurse them
    back to health again;
As long as healing hands are wanted, you'll find the
    nurses of the Corps;
On ship, or plane, on transport train, at home or on a
    far off shore;
With loyal heart we do our part, for the Army and the
    Army Nurse Corps.

Copyrighted 1944 by MCA Music; Lou Singen, Composer;
Hy Zaret, Lyrics.

---

he pinned his own flight surgeon's wings on the honor graduate, Geraldine Dishroon. As the first to receive the wings, she was designated the first flight nurse (Box 1-2).

During World War II, fixed-wing aircraft transported 1.5 million patients with educated flight nurses in attendance.[4,9] More than 1600 nurses were decorated for meritorious service and bravery under fire. By the end of the war, 201 nurses were dead and 16 were missing.

After World War II, flight nurse training was conducted by the Air Force. Flight nurses were activated for service during both the Korean and Vietnam Wars.

BOX 1-2 **Flight Nurses's Creed**

I will summon every resource to prevent the triumph of death over life.
I will stand guard over the medicines and equipment entrusted to my care and ensure their proper use.
I will be untiring in the performance of my duties, and I will remember that upon my disposition and spirit will in large measure depend the morale of my patients.
I will be faithful to my training and to the wisdom handed down to me by those who have gone before me.
I have taken a nurse's oath reverent in man's mind because of the spirit and work of its creator, Florence Nightingale. She, I remember, was called the "lady with the lamp."
It is now my privilege to lift this lamp of hope and faith and courage in my profession to heights not known by her in her time, Together with the help of the flight surgeons and surgical technicians, I can set the very skies ablaze with life and promise for the sick, injured and wounded who are my sacred charges.
…This I will do, I will not falter, in war or in peace.

David N.W. Grant
Major General, USA
Air Surgeon

During the Korean and Vietnam Wars, the value of helicopter transport of the injured was recognized. Many of the physicians, nurses, and corpsmen who spent time in these wars believed in a role for helicopter transport in the civilian care of those who were injured or needed to be transported to another care facility.[6]

In 1972, St Anthony's Hospital in Denver established a civilian-based flight program staffed by nurses with critical care experience. Herman Hospital in Houston established a flight program in 1976 and added a physician to the flight team. Respiratory therapists (RTs) were added in 1984 by Intermountain Health Care in Salt Lake City along with other team members whose specific task was to transport patients with acute respiratory distress syndrome (ARDS) and patients with acute injury and critical illnesses who needed advanced respiratory support. RTs are now commonly found as a part of pediatric and neonatal teams.[44]

During the 1980s, a boom began in the development of hospital-based programs. At one point, more than 220 programs existed. The primary crew member is generally a registered nurse with either emergency or critical care nursing experience. Other members of the flight team include paramedics, other registered nurses, physicians, and respiratory therapists (Figure 1-7). Some flight programs continue to offer specialized flight teams, such as for maternal or neonatal care.

The practice of flight nursing evolved from the role of nursing care in the field and continues to develop based on the type of patients who need transport today. As we begin a new century, we must not forget our roots. Flight nursing is a dynamic component of transport and the key to safe competent patient care.

PARAMEDICS IN CRITICAL CARE TRANSPORT

The lineage of the paramedic can be traced back to the early volunteer ambulance squads organized to provide aid during World War I. These squads provided little more than transportation of the injured soldier, with squad members having only rudimentary first aid training.

World War II introduced the corpsman, who provided battlefield care to the wounded soldier. In the Korean conflict, the corpsman evolved into the field medic, whose rapid care and interventions included packaging the patient for helicopter evacuation.

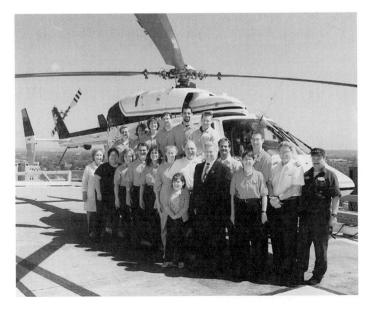

FIGURE 1-7 **University Air Care air medical transport crew.** (Courtesy University Hospital, Cincinnati, Ohio.)

During the Vietnam War, the medics were placed onboard the helicopters to provide rapid transport and immediate care.[2,13]

In 1966, significant advancements in civilian emergency medicine occurred in the United States. As a result of the number of traffic deaths, the US Congress passed the Highway Safety Act, which provided the impetus for the emergence of a nationwide system for prehospital emergency medical services (EMS).[2,13]

The federal Department of Transportation developed the first training course for emergency medical technicians (EMTs) in 1969, and plans were immediately underway to further develop an advanced life support provider, the emergency medical technician-paramedic (EMT-P).[2] These EMT and paramedic providers were trained in a variety of skills to provide initial stabilization of the acutely ill or injured and to continue this care during transport to a medical facility. The paramedic profession gained official recognition as a healthcare occupation in 1975, when the American Medical Association accepted and approved the EMT-P role.[13] Since these early beginnings, EMS has evolved to incorporate the use of paramedics within most ambulance systems, including most air medical transport programs (Figure 1-8).[12]

The first dual paramedic flight program in North America began in 1977 in Toronto with a single rotor-wing aircraft. This program continues to operate today with a paramedic-only team.[45,46]

Recently, associate and bachelor degree programs have become more common for paramedic education. The development of a critical care paramedic practice and the expanded scope of the paramedic practice have lead to the appropriately educated and trained paramedic-only critical care transport teams in the United States and throughout the world.[47]

SUMMARY

Patient transport has existed since patients needed movement from the battlefield to areas of safety so care could be rendered. Transport nursing originated through the work of nursing pioneers such as Florence Nightingale, Clara Barton, Marie Marvingt, and Laureate M. Schimmoler, whose theories and work became integral to patient care before and during transport over the past few centuries into today. As the principles of flight and transport nursing were incorporated into civilian care, hospital-based transport programs were started and staffed by nurses.

Paramedics have been involved in patient transport since the beginning of the century. Their role in critical care transport has continued to expand to critical care paramedics and flight paramedics.

In 1988, the US Department of Transportation published the Air Medical Crew National Standard Curriculum. This publication encompasses basic and advanced curriculum for the education and training of air medical transport teams. In 1990, the Commission for the Accreditation of Air Medical Service (CAAMS) began evaluating both helicopter and fixed-wing air medical transport services. In 1997, CAAMS changed to the Commission of Accreditation of Medical Transport Systems (CAMTS). As of April 2008, more than 150 accredited services exist.[48]

We must be familiar with and take pride in our origins as we forge into the future. Combining the expertise of many professions provides optimum patient care during all modes and phases of the transport process.

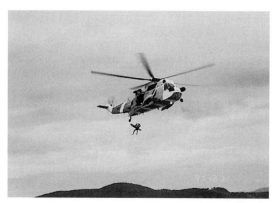

FIGURE 1-8   **Norwegian air medical helicopter.**

REFERENCES

1. Bader GB, Terhorst M, Heilman P, et al: Characteristics of flight nursing practice, *Air Med J* 14(4):214-218, 1995.
2. Browne B, Jacobs L, Pollack C: *Emergency care and transportation of the sick and injured*, ed 7, Sudbury, MA, 1999, Jones & Bartlett.

3. Carter G: The evolution of air transport systems: a pictorial review, *J Emerg Med* 6:499-504, 1986.

4. Donahue P: *Nursing: the finest art*, ed 2, St Louis, 1996, Mosby.

5. Eisenberg M, Pantridge J, Cobb L, et al: The revolution and evolution of cardiac care, *Arch Intern Med* 12(26):1-15, 1996.

6. Hackel A: History of medical transport systems. In McClosky K, Orr R, editors: *Pediatric transport medicine*, St Louis, 1995, Mosby.

7. Holleran RS: *Prehospital nursing: a collaborative approach*, St Louis, 1994, Mosby.

8. Zoll: *M series CCT defibrillator,* available at http://www.zoll.com/product.aspx?id=384, retrieved May 2008.

9. Lee G: History of flight nursing, *J Emerg Nurs* 13(4):212, 1987.

10. McNab A: Air medical transport: "hot air" and a French lesson, *J Air Med Trans* 11(8):15-16, 1992.

11. Porter R: *The greatest benefit to mankind: a medical history of humanity*, New York, 1999, Knopf.

12. Rau W: 2000 Annual transport statistics, *AirMed* 6(4):17-20, 2000.

13. Sanders M: *Mosby's paramedic textbook*, St Louis, 1994, Mosby.

14. Clark DY, Stocking J, Johnson J, editors: *Flight and ground transport nursing core curriculum*, Greenwood Village, CO, 2006, ASTNA.

15. McFarland RA: *Human factors in air transportation*, New York, 1956, McGraw-Hill Book Co.

16. Link MM, Coleman HA: *Medical support of the army air forces in World War II*, Washington, DC, 1955, Society for Military History.

17. Royal Flying Doctor Service: *Our history,* available at http://www.flyingdoctor.net/Our-History.html, retrieved April 2008.

18. Royal Flying Doctor Service: *What we do,* available at http://www.flyingdoctor.net/What-We-Do.html, retrieved April 2008.

19. Hutchinson I: *Air ambulance: six decades of the Scottish Air Ambulance Service*, Erskine, 1966, Kea.

20. Lam DM: Marie Marvingt and the development of aeromedical evacuation, *Aviat Space Environ Med* 74(8):863-868, 2003-2008.

21. www.aviation-ancienne

22. Lam DM: Marie Marvingt and the development of aeromedical evacuation, *Aviat Space Environ Med* 74(8):863-868, 2003.

23. Ontario Ministry of Natural Resources: *History of bush flying,* available at http://www.mnr.gov.on.ca/en/Business/AFFM/2ColumnSubPage/STEL02_165922.html, paragraph 45, retrieved May 2008.

24. *Air ambulance history,* available at http://www.100yearsofnursing.ca/english/content/SK_19.html, retrieved April 2008.

25. The Encyclopedia of Saskatchewan: *Air ambulance,* available at http://esask.uregina.ca/entry/air_ambulance.html, retrieved April 2008.

26. Schaefer Ambulance Service: *Air and ground ambulance service,* available at http://www.schaeferamb.com/air/index.htm, retrieved April 2008.

27. www.amerf.org, retrieved April 2008.

28. Helis: *Helicopter history site,* available at http://www.helis.com/introduction/prin.php, paragraph 6, retrieved May 2008.

29. *Focke-Achgelis Fa 223 "Drache,"* available at http://www.aviastar.org/helicopters_eng/focke_drache.php, paragraph 2, retrieved May 2008.

30. *History of the helicopter: Heinrich Focke Fa 61,* available at http://www.century-of-flight.net/Aviation%20history/helicopter%20history/Focke.htm, paragraph 10, retrieved May 2008.

31. *History of the helicopter,* available at http://inventors.about.com/od/hstartinventions/a/helicopter.htm, paragraph 5, retrieved May 2008.

32. *WWII helicopter evacuation,* available at http://www.olive-drab.com/od_medical_evac_helio_ww2.php, paragraph 2, retrieved May 2008.

33. Horn CJ: *Military innovation and the helicopter: a comparison of development in the United States Army and Marine Corps, 1945-1965,* page 103/4 and reference 234 (PhD thesis), available at http://www.ohiolink.edu/etd/send-pdf.cgi?osu1054563128, retrieved April 2008.

34. Rega: *Milestones in Rega's history,* available at http://www.rega.ch/en/dateien/medien/PDF_Meilensteine_en_07.pdf (page 1), retrieved April 2008.

35. Rega: *Milestones in Rega's history,* available at http://www.rega.ch/en/dateien/medien/PDF_Meilensteine_en_07.pdf (page 2), retrieved April 2008.

36. Rega: *Five Rega principles,* available at http://www.rega.ch/en/dateien/medien/PDF_Kernsaetze07_en.pdf, retrieved April 2008.

37. Forrest General Hospital: *FGH history,* available at http://www.forrestgeneral.com/story/history.php, retrieved May 2008.

38. Gonsalves D: Historical background of emergency medical services in the United States, *Emerg Care Q* 4(3):77, 1988.

39. *Einsatzzahlen,* available at http://www.rth.info/einsatzzahlen/einsatzzahlen.php, retrieved April 2008.

40. Flight for Life Colorado: *Helicopters (rotor wing),* available at http://www.flightforlifecolorado.org/index.php?s=40, retrieved May 2008.

41. *Christophorus 1,* available at http://www.oeamtc.at/netautor/pages/resshp/anwendg/1081946.html, retrieved May 2008.

42. *STARflight,* available at http://www.starflightrescue.org/History/History.htm, retrieved May 2008.

43. *Intermountain healthcare,* available at http://intermountainhealthcare.org/xp/public/lifeflight/aboutus/history.xml, retrieved May 2008.

44. *Intermountain healthcare,* available at http://intermountainhealthcare.org/xp/public/lifeflight/aboutus/teams/respiratory.xml, retrieved May 2008.

45. Ornge: *Backgrounder,* available at http://www.ornge.ca/news/Ornge-Backgrounder.pdf.

46. Ornge: available at http://www.ornge.ca/news/Ornge-YIR-2006.pdf, retrieved April 2008.

47. CAMTS: 2006 *Accreditation Standards,* ed 7, Standard number 02.05.05 (3).

48. CAMTS: available at http://www.camts.org/content/view/73/71/, retrieved March 2008.

PREPARATION FOR PRACTICE

Reneé Semonin Holleran, Sally Houliston

Critical care patient transport requires skilled and experienced personnel to meet the needs of complex cases in a challenging environment. It also necessitates clinical competency, critical thinking skills, and flexibility. The education, clinical proficiency, and knowledge needed to provide this care both before and during transport must be diverse and comprehensive. Transport teams vary and may be composed of registered nurses, paramedics, physicians, respiratory therapists, or others, as dictated by patient needs. Although no central reporting agency makes up a transport team, most teams within the United States continue to be staffed by registered nurses and paramedics.[4,15] However, all team members must possess some basic information: for example, aircraft safety, use of radios or communication devices, and survival training. The transport team staffing and education should be commensurate with the mission statement and scope of care of the medical transport service. The transport vehicle, by virtue of how it is staffed and medically equipped, becomes a patient care unit specific to the needs of the patient. The team that transports that patient must be appropriately educated and trained on patient management before and during the transport process.[4,16]

The make-up of a transport team varies across the world. The Commission on Accreditation of Medical Transport Systems (CAMTS)[4] defines team members on the basis of the mission of the transport. Table 2-1 describes the different types of missions and teams that may be involved in transport with use of the CAMTS definitions.

QUALIFICATIONS FOR TRANSPORT PRACTICE

TRANSPORT NURSE

The registered nurse has had a role in patient transport and the prehospital environment for numerous years. Discussion continues about what qualifications a nurse should have to practice. States, local emergency medical services (EMS) regulations, and even some national EMS and physicians associations have provided input into transport nursing practice. The Air and Surface Transport Nurses Association (ASTNA)[1] developed a position paper that addresses some of these issues. The preparation for patient care required to practice nursing, along with the appropriate experience and education, provides a sound foundation for practice in the prehospital and transport environments. However, that preparation rarely includes the skills needed to deliver patient care in the prehospital environment. ASTNA supports that State Boards of Nursing, or in other countries, the equivalent regulatory bodies for the profession

TABLE 2-1	**Transport Team Definitions**
Mission	**Definition**
Critical care	Critical care is defined as transport from a scene or clinical setting of a patient whose condition warrants care commensurate with the scope of practice of a **physician** or **registered nurse.**
Advanced life support	Advanced life support mission is defined as transport from an emergency department, critical care unit, or scene of a patient who needs care commensurate with the scope of practice of an **EMT-P.**
Basic life support	A basic life support is defined as the transport of a patient from an emergency department or scene who requires care commensurate with the scope of practice of an **EMT-B.**
Specialty care	These team members have a specific specialty and are added to the regularly scheduled transport team (e.g., neonatal, pediatric, perinatal, or IABP transports).

EMT-P, Emergency medical technician-paramedic; *EMT-B,* Emergency medical technician-basic; *IABP,* Intra-aortic balloon pump.

BOX 2-1	**Qualifications for Transport Nurses**

- Registered nurse (with appropriate state/provincial licensure)
- Minimum of 2 years of critical care or emergency department experience
- Specialty certification commensurate with previous experience (CEN, CCRN, CFRN, or CTRN within 2 years of hire)
- Basic cardiac life support or equivalent
- Age-specific advanced cardiac life support (ACLS or PALS)
- Transport nurse advanced trauma course (TNATC), advanced trauma life support course (ATLS), or equivalent
- Objective assessment of the transport nurse applicant's qualifications for transport based on, but limited to, the following characteristics:
  - Educational and experiential background
  - Technical and clinical competence
  - Leadership skills
  - Critical thinking skills
  - Proficient communication and interpersonal skills
  - Appreciation of public and community relations

CEN, Certificate for Emergency Nursing; *CCRN,* Critical Care Registered Nurse; *CFRN,* Certified Flight Nurse; *CTRN,* Certified Transport Registered Nurse; *ACLS,* advanced cardiac life support; *PALS,* Pediatric Advanced Life Support; *TNATC,* Transport Nurse Advanced Trauma Course; *ATLS,* Advanced Trauma Life Support.

of nursing. ASTNA seeks recognition by state EMS agencies or their equivalent for the unique role of a registered nurse to practice in the prehospital environment. The registered nurse who practices in the prehospital and transport environment must be properly prepared to deliver patient care safely and competently in this exceptional and challenging environment.[1, 17]

The ASTNA published a specific position paper that recommends the qualifications a transport nurse should have when hired. These qualifications are summarized in Box 2-1.[2]

TRANSPORT PARAMEDIC

The International Association of Flight Paramedics (IAFP; formally the National Flight Paramedics Association) proposes that the paramedic functions well in the air medical and critical care transport environment.[6] However; some confusion has been seen because of the several definitions of paramedic practice in the transport environment. Most definitions are determined by the area of the country (and even the world) in which the paramedic practices. The certified flight paramedic examination was developed to help clarify what preparation is necessary for an advanced role as a paramedic performing air medical and critical care ground transport. Box 2-2 provides a summary of the IAFP's recommendations for both the flight paramedic and the certified flight paramedic.[6]

BOX 2-2	Qualifications for a Transport Paramedic

- Minimum of 3 years experience in the field as an EMT-P working as an Advanced Life Support Provider
- Minimum of 5 years basic paramedic practice after graduation for the certified paramedic
- Basic Life Support
- Advanced Cardiac Life Support
- Basic Trauma Life Support
- Prehospital Trauma Life Support or Advanced Trauma Life Support audit
- Pediatric Advanced Life Support
- Neonatal Resuscitation Program

PREPARATION FOR PRACTICE

The CAMTS standards provide an outline for the Initial Training Program Requirements for each of the mission types (air or ground) for transport programs.[4] These requirements provide a strong framework on which a program's initial orientation and continuing education are built. A summary is found in Box 2-3.[4]

A comprehensive orientation can be provided in numerous ways. With use of adult learning principles, an educational program can be designed that uses self-directed learning packets, traditional lecture with discussion, or case scenario teaching, to name a few techniques.[3-5]

BOX 2-3	CAMTS Initial Training Program Requirements

Didactic Component

- Advanced airway management
- Altitude physiology/stressors of flight
- Anatomy, physiology, and assessment for adult, pediatric, and neonatal patients (specific to program's scope of care)
- Transport vehicle (aviation and road) orientation/safety and in-transport procedures as appropriate
- Cardiac emergencies and advanced cardiac critical care
- Disaster and triage
- EMS radio communications
- Hazardous materials recognition and response
- Hemodynamic monitoring, pacemakers, automatic implantable cardiac defibrillator (AICD), intra-aortic balloon pump, central lines, pulmonary arterial and arterial catheters, ventricular assist devices, and extracorporeal membrane oxygenation (ECMO)
- Human factors: crew resource management, air medical resource management
- Infection control
- Mechanical ventilation and respiratory physiology for adult, pediatric, and neonatal patients (specific to program's scope of care)
- Oxygen therapy in the medical transport environment: mechanical ventilation and respiratory physiology for adult, pediatric, and neonatal patients
- Pediatric medical emergencies
- Pediatric trauma
- Pharmacology

- Quality management
- Respiratory emergencies
- Scene management/rescue/extrication
- Survival training
- Didactic education that is mission specific and specific to scope of care and patient population
  - Burn emergencies (thermal, chemical, and electrical)
  - Environmental emergencies
  - Equipment education
  - High-risk obstetric emergencies (bleeding, medical, trauma)
  - Metabolic endocrine emergencies
  - Multitrauma (chest, abdomen, facial)
  - Neonatal emergencies (respiratory distress, surgical, cardiac)
- Toxicology

Clinical Component (on Basis of Program's Scope of Care)

- Critical care (adult, pediatric, neonatal)
- Emergency care (adult, pediatric, neonatal)
- Invasive procedures on mannequin equivalent for practicing of invasive procedures
- Neonatal intensive care
- Obstetrics
- Pediatric critical care
- Prehospital care
- Tracheal intubations (and alternative airway management)

In addition to the didactic information, a practical component of skills training is needed. This training should include various inpatient and prehospital care clinical experiences and an invasive skills laboratory.[4,5]

After the initial education and training is complete, the new transport team member needs to complete an internship or preceptorship, which provides further role definition, recognition of the need for additional education or training, and an opportunity to "put into practice" all the previous learning. Although evaluation is an ongoing process, a final evaluation during the orientation process assists new transport team members in assessing their experience and the need for any further education.

ADULT LEARNING PRINCIPLES

Incorporation of adult learning principles and the use of various teaching methods should be included in a comprehensive orientation program. Adult learning today is influenced by generational differences, technology advancements, and differing learning styles; these should be considered in development of any orientation or educational program for new team members. Adult learning also requires various educational techniques, including but not limited to: traditional lecture with discussion, case presentation/scenario-based teaching, internet-based learning, multimedia applications, simulation training, and self-directed learning packages.[8] In addition to the didactic component, transport nursing practice requires additional skills with a practical clinical component. These skills should include various prehospital care and inpatient clinical experiences in addition to simulation training with tools such as synthetic models and mannequins or computer simulations.[3,9,13]

Because of the variety of adult learning styles in today's education world and the knowledge that adult learners progress at a different pace, emphasis and due consideration are needed in evaluation of progress through the period of preceptorship. The duration of orientation and preceptorship for new team members varies according to the needs of the transport program and the individual member. After the initial education and training is complete, standard practice is for a new transport team member to participate in a period of preceptorship or internship.[2,7] This period allows for further role clarification and definition, provides an opportunity to put into practice all the learning from the initial education, and allows for recognition of the need for additional education or training.

COMPETENCY-BASED EDUCATION

Competency-based learning is a method of education that allows for flexibility, with building on previous knowledge. Competency-based instruction provides an opportunity for regular feedback and assessment of competency at the end of the various stages of the program, which provides positive response for progression through to the next stage and the ability to assess competency development as the transport nurse learns. An example is advanced airway management skills. The Plan is an outline of requirements for competency in advanced airway skills. The orientation member then initiates the plan (Do). An Assessment of the member's ability to perform advanced airway management is done; the Plan is then modified. Evaluation is continuous. Figure 2-1 illustrates the use of this model.

ASTNA[2,7] has developed a list of the minimal competencies that are recommended for nurses who practice in the transport environment. A summary of these competencies is found in Box 2-4.

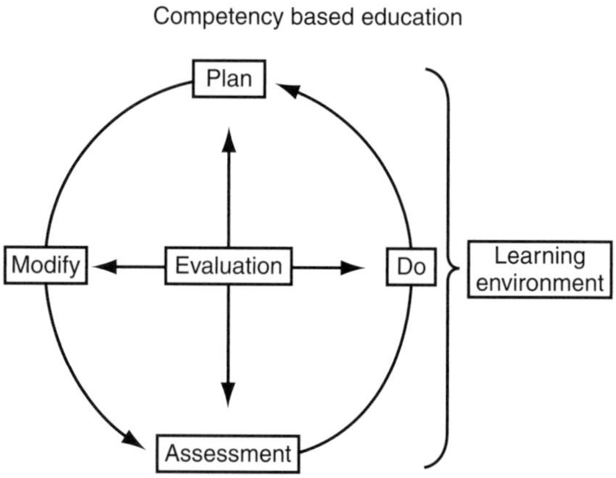

FIGURE 2-1   **Competency-based education model.**

BOX 2-4	**ASTNA Recommended Competencies for Transport Nurses**

- Advanced patient assessments skills to include anatomy, pathophysiology, assessment, and treatment for the age group and patients that are transported by the program (e.g., neonatal, pediatric, adult, geriatric):
  - Acute and chronic respiratory disease
  - Cardiovascular abnormalities
  - Surgical problems
  - Infectious diseases
  - Musculoskeletal abnormalities
  - Neurologic and spinal cord emergencies
  - Gastrointestinal emergencies
  - Genitourinary disorders
  - Integumentary disruption
  - Hematologic disorders
  - Metabolic/endocrine disorders
  - Genetic/disorders of dysmorphology
  - Disorders of the head, eyes, ears, nose, and throat
  - Trauma
  - Environmental and toxicological emergencies
  - Adult and child maltreatment
- Airway management (basic and advanced)
- Vascular access
- Medication administration
- Intra-aortic balloon pump management
- Ventricular assist device management
- Needle decompression
- Chest tube insertion
- Pericardiocentesis
- Pacing devices
- Immobilization skills
- 12-lead electrocardiographic (ECG) interpretation
- Arrhythmia analysis and treatment
- Invasive monitoring
- Fetal heart monitoring
- Radiographic interpretation
- Interpretation and treatment of clinical laboratory data
- Thermoregulation
- Psychologic/bereavement support and crisis intervention
- Transport equipment management

In addition, Johnson[7] has also developed a competency-based manual that provides several references and outlines for the orientation of transport personnel.

Each transport program, on the basis of the program's mission and scope of practice, has a standard of technical competencies and skills necessary for clinical practice. During the orientation period, new staff members are required to demonstrate competence in the specified requisites for progression to independent practice. Once demonstrated, these skill are built on by the novice practitioner and provide a continuing checklist for the expert for continuing professional development. Additional individual skill sets, or a blend of technical, interpersonal, and critical thinking as identified in a specific job description, need to be measurably shown by the end of the orientation program. These objectives may also form the basis for an annual performance development review or personal evaluations within the transport program. Feedback regarding performance from a variety of sources, including peer review, provides honest evaluation and is often powerful motivation for self development.

ASTNA recommends that clinical competencies be evaluated with use of written examinations, simulated practice/skills laboratories, transport preceptor/mentor supervised skills practiced during actual transports, case presentations, and oral examinations conducted by peers and the medical director. Staff meetings offer an excellent opportunity to teach both new and experienced transport personnel with use of actual transports.

Coaching, mentoring, and clinical supervision programs should be available to new transport team members. Mentors fulfill a different role than that of the preceptor. Mentors help new nurses in a role deepen their knowledge and develop professionally, whereas clinical supervision allows the practitioner to share clinical, organizational, developmental, and emotional experiences with another professional to enhance knowledge and skills.[18]

CONTINUING PROFESSIONAL DEVELOPMENT

Continuing professional development has a fixed portion of training determined by standards, regulations, and the transport program, including skills/technical training, occupational health and safety, and local and state requirements. Additional sources of continuing education may include current textbooks related to transport, professional journals, online discussion forums, and continuing education courses.

CAMTS RECOMMENDATIONS

CAMTS outlines specific components of transport education and skills that should be reviewed annually (see Box 2-5).[4]

In addition to these requirements, transport team members have a further responsibility to identify their own educational needs aside from any regulatory or accreditation standard requirements. As discussed previously, adult learners need a variety of experiences to learn and remain competent. Team members must maintain and continue to gain knowledge to meet patient needs and carry on the growth of the profession of transport nursing. This continuing education is an important part of the development and maintenance of expert practice in the field of transport nursing.

CLINICAL DECISION MAKING

Clinical decision making or clinical judgment is a process in which the clinician identifies, prioritizes, establishes plans, and evaluates data, which leads to the formation of a judgment to provide patient care.[5,10,11] In transport nursing, complex clinical decisions are made on a daily basis, in collaboration (see Figure 2-2) with other health professionals and transport team members. In dealing with increasing patient complexity and technological advancement, transport nurses must rely on sound decision-making skills to deliver up-to-date evidenced-based care and help facilitate positive patient outcomes.

REFLECTIVE PRACTICE

The use of reflective practice (application of learning experiences and current evidenced-based knowledge) in clinical decision making enhances patient care delivery. A higher level of learning is achieved by applying learned material to current situations. This application of reflective practice associated with learning from experience is an important strategy for health professionals who engage in continual

---

BOX 2-5   CAMTS Continuing Education/Staff Development

Didactic

- Hazardous materials recognition and response
- Human factors: crew resource management
- Infection control
- State EMS rules and regulations in relation to ground and air transport
- Stress recognition and management
- Survival training

Clinical/Laboratory

- Critical care (adult, pediatric, neonatal)
- Emergency/trauma care
- Invasive procedures laboratories
- Labor and delivery
- Prehospital experience
- Skills maintenance program documented to comply with number of skills required in a set period according to policy of the medical transport service (e.g., endotracheal intubations, chest drains)
- Clinical competency maintained by currency in the following or equivalent as appropriate for position description, mission statement, and scope of care:

- Basic Life Support (BLS): documented evidence of current BLS certification according to the American Heart Association (AHA)
- Advanced Cardiac Life Support (ACLS): documented evidence of current ACLS according to the AHA
- Advanced Trauma Life Support (ATLS): according to the American College of Surgeons, ATLS audit, ATLS for Nurse or Transport Nurse Advanced Trauma Course (TNATC)
- Pediatric Advanced Life Support (PALS) or Advanced Pediatric Life Support (APLS) according to the AHA and American College of Emergency Physicians (ACEP), or equivalent education
- Neonatal Resuscitation Program (NRP): documented evidence of current NRP according to the AHA or American Academy of Pediatrics
- Nursing certifications (such as CEN, CCRN, RNC, CTRN, and especially CFRN) are strongly encouraged; if required in position descriptions, certifications must be current

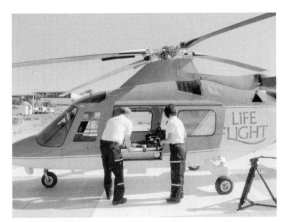

FIGURE 2-2 **Transport nurse and paramedic.**

learning.[12] The act of reflection is seen as a way of promoting the development of autonomous, qualified, and self-directed health professionals.

Engagement in reflective practice is associated with improvement in the quality of care, stimulation of personal and professional growth, and closing of the gap between theory and practice. If nurses do not think autonomously on a regular basis, they risk losing competence in their decision-making abilities.[14]

SUMMARY

Transport nursing requires experience, advanced skills, and continuing education so that the transport team is able to function autonomously and in collaboration with all others who may be involved in the transport process. Transport nursing occurs in diverse multidimensional situations in which patient care is delivered. The development of a sound orientation and strong preceptorship training program, in conjunction with continuing values-based professional development, provides the transport nurse with the skills and ability to care for patients in diverse and sometimes difficult situations. All of these experiences contribute to retaining a highly skilled nursing staff in a diverse environment.

REFERENCES

1. Air and Surface Transport Nurses Association (ASTNA): *Role of the registered nurse in the prehospital environment*, Denver, 2001, ASTNA.

2. Air and Surface Transport Nurses Association (ASTNA): *Qualifications, orientation, competencies, and continuing education for transport nurses*, Denver, 2003, ASTNA.

3. Bader GB, Terhorts M, Heilman P, et al: Characteristics of flight nursing practice, *Air Med J* 14(4):214-218, 1995.

4. Commission on Accreditation of Medical Transport Systems: *Accreditation standards*, ed 6, Anderson, SC, 2006, Commission on Accreditation of Medical Transport Systems.

5. Grossman S, Campblee C, Riley B: Assessment of clinical decision-making ability of critical care nurses, *Dimens Crit Care Nurs* 15(2):272-279, 1996.

6. Gryniuk J: The role of the certified flight paramedic as a critical care provider and the required education, *Prehosp Emerg Care* 5(3):290-292, 2001.

7. Johnson J: *Competency based orientation and continuing education for critical care transport*, Denver, 2007, Air and Surface Transport Nurses Association.

8. Knapp B: Competency: an essential component of caring in nursing, *Nurs Admin Q* 28(4):285-287, 2004.

9. Lamb D: Could simulated emergency procedures practised in a static environment improve the clinical performance of a critical care air support team (CCAST)? A literature review, *Intensive Crit Care Nurs* 23:33-42, 2007.

10. Miller M, Babcock D: *Critical thinking applied to nursing*, St Louis, 1996, Mosby.

11. Miller P, Epifianio P: Development of a prehospital nursing curriculum in Maryland, *J Emerg Nurs* 19(3):206, 1993.

12. National Health Service: *Example of a reflective practice tool*, available at http://www.wipp.nhs.uk/tools_gpn/toolu4_reflective.php, accessed April 5, 2008.

13. Paige J, Kozmenko V, Morgan B, et al: From the flight deck to the operating room: an initial pilot study of the feasibility and potential impact of true interdisciplinary team training using high fidelity simulation, *J Surg Educ* 64(6):369-377, 2007.

14. Pirret AM: The level of knowledge of respiratory physiology articulated by intensive care nurses to provide rationale for the clinical decision making, *Intensive Crit Care Nurs* 23:145-155, 2007.

15. Rau W: 2000 medical crew survey, *Air Med J* 6(5):17-22, 2000.

16. Rottman SJ, et al: On-line medical control versus protocol based prehospital care, *Ann Emerg Med* 30(1):62-68, 1997.

17. Shaner S, et al: Flight crew physical fitness: a baseline analysis, *Air Med J* 14(1):30, 1995.

18. Smith ME: From student to practicing nurse, *Am J Nurs* 107(7):72A-72D, 2007.

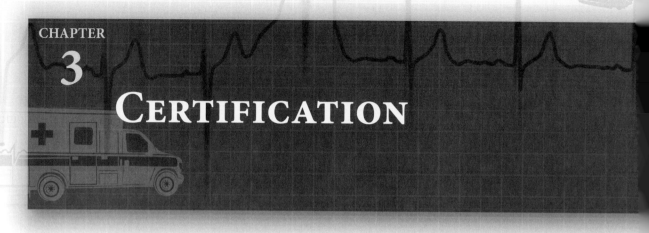

Reneé Semonin Holleran

Certification is defined by the American Board of Nursing Specialties as the formal recognition of specialized knowledge, skills, and experience demonstrated by achievement of standards identified by a nursing specialty to promote optimal health outcomes.[2,3] Certification in nursing first began in the 1940s. Since that time, the number of certifications offered in nursing and other healthcare-related professions has greatly increased.

Several studies have shown the value of certification.[6-10,12] The benefits of certification include increased job satisfaction, personal achievement, demonstration of knowledge of a specific body of nursing, commitment to the profession of nursing, increased credibility, indication of professional growth, enhancement in personal confidence in clinical abilities, and promotion of recognition from other health professionals.[6-10] The American Association of Critical Care Nurses in a study published in 2002 also found that certification has a significant impact on patient safety and patient care.[1]

Each certification has various requirements for one to sit for the examination. Examples include: years of experience in a particular specialty, number of hours of clinical practice, membership in a professional association, and licensing in a certain profession. Table 3-1 provides a summary of some of the certifications that may be used in transport nursing practice and the requirements for one to sit for the examinations.

The length of time that a nurse is certified varies among nursing specialties. How recertification is achieved also varies. Because of the growing trend that questions whether continuing education provides a measurement of competency; various methods other than continuing education are now being developed for recertification. Some certifications require a written examination as the only method of recertification, whereas others may require a certain number of hours worked in the specialty or completion of specific learning modules.

Variations also exist in the methods of test administration. Certifications in nursing are considered "high-stakes" certifications, which means that the examinations must be administered in a controlled environment and secured at all times. Feedback regarding the answers to questions cannot be given. At the present time, most certification examinations are administered in one of two formats: computer or paper and pencil. Paper and pencil examinations are generally offered during a national conference. However, most associations do provide an opportunity to schedule a paper and pencil test.

With computer-based examinations, the applicant must schedule a time before taking the examination, but the examination may be offered more frequently than paper-and-pencil tests. For example, the Certified Flight Nurse (CFRN) examination was offered two times a year as a paper and pencil

TABLE 3-1	Certification Examinations and Requirements[2,5]	
Certification	**Association**	**Requirements**
CCRN Examination available for neonatal, pediatric, or adult critical care nursing	AACN AACN Certification Corporation	1750 hours of direct bedside care (adult, neonatal, or pediatric). 875 hours must be accrued in the most recent year preceding the application.
CEN	BCEN	Two years of emergency nursing experience is recommended.
CFRN	BCEN With input from ASTNA	Two years of flight nursing experience is recommended.
CTRN	BCEN With input from ASTNA	Two years of critical care ground transport experience is recommended.
CPEN	BCEN	1000 hours in pediatric emergency nursing practice.

CPEN, Certified Pediatric Emergency Nurse; *AACN,* American Association of Critical-Care Nurses; *BCEN,* Board of Certification for Emergency Nursing.

test, but the computer-based version is now offered two times a day, 5 days a week (except holidays), 50 weeks of the year.

Certification examinations are primarily administered at a testing center that has contracted with the certifying organization. Computer-based examinations do not require computer experience, and most certifying examinations provide a tutorial before the examination.

The applicant is given an allotted time to take the examination. Computer-based examinations do allow the applicant to review questions, change answers, and skip questions to return to them later. The examination is composed of a set number of questions.

Most organizations also have a number of pretest questions in the examination. These questions are not counted into the final score; they are new questions that are being tried as statistically good questions to be used in the future. Many certifications that use computer-based testing also provide applicants with their scores before they leave the testing facility.

Preparation for a certification examination varies based on the examination. General information includes clinical experience and a review of information that may be presented on the test. Nursing specialties (e.g., transport nursing) have core curriculums that address the elements of that specialty. These books should be reviewed. Review courses

are also provided that may assist with examination preparation.

Other important information includes the location of testing sites and the types of identification that may be required for one to sit for the examination. This information is usually provided by the certifying organization before the applicant takes the examination. The information is available on the certification examination's web site or from the professional association that supports the examination.

With the vast overlap of knowledge among nursing specialties, nurses sometimes are unsure about which certification they should obtain. A point to consider is what knowledge is needed by the specialty one practices in. For example, the transport nurse may choose to take the Certificate for Emergency Nursing (CEN), Critical Care Registered Nurse (CCRN), CFRN, or Certified Transport Registered Nurse (CTRN). Each tests specific areas pertinent to transport nursing. For example, the CFRN addresses issues specific to flight nursing, such as landing zone and scene safety and aircraft operations.

TRANSPORT NURSING CERTIFICATION

Today, multiple certifications are available in nursing, including specialty and advanced practice certifications.[2] Transport nursing has two specialty certifications: Certified Flight Nurse (CFRN) and

Certified Transport Registered Nurse (CTRN).[4] Transport paramedics have the Flight Paramedic Certification (FP-C) examination.[5] In some states, additional certifications are required for nurses to practice. For example, in California, certifications are needed for the Mobile Intensive Care Nurse (MICN) or the Prehospital Health Professional (PHRN).

The CFRN and the CTRN were created through the work of the Air and Surface Transport Nurses Association (ASTNA; formally known as the National Flight Nurses Association [NFNA]) and the Board of Certification for Emergency Nursing. A member of ASTNA is appointed to the Board, and transport nurses are item writers for the examinations. Tables 3-2 and 3-3 contain summaries of the elements of each of the examinations.

ASTNA has published a Flight and Ground Transport Nursing Core Curriculum[10,11] that contains

TABLE 3-3	**CTRN Content List**	
Headings	**Topics**	**No. of Items**
Single-system emergencies	Cardiopulmonary	26
	GI/GU/OB	9
	Maxillofacial and orthopedic	8
Multisystem emergencies	Environmental	7
	General medical	9
Patient management	Patient care	10
	Advanced airway care	7
	Respiratory	5
	Shock/trauma	5
	Substance abuse/ toxicology	4
Safety issues	Safety	5
	Disaster management	3
	Survival	3
Professional issues	Legal	3
	Organizational issues	3
	Patient/community education	3

GI, Gastrointestinal; *GU,* genitourinary; *OB,* obstetric.

TABLE 3-2	**CFRN Content List**	
Topics	**Headings**	**No. of Items**
Single system emergencies	Cardiopulmonary	27
	GI/GU and OB	11
	Maxillofacial and orthopedic	8
	Neurologic	17
Multisystem emergencies	Environmental	9
	General medical	9
Patient management	Patient care	12
	Advanced airway care	9
	Respiratory	7
	Shock trauma	7
	Substance abuse/ toxicology	3
	Transport considerations	6
Safety issues	Safety	9
	Disaster management	3
	Survival	4
Professional issues	Legal	3
	Organizational issues	3
	Patient/community education	3

GI, Gastrointestinal; *GU,* genitourinary; *OB,* obstetric.

the knowledge needed for transport nursing practice. ASTNA also publishes review manuals and has other materials available for review for preparation for both the CFRN and the CTRN examinations.

Applicants must be sure that the certification organization is legitimate. Various certification programs offer examinations that are not psychometrically sound. To eliminate confusion, certifying organizations are now usually accredited.

FLIGHT PARAMEDIC CERTIFICATION

Although most air medical programs have expanded the flight paramedic's role to that of a critical care provider, some programs continue to provide basic paramedic-level care in the flight environment. This diversity in flight paramedic practice has clouded the definition of the profession. On one hand is a group of flight paramedics who define the practice as the ability to perform paramedic skills in the air medical environment; however, most flight paramedics define their practice as that of a critical care provider.

To combat this ambiguity and the lack of a nationally recognized flight paramedic examination, the National Flight Paramedics Association (NFPA; now the International Association of Flight Paramedics [IAFP]) introduced the FP-C examination. The FP-C examination was created on the premise that most flight paramedics function as critical care providers. Therefore, the certification process that defines the practice of the flight paramedic not only is based on an understanding of basic paramedic skills and flight physiology but also incorporates an understanding of critical care theory and practice. Specific recommendations for attaining and maintaining basic competencies are outlined in the NFPA position statement: "The role of the certified flight paramedic (FP-C) as a critical care provider and the required education."[7] Box 3-1 contains the NFPA's original position regarding the training necessary to pass the FP-C examination.

The title FP-C denotes an air medical professional with a broad expanse of knowledge. The FP-C examination process is not regionally specific. Regional practice and state laws are understood to direct the

---

BOX 3-1 | **Position of the NFPA Regarding the Training Necessary to Pass the Examination and Perform the Duties of a FP-C**

The NFPA believes the FP-C should have a minimum of 5 years of basic paramedic practice after graduation from a DOT-recognized paramedic training program before attempting to master the practice of flight medicine.

The NFPA believes the FP-C should maintain currency in the following certifications:

- Basic Cardiac Life Support
- Advanced Cardiac Life Support
- Basic Trauma Life Support
- Prehospital Trauma Life Support of Advanced Trauma Life Support audit
- Pediatric Advanced Life Support
- Neonatal Resuscitation Program

The NFPA believes initial didactic education for the FP-C should include content suitable to fill, at a minimum, the following number of hours in each area:

History, philosophy, and indications for air medical transport	1 hour
Industry associations and standards to include the standards of the Commission on Accreditation of Medical Transport Systems (CAMTS)	1 hour
Air medical outcome research, trauma systems, and trauma scoring	1 hour
Kinematics of trauma and injury patterns	1 hour
Aircraft: fundamentals, safety, and survival	3 hours
Flight physiology	1 hour
Stress management	1 hour
Advanced airway management techniques	2 hours
Radiographic interpretation	1 hour
Management of medical neurological emergencies	1 hour
Management of the critical cardiac case, to include pacemakers and invasive hemodynamic monitoring	8 hours
Intra-aortic balloon pump theory and transport considerations	8 hours
12-lead electrocardiographic (ECG) interpretation	8 hours
Management of the acute respiratory case, to include acid-base balance, ABG interpretation capnography, and ventilator management	6 hours
Management of septic shock	1 hour
Management of toxic exposures	1 hour
Management of the aortic emergency	1 hour
Management of hypertensive emergencies	1 hour

BOX 3-1	**Position of the NFPA Regarding the Training Necessary to Pass the Examination and Perform the Duties of a FP-C—cont'd**

Management of obstetric emergencies	3 hours
Management and delivery of the full-term or preterm newborn (neonatal resuscitation program and pediatric advanced life support are acceptable and encouraged alternatives)	16 hours
Management of the critical pediatric case	5 hours
Management of adult thoracic and abdominal trauma	2 hours
Management of neurological trauma	1 hour
Management of the burn case	1 hour
Management of pediatric trauma	1 hour
Management of environmental emergencies	1 hour
Trauma in pregnancy considerations	1 hour

Wherever appropriate, education should include information regarding radiographic findings, pertinent laboratory and bedside testing, and pharmacologic interventions.

The NFPA believes the FP-C should have initial and annual training in the indications, contraindications, desired effects, and adverse effects of the following skills. Furthermore, the NFPA believes that to ensure competency, the FP-C should have the opportunity to perform the skills in a laboratory setting.

- Rapid sequence induction intubation
- Pericardiocentesis
- Escharotomy
- Central venous access through subclavian, internal jugular, or femoral approach
- Chest tube thoracostomy
- Surgical cricothyroidotomy

The NFPA believes the FP-C should be given clinical exposure to critical care suitable to fill at a minimum the following number of hours in each area:

Labor and delivery	8 hours
Neonatal intensive care	8 hours
Pediatric intensive care	16 hours
Adult cardiac care (to include postoperative cardiothoracic surgery patients)	16 hours
Adult intensive care (to include medical and surgical patients)	16 hours

The NFPA believes the FP-C should maintain a minimum of 24 hours per year of continuing education in areas pertaining to critical care transport and care.

The NFPA believes the FP-C should maintain a minimum of 8 hours per year of patient contact hours in the following patient population areas (this time may be met through actual patient contact time during transports or through clinical time spent in the appropriate intensive care unit or specialty unit):

- Labor and delivery
- Neonatal intensive care
- Pediatric intensive care
- Adult cardiac care
- Adult intensive care
- Emergency/trauma care

The listed curriculum and minimum hours of content should not be considered endpoints for the FP-C. The IAFP (formally the NFPA) recognizes that individual learning styles and variances in transport program cultures and practices may require additional content to meet the needs of the individual FP-C provider.

flight paramedic's ability to perform certain procedures or administer specific medications. However, the IAFP does not believe that this precludes the necessity of the flight paramedic to maintain a basic knowledge of these skills or medications.

The Board for Critical Care Transport Paramedic Certification (BCCTPC) constructs and administers the FP-C examination. The examination is available via either paper and pencil or computer and currently consists of 125 questions. The focus of the examination is on the knowledge level of experienced paramedics who work with flight or critical care transport teams. The examination is not meant to test entry level knowledge. Table 3-4 contains a summary of the types and numbers of questions that are on the examination at this time.

The FP-C demonstrates, through written or computer-based testing, the ability to provide care beyond what may be allowed within a specific locale. By adopting this philosophy, successful completion of the FP-C examination should be viewed as the pinnacle achievement in the flight paramedic practice. Successful completion of the FP-C examination denotes the ability of the flight paramedic to practice with equal proficiency and without regional discrimination in both prehospital and interfacility transport.

TABLE 3-4 **Examination Content for FP-C[6]**	
Question Category	**No. of Questions**
Trauma management	9
Aircraft fundamentals, safety, and survival	12
Flight physiology	10
Advanced airway techniques	5
Neurologic emergencies	10
Critical cardiac cases	20
Respiratory cases	10
Toxic exposures	6
Obstetric emergencies	4
Neonates	4
Pediatric	10
Burn cases	5
General medicine cases	16
Environmental	4

SUMMARY

Certification holds value for healthcare and healthcare providers in many ways. Certified transport team members demonstrate to the consumer and the employer that nurses and paramedics have achieved a certain level of knowledge in a specific area of transport care. Certification confirms pride in one's profession and in one's specialty.

REFERENCES

1. American Association of Critical Care Nurses (AACN): *New data reveals nurse certification key component of patient safety and recruitment and retention programs (white paper)*, Aliso Viejo, CA, 2002, American Association of Critical Care Nurses; available at http://www.aacn.org/AACN/mrkt.nsf/Files/PressRelease/$file/PressRelease.pdf, accessed May 29, 2008.
2. AACN: *American Association of Critical Care Nurses Board of Certification*, available at http://www.aacn.org, accessed June 18, 2008.
3. American Board of Nursing Specialties: *American nurses credentialing center*, available at www.nursingcertification.org, accessed May 3, 2008.
4. ANCC: *American nurses credentialing center*, available at www.nursecredentialing.org, accessed May 3, 2008.
5. ENA: *Board of certification of emergency nursing*, available at www.ena.org, accessed May 3, 2008.
6. Board for Critical Care Transport Paramedic Certification (BCCTPC): *Candidate handbook*, Snellville, GA, 2006, BCCTPC.
7. Certified Flight Paramedics: *Value and benefits of certification*, available at http://www.certifiedflightparamedic.org/cfp/benefits.htm, accessed May 4, 2008.
8. Byrne M, Valentine W, Carter S: The value of certification: a research journey, *AORN J* 79(4):825-835, 2004.
9. Niebuhr B, Biel M: The value of specialty nursing certification, *Nurs Outlook* 55:176-181, 2007.
10. Sechrist KR, Valentine W, Berlin LE: Perceived value of certification among certified, noncertified and administrative perioperative nurses, *J Prof Nurs* 22(4): 242-247, 2006.
11. York-Clark D, Stocking J, Johnson J, editors: *Flight and ground transport nursing core curriculum*, ed 2, Denver, 2007, Air and Surface Transport Nurses Association.
12. Wynd C: Current factors contributing to professionalism in nursing, *J Prof Nurs* 19(5):251-261, 2003.

4

MEMBERS OF THE TRANSPORT TEAM

Reneé Semonin Holleran, Frank Thomas, Jonathan D. Gryniuk, Debbie K. Martin

With the advent of advanced treatment methods and the delineation of specialties at specific tertiary care centers, the need for available critical care transportation has become an integral component of many healthcare systems. Transport may be needed to ensure that the patient is able to receive life-saving care. Critical care transport is a collaborative practice and process. The scope and mission of the transport program, state nursing boards, emergency medical services (EMS) agencies, and types of patients transported contribute to crew member configuration. However, in the United States, the primary member of most critical care transport teams is generally agreed to be the registered nurse. An important note is that the primary member may vary both in the United States and globally.[8,33,37,39]

The team approach has proven effective in providing a holistic method to patient transport. The goal of the transport team is to provide seamless patient care, maintain or enhance the level of care from the referring facility or agency, and render interventions as appropriate. This chapter provides an overview of some transport team members.

THE TRANSPORT NURSE (FLIGHT, PREHOSPITAL, SURFACE)

In 1998, the Emergency Nurses Association (ENA) and the National Flight Nurses Association (NFNA; now known as the Air and Surface Transport Nurses Association [ASTNA]) released a joint position paper that described the role of nursing in the prehospital environment. Both organizations believe that nurses who practice in the prehospital care environment need to be appropriately educated to function successfully in that role and that practice should be regulated by state boards of nursing in the state in which the transport nurse practices. Box 4-1 presents a summary of this position paper.

Bader et al[1] conducted a national survey to discover the characteristics of flight nursing practice. The study results showed that one third of flight nurses who participated in flight programs were prepared at the baccalaureate level (BSN) and had 10 to 15 years of nursing experience. Most flight nurses had either emergency or critical care experience, had completed a trauma course, and were verified in pediatric advanced life support (PALS) and prehospital trauma life support/basic trauma life support (PHTLS/BTLS) and certified in emergency nursing (CEN). If the flight nurses were members of a professional organization, they belonged to NFNA or ENA.[1]

Currently, four curriculums outline the recommended education and skills needed to practice transport nursing: the Transport Nurse Advanced Trauma Course (TNATC) from ASTNA; the Air Medical Crew National Curriculum, developed by the US Department of Transportation; the National Standard Guidelines for Prehospital Nursing from ENA; and the Flight and Ground Transport Nursing

BOX 4-1	**Summary of the ENA/NFNA Position Statement: The Role of the Nurse in the Prehospital Care Environment**

1. ENA and NFNA qualified practicing nurses in the prehospital environment should not be required to certify as emergency medical or flight medical technicians.
2. ENA and NFNA endorse the need for special educational requirements for nurses practicing in the prehospital environment. Nurses need focused education and subsequent maintenance of specifically identified and recognized prehospital knowledge and skill.
3. ENA and NFNA recognize that EMS personnel possess a specialized body of knowledge and skills. Collaboration and communication are needed.
4. ENA and NFNA support that state boards of nursing are the regulatory body of the profession of nursing.
5. ENA and NFNA seek recognition of registered nurses by state EMS agencies for their unique role in the prehospital care environment.
6. ENA and NFNA endorse a collaborative role for the delivery of prehospital care.
7. ENA and NFNA support the use of the National Standard Guidelines for Prehospital Nursing Curriculum as developed by ENA and collaborating EMS agencies as a foundation for designing a course to meet the state and local requirements to practice in the prehospital environment. Competency-based testing should also be used. ENA and NFNA also support the utilization of the Flight Nursing Principles and Practice, Air Medical Crew National Standard Curriculum in conjunction with Practice Standards for Flight Nursing as the basis for training and education.

From ENA and NFNA Position Statement: *Role of the registered nurse in the prehospital environment,* adopted 1987 and revised 1998, available at http://www.ena.org/services/posistate/data/rolreg/htm.

Please note this is a summary from the position statement. To obtain the entire document go to http://www.ena.org/services/posistate/data/rolreg/htm.

Core Curriculum,[38] developed by the Air and Surface Transport Nurses Association. In addition, ASTNA has published standards of practice that provide nurses with a framework for air and critical transport nursing practice. Box 4-2 contains a description of the professional standards for transport nurses.

In 2006, the Air Medical Physician Association published Principles and Direction of Medical Direction. This document provides foundations for the education, roles, and required skills for transport team members and the framework of medical direction in the transport of patients.

A few states have prehospital care courses that serve as bridge courses for nurses to meet the requirements for emergency medical technician (EMT) and paramedic certification. An example of this is the Prehospital Nursing Course (PNC) that has been proposed in Maryland.[23] The PNC contains various modules related to prehospital care, and nurses may challenge all but four of these modules. The remaining modules reflect specialized didactic and practical training that is integral to clinical paramedic practice. Specific topics required by such bridge courses include: disaster/

BOX 4-2	**Professionalism Standards**

The flight nurse practices autonomously within the scope of practice defined by each institution.

The flight nurse practices in accordance with the state Nurse Practice Acts, state regulations governing prehospital care, NFNA standards, and policies and procedures set forth by medical direction and institution.

The flight nurse assumes responsibility and accountability for actions.

The flight nurse identifies self to patients, significant others, and healthcare providers.

The flight nurse participates in the education of the healthcare team, clients and their significant others, and the community.

From Hepp H: *National flight nurses standards of flight nursing practice,* St Louis, 1995, Mosby.

triage, rescue/extrication, vehicle operation, and orientation/role socialization.

Optimally, transport nurses should be prepared to function in the prehospital care environment. Even if nurses are not first responders, they must be familiar with the potential hazards of scene work and how to keep themselves and others with whom they work safe. The prehospital environment is dynamic and unforgiving. Most nurses have limited or no experience in this environment before they begin their transport careers.

Bader et al[1] found that flight nursing practice consists of both critical care and emergency nursing skills. The procedures that flight nurses performed included intubation, thoracentesis, cricothyroidotomy, escharotomy, intraosseous insertion, cutdowns, chest tube insertion, central line insertion, high risk obstetric management, and transport of patients with intraaortic balloon pumps in place. The ability to perform the skills necessary to carry out these procedures depends on the transport program mission, scope of practice, medical direction, level of the crew training, and state boards of nursing or State Bureau of Emergency Medical Services.

Acquiring these technical skills and remaining competent in them can be accomplished through laboratory practice, realistic interactive simulators, and supervised patient care. Many critical care transport programs require that a specific number of procedures be completed in a designated period of time. Box 4-3 contains a summary of some of the procedures performed by critical care transport nurses.

BOX 4-3   Summary of Skills for Transport Nursing Practice

Airway Management
1. Intubation
   Oral
   Nasotracheal
   Digital/manual
   Intubating laryngotracheal mask
2. Cricothyroidotomy
   Needle
   Surgical
3. End-tidal CO_2 monitoring
4. Pulse oximetry

Ventilation Management
1. Needle decompression
2. Chest tube insertion
3. Open thoracotomy-assisting
4. Pericardiocentesis
5. Ventilator management

Circulation Management
1. Vascular access
   Central line placement
   Venous cannulation
   Arterial cannulation
   Intraosseous line placement
   Seldinger technique
2. Medication administration
   Fluids
   Blood

    Blood products
    Vasoactive drugs
    Experimental and research medications
3. Intraaortic balloon pump management/left ventricular assist device
4. Pacing devices
   Internal
   External
5. Vital sign monitors
6. Invasive line monitors
   Blood pressure
   Pulmonary catheters
   Intracranial monitors
7. Urinary catheters
8. Gastric catheters
9. ECG monitors
10. 12-lead ECG monitors
11. Temperature management
12. Wound care
    Control of hemorrhage
    Protection from contamination

Additional Skills
1. Pain management during transport
   Movement
   Motion sickness
2. Emotional care
3. Family care

Critical-thinking skills constitute one of the most important interventions transport nurses bring to the transport environment. Critical care transport nurses constantly question, analyze, and reevaluate all components in the transport process. Critical thinking involves the use of knowledge and skills to explore practice situations.[12,24] Critical-thinking skills include the nurse's ability to be autonomous and organized and to view practice situations in an in-depth comprehensive way to better understand the experiences of the air medical patient.[12,24] This unique competence was identified in Bader et al,[1] who stated that flight nurses were held accountable for these skills: "These complex skills included decisions regarding the administration and titration of medications, initiating therapeutic treatment based on physical assessment findings, communicating and documenting significant findings and performing follow-up activities."[1]

Transport nursing requires education, training, experience, and continuous evaluation of competence. Transport nurses must be physically and emotionally ready to meet the demands of patient care during transport.[37,38] Although some general characteristics of transport nursing do exist, the specific responsibilities and practice protocols depend on the type of service provided, the crew matrix, the type of vehicles used for transport, and state regulations. Box 4-4 summarizes general educational preparation for critical transport nursing practice.[28-30,38]

PARAMEDICS

Today, specially trained skills that had previously been reserved for the hospital setting have found their way into the paramedic's skill set. Most notably, after appropriate education, paramedics have shown their abilities to perform advanced procedures that have historically been areas of practice for physicians, nurses, or respiratory therapists. Rapid sequence induction (RSI), 12-lead electrocardiographic (ECG) interpretation, and administration of fibrinolytics are a few of the advanced practice skills successfully and appropriately performed by the trained paramedic.[2,5,7,9,11,13-18, 22]

Paramedics who perform these skills were once viewed as advanced practice paramedics in that they

---

BOX 4-4	**Summary of Educational Requirements for the Transport Nurse**

Registered nurse (some programs require multiple
   licensure with provision of care across the state line)
Advanced Cardiac Life Support (ACLS)
Pediatric Advanced Life Support (PALS)
Emergency Nursing Pediatric Course (ENPC)
Prehospital care orientation course (determined by
   state EMS agency)
or
Prehospital Registered Nurse Course
or
EMT/EMT-P certification
Certification in a nursing specialty
Certified Emergency Nurse (CEN)
Certified Critical Care Nurse (CCRN)
Certified Flight Registered Nurse (CFRN)
Certified Transport Registered Nurse (CTRN)
Trauma course
International Trauma Life Support (ITLS)
Prehospital Trauma Life Support (PHTLS)
Advanced Trauma Life Support (ATLS)
Transport Nurse Advanced Trauma Course (TNATC)
Trauma Nursing Core Course (TNCC)

---

performed skills outside those taught within the Department of Transportation's EMS curriculum. The paramedics of today not only are responsible for prehospital patient care but also can frequently be found transporting patients between medical facilities or working as allied healthcare providers within the hospital setting.[32] This broadened scope of responsibility has given rise to subspecialty groups of paramedics: the critical care paramedic and the flight paramedic (Figure 4-1).

CRITICAL CARE PARAMEDIC

The resource-scarce healthcare environment of the 1990s spurred an increase in the number of patients needing critical care transport and thus an increase in the need for competent critical care–trained transport providers. Born of this need was the concept of the critical care paramedic (CCP or CC-EMTP) who could complete transports that previously required supplementation with hospital staff. CCPs

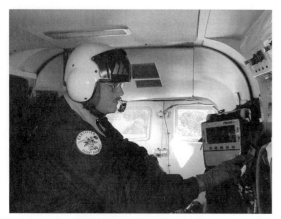

FIGURE 4-1   **Flight medic.**

receive training beyond that of "street" paramedics, which prepares them to appropriately assess and manage the patient who has already received significant medical interventions, including the use of advanced pharmacologic agents and the insertion of hemodynamic monitoring and assist devices.[26] Use of this new healthcare provider has shown promising results.[10]

Concerns have been raised regarding the ability of the CCP to use the critical-thinking skills that are often necessary in the management of the critical care case. However, the development of critical-thinking skills can be successfully instilled in the paramedic through an effective scenario-based approach to education and training.[14] Furthermore; no education is complete without the opportunity to apply newly learned skills in a clinical setting under direct observation of another skilled practitioner. Although a variety of CCP training programs offer a clinical practice component, no universal requirement has been established for inclusion of clinical training.[9,19-21]

Other concerns regarding the CCP have centered on the paramedic's ability to truly identify the critical nature of the patient's condition and ensure that appropriate resources are available during transport. Education and training, again, are the cornerstones to decrease this concern. Paramedics have shown their ability to correctly identify and plan for the transport of the critical care case after receiving appropriate education.[31] The CCP is generally partnered with either a critical care transport nurse

or respiratory therapist, which can further enhance the transport team.

Although a variety of commercial educational courses offer to train and graduate "critical care paramedics," an important note is that the use of the title CCP is not currently governed by any private, state, or federal agencies. Currently, no agreement exists on the content or length of CCP training programs.[31-36]

In 2008, the International Association of Flight Paramedics (IAFP) partnered with a nationally recognized university to complete a comprehensive survey to identify the skill set and education associated with critical care paramedic practice. The survey data have been collected and are being tabulated and analyzed to create a functional definition for the Critical Care Transport Paramedic (IAFP reference).

FLIGHT PARAMEDIC

The flight paramedic has played a pivotal role in the development of air medical transport. In 1970, the Maryland State Police instituted the first statewide EMS helicopter service. This multifaceted air transport, air rescue, and police program was staffed by emergency medical technician-paramedic (EMT-P)/police officers (Trooper Paramedic) and has remained in continuous operation to this day.[9,13]

In 1986, flight paramedics united to form the National Flight Paramedics Association (NFPA). The NFPA is now known as the International Association of Flight Paramedics (IAFP). The NFPA was formed to represent the global interests of flight paramedics within the air medical industry with an emphasis on safety and education. In 1990, the NFPA furthered its goals to promote quality within the industry by serving as a founding member of the Commission on Accreditation of Air Medical Services (CAAMS), now known as the Commission on Accreditation of Medical Transport Systems (CAMTS).

In 2005, the NFPA answered a global request for improved representation of flight paramedics from around the world by redefining their mission and adopting a new name: the International Association of Flight Paramedics (IAFP). Although the concept of the critical care paramedic is fairly new, the ability of the paramedic to function in this advanced capacity is not. Most air medical transport programs have used the flight paramedic in a critical care provider capacity since the early beginnings of air medical transport. Because of the complex nature of the cases transported by air medical programs, expanding the role of flight paramedics beyond that of their ground counterparts quickly became necessary. Additional responsibilities, such as surgical airway management, use of anesthetic agents to facilitate intubation, and the use of portable ventilators, became necessary to optimize the care of the critically ill and injured patients during air transport. A host of other skills followed as flight paramedics proved their ability to grasp and maintain competency in skills previously afforded to physicians and advanced practice nurses. These skills commonly include pericardiocentesis, chest tube insertion, escharotomy, and insertion of central venous access devices.

With advances in medical care came the need to maintain care of increasingly complex cases, which required a critical care–like setting during transport. Invasive hemodynamic monitoring, administration of blood products, initiation and titration of vaso-active and sedative medications, and analysis of a variety of laboratory data through portable devices became an integral part of air medical transport.[12] Today, it is not uncommon to find flight paramedics trained in monitoring and managing patient populations from the adult cardiac patients with an intra-aortic balloon pump or a left ventricular assist device to the preterm infant undergoing extracorporeal membrane oxygenation.[1,6,16]

RESPIRATORY THERAPIST

Respiratory therapists (RTs) typically work in hospitals, where they perform assessments, diagnostics, intensive critical care procedures, and patient interventions for all patient populations, including the neonate and the elderly. They also function as a vital part of a hospital's lifesaving response team.

Today, respiratory therapists are members of both air and ground critical care transport teams. The qualifications, education, and training for transport respiratory therapists are based on the scope of practice of the transport program and the program for which they may work.

A degree in respiratory care requires education in physics (gas laws), biology, pharmacology, chemistry,

and microbiology. A respiratory therapist possesses a skill base of more than 100 clinical interventions, including arterial line insertion, chest tube insertion, intubation, surgical airways, and medication administration (inhalation and parenteral). Clinical training includes the use of high technology medical equipment, such as mechanical ventilation, intra-aortic balloon pump, and pulmonary artery catheter monitoring.

The American Association of Respiratory Care (www.aarc.org) has a Surface and Air Transport members section that provides specific information about the roles of a transport respiratory therapist. The respiratory therapist, as a member of a transport team, should receive appropriate education and training to function in air or ground transport environments. This training should include safety, survival, and operating within individual transport vehicles.

This repertoire of education, skills, and clinical training makes the respiratory therapist an excellent critical care transport team member who is easily cross trained. Teams with a registered nurse (RN)/RT configuration contend that airway management is the first priority in prehospital and transport medicine and have found that specialists in airway maintenance and mechanical ventilation are extremely valuable.

PHYSICIANS

Traditionally, the training of a physician differs from the other transport team members. Physician training includes 4 years of premedical school, 4 years of medical school, a residency program that varies from 3 to 5 years, and a possible fellowship, which also varies in length from 2 to 3 years. Much of a physician's training centers on an understanding of basic science and differential diagnosis of disease processes. The physician team member can make a significant contribution to the care of the critically ill or injured patient who needs transport. Because of their training, physicians can be of great assistance in delineating the causes and, therefore, the required treatment of a medical condition.

A physician involved in a critical care transport program can function in one of three roles: (1) as a transport crew member; (2) as a provider of medical direction; or (3) as the physician medical director.[3,4,6,8]

FLIGHT PHYSICIAN CREW MEMBER

With the recent proliferation of for-profit air transport services, less than 6% of the flight programs are believed to use a physician as a crew member.[3,4] Most of these physician crew members represent physicians in residency or fellowship training. Only a small number of programs fly with attending-level physicians.

The need for or benefit of having a physician as a transport team member has been and continues to be a hotly debated subject.[5,7,25] The level of expertise of transport physicians may vary from that of an intern to that of an experienced board-certified physician specialist.[5,7] The selection of physician experience depends on the specific program. Unlike the flight nurse certification examination (CFRN), no certification test is available for flight physicians. However, the Commission on Accreditation of Medical Transports Systems (CAMTS) and the Association of Air Medical Physicians do provide educational and clinical recommendations for physicians involved in critical care transport (Box 4-5).[6,8]

BOX 4-5   CAMTS Recommendations for Medical Directors

The medical director of the program is a physician who is responsible for supervising and evaluating the quality of medical care provided by the medical personnel. The medical director ensures, by working with the clinical supervisor and by being familiar with the scope of practice of the transport team members and the state regulations in which the transport team practices, competency and currency of all medical personnel working with the service.

The medical director should be licensed and authorized to practice in the state or states in which the transport services are based.

The medical director should have experience in those areas of medicine commensurate with the mission statement of the medical transport service.

The medical director should be experienced in both ground and air emergency medical services and has received medical director education. The physician should be current and demonstrate competency or provide documentation of equivalent experiences directed by the mission statement and scope of care. If a physician is boarded in an area appropriate to the mission and scope of the service, specialty certifications are required as pertinent to the program's scope of care. These certifications include:

1. Advanced Cardiac Life Support (ACLS)
2. Advanced Trauma Life Support (ATLS)
3. Neonatal Resuscitation (NRP)
4. Pediatric Advanced Life Support (PALS) or Advanced Pediatric Life Support (APLS)
5. Patient care capabilities and limitations
6. Infection control
7. Stress recognition and management
8. Altitude physiology/stressors of flight if involved in rotor-wing or fixed-wing operations
9. Ground ambulance rules/regulations/driver safety course
10. Appropriate utilization of medical/ground interfacility services
11. Emergency Medical Services
12. Hazardous materials recognition and response
13. The medical director should demonstrate continuing education in transport

The medical director is actively involved in the quality management program (QA).

The medical director is actively involved in administrative decisions that affect medical care for the service.

Medical Control Physicians: On-line medical control physicians (who are trained and identified by the service) should have the appropriate knowledge base and experience sufficient to ensure proper medical care and medical control during transport for all patient types served by the transport services.

One advantage of physicians as medical flight crew members is that medical protocols, or standing orders, may be less necessary to have in existence.

PHYSICIAN MEDICAL CONTROL

In programs in which physicians are not used as transport team members, control of medical direction of the transport team is often provided by assigning a physician online responsibility for the actions of the transport team. This medical direction physician has the responsibility of overseeing that the correct team (i.e., adult, pediatric, or neonatal), equipment (i.e., advanced life support [ALS], basic life support [BLS], or specialized), and mode of transport (i.e., helicopter, fixed wing, or ground) are selected to meet the patient's transport medical needs and that appropriate medical backup is available to the nonphysician flight team.[24] For most transport systems, physician medical control falls under the oversight of emergency trained physicians. However, for patients who need specialty transports, medical direction often occurs under the oversight of specialty trained physicians (i.e., neonatologist, pediatric or adult critical care trained physicians).

Proper medical direction occurs when the physician does one of the following: (1) makes an inquiry on the patient's medical condition from the referring institution and relays that information to the transport team; or (2) provides online medical advice to the transport team.

PHYSICIAN MEDICAL DIRECTOR

The primary responsibility of the physician medical director is to provide administrative medical oversight and medical quality assurance over the transport program. Box 4-6 contains the position statement of

---

BOX 4-6 **Medical Direction and Medical Control of Air Medical Services Position Statement of the Air Medical Physician Association**

Approved by the AMPA Board of Trustees, Revised April 2002

Medical Direction

The Air Medical Physician Association believes that all air medical services require the active involvement and participation of a physician Medical Director(s), who shall be responsible for supervising, evaluating, and ensuring the quality of medical care provided by the air medical transport team.

At all times, Medical Direction must be consistent with the following priorities. Safety of the crew, patient, and vehicle must always be the first priority. The second priority is the provision of appropriate patient care. Finally, after addressing safety and patient care, medical direction should be committed to the appropriate utilization of medical transport resources and cost-effective patient transport.

Responsibility and Authority of the Medical Director

The Medical Director of an air medical service shall:
1. Have the final authority over all patient care and clinical aspects of the air medical service.
2. Oversee and ensure that:
   a. Medical personnel have adequate training and qualifications to deliver appropriate medical care.
   b. Appropriate medical equipment and supplies are available.
   c. Appropriate vehicle selection is made for transport.
   d. Patients are transported to appropriate destinations.
3. Have the responsibility and authority to develop and implement medical care policies and procedures and clinical standards commensurate with the scope of care of the air medical service in accordance with applicable laws and regulations.
4. Participate in the determination of the qualifications, hiring, training, continuing education, and competency evaluation of all air medical service medical personnel.
5. Have the authority to restrict the patient care activities of any medical crew member who does not meet the specified training program or whose performance is inconsistent with established policies, procedures, patient care protocols, or clinical standards of care.

(Continued)

BOX 4-6	Medical Direction and Medical Control of Air Medical Services Position Statement of the Air Medical Physician Association—cont'd

6. Establish criteria to ensure that patients are transported to appropriate destinations.
7. Be involved in any/all air medical service administrative decisions that may affect patient care.
8. Be actively involved in the air medical service continuous quality improvement (CQI) program.
9. Serve as a liaison to the medical community served by the air medical service.
10. Coordinate the orientation and training of any physicians providing on-line or off-line medical control for the air medical service with regard to the program policies, procedures, patient care protocols, and clinical standards.
11. Help resolve disputes regarding medical direction/control and patient care issues.

Qualifications of the Medical Director

The Medical Director of an air medical service shall:

1. Be licensed and authorized to practice medicine or osteopathy in the jurisdiction(s) that serves as a base for the air medical service.
2. Be actively involved in the care of critically ill or injured patients.
3. Have the educational experience and exhibit expertise in those areas of medicine commensurate with the scope of care of the air medical service or utilize consultant specialty physicians as indicated.
4. Be experienced and knowledgeable in aspects of air and ground patient transport commensurate with the scope of care of the air medical service. These areas shall include, but are not limited to:
   a. Program safety.
   b. In-flight patient care capabilities and limitations.
   c. Altitude and flight physiology and the clinical stresses of flight.
   d. Appropriate utilization of air medical services.
   e. Biomedical equipment appropriate to the transport environment.
   f. Infection control.
   g. Stress recognition and management.
   h. Hazardous materials recognition and response.
   i. Any applicable statutory laws, rules, or regulations that may impact patient care.

Obligations of the Air Medical Service

The qualifications, responsibilities, and authority of the Medical Director should be specified in a written agreement between the physician and the air medical service. The air medical service must empower their Medical Director with the authority and necessary resources commensurate with the responsibilities identified, which should include:

1. A job description detailing the Medical Director's authority, responsibility, and expectations.
2. Compensation for professional services.
3. Indemnification for actions and duties as Medical Director of the air medical service.
4. Personnel support, equipment, and supplies.

Medical Control

The Air Medical Physician Association believes that all air medical transports require physician medical control and that the responsibility for ensuring appropriate medical control rests with the Medical Director(s) of the air medical service.

The Medical Director has the final authority over all patient care aspects of the air medical service, which includes medical control for all transports. The Medical Director may, however, delegate the responsibility and authority for medical control to other qualified individuals.

The Medical Director is responsible for selecting, orienting, and ensuring the competency of any medical control physician. Orientation activities shall include review of the policies, procedures, patient care protocols, and in-flight patient care capabilities and limitations of the air medical service.

BOX 4-6	**Medical Direction and Medical Control of Air Medical Services Position Statement of the Air Medical Physician Association—cont'd**

Appropriate medical control must take into consideration the medical care requirements of the individual patient and a thorough knowledge of the scope of care that can be provided by the medical transport team. The scope of care for each air medical service is based upon the patient care capabilities of the transport personnel, available medical equipment, formulary, and the capabilities and limitations of their transport vehicles.

Medical control physicians must have the experience and knowledge to ensure that appropriate medical control and medical care is rendered and consistent with the scope of practice and the mission of the air medical service. If the experience of the medical control physician in a particular clinical area is insufficient to ensure appropriate care, the medical control physician should seek suitable and timely consultation.

Method of Medical Control

Medical control may be accomplished in one of three ways: on-line, off-line, and visually. On-line medical control represents direct real-time voice communication between the medical control physician and the transport team. During off-line medical control, there is no direct contact between the transport team and the medical control physician. Patient interventions follow written medical protocols or standing orders provided by the Medical Director, medical control physician, referring physician, or receiving physician. Visual medical control occurs when a medical control physician is physically present during the transport.

Responsibility and Authority for Medical Control
Interhospital Patient Transfers

While medical control for interfacility transfers may be assumed by the transferring physician, receiving physician, or the Medical Director (or designee) of the air medical service, AMPA believes that medical control should remain the responsibility of the Air Medical Director or his/her designee. Any variation from this standard should be specified in a patient transfer agreement or at the time of request for air medical transport.

Prehospital Patient Transfers

While medical control for prehospital transfers may be assumed by the receiving physician, EMS base station, or air medical service Medical Director (or designee), AMPA believes that medical control should remain the responsibility of the Air Medical Director or his/her designee.

---

the Air Medical Physicians Association (AMPA), entitled Medical Direction and Medical Control of Air Medical Services (2002). This statement provides a description of the responsibilities and authority of the medical director, qualifications of the medical director, obligations of the air medical service to the medical director, and a discussion of medical control.

Specifically, the physician medical director's role includes but is not limited to: (1) establishing medical protocols or guidelines; (2) ensuring adequate medical crew member training; (3) providing oversight of medical control physicians; (4) providing quality assurance oversight for the medical care rendered by the transport service; (5) providing support for medical crew members; and (6) assisting in the clarification and resolution of transport issues that may arise from the referring or receiving agency.

Establishing Medical Protocols

For the transport service that does not routinely use physicians as transport team members, the medical director is responsible for establishing medical protocols or guidelines that enable transport nurses to initiate care treatments and procedures considered outside their hospital-based nursing practice. Although the transport medical physician director may not directly write these protocols, the transport medical physician is ultimately regarded as responsible for the content and accuracy of these protocols. When confusion in treatment results, the team members, in conjunction with the medical director, should develop new policies, protocols, or guidelines that govern future medical care.

Ensuring Adequate Training

The medical director is actively involved in the development of training that ensures the transport team members can meet the expected level of medical care as it relates to the transport environment. Prospective training occurs through introduction courses to emergency and critical care transport. Such training includes, but is not limited to, altitude physiology, transport medical care, and procedures. In addition to the initial training, the medical director must provide continuous training and updating of the transport team members regarding new innovations in patient care. Often this education occurs during staff meetings where new information can be presented. Retrospective review of transport care provides immediate feedback for reinforcing or modifying care delivered by the transport team members.

Oversight of Medical Control Physicians

One role of the medical director is to ensure that physicians who provide medical control are educated to the mission and capabilities of the transport service. Clinical discrepancy between medical control and medical flight team members can arise. Under these circumstances, the medical director provides clarification to both parties as to the recommended standard of practice for the transport service. Likewise, control physicians can determine whether additional training may be necessary for selected crew members. Contacting the medical director regarding these training issues ensures that proper steps can be taken by the medical director to reduce medical mishaps.

During the transport, the control physician serves as the sounding board and provides medical support to the transport crew members. This support may be done before transport so the physician can provide the transport crew members with valuable information regarding the patient's status and with possible diagnostic or therapeutic suggestions. This support can also be provided during the transport, when the transport team recognizes that additional medical input may be beneficial in diagnosing or providing care to the patient.

After the transport, the transport team may wish to discuss the possible diagnostic and therapeutic options related to the patient's condition. Such interactions are beneficial because the transport crew members gain additional insight and the medical director recognizes any need for additional transport team training.

Quality Assurance Oversight

One of the most important roles of the medical director is to provide quality assurance of the medical care provided by the medical team, with use of a retrospective analysis of patient care during weekly or monthly staff meetings. During these meetings, patient charts are reviewed and reinforcement of current policies and procedures is made. In addition, particular problems that may have arisen from these policies and procedures are presented. The discussion that ensues allows all transport team members an opportunity to develop the best possible method for patient care in the future.

Psychologic Support of Medical Crew Members

Medical flight crew members are a highly trained group of individuals who have high expectations of themselves. Despite their training, these crew members are often put into circumstances in which the patient's condition may not be salvageable. When a patient dies after heroic attempts by the flight crew, some element of posttraumatic stress always results. The medical director, in conjunction with the nurse manager and program manager, is a key element in helping to reduce and alleviate these stresses.

Resolving Conflict with the Referring or Receiving Physician

Conflict can arise among transport team members, particularly when a nurse, paramedic, or respiratory therapist and a physician disagree about patient treatment. Most often, such conflict is a result of a difference in perspectives. When such conflicts occur, the team member and the physician should work together to resolve the issue. Physicians must attempt to understand transport team members' concerns as they relate to the delivery of patient care. Likewise, the transport team member must recognize that the physician may have a different perspective of the issue as it relates to patient treatment. The best patient care results from a collaborative effort between the team member and the physician. Medical directors can serve as a go-between to resolve these conflicts.

COMMUNICATION SPECIALISTS

Communication is the first step in the transport process. The National Association of Air Medical Communication Specialists (NAACS) has developed a description of the role of the communication specialist in the transport process. In addition, Operational Control has become an integral component of communications and the transport process. More components of the role of the Communication Specialist, particularly specific functions, are discussed in Chapter 8.

The communication specialist is responsible for obtaining patient information, along with Operational Control initiation of the transport, the following transport (air or ground), and notification of appropriate personnel before, during, and after the transport process. In addition, many communication centers serve as contact areas for transport team members and their friends and family, and other hospital personnel. The transport team must always remember that the communication specialist is the "voice" of the transport team. The communication specialist should be treated as a team member and included in decision making and stress management.

Communication specialists play a major role in the transport process and are integral members of the transport team.

PILOT CREW MEMBER

Transport team and pilot interactions play a critical role in the performance of air medical teams. Team-level and organization-level factors may enhance or impede the ability of well-trained individuals to work together effectively and efficiently. Each team member's position must be clearly stated and defined, which establishes structure and determines the flow of communication.

The National EMS Pilots Association (NEMSPA) is the association dedicated to pilots involved in

patient transport. NEMSPA is focused on improving the quality and safety of air medical transport (www.nemspa.org).

PILOT-IN-COMMAND QUALIFICATIONS

The pilot-in-command (PIC) is responsible for the safety of the aircraft, crew, and passengers. The pilot is accountable for nonmedical aspects of the flight and has final authority in all flight-related issues. CAMTS[8] outlines the PIC qualifications for both rotorcraft-helicopter and fixed-wing aircraft. These qualifications are summarized in Box 4-7.

The responsibility of the PIC is to create an atmosphere in which crew participation can flourish. The PIC must help maintain a balanced predictable environment while responding to changing situations. This responsibility implies that shifts of balance occur and that each crew member should understand that they have the responsibility to participate fully and professionally in every flight.

If the PIC has not succeeded in establishing a comfortable atmosphere of open participation, the flight team will not verbally communicate any concerns or discomforts. The PIC must establish clear leadership and command authority and appropriately apply the use of authority based on the current situation. The pilot must command respect but at the same time create an atmosphere conducive to crew participation.

Flight crew members assist in flight-related duties as outlined by the individual program or vendor's policies or general operations manual and as reinforced by the PIC. Flight team members offer assistance in a variety of flight duties. Some of their contributions include air or ground traffic sightings, hazard and obstacle sightings, obstacle avoidance procedures (landing zones), cargo (medical equipment) securing, passenger briefing, radio monitoring, and minor participation in the computation of weight and balance requirements.

When time and safety permit, the pilot may also assist the flight team by helping load and unload patients. In addition, the pilot can transport needed medical equipment to the flight team and relay medical information to the receiving hospital.

BOX 4-7	**CAMTS Rotor-Wing and Fixed-Wing Aircraft Pilot in Command Qualifications**

Rotorcraft-Helicopter Pilot-in-Command

Must possess at least a commercial rotorcraft helicopter and instrument helicopter rating.

Must possess 2000 total flight hours with a minimum of 1500 helicopter flight hours prior to assignment with a medical service with the following stipulations:

1. At least 1000 of those hours must be as the PIC in the rotorcraft.
2. At least 100 of those hours must be night-flight time as PIC.
3. A minimum of 500 hours of turbine time to 1000 hours of turbine time strongly encouraged. Pilot training should at a minimum consist of the following and be verified by written criteria, outlines, or curriculum.

Use of Federal Aviation Administration (FAA)–approved training devices and simulators along with mission-specific scenario-based training should be encouraged at initial and recurrent training cycles.

Airline Transport Pilot (ATP) certificate strongly encouraged.

Fixed-Wing Pilot-in-Command

Must possess 2000 airplane hours prior to assignment with a medical service with the following stipulations:

1. At least 1000 of those hours must be as a PIC in an airplane.
2. At least 500 of those hours must be in multiengine airplane time as PIC (not required of single-engine turbine aircraft).
3. At least 100 of those hours must be night flight time as PIC.

PIC must be ATP rated; Second in Command (SIC) is strongly recommended to be ATP rated and must complete an operator-approved SIC training.

To optimize program safety, an expectation of safety must override all other considerations. The adage "all to go, one for no" reflects the expectation that only one crew member can turn down a flight for safety concerns. The result is that a program's safety environment must support such decision making. Although administrative request for justification is reasonable, unjust consequences toward pilots or other transport team members should not exist for turn downs/flight aborts. Team members should feel safe to prioritize decision-making on the basis of established safety practices, program minimums, and previous flight experience.

The bond between established crew members and the air medical staff could become quite strong. The eight goals for a successful relationship between the pilot and transport team members (personal communication from Dr Michelle North in June 2002) are as follows:

1. Communicate positively.
2. Direct assistance as needed.
3. Announce decisions clearly.
4. Offer assistance.
5. Acknowledge the actions of others.
6. Be specific.
7. Know and understand the team's aviation roles and responsibilities.
8. Be vigilant in understanding the interaction between the crew members, the machine, and the environment.

PROGRAM DIRECTOR

In most critical care transport programs, the program director is responsible for coordinating the administrative activities of the transport service. The program director may be a registered nurse, physician, pilot, paramedic, or hospital administrator.[27] CAMTS has recommendations on the qualifications of the program administrator, which are listed in Box 4-8.[8]

The major responsibilities of the program director include formulating administrative policies, directing continuous quality improvement activities, managing vehicle contracts and vendors, maintaining the communications system, preparing and monitoring components of the budget, participating in strategic planning and marketing, serving as a resource for problem solving, and serving as community liaison.[21]

BOX 4-8	CAMTS Management Recommendations

Commitment to medical transport service.

Well-defined line of authority with clear reporting mechanisms to upper level management.

An organizational chart that defines how the transport service fits into the governing/sponsoring institution, agency, and cooperation.

All personnel understand chain of command.

Disciplinary policies.

Written policies and procedures indicate what therapies can be performed without on-line medical direction.

Encourages ongoing communications between patient care personnel, communications personnel, pilots, mechanics, and ground personnel.

Marketing activities.

Management assures an appropriate utilization review process.

Oriented to Federal Air Regulations (FARs) that are pertinent to air medical program and regulations that pertain to ground ambulance services.

The Association of Air Medical Services (AAMS) offers a Medical Transport Leadership Institute whose mission is to enhance the management of medical transportation services. This 2-year program offers courses in human resource management, leadership and administration, financial operations, program development, and asset management.[21] Program directors, medical crew supervisors, operators, lead pilots, and other leadership personnel in critical care transport are provided with a framework to strengthen or develop their leadership and administrative skills. A graduate level program is also offered, which expands on foundational concepts, providing further opportunity for interactive dialogue and problem solving. Networking with proven transport industry leaders is a daily occurrence at all levels and provides excellent opportunity for participants to realistically hone their acquired skills.

Each critical care transport program dictates the role of the program director. The transport team must know and understand the director's role in the program and the program's organizational chart and how the transport team functions in the program.

SUMMARY

For effective patient transport, multiple resources are necessary. The mission of the transport service designs the transport team and defines the roles of all disciplines involved. The patient and the patient's needs determine the members of the team. Patient transport depends on organized professional components, cohesively working together to ensure both safe and competent patient care.

REFERENCES

1. Bader GB, Terhorst M, Heilman P, et al: Characteristics of flight nursing practice, *Air Med J* 14(4):214-218, 1995.
2. Banerjee S, Rhoden WE: Fast-tracking of myocardial infarction by paramedics, *J Royal Col Phys London* 32(1):36-38, 1998.
3. Baxt W, Moody P: The impact of a physician as part of the aeromedical pre-hospital team in patients with blunt trauma, *JAMA* 257(23):3246-3250, 1987.
4. Baxt W, Moody P, Ireland HC: Hospital-based rotorcraft aeromedical emergency care services and transport: a multicenter study, *Ann Emerg Med* 14(9):859, 1985.
5. Bledsoe B, Benner R: *Critical care paramedic,* Upper Saddle River, NJ, 2006, Pearson Prentice Hall.
6. Blumen I, editor: *Principles and direction of air medical transport*, Salt Lake City, 2006, Air Medical Physician Association.
7. Certified Flight Paramedic Exam: *Outline of subjects*, available at http://www.certifiedflightparamedic.org/cfp/docs/examoutline.pdf, accessed August 2008.
8. Commission on Accreditation of Medical Transport Systems: *Accreditation standards*, ed 6, Anderson, SC, 2006, CAMTS.
9. Critical care transport program (CCEMTP): *University of Maryland Baltimore Campus*, available at http://ehs.umbc.edu/CE/CCEMT-P/CCEMTP.html, accessed August 2008.
10. Crowley RA, et al: An economical and proved helicopter program for transporting the emergency critically ill and injured patient in Maryland, *J Trauma* 13:1029-1038, 1973.
11. Domier R, et al: The development and evaluation of a paramedic-staffed mobile intensive care unit for interfacility patient transport, *Prehosp Disaster Med* 11(1):37-43, 1996.
12. Edwards SL: Critical thinking, *Nurse Educ Pract* 7: 303-314, 2006.

13. Florida Emergency Medical Services (EMS) Advisory Council: *State EMS medical directors report,* available at http://www.doh.state.fl.us/demo/EMS/EMSSAC/October2007EMSACMinutes.pdf, accessed August 2008.

14. Hatley T, et al: Flight paramedic scope of practice: current level of breadth, *J Emerg Med* 16(5):731-735, 1998.

15. Holmes E: *A brief history of aeromedical helicopters, soundings,* available at http://users.exis.net/-eholmes/soun-index.html, accessed August 2008.

16. International Association of Flight Paramedics: *FP news,* available at http://www.flightparamedic.org/docs/May08nwsltr.pdf, accessed August 2008.

17. Janing J: Assessment of a scenario-based approach to facilitating critical thinking among paramedic students, *Prehosp Disaster Med* 12(3):215-221, 1997.

18. Lee A, et al: Interhospital transfers: decision-making in critical care areas, *Crit Care Med* 24(4):618-622, 1996.

19. Lupton B, Pendray M: Regionalized neonatal emergency transport, *Semin Neonatol* 9:125-133, 2004.

20. McDonald CC, Bailey B: Out-of-hospital use of neuromuscular blocking agents in the United States, *Prehosp Emerg Care* 2(1):29-32, 1998.

21. Medical Transport Leadership Institute: *Association of air medical services,* available at http://www.aams.org, accessed July 19, 2002.

22. Michigan Society of Medicine EMS: Ad-*hoc committee on critical care transport, instructors/coordinators,* available at http://www.emgint.org/cct/draft.htm, accessed November 7, 2000.

23. Miller P, Epifianio P: Development of a prehospital nursing curriculum in Maryland, *J Emerg Nurs* 19(3):206, 1993.

24. Miller M, Babcock D: *Critical thinking applied to nursing,* St Louis, 1996, Mosby.

25. Murphy-Macabobby M, et al: Neuromuscular blockade in aeromedical airway management, *Ann Emerg Med* 21(6):664-668, 1992.

26. Pace SA, Fuller FP: Out-of-hospital succinylcholine assisted endotracheal intubation by paramedics, *Ann Emerg Med* 35(6):568-572, 2000, available at http://www.hlth.gov.bc.ca/bcas/bcasqual.html.

27. Pons S, Notterman DA: Roles of the medical program directors. In McClosky K, Orr R, editors: *Pediatric transport medicine,* St Louis, 1995, Mosby.

28. Rhee K, Burney RE: Is a flight physician needed for helicopter emergency services? *Ann Emerg Med* 15(2): 174, 1986.

29. Semonin Holleran R: *Prehospital nursing: a collaborative approach,* St Louis, 1994, Mosby.

30. Shaner S, et al: Flight crew physical fitness: a baseline analysis, *Air Med J* 14(1):30, 1995.

31. Shoestring Graphics and Printing: *Critical care paramedic protocols,* available at http://www.ssfx.com/CP2020/medtech/procedures/protocols/htm, accessed August 2008.

32. Southwest MedEvac Homepage: *Patient care,* available at http://swmedevac.com/homestart.htm, accessed August 2008.

33. Telelz D, Balazs K, Young L: Prehospital transport-air medicine. In McClosky K, Orr R, editors: *Pediatric transport medicine,* St Louis, 1995, Mosby.

34. Spencer C: Critical thinking in nursing: teaching to diverse groups, *Teaching Learning Nurs* 3: 87-89, 2008.

35. University of Iowa Hospitals and Clinics: *Critical care paramedic (CCP) provider course,* available at http://www.uihealthcare.com/depts/emslrc/courses/CCP%20Iowa%20City&2008.pdf, accessed August 2008.

36. Weaver WD, et al: Prehospital-initiated vs. hospital-initiated thrombolytic therapy: the myocardial infarction and intervention trial, *JAMA* 27(6):426, 1993.

37. Wilson P: Safe patient transport: nurses make a difference, *Nurs Times* 94(26):66-67, 1998.

38. York-Clark D, Stocking J, Johnson J: *Flight and ground transport nursing core curriculum,* Denver, 2006, Air and Surface Transport Nurses Association.

39. Zempsky WT, Haskell G: Paramedics as allied health care providers in the pediatric emergency department, *Ped Emerg Care* 14(5):329-331, 1998.

General Principles of Practice

CHAPTER

5

TRANSPORT PHYSIOLOGY

Reneé Semonin Holleran

Patient transport requires an understanding of physiologic stresses that may occur. Understanding the concepts of transport physiology is crucial because they are the basis for the special skills used in transporting patients within the air medical environment via fixed-wing or rotor-wing aircraft.

This chapter on transport physiology includes a discussion on gas laws and their potential effect on patients and the transport team. It also includes information about the physiologic stresses of transport and effects on the patient and team during air medical transport.

THE GAS LAWS

For optimal patient care in the air medical environment, transport personnel must possess in-depth knowledge of altitude physiology and the effects on the patient during transport. Altitude physiology exemplifies the concepts of the gas laws; the primary concern is the relationships among the interdependent variables of temperature, pressure, volume, and mass of gases. Before the gas laws are addressed, those factors that influence the behavior of gases need to be considered. The four basic variables that affect gas volumetric relationships are temperature, pressure, volume, and the relative mass of a gas or the number of molecules. These variables (T, P, V, and n) are defined as follows[4,25]:

1. *Temperature* (T), when expressed in degrees kelvin (K), indicates the level of energy of a gas sample and is referred to as absolute temperature, converted from temperature Celsius (°C) or Fahrenheit (°F).
2. *Pressure* (P), defined as absolute or total exerted pressure, is conventionally expressed in atmospheres (torr) or as a given column of mercury in millimeters (mm Hg) or of water balancing the pressure in centimeters (cm H_2O).
3. *Volume* (V) is expressed in cubic units, such as cubic meters (m^3), cubic centimeters (cm^3), or in liters (L).
4. *Relative mass* of a gas or number of molecules (n) or ions is expressed in gram molecules (the molecular weight of the substance in grams).

Gas laws govern the body's physiologic response to barometric pressure changes by these four variables. When the transport team is caring for the air transport patient, these changes become particularly important on ascent and descent.

BOYLE'S LAW

Boyle's law, which originated from experiments conducted by Robert Boyle in 1662, states that at a constant temperature, the volume of gas is inversely proportional to its pressure. This law applies to all gases and may be expressed as follows[31]:

$$P_1 \times V_1 = P_2 \times V_2 \text{ or } P_1/P_2 = V_2/V_1$$

where V_1 is initial volume, V_2 is final volume, P_1 is initial pressure, and P_2 is final pressure

Thus, at a constant temperature, the volume of a gas is inversely proportional to the pressure. The gas in a balloon, for example, expands as the balloon ascends.

DALTON'S LAW (LAW OF PARTIAL PRESSURE)

Dalton was a chemist who observed in 1803 that the total pressure of a mixture of gasses is equal to the sum of the partial pressures of each gas in the mixture. Dalton's law is expressed in the following formula:

$$P = P_1 + P_2 + P_3 + \ldots P_n$$

P is the total pressure of the gas mixture, and P_1, P_2, and P_3 are partial pressures of each gas in the mixture.

The partial pressure of each gas in the mixture is derived from the following equation[31]:

$$P_1 = F_1 \times P$$

where P_1 is the partial pressure of gas 1, F_1 is the fractional concentration of gas 1 in the mixture, and *P* is the total pressure of the gas mixture.[31]

In other words, gases in a mixture exert pressure equivalent to the pressure each would exert if present alone in the volume of the total mixture. Thus, each gas present in a mixture exerts a partial pressure equal to the fractional concentration (by volume) multiplied by the total pressure.[4,25]

A mathematical illustration of Dalton's law is shown in the following example, in which the partial pressure of oxygen (PO_2) at sea level is calculated:

$$PO_2 = 20.95 \ (21\%) \times 760 \text{ mm Hg} = 159.6$$

Barometric pressure, or atmospheric pressure, is the pressure exerted against an object or a person by the atmosphere (Table 5-1). At sea level, this pressure is 15 psi. Increased altitude results in decreased barometric pressure. Barometric pressure multiplied by the concentration of a gas is equal to the partial pressure of the gas.[3,31]

$$\text{barometric pressure} \times \text{gas concentration}$$
$$= \text{gas partial pressure}$$
$$760 \text{ mm Hg} \times 21\% \ O_2{}^a = 159.6 \text{ mm Hg } PO_2$$

---

[a]Note: Oxygen concentration remains at 21%, regardless of altitude. However, oxygen availability decreases with altitude because the oxygen molecules are farther apart, which could potentially result in hypoxia.

TABLE 5-1	**Stages of Hypoxia and Its Effects**			
	Indifferent Stage	**Compensatory Stage**	**Disturbance Stage**	**Critical Stage**
Altitude (thousands of feet)	0-10	10-15	15-20	20-25
Symptoms	Decrease in night vision	Drowsiness Poor judgment Impaired coordination Mistakes in judgment	Physiologic responses no longer compensate for oxygen deficiency Peripheral vision and central vision is impaired Impaired coordination Decreased sensation of pain Impaired judgment	Mental confusion Incapacitation Seizures Unconsciousness Cardiovascular collapse Death

CHARLES' LAW

An additional development in the early formulation of the laws of ideal gases came from the French physicist Jacques Charles who concluded that, "When pressure is constant, the volume of a gas is very nearly proportional to its absolute temperature." This law is expressed as follows[31]:

$$V_1/V_2 = T_1/T_2 \text{ or } V_1/T_1 = V_2/T_2$$

where V_1 is initial volume, V_2 is final volume, T_1 is initial absolute temperature, and T_2 is final absolute temperature.

Thus, the volume is directly proportional to the temperature when expressed on an absolute scale with all other factors constant (P and n are constant).[4] Consequently, if a mass of gas is kept under a constant pressure as the absolute temperature of the gas is increased or decreased, the volume increases or decreases accordingly.[7]

The motion of the molecules in a gas is directly related to temperature. A decrease in the temperature of a gas causes the molecules to move more slowly, whereas an increase in the temperature causes a faster motion. The relationship shows that when a greater force is exerted, the volume expands. An example is a can of shaving cream put into a fire; one can then watch Charles' law at work. Carrying out this experiment is not recommended.

Charles' law describes how gas volume is affected by temperature when pressure remains constant. However, because human body temperature is generally constant, the law has a limited effect on human physiology.[31]

GAY-LUSSAC'S LAW

Gay-Lussac's law is often combined with Charles' law because it, too, deals with a directly proportional relationship between pressure and temperature. Gay-Lussac's law expresses the same relationship but is stated as follows:

$$P_1/T_1 = P_2/T_2$$

where V and n are constant. Thus, the pressure of a gas when volume is constant is directly proportional to the absolute temperature for a constant amount of gas.[4] For example, the pressure in an oxygen tank decreases as the temperature decreases.

HENRY'S LAW

Henry's law deals with the solubility of gases in liquids. The law states: "The quantity of gas dissolved in 1 cm^3 (1 mL) of a liquid is proportional to the partial pressure of the gas in contact with the liquid." The absolute amount of any gas dissolved in liquid under conditions of equilibrium is dependent on the solubility of the gas in the liquid and the temperature, in addition to the partial pressure of the gas.[31] A simpler interpretation is that the weight of a gas dissolved in a liquid is directly proportional to the weight of the gas above the liquid.[7,39] An ideal example is a can of soda (i.e., a carbonated soft drink) that is opened immediately after it has been dropped. The soda was bottled with an equilibrium established between the soda and the gas in the can. When the can is opened, the pressure of the gas above the soda is drastically reduced, which releases the gas within the soda as bubbles. A further example of this law is decompression sickness. When a scuba diver ascends too rapidly from a deep dive, nitrogen bubbles can form in the blood and cause one form of decompression sickness.

GRAHAM'S LAW (LAW OF GASEOUS DIFFUSION)

Graham's law states that the rate of diffusion of a gas through a liquid medium is directly related to the solubility of the gas and inversely proportional to the square root of its density or gram molecular weight.[8] Gases move from a higher pressure or concentration to a region of lower pressure or concentration.[b] Examples are simple diffusion or gas exchange at the cellular level.[31]

STRESSES OF TRANSPORT

Multiple stresses that may be caused by air medical transport have been identified. According to the US Air Force,[3,29,33] which has done the most research on the subject of stresses related to flight, the eight classic stresses of flight are as follows:

- Hypoxia
- Barometric pressure changes
- Thermal changes
- Decreased humidity
- Noise
- Vibration
- Fatigue
- Gravitational forces

---

[b]Note: Carbon dioxide is 19 times as diffusible as oxygen. Hence, the uptake of carbon dioxide occurs 19 times faster than the uptake of oxygen.

Additional stresses related to transport include the following:

- Spatial disorientation
- Flicker vertigo
- Fuel vapors

HYPOXIA

Within the air medical environment, different types of hypoxia are found. An understanding of the terms hypoxia, hypoxemia, and hypercapnia is essential to establish a foundation of knowledge about the effects of decreased partial pressure of oxygen.

Hypoxia is a general term that describes the state of oxygen deficiency in the tissues. It refers to a decrease in tissue oxygen or an oxygen supply inadequate to meet tissue needs.[1,3,16,34] Hypoxia disrupts the intracellular oxidative process and impairs cellular function.[23,34]

Many factors may interfere with a blood cell's ability to carry oxygen to the body. Anemia, altitude, alcohol, medications, carbon monoxide poisoning, and heavy smoking can all decrease the blood's ability to absorb and transport oxygen.

Hypoxemia refers to a decrease in arterial blood oxygen tension (PaO_2). A normal PaO_2 does not guarantee adequate tissue oxygenation; conversely, a low PaO_2 may not indicate tissue hypoxia and may be clinically acceptable.[1,34]

Hypercapnia refers to an increased amount of carbon dioxide in the blood.[34]

Four Stages of Hypoxia

Four stages of hypoxia need to be considered in examination of its effects on human pathophysiology. These four stages are divided by altitude. The first stage is the *indifferent stage*. The physiologic zone for this stage starts at sea level and extends to 10,000 ft. In this stage, the body reacts to the lessened availability of oxygen in the air with a slight increase in heart rate and ventilation. Night-vision deterioration occurs at 5000 ft. The second stage is the *compensatory stage*, which occurs from 10,000 to 15,000 ft. In this stage, the body attempts to protect itself against hypoxia. Increases in blood pressure, heart rate, and depth and rate of respiration occur. Efficiency and performance of tasks that require mental alertness become impaired in this stage. The third stage is the *disturbance stage,* which occurs between 15,000 and 20,000 ft. This stage is characterized by dizziness, sleepiness, tunnel vision, and cyanosis. Thinking becomes slowed, and muscle coordination decreases. The *critical stage* is the fourth stage of hypoxia. This stage occurs between 20,000 and 30,000 ft and features marked mental confusion and incapacitation followed by unconsciousness, usually within a few minutes.[20,21,23,26] Table 5-1 contains a summary of the stages of hypoxia and its effects on humans.

Types of Hypoxia. On the basis of the physiologic effects elicited on the body, hypoxia can be divided into four different types: hypoxic hypoxia, hypemic hypoxia, stagnant hypoxia, and histotoxic hypoxia.

Hypoxic hypoxia is a deficiency in alveolar oxygen exchange. A reduction in PO_2 in inspired air or the effective gas exchange area of the lung may cause oxygen deficiency. The result is an inadequate oxygen supply to the arterial blood, which in turn decreases the amount of oxygen available to the tissues.[3,21,23] Decreased barometric pressure at high altitudes causes a reduction in the alveolar partial pressure of oxygen (PaO_2). The blood oxygen saturation, which is 98% at sea level, is reduced to 87% at 10,000 ft and 60% at 22,000 ft. This reduction in the amount of oxygen in the blood decreases the availability of the oxygen to the tissues and causes an impairment of body functions.[34] Hypoxic hypoxia is also referred to as altitude hypoxia because its primary cause is exposure to low barometric pressure. Hypoxic hypoxia interferes with gas exchange in two phases of respiration: ventilation and diffusion. During the ventilation phase, a reduction in PaO_2 may occur. Specific causes include breathing air at reduced barometric pressure, strangulation/respiratory arrest/laryngospasm, severe asthma, breath holding, hypoventilation, breathing gas mixtures with insufficient PO_2, and malfunctioning oxygen equipment at altitude. Causes of reduction in the gas exchange area include pneumonia, drowning, atelectasis, emphysema (chronic obstructive pulmonary disease), pneumothorax, pulmonary embolism, congenital heart defects, and physiologic shunting. Some causes of diffusion barriers are pneumonia and drowning.[3,21,23]

Hypemic hypoxia is a reduction in the oxygen-carrying capacity of the blood. If the number of red blood cells per unit volume of blood is reduced, as from various types of anemia or from a loss of blood, the oxygen-carrying capacity and thus the oxygen content of the blood are reduced.[34] Even with normal ventilation and diffusion, cellular hypoxia can occur if the rate of delivery of oxygen does not satisfy metabolic requirements.[1,23,34] Hypemic hypoxia interferes with the transportation phase of respiration and causes a reduction in oxygen-carrying capacity. Specific causes of hypemic hypoxia include anemia, hemorrhage, hemoglobin abnormalities, use of drugs (e.g., sulfanilamides, nitrites), and intake of chemicals (e.g., cyanide, carbon monoxide).[23,31] Carbon monoxide is significant to air medical crews because it is present in the exhaust fumes of both conventional and jet-engine aircraft. It is also present in cigarette smoke and any fire or smoke situations. Carbon monoxide binds with hemoglobin 200 times more readily than does oxygen and displaces oxygen to form carboxyhemoglobin.[23,31]

Stagnant hypoxia occurs when conditions result in reduced total cardiac output, pooling of the blood within certain regions of the body, a decreased blood flow to the tissues, or restriction of blood flow.[6,23] Stagnant hypoxia interferes with the transportation phase of respiration by reducing systemic blood flow. Specific causes include heart failure, shock, continuous positive-pressure breathing, acceleration (g forces), and pulmonary embolism. A reduction in regional or local blood flow may be caused by extremes of environmental temperatures, postural changes (prolonged sitting, bed rest, or weightlessness), tourniquets (restrictive clothing, straps), hyperventilation, embolism by clots or gas bubbles, and cerebral vascular accidents.[23,31]

Histotoxic hypoxia (tissue poisoning) occurs when metabolic disorders or poisoning of the cytochrome oxidase enzyme system results in a cell's inability to use molecular oxygen.[23,31] Histotoxic hypoxia interferes with the utilization phase of respiration because of metabolic poisoning or dysfunction. Specific causes include respiratory enzyme poisoning or degradation and the intake of carbon monoxide, cyanide, or alcohol.[23,31] Carbon monoxide can cause both hypemic and histotoxic hypoxia.

Effective Performance Time and Time of Useful Consciousness.   These two terms are frequently used synonymously but are not interchangeable. *Effective performance time* (EPT) denotes the amount of time an individual is able to perform useful flying duties in an environment of inadequate oxygen.[20] *Time of useful consciousness* (TUC) refers to the elapsed time from the point of exposure to an oxygen-deficient environment to the point at which deliberate function is lost.[6,29] EPT more accurately refers to critical (functional) performance than does TUC. With the loss of effective performance in flight, an individual is no longer capable of taking the proper corrective or protective action.[23] Thus, for air medical personnel the emphasis is on prevention.

In addition to altitude, factors that influence TUC are rate of ascent and an individual's physical fitness, physical activity, temperature, individual tolerance, and self-imposed stresses, such as smoking, intake of alcohol and medication, and fatigue.[6] Another factor that dramatically reduces both EPT and TUC is rapid decompression, which occurs when a quick loss of cabin pressure occurs in a pressurized aircraft at high altitudes. On decompression at altitudes above 10,058 m (33,000 ft), an immediate reversal of oxygen flow in the alveoli takes place, caused by a higher PO_2 within the pulmonary capillaries, which depletes the blood's oxygen reserve and reduces the EPT at rest by up to 50%. Exercise also reduces the EPT considerably.[23,31,34] Table 5-2 presents altitude and time of useful consciousness.

Causes.   Hypoxia has the three following causes: 1, high altitude; 2, hypoventilation; and 3, pathologic condition of the lung.

Characteristics.   The onset of hypoxia may be gradual or insidious. Intellectual impairment occurs, demonstrated by slowed thinking, faulty memory of events, lessened immediate recall, delayed reaction time, and a tendency to fixate.

Early Signs and Symptoms.   The individual symptoms of hypoxia can be identified in subjects under safe and controlled conditions in an altitude chamber. Once recognized, these symptoms do not vary dramatically in similar time exposures or among subjects. Hypoxia can be classified by objective signs (those perceived by an observer) or subjective symptoms (those perceived by the subject).[23] Signs and symptoms that appear on both lists in Box 5-1 may be seen by observers and recognized by the hypoxic subject when they occur.[3,11,18,21,35]

Cyanosis has been determined to be an unreliable sign of hypoxia because the oxygen saturation must be less than 75% in persons with normal hemoglobin levels before it is detectable.[3,31,36,38]

TABLE 5-2 **Average Time of Useful Consciousness for Nonpressurized Aircraft**	
Altitude (in ft)	**Time**
18,000 and lower	30 min
25,000	3-5 min
30,000	90 sec
35,000	30-60 sec
40,000 and higher	15 sec or less

BOX 5-1	**Signs and Symptoms of Hypoxia**

Objective Signs	**Subjective Symptoms**
Confusion	Confusion
Tachycardia	Headache
Tachypnea	Stupor
Seizures	Insomnia
Dyspnea	Change in judgment
Hypertension	or personality
Bradycardia	Dizziness
Arrhythmias	Blurred vision
Restlessness	Tunnel vision
Slouching	Hot and cold flashes
Unconsciousness	Tingling
Hypotension (late)	Numbness
Cyanosis (late)	Nausea
Euphoria	Euphoria
Belligerence	Anger

Treatment. The treatment for hypoxia is administration of 100% oxygen. The type of hypoxia needs to be determined so that treatment can be administered accordingly. The following are required steps for transport team members:

1. **Administer supplemental oxygen under pressure.** Provision of adequate supplemental oxygen is the prime consideration in the treatment of hypoxia. Consideration must be given to the altitude and the cause of the oxygen deficiency. Equipment malfunction or altitude exposure above 12,192 m (40,000 ft) cannot be corrected without the addition of positive pressure.[c] The physiologic requirements for breathing are as follows:

Normal	Positive pressure
Inspiration—active	Inspiration—passive
Expiration—passive	Expiration—active

The proper method of positive pressure breathing is as follows:

Inhale slowly → Pause → Exhale forcibly → Pause

2. **Monitor breathing.** After a hypoxic episode, the resulting hyperventilation must be controlled to achieve complete recovery. A breathing rate of 12 to 16 breaths per minute or slightly lower aids recovery.
3. **Monitor equipment.** The most frequently reported causes of hypoxia are lack of oxygen discipline and equipment malfunction. A conscientious preflight check of equipment and frequent in-flight monitoring reduce this hazard. Inspection of oxygen equipment when hypoxia is suspected may detect its cause. Ground-transport team members must also conduct the same careful inspection of their equipment before and after transport to prevent any problems with their oxygen-delivery system during transport. Correction of a malfunction should bring immediate relief of the hypoxic condition. If treatment for hypoxia does not remedy the situation, oxygen contamination should be suspected.

Use of an alternative oxygen source, such as the emergency oxygen cylinder or portable assembly, should be considered. Descent should be initiated as soon as possible, and the contents of the oxygen system should be analyzed.

4. **Descend.** Increasing the ambient oxygen pressure by descending to lower altitudes, particularly below 3048 m (10,000 ft), is also beneficial. Descent to a lower altitude compensates for malfunctioning oxygen equipment that may have caused the hypoxia.[23,26,38,39]

The primary treatment of hypoxia for any patient being transported is prevention. The transport team must remember that the patient's condition is already compromised and that stresses related to transport increase the risk of patient hypoxia unless the transport team continuously monitors the patient and accurately anticipates the oxygen needs of the patient during transport.

HYPERVENTILATION

Hyperventilation at altitude is an important consideration for air medical personnel and also for the air medical patient. Hyperventilation is of concern because it produces changes in cellular respiration. Although the causes are unrelated, the symptoms of hyperventilation and hypoxia are similar and often result in confusion and inappropriate corrective procedures. Despite increased knowledge, training, and improved life-support equipment, both hypoxia and hyperventilation are hazards in flying and diving operations.[23] *Hyperventilation* is an abnormal increase in the rate and depth of breathing that upsets the chemical balance of the blood[31]; it is commonly caused by psychologic stress (e.g., fear, anxiety, apprehensiveness, and anger) and environmental stress (e.g., hypoxia, pressure breathing, vibration, and heat). Certain drugs such as salicylates and female sex hormones also cause or enhance hyperventilation, and any condition that creates metabolic acidosis results in hyperventilation at high altitudes.[3,23,31]

Treatment

At high altitudes, hyperventilation and hypoxia are treated in the same way because of similarities in the

---

[c]Positive-pressure breathing is the opposite of normal breathing.

signs and symptoms. The following steps describe the treatment:

1. Administer 100% oxygen.
2. Begin positive-pressure breathing, which is the same as supplemental oxygen under pressure.
3. Regulate breathing and watch for hyperventilation.
4. Check equipment.
5. Descend.

The treatment for hyperventilation in the air medical patient is administration of oxygen. If treatment is successful, the amount of oxygen in the blood increases. Oxygen transfers from air to blood 20 times more slowly than carbon dioxide, and carbon dioxide transfers 20 times faster from blood to air than oxygen, which explains why the amount of carbon dioxide in the blood is directly associated with ventilation. When a patient is hyperventilating from anxiety, the act of putting a mask on the face to administer oxygen probably heightens the anxiety and increases tidal volume. Tidal volume must be reduced.[31] More favorable responses can be obtained by talking to patients to distract them, identifying causes of hyperventilation, and suggesting specific exercises to reduce respiratory rate. Several helpful exercises are:

1. The patient should count to 10 slowly while exhaling.
2. The patient should inhale and exhale only 10 times per minute.
3. Using a watch with a second hand, the patient should set a respiratory rate between 10 and 12 breaths per minute.
4. The air medical team member can provide counter pressure by suggesting isometric or active-passive exercises[5] that cause the patient to hold the breath and reduce the respiratory rate.

BAROMETRIC PRESSURE

Boyle's law states that at a constant temperature, the volume of a gas is inversely proportional to the pressure. On ascent, gases expand; on descent, gases contract. Therefore, trapped or partially trapped gases within certain body cavities (e.g., the gastrointestinal [GI] tract, lungs, skull, middle ear, sinuses, and teeth) expand in direct proportion to the decrease in pressure.[3,11,12,15,16,19,20,26,34]

Middle Ear

The *middle ear cavity* is an air-filled space connected to the nasopharynx by the eustachian tube. The eustachian tube has a slit-like orifice at the throat end that allows air to vent outward more easily than inward. During ascent, air in the middle ear cavity expands but normally vents into the throat through the eustachian tube when a pressure differential of approximately 15 mm Hg has been reached. A mild fullness is usually detected but disappears as equalization occurs. This constitutes the *passive process.*[6] On descent, however, a different situation exists. The eustachian tube remains closed unless actively opened by muscle action or high positive pressure in the nasopharynx. If the eustachian tube opens, any existing pressure differential is immediately equalized. If the tube does not open regularly during descent, a pressure differential may develop. If this pressure differential reaches 80 to 90 mm Hg, the small muscles of the soft palate cannot overcome it, and either reascent or a maneuver that is not physiologic is necessary to open the tube.[10,22] On descent, equalization of pressure in the middle ear can be accomplished by performing the Valsalva's maneuver, yawning, swallowing, moving the lower jaw, topical administration of vasoconstrictors, or use of a bag-valve mask. These procedures are examples of the *active process.*

Gum chewing is not recommended as a method of pressure equalization because it causes swallowing of air, thereby causing gastric distention and discomfort.

Barotitis Media.   *Barotitis media,* frequently referred to as an ear block, results from failure of the middle ear space to ventilate when going from low to high atmospheric pressure (i.e., on descent).[11,22] Pressure in the middle ear becomes increasingly negative, and a partial vacuum is created. As the pressure differential increases, the tympanic membrane is depressed inward and becomes inflamed, and petechial hemorrhages develop. Blood and tissue fluids are drawn into the middle ear cavity, and if equalization with ambient pressure does not take place, perforation of the tympanic membrane occurs. Severe pain, tinnitus, and possibly vertigo and nausea can accompany acute barotitis.[22] Priority is placed on patient briefing before flight and adequate instructions for air medical crews. The ears should be cleared on descent with the methods previously described. Patients who are sleeping should be awakened before descent so they can clear their ears in the normal manner.

Patients with colds or upper respiratory tract infections must be closely monitored during both ascent and descent for swollen eustachian tubes, a condition that interferes with normal equalization procedures.[3,22] Air medical crew members with upper respiratory tract infections should not fly.

If an ear block occurs, mild vasoconstrictors should be administered early, and the plane should reascend to a higher altitude until symptoms lessen or the patient's ear block clears. If patients have ear pain during ascent, which rarely occurs, air medical personnel should not have them execute a Valsalva's maneuver because that would only aggravate the problem; instead, personnel should have them swallow or move their jaw muscles or administer to them a mild vasoconstrictor.[6] Either the Politzer's bag or a source of compressed air may be used. A patient's nose should be sprayed with a decongestant solution to attain maximal shrinkage of the mucosa. For the Politzer's bag method, the olive tip is placed in one nostril, the nose is compressed between the air medical crew member's fingers, and the patient is then instructed to say "kick, kick, kick" while the bag is squeezed, thereby increasing the pressure in the nasopharyngeal cavity to the point at which the eustachian tube is opened and the middle ear space ventilated.[11,22]

In review, the treatment is as follows:

1. Patient performs Valsalva's maneuver.
2. Crew member administers vasoconstrictor spray.
3. Crew member administers Politzer's bag or bag-valve mask.
4. Aircraft reascends.

Delayed Ear Block. A *delayed ear block,* which occurs after the flight is terminated, results from breathing 100% oxygen during flight. As the ears clear during descent, 100% oxygen is forced into the middle ear cavity.[22] In addition, the absorption of oxygen by the middle ear and mastoid mucosa also contributes to the relatively negative pressure in those cavities. The patient may be symptom-free immediately after flight, but if the oxygen in the middle ear is not replaced with air, the surrounding tissues absorb it, creating a negative pressure within the cavity. Delayed barotitis media occurs when oxygen absorption is the primary factor in the development of a pressure differential.[11,22] This condition causes a tightness or "stopped-up" sensation in the ears and slight to possibly severe pain. To prevent delayed ear problems, the patient should perform the Valsalva's maneuver periodically after the flight.[22] However, if a flight is completed in the late-evening hours or during the night and the individual retires a short time later, a significant pressure differential may develop during sleep because of the combined effects of oxygen absorption and infrequent swallowing.[10] Patients who are maintained on 100% oxygen during flight are especially susceptible to this problem.[22]

Flight crew members who continue to have ear pain after flight can treat it with decongestants and analgesics. If symptoms persist, flying at high altitudes should be avoided until the symptoms subside. If the team member has had a ruptured tympanic membrane, several days to weeks may be needed before it heals and they should not fly until cleared.[3]

Barosinusitis (Sinus Block)

The sinuses usually present little problem when subjected to changes in barometric pressure. Because a free flow of air exists between the sinus cavities and the exterior, the sinuses automatically equalize with ambient pressure when the air in them expands or contracts.[22]

Barosinusitis is an acute or chronic inflammation of one or more of the paranasal sinuses produced by the development of a pressure difference, usually negative, between the air in the sinus cavity and that of the surrounding atmosphere.[10] Common causes of barosinusitis are colds and upper respiratory tract infections. Patients with such problems should be closely monitored during ascent and descent.[22]

The symptoms of barosinusitis are usually proportional to its severity and may vary from a mild feeling of fullness in or around the involved sinus to excruciating pain. Pain can develop suddenly and be incapacitating.[11] Another symptom is possible persistent local tenderness. The immediate treatment for barosinusitis is to reascend until the pressure within the sinus equals the cabin pressure, administer vasoconstrictors to reduce swelling, and descend as gradually as possible to afford every opportunity for pressure equalization.[22]

Barodontalgia

Barodontalgia, or aerodontalgia, is a toothache that is caused by exposure to changing barometric pressures during actual or simulated flight.[11,22] The precise cause of barodontalgia has not been determined; however, exposure to reduced atmospheric pressure is obviously a significant factor. This exposure is evidently a precipitating factor, with disease of the pulp the primary cause. Pressure changes do not elicit pain in teeth with normal pulps, regardless of whether a tooth is intact, carious, or restored.[11,22]

Some pathologic conditions may cause no symptoms at ground level but be adversely affected by a change in barometric pressure. Barodontalgia commonly occurs during ascent, with descent bringing relief.[6] Moderate to severe pain that usually develops during ascent and is well localized generally indicates direct barodontalgia. The patient or crew member is frequently able to identify the involved tooth. This condition can usually be prevented by high-quality dental care with an emphasis on slow careful treatment of cavities and the routine use of a cavity varnish. Indirect barodontalgia is a dull poorly defined pain that involves the posterior maxillary teeth and develops during descent.[11] If patients have tooth pain during descent, especially involving the upper posterior teeth, they may have barosinusitis and should be treated accordingly.[22]

A crew member who undergoes dental treatment involving deep restorations should be restricted from flying for 48 to 72 hours after treatment to allow time for the dental pulp to stabilize.[11,22]

Gastrointestinal Changes

Gas contained within body cavities is saturated with water vapor, the partial pressure of which is related to body temperature. In determining the mechanical effect of gas expansion, one must account for the noncompressibility of water vapor, which causes wet gases to expand to a greater extent than dry gases.[3,13,39,40] The stomach and intestines normally contain a variable amount of gas at a pressure that is equivalent to the surrounding barometric pressure. On ascending to high altitudes, however, the gases in the GI tract expand. Unless the gases are expelled by belching or the passing of flatus, they may produce pain and discomfort, make breathing more difficult, and possibly lead to hyperventilation or syncope.[39,40] Severe pain may cause a vasovagal reaction that consists of hypotension, tachycardia, and fainting. Abdominal massage and physical activity may promote the passage of gas. If this treatment is unsuccessful, a descent should be initiated to an altitude at which comfort is achieved.[13] Because the possibility of decompression does exist, however, certain precautionary measures should be taken to reduce the chances of GI gas-expansion difficulties. Such measures include avoiding hasty and heavy meals before flight, such as gas-forming foods, carbonated beverages, and foods that are not easily digested.[39,40] Normally, the average GI tract has approximately 1 L of gas present at any one time. Wet gas expands its original volume at 9000 ft.

One useful example is a pediatric patient with abdominal distention. Gas expansion in the abdominal cavity, if untreated, can increase to such a volume as to raise the diaphragm. With diaphragmatic crowding, lung volume and expansion are decreased. If this distention is large enough, the great blood vessels in the area are compressed, which alters the blood supply to vital organs.[39,40]

Patients with ileus (bowel obstruction) or recent abdominal surgery should have a gastric tube placed before transport. The gastric tube should not be clamped but should be vented for ambient air or low intermittent suction during transport. After abdominal surgery, pockets of air may remain in the abdominal cavity. For this reason, general recommendations are that patients not be transported by air until 24 to 48 hours after the surgery. Patients who have undergone colostomy should be advised to carry extra bags because of more frequent bowel movements that result from gas expansion.[22] Colostomy bags should be empty and properly vented before air medical transport. Penetrating wounds allow ambient air to travel along the wound tract. According to Boyle's law, penetrating wounds to the eyes, neck, thorax, abdomen, and lower extremities can cause the introduction of emboli, in addition to irreparable damage to nerves and surrounding tissues.

THERMAL CHANGES

An increase in altitude results in a decrease in ambient temperature. As a consequence, cabin temperature fluctuates considerably depending on the temperature outside the aircraft.[3] The ratio of altitude to temperature is fairly constant from sea level to approximately 35,000 ft. Temperature decreases by 1°C for every 100-m (330-ft) increase in altitude. From flight level (FL) 350 to FL 990, the temperature fluctuates ± 3°C to 5°C. The temperature remains relatively isothermic at approximately −50°C from FL 350 to FL 990.[28,30] Vibration and thermal change, depending on whether the change is to greater heat or more cold, can have either an antagonistic or a synergistic effect. The body's primary response to heat exposure is vasodilation and activation of cooling mechanisms. Exposure to cold and vibration stimulate vasoconstriction and decreased perspiration.[3] Exposure to whole-body vibration appears to interfere with the normal human cooling responses in a hot environment by reducing blood flow and decreasing perspiration.[28] Turbulence can be produced by high and low temperature changes in the air. Turbulence increases stress during flight by promoting fatigue and increasing one's susceptibility to motion sickness and disorientation.

The transport team must also keep in mind that some medications can also interfere with maintenance of a constant body temperature. Sedatives, analgesics, some psychoactive agents, and neuromuscular blocking agents are only a few examples of the medications that can place the patient at risk for problems with body temperature regulation.

Both hyperthermia and hypothermia increase the body's oxygen requirement. Hyperthermia increases the metabolic rate, and hypothermia increases energy needs as a result of shivering, thereby increasing the body's oxygen consumption.[5] Air medical crews can facilitate maintenance of adequate body temperature with blankets, warm clothing, and warm liquids.[3,28] An additional way to facilitate thermoregulatory control is with a first-aid thermal blanket, which is sometimes called a space blanket.

DECREASED HUMIDITY

Humidity is the concentration of water vapor in the air; as air cools, it loses its ability to hold moisture. Because temperature is inversely proportional to altitude, an increase in altitude produces a decrease in temperature and, therefore, a decrease in the amount of humidity. The fresh-air supply is drawn into the aircraft cabin from a very dry atmosphere.[5] Before takeoff, small amounts of moisture are present in the cabin air from clothing and other items on board that retain moisture, in addition to expired air from crew members, patients, and other passengers. As the aircraft altitude increases, the air exhausted overboard carries away trapped moisture. Eventually, all the original moisture is lost. The only moisture that remains is supplied by crew members, patients, other passengers on board, and the fresh-air system.[3,6] For example, on a typical flight of a military jet aircraft known as a C-141 Starlifter, which is a high-speed, high-altitude, long-range aircraft used for troops, cargo, and air medical transport, less than 5% relative humidity remains after 2 hours of flying time. Relative humidity decreases to less than 1% after 4 hours.[3,6,25] Propeller-type aircraft are not as dry inside because they do not fly as high; the lowest relative humidity levels reached on typical propeller aircraft flights range from 10% to 25%.[6] Patients and air crew members may become significantly dehydrated because of the decreased humidity at high altitudes. The ventilation systems on aircraft draw off what little moisture there is and contribute further to the decrease in the percentage of humidity. For a healthy person, low humidity results in nothing more than chapped lips, scratchy or slightly sore throat, and hoarseness. Steps that the medical crew member can take to minimize problems caused by decreased humidity include mouth care, use of lip balm, and adequate fluid intake.[5] Patients who receive in-flight oxygen therapy are twice as susceptible to dehydration because oxygen itself is a drying agent. Humidified oxygen should be used on extended patient transports. The transport team must be certain that when humidifiers are used, they are changed often to prevent contamination.

Patients who are unconscious or unable to close their eyelids must be provided with eye care. The administration of artificial tears and the taping shut of lids prevent corneal drying. Before transport, patients with compromised conditions predisposed by age, diet, or preexisting medical or surgical complications need special consideration with respect to decreased humidity.

Transport team members should also maintain adequate fluid intake to prevent dehydration. Water or other appropriate liquids need to be available during both air and ground transport. [14]

NOISE

Sound is any undulatory motion in an elastic medium (gaseous, liquid, or solid) capable of producing the sensation of hearing. Normally, the medium is air.[18,24,27] *Sound waves* are variations in air pressure above and below the ambient pressure.[21,31] Sound is described in terms of its intensity, spectrum, and time history. The *intensity* of a sound wave is the magnitude by which the pressure varies above and below the ambient level. It is measured with a logarithmic scale that expresses the ratio of sound pressure to a reference pressure in decibels (dBs), which are the units used to describe levels of acoustic pressure, power, and intensity.[27,29,30] The *spectrum* of a sound represents the qualities present distributed across frequency. The frequency of periodic motion (e.g., sound and vibrations) is the number of complete cycles of motion taking place in a unit of time, usually 1 second. The international standard unit of frequency is the hertz (Hz), which is 1 cycle per second.[27] *Pressure-time histories* describe variations in the sound pressure of a signal as a function of time. The frequency content is not quantified in pressure–time histories of signals, so analytic techniques must be applied to the signal to obtain frequency or spectrum characteristics.[27]

Theoretically, sound waves in open air spread spherically in all directions from an ideal source. As a result of this spherical dispersion, the sound pressure is reduced to half its original value as the distance is doubled, which is a 6-dB reduction in sound pressure level.[27] Hence, a number of factors are involved in the creation of sound. In relation to the definition of sound, it is usually easier to think of sound as comprising intensity, which is commonly thought of as merely loudness, in decibels; frequency, in cycles per second and pitch; and duration.

Thus, noise, which is dependent on sound, can more easily be defined. *Noise* may be defined subjectively as a sound that is unpleasant, distracting, unwarranted, or in some other way undesirable.[21,27] The human hearing mechanism has a wide range and is fairly tolerant, but at times in an aircraft this tolerance is exceeded, with the following potential effects:

- Communications in the form of speech and other auditory signals inside the aircraft or air-to-air or air-to-ground may be degraded.
- The sense of hearing may be temporarily or permanently damaged.
- Noise, acting as a stress, may interfere with patient care and safe transport.
- Noise may induce varying levels of fatigue.[21,27]

The A-level of a decibel (dBA) is a unit of noise measurement that correlates most closely with the way a human ear accommodates sound or noise. The dBA is a single measurement that incorporates both amplitude and the selective frequency response features that most closely parallel those of the human ear. When ambient noise levels exceed 80 to 85 dBA, a person must usually shout to be heard.[21,27] Essentially, unprotected exposure to noise can produce one or more of the following three undesirable auditory effects: interference with effective communication, temporary threshold shifts (auditory fatigue), or permanent threshold shifts (sensorineural hearing loss).[21,27] Auditory fatigue incurred by noise is frequently accompanied by a feeling of "fullness," high-pitched ringing, buzzing, or a roaring sound in the ears (tinnitus). Tinnitus usually subsides within a few minutes after cessation of the noise exposure; however, for some individuals, the tinnitus may continue for several hours.[5] Most of the truly significant forms of undesirable response to acoustic noise, such as nausea, disorientation, and excessive general fatigue, are associated with only very intense noise, which air medical personnel rarely encounter during normal airlift operations.[21,25] Other hazards of exposure are loss of appetite and interest, diaphoresis, salivation, nausea or vomiting, headache, fatigue, and general discomfort.

Noise in the transport environment also impairs the ability of the transport team to perform patient assessment before and during transport. Aircraft noise, sirens, and traffic and crowd noise can interfere with the evaluation of breath sounds, auscultation of blood pressure, or even the obtaining of patient information. Propeller aircraft noise is a loud tonal noise from piston or turbo propeller engines in the cabin. A beating noise may occur when the tonal noises from two propellers are at similar levels but differ slightly in frequency. Rotorcraft cabin noises can come from impulsive, periodic, and broadband noises from rotors and structures such as the gearbox. The noise from a helicopter contains both high-level and low-frequency noise. Jet aircraft also produce high frequency-level noise that increases with lift-off and climbing out.[27]

Transport team members need to rely on monitoring devices to measure patient blood pressure and monitor oxygen saturation, tube placement, and overall perfusion. Visible signs of distress or discomfort such as increased respiratory rate, changes in skin color, and grimacing may provide additional information about a patient's condition and comfort in a noisy transport environment.

Table 5-3 provides an example of the numbers of decibels that result from certain sources. Whenever the noise cannot be controlled at a desirable level,

TABLE 5-3	**Decibels and Source**
Decibels	**Source**
60	Normal conversation at 1 meter
80	Garbage disposal
88	Propeller aircraft flyover at 1000 feet
90	Noisy factory
	Cockpit of light aircraft
103	Jet flyover at 1000 feet
117	Jet on runway in preparation for takeoff
110-130	Construction site during pile-driving

ear protection devices that attenuate the noise on its way from the surrounding air to the tympanic membrane must be worn, whether in an aircraft or ground transport vehicles. Such devices include helmets, earplugs, and earmuffs. Because effectiveness can vary considerably depending on a device's basic performance and personal fit, all transport team personnel should be carefully instructed regarding quality and size selection and techniques for use.[31] Earplugs are inert devices, and headsets and earmuffs are occluding devices. Earplugs must fit tightly to offer the maximum allowable attenuation; the only requirement for using airtight earplugs during flight operations is that the plugs be removed before descent. Pressure changes that result from decreased altitude tend to pull the plugs inward toward the tympanic membrane.[5] Transport team members should have their hearing evaluated on a yearly basis.

The Commission on Accreditation of Medical Transport Systems[5] requires that all rotor-wing (RW) personnel wear helmets during patient transport operations. This requirement should help decrease the risk of hearing damage related to RW transport and will hopefully improve team member communications during transport.[5]

A patient's hearing, particularly that of an unconscious patient, needs to be protected during transport. Therefore, a headset or earmuffs should be placed on all patients.

VIBRATION

Vibration is the motion of objects relative to a reference position (usually the object at rest) and is described relative to its effect on humans in terms of frequency, intensity (amplitude), direction (with regard to anatomic axes of the human body), and duration of exposure.[27,32,39,40] Most vehicles contain two principal sources of vibration: the first originates within the vehicle (specifically, the power source), and the second comes from the environment, which encompasses the terrain over which the land vehicle travels, the turbulence of the air through which the aircraft flies, or the status of the sea in which the ship sails.[27,32,39,40] Thus, both air and ground vehicles cause vibration.

Helicopter vibration occurs with broadly similar intensity in all three axes of motion. Large differences in the amplitudes of specific harmonics in different modes of light may exist, but the overall amplitude of vibration tends to increase with airspeed and with the loading of the aircraft. Vibration is usually worse during transition to the hover position.[27,32,39,40]

In fixed-wing aircraft, any vibration from the power source is usually at a higher frequency than in helicopters. The main source of vibration encountered in fixed-wing aircraft is the atmospheric turbulence through which the aircraft flies. In consequence, the most severe vibration usually occurs during storm-cloud penetration or during high-speed low-level flight. The response of the aircraft as a whole to atmospheric turbulence is determined by the aerodynamic loading on the wings. An aircraft with a large wing area relative to its weight undergoes greater amplitude low-frequency excursions from level flight as a result of turbulence.[27,32,39,40]

Resonance frequencies of body structures produce a more pronounced effect than nonresonant frequencies.[27] Vibration between 1 and 12 Hz has been firmly established to cause performance decrement in the cockpit. For example, low-frequency vibration can induce motion sickness, fatigue, shortness of breath, and abdominal and chest pain.[27] Research has established that a human's sensitivity to external vibration is highest between 0.5 and 20 Hz because the human system absorbs most of the vibratory energy applied within this range, with maximal amplification between 5 and 11 Hz. The most physiologically harmful frequencies lay between 0.1 and 40 Hz.[18]

When the human body is in direct contact with a source of vibration, mechanical energy is transferred, some of which is degraded into heat within those tissues that have dampening properties. The response to whole-body vibration is an increase in muscle activity to maintain posture and possibly to reduce the resonant amplification of body structures. This response is reflected in an increase in metabolic rate under vibration and a redistribution of blood flow with peripheral vasoconstriction. The increase in metabolic rate during vibrations is comparable with that seen in gentle exercise. Respiration is increased to achieve the necessary increase in elimination of carbon dioxide (CO_2).[27] Disturbances in dynamic visual acuity, speech, and fine-muscle coordination result from vibration exposure.[27] The effects of vibration on the body can be reduced by attention to the source of vibration, modification of the transmission pathway, or alteration of the dynamic properties of the body.[27] Pain from injuries such as fractures or disease states can be increased, which causes the need for additional analgesia and sedation. Sensors, electrodes, leads, endotracheal tubes, and intravenous lines may become disconnected or dislodged. Vibrations then could make replacement of these during the transport difficult.[18]

Vibrations can also interfere with transport equipment such as cardiac and blood pressure monitors. The equipment should be secured in the transport vehicle in a manner least conducive to vibrations.

Aircraft manufacturers have eliminated severe vibrations by improving designs and materials; however, some vibrations still occur as a result of engine operation, flap and landing gear extension and retraction, and general aircraft movement. To minimize reactions to vibrations in either air or ground transport vehicles, transport crew members should properly secure patients, encourage and assist them with position changes, and provide adequate padding and skin care.[27]

FATIGUE

All of the many operational stresses of transport may induce fatigue to some degree. Fatigue is an inherent stress of transport duties. Erratic schedules, hypoxic environments, noise and vibration, and imperfect environmental systems eventually take their toll; therefore, in transport, fatigue is always a potential threat to safety.[3,39]

Fatigue is the end product of all the physiologic and psychologic stresses of flight associated with exposure to altitude.[6,30,39,40] Fatigue can also result from self-imposed stressors whether the transport is by air or ground. Box 5-2 shows self-imposed stresses that can have disastrous results.

G FORCE

In terms of practical application for civilian air medical transports, the effects of g force are limited and, in most cases, negligible.

BOX 5-2	**Factors That Affect Tolerance: DEATH**

Factors that affect tolerance to the stresses of flight can be summarized by the acronym DEATH.

D = Drugs. Use of over-the-counter drugs and antihistamines, misuse of prescription drugs, and use of stimulants such as caffeine can cause insomnia, tremors, indigestion, and nervousness.

E = Exhaustion (fatigue). Exhaustion can lead to judgment errors, limited response, falling asleep on the job, narrowed attention, and change in circadian rhythm.

A = Alcohol. Use of alcohol can cause histotoxic hypoxia, affect the efficiency of cells to use oxygen, interfere with metabolic activity, and result in a hangover.

T = Tobacco. Besides exposure of the body to nicotine, tar, and carcinogens, smoking of two packs of cigarettes per day results in 8% to 10% of the body's hemoglobin being saturated with carbon monoxide.

H = Hypoglycemia (diet). Poor dietary intake can cause nausea, judgment errors, headache, and dizziness.

For an examination of force as a stress of flight, an understanding of mass, speed, velocity, and acceleration is helpful to clarify the concepts of exerted forces.

Speed is the rate of movement of a body without regard to the direction of travel.

Velocity is the rate (magnitude) of change of distance and direction of travel of an object and is, therefore, a vector quantity. The velocity of a body changes if its speed or direction of travel changes. Velocity is expressed as the rate of change of distance in a specified direction.

Acceleration is the rate of change of velocity of an object, and like velocity, it is a vector quantity.[2,11]

Weight is the force exerted by the mass of an accelerating body.[2,11]

Mass is a measure of the inertia of an object (e.g., its resistance to acceleration).[2]

Newton's three laws of motion define the relationship between motion and force.[2]

Newton's First Law of Motion: Unless it is acted on by a force, a body at rest will remain at rest and a body in motion will move at a constant speed in a straight line.

Newton's Second Law of Motion: When a force is applied to a body, the body accelerates, and the acceleration is directly proportional to the force applied and inversely proportional to the mass of the body.

Newton's Third Law of Motion: For every action, there is an equal and opposite reaction.

Two types of acceleration must be considered: linear acceleration and radial acceleration. *Linear acceleration* is produced by a change of speed without a change in direction. In conventional aviation, prolonged linear accelerations seldom reach a magnitude that could produce significant changes in human performance because most aircraft do not exert sufficient thrust to produce extended changes in linear velocity. However, significant linear accelerations that last 2 to 4 seconds are produced during catapult-assisted takeoffs and arrested landings and when reheat is engaged in certain high-performance aircraft. Large prolonged linear accelerations occur during the launching of spacecraft and during slowing on reentry into the Earth's atmosphere. *Radial acceleration* is produced by a change of direction without a change of speed. Such accelerations occur when the line of flight is changed. Aircraft maneuvers are, by far, the most common source of prolonged acceleration in flight. Accelerations on the order of 6g to 9g or more can be maintained for many seconds by circular flight in agile military aircraft.[2,11]

When the main interest is the effect of acceleration on humans, the direction in which an acceleration or inertial force acts is described with the use of a three-axis coordinate system (X, Y, and Z), in which the vertical (Z) axis is parallel to the long axis of the body. Considerable confusion can result if a clear distinction is not made between the applied acceleration and the resultant inertial force because these, by definition, always act in diametrically opposite directions.[2,11]

Aircraft Motion

Because space is three-dimensional, linear motions in space are described with reference to three linear axes, and angular motions with three angular axes. In aviation, customary terms are the longitudinal (fore-aft), lateral (right-left), and vertical (up-down) linear axes and the roll, pitch, and yaw angular axes.[9]

Linear Axes	Angular Axes
Longitudinal axis (fore-aft)	Axis of roll
Lateral axis (right-left)	Axis of pitch
Vertical axis (up-down)	Axis of yaw

The relationship of this three-axis system with its action on humans is illustrated in Table 5-4.

Long-Duration Positive Acceleration. The crews of agile aircraft are frequently exposed to sustained positive accelerations ($+g_z$) with changes in the direction of flight, either in turns or in recovery from dives. Exposure to positive acceleration usually causes deterioration of vision before any disturbance of consciousness. For example, exposure to $+4.5\ g_z$ typically produces complete loss of vision, or "blackout," but hearing and mental activity remain unaffected. Exposure to a positive acceleration stress somewhat greater than that required to produce blackout results in unconsciousness. At moderate levels of acceleration ($5g$ to $6g$), blackout precedes loss of consciousness, but at higher accelerations, unconsciousness occurs before any visual symptoms occur.[2]

Long-Duration Negative Acceleration. Flight conditions that cause negative accelerations ($-g_z$) are outside loops and spins and simple inverted flight and recovery from such maneuvers. Tolerance for negative acceleration is much lower than that for positive acceleration, and the symptoms produced by even $-2\ g_z$ are unpleasant and alarming. Furthermore, low levels of negative acceleration produce serious decrements in performance.[2,3,11]

Long-Duration Transverse Acceleration. Accelerations of long duration acting at right angles to the long axis of the body ($+g_x$) rarely occur in present-day conventional flight. They are usually confined to catapult launches, rocket-assisted and jet-assisted takeoffs, and carrier landings, although forces in excess of $-2\ g_x$ may build up during flat spins. However, the forces in these maneuvers are small relative to human tolerance and do not cause problems.[2,3,11]

The definitions of the effects of g forces given here are applicable to high performance aircraft, mostly

TABLE 5-4	**Three-Axis Coordinate System for Describing Action on Humans Regarding Direction of Acceleration and Inertial Forces**		
Direction of Acceleration	**Direction of Resultant Inertial Forces**	**Physiologic and Vernacular Descriptors**	**Standard Terminology**
Headward	Head-to-foot	Positive g Eyeballs down	$+g_z$
Footward	Foot-to-head	Negative g Eyeballs up	$-g_z$
Forward	Chest-to-back	Transverse A-P-G Supine g Eyeballs in	$+g_x$
Backward	Back-to-chest	Transverse P-A-G Prone g Eyeballs out	$-g_x$
To the right	Right-to-left	Left lateral g Eyeballs left	$+g_y$
To the left	Left-to-right	Right lateral g Eyeballs right	$-g_y$

fighter-type, and to emergency situations. The longitudinal axis is most important in air medical transports. However, the effects of g forces are usually encountered only with forces greater than 1.5 *g*.

CABIN PRESSURIZATION

The pressure environment that surrounds the Earth can be divided into the four following zones: the physiologic zone, the physiologically deficient zone, the space-equivalent zone, and space. These zones are characterized according to their physiologic effects as follows:

> *Physiologic zone:* From sea level to altitudes up to 10,000 ft.
> *Physiologically deficient zone:* Altitudes from 10,000 to 50,000 ft.
> *Space-equivalent zone:* Altitudes from 50,000 to 250,000 ft.
> *Space:* Altitudes beyond 250,000 ft.

In the physiologic zone, humans are well adapted. Although middle ear or sinus problems may be experienced during ascent or descent in this zone, most physiologic problems occur outside this zone and when proper protective equipment is not used. In the physiologically deficient zone, protective oxygen equipment is mandatory because the decrease in barometric pressure results in oxygen deficiency and causes altitude hypoxia.[12,13] Additional problems may result from trapped and evolved gases. Travel in the space-equivalent and space zones requires either a sealed cabin or a full-pressure suit.

In general, the most effective way to prevent physiologic problems is to provide an aircraft pressurization system so the occupants of the aircraft are never exposed to pressures outside the physiologic zone. In cases in which ascent above the physiologic zone is necessary, protective oxygen equipment must be provided.[12,13] Aircraft pressurization consists of increased barometric pressure within crew and passenger compartments, which reduces the cabin altitude, creating near-the-Earth atmospheric conditions within the aircraft.[6] Commercial passenger aircraft normally pressurize to the equivalent of 5000 to 8000 ft, with the aircraft ascending a bit over 40,000 ft

(FL 400).[12,13,15] The conventional method, used in virtually all current aircraft, is to draw air from outside the aircraft, compress it, and deliver it into the cabin. The desired pressure is maintained within the cabin with control of the flow of compressed gas out of the cabin and to the atmosphere. The continuous flow of air ventilates the compartment; in most aircraft, this flow of air also controls the thermal environment within the cabin.[20] (Pickard and Gradwell)

The difference between the absolute pressure within an aircraft and that of the atmosphere immediately outside an aircraft is called the *cabin differential pressure.* Differential pressure is frequently controlled so that it varies with aircraft altitude.[17] The two principal aircraft pressurization systems, isobaric and isobaric-differential, are described as follows[13]:

Isobaric system: Isobaric control maintains a constant cabin pressure while the ambient barometric pressure decreases. Many military and civilian aircraft are equipped with isobaric pressurization systems. This pressurization increases the comfort and mobility of the passengers, negates the necessity for the routine use of oxygen equipment, and minimizes fatigue.

Isobaric-differential system: Tactical military aircraft are not equipped with isobaric pressurization systems because the added weight severely limits the range of the aircraft and the large pressure differential increases the danger of rapid decompression during combat situations. Instead, these aircraft are equipped with an isobaric-differential cabin pressurization system. The isobaric function controls cabin pressure until a preset pressure differential is reached. With continued ascent, the preset differential is maintained. Thus, the apparent cabin altitude progressively increases as the aircraft ascends.

In air medical transports, cabin pressurization is especially important. Not only does it protect the occupants from the physiologic hazards of altitude, but it also provides more effective control of cabin temperature and ventilation, promotes greater mobility and comfort, and reduces fatigue. Cabin pressurization does not eliminate all problems, however. Cabin pressure can be lost as a result of structural failure, such as a window or a door blowing out, or through a mechanical malfunction of pressurization equipment.[6]

DECOMPRESSION

A loss of cabin pressure is referred to as *decompression*. Aircraft decompression can be slow and gradual, over a period of several minutes, or it can be sudden, within a matter of seconds.[6,29] The risk of injury from decompression increases in proportion to the ratio of the area of the defect to the volume of the cabin and to the ratio of cabin pressure before and immediately after the decompression.[16,31] The following factors control the rate of decompression[17,18]:

- Volume of the pressurized cabin: The larger the cabin, the slower the rate of decompression if all other factors are constant.
- Size of the opening: The larger the opening, the faster the rate of decompression. The most important factor is the ratio between the volume of the cabin and a cross-sectional area of the opening.
- Pressure differential: The initial pressure gradient between the initial cabin pressure and the initial ambient pressure directly influences the rate and severity of decompression. The greater the differential, the more severe the decompression.
- Pressure ratio: Time is directly related to the pressure ratio between the cabin and ambient pressures. The greater the ratio, the longer the decompression.
- Flight pressure altitude: The altitude at which decompression occurs relates directly to the physiologic problems that occur after the incident.

Box 5-3 illustrates the physical characteristics of decompression.

The physiologic effects of rapid decompression are hypothermia, gas expansion, hypoxia, and decompression sickness. Hypoxia is by far the most important hazard of cabin decompression of an aircraft flying at high altitudes.[17,31] The rapid reduction of ambient pressure produces a corresponding drop in the PO_2 and reduces the alveolar oxygen tension. A twofold to threefold performance decrement occurs, regardless of altitude. The reduced tolerance for hypoxia after decompression is caused by: (1) a reversal in the direction of oxygen flow in the lungs;

BOX 5-3 | **Physical Characteristics of Decompression**

Slow Decompression

Onset is insidious and gradual and can occur without detection. Signs and symptoms are the same as for hypoxia. Decompression can be determined by checking the cabin altimeter.

Rapid Decompression

Onset is immediate, in 1 to 3 seconds, and is accompanied by noise, flying debris, and fog.

Noise

When two different air masses collide, a sound is heard that ranges from a swish to an explosion.

Flying Debris

On decompression, rapidly rushing air from a pressurized cabin causes the velocity of airflow through the cabin to increase rapidly as the air approaches the opening. Loose objects, such as maps, charts, and unsecured medical equipment, can be extracted through the orifice. Dust and dirt hamper vision for a short period of time.

Fog

During rapid decompression, both temperature and pressure suddenly decrease. This decrease reduces the capacity of air to contain water vapor and causes fog. The dissipation rate of fog is fairly rapid in fighter aircraft but considerably slower in larger multiplace aircraft.

Modified from Chase NB, Kreutzman RJ: Army aviation medicine. In DeHart RL, editor: *Fundamentals of aerospace medicine,* Philadelphia, 1985, Lea & Febiger; and Heimbach RD, Sheffield PJ: Decompression sickness and pulmonary overpressure accidents. In DeHart RL, editor: *Fundamentals of aerospace medicine,* Philadelphia, 1985, Lea & Febiger.

(2) diminished respiratory activity at the time of decompression; and (3) decreased cardiac activity at the time of decompression.[13,17,31]

Crew members and passengers must protect themselves from the potential physiologic hazards caused by loss of cabin pressure. Because hypoxia is the most immediate hazard, all occupants must breathe 100% oxygen. Air medical personnel must first ensure that they are breathing 100% oxygen before attempting to assist their patients. Patients who already have oxygen deficiencies, such as patients with coronary disease, anemia, or pneumonia, must be closely monitored after decompression. After the prevention or correction of hypoxia, descent is made to an altitude below 10,000 ft if possible.[31]

DECOMPRESSION SICKNESS

The first human case of decompression sickness was reported in 1841 by M. Triger, a French mining engineer who noticed symptoms of pain and muscle cramps in coal miners who had been working in an air-pressurized mine shaft.[13,15,31] Because tunnel workers were first to have the syndrome now known as decompression sickness, early terminology describing this disorder was related to that occupation; hence, the names *caisson disease* and *compressed-air illness.*[13,15,31]

A distinct difference is found between compressed-air illness and *subatmospheric decompression sickness,* although they share the same colloquial nomenclature for the common manifestations. Classically, the main manifestations are limb pain (the bends), respiratory disturbances (the chokes), skin irritation (the creeps), various disturbances of the central nervous system (the staggers), and cardiovascular collapse (syncope). These symptoms of subatmospheric decompression sickness virtually always subside or disappear during descent to ground level. Rarely, however, does recovery occur after recompression to ground level, and in some cases, the severity of the symptoms may increase, accompanied by a generalized deterioration in the individual's condition, which is known as *postdescent collapse.*[31]

Although the finer points of the pathologic processes that underlie some of the manifestations of altitude decompression sickness remain unknown, the basic mechanism is supersaturation of the tissues with nitrogen.[13-18] Because the partial pres-

sure of nitrogen in the inspired air falls with ascent to higher altitudes, nitrogen is carried by the blood from the tissues to the lungs, where it exits the body in the expired gas. In addition, because the solubility of nitrogen in the blood is relatively low and some tissues contain large amounts of nitrogen, the rate of fall of the absolute pressure of the body tissues, which is associated with the ascent in altitude, is greater than the rate of fall of the partial pressure of nitrogen in the tissues. These tissues therefore become supersaturated with nitrogen. In certain circumstances, supersaturation gives rise to the formation of bubbles of gas, the main constituent of which is initially nitrogen, in specific tissues of the body. Gas exchange is the governing mechanism in the formation of the bubbles, and these bubbles subsequently grow in size through the diffusion of nitrogen and other gases such as oxygen and carbon dioxide from surrounding tissues.

The driving pressure for bubble formation in a fluid is the difference between the partial pressure of the gas dissolved in the fluid and the absolute hydrostatic pressure.[31] Henry's law can be applied as follows: The amount of a gas that dissolves in a solution and remains in that solution is directly proportional to the pressure of the gas over the solution. Nitrogen is metabolically inert. At sea level, the amount of nitrogen dissolved in the body tissues and fluid is in equilibrium with the ambient pressure. At higher altitudes, nitrogen evolves in a manner similar to the formation of bubbles in a carbonated beverage when the bottle cap is removed. Decompression sickness is not usually encountered below a pressure altitude of FL 250.[6] The clinical manifestations of decompression sickness are shown in Box 5-4.[31]

In a small number of cases, circulatory collapse or postdecompression collapse may occur. The clinical symptoms vary. Typically, the patient becomes anxious, develops a frontal headache, and feels sick. Facial pallor, coldness, and sweaty extremities may occur, and peripheral cyanosis almost always occurs. General or focal signs of neurologic involvement, such as weakness of the limbs, apraxia, scotomata, and convulsions, may occur. Arterial blood pressure is generally well maintained until late in the development of the illness. Finally, in the worst cases, coma super-

| BOX 5-4 | **Clinical Manifestations of Decompression Sickness** |

Skin

Paresthesia (numbness or tingling sensation)
Mottled or diffuse rash of short duration
Itching
Cold or warm sensations

Joints

"Bends" pain (mild to severe) in muscles and joints, caused by nitrogen bubbles in the joint space
Pain is mild at onset, becomes deep and penetrating, and eventually becomes severe
Pain usually affects (in order) knee, shoulder, elbow, wrist or hand, and ankle or foot
Pain increases with motion

Lungs

"Chokes" (rare in both diving and aviation)
Deep sharp pain under sternum
Dry cough

Inability to take a normal breath
Attempted deep breath causes coughing (frequently paroxysmal)
Condition progresses to collapse if exposure to altitude is maintained
"False chokes" (caused by breathing cold dry oxygen, which dries the throat and causes irritation and a nonproductive cough)

Brain

Visual disturbances
Headache
Spotty motor or sensory loss, or both
Unilateral paresthesia
Confusion
Paresis
Seizures

---

venes. Recovery can occur at any stage, but in the past, it has been rare once coma has developed.[13,15-18,31]

In addition to supersaturation of the tissues with nitrogen, other factors that influence susceptibility are the rate of ascent, altitude, time of exposure, reexposure to high altitude, body fat, age (if greater than 40 years), exercise before and after flight, presence of infection, and alcohol ingestion.[13,17,18,31]

The primary treatment of decompression sickness that arises at high altitudes is recompression to ground level as rapidly as possible. Breathing 100% oxygen also relieves the tissue hypoxia produced by the reduction of local blood flow. The actual management of a case of serious decompression sickness depends on geographic location and the availability of a suitable hyperbaric chamber. Therefore, the order of preference of available treatment is as follows[13,15,18,37]:

1. Immediate hyperbaric compression with or without intermittent oxygen breathing should be administered.
2. Where no chamber facility exists, air medical personnel should treat circulatory collapse and arrange for early transfer to a hyperbaric chamber where this facility is available at a reasonable time or distance (less than 6 hours

of travel time). Surface transport is preferable; flight to a suitable chamber should be at an altitude below 1000 ft if possible and not higher than 3000 ft.
3. Air medical crew members should administer full supportive treatment for circulatory collapse if no possibility exists of transfer within a reasonable time to a hyperbaric chamber.

Transport team members should not fly for at least 12 hours after diving.

ADDITIONAL STRESSES OF TRANSPORT

SPATIAL DISORIENTATION

Spatial disorientation is described as an individual's inaccurate perception of position, attitude, and motion in relation to the center of the Earth.[3] When persons experience spatial disorientation, they cannot correctly interpret or process the information they are given by their senses. Spatial disorientation primarily occurs during air transport.

During flight, the following three systems are involved in maintenance of equilibrium: the visual, the vestibular, and the proprioceptive. These systems combine to allow the appropriate interpretation of input. However, the visual system plays the most important role.

Spatial disorientation can cause the following visual illusions[3,39,40]:

- Cloud formations being confused with the horizon or ground.
- Water or desert appearing to be farther away than it is.
- During night flight, the perception that another aircraft is moving away when it is actually getting closer.

These visual illusions can cause significant motion sickness, which may render pilots or transport team members incapable of performing their duties or providing patient care. Spatial disorientation can also lead to misinterpretation of a landing area and result in a crash.

To prevent spatial disorientation, transport team members should use proper scanning techniques, never stare at lights, get adequate rest and nutrition, and provide conscious patients with a tactile reference during transport.

FLICKER VERTIGO

Flicker vertigo can occur when transport team members and patients are exposed to lights that flicker at a rate of 4 to 20 cycles per second.[3,39,40] Flicker vertigo can cause nausea and vomiting. In severe cases, it can cause seizures and unconsciousness.

Flicker vertigo commonly occurs when sunlight flickers through the rotor blades of a helicopter or an airplane propeller. It has also been triggered by light from rotating beacons against an overcast sky.

Transport team members or patients with a history of seizures are at risk for flicker vertigo. Wearing of a hat with a bill and sunglasses can prevent flicker vertigo. Adequate rest and stress management may also decrease the risk.

FUEL VAPORS

Both ground and air transport can expose transport crew members and patients to fuel vapors. Jet fuel, diesel fuel, and gasoline are a few examples of what may be used in transport vehicles. Exposure to fuel

vapors can cause altered mental status, nausea, and eye inflammation.[39,40]

Fuel vapors may be an indication of a problem in the transport vehicle and, when detected, should be immediately reported by the transport team. Adequate ventilation can help decrease the effects of exposure.[39,40]

SUMMARY

To become an effective healthcare provider in the transport environment, each transport team member must be thoroughly familiar with the effects of the stresses of transport on the human body. Implementation of correct interventions is an essential responsibility of each team member to minimize the effects of the stresses of transport.

TRANSPORT PHYSIOLOGY CASE STUDY

A 70-year-old man with a history of a nonembolic stroke is being transported via rotor-wing aircraft for treatment of sepsis. His vital signs are blood pressure 84/59 mm Hg, pulse rate 120 bpm (sinus tachycardia), respiratory rate (intubation on transport ventilator) 14 bpm, and rectal temperature 97°F.

He has been prepared for transport in a BK 117. When the pilot begins to turn the rotors, the flight nurse notices that the patient's eyes are blinking rapidly and he begins to have a generalized tonic-clonic seizure. The monitor shows ventricular fibrillation, but a pulse can be palpated.

The transport nurse asks the pilot to stop the engines so that the team may obtain resuscitation assistance from the referring hospital personnel. As the rotors slow down, the patient's seizure activity ceases. After a quick evaluation and administration of 2 mg of lorazepam, the transport team prepares to leave again. Once again, with the turning of the rotors, the patient has the same symptoms.

This time, the transport nurse covers the patient's eyes with a towel and the seizure activity ceases. The team keeps the patient's eyes covered throughout the transport without further seizure activity.

DISCUSSION

Although flicker vertigo is not a common condition, sunlight flickering through rotor blades can trigger seizure activity in persons with seizure disorders or neurologic disorders that may place a patient at risk for seizures. This patient had had a recent stroke. Other clues that made the transport nurse consider flicker vertigo as the cause of this man's seizures are as follows:

- *The patient care platform positioned the patient's face in front of a window.*
- *The day was sunny.*
- *The activity ceased when the rotor blades stopped and began again with start-up.*

REFERENCES

1. Alspach JG, editor: *Core curriculum for critical care nursing*, ed 6, Philadelphia, 2006, Saunders Elsevier.
2. Banks RD, Brinkley JW, Allnutt R, et al: Human response to acceleration. In Davis J, Johnson R, Stepanek J, et al., editors: *Fundamentals of aerospace medicine*, ed 4, Philadelphia, 2008, Wolters Kluwer/Lippincott Williams & Wilkins.
3. Blumen IJ, Callejas S: Transport physiology: a reference for air medical personnel. In Blumen I, Lemkin DL, editors: *Principles and direction of air medical transport*, Salt Lake City, 2006, Air Medical Physicians Association.
4. Burton GG, Helmholz HF: Gas laws and certain indispensable conversions. In Burton GG, Hodgkin JE, editors: *Respiratory care: a guide to clinical practice*, ed 2, Philadelphia, 1984, JB Lippincott.
5. Commission on Accreditation of Medical Transport Systems (CAMTS): *Accreditation standards*, ed 7, Anderson, SC, 2006, CAMTS.
6. Department of the Air Force: *Aeromedical evacuation*, US Air Force Pamphlet No 164-2, Washington, DC, 1983, USAF.
7. Egan DF, Spearman CB, Sheldon RL: Gases, the atmosphere and the gas laws. In Scanlon CL, Spearman CB, Sheldon RI, editors: *Egan's fundamentals of respiratory therapy*, ed 4, St Louis, 1982, Mosby.
8. Gillingham KK, Wolfe JW: Spatial orientation in flight. In DeHart RL, editor: *Fundamentals of aerospace medicine*, Philadelphia, 1985, Lea & Febiger.
9. Glaister DH: The effects of long-duration acceleration. In Ernsting J, King P, editors: *Aviation medicine*, ed 2, London, 1988, Butterworth.
10. Hanna HH, Yarington CT: Otolaryngology in aerospace medicine. In DeHart RL, editor: *Fundamentals of aerospace medicine*, Philadelphia, 1985, Lea & Febiger.
11. Hawkins FH: The aircraft cabin and its human payload. In Orlady HW, editor: *Human factors in aviation*, ed 2, Aldershot, England, 1993, Avebury Technical.
12. Heimbach RD, Sheffield PJ: Decompression sickness and pulmonary overpressure accidents. In DeHart RL, editor: *Fundamentals of aerospace medicine*, Philadelphia, 1985, Lea & Febiger.
13. Heimbach RD, Sheffield PJ: Protection in the pressure environment: cabin pressurization and oxygen equipment. In DeHart RL, editor: *Fundamentals of aerospace medicine*, Philadelphia, 1985, Lea & Febiger/Lippincott Williams & Wilkins.
14. Kenefick RW, Cheuvront SN, Castellani JW, et al: Thermal stress. In Davis J, Johnson R, Stepanek J, et al., editors: *Fundamentals of aerospace medicine*, ed 4, Philadelphia, 2008, Wolters Kluwer.
15. Kizer K: Diving medicine. In Auerbach P, editor: *Wilderness medicine*, ed 4, St Louis, 2001, Mosby.
16. Macmillan AJ: Decompression sickness. In Ernsting J, King P, editors: *Aviation medicine*, ed 2, London, 1988, Butterworth.
17. Macmillan AJ: The pressure cabin. In Ernsting J, King P, editors: *Aviation medicine*, ed 2, London, 1988, Butterworth.
18. Martin TE: Clinical aspects aeromedical transport. *Curr Anaesth Crit Care* 14:131-140, 2003.
19. Neubauer JC, Dixon JP, Herndon CM: Fatal pulmonary decompression sickness: a case report, *Aviat Space Environ Med* 59(12):1181-1184, 1988.
20. Pickard JS, Gradwell DP: Respiratory physiology and protection against hypoxia. In Davis JD, Johnson R, Stepanek J, et al., editors: *Fundamentals of aerospace medicine*, ed 4, Philadelphia, 2008, Wolters Kluwer/Lippincott Williams & Wilkins.
21. PilotFriend: *Aviation medicine: effects of altitude*, available at http://www.pilotfriend.com/aeromed/medical/alt_phys.htm, accessed June 10, 2008.
22. Phelan JR: Otolaryngology in aerospace medicine. In Davis J, Johnson R, Stepanek J, et al., editors: *Fundamentals of aerospace medicine*, ed 4, Philadelphia, 2008, Wolters Kluwer/Lippincott Williams & Wilkins.
23. Raymann RB: Air crew health care maintenance. In DeHart RL, editor: *Fundamentals of aerospace medicine*, Philadelphia, 1985, Lea & Febiger.

24. Rood GM: Noise and communication. In Ernsting J, King P, editors: *Aviation medicine*, ed 2, London, 1988, Butterworth.

25. Sharp GR: The Earth's atmosphere. In *Aviation medicine*, London, 1978, Trimed Books.

26. Sheffield PJ, Heimbach RD: Respiratory physiology. In DeHart RL, editor: *Fundamentals of aerospace medicine*, Philadelphia, 1985, Lea & Febiger.

27. Smith SD, Gooman JR, Grosveld FW: Vibration and acoustics. In Davis, JR, Johnson R, Stepanek J, et al., editors: *Fundamentals of aerospace medicine*, ed 4, Philadelphia, 2008, Wolters Kluwer/Lippincott Williams & Wilkins.

28. Spaul WA, Spear RC, Greenleaf JE: Thermoregulatory response to heat and vibration in men, *Aviat Space Environ Med* 57(11):1082-1087, 1986.

29. Spoor DH: The passenger and the patient in flight. In DeHart RL, editor: *Fundamentals of aerospace medicine*, Philadelphia, 1985, Lea & Febiger.

30. Sredl D: *Airborne patient care management: a multidisciplinary approach*, St Louis, 1983, Medical Research Associated Publications.

31. Stepanek J, Webb JT: Physiology of decompressive stress. In Davis JR, Johnson R, Stepanek J, et al., editors: *Fundamentals of aerospace medicine*, ed 4, Philadelphia, 2008, Wolters Kluwer/Lippincott Williams & Wilkins.

32. Stoot JR: Vibration. In Ernsting J, King P, editors: *Aviation medicine*, ed 2, London, 1988, Butterworth.

33. United States Air Force School of Aerospace Medicine: *Flight nurse handouts*, June 1995.

34. Ward J: Oxygen delivery and demand, *Surgery* 24(10):354-360, 2006.

35. Welch BE: The biosphere. In DeHart RL, editor: *Fundamentals of aerospace medicine*, Philadelphia, 1985, Lea & Febiger.

36. Wilson LM, Price SA, editors: Respiratory pathophysiology. In *Pathophysiology: clinical concepts of disease processes*, ed 6, St Louis, 2003, Mosby.

37. Wirjosemito SA, Touhey JE, Workman WT: Type II altitude decompression sickness (DCS): U.S. Air Force experience with 133 cases, *Aviat Space Environ Med* 60(3):256-262, 1989.

38. Woodward GA, editor: *Guidelines for air and ground transport of neonatal and pediatric patients*, Elk Grove Village, IL, 2007, American Academy of Pediatrics.

39. Wofford MH, Frakes M, Mayberry R, editors: *Transport nurse advanced transport course*, ed 4, Denver, 2006, Air and Surface Transport Nurses Association.

40. York Clark D, Stocking J, Johnson J: *Flight and ground transport nursing core curriculum*, Denver, 2007, Air and Surface Transport Nurses Association.

EXTRICATION AND SCENE MANAGEMENT

Reneé Semonin Holleran

COMPETENCIES

1. Perform an initial scene evaluation to identify safety hazards.
2. Use the appropriate personal protective equipment.
3. Ensure that a patient has undergone decontamination before transport.
4. Identify who to call when hazardous materials have been spilled.
5. Demonstrate how to preserve evidence.

Extrication and scene management are important concepts for the transport team to thoroughly understand. Extrication, scene management, and hazardous material management exercises should be included in annual training for all transport personnel. The training officer of the local fire department or rescue team is an excellent resource for either joint agency training or training exclusively for transport personnel.

Air medical personnel are frequent participants in patient care in prehospital settings. Often, the rescue helicopter has been preceded by rescue personnel who have already freed trapped victims and secured them to backboards or triaged and decontaminated those exposed to hazardous substances. However, when extrication is prolonged or the helicopter is a first responder, air medical transport teams may need to use scene management and extrication skills. An important note is that only transport team members with the appropriate training and appropriate personnel protective equipment should participate in extrication. Technical rescues (including vehicle extrication, hazardous materials response, trench collapse, confined space, and rope rescue situations) for technical or heavy rescue companies are generally "high risk, low frequency" events that require coordinated, equipped, trained, and competent rescue personnel.

Most citizens and unskilled rescuers immediately rush to the victims. However, doing so can result in direct injury or exposure and contamination to both rescuers and victims and may delay the extrication and patient transport. Placement of a contaminated patient in a transport vehicle will result in that vehicle being taken out of service for decontamination.

SCENE MANAGEMENT

The following are scene management guidelines[3,8]:

1. Evaluate the situation for potential safety hazards (e.g., utilities, gasoline, propane, fuel oil, water, sanitary systems, movement of vehicles, or release of high-pressure systems).
2. Secure the accident scene.
3. Wear personal protective equipment (PPE) appropriate to the hazards on the scene (e.g., gloves, goggles, or self-contained breathing apparatus [SCBA]).
4. Gain access to the patient.
5. Provide life-sustaining care to the patient.
6. Disentangle the patient from the vehicle.
7. Prepare the patient for removal from the accident scene (e.g., place cervical collar).
8. Remove the patient.
9. Prepare the patient for transport to the hospital.
10. Provide the patient with treatment en route.

When the rescue involves wilderness or back country rescue, the TOMAS mnemonic should be applied[3]:

T: Terrain (exposure, cliffs, water, forest, vegetation, hiking terrain, snow).
O: Obstacles (trees, loose rock, debris, wires, daylight, rotor wash, blade clearance).
M: Method (type of insertion and location, landing near or remote from patient, hover load).
A: Alternatives (wait for search and rescue [SAR], ferry SAR personnel, relocate patient, no go/abort mission).
S: Safety (first, last, always).

Scene evaluation begins when the communications center obtains information about possible problems and circumstances the rescuers may confront. The communication specialist should continue to seek information that could aid the rescuers throughout the incident, such as time of day, weather conditions, location, terrain, and number of victims. Information about fire, spilled fuel, toxic chemicals, overturned or entangled vehicles, and downed electrical lines should also be related to the communication specialist.

The general rule is to never compromise the rescuers to aid the victims. Even with appropriate protective equipment, rescuers are at risk of injury.[14] The utility company should secure downed electrical lines; the fire department contains and controls hazardous materials. The rescuer should read placards on heavy trucks or read the manifest in the truck cab to determine the presence of any toxic or radioactive materials.

Scene security is usually provided by law enforcement personnel. Onlookers and the media should be kept well back from the operation. The area should be appropriately secured by the referring agencies.[6]

Proper placement of the helicopter is essential to avoid a second incident or hazard to personnel on the scene. The pilot retains the ultimate responsibility for landing the helicopter safely. Figure 6-1 shows a photograph of a tail rotor that was damaged when a vehicle drove under it in the dark and caused severe damage that put the aircraft out of service. Chapter 9 discusses scene landing recommendations.

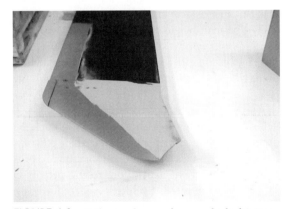

FIGURE 6-1   Tail rotor damage from a vehicle driving under it at a scene at night. Aircraft was out of service until the tail rotor was changed at the scene.

EXTRICATION[7,8]

The transport team may enter a vehicle, once it is stabilized and deemed safe, through the car doors or by breaking out the glass and crawling through the windows. The transport team should not enter a vehicle unless trained or directed by a trained individual. Although one side of a vehicle may be crushed beyond recognition, the opposite-side car door may be operable. If the vehicle is lying on its side and access is gained through the top-side car door, rescue crews should stabilize the vehicle before entry to prevent any unexpected movement. Any unanticipated vehicle movement is both unacceptable and unsafe for rescuers and occupants.

Once inside the vehicle, the rescue team must perform rapid triage. Initial emergency treatment before extrication is extremely limited. Usually the initial-entry rescuer brings in a rigid cervical collar, a pocket facemask, and trauma dressings. The objectives are to: 1, establish and maintain an airway with cervical spine protection with either the chin-lift maneuver or the jaw-thrust maneuver; 2, provide artificial ventilation (if oxygen is used, caution must be exercised because an inadvertent spark can ignite fuel-saturated clothing); 3, control external hemorrhage; and 4, provide cardiopulmonary resuscitation (CPR). CPR is not effective unless the patient is supine and on a firm surface; therefore, rapid extrication of the patient is needed for effective CPR. Patients who are apneic, pulseless, or unconscious or who have ineffective breathing must be removed quickly from the vehicle while manual cervical spine protection is maintained.

The basic principle of extrication is that the rescuers should remove the vehicle from the victim rather than the other way around. If the vehicle is on its side, the extrication is performed through the roof. If the vehicle is on its wheels or roof, extrication is conducted through the doors. Rescue personnel inside an upright vehicle should first unlock the doors and use interior handles while their partners use exterior handles to open the doors. Before proceeding with patient extrication, rescue personnel should always ensure the vehicle's emergency brake is engaged, the key/engine is turned off, the transmission is placed in park, and, whenever possible, the vehicle's battery is disconnected.

Once the doors are open, victims can be secured to short backboards that provide spinal column immobilization. Further obstacles to extrication may occur. Typically, a victim's thorax becomes wedged between the forward-displaced seat and the rearward-displaced steering wheel/column, or a victim's feet and legs become trapped under the downward-displaced dashboard and the accelerator or brake pedal. A quick option to create more room between the victim, the seat, and the steering wheel is to manually slide the seat back, if it remains operational. Multiple rescuers should control the seat and the patient to avoid unnecessary movement and possible risk of further injury.

The victim must be completely immobilized if the seat has been torn from the mechanical track. When the seat tracks snap, a series of physically jarring pops usually occurs that could substantially compromise an injured victim's condition.

Pulling the steering wheel usually disentangles the victim's legs and feet because it concurrently lifts the dashboard up and forward.

If the vehicle is resting on its side and has been stabilized, extrication can be achieved by cutting an upside-down U in the roof. The vehicle should be stabilized in the side position, the occupants should be warned of the very loud noise about to begin, and a heavy aluminized blanket should cover the occupants for their safety. After the three-sided U-shaped cut of the roof is made, the metal flap should be folded down to provide a smooth edge to move the victims across on their way out.[7]

AIR BAGS

Rescuers must also be aware of the hazard of air bags. Most recently built cars are equipped with these safety devices. Studies have documented the effectiveness of air bags in decreasing serious injuries to drivers and passengers.[1,7,10] However, air bags can also cause injuries such as facial abrasions and lacerations and contusions to the chest and upper extremities.[1,8,10]

Undeployed air bags may be a potential hazard to the rescuer and can cause injuries similar to those reported in accidents in which the air bag has deployed.

If the air bag has not been deployed, the rescuer should observe the following precautions[1,8,10]:

1. Disconnect or cut both battery cables. Always cut or disconnect the negative side first. Secure both cables so they do not spring back and touch each other or the battery.
2. Avoid placing personnel or objects in front of the air bag deployment path.
3. Do not mechanically displace or cut through the steering column until the system has been deactivated. Charts are available that indicate how long the airbag may take to deactivate. Some may take up to 30 minutes.
4. Do not cut or drill into the air bag module.
5. Do not apply heat in the area of the steering wheel hub.
6. Be aware of other air bags within the vehicle (e.g., the side air bag).

AIRCRAFT CRASH

The crash of even a light aircraft requires the response of a variety of emergency service units, including fire, rescue, emergency medical service (EMS), and law enforcement. For quick and effective response, the person who reports a crash must provide as much information about the incident as possible.

The following information should be obtained by communication center personnel and relayed to responders:

1. The time of the crash.
2. The type of aircraft (e.g., small passenger plane, commuter aircraft, large commercial jet, military transport plane, military fighter aircraft, or helicopter).
3. The number of engines, if known.
4. Whether the wreckage is on fire.
5. Whether a parachute was observed.
6. The number of occupants of the aircraft, if known.
7. Identification numbers and markings of the aircraft. Military aircraft are marked "US Air Force," "US Navy," and so forth. Commercial aircraft show the name of the carrier. Private aircraft may have a combination of letters and numbers that constitute the identification number.
8. The status (e.g., on fire, damaged, or collapsed) of any structures struck by the aircraft or its components.
9. The status of people in those structures, if known.
10. Vehicles that were struck by the aircraft or parts of it and the status of any persons inside the vehicles, if known.
11. Structures that appear to be endangered by encroaching fire, spilled fuel, military ordnance, and so on.

If the transport team arrives at the crash site before emergency service units, team members must proceed with caution. Survivors of the crash or persons who have been ejected or who have parachuted from the aircraft may be lying on the roadway leading to the crash site. If the aircraft is military, crew members must avoid both the front and rear ends of any externally mounted tanks or pods because these may be containers for missiles or rockets. The crew must be careful not to disturb any armament thrown clear of the aircraft; it may explode if improperly handled. No one should move body parts or components of the aircraft unless movement is necessary to care for injured persons. When emergency service units arrive on the scene, the transport team should report to the officer-in-charge everything known about the incident and the locations of any injured persons who have been assisted.

BUS CRASH[8]

STOPPING THE ENGINE

Buses equipped with diesel engines do not need electrical power once they have been started. If possible, the rescuers should stop the engine by using the emergency stop button located on the driver's left-hand side switch panel. If the engine does not stop with this button, a crew member should discharge CO_2 into the engine air intake located at the left rear corner of the coach, discharging the agent inward and toward the front of the coach. Dry chemical should not be used. Not all buses may be equipped this way.

ENTERING THE COACH

The rescuers should enter the coach through the front door if possible, but only after the vehicle is stabilized. Door unlocking and unlatching mechanisms can be found under the right-side wheel well, behind the front medallion, or to the left of the driver's seat, depending on the make and model of the bus. If the rescuers cannot enter through the front door, they can enter the bus through the windshield by removing the rubber locking strip from around the pane and then removing the pane. To enter the restroom (if the bus is equipped with one), the rescuers should open the small flap at the right rear window and lift the latch bar to open the window.

If the bus is lying on its side, entry may be possible through a roof access hatch or rear emergency window. Bus accidents are likely to overwhelm local rescue resources because of the high number of potential victims. Rescuers should be prepared to perform triage on passengers who remain inside the bus with the Simple Triage and Rapid Transport (START) triage system (RPM: Respirations, Pulse, and Motor) or an appropriate alternative. Removal of patients on stretchers requires a coordinated team effort to prevent further injury to patients or risk of injury to rescuers.

THE AIR SUSPENSION SYSTEM

The transport team must remember the warning to not place heads or extremities under any portion of the coach until it is securely stabilized.. The air suspension system bellows may deflate without warning, in which case the body of the coach may drop suddenly to within inches of the roadway.

ELECTRICAL EMERGENCIES[12]

High voltages are common on roadside utility poles. Wooden poles are sometimes used to support conductors of as much as 500,000 V. Energized downed lines may or may not arc and burn. No assurance can be given that a dead line at the scene of a vehicle accident will not become energized again unless it is cut or otherwise disconnected from the system by a representative of the power company. When an interruption of current flow is sensed in most power distribution systems, automatic devices restore the flow two or three times over a period of minutes.

The dispatcher should advise the power company of the exact location of the accident and the number of the power pole. The rescue team member designated to control bystanders should order spectators and nonessential personnel to leave the danger zone. The power company is responsible to ensure all power has been disconnected from energized lines. Depending on the distances between poles, the danger zone may be as large as 600 ft by 1500 ft. Any rescuer should stop the approach immediately if a tingling sensation is felt in the legs and lower torso. This sensation signals energized ground; current is entering through one foot, passing through the lower body, and leaving through the other foot. This current flow is possible because of the condition known as *ground gradient,* which means the voltage is greatest at the point of contact with the ground and then diminishes as the distance from the point of contact increases.

If a tingling sensation is felt, the proper procedure is to bend one leg at the knee and grasp the foot of that leg with one hand, turn around, and hop to a safe place on one foot. This maneuver ensures that the body does not complete a circuit between sections of ground energized with different voltages. The rescuer and the transport team should then stand by in a safe place until a representative of the power company can cut the lines or otherwise disconnect them from the power distribution system. The crew member who controls access to the scene must discourage ambulatory accident victims from leaving their vehicles until conductors that are either touching or surrounding the wreckage can be deenergized.

METAL OR CONDUCTING FENCES

A lethal current can be conducted through a chain-link fence for some distance. If working near or climbing a chain-link fence that may be energized by a downed conductor is necessary, a crew member should not approach the fence with arms extended and fingers pointing forward. If contact is made with an energized fence, the current will cause the person's fingers to curl around the fence mesh and hold the person in place.

If a fence is thought to be energized, personnel should stay a safe distance away and establish a safe perimeter and then wait for the power company to secure the area and contain the power.

The proper approach to the fence is with arms extended and the backs of hands facing forward.

If the fence is energized, the current will cause the person to be repelled backward.

HAZARDOUS MATERIALS EMERGENCIES[11,14]

Emergencies that involve hazardous materials occur in all areas of the United States, and transport teams are likely to be involved in the care of those who have been injured. When a hazardous material can be identified from a number or by name, emergency service personnel may obtain advice about the emergency from agencies that assist in the management of hazardous materials (Box 6-1). Agencies such as the Chemical Transportation Emergency Center (CHEMTREC) and the US Department of Transportation can offer specific information.

However, not every transport vehicle is marked with a placard that identifies the specific materials on board. Many have placards that identify only the category of material carried. CHEMTREC should be called for advice if a placard that identifies

the material with a four-digit number is noted (Figure 6-2).

Suggested procedures for transport teams that respond to the scene of a hazardous material transport emergency are as follows:

1. Land the aircraft uphill and far enough away from the scene to prevent rotor wash from spreading hazardous materials. Pilots should avoid flying over the top of hazardous materials areas.
2. Keep out of low areas in which heavier-than-air vapors can accumulate. Hazardous Materials crews will establish "Hot," "Warm," and "Cold" zones of operation. Helicopter EMS crews should always stage in the Cold zone to prevent risk of personal injury or contamination of the aircraft. Only hazardous materials responders trained to the technician or operations levels should operate in the Warm zone, and only those trained to technician level should work in the Hot zone. Rescuers should wear PPE that is appropriate for the situation, including respiratory and

---

BOX 6-1   Agencies That Assist in Hazardous Materials and Potential Rescue Incidents

Federal Agencies
Environmental Protection Agency (EPA)
Department of Transportation (DOT)
National Response Center (NRC)
United States Coast Guard (USCG)
Centers for Disease Control and Prevention (CDC)
Federal Aviation Administration (FAA)
United States Armed Forces (Army, Navy, Air Force, Marines)
US Department of Energy (DOE)

Regional and State Agencies
State EPA
State health departments
National Guard
State police
State emergency management agencies

Local Agencies
Emergency management
Fire service (HAZMAT units)

Poison control and information center
Law enforcement agencies
Public utilities
Sewage and treatment facilities

Commercial Agencies
American Petroleum Institute
Association of American Railroads (AAR) and Hazardous Materials Systems
Chemical Manufacturers Association
HELP (Union Carbide's emergency response system for company shipments)
Chevron (provides assistance with Chevron products)
Railway industry
Local industry
Local contractors
Local carriers and transporters

HAZMAT, Hazardous material.
From Sanders MJ: *Mosby's paramedic textbook*, St Louis, 2007, Mosby.

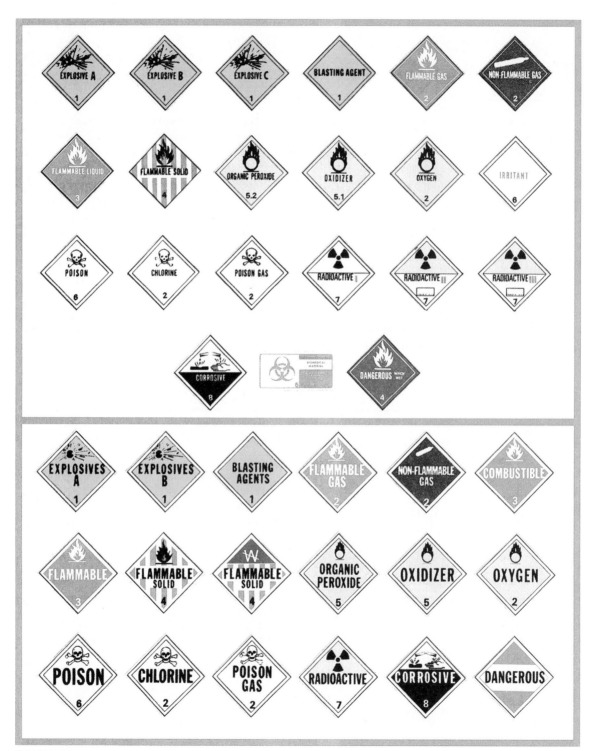

FIGURE 6-2   **Hazardous materials warning placards and labels.** (From Sanders MJ: *Mosby's paramedic textbook,* ed 3, St Louis, 2007, Mosby.)

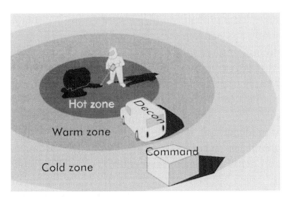

FIGURE 6-3 Safety zones for hazardous materials incident. (From Sanders MJ: *Mosby's paramedic textbook,* St Louis, 1994, Mosby.)

splash protection, as dictated by the nature of the hazardous material. Flight suits and flight uniforms are classified as Level D protection, the lowest level protection possible (Figure 6-3).

3. If the vehicle is on fire, be aware that some corrosive materials react violently with water. Attempt to extinguish a small fire with dry chemical or CO_2. Extinguish a large fire with water spray, fog, or foam. Fight the fire from the maximal distance that hose streams allow. Stay away from the ends of tank vehicles. Cool down uninvolved containers exposed to heat. Contain large amounts of spilled materials with dikes for later pick-up by personnel qualified in decontamination procedures.

In the event that someone has had contact with a dangerous substance, these procedures should be followed by personnel trained in decontamination:

1. Move the person to a safe place in fresh air.
2. Support respiration if the person is breathing with difficulty. Administer oxygen if it is available.
3. Initiate pulmonary resuscitation efforts if the person is not breathing.
4. Initiate CPR efforts if the person's breathing or heartbeat has stopped.
5. If skin surfaces (or eyes) have been in contact with a dangerous substance, begin flushing immediately with plenty of running water. The person may also be washed with water and a mild detergent.[7]

6. Strip away contaminated clothing and shoes while flushing with water. A properly decontaminated victim should have all clothing removed, including undergarments, and be given a disposable coverall or blanket to wear when decontamination is completed.
7. Continue to flush the exposed skin surfaces (or eyes) until reasonably certain all traces of the dangerous substance have been removed.
8. Isolate contaminated clothing and shoes.
9. Decontamination procedures must meet Occupational Safety and Health Administration (OSHA) requirements 29 CFR 1910.120.[11]
10. Never put any one in a transport vehicle who has not undergone proper decontamination.

DECONTAMINATION

The following steps have been recommended for use when a person needs decontamination after exposure to a hazardous material.[11] The decontamination corridor is called the Warm zone and is located between the Hot and Cold zones. This zone should be the only point of entry and exit to the Hot zone:

1. An entry point should be established for the "dirty" victims and rescuers to remove their clothing.
2. Surface decontamination should be performed with plenty of water unless the contaminant requires another decontaminant.
3. PPE should be removed and stored.
4. Other clothing may have to be removed, depending on the level of contamination.
5. Contaminated personnel and victims should be washed at least twice. Whenever possible, warm water with detergent should be used for decontamination.
6. The victims and personnel should be medically evaluated.
7. Injured individuals should be transported for definitive care.
8. The decontamination site must be cleaned up and contaminated materials disposed of.
9. All equipment that has been used should be decontaminated and cleaned.
10. Contaminated clothing should never be taken home and cleaned or transported with the patient. Remember that clothing may be evidence.

EXPLOSIVE MATERIALS EMERGENCIES[5]

An increase has been seen in the number of injuries and deaths caused by explosives. Between 1980 and 1990, 12,261 bombings occurred in the United States. Pipe bombs caused most injuries. Although transport teams are generally not first responders unless they have received appropriate education and training, they may inadvertently find themselves exposed to this situation or may be called to transport patients who have been injured.

The injuries that result from explosive materials include both blast and thermal injuries.[5,9,12] Three classes of explosives are discussed in the following paragraphs.

Class A explosives are the most hazardous types of explosives. They include dynamite, desensitized nitroglycerine, lead azide, mercury, fulminate, black powder, blasting caps, detonators, detonating primers, and certain smokeless propellants.

Class B explosives have a high flammability hazard and include most propellant materials.

Class C explosives include manufactured materials that contain limited quantities of Class A or Class B explosives as one of their components, such as detonating cord, explosive rivets, and fireworks. Class C explosives normally do not detonate under fire conditions.

A vehicle with a placard that indicates the presence of Class A or Class B explosives or blasting agents that is involved in an accident or fire is a potential danger. Traffic must be stopped in all directions, the area of nonessential personnel cleared for 2500 ft in all directions, and access denied to all persons not essential to firefighting or the rescue operation.

RADIOACTIVE MATERIAL EMERGENCIES[11,12,14]

The degree of hazard varies greatly depending on the type and quantity of the radioactive material. External radiation can result from exposure to unshielded radioactive material. Internal radiation contamination can result from inhalation, ingestion, or skin absorption. Runoff from fire control or dilution activities can cause water pollution and thus spread the probability of contamination. Although some radioactive materials may burn normally, they do not ignite rapidly.

If only the yellow, black, and white "Radioactive Material" placard is visible and the material being carried cannot otherwise be identified, people not essential to the firefighting or rescue operation should be kept at least 150 ft upwind of the area; greater distances may be advised by the radiation authority. A rescuer must enter the spill area only to save a life and, when entry is necessary, should stay only the shortest possible time. The rescuer must wear full PPE and a positive-pressure breathing apparatus. Persons and equipment exposed to the radioactive material must then be detained until the radiation authority arrives or other instructions are received.

If the vehicle is on fire, damaged containers should not be moved; undamaged containers may be moved if it is possible to do so safely. The crew should attempt to extinguish any small fire with dry chemical, CO_2, water fog, or foam.

Ensure that the victim has undergone appropriate decontamination before being placed in any transport vehicle. If the victim is not appropriately decontaminated, both the team and the transport vehicle can be contaminated if they are not protected. If the transport vehicle is contaminated, it needs to be taken out of service and decontaminated according to decontamination codes and guidelines.[5,9]

LIQUIFIED PETROLEUM GAS LEAK: NO FIRE

Quick action is necessary when a leak develops in a liquefied petroleum (LP) gas transport vehicle or a large LP-gas storage vessel. A large leak can produce a significant vapor cloud, and the heavier-than-air gas can easily ignite. Vapor releases are usually invisible, and not all LP gas is odorized.

As emergency service units arrive, firefighters set up large-diameter hose lines and take positions from which they can apply water to the sides of the tank. The officer in charge establishes a danger zone around the leaking container that should extend for at least 2000 ft from each end of the vessel and for at least 1000 ft from each side. Police officers evacuate the danger zone and deny access to all nonessential personnel until the emergency is over. If a transport team is the first to arrive, a member should first request that police close access roads and then alert the gas, electric, and telephone companies.

When hose lines are in position, the firefighters disperse the gas by directing water spray across the vapor path. The crew should remain behind the protective spray so that they are protected if the vapors ignite unexpectedly. No one should enter the vapor cloud. The gas company or plant operating personnel stops the flow of gas, if possible.

As utility company personnel arrive, the gas company representative shuts off the gas supply. The power company representative shuts off electricity to the surrounding buildings. The telephone company representative should disconnect the telephone service to buildings. A ringing telephone can trigger an explosion of flammable vapors.

REACTION VESSEL EMERGENCIES

Reaction vessels are steel kettles in which chemicals and other products are combined during a manufacturing process. Essentially "mixing bowls," these vessels can range in capacity from a few hundred to several thousand gallons. Some are simple, open, stainless steel vats with hinged lids; others are thick-walled vessels that can be sealed, pressurized, and heated. Large reaction vessels have manholes several feet in diameter, and others have elliptic openings as small as 12×16 inches. Mixing vessels have agitators, or "beaters," similar to those provided with a kitchen mixer. The edges of the beaters usually come to within a few inches of the vessel wall, and the rescue of a worker behind the beaters (in relation to the manhole) can be a difficult task.

Injury may occur when a worker fails to follow the established shutdown procedure, enters the vessel, and comes into contact with a hazardous material or a moving beater. A worker may fall and be injured while working inside the vessel. If any doubt exists about the quality of the air within the structure, rescuers should wear self-contained breathing units and a full set of protective clothing. Rescuers not certified in confined space rescue should attempt nonentry retrieval of victims via tag lines or other means without physically entering the confined space.

The rescuer should consult with the plant safety engineer or manager at the vessel location. If a knowledgeable person is not present (as in a multiple-injury situation), the Confined Space Entry Permit, which should be displayed near the entrance to the vessel, should be located. From the permit, the rescuer should be able to determine the following:

1. Any requirement for special protective clothing.
2. The frequency with which the atmosphere should be analyzed for oxygen concentration.
3. The frequency with which the atmosphere should be checked for explosive vapors.
4. The threshold limit value of any toxic material present.
5. The explosive limits of any flammable materials.
6. What chemicals were in the vessel before shutdown.
7. Any requirement for use of nonsparking tools.
8. The frequency with which radiation levels should be checked.
9. Any requirement to use safety harnesses.
10. Any requirement for standby personnel.
11. The type of respiratory protection required.
12. Any requirement for lifelines.

Plant personnel should close feed valves and charging chutes. A rescuer or other responsible person should be assigned to guard the valves and chutes to ensure that they are not inadvertently opened during the rescue operation.

Plant personnel deenergize the agitator power drive by opening the main disconnect switch and installing a lockout device. The padlock key should be secured until the rescue operation is over.

A rescuer should never be satisfied with someone's assertion that the agitator is shut off. If any doubt exists that the agitator is inoperative, the rescuer should have plant personnel remove drive belts or chains, or otherwise immobilize pulleys or flywheels. Appropriate lock-out tag-out kits should be used when available to prevent equipment or machinery from being reenergized.

CONSTRUCTION SITE EMERGENCIES

If a transport team member is near a piece of construction equipment when aiding a sick or injured operator and the engine of the machine is still running, the team member should not touch any of the operating levers, pedals, or other controls but should ask another operator to shut down the engine. If the injured operator can communicate, the transport team member should ask how to shut down the machine.

If another operator is not available and the sick or injured operator cannot provide instructions in the shutdown procedure and if the equipment is gasoline-powered, the medical team member should turn the key or master switch to the "off" position. If this does not stop the engine, the cable can be disconnected from the negative terminal of the battery. If the equipment is diesel-powered and has a level-type throttle control, pushing the lever all the way forward past the idle position and then turning the key or throwing the master switch to the "off" position will disrupt the electrical circuit to the engine.

RAILROAD INCIDENTS

Grade-Crossing Accident

In the event of an accident at a railroad crossing, the communication specialist should contact the railroad dispatcher with a request to stop all trains that are headed for the crossing.

Stopping the Train

The engineer of a train that is traveling at 60 mph has approximately 1 second to determine whether a collision is imminent and activate the emergency-braking system. The train will travel a distance of 7920 ft (1.5 miles). After the engineer applies the emergency brake, a train will continue for two thirds of a mile before stopping, even when traveling at only 30 mph.

To stop a train before it reaches a grade crossing, a person should be designated to go down the tracks to a point 1.5 to 2 miles from the grade crossing and swing a lighted flare slowly back and forth horizontally at right angles to the track. This stop signal is used by all railroads. The locomotive engineer should acknowledge the signal with two whistle blasts and then stop the train. The engineer might either misinterpret or disregard other signs and not stop the train. A flare can be waved day or night. If a flare is not available, a flashlight, battery-powered hand light, or lantern can be waved at night; a flag or other brightly colored object can be used during daylight.

In response to a derailment, the transport team should quickly assess the situation, report initial observations to the communication specialist, and request that the railroad dispatcher be notified of the incident. The railroad dispatcher arranges to halt rail traffic; dispatch railroad police, rescue, and clean-up crews; and notify railroad officials.

If the derailed train can be approached safely, the train conductor should be in or near the caboose. The conductor is in charge of the train and has documents that show whether the train is carrying hazardous materials.

The rescuers should not go under any derailed cars that are piled high to reach the caboose when passing close to the wreckage. A precariously perched car can come plunging down without warning.

If the conductor and other train members are incapacitated, the crew member can look in the documentation drawer in the caboose for information about the train cargo. Car movement waybills and a consist should be available. *Waybills* are documents that describe the cargo and identify the shipper and receiver. The *consist* is a car-by-car listing of the contents of each rail car.

When searching for injured crew members in the locomotive, the crew will observe forward and rear cabin doors. If access cannot be achieved by opening these doors inward, a rescuer can come in through the sliding cabin windows. The entire cabin area, including nose section, boiler room, and electrical power transmission areas, should be searched for injured persons.

Electric locomotives operate from an overhead electricity system that carries an 11,000-V alternating current. The overhead power must be disconnected by pressing the Pantograph Down button in the locomotive control cab. Rescuers must be aware that a derailed electric locomotive with a Pantograph that remains in contact with overhead wires poses the same electrocution threat as power lines that rest on a vehicle if rescuers contact the locomotive and the ground at the same time.

Steam generators are powered by diesel fuel. Fuel shutoff controls are located on each side of the car body under a cover plate marked Fuel Shut Off. The rescuer should lift the plate and pull the ring straight out 2 inches; the generator will stop running within 1 to 2 minutes.

Searching the train for injured passengers requires sliding open the side or end car doors or entering through an emergency window. The crew should check the entire car, including the toilet and baggage areas.

Side-entry doors on passenger cars may be locked and require tools to open. Side doors that slide in the car body panels have electric locks. The conductor and crew members have a skeleton key necessary to open this type of door latch. Access through dual-paned emergency exit windows is accomplished by shattering the outer tempered glass with a heavy, sharp, pointed tool, removing the inner window's rubber molding, and using a pry bar to remove the inner Lexan window.

UNDERGROUND EMERGENCIES

MINE EMERGENCY

In the event of a response to a mine emergency, the medical team should report directly to the mine office for instructions and follow those instructions explicitly.

CAVE EMERGENCY
Preemergency Activities

The medical team should identify cave-rescue specialists, speleologists, and local cavers in the area, catalog their qualifications, and establish procedures for contacting them at the time of a cave emergency.

Rescue equipment and medical supplies should be streamlined. Suggested equipment for cave rescue includes the following[2,4]:

1. Helmet-mounted light with 24 hours of light.
2. Helmet with a chin strap and headlight attachment.
3. Warm clothes and gloves that are waterproof and allow mobility.
4. Lug-soled boots that are light and drain water.
5. Specialized caving rope.
6. A litter that can fit through tight spaces.
7. Wetsuits, when water is expected in the cave.
8. Harnesses and rings resistant to chemicals and water.
9. Equipment to divert water from the victim and rescue crew.
10. Warm food and drink.

The medical crew should participate in cross-training programs so agency rescue personnel can become familiar with cave-rescue techniques, and the administrator should develop a continuing education program so rescue personnel can practice rescue techniques in real cave settings.

Care for an Injured Person During Cave Rescue

Caring for victims in a cave presents the medical crew with difficult challenges. Care must be provided in the dark and in muddy conditions. The transport team must be properly trained and experienced before they attempt any cave rescue.

The rescuer should carefully remove the victim from water or water spray, conduct a primary survey for life-threatening problems, and provide basic life support as necessary. The rescuer should remove the victim from drafts, if possible, and if not, should shield the victim with equipment or personnel. Heat loss to the ground can be prevented by placing a ground cover, blanket, articles of clothing, or rope under the victim. Heat loss to the surrounding air can be prevented by replacing the victim's wet clothes with dry clothing that is brought in or worn by the rescuers.

TRENCH COLLAPSE[7]

Workers and emergency service personnel can be buried under tons of earth when unsupported trench walls collapse. Sheeting and shoring a trench is a labor-intensive task but absolutely necessary if a rescue operation is to be carried out safely.

The steps to be followed in case of a trench collapse are as follows:

1. Determine who is in charge.
2. Assess the immediate injury problem. Determine whether the rescue team will operate in rescue mode or recovery mode; if the patient is obviously deceased, lives of rescuers should not be risked and all operations should proceed slowly and methodically to prevent unnecessary harm or injury to rescuers.
3. Determine how many people are buried.
4. Determine where people are buried. (Look for tools, clothing, personal belongings, heavy equipment, machinery, or pipe locations. If an open pipe end is near the location of the trench collapse, victims may have dived into open pipe ends before being buried. If the pipe can be accessed safely through an access point, rescuers should attempt communication inside the pipe to check whether victims may be inside the pipe.)
5. Assess on-the-scene capabilities of emergency medical services.
6. Request additional resources, if needed.

Hazard-control measures that can be taken include the following:

1. See that rescuers are protected.
2. Control traffic movement. All heavy equipment on scene must be parked, turned off, and locked-out and tagged-out. Heavy equipment should never be used during a rescue situation to dig out the patient.
3. Control spectator movement.
4. Make the trench lip safe.
5. Ventilate the trench.
6. Position a safety observer.
7. Make the trench safe.
8. Provide a second means of egress from the trench with ladders placed at opposite ends of the collapse site.
9. If the trench cannot be made safe, dig to the angle of repose.

Once access to the trapped victims has been achieved, the rescuers can dig them out by hand and remove the mechanisms of entrapment. First, a rescuer should uncover each victim's head and chest and initiate emergency care measures. When all the victims have been assessed and the ABCs (airway, breathing, circulation) have been treated, the rescuers can work to free them completely. Then, as the victim is freed, the victim should be secured to a backboard before being removed from the trench.

WELL EMERGENCIES

Deep wells have shafts that may penetrate the earth for several hundred feet. Depending on the diameter of the shaft, a person who falls into a deep well may become wedged only a few feet from the surface or may go all the way to the bottom. In most cases, rescue (or recovery) is possible only when a parallel shaft is drilled and a horizontal tunnel dug, through which rescuers can pass from the shaft to the well. Well emergencies should be treated as high-angle vertical confined space rescues.

Many conditions add to the danger of well emergencies. In shallow wells, the atmosphere may be oxygen deficient. Heavier-than-air toxic gases may be present at the bottom of the well. Methane gas may present the threat of an explosion. Water in the well may cause the victim to drown. Unstable shaft walls may collapse during a rescue operation.

All of these conditions warrant special precautions. To guard against possible shaft-wall collapse, the rescuer should place ground pads (sheets of 4 × 8–foot plywood) around the shaft opening. The pads distribute the weight of the rescuers and equipment and minimize the possibility of a cave-in. The possibility of an oxygen-deficient atmosphere must be anticipated if the victim at the bottom of the shaft is unconscious or incoherent. The rescuer should ventilate the well by having fresh air blown down the shaft. To reach the victim, the rescuer should put on a safety harness that is secured to a lifeline or a harness that is formed with the end of a lifeline.

The victim, when reached, should be secured in a harness attached to a lifeline or in a harness formed with the end of another lifeline. Whenever time, manpower, and resources allow, backup or secondary entry teams should be ready to enter the confined space to assist primary entry teams. If the rescuer cannot climb out, the ground-level rescuers should hoist the rescuer from the shaft with their lifelines. All rescuers should have a dorsal back-up line attached for emergency use. Before rescuers are lowered into the well shaft, atmospheric monitoring within the well should occur to determine whether the environment has had sufficient oxygen content for the victim to remain viable. All confined-space environments should be considered hazardous and treated as if a low oxygen environment exists; therefore, rescue teams with supplied air systems should always use supplied air for rescuers who serve as entrants into the confined-space environment. If a significantly low oxygen reading is obtained and no communication is occurring between the victim and rescuers, the patient may be deceased and recovery mode should be considered. Ventilation of the well shaft decreases the hazard risk to rescuers and may lead to improved patient outcomes. Whenever possible, rescue teams should use mechanical advantage systems to hoist and lower rescuers and victims into below-grade openings. Depending on well shaft diameter and patient condition, rescuers should attach a rescue harness to the victim for simultaneous extrication. Standard operation for confined space rescue is that, whenever possible, the rescuer is removed before the patient to avoid having the victim become stuck or wedged between the rescuer and the egress point. For rescuers with limited air supply, this could result in a potentially deadly situation.

Rescuers who set up lights to illuminate the shaft of a wet well must be sure the lights are tightly secured. If a lamp falls into the well during the rescue operation, it could electrocute victims and rescuers.

LAW ENFORCEMENT–RELATED SITUATIONS

Law enforcement officials expect the cooperation of other emergency personnel with a police emergency.

Bomb Threat

In the event of a bomb threat, the transport team should report the location and give an accurate description of the object to the command post or control point; this information should then be relayed immediately to the police, fire departments, and rescue units. The information should be relayed via telephone even if a two-way radio is available because radio transmission energy can cause detonation of an electric blasting cap. The object should never be touched or otherwise disturbed. Doors and windows should be opened to minimize primary damage from the blast and secondary damage from fragmentation.

Firearm Emergency

A weapon found at the scene of an emergency must be left in the exact position in which it was discovered. Rescuers should assume the weapon is loaded and in operating order even if it appears otherwise. Law enforcement officers should be called.

If the weapon must be moved for any reason before police officers arrive, a medical crew member may assume responsibility for moving and safeguarding the weapon or should delegate the responsibility to a trustworthy person. Only one person should handle the weapon until it can be turned over to the police officers. If a camera is available, a photograph can be taken of the weapon in place, with reference points, such as doors, windows, furniture, and so on, that will help investigators accurately place the weapon included in the picture. A photograph that shows only the weapon is useless. The crew member should pick up the weapon with the grips held between the fingers. Although this seems inconsistent with the policy of preserving fingerprints, it is the safe way to handle a handgun. Recognizable fingerprints cannot usually be recovered from checked grips. The crew member should not attempt to clear or unload the weapon. The number of live and expended rounds in a revolver, their position in the cylinder, and the status of the round under the hammer all may be important to investigators. When carrying the weapon, the person should keep the barrel pointed in a safe direction, preferably skyward.

EVIDENCE PRESERVATION[13]

Many investigations have been seriously hindered because emergency service personnel inadvertently disturbed or destroyed articles of evidence at the scene of a crime. Investigators look at everything, and even something that seems of little importance may be a valuable piece of evidence to law enforcement personnel.[13]

CRIME SCENE EVIDENCE

The transport team must keep unauthorized persons from the crime scene and not touch, kick, or otherwise move anything unless necessary during the rescue or during efforts to care for victims. Mental notes of possible clues, such as the position of a weapon, overturned furniture, or pooled blood, are helpful. As soon as rescue or emergency care activities are complete, observations can be shared with the investigating officers.

VEHICLE CRASH SCENE EVIDENCE

Among the items of significance to accident investigators are tire marks, runoff from radiators and crankcases, blood, broken glass, vehicle trim, motor parts, and even clods of dirt turned up by a vehicle's wheels. To assist police investigators at the scene of a vehicle accident, the transport team should first rope off the crash site so physical evidence can be preserved in place and then keep spectators from picking up or moving pieces of debris.

LAW ENFORCEMENT OFFICER

If responding to assist a wounded or injured officer, the transport team should report to the senior officer. No one should approach the wounded or injured officer until the officer–in-charge indicates it is safe to do so. If assessment and initial care efforts are unsafe to carry out on the spot, the officer should be moved to a safe place in such a manner that injuries are not compounded.

SUMMARY

Although the transport team may not be directly involved in extrication or rescue activities, crew members should be prepared to help the rescue effort and not endanger themselves so that they are unable to help the injured after they are rescued. Scene management of various incidences should be a component of all transport teams.

Air and ground transport teams can offer additional medical care and rapid transport to those injured in all types of incidents. Only transport teams that have had appropriate training, carry the correct equipment, and have experience performing rescues should be the rescuers. Without the proper equipment and training, the rescue crew may find themselves in need of rescue.

REFERENCES

1. Antosia RE, Partridge RA, Virk AS: Air bag safety, *Ann Emerg Med* 25(6):794-798, 1995.
2. Cooper DC, LaValla PH, Stoffel RC: Search and rescue. In Auerbach P, editor: *Wilderness medicine*, ed 5, Philadelphia, 2007, Mosby.
3. Grissom C, Thomas F, James B: Medical helicopters in wilderness search and rescue operations, *Air Med J* 25(1):18-25, 2006.
4. Hudson SE, McCurley LH: Caving and cave rescue. In Auerbach P, editor: *Wilderness medicine*, ed 5, Philadelphia, 2007, Mosby.
5. Karmy-Jones R, Kissinger D, Golocovsky M, et al: Bomb-related injuries, *Mil Med* 159(7):536-539, 1994.
6. Kramer A, Evans J: Ambulance operations and special response situations. In Holleran RS, editor: *Prehospital nursing: a collaborative approach*, St Louis, 1994, Mosby.
7. Martinette CV: *Trench rescue awareness, operations, technician*, Boston, 2008, Jones & Bartlett.
8. Moore RE: *Vehicle rescue and extrication*, St Louis, 2006, Mosby Jems.
9. Mellor SG: The relationship of blast loading to death and injury from explosion, *World J Surg* 16(5):893-898, 1992.
10. National Highway Transportation and Safety Administration: *Emergency rescue guidelines for air bag equipped vehicles*, available at http://www.nhtsa.dot.gov, accessed June 2008.
11. Occupational Safety and Health Administration: *Hazardous materials, standard number 1910.120*, available at http://www.osha.gov, accessed June 2008.
12. Sanders MJ: *Mosby's paramedic textbook*, ed 3, St Louis, 2007, Mosby.
13. Sharma BR: Clinical forensic medicine-management of crime victims from trauma to trial, *J Clin Forensic Med* 10: 267-273, 2003.
14. Welles WL, Wilburn RE, Ehrlich JK, et al: New York hazardous substance emergency events surveillance: learning from hazardous substances releases to improve safety, *J Hazardous Materials* 115:39-49, 2004.

DISASTER MANAGEMENT

Catherine Janson Hesse

COMPETENCIES

1. Define a disaster and what constitutes disaster planning and disaster management.
2. Describe natural and manmade disasters and potential medical crew integration with each.
3. Describe the organizational differences between a hospital-based disaster and the Hospital Incident Command System and a local/regional disaster and the Incident Command System/Unified Command.
4. Describe the lessons learned in recent disaster events and potential resources critical care transport teams might provide during the immediate, intermediate, extended, and demobilization/system recovery stages of a large scale disaster.

*D*isasters are events or processes that typify chaos and cause widespread destruction and distress to the population and communities who are affected. These events or processes may be natural, such as an earthquake, hurricane, or flood; or manmade, such as acts of terrorism or failure of bridges, buildings, or power plants, particularly nuclear.

A disaster is usually broken down into discrete and separate stages: immediate, intermediate, extended, and demobilization/system recovery. These stages provide a simple structure for the initial incident, as it gets underway, continues in intensity, and finally dissipates.

Disaster management, including planning, preparation, training, and actual response, is a complex task that necessitates a shift in the paradigm of using "the greatest number of resources for the greatest good of each individual patient to the allocation of limited resources for the greatest good of the greatest number of casualties."[1]

TABLE 7-1	**Phases of Disaster Management**
Phase	**Description**
Mitigation	Various efforts to prevent or reduce the effects of a disaster when they occur (e.g., building levies in a flood plain). Personal mitigation involves an assessment of personal and family risks related to a disaster (e.g., building a house on stilts when living near a flood plain).
Preparedness	Development of a plan of action when a disaster strikes (e.g., a communication system, mutual response, stockpiling equipment). These actions are the same on a personal level as well.
Response	Mobilization of appropriate personnel equipment, including search and rescue.
Recovery	Recovery involves efforts to return the affected area and individuals to their previous states. Recovery begins when the immediate threat to life has subsided. It may also include relocation to another place (e.g., moving away from the flood plain).

Adapted from Irving RACES/ARES Organization: *Emergency management,* available at http://www.irvinggraces.org/Emergency_Preparedness, accessed June 2008.

Disaster management has also been described in four phases: mitigation, preparedness, response, and recovery. These phases encompass both professional and personal activities. The phases are summarized in Table 7-1.

The variety of disasters and casualties typically overwhelms hospitals and local/regional healthcare systems, making it absolutely necessary for hospitals and emergency systems to plan, drill, and provide personnel, supplies, and systems to control and care for almost any eventuality. A critical resource, the transport team, should be part of this algorithm, not only to provide air or ground medical transport, but also to initial rescue and triage, short-term and long-term medical stabilization, and possibly long-term support of any department or agency that needs assistance. This finite resource should be available to both hospitals and regional disaster systems and be well known to both as a potential source of assistance. Air and ground medical resources should be readily available via an established network of communication channels, including use of a trigger mechanism for notification and activation.

Disasters continue to affect greater numbers of the population. In 2003, 255 million people were affected by disasters, a 180% increase from 1990.[5] This number is expected to increase from the combination of population growth, poverty, and environmental degradation. Terrorism is also expected to add to these numbers. History has shown that war is periodic; however, terrorism continues to be a visible and effective mechanism for various groups to gain attention and destabilize governments and countries. Whether it is natural or manmade, any disaster has the potential for overlap failures as a result of disruptions in power, loss of critical infrastructure, or the release of chemicals or bacteria into the environment from leaks or explosions.

All resources in a disaster situation should be examined, studied for potential use, and integrated into a tested and workable algorithm. A mechanism for activation of these resources should be created and used when necessary. Therefore, integration of the air or ground medical crew into the disaster management algorithm of hospitals and communities is essential as part of the preplan and ongoing work to control and contain disaster incidents.

TYPES OF DISASTERS

NATURAL DISASTER

Natural disasters are catastrophic events that occur worldwide. They cause both physical and property damage and overlap disruption of the communication, transportation, and healthcare infrastructure on which humans have come to rely. Disasters often occur when climate hazards and population vulnerability converge, such as coastal dwellers subject to tsunami. During the last 20 years, natural disasters have caused the deaths of more than 3 million people and the destruction of more than $50 billion in property damage.[5] In addition, higher concentrations of the population have relocated near risk zones (floodplains, coasts, earthquake faults), exposing them to both the hazard and the resulting overlap infrastructure failure.

Natural disasters are atmospheric, hydrologic, or geologic and may be classified into five types: earthquake, hurricane, tornado, flood, and fire. Almost every state in the United States can expect one or more of these potential hazards at some time in the future. Health impacts of these natural disasters may include: moderate to severe injury, poor nutritional status, respiratory and gastrointestinal (GI) disease from exposure and overcrowding, impacts to mental health that may be permanent, and water-borne illness from the release of chemicals and sewage into drinking water supplies and waterways.[9] All have the potential for death, irreversible mental or physical injury, disruption of critical services, and slow recovery back to the predisaster state. In addition, drought, extreme temperature, windstorm, avalanche, and landslide are less frequent but still lethal natural disasters that occur worldwide. The critical stage in a disaster is the immediate phase; the ability of an institution or community to adequately respond with appropriate resources. For example, drought may have long-term effects for decades and cause crop damage, land deforestation and destruction, and the inability to provide food and water for a significant part of the population. However, the onset and duration of a drought are far more insidious than the immediate destruction caused by a tornado. Drought and tornados both cause injury and property damage, yet the initial severity and long-term consequences may differ. Both pose unique challenges to the community and to the responders charged with disaster management.

The transport team has the potential to provide assistance in a natural disaster; however, early response during a severe storm or fire may be impractical because of poor flying or driving conditions. In addition, social unrest after disaster has the potential for unsafe conditions, whether in the air or on the ground. Rioting, looting, and gunfire that

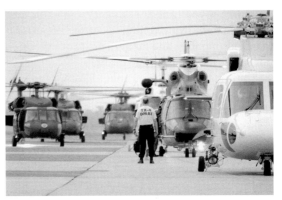

FIGURE 7-1 **Helicopter flight line, Hurricane Katrina.**

occurred during Hurricane Katrina exposed rescue workers to additional harm (Figure 7-1). Both air medical and National Guard helicopters were fired on during early rescue efforts, compromising crew and victim safety and causing some to suspend operations all together.[7] The abrupt termination of relief efforts added additional strain to an already tenuous situation, with the removal of assets when they were most needed by the population.

DISEASE-RELATED DISASTER (EITHER NATURAL OR MANMADE)

Communicable disease is often catastrophic and accounts for the deaths of millions of people annually. The Centers for Disease Control estimate that in the last 100 years, four pandemics alone have occurred: in 1889, 1918, 1957, and 1968, with the last 3 years virus-containing gene segments closely related to avian influenza.[3] Disease may be further classified into *naturally occurring* outbreaks, such as measles, mumps, and meningococcal disease; *emerging* diseases, such as severe acute respiratory syndrome (SARS) and avian flu; and *bioterrorism*.[3] The circumstances of infection may vary to include type of disease, scale of exposure, transmission method (droplet or contact), and whether the spread is intentional. Identification, response, containment, and prevention of further spread of any disease is critical, especially if it creates a disaster-like scenario with large numbers of victims. The recommendation for any rescue personnel is to identify endemic and epidemic diseases common to the area and review the living conditions of the population to include numbers and the availability of safe water, sanitation, food, shelter, and healthcare.

The Department of Public Health and the Centers for Disease Control have the duty to educate healthcare providers on disease recognition and early reporting to public health agencies, especially if large numbers of victims with similar symptoms are seen in emergency departments. In addition, containment and quarantine with mass prophylaxis may be necessary to keep the exposure controlled. This situation may present in either a healthcare facility or a community-wide outbreak. Separate Infectious Disease Emergency Response plans and teams are available to either contain the outbreak or be integrated into established systems to provide expert help and guidance.[3]

Critical care transport teams are an excellent resource during a widespread epidemic. Before any response or contact with patients, the crew must confirm that decontamination and isolation of the patient has occurred to protect the transport team from spread of infection. Furthermore, personal protective equipment (PPE) should be manageable and appropriate for the crew. For example, a self-contained breathing apparatus (SCBA) plus gear is not practical or safe in an aircraft; therefore, patients who need this form of isolation should not be flown. Ideally, respiratory or contact isolation is the most manageable form of PPE for a flight or ground crew and should not interfere with patient, crew, or pilot safety and the ability to work in a small enclosed space, such as a helicopter or ambulance.

Transport programs should create and follow decontamination policies and procedures that support crew, pilot, and patient safety. A predeparture discussion that is oriented to potential unusual situations should be focused on safety. In addition, a general consensus made by transport team members and the pilot or driver of whether to take a request with unusual circumstances should be part of the predeparture discussion and supported by the crew and their administration. Any identified issues made by a team member should not be discounted, even if the opinion is a minority one.

MANMADE DISASTER

Manmade disasters have similar potential for injury, especially if terrorism is the root cause of the disaster. Engineered intentional chaos and destruction is often successful, especially if the weapon is designed to maim or cause widespread panic or is placed in an area of high population density.

Manmade disasters may be classified as *biologic* (anthrax, plague); *chemical, blood, and nerve agent–related* (blister agents, cyanide, and sarin), or *nuclear*.[5] Biologic agents are further classified by the Centers for Disease Control into three categories on the basis of virulence and ability to spread from person to person. *Category A* agents are of highest concern; they pose risks to national security and safety because of high mortality rates and ease of dissemination. Anthrax, plague, and botulism are among Category A agents. *Category B* agents are moderately easy to disseminate, are less lethal, and tend to tie up healthcare resources in efforts to identify and treat the disease. Brucellosis and ricin are classified as Category B agents. *Category C* agents are emerging pathogens that are easily available and have the potential for high mortality rates and major health impacts; hantavirus and lethal influenzas are examples of Category C agents.[5]

Chemical, blood, and nerve agents are difficult to acquire, are often military in origin, and should indicate to first responders and air or ground medical crews that a terrorist-related event has occurred. Hazardous materials (HAZMAT) incidents are not considered intentional unless the method of delivery or exposure is engineered. First responders should be aware that incidents such as these have issues with scene safety and crowd control. Concise information regarding the agent used should be released to the first responders and air or ground crews by the Incident Commander on scene. Preparation that includes drugs and equipment needed should be made on the basis of the agent, the symptoms, and the number of victims at the scene.

Finally, nuclear disasters may be intentional, such as the deliberate use of nuclear or hospital waste materials in a bomb, or unintentional, such as a reactor incident. Both types of nuclear incidents cause complex injuries that may present immediately or have delayed symptoms and onset. *Acute radiation syndrome* (ARS) is the technical term for an acute illness that often takes hours to weeks to run its course. Survivability is determined by the victim's exposure in rads; any exposure of less than 100 rads is survivable, doses of more than 200 rads are possibly survivable, and doses of more than 800 rads are improbable.[5] Immediate consideration for the first responder or air or ground medical crew is critical if contamination has occurred. Clothing or radioactive material should be removed immediately as it poses some risk to rescue personnel. However, an irradiated victim who has been decontaminated poses no risk to first responders, so the initiation of airway, breathing, and circulation (ABC) measures should be done without delay.[5]

The challenge for the first responder is always to decipher whether the incident is accidental or intentional and, if a disease agent is used, whether the outbreak is natural or intentional in nature. For example, a large salmonella outbreak may be a simple food-borne illness from improperly cooked food at a restaurant. However, salmonella was used in the 1990s to deliberately contaminate and sicken a small community in Oregon to engineer the outcome of an election.[5] At the other end of the disease spectrum, a smallpox outbreak should be a red flag to first responders; it would signify a deliberate act of terrorism because the last known case occurred in 1978 and stockpiles of the virus only exist in secure laboratories worldwide.[3] First responders and air or ground transport teams should have a general working knowledge of disease and biologic, chemical, and radiologic agents to better understand the hazards and dynamics of the incident before arrival. Written charts should be created and made available to each air or ground crew member to describe the type of exposure, the symptoms, and any PPE or decontamination procedures necessary.

Other manmade disasters, either intentional or unintentional, include failures of bridges, cranes, elevated or tunneled roadways, and power plants, including nuclear accidents. The 2007 failure of the I-35 bridge in Minneapolis is an excellent example of an unintentional manmade disaster. Thirty-one people were caught during rush hour traffic on a bridge that collapsed, resulting in a high fatality rate. Air and ground transport teams were used on the scene to triage and airlift patients to local hospitals.

The air or ground transport team is an excellent resource in such incidents; however, careful attention should be paid to team and pilot or driver safety before arrival. Any exposure-related situation should not affect the rescuer; the patients involved must be decontaminated, and appropriate PPE for the air or ground environment should be issued before patient contact.

The initial confusion present at a disaster can produce additional risk for air medical crews. The convergence of multiple units and the involvement of multiple agencies can lead to communication breakdown and potential hazards. The crew should remember that the presence of multiple casualties and debris may overwhelm other responders and scene safety may be compromised.

Air medical communication centers should attempt to establish contact with the Mass Casualty Incident (MCI) command center and respond in an appropriate manner. They should *not* respond without being specifically requested.

Effective command and control of the MCI may take some time to establish. During the initial response, in particular, the air medical transport team should take extra precautions to ensure that safety is not compromised. Pilots should make certain that ground personnel select, prepare, and control the landing zone (LZ) in accordance with normal procedures. The need for thorough aerial and even ground reconnaissance should be considered to avoid conflict with disaster operations.

Air medical teams can and should offer and advise the MCI commanders about the full capabilities of their aircraft. Aircraft, especially helicopters, may be used for many roles, including: 1, transport of equipment and personnel to the MCI site; 2, transport of patients to or between hospitals; and 3, provision of aerial surveillance for the MCI coordinators.

THE HOSPITAL INCIDENT COMMAND SYSTEM

The *Hospital Emergency Incident Command System* (HEICS) was first used in the 1980s as a foundation for 6000 hospitals across the United States to prepare and respond to disasters. This system was updated in 2006 and changed to the *Hospital Incident*

Command System (HICS), which added features and updates to HEICS.[2] HICS is designed to be consistent with the Incident Command System (ICS) and National Incident Management System (NIMS) by strengthening hospital disaster preparedness in conjunction with community response agencies, with the goal that hospitals and the community must work together and use similar disaster management principles, chain of command, and communication language.[2]

The foundation of HICS includes: a predictable chain of command, accountability of position and team function, action checklists, and the use of common language in communication. This foundation was further enhanced in 2006 with the addition of job action sheets, scenario-specific planning guides, and incident response guides to assist personnel in thinking outside the box. The system attempts to provide the hospital with clear and concise instructions so that drilling and actual practice becomes second nature.

Basic roles are outlined in HICS and include the Incident Commander, whose role is always activated in an incident regardless of its nature. Other roles include the Operations Section Chief, who is responsible for tactical operations including patient care; the Planning Section Chief, who collects information and maintains resource status; the Logistics Section Chief, who provides support and resources to meet the objectives set forth by the Incident Commander; and finally, the Finance/Administration Section Chief, who reviews and monitors cost of the operation.

The HICS organizational chart is designed to expand and contract on the basis of the size of the hospital and incident (Figure 7-2). Hospitals across the United States have adopted HICS as part of their Joint Commission accreditation guidelines and have successfully integrated the updated job action sheets into their hospital emergency management programs. HICS also may be tailored to hospital size and be further modified, as needed.

Trauma Centers have been further charged by the American College of Surgeons to integrate the trauma team into the organizational HICS chart. This integration is best accomplished with a Trauma Surgeon and Trauma Program Manager or Nurse Practitioner as frontline triage officers who determine the resources needed for trauma cases. Transport teams can be tasked to perform rapid triage and assist in identifying trauma victims who need expert immediate care. Integration of individuals and specialties into the organizational chart, such as the air or ground medical crew, supports a well-developed hospital disaster management plan that uses resources efficiently.

INCIDENT COMMAND SYSTEM/UNIFIED COMMAND

The *Incident Command System* (ICS) and the *Unified Command* (UC) are the primary on-scene incident management concepts used in the field to allow responders to adopt an integrated organizational structure flexible enough and equal to the demand of any single incident without jurisdictional boundaries. The primary goal of the ICS/UC is commanding, controlling, and coordinating the efforts of different agencies to protect life, property, and the environment.

This plan was developed in the 1970s as a result of problems identified during wild land fires in Southern California. The original name was Firefighting Resources of California Organized for Potential Emergencies (FIRESCOPE).[2] At the time, unclear lines of authority and nonstandard terminology were used between agencies. A lack of consolidated action plans made on-scene organizational work difficult. The ICS was designed to streamline the organizational chart; establish immediate priorities, specifically the safety of the responders; stabilize the incident; determine incident objectives; and monitor the organization of the responders.[2] This design allowed for multiple agencies, all responding together, to work cohesively, communicate effectively, and manage the mission. The major advantages of the ICS system are prevention of chaos and individuality, injury, further damage, and unnecessary prolongation of the incident.

The UC brings together the incident commanders from all major organizations to coordinate an effective response and at the same time allow the incident commanders to continue to manage their own jurisdictional responsibilities. The UC links all organizations

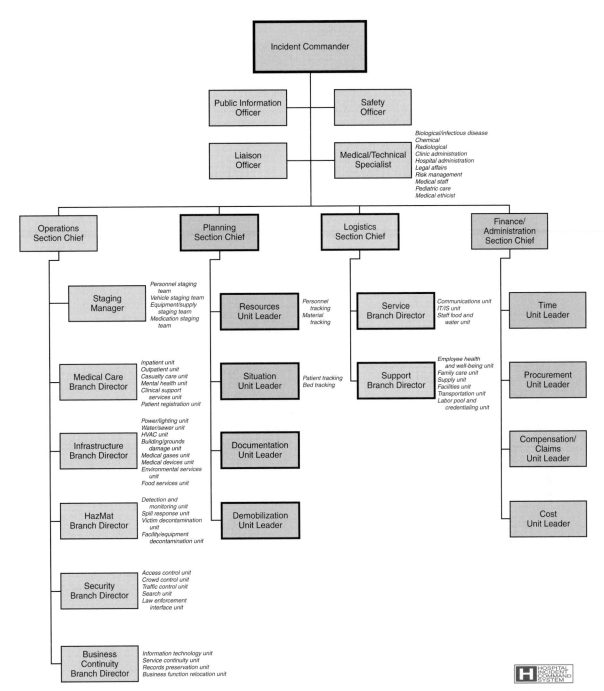

FIGURE 7-2 **HEICS framework.** (Available from www.hallrender.com/library/newsletters/135/241743PHLso06.pdf Accessed June 2008.)

that respond to a disaster for the purpose of creating an integrated response team that then shares common incident objectives and priorities.

The UC is responsible for overall management of the incident. The UC is determined on a case-by-case basis and may change during the course of the incident to account for changes in the situation. To be effective, the UC organizational efforts should limit group members. In addition, each member of the UC must agree on common incident objectives and priorities and be able to sustain a 24/7 commitment to the incident until the incident is cleared. Finally, the UC must have the authority to spend funds or acquire resources as needed to manage the incident and support responders and the injured.

The following list outlines the steps in implementing the ICS/UC in a disaster event:

- Incident occurs.
- Local fire departments, police, volunteers, and bystanders respond.
- Local responders (fire and ambulance) immediately organize into the incident command structure, with the senior first responder on scene (such as first arriving lieutenant on the engine) assuming the incident commander role.
- As more senior personnel arrive or the agency with the primary responsibility arrives, the incident commander turns over the command to these new personnel, giving a full briefing and notifying *all* staff of the change in command.
- If the incident becomes multijurisdictional, the responders integrate into the ICS structure and establish the UC to direct the expanded organization.

This structure exists until the incident is cleared. Postdisaster personnel in a large incident are involved in cleanup, morgue detail, and infrastructure evaluation and repair to return the community to the predisaster state.

TRIAGE

Triage is designed to provide the greatest good for the greatest number of patients. The key to effective triage is optimal utilization of available resources

to treat the majority of patients at hand. During a disaster, resources must be allocated to benefit the most patients. Triage, therefore, must be rapid, with the determination of severity and the need for care decided on quickly.

Several different triage methods are available for the first responder to review and use depending on hospital or community preference.

- START: Simple Triage and Rapid Treatment. Simple algorithm and flow chart used in the prehospital setting, characterized by rapid decision making on the basis of the ability to walk. Expectant status is well-defined.
- Color-Coded Disaster Triage. Black: expectant. Red: emergent. Yellow: urgent. Green: not urgent. Often seen as part of disaster management "tags" used to classify and identify victims.
- MASS: Move, Assess, Sort, Send.
- ID-ME: Immediate, delayed, minimal, and expectant.[5]

Each system of triage and classification embodies the principles of quick primary assessment, with rapid determination of potential for survival, need for intervention, and likelihood of death. The triage method chosen by first responders or air medical crews must be frequently drilled and should provide the ideal basis for decision making under stress and in difficult circumstances.

SECONDARY TRIAGE
One of the problems faced by air medical transport teams during disaster response and even routine MCI situations is the presentation of multiple red-tagged or immediate priority cases. Existing triage system in use in the prehospital environment is designed for rapid initial sorting. The START system, for example, has seen an accuracy rate of only 78% in recent exercises.[2,7] Many systems also do not have a demonstrated ability to predict survival outcomes. When air medical resources are limited, priority must be given to the patients with the best chance of survival.

One method to assure that the most appropriate patients are transported via air is for the team to perform a brief secondary triage of the patients presented for transport. The team examines the patients presented as red tags/immediates and performs a quick primary assessment. If the number of immediates is large, only the patients who are considered by the triage officer for immediate loading are reassessed. The injuries, vital signs, and care levels available are assessed to determine whether these cases are the highest priority. If an immediate intervention (i.e., airway maneuver) stabilizes the patient's condition, the patient is then at a lower priority for transport. If the injuries are likely terminal or the resources needed for stabilization are unavailable at the receiving center, the patient is also left for later transport. These additional primary assessments should result in the transporting first of patients with immediate care needs and viable outcomes, thereby optimizing the resources available in the best possible manner.

AIR/GROUND TRANSPORT TEAM STRUCTURE

Transport teams are generally set up as hospital-based or freestanding programs. Both types of programs have the ability to integrate into a hospital or community.

Traditional *hospital-based programs* are usually affiliated with large teaching facilities and have the advantage of immediate access to hospital resources, equipment, and blood. Transport teams in this situation typically are a part of the hospital disaster algorithm and may have their own place in the HICS organizational chart. The challenge for the hospital-based transport program is transitioning into the ICS system, drilling with fire, police, and ambulance providers. Ideally, collaboration should be part of the community preplan and be tasked to drill as often as the community organizes these events. Key components of this type of disaster management algorithm should be access to the hospital transport program via a trigger mechanism in a central dispatch, role in the ICS structure, and familiarity of the crew to different scales of events and the reporting structure and roles of each.

Freestanding programs typically have the advantage of alignment with the community in which they provide air or ground medical support. Usually, these programs have direct links to a central dispatch and are part of the ICS structure as a rule. These freestanding programs most likely plan and drill with community police, fire, and ambulance personnel regularly and are familiar with the ICS/UC structure.

The freestanding program challenge is to integrate into a hospital disaster situation and HICS. A likely scenario is back-to-back transports into a facility during an incident. The team may assume the responsibility of staying with the patient and assisting the physician or nursing staff with stabilization if the incident is straining emergency department resources. Another scenario is a major incident near a small community hospital with the next closest hospital hundreds of miles away. In this situation, the air or ground medical crew might be dispatched to the facility and be integrated into HICS as frontline triage personnel. They then provide this care until the incident is cleared or all patients are deemed stable or transferred out. The hospital administration needs to recognize the freestanding program as an untapped resource and be willing to integrate the team in the HICS structure on the basis of the skill set of the crew.

Both types of air or ground medical programs should be recognized as a resource and be used by both the hospital and the community during a disaster. Transport teams are highly trained and adaptable to the needs of the community.

RECENT DISASTERS AND LESSONS LEARNED

SEPTEMBER 11, 2001

The loss of the World Trade Center (WTC) on September 11, 2001, became a pivotal incident in US history. Modern travel, public gatherings, concerts, and crowds will never have the pre-9/11 freedom and ease that was once known. Today, inspection, search, and seizure are the norm. The American public has adapted uncharacteristically well to the shift in what was previously known and held as personal freedom. Terrorism on US soil was thought to be impossible, especially an incident of this size. The loss of life, especially to first responders, continues to be an American tragedy.

The actual collapse of the WTC caused a chain reaction of devastation. Five adjacent buildings either collapsed immediately or were so badly damaged that they were demolished soon after 9/11. Fifty-six other structures also suffered damage, mainly from falling debris and the tornado force winds created by the mass of the falling WTC. Seismographs registered earthquakes of 2.1 and 2.3 at 21 miles away.[8] The zone of destruction, the casualties, and the sheer amount of smoke and debris were immense.

The events and destruction continue to be analyzed. Planning for an event of this magnitude was never anticipated, and communities still grapple with the potential that events of this size may occur again.

Primary lessons learned are also of consideration. First responders encountered an extremely hazardous building, of immense size, with an aviation-fueled fire burning above them. The urgency to rescue potentially thousands of trapped WTC employees was paramount. Communication was disjointed. WTC employees were seen and heard falling from various levels of the buildings, sometimes injuring the rescuers below. The relatively short time between jetliner impact and total destruction was less than 2 hours, which was not enough time for first responders to assess, communicate, gather resources, and execute a rescue plan for almost 3000 people. For days after the collapse, rescuers, volunteers, and fire personnel arrived and began to dig, without PPE. Firefighters, police officers, and private sector workers initially had no masks. No central organization or distribution point was created to distribute masks until the Occupational Safety and Health Administration (OSHA) was called in on September 20, a full 9 days after the WTC collapse, to evaluate the situation. PPE then was emergently issued; however, exposures to lead, mercury, dioxin, and asbestos were already at high levels from inhalation and dermal routes.[8] OSHA elected to not slow down rescue operations and issued half face masks to the large number of rescue personnel. By most accounts, these masks were either used improperly or thrown away. In contrast, workers at the Pentagon site were escorted off the premises if proper PPE was not worn.[4] By 2006, almost 8000 New York City firefighters, rescue personnel, and police officers were ill, presumably from the toxic combinations of debris that had been inhaled after 9/11.[4]

LESSONS LEARNED

First responders and air or ground medical crews should be aware of the following in a large scale disaster:

- Anything is possible, and the first responder should be aware that previously held beliefs

on disaster size and magnitude should not be generalized to current events.
- Rescue personnel should be aware that they may be at risk from secondary acts of terrorism. A high index of suspicion should always accompany a scene of this nature.
- Safety is paramount. PPE should always be worn, and its use should not interfere with the ability to work.
- The ICS system should be adopted immediately, as should the UC, if multiple jurisdictions are involved.
- Scene safety and crowd control should be handled by the jurisdiction most equipped to provide it.
- Air or ground medical crews are a critical resource; however, scene safety may dictate that helicopter arrival is impractical.

The air or ground medical crew theoretically might have been an asset to the victims of 9/11; however, the rapid destruction of the buildings and congestion of the New York City area made integration of an air medical crew into a scene of this nature improbable. In the future, any disaster or drill of this magnitude should immediately trigger the activation of local resources, including air and ground transport teams capable of deploying flexible, skilled, and highly mobile personnel.

HURRICANE KATRINA

A Category 5 storm has always been a possibility in the Gulf States. August 2005 provided a proving ground for the Federal Emergency Management Agency's (FEMA) preparation and experience.

New Orleans is inconveniently situated at about sea level and below the water line of the Mississippi River. A system of large levees protect it from flooding and storm surges. In addition, a series of pumps and waterways protect the city from yearly flooding, all dependent on working power sources and constant monitoring. A large percentage of the population is poor and without means of transportation. In August 2005, the hurricane count had already broken records for sheer numbers of storms, and when a large storm began heading towards the Gulf coast, the city of New Orleans and various agencies began to evaluate resources and mechanisms for evacuation. No one expected that the storm would break the Category 5 level, the highest level based on wind speed.

The events of the day that preceded the storm are possibly the most critical lessons learned after 9/11. Local, state, and federal officials did not anticipate the power of the storm or the resources needed to manage the extreme challenges of the area. After storm landfall, state and local officials knew that the devastation was serious but lacked the interagency communication to coordinate a response. Federal officials arrived and attempted to assume the responsibilities generally performed by state and local authorities. All of this was done without prior planning or a functioning state or local incident command structure to assist with Federal efforts, which left an ineffective federal agency, with no real-time situational awareness or communication with local officials, and numerous agencies that performed overlap functions. Bureaucratic demands consumed valuable time. As a result, many agencies took independent action, which created confusion and duplication of efforts. Evacuation of thousands of people proved impossible, and the decision was made to use the Superdome for an emergency shelter. Lack of supplies and sanitation, civil unrest, and large numbers of ill people amplified problems, which made for a disorganized and dangerous situation. The dead were left unattended and in public, for the population to see. Quickly, victims began to feel that not enough had been done to care for and protect them during one of the largest hurricanes in modern times.

The damage to New Orleans was severe and consisted of both natural and manmade overlap failures.

- Wind damage caused power line failure from fallen trees.
- Water damage caused a tidal surge into the city from Lake Ponchartrain, with 8 to 12 ft of water into several communities.
- Levees failed and caused flood waters to inundate neighborhoods without warning.
- Movement of debris damaged homes and electrical equipment.
- Transformers were damaged, and water forced cooling oil out of systems, which caused overheating.

- Salt water caused failures as a result of corrosion.
- Generators were often housed in basements or on first floors and were flooded rapidly.
- Propane-powered generators at communication tower sites could not be refueled, which caused failures.
- High traffic volume with every communication source, including telephones, the 911 system, cell phones, and voiceover Internet phones (VoIP), created failures.[10]

The lessons learned are summarized:

- Agencies should be organized, trained, and equipped to perform their response roles, without overlap.
- Awareness of the National Preparedness Goals should be hardwired.
- The Department of Defense's role should be defined, and activation should be rapid.
- A self-healing, duplicative, and redundant communication system should be available to every first responder and agency in large scale disasters.
- Logistics should be transparent and encompass supplies, transport of rescue personnel, and evacuation.
- Mass evacuations should be done prior to storm landfall, before conditions arise that prevent vehicles or aircraft from entering an area.
- The Department of Public Health should be coordinated into any disaster to provide for adequate human services, supplies, and assistance.
- Temporary and long-term housing should be coordinated between the American Red Cross and the Department of Homeland Security. Mass care and sheltering during disasters should be a primary and initial focus.
- Foreign disaster assistance should be reviewed and used. One hundred and fifty-one countries offered assistance and relief; unfortunately, the United States did not have the mechanisms in place to accept the assistance because of bureaucratic red tape.[10] Countries who are willing to assist the United States should have no barriers to deliver goods or manpower in a disaster.

- Nongovernmental and volunteer contributions should be integrated into the broader effort. Private ambulances and air or ground medical resources should be given local resource support for their involvement before national disasters of any kind.

The lessons learned did prompt FEMA to issue a request for proposals the following year to provide ground ambulance, air ambulance, and Para transit services after a nationally declared disaster. FEMA initially issued this request for the Gulf and Atlantic states and fully intends to issue requests for the rest of the United States. The contractor agreement stipulates that 100 ground ambulances and 25 air ambulances and Para transit vehicles, with a combined capability to move 3000 individuals, should be able to be deployed within 6 hours and arrive within 24 hours at a disaster site.[6]

One of the other major lessons learned by air medical crews responding to Katrina and other natural disasters is the need for personal preparedness. Crews who live in the immediate vicinity of the disaster must have plans that enable them to immediately respond without worrying about personal responsibilities. A family care plan should be implemented, including care for children during the unscheduled prolonged duty period. Pets need to be included in these care plans. Some jurisdictions have off-duty personnel check on homes and families of the duty crews before they report in for duty, which ensures all families and pets are safe.

Natural disasters also often cause crews to be on duty for extended periods. Emergency Medical Services (EMS) crews who were deployed immediately after Katrina made landfall worked nonstop for 24 to 48 hours. They were unable to return to their stations for rest or refreshment. Personal hygiene then became an issue because of lack of personal supplies and available resources.

Transport teams should consider preparing a small kit for such emergencies. A change of uniform, socks, undergarments, toiletries, food, water, and medications for at least 72 hours should be available. A list of recommended items is shown in Box 7-1. These basic preparations can help the crew maintain their own comfort when they are in continuous operation. The transport team should not plan on the disaster response organizations having food and rest stations set up immediately, so self-sufficiency is important. Key points in the preparation of any disaster or survival kit should be immediate availability

---

| BOX 7-1 | **Sample 72-Hour Pack** |

Hat with sun protection	Personal medications in original bottle (1 month supply)
1 Pair socks	1 Sewing kit
1 Pair underwear	1 Towel
1 T-shirt	1 Washcloth
1 Pair gloves, leather	1 Insect repellent
1 Set rain gear	1 Pair of sunglasses
1 Flashlight/headlamp	1 Set spare of glasses/contacts, contact supplies
1 Leatherman/Gerber	1 Sunscreen (minimum SPF 15)
1 Lighter or waterproof matches	1 Watch
1 Writing set, including notepad, pen/pencil	1 Stethoscope
1 Identification set: drivers license, passport, money, credit cards	1 Bandage/utility scissors
	1 Roll of toilet paper
1 Toiletry kit: sanitary napkins, shaving gear, nail clippers, shampoo, soap, toothbrush and toothpaste, foot powder, hair comb or brush	3 Days worth of personal food
	1 Mess kit, eating utensils
	1 Quart of water
	1 Bottle of water purification tablets/water filter
	1 Personal first aid kit

(Adapted from AK 1 DMAT Team.)

to the owner, reliable contents that are checked frequently, and easy access before deployment, during a flight, or after a crash. Any survival pack that is large, bulky, heavy, or otherwise difficult to access immediately is worthless, and efforts should be made to carry less and possibly keep in a small attached pack, in a flight suit leg pocket or uniform pocket.

SUMMARY

Air and ground medical crews are a critical resource in a disaster situation. They should be involved in hospital and community disaster planning and management efforts. Roles should be assigned to crews to take advantage of their expanded nurse, paramedic, or specialty training and transport abilities. At any level of response, whether federal, state, or local, air and ground critical care teams are a valuable resource of highly trained, mobile, and flexible healthcare providers.

REFERENCES

1. American College of Surgeons: Statement on disaster and mass casualty management, *Bull Am Coll Surg* 88(8): 2003.
2. California Emergency Medical Services Authority: *Hospital incident command guidebook,* Sacramento, CA, 2006, California Emergency Services Authority.
3. Chin J: *Control of communicable diseases,* ed 17, Washington, DC, 2000, American Public Health Association.
4. DePalma A: *Air masks at issue in claims of 9/11 illnesses,* available at http://www.nytimes.com/2006/06/05/nyregion/05masks.html, accessed February 2008.
5. Emergency Nurses Association: *Trauma nursing core course,* ed 6, Des Plaines, IL, 2007, Emergency Nurses Association.
6. Garza M: *Government solicits national ambulance provider for disaster response,* available at http://www.jems.com/newsandarticles/articles/GovernmentSolicitsNationalAmbulance, accessed February 2008.
7. US Department of Homeland Security: *Hurricane Katrina: EmergencyNet News Real-Time reports analysis by the Emergency Response and Research Institute,* available at http://www.emergency.com/2005/katrina2005.htm, accessed April 2008.
8. Varchaver N: The tombstone at ground zero, *Fortune* 157(6): 2008.
9. Watson JT, Gayer M: *Epidemics after natural disasters,* available at www.cdc.gov/ncidod/EID/13/1/1.htm, accessed February 2008.

10. The White House: *Chapter five: lessons learned,* available at http://www.whitehouse.gov/reports/katrina-lessons-learned/chapter5.html, accessed February 2008.

BIBLIOGRAPHY

American College of Surgeons: *Resources for optimal care of the injured patient 2006,* Chicago, 2006, American College of Surgeons.

American College of Surgeons: Statement on disaster and mass casualty management, *Bull Am Coll Surg* 88(8): 2003.

California Emergency Medical Services Authority: *Hospital incident command guidebook,* Sacramento, CA, 2006, California Emergency Services Authority.

Chin J: *Control of communicable diseases,* ed 17, Washington, DC, 2000, American Public Health Association.

DePalma A: *Air masks at issue in claims of 9/11 illnesses,* available at http://www.nytimes.com/2006/06/05/nyregion/05masks.html, accessed February 2008.

Emergency Nurses Association: *Trauma nursing core course,* ed 6, Des Plaines, IL, 2007, Emergency Nurses Association.

Garza M: *Government solicits national ambulance provider for disaster response,* available at http://www.jems.com/news_and_articles/articles/Government_Solicits_National_Ambulance, accessed February 2008.

Holleran RS, ASTNA: *Air and surface patient transport: principles and practice,* ed 3, St Louis, 2002, Elsevier Health Sciences.

The White House: *Chapter five: lessons learned,* available at http://www.whitehouse.gov/reports/katrina-lessons-learned/chapter5.html, accessed February 2008.

US Department of Homeland Security: *Hurricane Katrina: EmergencyNet News Real-Time reports analysis by the Emergency Response and Research Institute,* available at http://www.emergency.com/2005/katrina2005.htm, accessed April 2008.

US Department of Labor, Occupational Safety and Health Administration: *What is an Incident Command System/Unified Command System,* available at http://www.osha.gov/LTC/etools/ics, accessed February 2008.

US Department of Labor, Occupational Safety and Health Administration: *How do responders prepare for ICS/UC implementation? Incident Command System,* available at http://www.osha.gov/SLTC/etools/ics, accessed February 2008.

Varchaver N: The tombstone at ground zero, *Fortune* 157(6): 2008.

Watson JT, Gayer M: *Epidemics after natural disasters,* available at www.cdc.gov/ncidod/EID/13/1/1.htm, accessed February 2008.

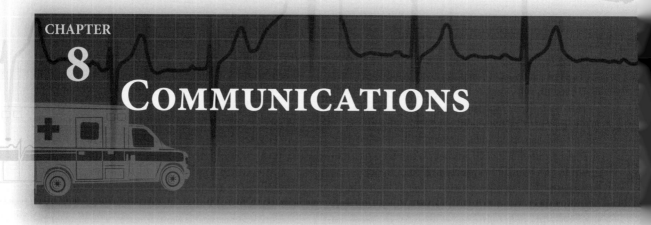

Reneé Semonin Holleran

COMPETENCIES

1. Demonstrate knowledge about communications systems and their use in patient transport.
2. Apply appropriate communication skills before, during, and after transport.
3. Demonstrate the use of appropriate communication equipment to provide safe and competent patient transport.

Communication encompasses more than the use of a radio or telephone; it is a total system that ensures the smooth operation of routine daily patient transports while guaranteeing optimal patient care and transport team safety (Figure 8-1). No one perfect communications system exists for all transport programs. The communications system must meet the present and future needs of the program it serves.

All transport team members must have good communication skills and know how to operate any equipment they may use for communication.[5] Communication equipment is influenced by the geographic location of the program and the education and training of those who use the equipment.

All communication needs to be HIPAA (Health Insurance Portability and Accountability Act of 1996) compliant. Team members must remember that radio and verbal communications can be easily overheard and cause a breach of patient confidentiality.[1,5]

COMMUNICATION CENTERS

Communication centers are an integral part of all transport programs. Multiple models are currently used for transport programs and include a dedicated center that is a part of a transport program; local emergency medical services (EMS) or fire dispatch centers that may coordinate transports and communication; security personnel or unit personnel at hospital-based programs that may provide communication services; and

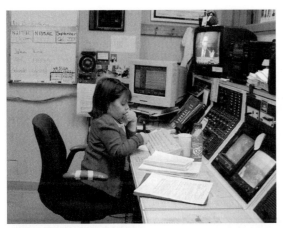

FIGURE 8-1 Communications Center, University Air Care, Cincinnati. (Courtesy Rose DeJarnette and John Robinson.)

the transport service that may have a centralized dispatch center, which may actually be in a different state than the program. The Commission on Accreditation of Medical Transport Systems Standards dictates that a communication specialist must be assigned to receive and coordinate all requests for the medical transport service.[2] The Federal Aviation Regulation (FAR) 135.79 requires that the Part 135 certificate holder must have procedures established for locating each flight for which a Federal Aviation Administration (FAA) flight plan is not filed.[3]

THE COMMUNICATIONS SPECIALIST

The complexities of organization of a communications system are unique with respect to its operation. Beyond dealing with electronic hardware and computer software, the program is faced with one of the most challenging of tasks: dealing with people.

Humans are both the strongest and the weakest points in a system. People represent a broad spectrum of personalities and opinions, and no two individuals are quite the same. A communications center, communications specialist, and communication skills are mandatory to ensure a safe transport operation.

ROLES AND RESPONSIBILITIES

The *communications specialist* (CS) is designated to coordinate requests for aircraft and ground responses.

The title assigned to the person with the CS function varies from program to program. The only limitation is that the FAA uses the term *dispatcher* to designate a person who has the decision-making role of whether or not an aircraft takes off. Unless this is the case with a program, another title should be used.

The CS is responsible for coordinating intraagency and interagency communications that pertain to any phase of a transport, from a request to hospital admission. The role of the CS is to serve as a facilitator for the smooth integration of all the resources at the program's disposal, with the dual objectives of program safety and excellent patient care.

The CS must perform a variety of tasks. These include the following[7]:

- Listening intently.
- Asking appropriate questions.
- Accurately confirming what was said.
- Reading maps (including using computer mapping software).
- Using spelling and professional grammar skills.
- Using medical, aviation, and EMS terms.
- Setting, evaluating, and resetting priorities.
- Providing customer service and good public relations.

SELECTION

Applicants for CS positions should be screened as thoroughly as applicants for transport team positions. Just as all persons who desire to be part of a transport team are not suited for the work, all persons who desire to be a CS may not be suited to the type of stress inherent in the job.[8,10]

The decision about whom to hire as a CS must be determined by each individual program. Certain minimal educational requirements must be met in any case, but some controversy has arisen about background requirements. Areas of controversy include the following:

1. Should the CS have medical field experience? If so, at what level and how much?
2. Should the CS have communications center experience? If so, what type of experience is acceptable, and how much experience is necessary?

Neither medical field experience nor communications center experience alone qualifies a person to be a CS; neither does being a friend or relative of someone employed by the program.

The Commission on Accreditation of Medical Transport Systems (CAMTS) recommends that certifications, such as emergency medical technician (EMT), emergency medical dispatcher (EMD), and National Association of Air Medical Communication Specialists (NAACS) Certified Flight Communications Course, be encouraged and actually required by some transport programs.[2]

TRAINING

Regardless of the background of the CS applicant, the person must be trained as a communications specialist. The CAMTS standards that address communications state that the training of the designated communications specialist be commensurate with the scope and responsibility of the Communications Center personnel. Box 8-1 contains a summary of the initial training.

The NAACS has developed a specific course to train and educate the CS. The components of this course are summarized in Box 8-2.

Training must be an ongoing process to ensure currency and proficiency. During training, the CS should be given a variety of situations, be allowed

---

BOX 8-2   Summary of the NAACS Training Course

Postaccident incident plan (PAIP)
Flight following
Radio communications skills
Aviation weather
Aircraft emergencies
Medical terminology
Navigation and map usage
Customer service/public relations
Air medical crew resource management
Stress management
FAA

---

to make decisions, and discuss why decisions were made. Just as many transport teams use their "worst transports" to teach others, the "worst communication situations" presented and discussed with new CSs may assist them in future work.

TESTING

The CS should undergo periodic testing on all elements of the position. The CS has the responsibility to know everything about the program and be able to use that information at a moment's notice with a high degree of accuracy. In terms of communications

---

BOX 8-1   Summary of CAMTS Initial Training of Communication Specialists

1. Medical terminology and how to obtain patient information.
2. Knowledge of emergency medical system, including roles and responsibilities of various levels of training.
3. State and local regulations that govern the EMS systems in which the transport service operates.
4. Familiarization with equipment used in the prehospital environment.
5. Knowledge of Federal Aviation regulations and Federal Communications Commission regulations pertinent to medical transport services.
6. General safety rules and emergency procedures pertinent to medical transportation and flight following procedures.
7. Navigation techniques/terminology and flight following and map skills.
8. Weather interpretation.
9. Radio frequencies used in medical and ground EMS.
10. Assistance with hazardous material response.
11. Stress recognition and management.
12. Customer services.
13. Quality management.
14. Air medical crew resource management.
15. Computer literacy and software training.
16. Postaccident incident plan (PAIP).

procedures, the goal is 100% accuracy. For example, many programs periodically practice downed aircraft or communication loss exercises.

DRESS CODE

Proper attire for communications personnel is a matter of preference for each program. Wearing of a uniform provides an appropriate display to the public and ensures that the CS is viewed as a part of the transport team.

COMMUNICATIONS OPERATIONS

OPERATIONAL CONTROL

Operational control (OC) requires that the certificate holder be responsible for all aspects of flight operations. The FAA recognized the challenge of maintaining Part135 operational control with different companies joined together to provide separate services. The responsibility and authority of operational control should never be in question, and the FAA provided guidance with order 8900.4. Flight operations consist of crew member training, currency and certification, aircraft maintenance and airworthiness, "weather minimums, proper aircraft loading, center of gravity limitations, icing conditions, and fuel requirements," and flight locating requirements.[11]

ROLES AND RESPONSIBILITIES

The FAA has compartmentalized operational control duties into two tiers. The OC responsibilities for *tier I* consist of "assignment of crew and release of aircraft to revenue service."[3] Tier I also requires management to verify and maintain the level of quality of employees. *Tier II* represents the daily operations or how a specific flight is conducted. Generally, these duties are performed at a management level, but they may be delegated without removing responsibility from the certificate holder.

COMMUNICATION ENVIRONMENT

A major aspect of any communications program is the physical environment of the communications center.[6] Following are some major considerations in the planning process for a communications center.

LOCATION

Whether located in a hospital, at an airfield, or within a separate facility, the communications center should be in an area with little pedestrian traffic. Physical inaccessibility and program policy discourage casual visitors. A system should be in place to ensure that the communication specialist is not disturbed while involved with a medical mission. A signal device or even locking the door during dispatch may assist.

SEISMIC STABILITY

In some areas of the United States and the world, the structural and functional integrity of the facility in the face of a major seismic disturbance is a very real concern and should be discussed with the facility's architect. That seismic stability is part of the design of the facility should not be taken for granted.

SECURITY

The level of security needed for a given communications center varies considerably, depending on its location. A steel door with a deadbolt lock should be considered the minimal level of security. Numerous high-technology security systems may be acquired; the level of security attained ultimately is a function of the budget.

Security does not end with a locked door. Additional security issues are fire alarm and fire suppression systems. Although the communications center may meet current local fire codes, one must remember that most fire codes are minimal, not maximal, requirements for protection. Stricter safeguards than those required by the code are permissible. For more detailed information, one should contact the local or state fire marshal.

EMERGENCY ELECTRICAL POWER

Each communications center should have its own emergency power supply. Although an independent source of electrical energy is preferable, hospital-based communication centers commonly receive emergency power from the hospital's emergency generator. However, independent communication centers must be sure that they have a back-up power source and be aware of its location.

An electrical generator of sufficient capacity for a given communications center should be located nearby. This generator may be powered by diesel fuel, gasoline, or natural gas, depending on which type of fuel is most economic in a given locale. Consideration should also be given to the use of alternative energy sources abundant in the region, such as sunlight, wind, or hydroelectric power. The technology for these alternative energy sources is available, and calculation of economies for the program is possible when these energy sources are used.

Emergency power must also be instantly available for remote transmitter/receiver sites.

WIRING ACCESS

Each communications center includes enough wiring and cables to stretch the length of several football fields. These wires, which are vital to the operation of the system, should be readily accessible, and the function of each wire should be readily identifiable. This may be accomplished either by running all wiring underneath a raised floor or by terminating all wiring into a utility room behind the wall where the console is located.

LIGHTING

Whether the communications operations center has the appearance of an office or resembles a combat information center on a ship is a matter of preference. The CS must be able to clearly see everything that must be done. Emergency lighting must come on the instant that power is lost, even if this is only for a short duration.

HEATING, VENTILATION, AND AIR CONDITIONING

Heating, ventilation, and air-conditioning systems should be engineered with local geographic weather conditions in mind.[4] These systems not only keep personnel comfortable but also help prevent equipment from malfunctioning.

CONSOLE LAYOUT AND DESIGN

Once a custom console is built and installed, it is costly to alter; therefore, consoles should be designed carefully, with use of full-scale plans and even cardboard mock-ups. In addition, a console should be designed to be ergonomically functional. The CS must be able to see and reach all portions of the console without twisting, craning, stretching, or squinting. The seat for a console must roll, swivel, tilt, and be comfortable while providing good lumbar support.

The communication area should be ergonomically designed. Information is available, and experts can assist with the design of a communication center to prevent work-related injuries.

ACOUSTIC INSULATION

The amount of insulation necessary to render the communications center oblivious to the external environment varies with the location of the center. Enough insulation should be used to deaden the noise from an aircraft engine 100 yd away at ground level. A communications center located deep within a building or above or below ground level is probably not as sensitive to external street or airfield noise.

RESTROOM FACILITIES

Each communications center should be equipped with full restroom facilities, including a toilet, sink, and shower. Depending on the schedule and program volume, the CS may not have the time to go elsewhere to use restroom facilities and certainly should not have to leave the communications center during a tour of duty.

LOUNGE AREAS

A room adjacent to the operations room of the communications center that the CS may use during down time is useful. This room may contain a couch, chair, coffee table, television, and multimedia player. The CS should not be in this room while a transport is underway. Whether such a lounge area is available in a given program depends both on policy and space constraints. The lounge might also contain the kitchen area or dormitory area, or both.

CREW REST AREA

The existence of a crew rest area with lounge chairs or bedrooms depends on program policy, shift schedules, program volume, and the number of personnel on duty. Sleeping while on duty is a controversial topic, and its appropriateness for specific types of personnel must be evaluated by each individual program.

KITCHEN EQUIPMENT

A small kitchen and pantry area is necessary to have in communications centers in which the CS is not able to leave. This area should include a small refrigerator and freezer, a small microwave oven, a coffee maker, and cabinet and counter space.

STORAGE

A secure storage area should be provided for communications center supplies, backup equipment, and archives. This space should not be shared with other departments. Some communication centers are also used to store disaster supplies because of their central location.

DECORATION

The decor of the communications center should be pleasant, easy to maintain, and in keeping with the character of the organization. An excellent idea is for the personnel who work in a given area to have input into its decor. Some communication centers have windows that allow viewing of the transport aircraft.

ALTERNATIVE SITES/BACKUP EQUIPMENT

An alternative site and backup equipment should be identified and prepared by every transport program. A plan of action to deal with such a scenario should it ever occur should be annually reviewed. Each communications center must be able to continue operations at an alternative site with backup equipment if for any reason the primary communications center becomes inoperable.

Plans should also be in place for rapidly repairing or replacing any piece of essential equipment in the communications center.

EQUIPMENT

Selection of equipment for a communications center should be made on the basis of the mission of the transport program, present and anticipated needs, functions, durability, reliability, expendability, serviceability, and, last but not least, cost.

For a decision about a given piece of equipment, a program should prioritize these factors, add any others that are applicable, and then determine the most cost-effective choice. The most costly item is not always the best item. However, also worth noting is that you get what you pay for.

TELEPHONES

Each communications center must have at least one dedicated line for the medical transport service.

Emergency telephone lines should not go through a switchboard; instead, they should be dedicated central office lines, so that if the switchboard fails, the communications center still has telephone communications. The number of incoming local and wide area telephone service lines should be based on the size of the service area and the projected volume of calls. Phone lines can be added relatively quickly when needed.

All calls made with use of emergency phone lines should be recorded, as should any outgoing call that pertain to requests for assistance or notifications.

Telephones today are available with a wide variety of features that may prove useful in a given operation. These features include speed dialing, memory banks of phone numbers, call queuing, hands-free operation, automatic redial, and so on.

Today, both wired and wireless communication systems are routinely used. Cellular phones are used by many transport services. However, their use should be guided by Federal Communications Commission (FCC) regulations on air medical transport vehicles. The FCC prohibits the use of cell phones in flight per FCC Code of Federal Regulations, part 22, subpart H, section 22.925. Cell phone use during ground transport should never interfere with patient care or safe driving.

Satellite phones may available as independent hand-held devices or as part of the aircraft. The satellite tracking systems discussed in Chapter 13 (Transport and Technology) come with satellite phone communication. Both CS and transport team members need to be educated as how to use them.

RADIOS

Radios continue to be the key hardware elements in a medical transport communications system. The crucial role of communication was especially recognized September 11, 2001, and during disasters such as hurricane Katrina. The radio

BOX 8-3	Radio Bands

VHF high-band FM (148-174 MHz): The radio signal in this band follows a straight line.

VHF low-band FM (30-50 MHz): The radio signal in this band follows the curvature of the Earth and has the greatest range.

VHF AM (118-136 MHz): This band is typically used for aviation-related communications.

UHF (403-941 MHz): These ultra-high frequencies have limited range and are most often used between ground units and base stations. They can be used for air-to-ground and ground-to-air communications for relatively short distances that fluctuate with the terrain.

800 MHz: Digital communication controlled by computers. They allow multiple agencies to communicate with each other and have higher frequency, less noise, and greater penetration outside of buildings.

AM, Amplitude modulation; *FM,* frequency modulation; *MHz,* megahertz; *VHF,* very high frequency; *UHF,* ultra-high frequency.

frequencies on which a program operates are assigned by the FCC on the basis of recommendations by the state chapter of Associated Public Safety Communications Officers, to which it has delegated responsibility for frequency coordination. The FCC issues licenses and assigns call letters. A program's assigned frequencies may be found in several radio bands (Box 8-3).

Included in the ultra-high frequency (UHF) spectrum are the so-called MED channels. *MED channels* are a set of 10 paired frequencies set aside by the FCC for the exclusive use of EMS units. The channels from MED 9 to MED 10 are frequency allocation channels used in metropolitan regions where UHF traffic is high. To use such a channel, an EMS unit calls the frequency allocation center, usually located in a fire department or ambulance service communications center, and requests assignment to a channel for the purpose of speaking with a specific hospital. The unit is then assigned an open channel or is told to stand by until one is available (Box 8-4).

BOX 8-4	MED Channel Frequencies

463.000/468.000 MHz (MED-ONE)
463.025/468.025 MHz (MED-TWO)
463.050/468.050 MHz (MED-THREE)
463.075/486.075 MHz (MED-FOUR)
463.100/468.100 MHz (MED-SIX)
463.150/468.150 MHz (MED-SEVEN)
463.175/468.175 MHz (MED-EIGHT)
462.950/467.950 MHz (MED-NINE)
462.975/467.975 MHz (MED-TEN)

The 800-MHz range has been assigned by the FCC because of overcrowding. These frequencies have a limited range because the signals are more line directed than the UHF and very–high frequency (VHF) spectrum.

Some programs have their own private VHF assigned to them. Others may choose to use one of the existing UHFs allocated for EMS use nationwide. The same rules and principles apply to use of any of them.

Since 9/11 and natural disasters as hurricane Katrina, a concerted effort has been made to make emergency and disaster management agencies interoperable. The advent of five mutual aid channels in the 800-MHz spectrum allows agencies from anywhere in the country to communicate to the incident command or units on the scene. One drawback has been that some agencies have given these frequencies different names, thus creating a myriad of names for the same channel (Box 8-5).

The several basic types of radio systems are as follows[3,5,6,9]:

1. *Simplex system:* The simplex system has the ability to transmit in one direction at a time with a single frequency.
2. *Full duplex system:* The full duplex system has the ability to transmit and receive simultaneously with two frequencies (typically UHF).
3. *Half duplex system:* The half duplex system has the ability to transmit or receive in one direction at a time with two frequencies (typically UHF high-band).
4. *Multiplex system:* The multiplex system has the ability to transmit from two or more sources over the same frequency.

BOX 8-5	New Mutual Aid Frequencies: Names and Renaming

Federal Standard

Mutual aid 1	866.0125
Mutual aid 2	866.5125
Mutual aid 3	867.0125
Mutual aid 4	867.5125
Mutual aid 5	868.0125

State of Ohio

| Air Med 1 | 867.0125 |
| Air Med 2 | 868.0125 |

Hamilton County, Ohio

I Call	867.0125
I TAC 1	866.5125
I TAC 2	867.0125
I TAC 3	867.5125
I TAC 4	868.0125

A repeater system is a type of half duplex system that involves a base station repeater at an elevated site remote from the communications center. This system is particularly useful in regions with mountainous terrain. A repeater system receives a signal on one frequency and instantly retransmits it on a second frequency to the other radios in the system, extending the communications center's range. The process is reversed when the repeater receives signals coming into the base station.

Radio Use

All members of the transport team must know how radios work. Kane[5] notes that each team member must know how to properly use radios under normal circumstances, how to troubleshoot a radio under abnormal circumstances, and how improper use of a radio could make a straightforward call complex, stressful, and potentially unsafe.

Phone-Radio or Radio-Phone Patch

With a phone-radio or radio-phone patch, special circuits in the radio console permit a radio and telephone to be linked together, one direction at a time, so that the medical crew can speak to a person who is not in the communications center and vice versa. This capability is useful for programs that require voice contact with a medical control physician and for occasions when a member of the medical crew needs to speak with the receiving physician. These optional circuits can be included when the radio console is purchased, or they can be added at a later date.

Programs that use a phone-radio or radio-phone patch have found that radio-like procedures must be used because transmissions are simplex. At times, this presents problems when patched through to persons who may not understand the system. Cellular telephones have supplanted this feature in many programs.

Squelch Control

Nearly all radios have squelch control, which is accessed by turning the knob until static is heard and then turning it in the opposite direction just past the point where the static ends. This adjustment is best made before the radio is used.

Continuous Tone Controlled Subaudible Squelch. Continuous tone controlled subaudible squelch circuits (CTCSSs) act as a filter to other users of the radio's frequency. Only users of radios with the same tone-control frequency setting normally hear each other. This feature may be disabled when the tone of a transmitting radio is unknown or different or the radio operator wishes to monitor the entire frequency. *Private line* and *channel guard* are proprietary names for continuous tone controlled subaudible squelch.

PAGERS

Most programs have a need for transport crews to carry personal pagers. The communications center should have its own paging encoder rather than use pagers that are accessed by dialing a telephone number. Telephone pagers have a lag time of up to several minutes, depending on the volume of pager calls in a given region. Direct encoding both speeds crew response time and results in long-term savings. A variety of pagers are available that can beep, buzz, vibrate, speak, or even display alphanumeric messages.

Two-way paging with use of satellite communications allows voiceless pages to be sent and an acknowledgment to be received with use of data terminals. PTT (Push to Talk) provides nation-wide service that combines instant communications with bases that use multiple transmitters across the country to provide service. These units offer global positioning system (GPS)–enabled tracking for aid in locating aircraft or staff should a precautionary landing need to be made and the staff leave the aircraft for some reason. The units can be left on the aircraft; they are not transmitting in the air, they are being pinged by the transmitters in the service area.

An extremely detailed needs assessment should be undertaken by qualified technical personnel before the implementation of any radio system. A program is ill-advised to purchase a system identical to that of another program on the basis of their satisfaction with it.

Headsets, Microphones, and Foot Switches

The use of headsets rather than microphones should be considered in busy communications centers. When used in conjunction with a foot switch, a headset leaves the CS's hands free, which is particularly desirable in operations in which only one CS is on duty.

When microphones are used, they should be the type that filters out background noises. A microphone placed on a bracket or gooseneck fixture attached to the console is preferable because it leaves the desktop space clear. When a headset microphone is used, it should be fairly close to the lips; proximity to the lips varies because of the varying speech characteristics of different people.

Logging Recorders

The CAMTS standards state that communication centers must have a system that records all incoming and outgoing telephone and radio transmissions with time recording and playback capabilities. These recording should be kept a minimum of 90 days.

All business-related telephone calls and all radio transmissions should be recorded. A program may elect to use an audiocassette logging system, digital audiocassette, VHS audiotape, or a reel-to-reel logging system.

Digital recording devices now allow recordings that can be accessed from personal computers and allow computer files of conversations to be sent along with e-mail attachments for education and clarification purposes. These digital files can be stored on many multimedia devices.

Cassette systems are more suitable for low-volume low-traffic operations. Cassette loggers typically limit the program to three recorded channels, with a fourth channel allocated for injection of the time signal. Most programs need a greater capacity than this.

Traditional reel-to-reel loggers are expensive; however, VHS and digital technology have reduced the cost and size of past generations of reel-to-reel recorders. The tapes for the reel-to-reel system are also expensive, but they are reusable. Currently available technology permits the contents of a 24-hour tape to be compressed and stored on a cassette for future reference. A program might elect to store several days of recording on reels, but this is costly and creates a storage problem.

If the program's budget permits, a dual logger should be purchased. A dual logger provides the redundancy needed in a communications center and permits playback of older tapes while still recording in real-time.

Short-Term Playback Devices

Short-term playback devices, through the use of either a continuous loop of recording tape or digital technology, record the last several minutes of telephone or radio traffic for review by the CS when needed. This device enables the CS to double-check any recent conversation at the touch of a button.

Computers and Peripherals

Computers are an integral part of the well-equipped communications center. What a computer can do for a program is limited primarily by imagination and budget.

Needs should be assessed before any computer system is purchased. First, what the program wishes the computer system to do should be decided; second, finding the appropriate software is necessary; and finally, a computer system should be selected that has the speed and power to accomplish the task.

A wide variety of software is available to aid in communications before, during, and after transport. Computer-aided dispatch programs can allow the CS and other transport team members to input data about the transport and the patient and keep track of data regarding medical procedures, transport times, delays, and downtimes. In addition, this software can also be used for billing and production of revenue.[7]

The communication center must also have access to the Internet to allow communication outside of the program. Internet access also allows the program to keep up-to-date information pertinent to transport such as weather conditions or selected patient data.

MOBILE DATA TERMINALS

Mobile data terminals are small computer terminals that are attached to a radio and have the ability to send data to and receive data from the base station or another mobile data terminal. These systems vary in complexity and require a dedicated radio frequency for their use.

WEATHER RADAR

All pilots have access to FAA Flight Service weather information. Although the FAA generally does an excellent job, its reports may not be as up-to-the-minute as desired at a given point in time. New weather tools are constantly being introduced. Great examples are available at http://weather.aero/hems/.

Weather radar display systems are available through several commercial services. These systems may be connected to the National Weather Service radar site in the region via telephone line or computer modem. All weather radar display systems provide displays and printouts of excellent quality. The display should be installed where the pilots have access to it. If the pilot needs an update while airborne, the CS should also have access to it. This situation may not be a problem if the aircraft has its own weather radar. If a program has a computer-driven system, the CS can access the weather report from the communications center. An alternative to the phone-line system is to place a remote monitor in the communications center.[3]

FAX MACHINES

A fax machine is an indispensable tool in a communications center. Fax machines today are multifunctional and operate scanners and copiers.

UNINTERRUPTIBLE POWER SUPPLY

An *uninterruptible power supply* is a device that provides steady electrical current to sensitive electronic equipment in the event of a power drop-off or surge and serves as a battery backup for a finite period of time until power is restored. An uninterruptible power supply is essential when computers are used for important tasks. These devices can support an operation for periods that range from a few minutes to several hours. Support for longer periods of time costs more money.

CLOSED-CIRCUIT TELEVISION/ WEB CAMERAS

The CS may need to have access to video scanning of the helipad or hangar ramp. Such scanning serves as a security system and enables the CS who does not have direct visual contact with the program's parked aircraft to see what is occurring. Television monitors are available that may serve as a computer screen or as a video monitor by pressing a button, thus reducing the cost to the program. Web cameras also may be used to monitor aircraft and other areas of the transport service.

CLOCKS

Each communications center should have several clocks, which may be analog, digital, or a mix of both types, all of which remain synchronized to reduce confusion in times that are given during transport. At least one good-quality battery-operated clock should be available to provide backup during power failures. Air medical crew members should familiarize themselves with the military time system used in aviation. Programs that operate in more than one time zone may wish to keep parallel sets of clocks in operation to avoid confusion in calculating arrival times (Box 8-6).

STATUS BOARD

Every communication center must have a status board that displays, for each aircraft and ground vehicle, their assigned aircraft (N) numbers, the crew on board, and its current status. Any type of board, from a chalkboard to an elaborate electronic device, may be used. Some status boards are integrated in the software used by the transport program.

BOX 8-6	**24-Hour Clock**						
AM							
	1:00	0100	4:00	0400	7:00	0700	10:00	1000
	2:00	0200	5:00	0500	8:00	0800	11:00	1100
	3:00	0300	6:00	0600	9:00	0900	Noon	1200
PM							
	1:00	1300	4:00	1600	7:00	1900	10:00	2200
	2:00	1400	5:00	1700	8:00	2000	11:00	2300
	3:00	1500	6:00	1800	9:00	2100	Midnight	2400 (0000)

MAPS

Technology has vastly improved "finding" EMS providers and referring hospitals. Mapping software is available that allows the CS to point and click on selected response sites, displaying coordinates for navigational purposes. GPS devices allow EMS to provide exact location information to both the communication center and the transport team. Many transport programs actually create web sites with information about common destinations (hospitals, predesignated landing areas), which could save time and also affords an opportunity to review helipads and landing areas. An example of a web site that shares this type of information is Western Helipads, which was developed between two transport programs in northern Utah. This site can be accessed at http://www.western.pad.info.

An important point to remember is that technology is generally only as good as the operator, so CS, pilots, and transport team members must know how to use a map. An aviation sectional map or maps of the program's normal area of operations should be available in the communications center and on board transport vehicles. A compass radial overlay with a center string attached should be affixed to the map, centered over the base of operations for back up if systems go down or are not functioning. A heavy dark line that radiates from base operations should be drawn on the map and marked off in 10-mile increments. This map enables the CS to rapidly obtain a heading and distance to a given point.

A street map should also be included of the metropolitan area around the base of rotary-wing operations as they are called on to precede directly to the scene. This map should be modified, as previously mentioned.

Topographic maps that show variation in terrain contour and various other maps that may be obtained from state or county highway departments prove useful in the communications center.

ROLODEX

A Rolodex may serve as the primary reference device in an office. It is inexpensive, consumes no energy, and is 100% reliable in operation. Computerized communications centers must have one on hand as part of backup inventory. Rolodexes are available in several different sizes and configurations.

CARDEX

A Cardex is a book similar to a Rolodex in that it has a separate card for each hospital in the service area. Information included in a Cardex should be updated and dated, and each card should include landing zone information and all telephone numbers. Although many communication centers are now computerized, a written back-up system is imperative in the event of a power failure or data loss.

REFERENCE MATERIAL

There is no limit to the amount of useful reference material that should be available in the communications center. Available reference materials should include telephone books, aviation material, medical information, hazardous materials data, and anything else thought to be useful by a particular program.

SERVICE CONTRACTS

A service contract should be purchased for all equipment selected for inclusion in a communications center. Service contracts usually result in long-term savings and more efficient operations because of decreased downtime of equipment. Before any purchase is made, a program should determine whether a vendor is able to support the operation with a loaner piece of equipment if the program does not have backup equipment.

The Commission on Accreditation of Medical Transport Systems[2] lists the components that a communication center must contain. Box 8-7 lists these components.

POLICIES AND PROCEDURES

A detailed policy and procedures manual is necessary for any organization that wishes to function in a systematic effective manner. The communications center manual must be a part of the program's overall policy and procedures manual. When the communications center manual is written, it should be carefully integrated with existing policies and procedures to minimize potential conflicting instructions to the CS.

The manual must cover all aspects of operation that have anything to do with communications. Each segment of the manual should be extremely detailed so that if a question arises about a specific item, it can be resolved by referring to the manual.

COMMUNICATING

RADIOS
Language
To effectively communicate within a program, standardized terminology should be used so that meanings are not lost or misinterpreted.

In general, communication in plain language is preferable to use of various codes; this precludes errors caused by misunderstanding of a garbled coded transmission. Because of the broad area over which an air medical program operates, knowledge of codes for each of the many jurisdictions in the program's service area would be extremely difficult.

Speaking
When initiating a radio transmission, a transport team member should begin with the name or call sign of the unit being called, followed by the member's own name or call sign. When older radio systems and poorly maintained new systems are used, the speaker, when keying the microphone, should pause for a second before speaking to allow the radio to reach its maximal output level. This practice helps prevent the frequent problem of incomplete messages being received. Another cause of this problem is speaking before keying the microphone.

The speaker should talk at a normal level; yelling into the microphone distorts the transmission. The speaker should know what to say before keying the microphone; speak clearly and concisely with-

---

BOX 8-7 | **Components of a Communication Center**

At least one dedicated phone line.

A system for recording all incoming and outgoing telephone and radio transmissions, which should be stored for 30 days, with time recording and playback capabilities.

Capability to notify the transport team and online medical direction for a request and during transport.

Back-up emergency power when power outages occur.

A status board to follow transport vehicles and show who is on the transport teams, weather status, and so on.

Local aircraft service area maps and navigation charts.

Road maps available for ground transport.

Communication Policy and Procedures manual.

From Commission on Accreditation of Medical Transport Systems: *Accreditation standards*, ed 5, Anderson, SC, 2006, The Commission.

out irrelevant comments; attempt to control the voice level and intonation even when under stress; try to avoid transmissions that reflect disgust, irritation, or sarcasm; and avoid the use of profanity at all times. Radio transmissions are a measure of a program's professionalism, and both the media and a large population of citizens with scanners hear every word that is said on the radio.

Transport team members must know how to properly operate the two-directional radio-intercom switch commonly found on headset cords in aircraft or ground vehicle. Many transport team members have been embarrassed when personal conversations or comments less than socially acceptable were broadcast over a wide area. This problem occurs less often in programs that operate pressurized aircraft, in which transport team members may not use a headset system.

Intracrew communications are also important. The pilot should keep the medical crew informed of any developments in a clear complete message that leaves no doubt about what is happening. The following two anecdotes illustrate this point; although the incidents are somewhat humorous now, the crews involved did not think so at the time. In the first incident, the crew received a badly scrawled note from the pilot, pushed through an opening behind his seat, just as the helicopter began an unexpected banking turn. The note read "I can't talk." The crew members looked at each other, each thinking that the pilot had had a cerebrovascular accident. They were about to become upset when the aircraft resumed straight and level flight. The pilot came on the intercom and explained that he could not talk on the medical radio, that he had spoken to approach control, and that he was returning to base for another aircraft. A more complete written message or advance warning on the intercom could have prevented a tense few moments for the crew.

In the second incident, the pilot of an outbound aircraft observed a transmission chip light blink on. In accordance with company policy, he immediately began a descent in preparation for landing. He told the crew "We're going down." The crew prepared themselves for a hard landing, and then began a vigorous discussion over the use of the one pillow on board. A normal landing was made, the mechanic arrived and corrected the problem, and the aircraft returned to its base. Once again, a more complete explanation would have prevented these tense moments.

During a flight, the pilot of an airport-based aircraft communicates with each of the following, in addition to the CS: ground control, airport tower departure control, air route traffic control center, approach control, airport tower, and ground control again.

Hospital-based rotorcraft may or may not be near an airport but will be in communication with the appropriate segments of the air traffic control system and the program's own communications center. In either case, only the pilots should communicate with air traffic control. Aircraft on scene flights also speak with units already on the scene.

Sterile cockpit (not speaking except in case of an emergency) must be practiced during takeoff and landing and any other critical phases of flight. Radio traffic should always be kept to a minimum to avoid unnecessary distractions, whether transporting via air or ground.

Transport teams in programs with multiple aircraft should also be aware that nonessential interaircraft conversations may make a telephone conversation or receipt of an essential transmission from another unit difficult for the CS.

If a team member asks the CS to make a telephone call, a minute or so should be allowed to pass before transmitting again to avoid interrupting the call.

If either party is having difficulty making a word understood, then that person should spell it using the phonetic alphabet (Box 8-8).

TELEPHONES

Often, a requesting party's first impression of a program is created by the CS who answers the telephone. A courteous manner combined with comprehensive knowledge of the program helps give the caller the impression that the program is staffed by competent professional personnel.

MEDICAL DIRECTION

Programs that operate with nurses or paramedics are included under medical direction regulations that

BOX 8-8	Phonetic Alphabet and Numbers[3]

Phonetic Alphabet

A – Alpha
B – Bravo
C – Charlie
D – Delta
E – Echo
F – Foxtrot
G – Gulf
H – Hotel
I – India
J – Juliet
K – Kilo
L – Lima
M – Mike
N – November
O – Oscar
P – Papa
Q – Quebec
R – Romeo
S – Sierra
T – Tango
U – Uniform
V – Victor
W – Whiskey
X – X-ray
Y – Yankee
Z – Zulu

Phonetic Numbers

1 – WUN
2 – TOO
3 – TREE
4 – FOW-ER
5 – FIFE
6 – SIX
7 – SEV-EN
8 – AIT
9 – NIN-ER
0 – ZEE-RO

From FAA: *Federal Aviation Administration*, available at http://www.faa.gov, accessed June 2002.

vary from state to state. Whether communicating with their medical direction physician via radio, radiophone patch, satellite, or cellular phone, the medical crew should follow the medical reporting format used in the region. All reports should be to-the-point. Any treatment order received should be acknowledged by repeating the order verbatim.

FACE-TO-FACE

Of particular importance to the success of a program are interpersonal communications among all program personnel. An understanding of the problems and stress inherent to each position tends to foster patience. Cross-orientation sessions between transport team members and communications personnel are useful in creating this understanding. Anyone who works in a program is going to have an occasional bad day, and colleagues must be able to deal with this circumspectly.

Successful working relationships frequently lead to personal friendships. Social events within programs also tend to relieve stress and improve working relationships.[5]

ON PAPER OR ONLINE

In this litigious age, everything that occurs must be documented. "If it is not written down, then it did not happen" is a concept pursued by attorneys who specialize in the field of malpractice. Programs may use paper forms, computer documentation, or both.

All forms used by the program should be filled out assiduously. If requested information does not apply, a line should be drawn through the space or the letters NA (not applicable) should be inserted. For computer-based documentation, the NA should be checked.

When forms to be used in the program are created, an attempt should be made to minimize the number of times that any one piece of information must be documented. If the originals do not have separate destinations, forms should be consolidated. Communications forms and documentation should have the same flow as those used by the transport team to make documentation of what the CS says easier for the transport team member.

A 6-month supply of most forms should be adequate as long as a new supply is ordered before the previous supply is finished. All forms and methods of documentation should be evaluated periodically to determine whether they are still functional.

Programs must have a means of communication, whether written or web-based. All transport team members must be aware of how to access policies and procedures and the flow of information within a program.

WITH THE MEDIA

Local news media usually have a high level of interest in the activities of any transport program. The CS must be able to politely, but firmly, deal with their calls when they interfere with operations. The CS must be aware of program policy with respect to giving out information and should refer the caller to the appropriate person if this is dictated by policy.

Establishing a good rapport with the local media is essential. Many people have strong negative feelings about certain aspects of the news media. A decision may be reached within a program to notify the media of the types of events in which they usually express interest, time permitting. The transport operation always comes first.

EMERGENCY PROCEDURES

The operational procedures section of the policy and procedures manual should include a subsection that deals with procedures to be followed in the event of any unscheduled event that affects the use of the aircraft or directly involves the aircraft.

POSTACCIDENT INCIDENT PLAN

Every transport program must have a written plan in the event of an incident such as a vehicle accident. Each program should identify which incidents trigger this plan. The *Postaccident Incident Plan* (PAIP) must be easily identified, readily available, and understood by all of the transport team members. CAMTS[2] recommends that at a minimum the plan should include: a list of personnel to notify in order of priority; consecutive guidelines to follow in attempts to communicate with the aircraft or ambulance, initiate search and rescue or ground support, have a back-up plan for transporting the patient or team, and have an aviation individual identified as the scene coordinator to coordinate activities at the crash site; preplanned time frame to activate the PAIP for overdue vehicles; a method to ensure accurate

dissemination; coordination of transport of injured team members; procedure to document all notifications, calls, and communications and to secure all documents and tape recordings related to the incident; procedure to deal with releasing information to the press; resources available for critical incident stress management (CISM); and a process to determine whether the program will stay in service.

MASS-CASUALTY INCIDENTS

Most transport programs are undoubtedly a part of any mass-casualty incident plan developed in the program's service area. Copies of the program's roles in these situations should be immediately accessible to the CS.

UNSCHEDULED EVENTS

Detailed contingency plans must exist for various emergencies that involve the program's aircraft and ground vehicles. These plans must be immediately accessible to the CS.

DRILLS

The CS should participate in practice exercises, both scheduled and unscheduled, that relate to various emergencies that might occur. These practice exercises reinforce the CS's knowledge of the procedures and test the procedures for weak spots.

CRITICAL-INCIDENT STRESS MANAGEMENT

Each program should have a critical-incident stress-management plan in place in the event of the loss of an aircraft and its crew. The CS on duty at the time must be included in this plan. The CS will experience all the same feelings of grief and loss as the other program members, and more. The CS may believe that he or she could have done something more or failed to do something and, thus, take on unwarranted feelings of guilt. Unless a CS receives some type of stress management immediately, this CS may be lost to the program at some point in the future.

AIRCRAFT RADIOS

Each medical crew member should be familiar with the operation of the radios used in the program's aircraft. Some aircraft may have more than one radio, thus permitting the medical crew to communicate with someone on the ground while the pilot talks to someone else.

Other aircraft have one radio and two control heads, one for the pilot and the other for the medical crew. The medical crew member should check with the pilot before using the radio to be certain that the pilot has no need of it at the time.

Portable Units

A program may elect to provide transport members with portable handheld radios for use on the ground outside the aircraft. These radios are particularly useful for programs that do emergency scene flights, and they are also useful during transfer flights for alerting the pilot to the imminent return of the crew with the patient.

Cellular and satellite phones may also be used by transport team members for communication.

SUMMARY

The communications center of a transport program is the foundation of a successful venture. Planning and implementation of a communications center must be organized, logical, and cost-effective. The program's mission, philosophy, and resources must be continually evaluated to ensure the quality of its communications.

REFERENCES

1. American Academy of Pediatrics: *Air and ground transport of neonatal and pediatric patients*, ed 3, Elk Grove, IL, 2007, American Academy of Pediatrics.
2. Commission on Accreditation of Medical Transport Systems: *Accreditation standards*, ed 7, Anderson, SC, 2006, CAMTS.
3. FAA: *Federal Aviation Administration*, available at http://www.faa.gov, accessed June 2008.
4. Hawsey KO, Lee A: "This is a drill": overdue aircraft drill for a postaccident/incident plan, *Air Med J* 20(5):15-17, 2001.
5. Kane D: Communications. In York-Clark D, Stocking J, Johnson J, editors: *Flight and ground transport nursing core curriculum*, ed. 2, Denver, 2006, Air and Surface Transport Nurses Association.
6. Illman P: *Pilot's communication handbook*, ed 5, New York, 1998, McGraw-Hill.
7. NAACS: *National Association of Air Medical Communications Specialists*, available at http://www.naacs.org, accessed June 2008.
8. Rau W: 2000 Communications survey, *Air Med J* 6(2):22-26, 2000.
9. Sholl S, Morse AM, Broome R, et al: Communications. In Blumen IJ, editor: *Principles and directions of air medical transport*, Salt Lake City, 2006, Air Medical Physicians Association.
10. Yocum K: A new look at hiring communication specialists, *Air Med J* 5(2):132-134, 1999.
11. FAA: *FAA document N 8000.347, order 8400.10*, appendix 1, vol 3, chapter 6, section 5, dated 12/28/2006, Washington, DC, 2006, FAA.

SAFETY AND SURVIVAL

Gordon H. Worley

COMPETENCIES

1. Identify the safety risks related to air and surface patient transport and methods to reduce those risks.
2. Describe the medical transport industry's safety initiatives to improve safety and reduce accident rates.
3. Describe safe operations around helicopters, fixed-wing aircraft, and ground transport vehicles.
4. Understand and use Air Medical Resource Management.
5. Correctly perform emergency procedures, including emergency egress.
6. Identify the components of a Postaccident Incident Plan.
7. Identify the priorities in a survival situation and perform basic survival skills, including shelter building, fire building, water procurement, and signaling.

"Safety does not just happen, it is not a specific event or a 'thing' — it is an attitude."
Dr. Ira Blumen and the UCAN Safety Committee, 2002[6]

Most chapters in this book contain information intended to help the air medical or ground transport crew member provide care for the critically ill or injured patient. This chapter is different; its purpose is to encourage the development of a safety attitude. It seeks to foster an active awareness and commitment to safety in every aspect of every mission. In short, it is devoted to taking care of the transport team member.

A safety culture must exist within every transport program. Each member of the program must accept that they contribute directly to a safe environment. Every individual, whether they are a nurse, paramedic, physician, respiratory therapist, emergency medical technician (EMT), pilot, mechanic, communications specialist, or administrator, must accept personal responsibility for safety and be a safety advocate.

DEFINITION OF SAFETY

Webster's Dictionary defines *safety* as "... the state of being safe from the risk of experiencing or causing injury, danger or loss." Few human endeavors are completely safe from risk. The medical transport environment by its nature presents a wide range of potential risks. Medical transport exists at the unique interface of aviation, public safety, emergency medicine, and critical care medicine, all of which are complex technologic and human systems. In any complex system, human errors inevitably occur.[3] Effective risk management and safety programs recognize this and focus efforts on both reducing the rate of errors and, more importantly, reducing the consequences of the errors that do occur.

Safety may best be defined in the medical transport setting as: identifying risks and managing them in such a way as to eliminate or significantly reduce the possibility of accident or injury. The following sections explore some of the significant risks associated with air and ground medical transport and identify what has been, and is being, done to manage these risks and improve safety in the transport environment.

HAZARDS IN THE TRANSPORT ENVIRONMENT

Note: The use of the term *accident* in the following discussion reflects its use by the National Transportation Safety Board (NTSB) for an event "... in which any person suffers death or serious injury, or in which the aircraft receives substantial damage."[10] This does not suggest that these tragic events are or were unavoidable. Most, if not all, of the accidents discussed had controllable factors that could have potentially prevented the occurrence or lessened the severity of the event.

AIR MEDICAL ACCIDENTS

The first hospital air medical program was established in 1972. In the following years, the air medical industry underwent tremendous growth, from that one program in 1972, to 32 in 1980, and 101

by 1985.[6] With this growth came the realization that air medical helicopters had an accident rate far greater than that of helicopters engaged in general aviation.

From 1980 to 1985, the helicopter emergency medical services (HEMS) industry had an estimated accident rate of 12.3 accidents/100,000 patients transported. The accident rate for nonscheduled turbine-powered air taxi helicopter operators, a comparable non-HEMS population, was 6.9/100,000 for the same time period.[47] In 1988, the NTSB released the results of its investigation of 59 Emergency Medical Services (EMS) accidents that occurred between 1978 and 1986. The study concluded that weather-related accidents were the most common and most serious type of accident experienced by EMS helicopters.[47]

The 1990s showed continued growth in the air medical industry, from an estimated 174 HEMS programs operating 232 helicopters in 1990 to 225 programs operating 360 helicopters in 1999.[6] In 1990, one accident occurred with no fatalities. During the next 5 years, an average of 5.5 accidents per year occurred. In 1996, only one HEMS accident again was seen, this one fatal, and three were seen in 1997. During the period from 1998 to 2001, the accident rate increased sharply to an average of 10.8 HEMS accidents per year.[6] A review of 121 air medical accidents from the late 1970s through the late 1990s found weather-related accidents to be the most common type, with an increase of 10% from the 1980s to the 1990s.[22-24]

In 2002, the Air Medical Physicians Association (AMPA) released *A Safety Review and Risk Assessment in Air Medical Transport*, which examined HEMS accidents from 1980 to 2001.[6] This report looked not only at the total yearly numbers of accidents but also at accident, injury, and fatality rates as functions of the number of EMS aircraft operating, the number of patients transported, and the estimated total flight hours for each year. The analysis showed a generally decreasing trend in number of HEMS accidents per 100,000 patient transports from the high in 1982 of 24.9/100,000 (a higher rate than that calculated by the NTSB in 1988) to a low in 1996 of 0.57/100,000. The average for the last 5 years of the study (1997 to 2001) was 4.6/100,000 patient transports. The most common recurrent factors in HEMS accidents were again found to be poor weather conditions and operations at night.

In 2003, the year after the publication of the AMPA study, there were 18 HEMS accidents, four of which were fatal. The year 2004 had 13 accidents, and 2005 had 17, with six fatal accidents each year. In January 2006, the NTSB released an Aviation Special Investigation Report that examined 55 EMS aircraft accidents that occurred between January 2002 and January 2005, 41 of which were helicopter accidents.[48] The investigation identified these recurrent safety issues:

- Less stringent requirements for EMS operations conducted without patients on board.
- A lack of aviation flight risk evaluation programs for EMS operations.
- A lack of consistent comprehensive flight dispatch procedures for EMS operations.
- No requirements to use technologies such as terrain awareness and warning systems (TAWS) and night vision imaging systems (NVIS) to enhance EMS flight safety.

Also in 2006, Baker et al[5] reviewed HEMS accidents for the period from 1983 to 2005 to determine the factors related to fatal outcomes. They concluded that accidents that occur at night or in bad weather or that result in a postimpact fire have a higher risk of being fatal.[5]

In 2006, a total of seven HEMS accidents occurred, three with fatalities, and in 2007, six accidents occurred, two of which were fatal. The year 2008 brought the worst year in the industry's history for fatal accidents, with a total of 12 HEMS accidents from January to November 2008, including the first-ever mid-air collision of two helicopter air ambulances (included in these totals as two accidents). Nine of these accidents were fatal, claiming a total of 29 lives, including five patients.[11,26,46] In 2008, 264 HEMS programs were in the United States, operating 699 helicopter bases and a total of 840 helicopters,[4] more than twice the number of aircraft in operation in 1999. Figure 9-1 summarizes accidents from January 1980 to November 2008.

Fixed-wing air medical accidents have not been as well studied as HEMS accidents. In 2008, 108 air medical programs listed in the Atlas and Database of Air Medical Services (ADAMS) operated a total of 292 fixed-wing aircraft.[4] Sixty-two of these programs operated both fixed-wing aircraft and helicopters. A review of accident data from 2002 to November 2008 showed a total of 14 accidents from 2002 to 2006, six of which were fatal. In 2007, six fixed-wing air medical accidents occurred, four of which were fatal; none were found in 2008.[11,26,45,48]

The data presented do not pretend to paint the whole picture of accident risk in air medical transport. The actual rates and the causes of air medical accidents are continuing topics of intense study and

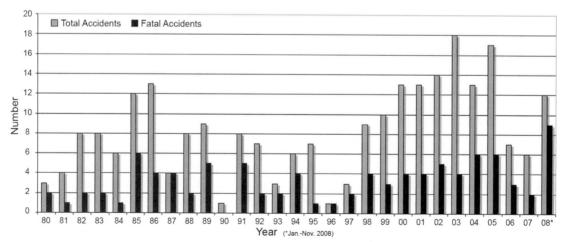

FIGURE 9-1   **Helicopter EMS accidents January 1980 through November 2008.**[6,7,11,26,45]

debate.[3] Although specific numbers and root causes may not always be clear, what is clear is that we continue to have accidents and that patients and flight crews continue to be injured and killed. Also clear is that recurrent factors continue to be involved in air medical accidents, most notably operations at night and in inclement weather. We need to maintain a respect for these hazards and promote (and use) every tool and practice available to reduce the risks of flight in the HEMS environment.

GROUND AMBULANCE ACCIDENTS

The same level of attention paid to air medical accidents has not been paid to ground ambulance accidents. Unlike air medical accidents, which must be reported and are investigated by the NTSB, ground ambulance crashes are generally monitored on a state or local level, which makes consistent nationwide data difficult to obtain. In 2001, Kahn et al[30] published a review of all reported fatal US ambulance crashes from 1987 to 1997. The 339 fatal accidents resulted in 405 fatalities and 838 injuries. Those victims in the rear compartment who were unrestrained or improperly restrained had the most severe injuries and fatalities. Most of the crashes (202/339), and fatalities (233/405), occurred during emergency operations. The most common crash location was at an intersection.[30] The Centers for Disease Control (CDC) reported in 2003 on 300 fatal ambulance crashes that occurred from 1991 to 2003. These crashes resulted in the deaths of 27 on-duty EMS workers, 55 other occupants of the ambulances, and 275 occupants of other vehicles and pedestrians. Most of the EMS worker fatalities (60%) occurred in the front of the vehicle.[39]

These studies show that ground ambulance accidents also have recurrent contributing factors. Safety training programs should focus on awareness of these risks, safe driving, and proper use of safety equipment, such as seatbelts. Ground transport programs need to establish the same safety culture and have the same commitment to safety and risk reduction as air medical programs.

REDUCING THE RISKS

Since the 1980s, efforts have been made to reduce the risks of flight in the air medical environment. These efforts at risk reduction have taken many forms, from safety policies and procedures, to training and new technologies.

Critical Thinking, Decision Making, and the Human Factor

The probable cause for many of the accidents described previously is listed as *pilot error,* which is another way of saying the pilot made a bad decision, or a series of bad decisions, that resulted in the accident. Decision making in the aviation environment is a complicated process, with many factors that need to be considered. To be able to make good decisions, pilots and flight crew members need to have training in critical thinking and decision making in the HEMS environment and have access to decision-making tools.[29] These tools may be technologies, policies, algorithms, or other processes. No single tool or practice ensures a good decision, but used together they can be effective in helping pilots and crews make safe decisions. The human factor, the ability of the pilot and crew to make informed safe decisions, remains the single most important factor in ensuring safety in the medical transport environment.

Weather Minimums

From the beginnings of the industry, weather and impaired visibility (instrument meteorologic conditions [IMC]) have been recognized as a significant cause of accidents. The Commission on Accreditation of Medical Transport Systems (CAMTS) accreditation standards require that programs have minimum cloud ceiling and visibility limits for operations under visual flight rules (VFR).[12] In November 2008, the Federal Aviation Administration (FAA) released draft revisions to Operations Specification that pertained to HEMS operations. The revisions include higher VFR ceiling, visibility and obstacle clearance requirements when a "flight or sequence of flights includes a part 135 segment."[19] These new Operations Specifications became effective in February 2009. Each program's weather minimums must comply with FAA regulations, meet CAMTS requirements, and address the specific needs and hazards of the program's operating area. Once a program's weather minimums have been established, they need to be followed; "pushing the envelope" on minimums has been implicated in many weather-related HEMS accidents.

Another weather-related concern noted in the 2006 NTSB report was the lack of reliable information regarding weather conditions in many areas where HEMS programs operate, which increases the risk of an inadvertent entry into IMC. In an effort to find ways to reduce this risk, representatives of the HEMS industry, the FAA, and the University Center for Atmospheric Research (UCAR) conducted a HEMS Weather Summit in 2006. One result of this summit was the development of the Aviation Digital Data Service (ADDS) experimental HEMS Low Altitude Flight Tool (http://www.weather.aero/hems/). This online application is designed to enhance the safety of flight in the low altitude environment used by HEMS aircraft. It provides a visual representation of ceiling, visibility, convection, radar information, and geographic information system (GIS) data in areas between established weather reporting sites.[20,43]

Mission Planning and Risk Assessment

The safe completion of any medical transport mission starts with mission planning. The first step in mission planning is an assessment of the potential risks involved, which leads to a decision about whether or not the mission should be accepted. Once the decision has been made to accept the mission, other aspects of mission planning must occur, including weight and performance planning, fuel management, destination considerations, pilot and crew duty time, and clinical factors.

Operational risk assessment begins with a daily or shift evaluation, which takes into account factors that remain relatively constant during the day. These factors can include prevailing weather patterns, pilot and crew experience, and the availability of safety technologies (discussed subsequently). Another risk assessment should be performed at the time of each mission request, evaluating the time of day, current weather conditions, weather forecasts, pilot and crew fatigue, and other variables. Some programs have established operational control centers to assist pilots in assessing the risks of certain missions by having the mission request reviewed

and any identified risks evaluated by another individual (typically a senior pilot) before the request is accepted. Figure 9-2 shows an example of a computer-based risk assessment tool.

Risk assessment should be a fluid dynamic process. If conditions change as the mission progresses, then so should the risk assessment. Pilots and flight crews need to continuously observe and evaluate the mission environment and the potential risks. If changes in the mission environment can be anticipated, then decision thresholds and alternative plans can be discussed and decided on ahead of time.

Declined Missions

Although the pilot-in-command (PIC) has the ultimate responsibility for accepting or declining any mission request, all members of the flight team have the right, and the responsibility, to refuse to accept any mission where there is a legitimate safety concern. Each program should have a written policy for declining or aborting missions, so that individual crew members do not have to worry about disciplinary action or other negative action as a result of refusing to participate in a mission because of safety concerns.[1] The safety culture of the program should support the "Three to say go, one to say no" philosophy.

Air Medical Resource Management

Air Medical Resource Management (AMRM) is the operational practice of involving all members of the flight team (pilot and clinical crew members) in mission planning, decision making, and mission safety. It is the air medical industry's adaptation of *Crew Resource Management* (CRM), used in the commercial aviation industry and by the US Air Force. CRM grew out of several significant accidents that resulted from poor decision making on the part of airline pilots, in some cases over the objections of other flight crew members.[52] The PIC was traditionally the sole decision maker in an airline cockpit. The rest of the crew followed the PIC's instructions and did not offer input or question decisions. By encouraging crew members to pay attention, make suggestions, and voice concerns, CRM involves all of the crew members in the decision-making process. The PIC still has the ultimate authority and responsibility for

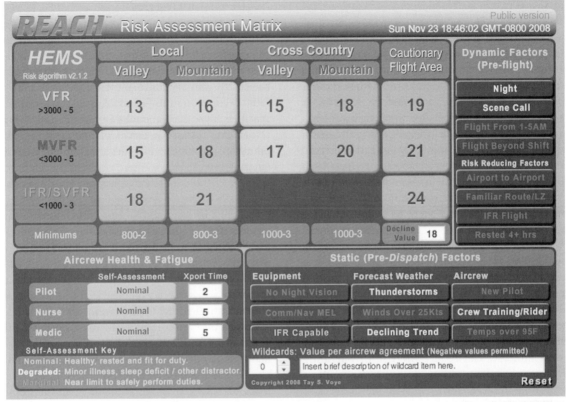

FIGURE 9-2 **A computer-based risk assessment tool.** This computer program takes into account weather conditions, operating area, pilot and crew experience, pilot and crew fatigue, safety technologies (IFR, NVG, etc), and other factors to provide an objective measure of the risk presented by any individual transport request. (Image courtesy of Tay S. Voye, 2008, available at http://www.hemsrisk.com.)

the aircraft, but other crew members are able to offer suggestions or, more importantly, question decisions they feel are unsafe or unwise.[52]

The essence of AMRM/CRM is teamwork, based on good communication between all crew members and the use of all available resources to maximize mission safety.[6] Mutual respect, trust, and an organizational culture that supports safety provide the best environment for effective communication and use of AMRM. AMRM classes should be a part of initial and recurrent training and should involve both pilots and clinical crew members in a group setting.

Helicopter Shopping

Fatal HEMS accidents have occurred when a HEMS program has accepted a mission that

had been declined by another provider.[46] The International Association of Flight Paramedics (IAFP, formerly the National Flight Paramedics Association [NFPA]) published a position paper in 2006 that addressed the problem of local agencies placing sequential requests to different air medical programs in an attempt to obtain a response to a mission request that had been declined by one provider (or multiple providers) for reasons of weather, landing zone availability, or other safety factors. This practice in commonly referred to a *helicopter shopping.*[28]

All programs need to educate the EMS agencies, dispatch centers, and hospitals in their service areas about the hazards of this practice and work with them to develop systems to prevent it. When any program declines a mission request, the reason should be clearly stated and communicated to any other program that may be asked to accept the mission. Air medical programs that serve the same areas should have interprogram communication pathways to permit each program to notify others when a mission is declined or to inquire whether another program has turned down a request. These pathways may include regional or national turndown reporting web sites or formal interprogram notification systems. If the nature of a flight request (location, etc) suggests that another program may have been contacted first, the dispatcher/communications specialist should inquire whether any other programs were contacted about the flight and the reasons for any declines.

SAFETY TECHNOLOGIES

All reviews of air medical accidents have identified the same two environments as significant contributing factors: operations at night and during bad weather. These two environments have one major factor in common: reduced visibility. A variety of technologies can reduce the risk of operating during reduced visibility conditions by supplying additional information about potential hazards in the flight environment. One of the recurrent safety issues identified in the 2006 NTSB report was the lack of requirements that air medical aircraft make use of these safety technologies to enhance flight safety.

Instrument Flight

Flight operations under *instrument flight rules* (IFR) are a common practice for fixed-wing aircraft but are less common in helicopter aviation. Many helicopter models used in air medical transport are not approved for instrument flight, except in emergency conditions. When operating under IFR, the pilot is flying under the guidance of the FAA air traffic control (ATC) system. The controller monitors the position of the aircraft on radar and provides routing instructions that keep the aircraft away from terrain and other air traffic.[51] For an IFR-capable aircraft and pilot, unexpected entry into IMC is an inconvenience, not an emergency. Many newer models of helicopters are designed and equipped to be IFR capable.

Night Vision Goggles

Night vision goggles (NVGs, also called night vision imaging systems [NVIS]) use an electronic system to amplify visible light and provide improved visibility during night operations. NVGs have been in use by the military for many years and have seen a rapid acceptance in the HEMS community in recent years. In 2008, the National EMS Pilots Association (NEMSPA) released a survey of 382 active HEMS pilots on the subject of NVG usage in the HEMS environment. The responses were overwhelmingly in favor of the use of NVGs in night HEMS operations.[41] NVGs are expensive and may necessitate that the aircraft be modified to be compatible with the system's lighting requirements.

Terrain Awareness and Warning Systems

One of the common scenarios in air ambulance accidents is loss of adequate visibility and subsequent controlled flight into terrain (CFIT). *Terrain awareness and warning systems* (TAWS) provide the pilot with a visual display of the terrain along the flight path and alert the pilot with visual and audible alarms if the aircraft flies too close to the terrain. Some of these systems also include a *traffic collision avoidance system* (TCAS), which provides information about the location of other nearby air traffic.

Satellite Tracking and Position Reporting

Automated flight following with a satellite-based tracking system provides the flight communications center with up-to-the-minute information regarding the position and status of the aircraft. In the event of an emergency situation, the exact position of the aircraft is always known. Many of these systems also permit satellite-based voice and data communications.

Crashworthy Aircraft and Vehicle Systems

Design changes to improve the crashworthiness of the airframe, fuel system, and seats in US military aircraft have shown improved crash survival rates.[32] Newer civilian and military helicopters are equipped with crashworthy landing gear, crashworthy fuel systems, and crash attenuating seats that absorb energy and reduce the g force applied to the occupant in a hard impact to improve occupant survival in a crash.[5] Changes in ground ambulance design to enhance safety have included improved seat and seatbelt/harness restraint systems for occupants of the rear compartment, ergonomic interior designs that permit easier access to the patient and supplies while remaining restrained, padded ambulance interiors, and back-up camera systems.

INDUSTRY SAFETY INITIATIVES

When the disturbing HEMS accident rates of the 1980s were identified, the air medical industry recognized the need to improve safety and reduce accident rates. A great emphasis has been, and continues to be, placed on improving air medical safety and risk management techniques. A number of organizations have launched programs and established standards designed to improve safety practices, enhance the safety consciousness of the industry, and reduce or eliminate errors of consequence.[3]

AIR AND SURFACE TRANSPORT NURSES ASSOCIATION

The Air and Surface Transport Nurses Association (ASTNA, formerly the National Flight Nurses Association [NFNA]) has long been a safety advocate and has published a series of position papers related to air medical safety. ASTNA is a professional nursing organization with a membership that includes transport nurses from throughout the United States and Canada. In 1988, the NFNA (ASTNA) published the position paper *Improving Flight Nurse Safety in the Air Medical Helicopter Environment*. In this paper, the organization endorsed many of the recommendations of the NTSB study published earlier the same year. The NFNA stated that "available knowledge and technology which could significantly enhance [a] flight nurse's safety in the air medical helicopter environment is not consistently applied and utilized in all air medical transport programs."[42] The position paper proposed several corrective measures. The proposals dealt with: (1) crew scheduling and rest periods; (2) the right of flight nurses to refuse to participate in a flight as a result of concerns for personal safety; (3) the need for programs to develop written protocols for the use of physical and pharmacologic restraints when combative or potentially combative patients are transported; (4) the need for programs to critically evaluate hot-loading and unloading policies and procedures and to ensure personnel assigned to hot load or unload do so only after proper training; and (5) the adoption of measures to maximize safety and reduce the potential of serious injury with use of helicopter design changes such as energy-attenuating seats, addition of shoulder harnesses to lap belts at each position in the aircraft, and development and installation of crash-resistant fuel systems in aircraft as soon as possible.

The 1988 NFNA position statement also dealt with specific in-flight duties to be performed by flight nurses to ensure a safe aviation environment. These responsibilities included: (1) securing equipment during flight; (2) use of seat belts and shoulder harnesses; (3) properly securing patients within the aircraft; (4) judicious use of night lighting; and (5) isolation of the pilot and controls from potential patient movement.

In 1998, the NFNA position paper was updated and expanded to include the following recommendations: (1) that flight nurses interact more with the PIC, participating in recurrent safety, premission, and postmission briefings; being taught how to report aircraft position; and undergoing crew member emergency training; (2) use of appropriate personal protective gear, including helmets, flame-resistant flight uniforms, and protective footwear; (3) stress-management programs to enhance flight nursing performance; and (4) use of back-up aircraft that are similar to the primary aircraft in the flight program.[42] These recommendations have since become part of routine operations for a large portion of the air medical industry.

In 2006, a third revision, *Transport Nurse Safety in the Transport Environment,* was published. It reinforced the positions stated in the first two editions of the paper and updated them to reflect the safety concerns of the medical transport industry in the early 21st century. The paper also expanded its focus to apply to transport nurses in all practice settings, including helicopter, fixed-wing, and ground patient transport.[1]

THE COMMISSION FOR ACCREDITATION OF MEDICAL TRANSPORT SYSTEMS

In 1990, the Commission for Accreditation of Medical Transport Systems (CAMTS) was established. The CAMTS accreditation standards require that "There is evidence that safety issues are addressed specific to the operational environment (i.e., weather, terrain, aircraft performance)." CAMTS standards also contain recommendations and requirements for weather minimums, safety management programs, accident/incident reporting, and pilot and flight crew training.[12]

THE AIR MEDICAL SAFETY ADVISORY COUNCIL

The Air Medical Safety Advisory Council (AMSAC) was organized by the Association of Air Medical Services (AAMS) in 2002 at the request of the FAA to address the increasing rate of air medical accidents. AMSAC is composed of representatives from AAMS, NEMSPA, ASTNA, FAA, National Aeronautics and Space Administration (NASA), insurance companies, and other industry groups. It serves as a forum to discuss the safety issues and concerns of the air medical community, including flight and duty time, fatigue countermeasures, minimum flight time standards, AMRM, data collection, accident/incident reporting, and shared critical maintenance information. A focus area for AMSAC has been the potentially negative effect of interprogram competition.[35]

VISION ZERO

In 2005, AAMS, in cooperation with many other organizations, launched the Vision Zero Initiative "to reduce and eliminate errors of consequence— those events within the transport medicine environment that result in serious injury or fatality"[3] by 80% in 10 years. The Vision Zero Initiative is intended to foster communication and cooperation between all aspects of the medical transport industry (safety organizations, professional associations, trade organizations, and regulatory agencies) to develop voluntary and regulatory measures to achieve the stated goals.[3]

VOLUNTARY SAFETY REPORTING

Voluntary safety reporting systems encourage individuals, transport programs, and aviation certificate holders to voluntarily report safety issues, concerns, and events. By submitting voluntary reports, programs and individuals may identify safety issues that affect more than just their program or agency and permit others to learn from their experience. The CONCERN Network (http://concern-network.org) is a voluntary reporting system whose purpose is "to increase awareness of safety hazards in the medical transport community." Transport programs submit reports of accidents or incidents, and bulletins are then distributed via e-mail to CONCERN Network subscribers and maintained in an online archive.[11] Transport team members may also submit anonymous reports. The FAA's Aviation Safety Action Program (ASAP) is designed to improve safety throughout the aviation industry. It allows participants to submit confidential reports that "identify actual or potential risks throughout their operations." All of the parties involved can then work together to develop or update operational practices to reduce the risk of accidents and other safety-related events.[18]

SAFETY MANAGEMENT

An effective comprehensive Safety Management System (SMS) should be a major part of all transport programs. The commitment to safety must include "… all disciplines and processes of the organization."[12] Safety needs to be a core component of the organizational culture of every transport program, from the CEO to the newest front-line employee.

The Accreditation Standards published by CAMTS list the components of a Safety Management System, which include[12]:

- Involvement of senior management.
- A safety committee.
- A nonpunitive system for employees to report hazards and safety concerns.
- A system to track, trend, and mitigate errors or hazards.
- A safety manual.
- Operational risk assessment tools.

- Ongoing safety training for all personnel (including managers).
- A system to audit and review organizational policy and procedures.
- A mechanism to ensure compliance with safety policies and procedures.

THE SAFETY COMMITTEE

The Safety Committee should be composed of representatives of all disciplines involved in the transport program: aviation, clinical, maintenance, communications, and administration. The committee should meet at least quarterly to address safety issues, practices, concerns, or questions. Reports of the committee's discussions and actions should be sent to the program's management and kept on file.

Other duties of the Safety Committee include planning and presenting annual safety training, interacting with the program's continuous quality improvement (CQI) and risk management systems, and tracking safety-related events. Information that results from the decisions and recommendations made by the Safety Committee should be communicated appropriately and, when indicated, incorporated into the program's policies, procedures, and operations.

SAFETY TRAINING
Operational Safety Training

All regular transport team members, and members of specialty teams who may also participate in transports, should receive regular operational safety training. Operational safety training should include air medical resource management (AMRM), mission planning, use of the program's operational risk assessment tools, aircraft and ground vehicle safety, emergency scene operations, and survival. In addition to scheduled didactic sessions, operational safety training should include regular aircraft or ground vehicle emergency drills.

Clinical Safety Training

Clinical safety training should review flight physiology and the stressors of flight, hazardous materials (HAZMAT) recognition and response, infection control, and the management of combative or violent patients. These subjects are addressed in detail in other chapters of this textbook. Other safety training topics may include employee wellness, injury prevention, and specific topics required by state, federal or local statutes.

Aircraft Safety Training

All flight crew members must be familiar with the aircraft in use by their program, including all regular and back-up aircraft operated by the program in which the crew member may be expected to fly. Specific items with which all crew members must be familiar for all aircraft include:

- Operation of seatbelts or harness.
- Operation of all doors and emergency exits.
- Emergency egress procedures.
- Emergency engine shutdown.
- Emergency communications.
- Oxygen and medical gas shut-off.
- Location and operation of onboard fire extinguishers.
- Location and use of other onboard emergency equipment, such as the survival kit, personal flotation devices, and aviation emergency oxygen systems.
- Hot-loading and offloading procedures and policies.

Ground Ambulance Safety Training

Ground ambulance safety should be a part of training of both ground and air transport providers. Air medical crews often are expected to transfer patients from an airport or other landing site to the hospital via ambulance. Ground vehicle safety training should include:

- Driver training (where applicable).
- Use of seatbelts by all crew members while the vehicle is in motion.
- Avoiding standing or kneeling in the patient compartment.
- Oxygen and medical gas shut-off.
- When to use red lights and siren (RLS) response.
- Securing equipment in the ambulance.
- Gurney operations and back/lifting safety.

Occupational and Workplace Safety Training

All crew members must be familiar with the safety procedures and requirements of the assigned workplace, whether in a hospital, at an airport, or at another location. Items with which all staff need to be familiar include the location and type of fire extinguishers, use of the fire extinguishers, the process for refueling aircraft or vehicles, HAZMAT or fuel spill response, electric and gas shut off, occupational injury or illness reporting, and site-specific procedures or practices, such as emergency evacuation routes.

Outreach Safety Education

Along with safety training for transport program staff, safety training and practice must be provided for first responders and others who may be asked to work around EMS aircraft. These personnel may include fire service, law enforcement, EMS, and park rangers or game wardens.

SAFETY IN THE TRANSPORT ENVIRONMENT

PERSONAL SAFETY

Personal safety is an important aspect of the safety attitude. For the individual crew member, personal safety is the mindset, habits, and daily practices that keep that individual safe. Each member of the transport team also bears the responsibility for the personal safety of others, including partner, pilot, patient, and fellow responders. For the transport service, personal safety means providing a safe work environment, appropriate personal protective equipment, and safety training and also involves establishing and following safety standards and policies. The best safety training and equipment in the world are of little value if not used properly, and safety standards cannot be effective if they are not followed.

Fitness Standards

The transport environment is physically challenging and requires that transport team members maintain a high personal level of both physical and emotional fitness. Requirements of each program vary, and no industry-wide formal guidelines exist.[53] Minimal physical requirements of any person working in the medical transport environment should include

the ability to work within the space limitations of the transport aircraft and vehicles operated by the program, to lift and carry a reasonable amount of weight, and to function in the typical work environments encountered by the program, such as scene calls. Transport team members must not have any preexisting conditions that could interfere with flexibility, strength, or cardiovascular fitness. Transport team members also must not have any condition that could cause altered mental or neurologic function.

Fatigue Policies

Studies on the effects of fatigue on performance have shown that they are similar to the effects of alcohol. Fatigue has been found to be a factor in a significant number of aviation mishaps and accidents. It should be addressed in the same fashion as other risks, especially during night operations.[52] Transport programs need to have policies in place to address crew fatigue. Crew members should have the right to call time out from flight duties if they or a fellow flight team member feel that continuing duty is unsafe because of fatigue, no matter what the shift length. No adverse personnel action or undue pressure to continue should occur.[2,12]

Pregnancy

Many women of childbearing age work in the transport setting. No existing industry standard is found regarding pregnancy employment policies.[17] The effects of high altitude, high noise levels, and vibration and the increased risk for injury in mishaps have been identified as potential risks to the fetus and maternal health.[36] Transport team members who are considering pregnancy should discuss these risks with their personal physician and program administration.

PERSONAL PROTECTIVE EQUIPMENT

The 1988 NTSB study recommended that air medical personnel who routinely fly EMS helicopter missions wear protective clothing and equipment to reduce the chance of injury or death in survivable accidents.[25] The ASTNA position papers have also endorsed the use of protective equipment. Protective equipment consists of helmets, fire-resistant uniforms, and boots.

Helmets

In the military, the use of flight helmets has been shown to protect significantly against head injuries.[15] Despite the obvious advantages afforded by flight helmets, acceptance in civilian air medical programs was not initially widespread. Reasons cited for not wearing helmets included high cost, uncertain benefit, and negative public relations.[33] However, a survey performed to determine the public's perception of helmet usage found that patients and family members positively viewed the use of helmets by air medical personnel.[50] In recent years, the use of helmets by EMS pilots and flight crew members has become the accepted standard.

The flight helmet must be approved for use in helicopters. The chinstrap should hold the helmet firmly in place, and the liner needs to fit comfortably. Some manufacturers use customized liners that are molded to the individual's head. The helmet visor should be kept in the down position as much as possible during flight.

Fire-Resistant Clothing

The goal of fire-resistant clothing is to minimize skin exposure to the intense heat of an aircraft fire. The uniform should have long sleeves and be made of a flame-resistant heat-resistant material such as Nomex. Flame-resistant fabrics are designed to withstand high temperatures for a brief period, usually less than 20 seconds, which permits the wearer to evacuate a burning aircraft or vehicle.[27] The fabric can reduce the risk or severity of tissue damage but does not prevent thermal injury to the skin.

Undergarments worn under the fire-resistant flight suit (including briefs, t-shirt, or long underwear) should be made of natural fibers, such as cotton, silk, or wool.[25] When exposed to flames, synthetic materials such as polyester or polypropylene melt and become embedded into the skin. The uniform should also fit to allow 0.25 inch of air space between the flight suit and undergarments. Nomex gloves protect the hands and should be considered by persons who wear fire-resistant uniforms.

Protective Footwear

Boots should protect the foot from punctures, lacerations, and thermal injuries and provide stability to the ankle on rough or uneven ground. Boots should be constructed of leather, or leather and Nomex, and extend several inches above the ankle. The sole should be thick and oil-resistant, and the boot should have a safety toe and shank. The boot should also have adequate ventilation to prevent moisture from being trapped.

Hearing Protection

The average sound level produced by a running helicopter is between 90 and 100 dB. The Occupational Safety and Health Administration (OSHA) regulations require employers to provide hearing-conservation programs for employees exposed to time-weighted average sound levels of 85 dB or greater. Hearing protection, such as earplugs, earmuffs, or the flight helmet, should be worn during high decibel exposures such as engine start-up, hot loading and unloading, extreme noise levels at some scenes, and around running aircraft at airports. Earplugs are smaller and less expensive, but noise protection varies with fit; custom-fitted earplugs provide the most noise reduction. Earmuffs offer more uniform protection but are more expensive, are not as easily carried or stored, and may be less comfortable than earplugs. A properly fitted flight helmet provides adequate hearing protection for most individuals and should be worn at all times while in flight. Active noise reduction (ANR, or noise canceling) circuitry or communications earplugs (CEP) can be added to most flight helmets to provide further noise attenuation.

PATIENT SAFETY

Along with the safety of the transport team, the safety of the patient being transported must be assured. The patient should be properly restrained in the transport vehicle and provided with appropriate hearing and thermal protection.[12] All patient care should be performed in a safe manner. Clinical decision making, patient treatment, and error reporting are all discussed elsewhere in this textbook, but each has a significant impact on patient safety. Keeping the patient safe should be an equally important part of the safety attitude.

OPERATIONAL SAFETY

AIRCRAFT SAFETY

Helicopter Safety

The most obvious component of the helicopter that presents a risk is the rotor system. The main rotor blades turn at approximately 400 rpm, with the rotor tips moving at more than 500 mph. At full speed, the main rotor blades create a disk that can be seen above the cabin. When the main rotor is spinning at lower speeds, such as during the start-up and shut-down phases, the blades can flap or sail with wind gusts, which may allow the blades to drop below shoulder level. The degree to which this presents a hazard varies by aircraft model and design, but the best precaution is to never approach or depart any helicopter during start-up or shut-down. The crouch position is advised for anyone approaching or departing the aircraft at other times while the blades are turning. When a helicopter lands on uneven ground or on a slope, the rotor disk comes closer to the ground on the uphill side. In this situation the aircraft should always be approached and departed from the downhill side in the crouched position, with constant attention paid to the terrain and the rotor disc. Program policy dictates whether patients are loaded into the aircraft with the rotor system turning, commonly referred to as *hot loading*. When loading or unloading patients and equipment, nothing should ever be carried above the head.

The tail rotor is potentially the most hazardous component of the helicopter. At a speed greater than 2000 rpm, it is nearly invisible. Aircraft manufacturers have worked to reduce the risks presented by the tail rotor by developing safer designs, such as the shrouded fenestron and no-tail-rotor (NOTAR) systems. A safety person should be designated at all unsecured landing sites to ensure that no one inadvertently walks near the tail rotor. Figure 9-3 shows an example of an aircraft with a shrouded fenestron tail rotor.

All persons who approach the helicopter must do so in full view of the pilot and should not proceed under the rotor disc without the pilot's permission. The safest approach zone for most helicopters is from the sides, at the 3 o'clock or 9 o'clock position (12 o'clock is the nose of the aircraft; Figure 9-4).

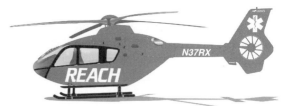

FIGURE 9-3   **Eurocopter EC-135 helicopter, showing its shrouded fenestron tail rotor system.** (Courtesy REACH Air Medical Services.)

Some aircraft models permit a safe approach from the front, depending on rotor or skid height and aircraft design. Flight crew members must be familiar with the safe approach zones for their program's aircraft. Those who work around the aircraft, such as EMS personnel, must be instructed to remain back from the aircraft after it lands and to approach only after being directed to do so by the pilot or a flight crew member and to never approach the aircraft from the rear.

The wind created by the moving rotor blades, referred to as *rotor wash,* can exceed 50 mph. In a hover and on the ground during the warm-up or cool-down stage, a rotor wash of approximately 25 mph can occur. Crew members should keep helmet visors down or wear protective glasses when operating around the running aircraft. All loose objects near the helicopter must be secured to prevent them from being blown away or ingested into the air intake of the helicopter's engine. Rotor wash also increases the wind-chill factor. An air temperature of 10°F combined with a 25-mph rotor wash creates a wind-chill temperature of −11°F.[8] Flight crew members need to consider this and take steps to protect the patient before loading. Other hazardous areas that should be avoided include the engine exhaust ports (the exhaust temperature is approximately 400°C) and the pitot tubes, used to measure the aircraft's airspeed and heated to prevent ice formation, which presents a burn hazard.

Fixed-Wing Aircraft Safety

Fixed-wing aircraft have their own set of safety requirements. The propellers carry the same risk of injury as the rotors on a helicopter, and jet engines present risks from both the engine exhaust and the

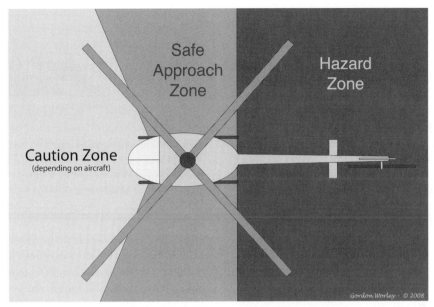

FIGURE 9-4   **Typical safe helicopter approach zones.**

possibility of aspiration into the engine intakes. No one should be allowed to approach the aircraft until the engines have been shut down. Many fixed-wing aircraft used as air ambulances have pressurized cabins, which permit flight at higher altitudes. All crew members need to be familiar with how to ensure that the hatches are properly sealed and with emergency procedures in the event of cabin depressurization.

Ground Ambulance Safety

Study results of ground ambulance crashes described previously show that the high-risk environments for ground ambulance operations are emergency responses and intersections. Regulations for emergency response with use of red lights and siren (RLS) vary from state to state, but generally the decision is left to the transport team. In deciding whether or not an RLS response is necessary, the safety of all involved needs to be considered. Ground vehicle safety and driver training programs need to provide guidance regarding when to operate in the RLS mode. Air transport programs should also educate their crews about when to use RLS in a ground vehicle. Use of proper safety equipment in ground vehicles should be just as important as in aircraft.

Seatbelts should be worn in both the front seat and the patient compartment, and all equipment should be properly secured.

DAILY PREFLIGHT PROCEDURES

At the beginning of each duty shift, the pilot and flight crew should complete an aircraft safety inspection. This inspection should include an overall walk-around inspection of the aircraft and a check of onboard safety equipment. The pilot and flight crew should also perform their respective daily checklists and ensure that the aircraft is ready to respond. The daily risk assessment should be performed, and the pilot should brief the crew regarding weather, expected maintenance or other issues related to the aircraft, and any specific mission-planning needs.

DISPATCH/COMMUNICATIONS

The 2006 NTSB report recommended that air medical programs be dispatched from a dedicated flight dispatch center, separate from any hospital or public safety dispatch center. The report also recommended expanding the role of the flight dispatcher/communications specialist to include specialized training in aviation weather, navigation, aircraft weight and balance planning, instrument approaches, and other aviation topics.[48] The intent of these recommendations was not to take any decision-making authority away from the pilot or flight crew but to provide a resource to the pilot for informed safe decisions. Communications and the role of the communications specialist are discussed in detail in Chapter 8.

An important safety consideration during the dispatch of a mission is that the communications specialist should provide the pilot with the information needed to make the decision regarding whether or not the mission can be safely accepted but should not include any patient-specific information. The initial notification of the pilot should include:

- Nature of the request (scene call versus interfacility transfer).
- Location of the request.
- Destination (if known).
- Patient weight (if known).
- Whether another aircraft or program has declined the request, and the reason for any such decline.
- Known weather or other hazards.

Once the pilot has evaluated the request and made the decision that the mission can be safely accepted, additional patient information may be communicated. An alternative method is to have the communications specialist contact the clinical crew separately and provide them with the patient information. The clinical crew should not discuss the patient with the pilot until a decision has been made as to whether the mission can be safely accepted. The clinical crew should under no circumstances pressure the pilot to accept a mission on the basis of patient needs if the mission has been declined for safety reasons.

HELIPAD/AIRPORT SAFETY

Hospital and off-site helipads should be designed to meet all applicable FAA and local regulations and should be able to safely accommodate the weight and size of the largest helicopter expected to use the helipad (Figure 9-5). Other helipad planning considerations include approach and departure routes, the location of the helipad relative to patient care areas, the provision of emergency exits, fire protection

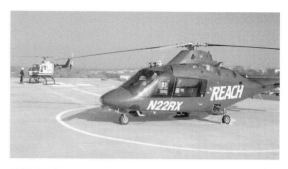

FIGURE 9-5   **Marked rooftop helipad with space for two aircraft.** (Photograph courtesy Denise Drinkhall.)

equipment, and helipad lighting.[38] Provisions also need to be made for snow removal, fuel/HAZMAT/biohazard spills, and general cleaning. The helipad should be secured and monitored to prevent access by unauthorized persons. All flight crew members should be trained in fire safety and should know the location of fire alarm boxes and fire extinguishers. Smoking should be prohibited around or near the aircraft.

Crew members of aircraft based at airports need to be familiar with the safety and security requirements of the airport, the location of fire extinguishers and other emergency equipment at the base, and the methods of reporting an emergency to the FAA control tower (if present), airport administration, and local authorities. Other safety considerations at airports include access to restricted areas, awareness of runway/taxiway safety, and operations around other aircraft.

IN-FLIGHT SAFETY

In-flight safety begins with pre-liftoff checks of the aircraft to ensure that all doors and outside cowlings are secure, that engine and other covers/tie downs have been removed, that shoreline electric cords have been disconnected, and that the aircraft is ready for departure. It also includes the use of safety equipment such as helmets, seatbelts, and shoulder harnesses during all phases of flight. At times, patient needs may necessitate that a crew member come "out-of-belt," but this should be done only while in level flight and with the approval of the pilot, and the belts should be reapplied as soon as possible.

Situational Awareness

Situational awareness refers to the maintenance of an active awareness of all aspects of the flight environment. This awareness includes scanning for other aircraft, listening to radio traffic, maintaining a sterile cockpit during critical phases of flight, and observing for hazards on approach to scenes or other unfamiliar landing areas. Crew members should always advise the pilot when they need to be "eyes in," with their attention focused inside the aircraft for patient care or other reasons.

Crew members should scan for other air traffic as much as possible, especially when no patient is on board. They need to report any obstacle or other air traffic, even though the pilot may have already seen it. Traffic or other hazards should be reported with use of clock position, with 12 o'clock being the nose of the aircraft and 6 o'clock being the tail. The location should further be identified as high, level, or low. One effective technique for scanning is the front-to-side method. This method involves starting with a fixed point in the center of the front windshield, slowly moving the field of vision leftward, returning to the center, refocusing, and then moving the eyes to the right. Other scanning techniques are available, and selection of one is a matter of preference, but the technique should involve some series of fixations. When the head is in motion, vision is blurred, and the mind does not register targets as easily.

Sterile cockpit refers to restricting all nonessential communications over the aircraft intercom system. Federal Aviation Regulations (FAR 135.100) require observance of sterile cockpit during all critical phases of flight. The critical phases of flight include taxi, takeoff, landing, and all other flight operations except cruise flight. Flight crew members should also attempt to maintain an awareness of the location of the aircraft along its flight path. Should a sudden emergency arise, quick communication of the aircraft's position may be necessary.

Flight Following

A crucial component of transport safety is having the location of the aircraft or vehicle known at all times, a process known as *flight following*. If an aircraft has any type of mishap that requires an emergency landing and the crew is unable to make a distress call, the flight following information permits the aircraft's position to be estimated with a high degree of accuracy. Typically, the communication specialist keeps abreast of the progress of the transport with periodic scheduled communications with the pilot or driver. Some programs use satellite-based real-time tracking systems that display the aircraft or vehicle location on a computer screen or map. Cellular telephones should not be used while in flight but may be used by ground transport teams to provide position/status reports.

When direct communications are not available, the pilot, driver, or crew should make contact with other transport program communications centers, emergency dispatch centers, airports, or hospitals along the flight or transport path and ask them to relay status reports. Flight following can also be requested from the FAA ATC system. Flight following with ATC has the added advantage of the aircraft being followed on radar by the controller.

Securing Patients and Equipment

The CAMTS accreditation standards specify that patients must be secured with a minimum of three cross straps that restrain the patient to the litter at the chest, hips, and knees. Patients who are loaded head forward should also be restrained with a shoulder harness. The belts need to be adjustable to accommodate patients with specific needs or injury locations. The patient must also be secured in such a way that they are isolated from the pilot and the controls. Pediatric patients should be restrained with an appropriately sized securing device. If a car seat is used, it must have an FAA approval sticker.[12]

Combative or potentially violent patients should be evaluated for the need for physical or chemical restraint before loading into the aircraft or vehicle. Physical restraints should be applied before takeoff. The use of physical or chemical restraints should be guided by program policies that are periodically reviewed and updated.

All bags and equipment must be secured while the aircraft or vehicle is in motion to prevent these objects from becoming projectiles and inflicting injuries to the patient or crew. Confirmation that all bags and equipment are properly secured should be a part of the pre-liftoff checks.

SCENE SAFETY

The EMS scene call environment is one of the most potentially hazardous aspects of air medical operations.[6] The number of variables is huge, and the flight crew has direct control over only a small portion of the operation. Situational awareness, attention to detail, communications skills, critical thinking abilities, and knowledge of program and local EMS policies all come into play during each scene response. Flight crew members who operate in the scene call environment should be familiar with the Incident Command System (ICS, also called the Incident Management System [IMS]), as it is used in their service area.[21]

Landing Zone Selection and Safety

Landing a helicopter at an unfamiliar location presents a variety of hazards. Each program should establish requirements for a suitable landing zone (LZ) for the program's aircraft. In general, the LZ should be at least 75 ft × 75 ft for daytime use and 125 ft × 125 ft or larger at night. Larger is always better. A useful way to determine whether a proposed LZ is suitable is the mnemonic HOTSAW (Box 9-1).

Although the pilot makes the ultimate decision about landing at any site, the initial selection and preparation of the landing zone are often the responsibility of the local fire department or EMS provider. Landing zone selection and preparation should be a part of routine outreach education provided to first responders. Training should also include a discussion of radio and visual communications procedures, use of eye and hearing protection, hot-loading procedures, and an aircraft-specific orientation.

Two-way radio contact should be established with the LZ coordinator as early as possible before arrival. The usual preference is to use a dedicated air-to-ground frequency for LZ communications, one that is not in use for other on-scene radio traffic. If a hazard is identified during approach or landing, the LZ coordinator needs to be able to notify the aircraft immediately. The pilot should perform a high reconnaissance,

BOX 9-1	HOTSAW: A Tool for Evaluation of Potential Landing Zones
Hazards	**Potential Hazards Within LZ** Rocks Downed timber Vegetation Fences Loose debris Vehicles
Obstructions	**Overhead Obstructions Along Flight Path Into or Out of LZ** Trees Hills Power lines Flag poles Buildings
Terrain	**Nature of LZ and Nearby Terrain Features** Elevation Uneven ground Creeks or ditches Surrounding terrain (mountains, cliffs, water, etc)
Surface/ Slope	**Nature of Surface** Character of surface: • Hard • Soft/muddy (risk of landing gear sinking) • Icy Loose surface materials that may blow in rotor wash: • Sand • Snow • Dirt • Dry vegetation Slope of ground
Animals	Domestic animals (horses, cows, dogs, etc) Wild animals Humans (bystanders and responders)
Wind/ Weather	Wind speed and direction Overall weather conditions (clouds, fog, height of cloud ceiling, precipitation, air temperature)

followed by a low reconnaissance, which allows the pilot and flight crew to observe for hazards before the final approach. If the pilot or crew detect a problem with the LZ, the landing should be aborted and the LZ coordinator informed of the issue. If the concern can be immediately corrected, then the site may be used. If the situation cannot be easily resolved, then a new LZ may need to be chosen.

An awareness of activities in and around the LZ is important at all times when the aircraft is on approach, on the ground, and departing. Ground personnel should only be allowed to approach the aircraft when directed to do so by the pilot or a flight crew member. On departing the scene, the flight crew should provide the LZ coordinator with a final report. A "thank you" to the ground crew for their help is always a good idea.

Multiple Aircraft Response

When more than one helicopter is on scene, or other aircraft are expected to land, clear communications must be maintained between the pilots of all aircraft and with the LZ coordinator. All air medical personnel on scene should remain in communication with their own pilot via radio and with the pilot or crew of any other helicopter on scene via direct radio contact, relay via their own pilot, or hand signals. Crew members should never approach or pass under or near the rotor disc of another aircraft without the knowledge and approval of the pilot of that aircraft.[49]

On-Scene Safety

Crew members must maintain an awareness of the hazards present in the prehospital setting. Unless specifically trained and authorized, transport team members should not participate in vehicle extrication or specialized rescue efforts. The extrication process should only be interrupted if immediate life-saving measures are needed, and then only if the procedure can be performed without unnecessary risk to the crew member or other rescuers. When responding to the scene of a violent crime, transport teams should always consult with law enforcement personnel to ensure the scene is safe before entering. When caring for a victim of a violent crime, care should be taken to disturb the scene no more than necessary to preserve possible evidence.

Hazardous Materials

Response to hazardous materials (HAZMAT) scenes must be done cautiously. The first priority is always the safety of the flight crew and aircraft. The LZ should be upwind of the incident and at a safe distance. Air medical personnel should not participate in the decontamination process for HAZMAT-exposed cases, regardless of any skills or experience the individual crew members may possess. HAZMAT-exposed cases should never be placed onboard the aircraft until they have undergone complete decontamination by a qualified HAZMAT team.

Postmission Debriefings

A preflight briefing is an important part of mission safety. A postmission debrief is equally, if not more, important. It permits the crew to come together and review the mission and identify issues or concerns about any aspect of the flight, including adequacy and accuracy of mission planning, operational safety and decision making, and clinical care of the patient. Debriefings can help to identify recurrent issues and mission-specific occurrences that need to be addressed. They may also identify risk factors that should be taken into account in the planning of subsequent missions.

IN-FLIGHT EMERGENCIES

An *in-flight emergency* is "a sudden unforeseen occurrence or incident requiring immediate action."[9] These events can range from the catastrophic failure of a critical aircraft component to a malfunction in an aircraft system that does not present an immediate risk but indicates that prompt action must be taken to prevent further problems. A common aviation description of how to manage an in-flight emergency is to *aviate, navigate, communicate.* The priorities are to maintain (or regain) control of the aircraft, decide on the next step, and select an appropriate emergency landing site (if indicated), and then report the emergency to the program communications center, ATC, or the local emergency dispatch center.[49]

The primary role of the flight crew member in an in-flight emergency situation is to serve as a resource to the pilot. Once the pilot has announced an emergency, the crew members should:

- Ensure sterile cockpit.
- Assist the pilot as needed or requested.
- Prepare self for an emergency landing: helmet strap tight, visor down, seatbelts snug.
- Prepare the patient for an emergency landing: position properly, secure/tighten seatbelts.
- Prepare the cabin for an emergency landing: secure equipment, shut off oxygen and inverter.
- Look for suitable emergency landing sites.
- Initiate emergency communications as directed by pilot.

Training in emergency procedures should be part of the safety training program, and proficiency should be demonstrated annually. Regularly scheduled emergency drills permit practice and increase familiarity with emergency procedures.

AIRCRAFT MECHANICAL EMERGENCIES

Mechanical emergencies involve a malfunction in some aspect of the aircraft's systems. Sensors are located in all of the aircraft's important systems to provide the pilot with a visual or audible warning if a problem occurs in that system. Some of these conditions can be managed in flight, and others require that the aircraft land to ensure safety. The pilot should inform the crew as soon as a potential mechanical emergency situation is identified and advise them whether or not an emergency landing is necessary.

AIRCRAFT FIRE EMERGENCIES

Aircraft fires can be divided into two broad categories: those that involve the engines and fuel system, and those that occur within the aircraft cabin. Engine fires usually trigger a warning light on the pilot's instrument panel and produce visible smoke. To confirm the presence of an engine fire on a helicopter, the pilot may put the aircraft into a gentle turn and ask the crew member on the side facing the inside of the turn to look back for a smoke trail. A confirmed engine fire is a serious emergency and requires that the affected engine be shut down. On twin-engine aircraft, emergency procedures should dictate that

the pilot request visual confirmation from the crew that the correct engine is being shut down before actually doing so. Some aircraft have built-in fire extinguishers in the engine compartments.

Smoke from an aircraft cabin fire can fill the cabin quickly and potentially incapacitate the crew. Fire extinguishers should be located within easy reach of all crew members. On larger aircraft in which the medical crew is separated from the pilot, a fire extinguisher should be located in each compartment. In the event of a cabin fire, the crew members should shut off the oxygen source, turn off the inverter, and close the windows and vents to prevent acceleration of the fire. If the fire is caused by medical equipment plugged into the aircraft power supply, the equipment should be turned off and unplugged and the inverter turned off. If smoke and heat become excessive, the crew should open windows or doors with discretion, fight the fire aggressively with the fire extinguisher, and prepare for an emergency landing.[37] Aircraft fire extinguishers are typically filled with halon, an inert gas that extinguishes fire by displacing oxygen. Halon extinguishers present the risk of asphyxiation when discharged in a closed space and should only be used in ventilated spaces. Fire extinguishers should only be discharged in the aircraft cabin at the direction of the pilot.

EMERGENCY COMMUNICATIONS

Emergency communications are ultimately the responsibility of the pilot but may be delegated to a crew member, depending on program policy. If a crew member is expected to make emergency radio calls, this responsibility should be clearly defined in the program's emergency procedures. Emergency radio calls should only be made at the direction of the pilot. All members of the flight team should be familiar with radio operations.

In the event of an emergency landing as a result of a serious situation (engine fire, etc), the term *Mayday* is used to ensure that the severity of the situation is clear to the receiving party and to indicate the need for additional assistance to respond to the emergency landing site (fire department, etc). A Mayday call indicates immediate serious distress and should only be used in a true emergency situation. The typical way to declare an emergency over the radio is: Mayday, mayday, mayday; (aircraft tail number/identifier) is making an emergency landing at (location) due to (nature of emergency).

In less serious situations that necessitate a precautionary landing, the appropriate description should be used, rather than a Mayday call. Include the location of the landing site and as much additional information as the circumstances dictate. In some situations, initial radio calls should be made to the local 911 emergency dispatch center. The local dispatch center may be easier to contact than the program's dispatch center and can rapidly mobilize any needed resources (fire department, ambulance, etc).

EMERGENCY LOCATOR TRANSMITTER

All EMS aircraft are required by the FAA to carry an emergency locator transmitter (ELT). The ELT is activated by an impact that exceeds $4g$ (4 times the force of gravity) and broadcasts a signal on one of the universal distress frequencies: 121.5 MHz, 243 MHz, or 406 MHz. The signal is received by the international COSPAS-SARSAT satellite system, and the information relayed to search and rescue (SAR) personnel. The radio signal generated by 121.5-MHz and 243.0-MHz ELTs does not pinpoint the position of the aircraft but gives rescuers a general area in which to begin a search. Newer 406-MHz ELTs transmit a digital signal that identifies the aircraft and contains global positioning system (GPS) position information.

As of February 1, 2009, the COSPAS-SARSAT system will no longer perform satellite-based monitoring of the 121.5-MHz or 243.0-MHz frequencies. After this date, 121.5-MHz and 243.0-MHz ELT distress signals will only be detectable by ground-based receivers or by other aircraft.[44] Existing 121.5-MHz/243.0-MHz ELTs will remain legal but will provide limited assistance for a downed aircraft, especially if the crash occurs in a remote location.

Flight team members should know the location of the ELT on all of their program's aircraft and how to ensure that it has been activated. If an impact does not automatically activate the ELT, it can be activated manually by following the directions on the front of the unit.

EMERGENCY LANDINGS

In an emergency or precautionary landing situation, in which a hard landing may be anticipated, flight crew members should assume the survival position before impact. They should sit upright with the knees together and feet approximately 6 inches apart. In forward-facing seats equipped with shoulder belts, one should hold the arms across the chest, forming an X with the forearms and grasping the shoulder harness. In forward-facing seats without shoulder belts, one should bend forward at the waist and encircle the knees with the arms. In aft-facing seats, one should sit upright with the head held against the seat head rest and the arms in a X across the chest. Crew members should keep a point of reference inside the cabin to maintain spatial orientation in case the aircraft comes to rest on its side or inverted.

EMERGENCY EGRESS

All crew members need to be prepared to manage the emergency evacuation of the crew and patient from all of the aircraft used by their program. After an emergency landing, disorientation is common, particularly if the aircraft is not upright. The only available route of egress may involve climbing up to a door or window, into the cockpit, over seats, or over other occupants of the aircraft. One should make a quick survey to reestablish spatial orientation and assess the condition of the aircraft, other crew members, and the patient. In night conditions or in smoke-filled cabins, spatial orientation can be maintained with the hand-over-hand method, where one hand is kept on a known reference point while a new reference point is selected with the other hand. After the aircraft has come to a complete stop, the aircraft should be exited by normal means when possible or by jettisoning doors, opening emergency exits, or using forcible means if necessary.[37]

Individual crew members should evacuate to a predesignated position, typically the 12 o'clock position off the nose of the aircraft, and evaluate the risk of fire and other hazards before attempting the rescue of injured or entrapped crew members or the patient. After a forced landing, a significant danger is fire. All crew members should be familiar with the emergency shutdown procedure for all aircraft in which they may be asked to operate and how to operate the fire extinguishers carried on the aircraft.

Emergency egress, aircraft evacuation, and emergency shutdown should be part of initial training for all crew members and should be practiced regularly. Crew members should keep in mind that they may need to perform postcrash emergency egress and evacuation when they themselves are injured. Practice and drills should include consideration of how to open emergency exits or perform emergency shutdown with only one arm and with other possible disabilities.

FORCED WATER LANDINGS

Air medical programs that frequently operate over large bodies of water need to ensure that all crew members are familiar with emergency egress procedures in the event of a forced water landing, or ditching. When flying over water, all flight team members should wear a personal flotation device (PFD). Aircraft PFDs should have an attached strobe light that automatically activates on contact with the water. Flight team members may consider wearing additional survival gear and signaling devices in a vest system. The ability to swim should be mandatory, and water egress procedures and open-water survival should be part of the training received by all flight team members. Each program should evaluate its risk of a water landing and provide specialized open-water survival equipment where appropriate.

In a ditching situation, jettisoning of doors and other emergency procedures should be performed under direction of the pilot. The sequence for emergency escape from an aircraft after a water landing is as follows:

Before Impact with the Water

1. Try to keep calm and concentrate on how you are going to get out.
2. Know which way the closest door is from your position.
3. Open or jettison doors as directed by the pilot.
4. Place one hand on a known reference point within the cabin.
5. Disconnect your ICS cable.
6. Place your other hand on the seatbelt buckle (do not release).

After Impact with the Water

7. Do not attempt to exit the aircraft until the rotor or propeller has stopped moving.
8. Helicopters almost always capsize after striking the water; do not attempt to exit the cabin until the aircraft is upside down.
   - Wait for the helicopter to all but fully fill with water.
   - Take a deep breath.
   - Release your buckle; you will immediately float.
   - Pull yourself towards the closest door and out.
   - Do not swim or kick; this increases the chance of becoming entangled and you may unintentionally kick other crew members.
   - Exhale slowly during ascent to the surface, to reduce the risk of pulmonary barotrauma.
   - If necessary, observe your air bubbles to determine which way is up.
9. Fixed-wing aircraft generally float for a few minutes.
   - Locate the safest exit route.
   - Open the appropriate door and crawl through.
   - Assist others in exiting.
   - Enter the water and move away from the fuselage before it sinks.
10. Do not inflate your life vest until outside and away from the aircraft.
11. If a helmet is worn, keep it on for insulation and visibility.

Open water survival is discussed in the Survival Basics section on the following page.

GROUND VEHICLE EMERGENCIES

All persons riding in the front seat of ground transport vehicle should wear their seatbelts at all times. Everyone in the patient compartment should remain in seatbelts as much as possible during patient care and stay in their seats with seatbelts secured at all other times. Programs should have response plans to address ground vehicle accidents, as well as aircraft accidents. All vehicles should be equipped with fire extinguishers, and emergency egress and evacuation training should be a part of annual training.

POSTCRASH RESPONSIBILITIES
Crew Responsibilities

After any crash or other accident, the crew should first ensure the safety of all on board the aircraft or vehicle. Then, the crew members should attend to any injuries that have occurred and attempt to contact help. Help may be the local emergency dispatch center, the program communications center, or the FAA. A 911 call from a cellular phone may be the easiest and most expedient way to accomplish contact help, if a cellular signal is found.

Missing or Overdue Aircraft or Ground Vehicle Procedure

The practice of flight or ground transport following should be a standard operating procedure in all transport programs. The communications specialist should maintain a constant awareness of the location of each aircraft or vehicle for which they are responsible. If a scheduled check in is missed, or arrival is overdue, the communication specialist should initiate the postaccident incident plan.

Postaccident Incident Plan

The *postaccident incident plan* (PAIP)[12] is a program policy document that outlines the responsibilities of the communication specialist and program administration in situations such as:

1. Unscheduled landing, which covers any emergency or precautionary landing.
2. Missing or overdue aircraft.
3. Declared aircraft emergency.
4. Confirmed aircraft accident.
5. Ground vehicle accident or emergency.

The initial response to a missing or overdue aircraft or vehicle should an attempt to locate the aircraft by contacting the FAA/ATC, EMS agencies, law enforcement agencies, other air medical programs, and airport facilities along the flight path. For other emergencies, the communications specialist should notify local fire and EMS resources of the incident and request a response to the emergency landing site. Provisions may be needed to continue the transport of the patient, in addition to management of the aircraft or vehicle emergency.

The PAIP should indicate which administrative personnel should be notified for each specific set of circumstances. In the event of an aircraft crash or other significant event, an administrative crisis team should be assembled. The members of this team and their duties should be clearly described in the PAIP. Emergency drills should be conducted on a regular basis, and the PAIP should be reviewed and updated regularly. A copy of the AAMS Postaccident Resource Document is contained in the appendices.

Critical Incident Stress Management

Any event that occurs that may have a stressful effect on the members of a transport program should be identified and the appropriate level of stress debriefing offered to the affected individuals. Critical incident stress and critical incident stress management (CISM) are discussed in more detail in Chapter 41.

THE SAFETY ATTITUDE REVISITED

The preceding sections of this chapter have discussed the historic and current safety records of the air medical industry and the initiatives, practices, and tools presently available to improve safety. These resources alone are not enough to prevent future tragedies. The vital component is the human factor. Every individual involved in medical transport must commit themselves to the development of a positive safety culture within their own program and throughout the industry. Each of us must stay informed about new safety practices and technologies and maintain an open mind about their use. Most importantly, we must each make good, safe, informed decisions about every aspect of every mission. We must all develop, maintain, and spread a safety attitude.

SURVIVAL BASICS

All medical transport crew members need to be prepared to face the possibility of a survival situation. The situation may result from an emergency landing in a remote location as a result of weather or mechanical issues or changes in the mission environment (such as weather deterioration while at a remote scene LZ). Ground transport vehicles may break down or be stranded by weather. Regardless of the cause, the essentials of survival remain the same.

The goal in a survival situation that involves a medical transport team and patient is survival until a rescue can be accomplished. Flight-following procedures provide the flight communications center with the general location of the incident. The emergency locator transmitter on the aircraft assists rescuers in locating the aircraft and crew. All air medical aircraft should be equipped with a complete survival kit, and all crew members should receive training in its use. Ground transport vehicles that operate in remote areas should also carry survival equipment. Crew members should be prepared to spend an unexpected 24 to 72 hours outdoors and be able to look after their own needs for that period.

PREPARATION AND PRIORITY SETTING

Successful survival strategy is based on two equally important concepts: preparation and priority setting.[14] In a survival situation, individuals who are both psychologically and physically prepared to survive and who can establish and address the priorities for their own survival needs have a much higher chance of surviving the situation.

Psychologic Preparation

The biggest threat to survival in any emergency situation is panic. Panic reduces the mind's ability to respond properly to a threat and leads to actions that may worsen the situation. Fear, anxiety, anger, and denial are all normal reactions to an emergency situation, but they need not lead to panic. Preparing oneself psychologically for a survival situation means developing a positive attitude about one's own abilities to manage such a situation. Practice and familiarity with the tools and skills necessary in a survival situation help to build self confidence and develop a positive "I can do this" attitude. The most valuable tool in one's survival kit is a mind that possesses a positive outlook.[31]

Psychologic preparation also involves preparing oneself for the possibility of being in a survival situation while injured or when others have been injured or killed in a crash. Practice and familiarity with survival skills, faith in the Search and Rescue (SAR) system, personal beliefs, and introspection can all help crew members to function and manage under such circumstances.

Physical Preparation

Physical preparation for survival consists of two primary areas: keeping oneself in good physical condition and the selection and carrying of the items needed for a survival situation. A good physical fitness routine is important for everyone, but the demands of a survival situation make good physical condition even more important.

Clothing and Personal Equipment

Clothing is the first line of defense against the environment and needs to be selected on the basis of the nature of that environment. Clothing should protect the wearer, be comfortable and practical, and meet the fire safety guidelines described previously. Garments should be layered; this method traps the most dead air, provides the best insulation, and allows adjustment as environmental conditions change.[8] Even if the weather appears mild, a jacket should be taken on all transports. Gloves and a warm hat or cap should be carried during cold weather. Warm-weather clothing should protect against the sun. Long sleeves and pants legs, together with head and eye protection, diminish water loss and heat exposure.

Personal equipment includes a personal survival kit and other items carried by the crew member. The most well-designed and comprehensive aircraft or vehicle survival kit is not of much use if it is not accessible because of damage to the aircraft, fire, or injury.[54] Each crew member should carry basic survival items on their person (see Box 9-1).

Priority Setting

To establish the priorities in a survival situation, follow the *Rule of Threes*. The average person can survive 3 minutes without oxygen, 3 hours without shelter in extreme conditions, 3 days without water, and 3 weeks without food.[25] Once safety and immediate medical concerns have been addressed, the Rule of Threes should guide priority setting. The two biggest killers in the outdoors are inadequate thermoregulation (lack of shelter) and dehydration (lack of water).[34] With this in mind, the immediate priorities should be finding or creating shelter, building a fire, taking steps to maintain hydration, and signaling by whatever means are possible.

SURVIVAL SKILLS

The subject of emergency survival cannot be covered fully in this brief section. Transport programs should conduct annual survival training to ensure that all crew members have the necessary knowledge and skills. Survival training should include hands-on practice with all of the items in the aircraft or vehicle survival kit and a review of survival strategies for a variety of environmental conditions, with emphasis on how to prepare for those that exist in the program's service area. Transport team members are encouraged to consult other sources of information to improve their individual survival knowledge and skills, including the references listed at the end of this chapter, other survival manuals, and outside survival classes.

Shelter

An emergency shelter should be as simple to construct as possible and provide protection from wind, rain, snow, sun, extremes in temperatures, and animals. The shelter should be big enough to protect all survivors and their survival equipment but not so large as to be difficult to construct or to heat. Shelter building should be practiced during survival training.

The aircraft or vehicle should be the first choice for an emergency shelter. If the aircraft or vehicle is used for shelter, ensure that it is stable and will not roll or tilt on the terrain or during adverse weather. Any holes should be patched with sheets, tarps, or space blankets. All windows and exposed metal should be insulated to reduce heat loss. Avoid sleeping on, or placing the injured on, exposed metal or directly on the ground. Aircraft are usually poorly insulated; in cold weather, construction of a shelter near the aircraft that can be heated with a fire may be a better choice.[8]

If the aircraft or vehicle is not available or safe, a shelter must be located or constructed. Natural shelters such as caves, rock overhangs, or large trees may be available. Look for potential hazards such as dead trees or tree limbs that may fall in a strong wind, rock slides, caves with other inhabitants (such

as bears, skunks, or cougars), and tall trees or rocks that may conduct lightning. If a shelter needs to be constructed, the first step is locating a suitable site. When selecting the site, attempt to[40]:

1. Stay as close to the aircraft or vehicle as possible.
2. Find a spot that is protected from the prevailing wind.
3. Avoid natural hazards such as overhanging tree branches, avalanche or rock fall chutes, and steep terrain.
4. Find a level spot that will stay dry; avoid dry stream beds that could flood.
5. Avoid low-lying areas that collect cold air.
6. Orient the door of the shelter towards the east, so that the morning sun will warm the shelter.

Shelters can be constructed with a variety of natural materials, supplies from the survival kit, and items from the aircraft or vehicle. Examples are shown in Figure 9-6. Natural materials that may be used for shelter construction include trees, branches, brush, logs, and rocks. In snow country, trench shelters are quick and easy to construct. Aircraft and vehicle parts that may be useful include doors (shelter panels), foam from seats or litters (insulation), and wiring (for tying or lashing). Large heavy-duty plastic trash bags are useful for constructing shelters. An individual can use one bag as a bivvy sack, or bags may be opened up and used as a tarp to build a lean-to. They can also be used to waterproof shelters constructed from brush or branches or to create a roof for a snow shelter. Mylar plastic space blankets are compact to store and effective at reflecting heat but tear easily and are noisy in windy conditions.[8] Corners, edges, and stress points on space blankets or plastic bags can be reinforced with duct tape.

Fire Building

A fire provides warmth, light, and a sense of security. If adequate clothing and shelter are available, a fire may not be needed for warmth. When the need is recognized, prepare the materials and start the fire before dark. Gather enough firewood to last through the night. Locate the fire so that it provides as much heat to the inside of the shelter as possible, and contain it within some type of boundary to prevent its

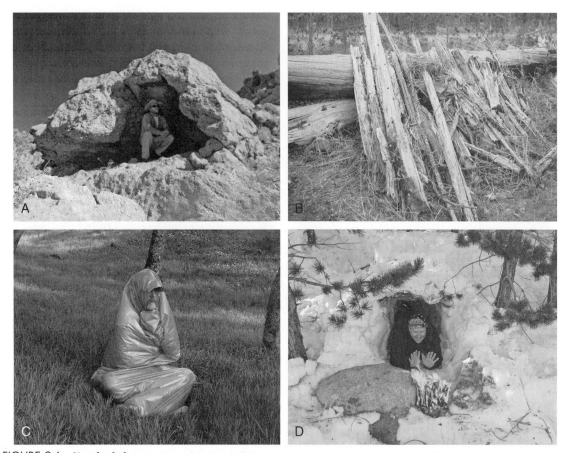

FIGURE 9-6   Simple shelters. A, Natural shelter: shallow cave in the desert; **B,** lean-to shelter made from natural materials; **C,** large heavy-duty plastic garbage bag may be used as a bivvy sack; and **D,** snow trench shelter.

spreading by accident. In high fire danger conditions, exercise caution when building any fire.

Many methods of fire building and many ways to start a fire can be used, including waterproof matches, lighters, and "metal matches," which create a shower of sparks when scraped with a steel edge (Figure 9-7). At least two reliable methods of starting a fire should be packed in the survival kit. Matches (even waterproof matches) should be stored in a waterproof match safe. Transport team members need to be familiar with the use of all of the fire starting tools carried in the survival kit.

The simplest way to build a fire is to create a teepee of small sticks or kindling over a pile of fine dry tinder. On damp ground or snow, build the teepee on top of a platform of large dry sticks. Use the available fire-starting equipment to create a flame in the tinder. As the tinder ignites and begins to set the small sticks on fire, slowly add small and progressively larger kindling to the fire. As the fire grows, larger pieces of wood may be added. Practice with the techniques of fire building should be a part of all survival training.

Hydration

Maintenance of adequate hydration is important in the survival setting. Each person should drink at least 1 to 1.5 L of water daily in temperate conditions. Extremes of temperature (hot or cold) and exertion can dramatically increase water requirements. A good rule of thumb is to drink enough water to produce at least 1 liter of urine every 24 hours.[40] Conserve available water stores by rationing until a water source

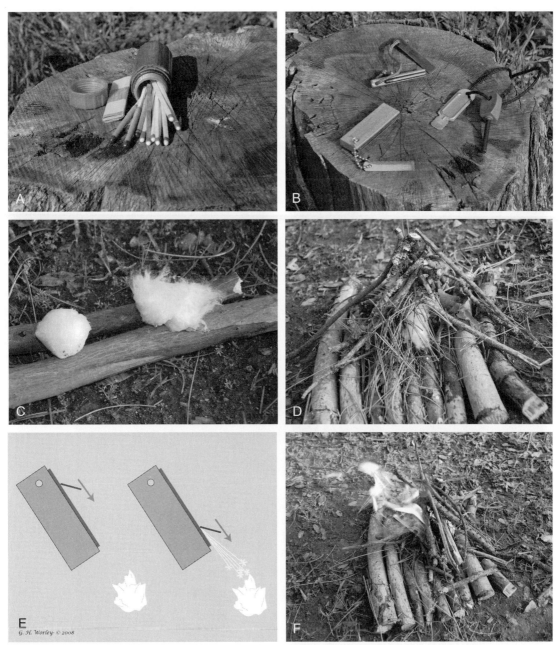

FIGURE 9-7 **Fire building. A,** Commercial storm-proof matches *(left)* and strike-anywhere kitchen matches, waterproofed with clear nail polish *(right)*, in a waterproof match safe. **B,** A variety of metal matches are available; all incorporate a piece of mish-metal that creates sparks when scraped with a steel edge. **C,** A cotton ball smeared with petroleum jelly makes effective tinder *(left)*; 6-8 will fit into a film can. To use, pull the cotton ball apart to expose the inner fibers *(right)*, which ignite easily.[34] **D,** Basic fire teepee with cotton ball tinder in the center. The tinder can be ignited with matches or a metal match. **E,** Hold the tip of the metal match about an inch from the tinder and scrape the mish-metal insert with the striker, directing the shower of sparks onto the tinder. **F,** As the fire builds, slowly add small and progressively larger kindling.

is located. All surface water must be purified before drinking by boiling, filtration, or using water-purification tablets to prevent gastrointestinal (GI) infection from bacteria, viruses, or parasites. GI infections can lead to vomiting and diarrhea and cause significant water loss and worsening dehydration.

In woodland environments, water can be collected with a transpiration bag (Figure 9-8). Place a plastic bag over a tree branch, ideally in the sun, with a small clean rock in one corner of the bag. The leaves or needles transpire water vapor, which then condenses and collects on the inside of the bag. Dew can be collected from leaves, plastic sheets, or the outside of the aircraft. If rain is expected, set up a method of catching the rainfall. Do not eat snow; this can cause substantial heat loss. Snow may be melted over a fire or by placing a canteen filled with snow in the sun or between the outer and inner layers of one's clothing. Protect water from freezing, keeping the container inside the shelter or under the outer clothing. In the desert, efforts to find and collect water may return less water than the amount that is lost in sweat. If

rescue can be expected shortly, conserve water by resting in a shaded location and minimizing water loss from sweating.

Signaling

Once basic needs have been met, signaling becomes the next priority. As soon as an aircraft is reported overdue, SAR resources are mobilized. SAR aircraft initially search for transmissions from the aircraft radio and ELT. If the aircraft radio and the ELT are not operational, other methods of signaling must be used. Signals in groups of three are recognized internationally as distress signals.[13] Visual signals should have as much movement and contrast with the environment as possible.

1. *Portable radios and cell phones:* Aviation portable radios should be tuned to the last known ATC frequency or the emergency frequency (121.5 MHz). Conserve the batteries, turning on the radio to transmit only when an aircraft is heard. Cellular phone service now covers an extensive area in North America; a cellular signal may be obtainable even in remote locations.

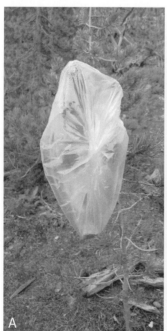
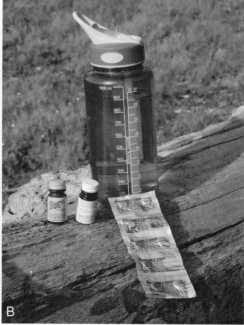

FIGURE 9-8   **Hydration. A,** Transpiration bag tied around a tree branch; and **B,** water purification tablets. Be sure to follow the manufacturer's instructions for each type.

2. *Smoke and fire:* In addition to providing warmth, the fire is a valuable signaling tool. At night, a fire can be visible for many miles. Smoke is an effective way to signal search-and-rescue aircraft during daylight. The addition of green leaves, grass, or water to the fire creates white smoke. The addition of oil, rubber, plastic, or pitchy wood creates black smoke. A can filled with sand and oil burns and generates black smoke for a long period of time. Use the color of smoke that provides the most contrast with the background.

3. *Flashlights, strobes, and flares:* A flashlight or a small lightweight strobe light can be an effective signal at night. Flares can be used if they are available in the aircraft but should be used with caution during high fire danger conditions. Many SAR aircraft are now equipped with night-vision goggle (NVG) technology. Even the smallest light is visible for many miles to searchers with NVGs.

4. *Signal mirror:* All crew members should practice signaling with the signal mirror. The preferred type of mirror is one made of laminated safety glass with a sighting hole in the center. Flash the mirror in the direction of any aircraft that can be heard, even if it cannot be seen. Other shiny objects such as CDs, cans, foil, or aircraft parts may be used as improvised signal mirrors.

5. *Clothing and other colored objects:* Brightly colored parkas, space blankets, plastic garbage bags, signal panels, or other items that provide a contrast with the colors of the surrounding environment are useful signals. These may be placed on the ground in a geometric pattern or waved to create maximal visibility.

6. *Whistle:* A plastic whistle provides an effective way to signal ground SAR units. Use of a whistle is much more efficient than shouting. The standard signal is three blasts, pause, three more blasts, then listen for a reply.

7. *Ground to air signals:* Signals may be created by piling debris, digging trenches, or stamping out patterns in snow or sand. The most easily recognized patterns are a large X or the letters S-O-S.

8. *Dyes:* Dyes are effective in water and on snow. Fine dyes should be used downwind.

Food

The need for food is a low priority during a survival situation of fewer than 4 to 5 days. Although not a direct threat to survival in the short term, depleted energy stores can have other negative effects, including depression and diminished problem-solving capabilities. In cold weather, lack of calorie intake can increase the risk of hypothermia.

Overland Travel and Navigation

The first rule in a downed aircraft situation is to stay with the aircraft; it is what searchers are looking for. Consider overland travel only in case of a clearly identified need, such as an injured person who needs immediate medical attention. Land navigation skills require training and practice. Cross-country travel should only be attempted by individuals who possess the necessary experience and skills and who have a clear picture of the route they need to follow to reach a location where help may be obtained. If the decision is made to leave the aircraft, leave a detailed note listing the number of survivors, their condition, the intended route of travel, and the intended destination. Mark the outbound route with visible markers, such as strips of brightly colored cloth or surveyor's tape, to permit retracing the route of travel (if necessary) and aid searchers in following the trail. In most situations, the best decision is to stay put and devote one's energy to shelter building, water procurement, and signaling.[40]

SPECIFIC ENVIRONMENTAL CONSIDERATIONS

Transport programs that operate in regions that have specific environmental conditions or seasonal weather patterns should conduct specialized survival training focused on those environments.

Water Landings and Open Water Survival

The process for emergency aircraft evacuation after a water landing is described previously in the In-Flight Emergencies section. After impact with the water, the first priorities are to evacuate the aircraft, account for all persons who were onboard, and move to safe location away from the sinking aircraft. A prearranged rendezvous spot should be part of the emergency evacuation plan. If the accident occurs close to shore, consider swimming towards the shore. Distances can be hard to estimate, and one can easily become exhausted when swimming against waves or current.

If the distance does not seem to be within the survivor's capabilities to swim, or if one of the survivors is injured, the best option may be to minimize heat loss with the heat escape-lessening posture (HELP) shown in Figure 9-9. Remain still and assume the fetal position, crossing your arms over your chest and bringing your knees up to your chest. A PFD must be worn when assuming the heat escape-lessening posture to stay afloat.[16] Surviving flight team members should huddle together to decrease heat loss. The flight helmet should be worn in the water; it provides insulation and improved visibility to searchers. Protect against salt and sun exposure by covering any exposed skin surface. Protection against hypothermia, care of the raft (if used), and signaling are the primary objectives in open-water survival.

Desert Survival

Desert areas can reach ambient temperatures of more than 120°F (50°C) during the day and drop to below freezing at night. Maintain an awareness of heat exposure and illness, minimize exertion, and rest in the shade as much as possible. Sheltering in the shade of the aircraft may be preferable to the interior during the daytime. Wear long sleeves and long pants, along with head and neck protection, sunglasses, and sunscreen. Water collection, hazardous plants and animals, and desert shelter construction should all be part of desert survival training.

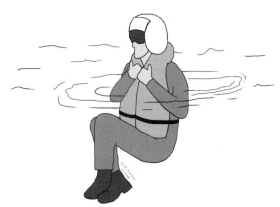

FIGURE 9-9   **Heat escape-lessening posture (HELP).**

Cold Weather Survival

Transport programs that operate in areas that have significant snowfall should conduct specialized winter survival training, including snow shelter construction, water procurement, fire building in winter conditions, and the use of any specialized equipment in the survival kit (tents, snowshoes, etc). Adequate clothing, sunglasses, and sunscreen should be worn or carried when operating in cold weather conditions.

International Survival Concerns

Flight teams who may cross international boundaries need to consider international survival concerns. Air medical team members should be aware of the climate and terrain of the areas that they fly over and of the final destination of the mission. Recognition of the need for additional survival equipment and food stores should be part of mission planning. In some countries, SAR resources are limited, and in many others, they are nonexistent.

PATIENT CARE IN A SURVIVAL SITUATION

In addition to looking after their own needs, a stranded transport team may also need to care for a patient or an injured team member. The first priority is to ensure the safety of everyone involved before starting medical care. Providing shelter and warmth for the injured should be a high priority and take precedence over everything except interventions to address life-threatening conditions. Ration patient care supplies, such as oxygen and intravenous (IV) fluids, and use battery-powered equipment to monitor the patient intermittently to conserve battery life. Mental and emotional preparation for an unfavorable patient outcome is also important, particularly if rescue is delayed.

SURVIVAL EQUIPMENT

Survival equipment should be carried on all air medical aircraft and on ground transport vehicles that operate in remote or severe weather settings. The specifics of the service area, climate, type of aircraft or vehicle, and time of year should all be considered in selection of survival equipment and supplies. The survival kit should be assembled and stored in a manner that affords easy access, ideally in

BOX 9-2	Survival Kits

Basic Personal Survival Equipment (Minimum Recommended List)

Flashlight or headlamp	Water bottle
Knife	Nylon cord
Plastic whistle	Sunglasses
Waterproof matches in match safe or other reliable method of fire starting	Space blanket or large heavy-duty plastic trash bag
Compass	Energy bars

Basic Aircraft Survival Kit

Flashlight or headlamp	Water-purification tablets or water filter
Plastic whistle	Water container
Waterproof matches in match safe	Nylon cord or rope
Second reliable method of fire starting (metal match, etc)	Space blankets or large heavy-duty plastic trash bags
Dry tinder (cotton balls/petroleum jelly)	Aluminum foil
Candle	
Knife	Signal mirror
Compass	Signal flares
Maps	Ax or saw
Insect repellant	Duct tape
Sunscreen	Pocket survival guide or card

Additional Aircraft Survival Kit Items (Depending on Operating Environment and Aircraft Type)

Tent	Appropriate additional clothing
Sleeping bags and pads	Tarps or plastic ponchos
Cook kit	Snowshoes
Stove	Snow shovel
Foodstuffs	Inflatable raft
Handheld GPS unit	Fishing kit
Strobe light	Canned smoke or smoke flares

the aircraft cabin. Flight crew members should carry basic survival equipment on their persons, in case the aircraft survival kit is damaged or inaccessible. Box 9-2 lists recommended items to be included in personal and aircraft survival kits.

SUMMARY

Safety should be the number one priority of all transport services. Safety is a pervasive attitude that must be supported by all transport team members.

Just as transport team members must be safe, they must also be prepared to survive. The goal in a survival situation that involves a medical transport team and patient is to survive until a rescue can be accomplished.

This chapter has provided an overview of two important transport concepts. Every individual, whether nurse, paramedic, physician, respiratory therapist, EMT, pilot, mechanic, communications specialist, or administrator, must accept personal responsibility for safety and be a safety advocate.

REFERENCES

1. Air and Surface Transport Nurses Association: *Transport nurse safety in the transport environment*, Greenwood Village, CO, 2006, ASTNA.

2. Air Medical Safety Advisory Council: *Recommended practice: medical crew rest guideli*nes, 2004, available at http://www.amsac.org/images/RecommendedPractice.pdf, accessed February 2008.

3. Association of Air Medical Services: *Vision zero whitepaper*, Alexandria, VA, 2005, AAMS, available at http://visionzero.aams.org, accessed February 2008.

4. Atlas and Database of Air Medical Services: *ADAMS annual public atlas*, ed 6, Buffalo, NY, 2006, ADAMS, available at http://www.adamsairmed.org/public_site.html, accessed November 2008.

5. Baker SP, Grabowski JG, Dodd RS, et al: EMS helicopter crashes: what influences fatal outcome? *Ann Emerg Med* 47(4):351-355, 2006.

6. Blumen IJ, et al: *A safety review and risk assessment in air medical transport*, Supplement to the Air Medical Physician Handbook, Salt Lake City, 2002, Air Medical Physicians Association.

7. Blumen IJ: *HEMS accidents: reasons, rates, risks and recommendations*, presented at the Critical Care Transport Medicine Conference, 2006, Las Vegas.

8. Bowman WD, Kummerfeldt P: Essentials of wilderness survival. In Auerbach PS, editor: *Wilderness medicine*, ed 5, Philadelphia, 2007, Mosby.

9. Castro R: *Emergency and pre-accident plans*, Alexandria, VA, 1988, Flight Safety Digest, Flight Safety Foundation, available at http://www.flight-safety.org/fsd/fsd_may88.pdf, accessed March 2008.

10. Code of Federal Regulations: *Title 49, Chapter VII: National Transportation Safety Board (49CFR830.2)*, Washington, DC, 2007, US Government Printing Office, available at http://www.access.gpo.gov/nara/cfr/waisidx/49cfr830.html, accessed March 2008.

11. Concern Network: *Concern Network archive*, Greenwood Village, CO, 2008, available at http://www.concern-network.org/concern-archive/, accessed November 2008.

12. Commission on Accreditation of Medical Transport Services: *Accreditation standards*, ed 6, Sandy Springs, SC, 2006, CAMTS.

13. Cooper DC, editor: *Fundamentals of search and rescue*, Sudbury, MA, 2005, Jones & Bartlett Publishers.

14. Craighead FC, Craighead JJ: *How to survive on land and sea*, ed 4, Annapolis, MD, 1984, Naval Institute Press.

15. Crowley JS, Licina JR, Bruckart JE: Flight helmets: how they work and why you should wear one, *J Air Med Transport* 11(8):19, 1992.

16. Department of the Army: *Survival, FM 3–05.70*, Washington, DC, 2002, US Government Printing Office.

17. Drew K: Should a pregnant flight nurse be allowed to fly? *J Air Med Transport* 10(7):11, 1991.

18. Federal Aviation Administration: *Flight Standards Information Management System (FSIMS)*, vol 11, Washington, DC, 2007, Aviation Safety Action Program (8900.1).

19. Federal Aviation Administration: *Operations specification A021, Helicopter Emergency Medical Services (HEMS) operations (draft revisions)*, Washington, DC, 2008, FAA.

20. Federal Aviation Administration: *Helicopter Emergency Medical Services (HEMS) use of the Aviation Digital Data Service (ADDS) experimental HEMS tool (8000.333)*, Washington, DC, 2006, FAA.

21. FEMA Emergency Management Institute: *IS-100 introduction to incident command system*, Washington, DC, 2007, available at http://training.fema.gov/EMIWeb/IS/is100.asp, accessed March 2008.

22. Frazer R: Air medical accidents: a 20 year search for information, *Air Med J* 8(5):33, 1999.

23. Frazer R: Air medical accidents involving collision with objects, *Air Med J* 20(3):13, 2001.

24. Frazer R: Weather accidents and the air medical industry, *Air Med J* 6(6):49, 2000.

25. Hawkins M: Personal protective equipment in helicopter EMS, *Air Med J* 13(4):1123, 1994.

26. Helicopter Association International: *U.S. Civil Helicopter Accident Database, 2008*, available at http://www.rotor.com/Default.aspx?tabid=598, accessed February 2008.

27. Holleran RS: Prehospital safety. In Holleran RS, editor: *Prehospital nursing: a collaborative approach*, St Louis, 1994, Mosby.

28. International Association of Flight Paramedics: *Position paper on helicopter shopping*, Snellville, GA, 2006, IAFP.

29. Isakov AP: Souls on board: helicopter emergency medical services and safety, *Ann Emerg Med* 47(4):357-360, 2006.

30. Kahn CA, Pirrallo RG, Kuhn EM: Characteristics of fatal ambulance crashes in the United States: an 11-year retrospective analysis, *Prehosp Emerg Care* 5(3):261-269, 2001.

31. Kibbee G: *Surviving the unexpected night out*, presented at the 20th National Conference on Wilderness Medicine, 2006, Big Sky, MT.

32. Krebs MB, Guohua L, Baker SP: Factors related to pilot survival in helicopter commuter and air taxi crashes, *Aviation Space Environ Med* 66(2):99-103, 1995.

33. Kruppa RM: Air medical safety, a follow-up survey, *J Air Med Transport* 8(10):10, 1991.

34. Lundin C: *98.6 degrees: the art of keeping your ass alive!* Salt Lake City, 2003, Gibbs-Smith Publishers.

35. MacDonald E, Heffernan J: An Air Medical Safety Advisory Council update, *Air Med J* 21(4):15-16, 2002.

36. Mason KT: Letter, *Air Med J* 13(6):242, 1994.

37. Mayberry RT: Medical air crew roles and responsibilities during aircraft emergencies, *Aero Med J* 3(4):16, 1988.

38. Militello PR, Ramzy AI: Safety by design, *J Air Med Transport* 9(8):15, 1990.

39. MMWR: Ambulance crash-related injuries among emergency medical services workers: United States, 1991-2002, *MMWR* 52(08);154-156, 2003.

40. Morton PM, Kummerfeldt P: Wilderness survival, *Emerg Med Clin North Am* 22: 475-509, 2004.

41. National EMS Pilots Association: *Helicopter Emergency Medical Services (HEMS) NVG utilization survey, 2008*, available at http://www.nemspa.org/Shared%20Documents/NEMSPA_NVG_Survey_0508.pdf, accessed November 2008.

42. National Flight Nurses Association: *Improving flight nurse safety in the air medical helicopter environment*, Park Ridge, IL, 1998, NFNA.

43. National Oceanic and Atmospheric Administration: *HEMS low altitude flight tool*, Kansas City, MO, 2008, available at http://www.weather.aero/hems/, accessed April 2008.

44. National Oceanic and Atmospheric Administration: *Satellite processing of 121.5/243 MHz emergency beacons to be terminated on Feb. 1, 2009 (NOAA 00-R312)*, Suitland, MD, 2000, available at http://www.sarsat.noaa.gov/121phaseout.pdf, accessed March 2008.

45. National Transportation Safety Board: *Aviation accident database and synopses*, 2008, US Department of Commerce, available at http://www.ntsb.gov/ntsb/query.asp, accessed November 2008.

46. National Transportation Safety Board: *Aviation accident report # FTW03FA082*, 2004, US Department of Commerce, available at http://www.ntsb.gov/ntsb/query.asp, accessed March 2008.

47. National Transportation Safety Board: *Safety study commercial emergency medical service helicopter operations*, Washington, DC, 1988, National Technical Information Service, NTSB/SS, US Department of Commerce.

48. National Transportation Safety Board: *Special investigation report on emergency medical services operations, aviation special investigation report*, Washington, DC, 2006, National Technical Information Service, NTSB/SIR, US Department of Commerce.

49. REACH Air Medical Services: *Rotor wing crew chief manual*, Santa Rosa, CA, 2006, REACH.

50. Ryan T, Studebaker B, Brennan G: Patient impression of the use of helmets by HEMS personnel [abstract], *J Air Med Transport* 11(10):65, 1992.

51. Springer B: The IFR bullet: can it kill our accident rate? *Air Med J* 24(1):29-31, 2005.

52. Winn W: *A safe ride to a soft bed*, available at http://www.williamwinn.com/, accessed February 2008.

53. Wraa CE, O'Malley JO: Flight nurse physical requirements, *J Air Med Transport* 11(10):17, 1992.

54. Wolfe K, Reidy M, Robinson J: A crash experience proves need for personal rescue packs, *Air Med J* 13(10):429, 1994.

Patient Care Principles

CHAPTER

10 PATIENT ASSESSMENT AND PREPARATION FOR TRANSPORT

Reneé Semonin Holleran, Denise M. Treadwell

COMPETENCIES

1. Obtain initial, focused, and comprehensive subjective and objective data through history taking, physical examination, review of records, pertinent laboratory values and radiographic or diagnostic studies, and communication with other healthcare providers, including prehospital and referring personnel.
2. Recognize and anticipate critical signs and symptoms related to the patient's illness or injury.
3. Perform critical patient interventions as indicated by the patient's illness or injury.
4. Identify flight operations specific to air ambulance transport that may impact the delivery of care and the safety of the patient and team.
5. Prepare the patient for transport via ground vehicle or rotor-wing or fixed-wing aircraft.
6. Identify and prepare for issues related to international transport.

The first half of this chapter presents an overview of patient assessment and preparation for transport, including identification of the indications for transport, communication, consent for transport, all the factors involved in a patient assessment, and steps to prepare the patient for transport. The second half of this chapter discusses necessary knowledge for all air medical teams in regards to flight operations with an emphasis on those pertinent to fixed-wing transport, including international transport.

The transport process begins with identification of the need to transfer a patient. In many cases, this step has been initiated by members of the referring agency, such as prehospital care providers or health-care providers in the transferring hospital.

Communication about the need for transport and the care the patient has received and will need from the transport team is an integral part of preparation. This communication begins before the transport team arrives, continues during transport, and concludes with patient follow-up information to the referring agency.

Patient assessment provides the transport team with an opportunity to identify problems and interventions needed before transport. Patient assessment also allows the transport team to anticipate and prepare for events that may occur during transport.

Patient assessment and preparation for transport are composed of multiple elements, including primary and secondary assessment, performance of critical interventions, and treatment of specific problems, such as pain management.

The transport environment is not always conducive to all of the components of patient assessment and preparation. However, the transport team must be familiar with all of these components of patient assessment and preparation so that they can perform the appropriate interventions necessary for safe and successful patient transport. Findings identified during the patient assessment may also be useful in determination of the most appropriate receiving facility and in advanced notification of anticipated therapies necessary immediately on the patient's arrival or shortly thereafter.

INDICATIONS FOR PATIENT TRANSPORT

Currently, no universal agreement exists on what is an indication for transport. Numerous research studies have identified reasons to transport patients, and national organizations have suggested indications for air medical transport, particularly rotor-wing transport.[8,12,47] In general, the need to move or transfer a patient is based on the severity of the patient's illness or injury, time, distance, terrain, weather, need for nursing and medical expertise or diagnostic procedures not available at the referring health facility, and

a request by the patient's family that the patient be transferred to another facility.[37,38,61,69]

TRAUMA PATIENTS

Numerous guidelines for air medical transport of trauma patients are available. Air medical transport of trauma patients is commonly accepted probably because of its relation to the history of helicopters, which were first used to transport injured patients from the battlefield and were subsequently used to transport trauma patients in the civilian population (see Chapter 1 for the history of air medical transport). In 2002, the National Association of Emergency Medical Services Physicians published extensive guidelines for air medical transport use.[65] Scoring systems have also been used to determine indications for patient transport. Some examples of these scoring systems are the trauma revised trauma score, the trauma triage rule, the Glasgow coma score, Glasgow motor score (GMR; score greater than 5), and the vehicular trauma checklist.

The American College of Surgeons (ACS)[12] continues to include recommendations for the transfer of injured patients in both their Advanced Trauma Life Support Course and their Resources for the Optimal Care of the Injured Patient. In addition, the ACS recommends that the trauma patient should no longer be transferred to the closest hospital but to the closest appropriate hospital, preferably a verified trauma center.[11] Some of the recommendations of the ACS are listed in Box 10-1.

PATIENTS WITH CARDIOVASCULAR AND MEDICAL EMERGENCIES

Most of the research related to the indications for transport involves trauma patients. The emergent transport of nontrauma patients from the scene is rarely practiced and has been shown to provide little to no benefit to the patient.[38] These patients are generally admitted to the local facility for immediate care and then transferred to a specialty facility as an interfacility transfer. Interfacility transfers allow for preliminary diagnoses, initial medical screening, and select diagnostic procedures before the transport. For cardiovascular patients, indications recognized for interfacility transfer include the need for cardiac critical care that is not available at the referring

| BOX 10-1 | ACS Criteria for Consideration of Transfer |

A. Critical Injuries to Level I or Highest Regional Trauma Center
1. Carotid or vertebral arterial injury
2. Torn thoracic aorta or great vessel
3. Cardiac rupture
4. Bilateral pulmonary contusion with PaO_2 to FiO_2 ratio less than 200
5. Major abdominal vascular injury
6. Grade IV or V liver injuries that necessitate > 6 U RBC transfusion in 6 h
7. Unstable pelvic fracture that necessitates > 6 U RBC transfusion in 6 h
8. Fracture or dislocation with loss of distal pulses
B. Life-Threatening Injuries to Level I or Level II Trauma Center
1. Penetrating injury or open fracture of the skull
2. Glasgow Coma Scale score < 14 or lateralizing neurologic signs
3. Spinal fracture or spinal cord deficit
4. More than two unilateral rib fractures or bilateral rib fractures with pulmonary contusion
5. Open long bone fracture
6. Significant torso injury with advanced comorbid disease (such as coronary artery disease, chronic obstructive pulmonary disease, type 1 diabetes mellitus, or immunosuppression)

ACS, American College of Surgeons; *PaO_2*, partial pressure of oxygen in arterial blood; *FiO_2*, fractional concentration of oxygen in inspired gas; *RBC*, red blood cells.
Note: An injured patient may undergo operative control of ongoing hemorrhage before transfer if a qualified surgeon and operating room resources are promptly available at the referring hospital.
From American College of Surgeons: *Resources for optimal care of the injured patient*, Dallas, 2006, ACS.

facility, cardiac catheterization, treatment for cardiogenic shock that may include insertion of a balloon pump, mechanical assistance devices, experimental medications, and organ transplant.[24,28,45,49] Research and case reports have shown that patients with cardiovascular emergencies tolerate the transport process well and have benefited from it.[45] For other non-trauma cases, indications for interfacility transfers are generally specific to the limited availability of specialty care and advanced equipment needed for the patient's condition at the referring facility.[5-7,21,59]

Loos, Runyan, and Pelch[59] developed a Medical Classification Criteria Tool (MCCT) modeled on trauma classification tools to assist in determination of the severity of illness and what resources may be needed for appropriate transport. The advantages of this tool include enhancement of communication between the referring and receiving facility and advanced notification of the severity of the patient's illness so that the receiving facility can be appropriately prepared. This tool can also be used to monitor the appropriateness of medical transfers. Box 10-2 details the MCCT.

The appropriateness of interfacility patient transfer is by and large measured by comparing the benefits of the transfer to the patient and the risks. The Acute Physiology and Chronic Health Evaluation (APACHE) score is often used in the critical care setting as a predictor of the patient's mortality.[21,72-74,80]

PREGNANT WOMEN AND NEONATES
Other patients who may need transfer and transport include pregnant women and neonatal patients. The transport of these patients requires specially trained and equipped medical teams.[2-4,71] Indications for the transport of pregnant women include placenta previa, fetal distress, maternal trauma, prenatal complications, and perimortem delivery. Indications for the transport of neonates include the age and weight of the infant and neonatal illness and injury that cannot be appropriately cared for at the referring facility.[13,61] Teams must be able to monitor for maternal and fetal distress and have additional training and experience to manage those conditions during the transport.

APPROPRIATE PATIENT TRANSFER
In 1986, the Consolidated Omnibus Reconciliation Act (COBRA) was implemented. This legislation, coupled with the 1990 Omnibus Reconciliation Act amendments to COBRA, furnishes guidelines, regulations, and penalties that govern patient transfer and transport. The implications of this law and its recent revisions are discussed in Chapter 36.

In transport of an ill or injured patient, transport services should provide: (1) a transport team with

BOX 10-2	Medical Classification Criteria Tool

Staff for Life Helicopter Service, University of Missouri Hospital and Clinics

Code blue: Cardiopulmonary arrest (nontraumatic source)
Class I: Life-threatening Illness or Unstable Vital Signs

A. Unstable airway

Acute respiratory distress (i.e., acute pulmonary edema, unconscious patient, patient needs recent intubation)

B. Patient needs ventilatory support (oxygen saturation, <80% via pulse oximetry)

C. Circulatory instability

Clinical signs and symptoms of shock

Symptomatic hypotension, <90 mm Hg systolic

Symptomatic hypertension, >200 mm Hg systolic or >110 mm Hg diastolic

Unstable or symptomatic cardiac rhythms

Uncontrolled chest pain

S/P arrest

Therapies to include but not limited to:

- Transvenous pacer
- Intraaortic balloon pump
- External pacer
- Vasopressor administration

D. GCS, <8 (i.e., acute mental status changes, status epilepticus)

Class II: Potentially Life-threatening Illness, but Vital Signs Currently Stable

A. Controlled pulmonary disease

B. Controlled or decreasing chest pain

C. Controlled acute cardiac dysrhythmias

D. S/P new-onset seizures

E. Vascular disorders

F. Thrombolytic therapy

G. Previously class I case that has been stabilized with treatment

H. GCS, 9-12

Class III: No Obvious Life-threatening Illness and Vital Signs Stable

GCS, Glasgow coma scale.

From Loos L, Runyan L, Pelch D: Development of prehospital medical classification criteria, *Air Med J* 17(1):14, 1998.

the experience necessary to perform an initial assessment and stabilize the patient's condition before and during transport; (2) staff who are capable of using the equipment and technology necessary to deliver care during transport to specific groups of patients, such as the critically ill or injured; and (3) the ability to demonstrate that the transport will make a difference in patient outcome.[8,10-14,21,27]

The American College of Emergency Physicians has developed guidelines for appropriate transfer and transport of ill or injured patients. These guidelines are summarized in Box 10-3. In addition, the American College of Critical Care Medicine has proposed its own recommendations for the transport of critically ill or injured patients. Box 10-4 contains a summary of these guidelines, which address both interhospital and intrahospital transport of patients. Boxes 10-5 and 10-6 provide recommendations from the Air Medical Physician Association (AMPA) for air medical transport in acute coronary syndromes and acute stroke syndromes.

Finally, in 1995, the Emergency Nurses Association (ENA) developed a document (revised July 2005) that provides guidelines for the transport of ill or

BOX 10-3	**American College of Emergency Physicians Guidelines for Transfer and Transport from Emergency Department to Another Facility**

1. The optimal health and well-being of the patient should be the principal goal of patient transfer.
2. Emergency physicians and hospital personnel should abide by applicable laws regarding patient transfer. All patients should be provided a medical screening examination (MSE) and stabilizing treatment within the capacity of the facility before transfer. If a competent patient requests transfer before the completion of the MSE and stabilizing treatment, these should be offered to the patient and documented. Hospital policies and procedures should articulate these obligations and ensure safe and efficient transfer.
3. The transferring physician should inform the patient or responsible party of the risks and the potential benefits of transfer and document these. Before transfer, patient consent should be obtained and documented whenever possible.
4. The hospital policies and procedures or medical staff bylaws should identify the individuals responsible for and qualified to perform MSEs. The policies and procedures or bylaws must define who is responsible for accepting and transferring patients on behalf of the hospital. The examining physician at the transferring hospital will use best judgment regarding the condition of the patient when determining the timing of transfer, mode of transportation, level of care provided during transfer, and destination of the patient.
5. Agreement to accept the patient in transfer should be obtained from a physician or responsible individual at the receiving hospital in advance of transfer. When a patient requires a higher level of care other than that provided or available at the transferring facility, a hospital with the capability to provide a higher level of care may not refuse any request for transfer.
6. An appropriate medical summary and other pertinent records should accompany the patient to the receiving facility or be electronically transferred as soon as is practical.
7. When transfer of patients is part of a regional plan to provide optimal care at a specialized medical facility, written transfer protocols and interfacility agreements should be in place.

From American College of Emergency Physicians: *Appropriate interhospital patient transfer,* Dallas, 2002, ACEP.

BOX 10-4	**Summary of American College of Critical Care Medicine Guidelines for the Transport of the Critically Ill or Injured Patient**

1. The benefits of transferring the patient should outweigh the risks.
2. The practitioner needs to be aware of the legal implications of patient transfer and transport.
3. Before the patient is transported, physicians and nurses at the referring and receiving facilities should be in contact, a decision should be made about the mode of transportation to be used, and a copy of all medical records relevant to the patient's care should be secured.
4. Accompanying transport personnel should include a minimum of two patient care providers and a vehicle operator. At least one care provider should be a registered nurse.
5. The equipment (including monitors) and medications necessary to manage the patient's airway, breathing, and circulation should be available. Communication equipment used during transport should also be available.
6. Continuous monitoring should take place during transport. At a minimum, ECG monitoring and monitoring of vital signs are required. Patients with specific problems may require additional monitoring, such as capnography and invasive monitoring.

Modified from the Guidelines Committee of the American College of Critical Care Medicine Society of Critical Care Medicine and the Transfer Guidelines Task Force of the American Association of Critical Care Nurses: *Guidelines for the transport of the critically ill patient,* 2004. Accessed from http://www.sccm.org. June 30, 2008.

| BOX 10-5 | **Appropriateness of Air Medical Transport in Acute Coronary Syndromes** |

Position Statement of The Air Medical Physician Association
Approved by the AMPA Board of Trustees, November 10, 2001

Background

Acute coronary syndromes are common reasons to utilize air medical transport. Regionalization of cardiac care to highly specialized centers, increasing use of invasive and time sensitive therapies, and efforts to minimize both the absolute time to therapy and the dangerous out of hospital time are significant drivers in improving cardiac care and for increasing the utilization of air medical transport.

AMPA Position Statement

The AMPA supports the use of air medical transport for adult patients with acute coronary syndromes requiring or potentially requiring urgent or time-sensitive intervention not available at the sending facility.

As outlined by the American Heart Association, acute coronary syndromes represent the spectrum of clinical disease presenting with syndromes ranging from unstable angina to Q-wave and non–Q-wave myocardial infarctions.

It is AMPA's position that the determination for the need for urgent or time-sensitive interventions is made by a physician, as documented on a written Certification of Medical Necessity.

Furthermore, AMPA acknowledges that scene air medical transport of acute coronary syndromes occurs routinely and supports that the medical necessity is determined by the requesting authorized provider based on regional policy and their best medical judgment at the time of the request for transport. AMPA supports that a receiving physician or the transport program medical director may complete the Certificate of Medical Necessity on scene transports.

The AMPA does not support the use of discharge ICD-9 codes or other methodologies that retrospectively determine medical appropriateness of acute coronary syndromes as this may adversely restrict access to appropriate care and may contradict the intent of EMTALA regulations. AMPA also believes that retrospective determination of medical appropriateness negates the regional, environmental, level of prehospital care, and situational issues that are important factors at the time of transport in determining medical appropriateness for air medical transport in acute and potentially acute coronary syndromes.

injured children. Unlike the documents previously mentioned, this document specifically addresses the needs of the ill or injured child. These guidelines are available from the ENA.

THE DECISION TO TRANSPORT

Several factors must be considered by referring personnel when they decide whether to transport a patient. The first factor to be considered is the appropriateness of transport, which was previously discussed. Identification of a suitable receiving facility is a second factor that must be considered. When choosing a receiving facility, referring personnel must look at the resources available at the receiving facility, such as specialized care staff, equipment, bed availability, and expertise. The location of the receiving facility is also an important consideration.

Another factor that should be considered in the decision of whether to transport a patient involves the existence of written policies and agreements among the receiving and referring agencies. The identification of centers that are capable of certain types of services and generation of triage guidelines could save precious time.

COMMUNICATION

Communication is probably one of the most important components in the preparation of the patient for transport. Communications center operations are discussed in Chapter 8. This discussion focuses on the communication process among personnel at the referring and receiving agencies (either a healthcare facility or an emergency medical services [EMS] agency).

Appropriateness of Medical Transport and Access to Care in Acute Stroke Syndromes

Position Statement of The Air Medical Physician Association
Approved by the AMPA Board of Trustees, October 23, 2004

Background

Acute coronary syndromes are common reasons to utilize air and ground medical transport. Regionalization of primary stroke centers and effects demonstrated by rapid access to stoke treatment centers providing thromlysis and systematized stroke care as well as advance interventional neuroradiologic treatment for acute stroke syndromes are significant drivers for increasing the utilization of air and ground medical transport.

AMPA Position Statement

The AMPA supports the use of air and ground medical transport for patients with acute stroke syndromes requiring or potentially requiring urgent or time-sensitive intervention only available at stroke treatment centers.

It is AMPA's position that the determination for the need for urgent or time-sensitive interventions is made by a physician or other qualified provider, as documented on a written Certification of Medical Necessity.

Furthermore, AMPA acknowledges that scene air medical transport of acute stroke syndromes occurs routinely and supports that the medical necessity is determined by the requesting authorized provider using standardized field identification and based on regional policy and their best medical judgment at the time of the request for transport.

The AMPA does not support the use of discharge ICD-9 codes or other methodologies that retrospectively determine medical appropriateness of acute stroke syndromes as this may adversely restrict access to appropriate care and may contradict the intent of EMTALA regulations. AMPA also believes that retrospective determination of medical appropriateness negates the regional, environmental, level of prehospital care, and situational issues that are important factors at the time of transport in determining medical appropriateness for air medical transport in acute and potentially acute stroke syndromes.

Communication should begin before the transport team arrives. Written policies, procedures, and triage guidelines should be in place at the referring agency. These documents should address the type of patient who should be transferred and the mode of transportation, the care that is needed before transport, whether or not passengers are allowed to accompany the patient and team during the transport, and the steps that need to be taken by the referring agency to prepare for the arrival of the transport vehicle. For example, if a helicopter will be transporting the patient, where will it land, who will meet it, and who will monitor it while the team prepares the patient for transport?

When initial contact has been made by the referring agency, information that should be provided for the transport team includes the patient's chief symptom, the indications for transport, interventions and their effects, and the patient's current condition.

The reason for the patient transfer should be clearly identified and documented. Some transport programs require signed documentation by the treating or accepting physician to certify the need for transport before they transfer the patient because of recent reimbursement issues, particularly from Medicare.

The patient's problem, age, and location must be communicated effectively so the most suitably trained and equipped transport team can be sent to provide care for the patient. For example, some areas of the United States have transport teams specifically designed to provide care for pregnant women, children, neonates, and critical care patients. As discussed previously, the equipment required by the patient's illness or injury might influence the clinical skills that may be needed during transport (e.g., an intraaortic balloon pump necessitates personnel who are trained in its use in the transport environment).

Once the transport team arrives, they can obtain additional information about the patient directly from the staff at the referring agency. When the transport team members arrive at the scene, they should identify the person in charge and offer assistance.

During the initial assessment and preparation of the patient for transport, transport team members communicate with referring individuals. The communication process is composed of both verbal and nonverbal behaviors, and one's attitude is an important intervention. Thus, the transport team should always involve those who have been caring for the patient with an attitude of respect and professionalism.

Any laboratory results and radiographic and diagnostic study results should be copied and sent with the patient. Technology continues to make some paperwork easier to transfer. For example, radiographic and diagnostic study results may be transmitted by means of telemedicine before the patient leaves the receiving facility. If the patient has any valuables, they must be accounted for. Valuables are sometimes easier left with a family member, but this may not be possible. Recording a list of what was brought with the patient and to whom it was given on arrival at the receiving facility may prevent problems. Clothing or other valuables are sometimes considered evidence and should be treated as such on the basis of evidence protocols.

CONSENT

Patients must consent to treatment and transfer. However, written or verbal consent for transport and for emergency treatment is not always possible to obtain directly from the patient or family. Consent for transport is usually implied. Implied consent is considered to be given only in an emergency situation, when the patient is incapacitated and in a life-threatening situation.[14,25]

Although the patient's consent is implied, the transport team should always explain to the patient and available family members all procedures and the transport process. If family members are available, they may be able to provide consent for treatment. If consent forms are part of the transport documentation, the transport team should ensure that they are transported with the patient. On interfacility transfers, the team may elect to leave a copy of the consent with the referring facility.

A TWENTY-FIRST CENTURY PATIENT TRANSPORT CHALLENGE

During the past few years, the closing of hospitals, the decrease in nursing and other healthcare providers, and the lack of funds to provide healthcare have created a unique crisis that has grave implications to patient transport.[79,92] Many facilities that in the past accepted patients without question have now adopted diversion policies, which means a decrease in available beds, longer waits for transfer, refusal of some patients, and diversion. The American College of Emergency Physicians has developed Guidelines for Ambulance Diversion.[9] Box 10-7 contains a summary of these guidelines.

BOX 10-7	**Guidelines for Ambulance Diversion**

- Identify situations in which a hospital's resources are not available (critical care beds, nursing staff) and temporary diversion is necessary.
- EMS systems and hospital personnel must be notified of such occurrences, and the notification must occur through a lead EMS agency or designated communication coordination center.
- The hospital's diversion status must be regularly reviewed.
- Policies and resources need to be in place to provide for the safe, appropriate, and timely care of patients who continue to enter the EMS system during the period of diversion.
- The EMS system and other appropriate personnel should be notified when the diversion status has changed.
- Explore solutions that address the causes of diversion and implement policies that minimize the need for diversions.
- Continuously review polices and guidelines governing diversion.

Modified from Brennan J: *Guidelines for ambulance diversion,* Irving, TX, 2006, American College of Emergency Physicians.
EMS, Emergency medical service.

Transport programs need to ensure that the patient has a receiving facility, bed assignment, and accepting physician. Diversion notification should also include all services that provide patient transport to prevent any undue delay in patient transfer and transport.

PATIENT ASSESSMENT

Primary and secondary assessment, identification of patient problems, and initiation of critical interventions provide a framework for preparing a patient for transport. Each of these tasks must be performed in an organized, rapid, and complete manner. Patient assessment is a continuous process that occurs before, during, and after transport.

ASSESSMENT OF THE PATIENT IN THE PREHOSPITAL CARE ENVIRONMENT

Assessment of the patient in the prehospital care environment can be an intense challenge. The location of the patient (e.g., trapped in a vehicle; Figure 10-1), the limited availability of personnel and equipment, and the nature of the illness or injury present potential barriers to prehospital patient assessment.

The environment in which the patient is located during the transport may also pose barriers to assessment. Noise, a lack of light and space, vehicle movement and the speed at which the vehicle is moving, and outside weather can make normal assessment maneuvers, such as auscultation, difficult to perform.

The type of vehicle used to transport the patient may pose additional barriers to patient assessment. Ground, helicopter, and fixed-wing vehicles each have specific limitations that may complicate the team's ability to assess the patient. Although equipment is now more portable, some pieces of equipment are still susceptible to movement and vibrations that could affect reliability when used for patient assessment. Noise hampers patient assessment no matter what mode of transport is used.

SCENE ASSESSMENT

Assessment of the patient before reaching the hospital begins with assessment of the scene, whether the transport team responds directly to the patient or to another facility. The transport team should assess the surrounding environment for hazards. Box 10-8 contains a summary of some of the hazards that may be encountered.

On arrival at the referring facility, the transport team should survey the resources that are available

FIGURE 10-1 **Primary and secondary assessments can be difficult to perform depending on patient location.** (Courtesy Stanford Life Flight.)

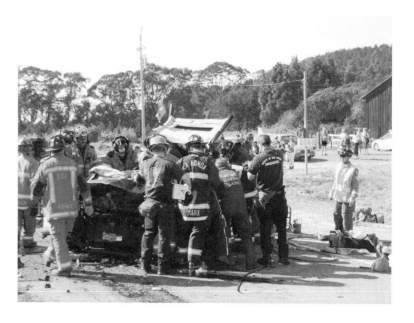

BOX 10-8	**Potential Environmental Hazards**

Hazards at the Scene

Wires
Uneven ground
Vehicles
Accident itself
People
Signs
Light poles
Water
Loose debris
Hazardous materials (HAZMAT)
EMS rescue apparatus
Fire
Smoke
Weather hazards
Heavy machines or construction equipment

Hazards at the Referring Facility

Buildings
People
Wires
Construction equipment
Shovels or other items used to clean landing zone area

to assist in preparing the patient for transport. Equipment and supplies necessary for patient stabilization may be limited, and thus, the team may need to bring additional equipment.

The principles of patient assessment used by the transport team are no different than those used when patients are assessed within the walls of a hospital. However, the prehospital environment dictates that the assessment be organized, direct, and rapid. Adaptation and flexibility are necessary when patient assessment is performed outside the hospital. Confined spaces, lack of light, noise, and equipment that may or may not be functioning can present challenges to patient assessment in the prehospital care environment.

HISTORY

Patient assessment begins with obtaining a history as the primary assessment is performed. The history of the illness or injury provides a guide for critical interventions, preparation of the patient for transport, and ongoing assessment during transport and also alerts the transport team to problems that may develop during transport. For example, the history of a patient who has multiple rib fractures and will be flown alerts the transport team to the potential for the development of a tension pneumothorax.

Generally, the transport team is given some information while en route to the patient. However, experience has shown that the situation on arrival may be quite different than that described beforehand.

General Principles of History Gathering

According to Henry and Stapleton,[50] "history is the patient's story of significant events related to and surrounding the present problem." Some general principles should be followed when gathering information related to the patient's illness or injury. One of these principles is that the patient's chief symptom or problem should be identified. If the patient is unable to provide this information, the transport team may obtain it from others at the scene (prehospital care providers, police, or bystanders), referring personnel (nurses or physicians), or any persons who may be with the patient. A survey of the scene by the transport team can also provide valuable information about what may have happened. If the patient is unconscious, the transport team should look for medic alert jewelry, syringes, medications, pill bottles, or information in the patient's wallet or purse.

A common mnemonic used to collect general history information is SAMPLE:

S Signs and symptoms reported.
A Allergies, alcohol, or substance abuse.
M Medications, including immunizations, particularly in a pediatric history.
P Past medical history, including illnesses and injuries.
L Last meal or intake.
E Events that led to the emergency and everything that has been done before the arrival of the transport team.

If the patient's chief symptom or problem is related to pain, the PQRST method is of use in collection of information on history. PQRST[43,46,50,57,58] represents the following:

P Provoking factors: What caused or causes the pain? Does anything relieve the pain or make it worse? What was the patient doing when the pain began?

Q Quality of the pain: Some of the words used to describe the pain may provide the nurse with clues to the origin of the pain. For example, patients who describe chest pain often use words such as "burning" or "crushing."

R Region and radiation: The patient should be asked to point to the area where the pain is felt. Pain patterns can provide the transport team with clues to the cause of the patient's pain and may help guide the management of the patient's pain.

S Severity: Numbering, such as from 1 to 10, can be used to describe the severity of the pain.

T Time: The patient should be asked to describe the temporal nature of the pain, such as how long it has been present and when or at what time of day it began.

The transport team may find a history difficult to obtain in the prehospital care environment as a result of obstacles such as the patient's inability to communicate because of illness or injury, the lack of witnesses to a particular event, or the absence of family members or significant others at the scene of the illness or injury.

When possible, and particularly when the patient is transported from a referring facility, as much information as possible should be collected and communicated with the receiving facility. At other times, particularly when patients are transported directly from the scene, much information may not be available. The transport team should keep in mind that history provides key information. History also alerts the nurse to problems that may develop during transport.

Trauma History

History gathering is different for the trauma patient than for the patient with a medical illness. The mechanism of injury generally triggers the trauma history. The transport team must find out when, where, and how the patient was injured. A complete

BOX 10-9	**Predictable Injuries That Result From Motor Vehicle Crashes**

Unrestrained Driver
Head injuries
Facial injuries
Fractured larynx
Fractured sternum
Cardiac contusion
Lacerated liver or spleen
Lacerated great vessels
Fractured patella and femur
Fractured clavicle

Restrained Driver
Caused by a Lap Restraint
Pelvic injuries
Spleen, liver, and pancreas injuries

Caused by a Shoulder Restraint
Cervical fractures
Rupture of mitral valve or diaphragm

Modified from McSwai N, Frame S, Salomone J: *Basic and advanced prehospital trauma life support,* ed 5, St Louis, 2003, Mosby.

description of the event is often limited. However, a general idea of the mechanism of injury provides clues regarding additional injuries and complications that may occur during transport. Box 10-9 describes predictable injuries that may occur as a result of motor vehicle crashes, as an example of taking a trauma history.[43,46,50,57,58]

In recent years, instant photographs, video recorders, and digital cameras have been used to provide information about the mechanism of injury.[67] Rescuers must use caution when taking photographs of the scene to prevent the violation of patient privacy laws or Health Insurance Portability and Accountability Act (HIPAA) regulations. Photographs should be of vehicles and property. Patient faces and deceased patients should generally not be photographed. Many transport services have strict HIPAA policies regarding disclosure of patient details, including the use of photographs; therefore, understanding of and strict adherence to company policies should be followed.[30,77] Dickinson, Krett, and O'Connor[30] reported that when photography was used to provide details related to a motor vehicle crash, receiving physicians altered perceptions about the patient's injuries in 46% of the cases. In addition, the receiving physician upgraded the severity of the motor vehicle crash after viewing the photographs in 22 of 26 cases (85%).

When obtaining the history of a trauma patient, the transport team should also gather information that describes the scene of the crash. Did the collision involve multiple victims? Are all of the victims accounted for? Were there fatalities? If the on-scene patients are unable to provide information about additional patients, the presence of schoolbooks, clothing, or toys may suggest that additional victims are present.[17]

History Related to Medical Illness

A patient's medical history begins with the chief symptom or current problem. The SAMPLE and PQRST mnemonics previously described can be of assistance when obtaining a medical history. The transport team should obtain history related to the present illness, including related signs and symptoms. Significant medical history and risk factors for a particular disease process (such as smoking and chronic obstructive pulmonary disease) can provide additional pieces of meaningful information.

Information about current medications should be provided. Drug interactions or the effects of not taking a scheduled medication may cause additional problems during transport.

Information about care initiated before the arrival of the transport team must be gathered. These data[50] should include initial physical findings, initial treatments and results, vital sign trends, medications given, laboratory results, radiographic or diagnostic study findings, electrocardiographic (ECG) interpretation, intravenous infusions administered, intake and output measurements, and status of family notification.

Diversity Assessment

Although the focus of patient care during the transport process is generally on critical needs, age, class, culture, ethnicity, gender, nationality, race, religion, and sexual orientation influence response to illness and injury. The transport team must take into consideration these factors when providing care and respect and, when possible, adapt the care to include the impact of diversity on response to illness, injuries, and the need to be transported.[28,31]

Awareness and knowledge of all patient diversity is impossible. However, the transport process can be a little less stressful for the patient, the family, and the transport team when the multiple factors that influence a patient's response to illness and injury are not ignored.

In 1997, the Emergency Nurses Association developed a Diversity Practice Model that can assist in approaching patient diversity.[33-36] The components of this model are summarized in Table 10-1. The use of this model may offer some added patient care information and help us recognize what makes us different and the same.

PRIMARY ASSESSMENT AND CRITICAL INTERVENTIONS

Primary assessment is based on assessment of the patient's airway, breathing, circulation, neurologic disability, and exposure. During the primary assessment, as patient problems are identified, critical interventions are initiated. The basic steps remain the same, whether at a scene or an interfacility transport.

Airway

The patient's airway is assessed to determine whether it is patent, maintainable, or not maintainable. For any patient who may have a traumatic injury, cervical spine precautions are used while the airway is evaluated. Assessment of the patient's level of consciousness, in concert with assessment of the airway status, provides the transport team with an impression of the effectiveness of the patient's current airway status (Box 10-10).

If an airway problem is identified, the appropriate intervention should be started. The decision to use a particular intervention depends on the nature of the patient's problem and the potential for complications during transport. Airway interventions are addressed in Chapter 11. Supplemental oxygen should be given to all patients before transport. Specific equipment, such as a pulse oximeter or CO_2 detector, help provide continuous airway evaluation during transport. The indications and the procedures for use of these devices are included in Chapter 12.

TABLE 10-1	**Diversity Practice Model**	
A	Assumption	What do we assume or take for granted about this individual or the community that they come from?
B	Beliefs or behaviors	How does my belief system affect the care I provide for this patient?
		Are my beliefs mirrored in the way I behave toward the patient? For example, a patient who may not have bathed for a long period of time may be viewed as homeless.
C	Communication	How does the patient communicate? Does the patient speak English? If not, is a translator available? Can the patient hear, see? Has the patient had an injury such as a stroke that impairs the ability to communicate or understand?
D	Diversity or identification of how the patient differs	Some diversity is visible, such as skin color, age, or ethnic background. Some is invisible, such as sexual orientation or class.
E	Education	Education involves learning about the patient's diversity.
	Ethics	Ethical decisions are influenced by one's diversity.

Emergency Nurses Association Diversity Task Force: *Approaching diversity: an interactive journey*, Des Plaines, IL, 1997, ENA.

BOX 10-10	**Summary of Primary Airway Assessment**

- Airway: Patent, maintainable, nonmaintainable
- Level of consciousness
- Skin appearance: Ashen, pale, gray, cyanotic, or mottled
- Preferred posture to maintain airway
- Airway clearance
- Sounds of obstruction

Pharmacologic Adjuncts for Airway Management. Specific pharmacologic agents have been found to be useful in prehospital airway management. These agents include those that provide sedation and amnesia and neuromuscular blocking agents that facilitate intubation. An in-depth discussion of the use of these medications is provided in Chapter 11.

Transport team members must remember when these medications are used, particularly if the patient received neuromuscular blocking agents; they then are totally dependent on the transport team. Measures to ensure patient safety and comfort, including keeping the patient warm and providing sedation and analgesia, must be provided by the team during transport.

Breathing

The assessment of ventilation begins with noting whether the patient is breathing. If the patient is apneic or in severe respiratory distress, immediate interventions are indicated. If the patient has any difficulty with ventilation, the transport team must identify the problem and proceed with the appropriate interventions. Emergent interventions may include decompression with a needle or insertion of a chest tube (Box 10-11). Ventilation interventions are discussed in Chapter 12.

BOX 10-11	**Summary of Primary Breathing Assessment**

- Rate and depth of respirations
- Cyanosis
- Position of the trachea
- Presence of obvious injury or deformity
- Work of breathing
- Use of accessory muscles
- Flaring of nostrils
- Presence of bilateral breath sounds
- Presence of adventitious breath sounds
- Asymmetric chest movements
- Palpation of crepitus
- Integrity of chest wall
- Oxygen saturation measured with pulse oximetry

Circulation

Palpation of both the peripheral and the central pulse provides information about the patient's circulatory status. The quality, location, and rate of the patient's pulses should be noted. The temperature of the patient's skin can be assessed along with the pulses. Observation of the level of consciousness helps evaluate the patient's perfusion (Box 10-12).

Active bleeding should be quickly controlled with interventions such as direct pressure. The transport team should observe the patient for indications of circulatory compromise. Skin color and temperature, diaphoresis, and capillary refill are appraised during circulatory assessment.

Intravenous access is obtained for administration of fluid, blood, and medications. Depending on the patient's location and the accessibility of veins, peripheral, central, or intraosseous access may be used. Fluid resuscitation must be guided by the patient's response.

Disability: Neurologic Assessment

Neurologic assessment includes assessment of the level of consciousness; the size, shape, and response of the pupil; and motor sensory function. The following simple method called AVPU may be used to evaluate the patient's level of consciousness:

A Alert.
V Responds to verbal stimuli.
P Responds to painful stimuli.
U Unresponsive.

Both the Glasgow and the Pediatric Glasgow Coma Scales provide assessment of the patient's level of consciousness and motor function and serve as predictors of morbidity and mortality after brain injury.[1,34]

If the patient has an altered mental status, the transport team needs to determine whether the patient has ingested any toxic substances, such as alcohol or other drugs, or may be hypoxic because of illness or injury. A patient with an altered mental status may pose a safety problem during transport. Use of chemical paralysis, sedation, or physical restraints may be necessary to ensure safe transport.[63]

Exposure

As much of the patient's body as possible should be exposed for examination, with the effects of the environment on the patient kept in mind. Discovery of hidden problems before the patient is loaded for transport allows the transport team to intervene and prevent potentially disastrous complications. Although exposure for examination has been emphasized most frequently in the care of the trauma patient, it is equally important in the primary assessment of the patient with a medical illness.

Team members should always look under dressings or clothing, which may hide complications or potential problems. Intravenous access can be wrongly assumed underneath a bulky cover. Clothing can also hide bleeding that occurs as a result of thrombolytic therapy or rashes that may indicate potentially contagious conditions (Box 10-13).

Once patient assessment has been completed, the patient needs to be kept warm. Hypothermia can cause cardiac arrhythmias, increased stress response, and hypoxia. Medications such as neuromuscular blocking agents interfere with the patient's ability to maintain a stable body temperature.

BOX 10-12	**Summary of Primary Circulation Assessment**

- Pulse rate and quality
- Skin appearance: Color
- Peripheral pulses
- Skin temperature
- Level of consciousness
- Urinary output
- Blood pressure
- Cardiac monitor
- Invasive monitor

BOX 10-13	**Summary of Exposure Assessment**

- Appropriate tube placement: Endotracheal tubes, nasotracheal tubes, chest tubes, nasogastric or orogastric tubes, and urinary catheters
- Intravenous access: Peripheral, central, and intraosseous
- Identification of injury; active bleeding; indication of a serious illness such as presence of purpura

If extended transport times are necessary, the team should reassess the patient's temperature during the transport.

Prevention of hypothermia should be considered a critical intervention, and methods to decrease the risk of heat loss initiated during the primary assessment should be initiated by the transport team. These include the following[48,51,66]:

- Covering the patient with blankets or an insulated layer.
- Limiting exposure when examinations are needed.
- Keeping the patient away from metal or anything that may draw heat away from the patient.
- Shielding the patient from wind rotor wash.
- Using warmed humidified oxygen and warmed intravenous fluids.

Equipment Assessment

Although the concept of equipment assessment has not been routinely included in previous descriptions of primary assessment, it is an important process that must be performed. Before the patient is transported, the transport team should ensure that the patient is wearing an appropriately sized cervical collar, that the chest tube drainage system is functioning, and that the patient is correctly restrained. The team should also confirm that the equipment in use is approved for continued use in the transport environment. This assessment of equipment helps prevent problems during transport that could potentially leave the patient at risk for further injury.

SECONDARY ASSESSMENT

Whether a secondary assessment can be performed depends on the patient's condition and the amount of time needed for transport. Lack of space in the transport vehicle, lack of light, and noise may interfere with the transport team's ability to perform a secondary assessment during transport.

Secondary assessment is done after the primary assessment is completed and involves evaluation of the patient from head to toe.[1,12,23,34] Patient data are collected by means of inspection, palpation, and auscultation during secondary assessment. Whether the patient has had an injury or is critically ill, the evaluator should observe, touch, and listen to the patient.

Secondary assessment begins with an evaluation of the patient's general appearance. The transport team should observe the surrounding environment and evaluate its effects on the patient. Is the patient aware of the environment? Is there appropriate interaction between the patient and the environment?

Additional systems that should be assessed include the integumentary (color, presence of wounds, temperature); head and neck (deformities, crepitus, pain); eyes, ears, and nose (drainage); thorax and lungs (chest movement and heart and breath sounds); abdomen; genitourinary; and extremities and back (Box 10-14).

PAIN ASSESSMENT

Determination of the amount of pain the patient has as a result of illness or injury is an important component of patient assessment. Physiologic indicators of pain include tachypnea, controlled respirations (splinting), tachycardia, hypotension, hypertension, nausea and vomiting, and diaphoresis. Behavioral indications of pain are crying, protective behavior, guarding, moaning, and self focusing.

Baseline data are collected about the pain the patient has so that the effectiveness of pain management can be assessed during transport. Pain relief is one of the most important interventions for out-of-hospital patient care providers.[16,29,44]

SCORING SYSTEMS

Scoring systems were initially developed to identify patients who were in need of critical care that was not available at referring facilities,[8,19] such as patients who needed to be transported to a level I trauma center. Scoring systems can be used in the field and for evaluation of patients who may need interfacility support. Scoring systems have most commonly been used for the trauma patient. These systems include the Prehospital Index Score, CRAMS Scale Score, Triage-Revised Trauma Score, and Baxt's Trauma Triage Rule. Little research has been done regarding triage scores and severity scores that can be used for other medical problems.[23,32,68,78,95]

| BOX 10-14 | **Summary of Secondary Assessment** |

Skin

- Presence of petechia, purpura, abrasions, bruises, scars, birthmarks
- Rashes
- Abnormal skin turgor
- Signs of abuse and neglect

Head and Neck

- Presence of lacerations, contusions, raccoon eyes, Battle's sign, or drainage from the nose, mouth, and ears
- In the infant, examination of the anterior fontanel
- Gross visual examination
- Abnormal extraocular movements
- Position of the trachea
- Neck veins
- Swallowing difficulties
- Nuchal rigidity
- Presence of lymphadenopathy or neck masses

Eyes, Ears, Nose

- Lack of tearing
- Sunken eyes
- Color of the sclera
- Drainage
- Gross assessment of hearing

Mouth and Throat

- Mucous membranes
- Breath odor
- Injuries to teeth

- Drooling
- Drainage

Thorax, Lungs, Cardiovascular System

- Breath sounds
- Heart sounds

Abdomen

- Shape and size
- Bowel sounds
- Tenderness
- Firmness
- Masses (e.g., suprapubic mass)
- Femoral pulses
- Pelvic tenderness
- Color of drainage from nasogastric or orogastric tube

Genitourinary

- Blood at meatus
- Rectal bleeding
- Color of urine in catheter

Extremities and Back

- Gross motor and sensory function
- Peripheral pulses
- Lack of use of an extremity
- Deformity, angulation
- Wounds, abrasions
- Equipment is appropriately applied (e.g., traction splints)
- Vertebral column, flank, buttock

PREPARING THE PATIENT FOR TRANSPORT

This section summarizes patient preparation for transport. More in-depth discussions about patient preparation are contained in the clinical care sections of this book. The patient is prepared for transport on the basis of information obtained from the primary and secondary assessment, the type of vehicle used for transport, the amount of time of the transport, and the problems that may develop in relation to the patient's illness or injury during transport. Patient preparation includes anticipatory planning;

anticipation of potential patient problems makes patient care easier and safer.

During the past 20 years, technology has markedly improved transport equipment. Continenza and Hill[27] recommend that the equipment meet the following criteria:

- It should be useful in the transport setting.
- It should be lightweight, portable, and perhaps fulfill several functions (Figure 10-2).
- It should be easy to clean and maintain.
- It should have a battery life or power source that lasts the length of the transport.

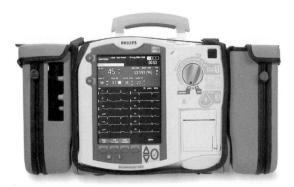

FIGURE 10-2   **Example of multifunctional monitor.**
(HeartStart MRx, courtesy Philips Healthcare, Andover, Mass.)

- It should have the ability to be used both inside and outside the transport vehicle.
- It should be able to withstand the stresses of transport, such as movement, altitude changes, mishandling (e.g., being dropped), water or fluid contamination, weather changes, and use by multiple persons.

Box 10-15 contains a generic list of equipment that may be used during transport. The types of patients cared for and the length of the transport dictate the amount and type of equipment carried by each service.

AIRWAY MANAGEMENT

Patient preparation begins with assessment and management of the patient's airway. The location of the patient may limit the type of airway management the team is able to provide. For example, if a patient is trapped in a vehicle, the team may have limited access for airway management.

Factors that may influence the decision about how to manage the airway include the nature of the patient's illness or injury, the amount of time of the transport, the room available in the transport vehicle, and the positioning of the crew in the transport vehicle.

If intubation has already been performed, tube placement and security should be evaluated. An unsecured endotracheal tube may be inadvertently removed during transport. In addition, movement of the endotracheal tube can cause mucosal damage, induce gagging and coughing, and increase the patient's intracranial or intraocular pressure.[93,95,96]

Oxygen should be administered to the patient. When available, additional monitoring equipment such as a pulse oximeter, CO_2 monitor, or apnea monitor should be used for continuous airway evaluation. These monitoring devices are discussed further in Chapter 12.

VENTILATION MANAGEMENT

A rapid focused assessment of the patient's ventilatory status should be performed as the patient is prepared for transport. If a chest radiograph has been obtained before arrival, it should be viewed to determine whether any pathosis exists. Breath sounds should be auscultated before the patient is placed in the transport vehicle because of noise interference.

If pneumothorax is suspected or is present on chest radiograph results, appropriate interventions should be initiated. If a chest tube or tubes are already in place, the nurse should check to see whether they are functioning. The drainage system may need to be changed so that it continues to function during transport.

If a portable ventilator is to be used, the patient's tidal volume, respiratory rate, and fractional concentration of oxygen in inspired gas (FiO_2) must be calculated before the patient is connected to the ventilator. Patients who are dependent on a ventilator may need to spend some time connected to the transport ventilator to ascertain whether they are able to tolerate the change.[24] Ventilator use is discussed in Chapter 12.

CIRCULATION MANAGEMENT

Initial care related to circulation management is directed at controlling any active bleeding. Bleeding can be controlled with direct pressure with application of gauze pads and elastic tape or bandages. Military antishock trousers (MAST) pants have been used in the past to help control bleeding but necessitate frequent monitoring during the transport because they may occlude distal circulation as a result of the effects of altitude in these air-filled chambered devices. The source and cause of the bleeding should be carefully evaluated before transport. Once the patient is "packaged," sheets and blankets can easily hide bleeding.

BOX 10-15	**Equipment for Transport**

A comprehensive list of equipment that needs to be stocked by transport services consists of a core set of supplies. The following equipment list serves as a guide, but it must be upgraded for special patient considerations and streamlined in the event of cost constraints.

Airway Equipment

Resuscitation bags (infant, child, adult)
All sizes of masks for bag-valve-mask ventilation
Nonrebreather masks
Pediatric
Adult
Nasal cannula
Oral and NP airways
Nebulizer setup
Portable suction unit
Tonsil suction
Suction catheters in the following sizes: 5/6F, 8F, 10F, 14F, and 18F
Magill forceps (pediatric and adult)
Laryngoscope handles (pediatric and adult)
Laryngoscope blades in the following sizes:
    Miller: 0, 1, 2, and 3
    MAC: 2, 3, and 4
Spare laryngoscope batteries and bulbs
Endotracheal tubes

Uncuffed		Cuffed		Endotrol
2.5	4.0	5.5	7.0	7.0
3.0	4.5	6.0	7.5	8.0
3.5	5.0	6.5	8.0	

Stylets
Benzoin, adhesive tape, and tracheostomy tape
End-tidal CO_2 monitor
PEEP valve
Pulse oximeter
Ventilator and filter and spirometer
Venturi mask
Aerosol mask for nebs
HMEs
Bipap mask
Alternate airways (laryngeal mask airway [LMA], Combitube, etc)
Cricothyrotomy tray
Tracheostomy tubes
Needle cricothyrotomy setup
Gastric tubes in sizes 5 to 18
Catheter tip syringe
Surgilube

Cardiothoracic Equipment

Cardiac monitor and supplies, including extra batteries
Defibrillator and supplies, including adult and pediatric paddles
Defibrillator pads
Multipurpose pads (defibrillator/pacer)
External pacer and supplies
Transvenous pulse generator and cable
Noninvasive blood pressure monitor
Manual blood pressure equipment (pediatric, adult, and obese)
Doppler scan
Pressure monitor and transducer and tubing kit
MAST pants (depends on state regulations)
Thoracotomy tray and drainage system
Chest tubes in sizes 12F to 36F
Chest tube dressing
Needle decompression supplies
Pericardiocentesis setup
Multiple adapters (Sims, connectors, small and large Y)

Intravenous Access Equipment

Intravenous solutions based on local protocols
Blood tubing
Minidrip tubing
Extension tubing
Intravenous needles (24 to 14 gauge)
Butterfly needles (27 to 19 gauge)
Intraosseous needles (15 and 18 gauge)
Rapid-infusion catheters
Triple lumen catheter set-up
Syringes of multiple sizes
Intravenous start packs
Razors
Arm boards
Laboratory blood tubes
Stopcocks
Pressure bag
Intravenous controllers or pumps and setup
Blood products and blood cooler

Medications

ACLS medications
Antianginal agents
Antiarrhythmics
Anticonvulsants

(Continued)

BOX 10-15	Equipment for Transport—cont'd

Medications—cont'd

Antiemetics
Antihistamines
Antihypertensives
Diuretics
Local anesthetics
Narcotics
Nasal decongestant
Neuromuscular blocking agents
Steroids
Tocolytics
Vasopressor agents

Miscellaneous

Oxygen
Stethoscope
Standard precautions equipment
Infectious waste management receptacles
Sharp object safety boxes
Instruments
Bandage scissors
Trauma scissors
Hemostats
Ring-cutter
Tape
Betadine solution
Dressing supplies (4 × 4s, elastic, bandages, cravats)
Eye shields
Burn cable and electrodes
Cervical collars
Cervical immobilization device
Pediatric transport board
Car seat
Isolette
Obstetrics delivery tray
Bubble bag
Stockinette cap

Stuffed toys
Pediatric dosage calculation references
Soft or leather restraints
Linen, blankets, towels
Flashlight
Cellular telephone
Satellite telephones
Two-way radio
Thermometer
Camera: instant, digital, video recorder
Documents
Directions and map to receiving facilities
Additional equipment specific to a particular type of service may include the following:

Ambulance

Immobilization devices (because space and weight are less of a consideration in an ambulance than in a helicopter or fixed-wing aircraft)
Backboard
Traction splint
Vacuum splints

Helicopter

Ear protection for the patient and crew
Survival bag stocked with necessary equipment in the event of an emergency landing

Fixed-Wing Aircraft

Certain bulk supplies (because of extended transport times)
Intravenous solutions, medication
Food and drink for the crew
Patient comfort kit (e.g., bedpan, urinal, urinary catheter)

Survival Equipment
Life Rafts
Life Vests

Intravenous access must be ensured. Whether one or two lines are inserted depends on individual protocols. However, access to the intravenous line is important for fluid replacement, blood administration, and medication administration.

When medications are infused, intravenous monitors may be used to ensure the appropriate delivery of medication. Medication concentrations and dosages should always be checked before a change is made in the equipment used. Some transport nurses have found that the easier method is to prepare medications with their own equipment and then make any changes in concentration and dosage, rather than transfer medication infusions that are currently infusing, particularly when their own equipment requires specific types of tubing.

Urinary catheters must be appropriately placed and affixed so that they are not pulled out with patient movement. Recommendations are that the catheter bag be emptied before the patient leaves the referring facility. The amount of urine emptied from the bag and its color should be recorded.

If invasive lines such as pulmonary or arterial catheters are in place, the transport team needs to check the patency and functioning of these lines. In some cases, transport monitors that offer specific readings during transport may not be available. The lines must be appropriately maintained and secured so that their functioning is not impaired. If a transport monitor is available, readings should be taken and recorded before, during, and after transport.

GASTRIC DECOMPRESSION

A gastric tube should be inserted to prevent the potential for aspiration and to provide gastric decompression during transport.[12] This procedure is not generally performed when a patient is transported directly from a scene, but it should be considered, particularly when the patient has undergone bag-valve-mask ventilation.

As with the urinary catheter, the gastric decompression tube must be appropriately placed and secured to prevent it from being removed. If the tube is not going to be placed on suction during transport, it should be capped so that it does not spill. If not connected to suction on fixed-wing transports with potentially higher altitudes, opening the gastric tube to gravity at fixed intervals may be necessary to prevent gastric distention. When possible, the patient's stomach should be drained before the tube is plugged. The amount of the drainage and its color should be recorded.

When patients undergo treatment for extensive gastrointestinal (GI) bleeding, such as that seen in the patient with liver disease, a specific type of gastric tube, such as the Sengstaken-Blakemore tube, may be in place. Traction must be maintained so that the tube continues to function properly. When this tube is present, the patient may be at risk for aspiration, asphyxia, gastric rupture, and erosion of the esophageal wall.[46,84] When the patient is transported, the airway should be secured with intubation, and the transport team must be prepared to intervene if any complications occur and to provide continued traction on the tube.

WOUND CARE AND SPLINTING

Wounds and splinting devices should be surveyed quickly, before the patient is moved. Hidden wounds may cause the patient discomfort and place the patient at risk for bleeding and long-term complications. Improperly placed splints or lack of splinting when indicated may also cause problems.

Several types of splints and splint devices are available for use in the patient being transported. The transport team must be familiar with the type of equipment that is used. Placement of the splint, potential complications of the device, and indications for removal are some examples of the kind of information needed. The neurovascular status of the extremity to which the splint is applied should be assessed and documented. Orthopedic and vascular emergencies are discussed in Chapter 19. Wound care is provided for patient comfort and protection. Dressing the wound helps control bleeding and keep it free of debris. If concern exists about additional bleeding or neurovascular compromise, the wound should be dressed in such a manner that continuous assessment is possible during transport. Any wet dressings are replaced with dry sterile dressings to prevent heat loss during transport.

The need for infection control is important to keep in mind when tending to the wounds of the patient being prepared for transport. Many patients being transported may have infected wounds that create a risk for the transport team and anyone else who may need to be transported in the vehicle. Appropriate decontamination procedures should be followed for both the transport team members and the vehicles.[87]

PATIENT SAFETY

An entire chapter in this textbook (Chapter 9) has been devoted to safety issues. In this section, we examine the safety measures that must be taken into consideration by the transport team when preparing the patient for transport. If the patient is combative, neuromuscular blocking agents and sedation may be indicated to ensure the safety of both the patient and the transport team.

A policy based on guidelines issued by the Food and Drug Administration should be in place regarding the use of restraints. These guidelines include the need to clearly document the necessity of the use of restraints during transport, follow local and state laws regarding the use of patient restraints, closely monitor the patient in restraints, carefully apply the restraining device, adjusting it properly to maintain body alignment and comfort, and consider restraints as a temporary solution.

When transporting a child, the child's size, weight, and state laws necessitate that restraint systems appropriate for a child be used. Devices that may be used include care beds, car seats, restraint systems, and transport boards. Any equipment that is used during transport needs to meet both federal and state standards.

PAIN MANAGEMENT

Pain management in the prehospital care environment is frequently not given priority consideration.[55] Several factors influence the use or lack of use of pain medications in the field, including the location of the patient, the nature of the patient's illness or injury, the possible masking of symptoms, and the effect of pain medications on the patient's vital signs. Movement, noise, changes in temperature, and fear may be contributing factors that cause or increase the patient's pain during preparation and transport.

Certain patient problems, such as chest pain related to myocardial infarction, have been dealt with outside of the hospital without any difficulty. However, acute pain, whether the result of trauma or other disease states, continues to be undertreated by healthcare professionals.[1,2,7,29,44,63]

In 1992, the United States Department of Health and Human Services published its *Clinical Practice Guidelines for Acute Pain Management: Operative or Medical Procedures and Trauma*. The need for appropriate pain management is emphasized in these guidelines. Although the prehospital management of pain is not directly addressed, these guidelines can easily be applied to the transport process.

The guidelines point out the following[1,2,7,29,44,63,86]:

The transport team should perform a brief assessment related to the patient's pain. The PQRST mnemonic previously described helps provide the nurse with a baseline description of the patient's pain. If the patient received medication before the team's arrival, information about the medication used and its effect on the patient should be included in the pain assessment.

Pain medications used for analgesia in the prehospital care environment need to be rapid in onset, short in duration, easy to administer, and easy to store.[78] The intravenous route is the quickest method of administration and has a rapid onset. However, intravenous access may not always be available. The transport team needs to be familiar with specific medications that can be used during transport to provide analgesia and sedation. This knowledge must include appropriate medication dosage, possible drug interactions, adverse reactions, and management of these adverse reactions.

Another important point to keep in mind regarding pain management during transport is that many patients have received neuromuscular blocking agents for safe transport, management of specific problems, or both. The transport team should pay particular attention to the needs of these patients for sedation and pain management because they are unable to let the flight team know when they are anxious or in pain.

Use of nonpharmacologic methods combined with conventional methods of pain management is also recommended for consideration for acute pain relief.[58] Nonpharmacologic methods that may be used by the transport team to help with pain management during transport include the following:

- Distracting the patient. For example, allow patients to look out the window if they are alert enough to do so. Also, a security object such as a stuffed toy may be of help to a child.
- Talking to the patient.
- Keeping the patient warm.
- Placing the patient in a comfortable position when possible.
- Describing everything that is going to occur.
- Allowing a family member to accompany the patient.
- Using therapeutic touch.

PATIENT PREPARATION: THE FAMILY

Any time a family member is ill or injured, a crisis is created in the family. The need to transfer the patient to a distant facility produces additional stress.

At times, the transport team does not have the opportunity to interact with the patient's family. Family members may not be present at the scene of the illness or injury, or they themselves may be injured. When family members are present, the team may be able to obtain a pertinent patient history from them.

The transport team should ensure that information is provided to the family before, during, and after transport of the patient. Policies and procedures that address when a family member may accompany an injured or ill family member should be in place. A discussion about family needs, how to care for the family, and when transport of a family member is appropriate is contained in Chapter 38.

DOCUMENTATION

Copies of any relevant documentation from the referring agency or EMS care providers should accompany the patient. If pictures of the scene of the accident are available, the transport team should bring them as well.[77] Customized charting software for use with laptop computers and handheld devices provides an efficient and thorough manner in which to document the patient assessment and record any changes or care provided during the transport. The documentation can then be downloaded into a centralize database that allows for storing and categorizing collected data. However the documentation is completed, the team must be able to leave copies with the patient at the receiving facility.

Copies of laboratory results, radiographic and diagnostic studies, and documentation by other healthcare providers should also accompany the patient. Consent forms, reasons for transport, and any other pertinent papers should be placed in the transport vehicle so that the team does not forget them when the patient arrives at the receiving facility. Remember to maintain patient confidentially when transporting or reviewing patient records.

Documentation by the transport team should reflect the reason the patient was transported; the interventions performed before, during, and after transport; and how the transport was completed. Strong and Thompson[79] found that the top 10 decisions made and documented during transport regarded fluid administration, immobilization, ventilation, oxygen administration, safety management, monitor use, intubation decisions, intravenous access, method of loading the patient (hot versus cold), and the use of neuromuscular blockade.

Documentation not only of what specific intervention was performed but also of how the decision was made is important. For example, why was the decision made to perform rapid sequence induction (RSI) to secure the patient's airway? If medications were administered for pain or arrhythmia management, did they have an effect on the patient and what was that effect?

The patient's chart is not only used to document interventions and their indications, but it is also used for continuous quality improvement and reimbursement of services. Documentation is an integral part of patient care. It must be clear, complete, and readable.

What is documented and who does the documentation are determined by the transport service and the specific standards. Nurses and paramedics have standards that describe their practice and provide guidelines for documentation (e.g., Air and Surface Transport Nurses Association [ASTNA], formerly called the National Flight Nurses Association [NFNA]).

PREPARATION FOR THE TRANSPORT OF THE BARIATRIC CASE

Obesity is an unhealthy epidemic in the United States that is rapidly spreading to other parts of the world. A patient is considered obese when body weight is 30% greater than ideal body weight.[75] Because of the increase in larger patients, the care of the bariatric patient has become a part of preparing a patient for transport. A bariatric patient includes patients who are overweight, obese, and morbidly obese and those who have had some sort of bariatric surgery.[81] The American Association of Operating Room Nurses (AORN) has developed weight categories by body mass index (summarized in Table 10-2).[56] The transport team must consider several issues in the care and preparation for the transport of the bariatric patient.

TABLE 10-2 **Weight Categories by Body Mass Index**	
Category	**BMI (kg/m²)**
Underweight	<18.5
Normal	18.5-24.99
Overweight	25-26.99
Mild obesity	27-30
Moderate obesity	>30
Severe obesity	>35
Morbid obesity	>40
Super obesity	>50

BMI, Body mass index.

SELECTION OF AN APPROPRIATE VEHICLE

The primary challenge involves whether a transport vehicle, particularly an aircraft, is capable of carrying an obese patient. Each transport program must have policies and procedures that address the weight and size of the patient that can be safely managed within the aircraft or even ground vehicles that are a part of a program. For example, a weight restriction may identify one limitation, but the girth of the patient can also impede safe and competent care in some transport vehicles.

Weight limitations may also be influenced by the weight of the transport team members, the equipment on board of the aircraft necessary to provide patient care, weather conditions, amount of fuel on board, location of the patient, and landing zone restrictions. Some transport vehicles do not have stretchers that can accommodate obese patients. Aircraft doors may not be wide enough to allow a patient into an aircraft. A patient may not be able to tolerate a position (e.g., laying flat) for loading into the aircraft.[20]

PATIENT ASSESSMENT AND INTERVENTION DIFFERENCES IN THE BARIATRIC PATIENT

Assessment of the bariatric patient is the same as for any patient who needs transport on the basis of primary and secondary assessments. The obese patient commonly has significant comorbid factors that must be considered by the transport team.

TABLE 10-3 **Comorbid Factors That May Accompany Obesity and Implications to Patient Care**	
Comorbid Factor	**Implications to Care**
Alveolar hypoventilation	Hypoxia may already be present in these patients. Sedation and pain medication may increase hypoxia.
Obstructive apnea	Patient may not be able to lay flat for loading or transport. Preexisting hypoxia can be increased as well if the patient must be flat for transport.
Gastroesophageal reflux	Patient is at greater risk for vomiting and aspiration. Can be aggravated if patient must be flat for loading, unloading, and transport.
Increased body tissue	Equipment may not obtain accurate readings. Pulse oximeters may be unreliable because of increased finger thickness and poorly transmitted light waves. Inappropriately fitting blood pressure cuffs do not provide accurate blood pressure readings. Low QRS voltage interferes with cardiac monitoring

These factors are summarized in Table 10-3 as are the implications for patient care.[15,18-20,22,31,56,62]

The most challenging issues that transport members face when caring for an obese patient is the management of the patient's airway, breathing, and circulation.[15,19,20,22,31,56,62] Because many obese patients are already hypoxic, the patient must undergo effective preoxygenation. Medications that are used to facilitate intubation that can further contribute to hypoxia must be carefully used (see discussion in Chapter 11). Limited neck mobility and mouth opening may also impair intubation success.

An obese patient can be difficult to ventilate with a bag-valve-mask device (BVM) because of reduced pulmonary compliance, increased upper airway resistance, and abnormal diaphragmatic position.[1,20] Gastroesophageal reflux also increases the risk of vomiting and aspiration with BVM ventilation. As previously pointed out, even if a patient does not require intubation or BVM ventilation, because of increased work of breathing related to body mass, many patients need to remain in a sitting position for adequate ventilation.

The cardiovascular system is challenged as well. Heart rate in a patient who is morbidly obese and nonhypertensive should be within normal limits, but the patient will have increased blood volume, stroke volume, cardiac output, and left ventricular function and lowered systemic vascular resistance related to the high metabolic activity of excessive fat. If the patient is hypertensive, these physiologic changes are more pathologic.[15,19,20,22,31,56,62] Fluid resuscitation and medication administration must be carefully calculated and monitored.

PREPARATION FOR TRANSPORT

The transport team must be familiar with physical and physiologic changes related to the bariatric patient. Airway, ventilation, and circulation management must be approached with the appropriate training, equipment, and monitoring devices. Preparation is key in prevention of complications.

Airway management must include equipment for a potential failed airway such as a laryngeal tracheal mask airway. Failed airway management is discussed in Chapter 11.

Excessive weight makes vascular access difficult. Alternative sites, such as central venous access, should be identified, and equipment available. However, this access should only be attempted by skilled persons. If intraosseous access is chosen, the size of the patient must be considered related to the length of the needles used.

Transport of the bariatric patient requires specialized equipment. Stretchers should be rated for the weight of the patient. These weight limits must be posted on the stretcher. In addition to ability to support the patient's weight, does the stretcher allow for safe restraint of the patient without impairment

of breathing? The head of the stretcher must allow for support of adequate ventilation.

Adequate personnel must be available to get the patient both in and out of the transport vehicle. Several commercial devices are now available that have been found to ease patient transfer from beds to stretchers. Some transport companies also have specially equipped vehicles to transport morbidly obese patients.

The care and transport of the bariatric patient present unique challenges to the transport team. The primary key to safe and competent transport is identification of the physiologic changes related to obesity, provision of care based on these differences, and preparation for the transport.

LABORATORY AND DIAGNOSTIC TESTING INTERPRETATION

LABORATORY TESTS

Laboratory and diagnostic tests can provide additional information about patient illnesses and injuries that may necessitate interventions before transport or could put the patient at risk for further problems during the transport process. Laboratory tests that may be of use to prepare for transport are summarized in Table 10-4. This list is not inclusive but does include some of the tests that may contribute to patient problems during the transport process.

CHEST RADIOGRAPH INTERPRETATION[1,64]

The chest radiograph can supply important information. A chest radiograph assists in confirmation of endotracheal tube placement and identification of injuries such as a pulmonary contusion or illnesses such as pneumonia that may causes problems with ventilation and oxygenation during transport, especially in the patient with thoracic trauma who may be at risk for pneumothorax. Altitude presents the risk of development of a tension pneumothorax for a patient with pneumothorax if the chest has not been properly decompressed (Figure 10-3).

Chest radiograph interpretation takes education and practice. Transport team members

TABLE 10-4	**Laboratory Tests Useful Transport: Tests and Values**
Laboratory Test	**Normal Values**
Arterial blood gases	pH: 7.36-7.44
	pCO_2: 34-44 mm Hg
	pO_2: 80-100 mm Hg
	HCO_3: 22-26
	O_2 saturation: 95% or greater
Hemoglobin	Male: 14-18 g/dL
	Female: 12-19 g/dL
Hematocrit	Male: 40.7%-50.3%
	Female: 36.1%-44.3%
Internationalized normalized ratio (INR)	2.0-3.0 standard therapeutic range
Platelet count	Adults: 150-400,000
	Children: 150-450,000
Potassium	3.5-5.0
Sodium	135-145

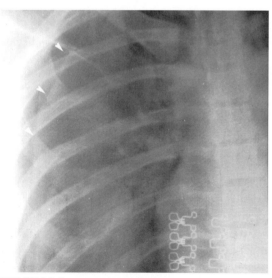

FIGURE 10-3   **Radiograph of pneumothorax.** (From Mirvis SE, Shanmuganathan K: *Imaging in trauma and critical care,* ed 2, Philadelphia, 2003, Saunders.)

should take every opportunity available to practice reading chest radiographs. The Transport Nurse Advanced Trauma Course (TNATC) provides an opportunity to interpret and discuss chest radiographs.

The following list provides a summary on how to interpret a chest radiograph:

- Identify that the chest radiograph is for the patient who is to be transported. Ensure that the proper labeling is on the film and that it is the most current and correct film.
- Ensure that the degree of penetration is adequate. On an anterior-posterior (AP) view, the intervertebral spaces should be possible to make out behind the heart.
- The medial ends of the patient's clavicle should be equally distant from the spine. If not, the patient is rotated.
- Adequate inspiration is determined by level of the diaphragm. The right hemidiaphragm should be at the level of the eighth or ninth posterior rib. Inadequate inspiration decreases the amount of air in the lungs and could mimic other conditions.
- The margins of all lung fields should be visible on the film. The top lung margin should extend to include the apices of the lungs. The bottom margins should include the costophrenic angle. The side margins should not crop off either side of the thoracic cage.
- The position of the patient in the radiograph should be noted.
- A systematic approach should be used to evaluate the:
  - Airway: Trachea is visible from the sixth cervical vertebrae to the third thoracic vertebrae where it divides at the carina into the right and left mainstem bronci. Normally, only the trachea and the two mainstem bronchi are visible on the chest radiograph.
  - Bones seen on the chest radiograph include: clavicle, ribs, sternum, and thoracic spine.
  - Cardiac: The lateral borders of the heart and mediastinum should be clearly visible from the diaphragm to the clavicles.

COMPUTED TOMOGRAPHIC SCAN INTERPRETATION[1,64]

The most common computed tomographic (CT) scans evaluated by the transport team are cranial CT scans. CT scans of the head can assist with the diagnosis of neurologic injury and evaluation of seizures and stroke symptoms. Just as with chest radiographic interpretation, evaluation of cranial CT scans takes education and practice. The CT scan should always be used in conjunction with a physical assessment.

A CT scan is created when radiographs pass through the body and are recorded in terms of different absorption values.[1] A denser body part absorbs more radiation. A CT scan can detect bleeding, fractures, and soft tissue injury.

Computed tomographic scan interpretation requires familiarity with the basic anatomy of the part of the body that is being scanned. For example, a healthy head CT scan shows the skull as white and the brain as gray in color. Dark areas within the brain indicate areas filled with fluid. These areas include the ventricles, cisterns, and the sagittal and transverse tissues. The cisterns are four fluid spaces in the brain and are visible on the CT scan.

A systemic review to cranial tomography includes the following[1,64]:

- Is the skull vault intact?
- Is the midline still in the middle and straight?
- Are only the usual densities present on the CT scan?
- Is the CT scan symmetrical about the midline?
- Is this the correct patient's CT scan?

When evaluating the brain in the CT scan, the following should be looked at:

- Gray-white differentiation.
- Shift: The falx should be in the midline, and the ventricles evenly spaced to the sides.
- Hyperdensity or hypodensity, which can occur with the presence of blood, calcification, or intravenous (IV) contrast.

Blood is bright white on a CT scan. It eventually is less white as the blood ages and breaks down. Figures 10-4, 10-5, and 10-6 show CT scans of a depressed skull fracture, an epidural hematoma, and a subdural hematoma, respectively.

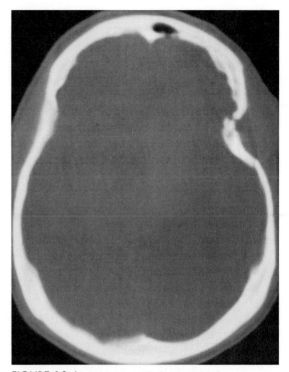

FIGURE 10-4   **Image reveals depressed left posterior frontal calvarial fracture.** (From Mirvis SE, Shanmuganathan K: *Imaging in trauma and critical care*, ed 2, Philadelphia, 2003, Saunders.)

PATIENT ASSESSMENT DURING TRANSPORT

The nature of the patient's illness or injuries and the initial interventions performed influence the assessment and management needed during air medical transport. Each of the clinical chapters in this textbook addresses the specific care needed during transport as a result of the patient's illness or injury. Some general principles of assessment and management during transport include the following:

- Transport team members should position themselves in the aircraft so that they can effectively manage the patient's airway, breathing, and circulation (ABCs).
- Airway equipment, including suction equipment, should be easily accessible.

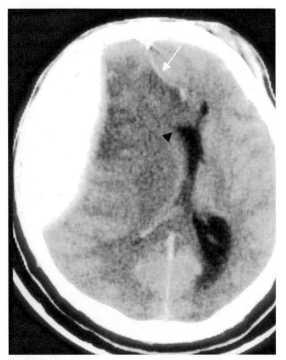

FIGURE 10-5   **Large right epidural hematoma.** (From Mirvis SE, Shanmuganathan K: *Imaging in trauma and critical care,* ed 2, Philadelphia, 2003, Saunders.)

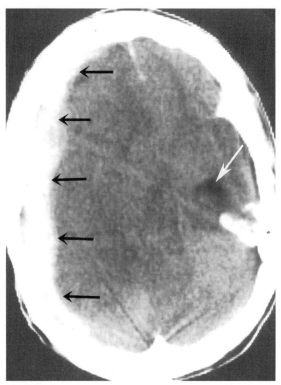

FIGURE 10-6   **Subdural hematoma (SDH).** CT scan image of large right convexity SDH *(arrows).* (From Mirvis SE, Shanmuganathan K: *Imaging in trauma and critical care,* ed 2, Philadelphia, 2003, Saunders.)

- All intravenous, central, or intraosseous lines should be accessible and functioning.
- All tubes and drainage systems should be functioning and secured to decrease the risk of dislodgement.
- If any question exists about cervical spine injury, the cervical spine should be immobilized for transport.
- A combative patient should be properly restrained, both physically and chemically, if indicated. If chemical restraint is chosen, the transport team needs to ensure that the patient receives adequate analgesia, sedation, and environmental control during the transport.
- All monitors should be placed within the transport team's field of vision.
- When indicated, wounds and injured limbs should remain exposed for inspection.

Assessment and preparation are the foundations of patient transport. Primary and secondary assessments provide initial information about the patient's current and potential problems. On the basis of these assessments, the transport team initiates appropriate interventions. Box 10-16 lists some of these interventions.[54]

Patient preparation includes not only obvious care but also anticipation of what may occur. In the prehospital care environment, resources are limited and anticipatory planning, safety, and prevention are key care interventions.

FIXED-WING PATIENT TRANSPORT

In fixed-wing aircraft patient transport, the transport team must pay critical attention to preflight preparation because of long periods of time typically spent on the ground and in flight. Fixed-wing aircraft transports usually entail lengthy periods

BOX 10-16	**Patient Care Interventions**

- Airway management
- Electrolyte and acid base management
- Drug management
- Neurologic management
- Respiratory management
- Physical comfort promotion
- Thermoregulation
- Tissue perfusion
- Psychologic comfort promotion
- Crisis management
- Risk management
- Lifespan care
- Information management

From McCloskey J, Bulechek G, Butcher H: *Nursing interventions classification (NIC),* St Louis, 2008, Mosby/Elsevier.

of patient care; thus, detailed preflight information must be obtained so that air medical personnel can make appropriate preparations for the transport. The aircraft should not depart to pick up the patient until all preflight preparations are complete. In addition to preparation for the medical aspects of the flight, the logistics and itinerary must be worked out and any other preflight information needed by the pilots must be obtained. The transport team and pilots should collaborate in gathering this preflight information and in coordinating the entire flight to ensure appropriate quality patient care.

In this section of the chapter, issues encountered by care providers in the fixed-wing transport environment are discussed. The following topics are covered: preflight preparation, federal aviation regulations, preparation for patient transport, patient "packaging," in-flight factors that influence patient care, air medical personnel resources, in-flight codes, and safety and emergency procedures. In addition, issues related to international transports and escort flights are highlighted.

PREFLIGHT PREPARATION

Preplanning by air medical personnel and the pilot is necessary if the patient transport is to go smoothly. Fixed-wing aircraft flight times are usually much longer than rotor-wing aircraft flight times and may vary greatly from service to service. Fixed-wing aircraft flight times may be as brief as 40 minutes within the state or as long as 3 to 6 hours within a particular region or across the country. In addition, transport distances may range from 150 to 500 miles for a propeller or turbopropeller aircraft to more than 500 miles for a jet. Once the patient transfer has been agreed on by a receiving physician and facility, the transport team should begin by obtaining information such as physician names, telephone numbers, and an accurate account of the patient's diagnosis and condition. This information will, it is hoped, ensure that the skills of the air medical personnel and the medical equipment available during transport are appropriate for the anticipated medical needs of the patient. In addition, logistic information such as patient and luggage weights, the number of family members who will ride along and their weights, and the "do not resuscitate" (DNR) status of the patient must also be obtained.

Preflight preparation also entails coordination of information with the pilot and appropriate authorities (e.g., Transportation Safety Administration [TSA], Customs and Immigration). Issues to be discussed should include location of airports, refueling and restroom stops, weight and balance issues, in-flight times to and from airports, ground ambulance times to referring and receiving facilities, ground unit resources, nutritional and fluid requirements, and disposal of wastes. The transport team must take into account in-flight and ground times when calculating the amount of IV fluids, medications, medical supplies, and oxygen that will be needed and when checking to ensure that medical equipment is fully charged.[1,46-50]

FEDERAL AVIATION REGULATIONS

Air medical services must actively participate in the daily aviation operations dictated by the Federal Aviation Administration (FAA) or national and international regulations specific to the operations of the air medical service in the country of residence, as applicable, to provide safety for all patients and care providers in the air transport environment. The fixed-wing air taxi certificate holder must comply with the appropriate Federal Aviation Regulations

(FARs). These regulations pertain to air traffic control, airports, visual and instrument flight rules, and aircraft operations.[39-42] Most air medical services must comply with the appropriate FARs, depending on who possesses the air taxi certificate.

The FAR Part 91 pertains to general operating and flight rules for aircraft flying in US airspace. The FAR Part 135 provides specific rules for air taxi operators and commercial operators. Most air medical services are regulated under Part 135 of the FARs because of the nature of transporting passengers or persons for compensation or hire.[39-42] In previous years, more than half of the fixed-wing transport programs in operation possessed their own FAR Part 135 certificate.[61] On the basis of an audit of their membership records conducted in 2008, the Association of Air Medical Services (AAMS) states that approximately 23% of current AAMS members have voluntarily reported holding their own Part 135 US Air Carrier Certificate for either rotor-wing operations, fixed-wing operations, or combined. A brief explanation of weather minimums, weight and balance, the term *lifeguard*, and ambient temperatures as they relate to FARs gives the transport team an understanding of how they can assist the pilot in complying with FARs and ultimately with safety.[88]

Weather Minimums: Visual and Instrument Flight Rules

The FARs define explicit weather minimums and rules that must be in effect for an aircraft to operate within consistent safety standards. Under FAR Part 135, air medical services operate under either Visual Flight Rules (VFRs) or Instrument Flight Rules (IFRs).[88] The pilot of a fixed-wing aircraft must comply with the appropriate rules that define flying limitations in adverse weather conditions.

The *VFRs* govern the procedures for conducting flight under visual conditions as interpreted by the pilot. *Flight visibility* is defined by the distance forward into the visible horizon, and the ceiling (vertical boundary) is the height above the ground or water to the base of the lowest (broken) layer of clouds.[39-42,88] FAR Part 91.155 addresses the basic VFR weather minimums that are maintained for the corresponding altitude and class airspace for all aircraft.[88]

The *IFRs* govern the procedures for conducting instrument flight when weather conditions do not meet the minimum requirements for flight under VFRs.[39-42,88] IFRs indicate that the pilot intends to navigate via instrumentation for at least a portion of the flight. Most programs that operate with fixed-wing aircraft have the capability to operate under IFRs. However, IFRs pose other limitations, such as the need to land at approved airports when instrument approaches are used; compliance with restrictions for takeoff, approach, and landing minimums; and plans in place in case of the need to use approved alternate airports.

Weight and Balance

Weight and balance requirements are important for rotor-wing and fixed-wing aircraft as specified in the airplane or rotorcraft flight manual. The manual contains aircraft performance data regarding maximum certified gross weights, center-of-gravity limits, and runway lengths that fixed-wing aircraft use for takeoff. Because fixed-wing airplanes (depending on the model) have fewer weight restrictions and more cabin space than rotor-wing aircraft,[73] family members and other persons frequently accompany patients on fixed-wing aircraft transports.

According to FAR Part 91.605, the pilot must ensure that the aircraft is loaded within weight and balance limits at all times.[39-42] Because the gross weight of the aircraft is predetermined by the airplane flight manual, the pilot is responsible for determining the daily operational weight, which is the weight of the aircraft, fuel, pilot, air medical personnel, and equipment. These calculations must be completed before taking off on a medical transport. Therefore, when in contact with the referring facility, air medical personnel should attempt to obtain the weights of patients and persons who will ride along. The pilot can benefit from early notification of the patient's weight, especially for the patient who weighs more than 300 lbs, and the weight of any additional passengers that may accompany the patient or any additional equipment that may be brought on board. The pilot has final authority for weight limitations and may decide that family members or other persons may not accompany the patient. In addition, the pilot may decide to decrease fuel loads, rearrange the seating of passengers, unload unnecessary equipment, leave behind unnecessary passengers and air medical personnel, or depart from an airport with a longer runway.

A second important weight and balance requirement is that aircraft be loaded within the center-of-gravity range or limitations.[39-42] Once the maximal weight has been determined, the weight distribution, or where the weight is placed in an aircraft, is critical for aerodynamic performance and safety while the aircraft is in flight.[39-42] The weight must be properly loaded fore and aft of the center of gravity, according to the manufacturer's airplane flight manual.

Lifeguard Status

Air ambulance services may declare *lifeguard* status for priority flights in the air traffic control system. Lifeguard affords the airplane priority when taking off or landing and should be used with extreme discretion. This status is only "intended for those missions of an urgent medical nature" (i.e., when a patient's condition is deteriorating or in full arrest) when a patient is on board or for the "portion of the flight requiring expeditious handling."[67] Lifeguard status is filed with a flight service station. Although landing and departing time differences are minimal at small airports, lifeguard status often achieves a tremendous time advantage at metropolitan and international airports. An air medical aircraft that is on lifeguard status may be allowed to take off or land ahead of multiple commercial and private aircraft, but this causes delays for these aircraft or extends their holding pattern time, costing thousands of dollars. Therefore, an air medical service must reserve lifeguard status for those times when it is absolutely necessary. Lifeguard status does not negate the need to comply with Transportation Security Administration reporting requirements.[91]

Ambient Temperatures

Several aircraft temperature considerations should be addressed before a flight commences because temperature can present potential problems in the air medical environment. The first consideration is the amount of time the aircraft will spend on the ground because air conditioning or heating cannot be left on for more than a few minutes during this time unless an auxiliary power unit is used. Unfortunately, auxiliary power units are usually not available at smaller airports, where most fixed-wing transports originate.

A second temperature consideration is evident at higher altitudes, at which the ambient temperature decreases. As the altitude increases, temperature decreases to the *tropopause*, which is the location at which the temperature reaches its lowest point and remains constant. The fuselage circumference of most air medical aircraft tends to be relatively small, and insulation of the walls is such that the walls and floor feel cool.[51] The cumulative effect of all of these factors is often a cooler environment in a fixed-wing aircraft.

A third temperature consideration is encountered when descending into tropical or humid climates. On descent, windows become fogged and other types of condensation occur inside the aircraft.

Additional Considerations

On the basis of investigative findings of recent air ambulance aviation incidents and accidents, the National Transport Safety Board (NTSB) has published recommendations to enhance safe operations.[67] Furthermore, the FAA has issued similar guidance.[39-42] Air ambulance services are encouraged to operate all flights within the regulations governing 14 Code of Federal Regulations (CFR) Part 135 flights, including positioning flight, especially when operated with visual flight rules (VFR) as opposed to instrument flight rules (IFR).[39-42] *Positioning flights* refer to flights that are conducted under 14 CFR Part 91 to optimally situate the aircraft. Weather minimums and crew rest requirements differ between Part 135 and Part 91 regulations, with Part 135 requirements being more restrictive. Part 91 flights may be done with medical team members on board, but flights with patients on board must be conducted in compliance with Part 135 regulations.

The recommendations and guidance also advocate air ambulance operators to develop flight risk evaluation programs. The programs should be part of the decision-making process and provide a methodology by which risks such as inclement weather, night-time flight operations, lack of visual cues commonly used along possible flight routes, lack of familiarity with landing zones or sites, pilot training and expertise, and compelling factors that influence the decision to take the flight are systematically evaluated before acceptance of each flight. Coupled with the flight risk evaluation program, comprehensive flight dispatch and flight following procedures performed by personnel with aviation experience may minimize undue risks and further enhance safe operations.

The proposed use of available technology, namely terrain awareness warning systems (TAWS), traffic collision avoidance systems (TCAS), and night vision imaging systems (NVIS), including but not limited to night vision goggles (NVGs), may greatly reduce the incidents or accidents experienced in EMS operations resultant of controlled flight into terrain. Conversely, the use of NVIS requires special training and is not considered practical in more ambient lighted areas such as populated or urban areas.[39-42,67] The addition of TAWS and TCAS units may be costly and weight and space prohibitive for some older airframes in operation.

PREPARATION FOR PATIENT TRANSPORT
Transferring and Accepting Physician and Facility

The transport team must ensure that an appropriate referral is arranged for the fixed-wing transport. Because additional time is usually available to preplan for an interfacility fixed-wing transport, the names of both the referring and the accepting physician should be documented for the transfer.

In 1985, Congress enacted the Consolidated Omnibus Budget Reconciliation Act (COBRA), which was amended in July and November 1990. COBRA protects indigent uninsured patients from being denied access to emergency care by hospitals or from being transferred inappropriately between hospitals on the basis of the patient's inability to pay.[76] This legislation requires that the referring hospital assume liability for the adequacy of stabilization before transport. COBRA also requires documentation before the transfer that the receiving hospital has been verified and that a receiving physician is willing to accept the patient. If a transfer is necessary for a patient whose condition is not yet stabilized, COBRA states that various conditions are to be met, including the following[76,82,85]: (1) the physician certifies in writing that, in his or her professional opinion, the benefits of the transfer outweigh the risks; (2) the transferring hospital treats the patient within its capacity, which minimizes the risks to the patient; (3) the receiving facility agrees to accept the patient and has available space and qualified personnel to provide appropriate medical treatment; (4) the transferring hospital sends to the receiving facility all medical records (copies) available at the time of transfer; and (5) the transfer is affected through qualified personnel and transportation equipment.

The transport team must often validate transfer information from the communications center. This information must be validated because these patients are transferred from towns, cities, and states in which air medical personnel are not necessarily familiar with the hospitals and physicians involved in the transfer.

Oxygen Requirements

Determination of in-flight and ground ambulance times from the referring to the receiving facility assists the flight nurse in calculating the amount of oxygen needed to meet the needs of the patient. The transport team must ensure sufficient oxygen to deliver 1.0 FiO_2 or to operate a ventilator, if needed, for 1 to 1.3 times the entire length of the patient transport.[19,26,70] In some patient transports, more time is spent on the ground than in flight. Time spent on the ground may be 90 minutes or longer. Therefore, all fixed-wing aircraft should carry a portable back-up oxygen tank in case the main system fails or the ground ambulance has no oxygen available. Some foreign countries do not carry oxygen in their ambulances (Table 10-5).

Patient Medical Equipment Requirements

Air medical services are improving fixed-wing aircraft standards by providing dedicated aircraft with custom medical configurations, which allows services to permanently secure ventilators, heart monitors, and other patient medical equipment. Equipment that is needed may be chosen on the basis of the mission

TABLE 10-5   Calculation of Oxygen Cylinder Time

$$\text{Time} = \frac{(\text{Pcylinder} \times \text{CF})}{V}$$

Cylinder	CF
D Cylinder	0.16
Jumbo D Cylinder	0.25
E Cylinder	0.28
G Cylinder	2.41
H Cylinder	3.14
K Cylinder	3.14
M Cylinder	3.14

CF, Conversion factor; *Pcylinder,* total pressure in cylinder is 500; *V,* flow rate in liters per minute.

From Oakes D: *Clinical practitioner's pocket guide to respiratory care,* Philadelphia, 2006, Health Educator Publications.

and the scope of care provided by the air medical service. For example, a service whose mission is critical care for children and adults should have appropriate transport equipment readily available. This equipment may include a heart and hemodynamic monitor, a noninvasive blood pressure (BP) monitor, a pulse generator, IV pumps, a pulse oximeter, an on-board suction device, a transport ventilator, an isolette, and a transport intraaortic balloon pump.

Medical equipment that requires battery power should also have auxiliary power capabilities that can use the aircraft's inverter. The transport team should always ensure that the inverter power source on the aircraft and ground ambulance works properly in case batteries should fail. Because many ground ambulances outside the United States do not have inverters, the transport team should have spare batteries available.

For example, with the improvement of medical transport equipment in recent years, the most critical patients who need the support of several different pieces of medical equipment may now be transported without difficulty. Transport equipment, including IV pumps, ventilators, intraaortic balloon pumps, fetal heart monitors, and other devices, has been designed and tested for the transport environment.

A portable suction unit should also be included in the standard equipment for fixed-wing transports. This unit provides the team with back-up equipment should the main suction system fail in the fixed-wing aircraft. The portable suction unit is also valuable during transport once the patient is removed from the aircraft at isolated or foreign airports.

Finally, transport services must comply with state licensure requirements for air medical aircraft, which include specifications about medical equipment that must be placed on the aircraft. Because these requirements vary from state to state, some aircraft may be required to carry additional equipment according to state regulations.

Patient Care Supplies and Medications

The aircraft must be stocked with adequate medical supplies and medications to provide the nursing care needed by the patient for the entirety of the transport. In addition to the required air ambulance equipment, extra supplies may be tailored to the anticipated needs of the patient. For example, if a patient needs breathing treatments while in flight, additional nebulizer setups and extra or multivial doses of the medication may be stocked. Also, because a patient who used intubation may need frequent suctioning, additional saline bullets and sterile suction catheters should be stocked on the aircraft.

Bedding and Linens

Because fixed-wing flights involve longer periods of patient care, comfort becomes a major issue. The traditional fixed-wing aircraft stretcher pads are hard, thin, and narrow and have limited flexibility. The transport team can plan ahead and attempt to use bedding, egg crates, or blankets on top of the stretcher to provide extra padding and create a softer surface. If an air mattress is to be used, air must be able to be released to prevent the mattress from rupturing in flight as a result of gas expansion at higher altitudes.

In addition, the transport nurse may stock extra pillows for use in supporting the head, neck, back, and knees and for positioning between knees and elbows and elevating extremities and feet. On longer flights, the team must pay greater attention to the patient's position. Patients, especially those who are comatose or paralyzed, may need to be turned to prevent skin breakdowns. The patient may be placed on a "turn" or "draw sheet" so that air medical personnel can reposition the patient more easily in flight. Passive range-of-motion exercises also decrease the risk of blood pooling, deep vein thrombosis, pulmonary embolus, and additional skin injury from immobility.

The transport team should also pay attention to their own immobility on long flights. Stretching exercises and increased fluid intake can help prevent circulatory problems.

Nutrition and Fluid Requirements

Adequate nutrition and fluids should be provided for all persons on board the aircraft. Depending on the transport time and the time of day, food may be catered for the patient, family, pilots, and air medical personnel. The team must choose the proper food or provide the specialized diet (e.g., a low-fat or diabetic diet) needed by the patient. Proper storage of the food and fluids is necessary. In addition, an adequate stock of fluids, such as juice, and plenty of water for the entire length of the transport should be available. Because of the longer in-flight times, higher altitudes, and stresses of flight, the nurse should provide sources for replenishing energy and preventing dehydration for all persons on board the aircraft. Emphasis should be placed on taking care of oneself in addition to the patient and other passengers during the transport.

Disposal of Contaminated Wastes

All air medical personnel must comply with Occupational Safety and Health Administration (OSHA) regulations regarding occupational exposure to blood-borne pathogens.[87] The air medical service must have an exposure-control plan. Policies, procedures, and equipment must be provided in the plan to comply with these regulations and protect employees from infectious diseases. Air medical personnel must follow infection control policies by observing standard precautions and stocking extra personal protective equipment, supplies, and cleaning agents for these long flights. Depending on the

flight distance and in-flight patient care times, the team must plan for the containment and disposal of contaminated needles, dressings, empty IV fluid bags, and human wastes according to OSHA regulations. A urinary catheter makes disposal of urine easy. The team must also plan for providing care and properly disposing of wastes should the patient have a bowel movement. Multiple large red isolation bags may be used to dispose of wipes, bedpans, and urinals.

Air medical personnel, pilots, and family members should plan to use restroom facilities before departure and during fuel stops. Some fixed-wing aircraft may have toilet facilities.

Required Ground Ambulance Capabilities

For fixed-wing transports, the transport team can never assume that a particular ground ambulance unit is available. The team must investigate the capabilities and resources of the ambulance that arrives at the airport. If the patient needs various kinds of medical equipment, inverter power should be available on the ambulance to power the equipment. The transport team should also assess the resources of the ambulance service to determine whether it can provide the appropriate basic life support or advanced life support services. In some countries, no resources may be available in the ambulance, in which case *all* medical equipment with adequate battery power, medications, and oxygen needed for the patient must be provided by the flight team.

PATIENT "PACKAGING" FOR TRANSPORT
Preparation

Preparation of a patient for a fixed-wing transport usually requires a thorough assessment, stabilization, and preparation process because of lengthy patient care times. In rare cases, the transport team may "swoop and scoop" the patient, primarily as a result of the patient's condition or when the patient is brought to the transport team at an airport. Most of the time, the team performs a rapid assessment at the referring facility and initiates patient care. A pre-flight plan helps minimize the amount of time spent on the ground before departure.

Loading Considerations

After ground transport to the aircraft, air medical personnel must plan to transfer the patient into the aircraft and secure the medical equipment. Because most aircraft doors are relatively narrow, the team must make the patient package as slender as possible. Once on the aircraft, equipment must be secured according to FAA regulations and placed in a position that permits continuous assessments while allowing the tubes and catheters to remain patent and accessible.

Numerous companies provide equipment for loading a patient into fixed-wing aircraft. Because of an increase in fixed-wing transports, these companies have developed and marketed stands, lifts, slides, and sleds to assist with loading and unloading patients through narrow fixed-wing aircraft doors. These loading devices have significantly eased the loading procedure, but more importantly, they assist with preventing excessive movement and potential injury to the patient during loading and unloading and work-related injuries for the pilot and air medical personnel.

Immobilization Equipment

Immobilization devices present unique challenges for loading a patient through a fixed-wing aircraft door and positioning the patient in the aircraft. Some aircraft doors are too narrow to accommodate standard backboards for loading patients into aircraft. For this reason, tapered backboards are suggested. The team must also prepare for patients who have other immobilization devices, such as a traction splint, in place. Loading the patient on the aircraft may be difficult because of the length of the splint. In addition, positioning the patient can present challenges.

Bulky dressings, splints, and the need to maintain a position of comfort for an injured extremity may make transfer of the patient smoothly through the aircraft door difficult. In addition, the patient needs to be positioned in the aircraft so that the extremity can be supported, while optimal positioning is maintained and access for nursing care is allowed.

As discussed previously, if air-filled splints are used on fixed-wing transports, the flight nurse must closely monitor distal circulation during flight and must be able to release air from the splint as needed to prevent patient injury as a result of gas expansion at higher altitudes.

In-Flight Factors That Influence Patient Care

Limited Space

The fixed-wing transport team must consider several issues that may not be factors in rotor-wing aircraft transport. Space may vary greatly from one aircraft to another. Propeller and turbopropeller aircraft tend to be more spacious than some of the jet models, which can be extremely important when patients need large advanced life support equipment or immobilization devices or when family members desire to accompany the patient.

Air Conditioner and Heater

In-flight climate-control systems may not meet most caregiver expectations. The thin walls and floor of the fuselage do not allow much space for thermal insulation. Therefore, the air conditioning may not adequately cool the airplane to the desired temperature on extremely hot summer days; and in the winter, some aircraft cabins may still feel cool when heaters are performing at maximum capacity. During fuel stops, most aircraft are dependent on the availability of a ground power unit to maintain comfortable cabin temperatures.

Extended Flight Times

Fixed-wing transports may involve longer flight times than generally appreciated with helicopter transfers. The patient should be assessed for risks related to the development of deep vein thrombosis (DVT) and pulmonary embolus (PE) often experienced with extended flight exposure. The effects of altitude combined with immobility places the patient at a greater risk of these complications. For any flights that involve lengthy flight times, the team should initiate measures to prevent the patient's development of DVT and PE, such as passive range of motion exercises and the use of anti-embolic stocking, and should evaluate the patient for the appropriateness of prophylactic pharmacologic measures.

Diversions

Because fixed-wing transport times are often longer than other types of patient transport, the potential for diversion of the flight is increased. Diversion can be prompted by mechanical problems, weather, or even a significant deterioration in the patient's status. Plans must be in place before transport to address diversion so that patient care is not jeopardized.

AIR MEDICAL PERSONNEL RESOURCES

One of the most critical factors for fixed-wing transports is the team's knowledge of available resources and how these resources can be accessed. The transport team must be familiar with medical control policies and procedures. Medical control may be extremely helpful to those involved with political situations, a patient whose condition is deteriorating, cardiac arrests that occur during the flight, interstate transports, and flights outside of the United States. The transport team must ensure that the air medical service has policies and procedures in place and must know how to contact the medical control to deal with these situations. In addition, the transport team must be able to use the resources of the communications center to contact the program director, clinical supervisor, or medical director as needed to assist with patient decisions and coordination of the patient transfer in emergency situations.

Medical Control

Most air medical services receive medical control services from the medical director and the designated medical control physicians. As discussed previously in this chapter, most fixed-wing aircraft flights are interfacility transports. Therefore, a physician referral has been made to transfer the patient to an accepting physician and facility. Before departure from the referring facility, a nurse may contact a medical control physician via telephone to discuss a patient's medical condition and request further orders as needed. Once the team is in the ground ambulance or in flight, the opportunities for telephone communication may be limited to satellite services, two-way pagers, or less-than-reliable cellular services.

Communication

The transport team should be familiar with all of the capabilities and aircraft communications of the communications center. The team should also become familiar with the various nonaviation radio frequencies for contacting the communications center and ground EMS agencies. In addition, air medical services should be encouraged to provide flight telephones or satellite telephones on the aircraft to initiate medical patching during the flight if the patient's condition deteriorates. Use of flight or satellite telephones is legal during flight, whereas use of cellular telephones or two-way pagers is illegal when airborne. Flight telephones are licensed and regulated by the Federal Communications Commission. Satellite telephones use global satellites for connection rather than the traditional cellular sites. When a flight or satellite telephone is available, the transport team can contact medical control during in-flight medical emergencies.

IN-FLIGHT CODES

The transport team faces unique challenges and must use decision-making skills when a patient goes into cardiopulmonary arrest during a fixed-wing aircraft transport. The air medical personnel should be apprised of the patient's current code status. In addition, before transport, the patient and family members who accompany the patient should be made aware of the risks of air medical transport and the potential for diversions should the patient's condition deteriorate.

The team must address four essential issues if a patient has a full cardiopulmonary arrest during the fixed-wing aircraft transport. The team must consider the following: (1) the service's policies and procedures for in-flight codes; (2) the decision to return, divert, or continue to proceed to the destination; (3) the availability of resuscitation equipment and medications; and (4) the endurance of the air medical personnel. After all of these issues have been weighed and deliberated, the team shall make the final decision in conjunction with medical control.

First, air medical personnel need to be well versed in the air medical service's policies and procedures for full codes on a fixed-wing aircraft transport. Every state has specific laws that deal with terminating resuscitation efforts in the prehospital arena. The program should have policies and procedures in place that relate to patients in full cardiopulmonary arrest and the actions that are required by air medical personnel in consultation with the service's medical control.

In addition, legal aspects of interstate and international transport may complicate the decision to terminate resuscitation en route or before reaching the destination. Therefore, some air medical services have a policy that a patient cannot be pronounced dead until the aircraft has landed, especially if the transport takes place outside the United States.[46]

Second, if the patient's condition deteriorates into a full code during any portion of the transport, the air medical personnel must weigh distance and time factors to decide literally in which direction to transport. This decision may be based on the distance and time to return to the referring facility or to the closest appropriate facility, on the availability of ground ambulances, and on overall patient status. The question for the air medical personnel is whether to divert the aircraft or continue to the final destination after weighing all these factors.

The third essential issue relates to the service's available resuscitation equipment and medications. This equipment may include oxygen, endotracheal tubes, advanced cardiac life-support medications, fluids, and the battery power on life-support equipment. Given the limited supplies available on fixed-wing aircraft, the transport team may need to make a decision based on the air medical team exhausting all of the resuscitation equipment.

Finally, the endurance of the air medical personnel on the transport should be considered, especially for transports that also require ground times in excess of 90 minutes. The air medical personnel may need to contact medical control and recommend ceasing resuscitation efforts if the patient does not respond to medical therapy on an extremely long flight.

"Do Not Resuscitate" Orders

Fixed-wing aircraft transport services may provide DNR transports at the family's request and not because of medical necessity. These flights are prescheduled with an air medical service, but again, the transport team should be familiar with DNR policies and procedures. Because various states have different definitions for DNR patients, services that conduct these types of flights should provide policies and procedures for air medical personnel.

SAFETY AND EMERGENCY PROCEDURES

Safety is the number one priority for any patient transport. In the fixed-wing aircraft transport environment, the transport team should receive initial and annual ongoing education regarding fixed-wing aircraft operations, regulations, and unscheduled aircraft emergencies. According to FAR 91.505 and 135.331, all flight crew members should receive emergency training for each aircraft type and model.[88-90] Because air medical personnel are considered passengers and not flight crew, an air medical service may not provide all the crew member emergency training requirements. All air medical personnel should receive safety education in potential in-flight emergencies and procedures appropriate for each kind and model of aircraft flown, which allows the air medical personnel to understand and assist the pilot with various procedures. According to Wright et al,[94] education regarding in-flight emergencies increases the confidence of air medical personnel and pilots and affects their ability to deal effectively with these emergencies before and after the emergency. At a minimum, education should be provided for dealing with the following emergencies: (1) fire during the flight; (2) electrical failure; (3) hydraulic failure; (4) slow or rapid decompression; (5) water ditching, if flying over water; (6) rapid egress procedures; and (7) survival procedures and available equipment. For further review of emergency procedures and survival, see Chapter 9.

INTERNATIONAL TRANSPORT ISSUES

Air Medical Service International Transports

The discussion of air medical transport no longer focuses only on domestic transports. International transports continue to increase for patients who need medical transport from one country to another. Although similarities exist between domestic and international air medical transports, there are many unique differences. This section focuses on some of the issues and obstacles that may be encountered with international transports, such as preflight preparation and logistics, documentation, language barriers, patient locations, ground ambulance times and resources, pilot and air medical personnel duty times, and medical equipment and supplies.[51-55]

Preflight Preparation and Logistics

Preflight preparation becomes extremely critical for international air medical transports. As with fixed-wing transports; extensive plans for the logistics must be completed by the entire team with the realization that the flights are often much longer than other air medical transports. Additional preflight plans must include customs, immigrations, international weather briefings, landing permits, refueling stops, ground handling, oxygen requirements, catering arrangements, medical equipment needs, and rest requirements.[38] Inadequate preparations or failure to notify the appropriate authorities only frustrate the air medical team and create enormous delays. In addition, meticulous attention should be given to obtaining as much accurate patient information as possible to prepare for the medical needs of the patient.[51-55] Because international transports of critically ill and injured patients may not be accomplished on some commercial airliners and many carriers now restrict the transport of stretcher-dependent patients, some air medical services conduct routine international transports. These programs have dedicated jets that are medically configured. In preparation for the worst-case scenario, these aircraft have redundant medical equipment and systems. These jets also offer lavatory facilities and auxiliary power units for maintaining a comfortable cabin environment and charging medical equipment during ground times of the transport.[38] Many aviation companies are able to assist an air medical service in preparation for international transport.

Documentation

Air medical personnel and pilots should always have the appropriate documentation for customs and immigration requirements on their person. This documentation includes passports, entry and exit visas, and immunization records.[33-36] International guideline charts are available to explain requirements for different countries.[1,51-55] The State Department can advise on the specific customs and immigration requirements for a country.

The Centers for Disease Control and the World Health Organization publish guidelines for required and recommended immunizations for each country. The patient and all accompanying passengers should also have the required customs and immigration papers. The transport company is held responsible for any fines or citations incurred from the lack of these required documents.

When planning for the flight, the appropriate documentation must also be verified for the patient and any passengers. Frequently the pilot organizes this information when filing the flight plan and making arrangements with customs.

As discussed previously, the team must document all assessment findings, care administered during the transport, and the patient's status throughout the transport as part of the medical record. Documentation must be done in a manner that allows the nurse to leave a copy of the chart with the patient when care is transferred to the receiving facility.

Language Barriers

When attempting to obtain an accurate patient diagnosis and discover the patient's medical condition and care needs, air medical personnel may deal with language barriers from the referring facility, physician, or family members that may require the use of a translator. Many long-distance telephone companies now offer translators fluent in multiple languages.[36] In addition, insurance companies and travel assistance companies that coordinate these international flights have resources available for translating patient information.

The medical director or clinical supervisor and the flight nurse involved with the flight must use the necessary resources to obtain patient information that is as accurate as possible, even if this delays the transport.[51] This information ensures that the skills of the air medical personnel and the available medical equipment are appropriate for the anticipated medical needs of the patient. In some cases, when transporting an American citizen back to the United States, the transport team may be able to obtain medical information by speaking directly with the patient or family members.

The air medical personnel must also plan for language barriers when arriving at the patient location and during the flight. An interpreter may be needed at the referring hospital or clinic to translate the medical terms, current treatment, and patient care needs.[36] In addition, the air medical personnel on the flight benefit from learning specific medical terms and words related to caring for the patient during the flight (e.g., terms related to current chest pain status and restroom needs).

Patient Location

International air medical transports may involve patients who are located not only in hospitals but also in clinics, private homes, trailers, hotels, physician offices, cruise ships or docks, and other locations that may never before have been encountered. The stability of the patient's condition on arrival may not be predictable; therefore, the flight nurse must prepare for the worst-case scenario. Patients who arrive at the airport by taxi may have had minimal care. The air medical personnel, being the only providers of advanced life support, have to initiate medical care.

Transport times should allow for a visit to the patient by the medical team at the referring facility. This time should involve a patient evaluation, obtaining medical records, and completing final arrangements. Each team member must always practice professional courtesy and obtain permission before entering the patient care area, examining the patient, and reviewing medical records. The transport team must keep in mind that medical care and local customs may influence their approach to the patient and the referring facility.

Ground Transport Times

Preflight planning must include an accurate calculation of the distance and ground times between the patient's location and the airport. Information such as traffic and road conditions may also be sought.[51-55] This information is extremely important

for calculating oxygen requirements for ventilation, battery life of equipment, and necessary supplies for the patient during transport.

Ground Ambulance Resources

Whether the patient is transported to the airport or the team is transported to the patient, the resources of the ground unit may be limited. The ambulance vehicle may be a private car, a taxicab, a suburban vehicle, a Volkswagen camper, a pickup truck with a camper shell, or an ambulance unit.[47] Some ambulances may be stripped to an empty unit with no oxygen source or suction equipment. Others may be elaborately stocked with supplies and medical equipment. In addition, the skills of the ambulance personnel that accompany the team and patient may vary widely, from a driver with no medical knowledge to emergency medical personnel, nurses, or physicians with varying degrees of skills.

Finally, one must consider the safety issues of the ground transport to and from the airplane. Road conditions, driving skills and compliance with traffic laws, the inability to secure equipment, and the lack of familiarity with the ground transport unit and local area by the medical team are a few of the concerns that may be faced during the ground transport. All of these issues contribute additional stresses to the international transport of patients.

Pilot and Air Medical Personnel Duty Times

Duty and rest times must be considered for each international transport for the pilot and air medical personnel. This issue is already addressed for pilots because they must comply with FAR Part 135.267 flight time limitations and rest requirements.[88] Therefore, during the preflight preparation, rest requirements must be calculated into the plan and arrangements made for relief pilots to assume flight duties at appropriate fuel stops or at the destination.

When making preflight preparations, air medical personnel should determine the length of the flight and patient care times and use judgment in scheduling adequate team breaks. Depending on the duty times of the flight and medical crew members, an overnight stay may be necessary to comply with crew rest and FAA requirements. This stay may involve the acquisition of lodging for each team member. Many times, these arrangements are easily facilitated with use of a handling agent in the country to which the patient is transferred; this agent can assist with hotel arrangements, aircraft refueling, catering, ground transportation, and any other needs of the team.

Rest for air medical personnel may be accomplished during the flight depending on available rest areas onboard the aircraft, with "members of the team sleeping in a rotation where the transport nurse or physician is always awake with the patient."[26,51] For extremely long transports, the air medical service may send a relief team of air medical personnel to a scheduled fuel stop to assume patient care. Programs should have policies that define when rests occur and when relief medical teams are required.

Medical Equipment and Supplies

As with preflight preparations for any fixed-wing aircraft transport, the transport team must ensure that plans are complete for international transports. The transport nurse must be meticulous in planning and arranging for adequate oxygen, medical equipment, batteries, supplies, bedding and linens, nutrition and fluids, and disposal of contaminated wastes. Remember that a greater potential for unexpected delays exists for these transports because of customs coordination, ambulance delays, and refueling stops. In addition, international transports may be of longer duration than other transports and to destinations with no stock of medical supplies or supplies incompatible with that of the air medical personnel. Therefore, air medical personnel should stock enough medical supplies and medications for twice the predicted time of transport.[1,51-55,74,82,83]

Many countries require special permits or have adopted specific requirements for the transport of certain medications. These requirements should be identified before the team's arrival to prevent any delays or confiscation of the medications needed to care for the patient. Medications should be kept in kits or medical packs and never carried in the team members' personal luggage.

Finally, the compatibility of medical equipment with foreign electrical current may need to be considered. The team may need to obtain several types of foreign adapters to convert the current so that monitors and suction units can be properly charged. The equipment manufacturer should be consulted on the ability to fully charge the equipment on differing hertz, or cycles per second, of foreign electrical currents.

ESCORT AND MEDICAL ASSIST TRANSPORTS ON COMMERCIAL AIRLINERS

One more form of patient transport, called a commercial medical *escort flight* or *medical assist transport,* should be discussed. Escorts may be either domestic or international transports. These transports are referred to as *commercial escorts.* A commercial escort is defined as the escort of a patient with a stable condition on a contracted aircraft or a commercial airliner with the airliner's approval with only one attendant who may be an emergency medical technician (EMT), emergency medical technician-paramedic (EMT-P), registered nurse (RN), or medical doctor (MD).[22] These flights may involve transporting a patient at the basic life support level who needs medical assistance, a critically ill or injured patient, or one who needs advanced life support or extensive nursing care.[46] The number and expertise of the accompanying attendants needed depends on the patient's condition, the ability to ambulate, and the length of the transport. In addition, when determining the medical escort team configuration, the requirements of the commercial airline must also be considered.[26]

With regard to preflight preparation and logistics for this type of transport, the flight nurse should ensure that all arrangements are complete and plan to address several unique obstacles. These issues include not only commercial air carrier regulations, documentation, airline oxygen requirements, oxygen adapters, and electrical power, but also privacy and nonstop flights. Because transport of a patient on a commercial airliner requires approval of the escort by the air carrier's medical desk and coordination that is not under the control of the air medical service, these arrangements may take several days to an entire week to complete.

Commercial Air Carrier Regulations

Regulations for transporting a patient on an airliner vary, depending on the patient's designated level and condition. Many commercial air carriers allow a patient in stable condition who needs limited care to sit in the first-class or business-class section for transport.[51] On the other hand, transfer of a critically ill patient may necessitate the purchase of multiple seats (6 to 12) in the business-class section or in the rear coach compartment of the airplane so the litter can be secured. Many airliners prohibit stretcher-bound patients. Most of the airliners that can accommodate patients that are unable to travel in a seated position have a dedicated patient litter that rests above the folded passenger seats and is bolted to the seat tracks.[74] Special arrangements should be made with each commercial airliner because each carrier has a different patient litter, loading and securing procedures, and quantity of medical oxygen available. The transport team should plan for the logistics of these escorts to ensure that the transport is completed smoothly.

In addition, provisions must be made for transporting medical equipment and supplies in such a way that they are readily available for the patient and yet secured according to the FARs. The equipment also should be organized in such a manner that it can be easily transferred and checked by customs and immigration authorities.

Documentation

The air medical personnel must organize all of the paperwork necessary for the entire transport, including the airline tickets, passports, itinerary, and customs documents. This documentation for the air medical personnel, patient, and family members must be readily available for customs and immigration authorities. Air medical personnel should always keep this paperwork on their person.

As with other transports, patient documentation must be completed and copies of the medical record must be left with the patient at the receiving facility.

Airline Oxygen Requirements

Each air carrier has a different procedure for obtaining oxygen and securing the O_2 tanks. The oxygen tanks routinely provided by most airliners deliver only 2 to 4 L per minute. Therefore, arrangements must be made to have extra oxygen tanks available for patients who require 100% O_2 or a ventilator. A minimum of 24 hours of notice is necessary, but frequently several days are needed to make such arrangements.[51-55,74] Many airliners charge additional fees to provide medical oxygen and may restrict the amount that can be secured because they have limited capacity to accommodate and secure larger oxygen tanks. In addition to having oxygen provisions during flight, the availability of oxygen within the terminals during layovers and plane changes must also be considered. The commercial airline may not have the ability to provide oxygen outside the aircraft and gate area.[74]

Oxygen Adapters

Particular attention should be given to the oxygen adapters and regulators available on each airliner. Most of this equipment is not compatible with air medical transport ventilator fittings. In addition, oxygen flow meters are often irregular. For instance, in some airliners, the O_2 outlet has three prongs.

Electrical Power and Adapters

The commercial air carrier's electrical power sources must be assessed and coordinated to power the medical equipment. A power source may be needed for transport ventilators, heart monitors, intravenous pumps, and suction equipment. As previously mentioned, the appropriate adapters must be obtained to convert the current in these foreign airplanes.

Privacy

Most commercial airliners have various rules pertaining to patients in critical condition. Their presence may offend or upset other paying passengers. Some airlines provide privacy for the patient by installing temporary curtains, but most of the time they are inadequate. Other airlines may require the patient be transported in a private medical suite.[82] Additional sheets or drapes may be necessary to provide adequate privacy for the patient.

Nonstop Flight

Every attempt should be made to make reservations on a nonstop flight for the patient transport.[51-55,82]

The nonstop flight eliminates the frustrations of making additional arrangements to get on and off of the airplane, to transfer the patient, and to provide documentation for customs and immigrations officials. In addition, plans must be made to organize all of the medical equipment, patient and family belongings, and luggage of air medical personnel for each transfer.

SUMMARY

Although many general principles of practice and patient care are identical in the rotor-wing aircraft, fixed-wing aircraft, commercial medical escort, and ground transport environments, differences do exist. First, one must focus on learning the safety and emergency procedures to be used in the fixed-wing aircraft. Second, because air medical transport on fixed-wing aircraft requires longer patient care times than other types of transport, the transport team must be meticulous in preplanning for the entire flight, coordinating resources, and providing care for all persons on board. Fixed-wing transport, both national and international, offers unique challenges to patient transport; to ensure safe and competent care, team members need to be appropriately selected and educated.

REFERENCES

1. Air & Surface Transport Nurses Association: *Transport nurse advanced trauma course*, Greenwood Village, CO, 2006, ASTNA.
2. Air & Surface Transport Nurses Association: *Standards for critical care and specialty ground transport*, Greenwood Village, CO, 2002, ASTNA.
3. Air & Surface Transport Nurses Association: *Standards for critical care and specialty rotor-wing transport*, Greenwood Village, CO, 2003, ASTNA.
4. Air & Surface Transport Nurses Association: *Standards for critical care and specialty fixed-wing transport*, Greenwood Village, CO, 2004, ASTNA.
5. Air Medical Physicians Association: *Medical condition list and appropriate use of air medical transport*, Salt Lake City, 2001, AMPA.
6. Air Medical Physicians Association: *Appropriateness of medical transport and access to care in acute stroke syndromes*, Salt Lake City, 2004, AMPA.
7. Alterman D: Consideration in pediatric trauma, *eMedicine* [www.emedicine.com], *Medscape J* 2008. Accessed June 30, 2008.
8. American College of Emergency Physicians: *Appropriate interhospital patient transfer*, Dallas, 2002, ACEP.
9. American College of Emergency Physicians: *Ambulance diversion*, Dallas, 2006, ACEP.
10. American College of Emergency Physicians: *Interfacility transportation of the critical care patient and its medical direction*, Dallas, 2005, ACEP.
11. American College of Surgeons: *Resources for optimal care of the injured patient*, Dallas, 2006, ACS.
12. American College of Surgeons: *Advanced trauma life support program for doctors*, Chicago, 2008, ACS.
13. Aoki B, McClosky K: *Evaluation, stabilization, and transport of the critically ill child*, St Louis, 1992, Mosby.
14. Association of Air Medical Services: *Recommended minimum quality standards for rotor-wing and fixed-wing standards*, Pasadena, CA, 1992, AAMS.
15. Baptiste A: Technology solutions for high-risk tasks in critical care, *Crit Care Nurs Clin North Am* 19:177-186, 2007.
16. Benevilli W, Thomas S, Brown D, et al: Safety of fentanyl during transport of trauma patients, *Air Med J* 14(3):156, 1995.
17. Benson J: *FDA safety alert: potential hazards with restraint devices*, Rockville, MD, 1992, Food and Drug Administration.
18. Binks A, Pyke M: Anaesthesia in the obese patient, *Anaesth Intens Care Med* 9(7):299-302, 2008.
19. Brink LW, et al: Air transport, transport medicine, *Pediatr Clin North Am* 40(2):452, 1993.
20. Brunette DD: Resuscitation of the morbidly obese patient, *Am J Emerg Med* 22(1):40-47, 2004.
21. Burney R, et al: Evaluation of hospital based aeromedical programs using therapeutic intervention scoring, *Aviat Space Environ Med* 6:563, 1990.
22. Bushard S: Trauma in patients who are morbidly obese, *AORN J* 76(4):585-589, 2002.
23. Campbell J: *International trauma life support*, ed 6, Upper Saddle River, NJ, 2008, Pearson Prentice Hall.
24. Chalfin D, et al: Impact of delayed transfer of critically ill patients from the emergency department to the intensive care unit, *Crit Care Med* 35(6):1477-1483, 2007.
25. Cohn H: Legal issues. In Neff J, Kidd P, editors: *Trauma nursing: the art and science*, St Louis, 1993, Mosby.
26. Commission on Accreditation of Medical Transport Systems (CAMTS): *Standards*, Anderson, SC, 2006, CAMTS.

27. Continenza K, Hill J: Transport of the critical child. In Blumer J, editor: *Pediatric intensive care*, St Louis, 1990, Mosby.

28. Crippen D: Critical care transportation medicine: new concepts in pretransport stabilization of the critically ill patient, *Am J Emerg Med* 11:551, 1990.

29. D'Arcy Y: Meeting the challenges of acute pain management, *Medscape Neurol Neurosurg MedScape J* (www.medscape.org). Accessed June 30, 2008.

30. Dickinson E, Krett R, O'Connor R: The impact of prehospital instant photography of motor crashes on physician perception and patient management in the emergency department, *Prehosp Disaster Med* 7(suppl 1), 1992.

31. Drake D, Dutton K, Engelke M, et al: Challenges that nurses face in caring for morbidly obese patients in the acute care setting, *Surg Obesity Related Dis* 1:462-466, 2005.

32. Emergency Nurses Association, Newberry L: *Sheehy's emergency nursing: principles and practice*, ed 4, St Louis, 2003, Mosby.

33. Emergency Nurses Association Diversity Task Force: *Approaching diversity: an interactive journey*, Des Plaines, IL, 1997, updated 2003, ENA.

34. Emergency Nurses Association: *Trauma nursing core course*, Des Plaines, IL, 2007, ENA.

35. Emergency Nurses Association: *Emergency nurse pediatric course*, Des Plaines, IL, 2004, ENA.

36. Emergency Nurses Association: *Diversity in emergency care*, Des Plaines, IL, 2003, ENA.

37. Emerman C, Shade B, Kubincanek J: Comparative performance of the best trauma triage rule, *Am J Emerg Med* 10(4):294, 1992.

38. Falcone RJ, et al: Is air medical scene response for illness appropriate? *Air Med J* 12(6):191, 193-195, 1993.

39. Federal Aviation Administration: *Code of federal regulations: title 14, aeronautics and space, parts 91 and 135*, Washington, DC, 2008, US Department of Transportation.

40. Federal Aviation Administration: *Code of federal regulations: subpart F 135.261-269*, Washington, DC, 2008, US Department of Transportation.

41. Federal Aviation Administration: *Code of federal regulations: subpart F 135.271-273*, Washington, DC, 2008, US Department of Transportation.

42. Federal Aviation Administration: *Public Helicopter Emergency Medical Services (HEMS) operations notice N 8000.318*, Washington, DC, 2006, US Department of Transportation.

43. Forgey WW: *Wilderness medical practice guidelines for wilderness emergency care*, Guilford, CT, 2006, Globe Pequot Press.

44. Frakes M, et al: Efficacy of fentanyl analgesia for trauma in critical care transport, *Am J Emerg Med* 24(3):286-289, 2006.

45. Gabram S, Piancentini L, Jacobs L: The risk of aeromedical transport for the cardiac patient, *Emerg Care Q* 2:72, 1990.

46. Hart M: Patient assessment, preparation and care. In *US Department of Transportation: Air medical crew national standard curriculum*, Washington, DC, 1988, US Department of Transportation.

47. Hart M, et al: Air transport of the pediatric trauma patient, *Emerg Care Q* 3:21, 1986.

48. Hatfield ML, Lang A, Han ZQ, et al: The effect of helicopter transport on adult patients' body temperature, *Air Med J* 18(3):103, 1999.

49. Hatlestad D, Van Horn J: Air transport of the IABP patient, *Air Med J* 21(5):42-48, 2002.

50. Henry M, Stapleton E: *EMT prehospital care*, Philadelphia, 2006, Saunders.

51. Holdefer WF, Diethelm AG, Tolbert FT: International air medical transport, part I: methods and logistics, *J Air Med Transport* 9(7):6, 1990.

52. Holdefer WF, et al: International air medical transport, part II: results and discussion, *J Air Med Transport* 9(8):8, 1990.

53. Holdefer WF, Treadwell D, Tolbert JT: International air medical transport, program profile, *Int Air Amb* 7:36, 1998.

54. Holdefer WF, Treadwell D, Moore S, et al: International air medical transport ventilator dependent patients, *Int Air Amb* 9:22, 1999.

55. Husum H, et al: Preventing post-injury hypothermia during prolonged prehospital evacuation, *Prehosp Disaster Med* 17(1):23-26, 2002.

56. Ide P, Farber E, Lautz D: Perioperative nursing care of the bariatric surgical patient, *AORN J* 88(1):30-58, 2008.

57. Kidd P: Assessment of the trauma patient. In Neff J, Kidd P, editors: *Trauma nursing: the art and science*, St Louis, 1993, Mosby.

58. Kitt S, et al: *Emergency nursing*, Philadelphia, 1995, Saunders.

59. Loos L, Runyan L, Pelch D: Development of prehospital medical classification criteria, *Air Med J* 17(1):13, 1998.

60. McCloskey J, Bulechek G: *Nursing interventions classification*, St Louis, 1996, Mosby.

61. McCloskey K, Orr R, editors: *Textbook of pediatric transport medicine*, St Louis, 1995, Mosby.

62. McCullough P, Silver M, Kennard E, et al: Impact of body mass index on outcomes of enhanced external counterpulsation therapy, *Am Heart J* 151(1):139. e9-139.3-13, 2006.

63. Mirski M, Hemstreet M: Critical care sedation for neuroscience patients, *J Neurolog Sci* 261(1):16-34, 2007.

64. Mirvis SE: Imaging in trauma and critical care, ed 2, Philadelphia, 2003, Saunders.

65. National Association of Emergency Medical Services Physicians: Guidelines for air medical dispatch, *Prehosp Emerg Care* 7(2):265-274, 2003.

66. National Flight Nurses Association: *Practice standards for flight nursing*, St Louis, 1995, Mosby.

67. National Transportation Safety Board: *NTSB adopts EMS special investigation report and issues new recommendations*, Washington DC, 2006, NTSB.

68. Neff JA, Kidd PS, editors: *Trauma nursing: the art and science*, St Louis, 1993, Mosby.

69. Newberry L: Directory of air medical services, *Air Med J* 20(6):41, 2001.

70. Oakes D: *Clinical practitioner's pocket guide to respiratory care*, Philadelphia, 2006, Health Educator Publications, Inc.

71. Ohning Bryan: Transport of the critically ill newborn, *eMedicine* [www.emedicine.com], *Medscape J*, 2006. Accessed June 3, 2008.

72. O'Malley RJ, Watson-Hopkins M: Monitoring the appropriateness of air medical transports, *AirMed J* 13(8):323-325, 1994.

73. Petri D, et al: Medically appropriate use of helicopter EMS: the mission acceptance/triage process, *Air Med J* 26:1, 2007.

74. Ridley S, Carter R: The effects of secondary transport of critically ill patients, *Anesthesia* 44(10): 2007.

75. Sanders MJ: *Paramedic textbook*, ed 3, St Louis, 2007, Mosby JEMS Elsevier.

76. Schneider C, et al: Evaluation of ground ambulance, rotor-wing and fixed-wing aircraft services, *Crit Care Clin* 8(3):543, 1992.

77. Sharp D: Flight crews' use of digital cameras, *Air Med J* 21(5):24-27, 2002.

78. Stewart R: Analgesia in the field, *Prehosp Disaster Med* 4(1):31, 1989.

79. Strong C, Thompson CB: Documentation of decision-making during air transport, *Air Med J* 19(3):77, 2000.

80. Surgenor S, et al: Survival of patients transferred to tertiary intensive care from rural community hospitals, *Crit Care* 5(2):100-104, 2001.

81. Szczensiak SL: Trauma in the bariatric patient. In McQuillan K, Makic MBF, Whalen E, editors: *Trauma nursing: from resuscitation through rehabilitation*, ed 4, Philadelphia, 2009, Saunders Elsevier.

82. Treadwell D: In case of emergency: selecting a qualified air ambulance provider, *URMIA J* 2007-2008: 61-66, 2007.

83. Treadwell D: *The commercial carry-on, insurance journal supplement: 17*, Bristol, UK, 2007, Voyageur Publishing & Events LAD.

84. Treger R: Singstaken-Blakemore tube, *eMedicine* [www.emedicine.com], *The Medscape J*, 2007. Accessed June 30, 2008.

85. United States Code: *Consolidation Omnibus Budget Reconciliation Act (COBRA) of 1985 (42USC139dd)*, as amended by the Omnibus Budget Reconciliation Acts (OBRA) of 1987, 1989, and 1990.

86. US Department of Health and Human Services: *Acute pain management: operative or medical procedures*, Washington DC, 1992, USDHHS.

87. US Department of Labor, Occupational Safety and Health Administration: *Occupational exposure to bloodborne pathogens*, 29 CFR part 1910.1030, Washington DC, 2006, US Department of Labor, Occupational Safety and Health Administration.

88. US Department of Transportation: *Guide for interfacility patient transfer*, Washington DC, 2003, NHTSA EMS Division.

89. US Department of Transportation: *Safety alert for operators SAFO 0600*, Washington DC, 2006, Flight Standards Service.

90. US Government Accountability Office: *Aviation safety: system safety approach needs further integration into FAA's oversight of airlines,* in Report to Congressional Requisiters, Washington DC, 2005, US Government Accountability Office.

91. US Transportation Safety Administration: *Standard security program: 3(12–5)*, Washington, DC, 2007, TSA.

92. Velianoff G: Overcrowding and diversion in the emergency department, *Nurs Clin North Am* 37(1):59, 2002.

93. Warren J, et al: Guidelines for the inter-and intrahospital transport of critically critical care, *Med* 32(1): 256-262, 2004.

94. Wright A, et al: The effect of an in-flight emergency training program on crew confidence, *Air Med J* 13(4): 127, 1994.

95. York Clark D, Stocking J, Johnson J: *Flight and ground transport nursing core curriculum*, Denver, 2006, Air and Surface Transport Nurses Association.

96. Zecca A, et al: Endotracheal tube stabilization in the air medical setting, *J Air Med Transport* 3:7, 1991.

AIRWAY MANAGEMENT

Michael Rouse, Michael Frakes

COMPETENCIES

1. Identify the indications for basic and advanced airway management.
2. Describe and use the universal emergency airway algorithm for airway management.
3. Identify the indications and contraindications for specific airway interventions.
4. Demonstrate the ability to perform alternative airway management.
5. Describe the pharmacology of advanced airway management.

Airway management is the first priority of patient care and often accounts for one of the most difficult clinical dilemmas encountered by transport personnel. The most common error in airway management is failure to anticipate the need for active intervention in patients at high risk for airway obstruction or respiratory insufficiency. Patients with a decreased level of consciousness, cardiopulmonary disease, head and neck injuries, and major traumatic injuries need quick decisive airway management, based on a sound knowledge of physiologic and anatomic principles, to prevent life-threatening complications during transport.

Many skills and much equipment are needed for control of the airway; however, the essential component of the airway management skill set is critical thinking. The transport team must know when to intervene, when not to intervene, how to intervene,

and how to avoid complications. In addition to critical thinking, the competent transport team member must also possess the technical skill to perform an intervention when it is indicated. Critical thinking skills are developed through experience and practice. Technical performance is improved through advanced instruction and practice. Transport team members must be familiar with alternative airway options and their risks and benefits when deciding on a particular airway management technique.

Any vehicle used for patient transport may be an unfavorable environment for airway management. Noise, vibrations, sudden movements, inadequate lighting, lack of assistive personnel, limited access to the patient, and the inability to position the patient for better airway management are only a few of the reasons that airway management can be difficult in the transport environment. Failure of transport personnel to properly secure the airway before transport can lead to further respiratory decompensation, which can hasten systemic failure or produce an unmanageable transport in which safety may be compromised. Safety must never become a secondary consideration for the transport. Therefore, the airway must be fully controlled before critical care transport, even at the expense of additional time spent at the scene or referring institution.[50]

This chapter describes assessment parameters, airway interventions, and methods of evaluation of the patient's airway and ventilation during transport. Therapies to restore breathing and circulation are discussed in later chapters.

PATHOPHYSIOLOGY

INDICATIONS FOR INTUBATION

The multiple indications for initiation of airway management include apnea, airway obstruction, airway protection, respiratory insufficiency, foreign body obstruction, metabolic acidosis, and respiratory failure.[2,8,23,59,90] Also, at times, the decision to intubate is made without an obvious reason except the anticipation of a problem during transport. For example, the size of the transport vehicle may dictate that the patient has a secure airway before transport.

Invasive airway management can be beneficial for patients with hemodynamically unstable conditions. When a patient is in shock, an imbalance exists between oxygen supply and demand. Oxygen consumption increases linearly with work of breathing, and respiratory efficiency declines as work of breathing increases. External ventilator control can reduce that oxygen demand while providing direct airway access to increase oxygen delivery.[59] Particularly in patients with septic or hypovolemic shock, early intubation may be extremely beneficial.[90]

Just as the transport nurse must maintain situational awareness by considering past events, the current situation, and likely future events, development of the patient care plan must also include determination of whether the need for airway intervention will develop over the course of the transport. The transport nurse must consider the likelihood of progressive obstruction from soft tissue swelling or the expansion of a hematoma or abscess, the likelihood

of worsening oxygenation or ventilation, and the possibility of hemodynamic deterioration. Although airway procedures can clearly be performed in many transport vehicles, the procedures are also not possible in some; resource and access limitations can be associated with procedures performed in a transport vehicle instead of a healthcare facility. The transport team must factor those considerations into the pretransport care plan.

For the transport provider, patient and provider safety also sometimes necessitates airway intervention. In some environments, management of aggressive behavior with physical restraint may be appropriate, but the transport environment, and particularly the air transport environment, may necessitate the use of sedation so deep that it leads to respiratory depression or the inability to protect an airway.

The transport team should never ignore the competence that experience brings. Also, although intubation is a life-saving procedure, it is not without the potential for the development of serious complications. These complications include soft tissue injuries to the mouth, dental injury, vocal cord injury, tracheal or bronchial disruption, right mainstem intubation, aspiration, the development of a pneumothorax, esophageal intubation, and cardiac dysrhythmias. Complications can also occur with the use of neuromuscular blocking agents, anxiolytics, and sedative hypnotics that are used to facilitate intubation.[8,50,63]

Much research on emergency airway management has been done during the last 20 years. In an effort to develop a fundamental approach to the emergency airway, the National Emergency Airway Management Course published emergency airway algorithms that use a clinical critical-thinking approach. The algorithms are intended as guidelines in the approach to the emergency airway.[8,93,94] Figures 11-1 through 11-5 contain the universal emergency airway algorithm, main emergency airway management algorithm, crash airway algorithm, difficult airway algorithm, and failed-airway algorithm. The different airway interventions that are presented in these algorithms are discussed throughout this chapter. These algorithms also provide a framework to develop quality management and research programs related to airway management in the transport environment.

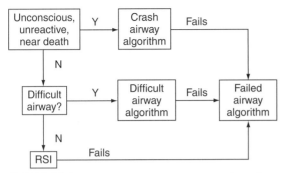

FIGURE 11-1 **Universal emergency airway algorithm.** (Reprinted from Walls R, Luten R, Murphy M, editors: *Manual of emergency airway management, a companion manual for the National Airway Management course,* Philadelphia, 2000, Lippincott Williams & Wilkins, available at www.theairwaysite. com. Accessed June 30, 2008.)

Selected Pathophysiology Related to Airway Management

Apnea can be the result of cardiac or traumatic arrest and is easily recognized and should be quickly treated. Initial basic airway management treatment begins with the insertion of an oral airway followed by adequate bag-valve-mask ventilations. This skill, although considered basic, requires maintenance of an adequate mask seal with one hand and provision of ventilations with the other. The mastery of bag-valve ventilation is the cornerstone of airway management and must be perfected by every emergency airway provider.

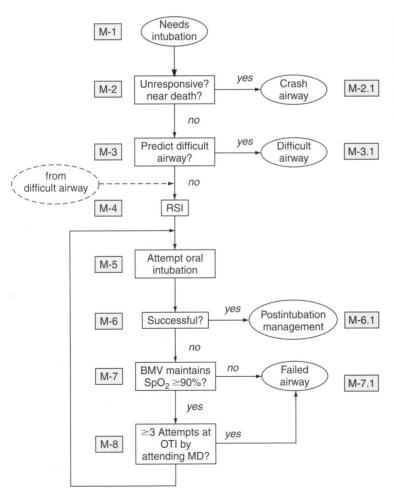

FIGURE 11-2 **Main emergency airway algorithm.** (Reprinted from Walls R, Luten R, Murphy M, editors: *Manual of emergency airway management, a companion manual for the National Airway Management course,* Philadelphia, 2000, Lippincott Williams & Wilkins, available at www.theairwaysite.com. Accessed June 30, 2008.)

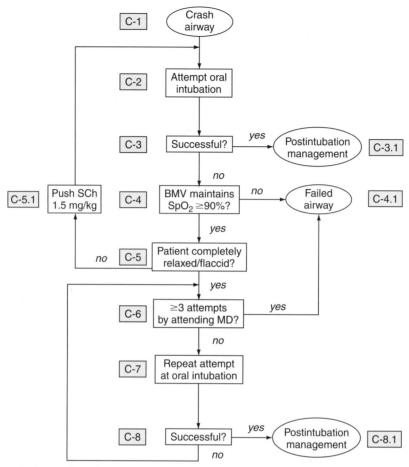

FIGURE 11-3   **Crash airway algorithm.** (Reprinted from Walls R, Luten R, Murphy M, editors: *Manual of emergency airway management, a companion manual for the National Airway Management course,* Philadelphia, 2000, Lippincott Williams & Wilkins, available at www.theairwaysite.com. Accessed June 30, 2008.)

Upper airway obstruction in the trauma patient is usually caused by the tongue, teeth, or blood. In the nontrauma patient, excessive secretions place the patient at risk for serious aspiration and an edematous epiglottis may obstruct the upper airway. Airway protection must be considered for the patient with actual or potential emesis and active bleeding.

The management strategies for the treatment of traumatic brain injury (TBI) have changed significantly since the previous editions of this text. No longer are patients mildly hyperventilated in an effort to reduce intracranial pressure (ICP). The understanding now is that hyperventilation reduces ICP by causing cerebral vasoconstriction and a subsequent reduction in cerebral

blood flow. Although early intubation to prevent the mortality that accompanies hypoxia is considered the standard of care for severe TBI, the effectiveness of this approach remains unproven.[8,90,93,94] Hyperventilation to a partial pressure of carbon dioxide in arterial blood (P_aCO_2) of 30 mm Hg in the patient with TBI today is reserved as a temporizing measure in patients with obvious clinical signs of herniation. Limiting the use of hyperventilation after severe TBI may help improve neurologic recovery after injury, or at least avoid iatrogenic cerebral ischemia.[8] The optimal CO_2 range appears to be 35 to 40 mm Hg or the lower limits of normocapnia. The use of quantitative capnometry can be a significant aid in confirmation of endotracheal tube placement but

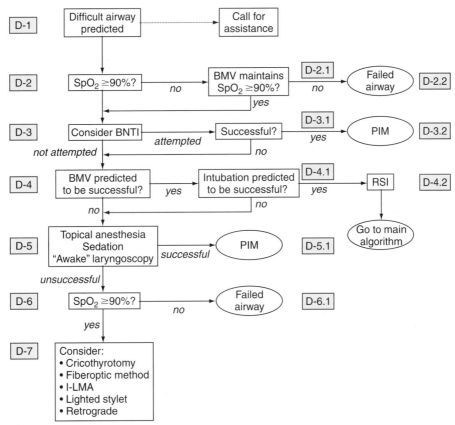

FIGURE 11-4   **Difficult airway algorithm.** (Reprinted from Walls R, Luten R, Murphy M, editors: *Manual of emergency airway management, a companion manual for the National Airway Management course,* Philadelphia, 2000, Lippincott Williams & Wilkins, available at www.theairwaysite.com. Accessed June 30, 2008.)

also aids in prevention of inadvertent severe hyperventilation in the patient with TBI.[8,24,26,33]

Respiratory insufficiency may be traumatic or nontraumatic in origin and involves disease of the lower airways, where actual gas exchange takes place. Traumatic respiratory insufficiency may result, for example, from a flail segment or pulmonary contusion. Nontraumatic conditions that cause respiratory distress include pulmonary emboli, congestive heart failure, adult respiratory distress syndrome, and status asthmaticus. Impending or potential airway compromise may be the most difficult situation to ascertain. Consideration must be given to the history of illness or injury, therapies used to treat the patient before the arrival of the transport team, the patient's response to the therapies, and transport time to the receiving

agency. A situation in which a patient has sustained burn trauma with an inhalation injury and circumferential burns of the neck and chest should leave the transport team with little doubt of the need for airway control. However, the transport team frequently encounters situations in which the potential for airway compromise is not as obvious. In these circumstances, the transport team must rely on subjective and objective assessment parameters and past experience to guide their judgment.

ASSESSMENT

Assessment of the airway is a two-part process. The primary survey is quick and crude; the secondary survey is slower and more refined. The primary survey

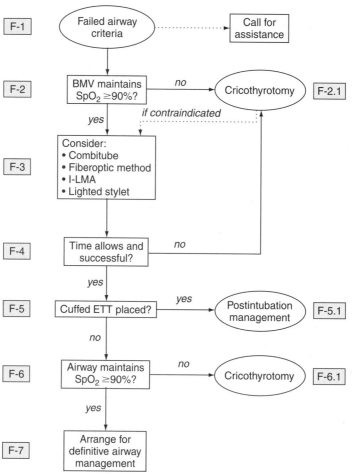

FIGURE 11-5   **Failed airway algorithm.** (Reprinted from Walls R, Luten R, Murphy M, editors: *Manual of emergency airway management, a companion manual for the National Airway Management course,* Philadelphia, 2000, Lippincott Williams & Wilkins, available at www.theairwaysite.com. Accessed June 30, 2008.)

begins with assessment of airway patency. The ability of the patient to speak with a clear unobstructed voice is strong evidence of both airway patency and protection. However, in the patient who has lost protective airway reflexes, the assessment stops, and immediate action is taken to establish airway patency. During the secondary survey, the transport team must determine whether airway patency and an appropriate level of oxygenation can be maintained throughout transport; an altered level of consciousness may indicate hypoxia. If in doubt, the transport team must initiate appropriate interventions. Initially,

the transport team assesses the patient by looking, listening, and feeling for spontaneous respirations. The mouth is opened and observed for obvious injuries and the presence of blood, teeth, the tongue, or foreign bodies obstructing the upper airway. The patient in the compensatory stage of shock may also have an increase in the rate, rhythm, and depth of respiration; pale, moist skin; and tachypnea and tachycardia caused by a stimulation of the sympathetic nervous system. Pallor, rather than cyanosis, is an indicator of shock for both adult and pediatric patients because sympathetic nerve stimulation causes blood to shunt from minor to major organs; the skin is considered a minor organ. Major organs are the heart and brain, and the body strives to maintain their oxygenation. The patient's general appearance may also provide assessment data. The use of accessory muscles, nasal flaring, and the position the patient assumes should all be noted. The patient with hypoxia may attempt to sit upright and appear anxious and apprehensive and subjectively report shortness of breath.

The neck should be observed for obvious injuries that may produce an expanding hematoma, edema, or subcutaneous emphysema. The position of the trachea and presence of jugular vein distention should also be noted.

The purpose of auscultation is identification of the presence of absent, decreased, or adventitious breath sounds. Absent or decreased breath sounds may be present with a pneumothorax or hemothorax. Adventitious breath sounds are auscultated with obstruction of upper or lower airway structures.

The chest wall should be palpated for tenderness, crepitus, subcutaneous air, and symmetry of movement. Percussion is not a practical tool in the field at a noisy scene. However, in a quiet environment, percussion, like palpation, can provide excellent information about the status of the underlying thoracic structures. The normal lung sound is resonant, a hemothorax is dull, and a tension pneumothorax is hyperresonant.

The history of mechanism of injury or progression of illness may also provide subjective and objective data and assist the transport team in determination of a course of action.

Pediatric patients should be assessed in the same manner as adults. However, children do not have the chronic diseases of adulthood and therefore have more efficient compensation. To the untrained or unsuspecting eye, the child who appears to be in mild respiratory distress may be severely ill. (See Chapter 33 for discussion of the pediatric patient.) Recognition that bradypnea and bradycardia are critical signs of impending respiratory failure in the pediatric patient is essential. Primary cardiac arrest in children is rare. Cardiac arrest is usually caused by respiratory failure, and interventions to support respirations also sustain the cardiac system. Therefore, early and aggressive airway management for children is mandatory.

Children with respiratory insufficiency may show general signs and symptoms of fatigue, restlessness, irritability, and confusion and may cling to their parents with anxiety and apprehension. A weak cry is also typical. Observation may also reveal nasal flaring and substernal, supraclavicular, or intercostal retractions. Skin color is an excellent indicator of oxygenation in children; skin that is pale, has a capillary refill time of greater than 2 seconds, is mottled, or is cyanotic represents distress in the nontrauma patient. In the pediatric trauma patient, cyanosis may not be seen as a result of hypovolemia. Cyanosis is the result of desaturated hemoglobin. Active bleeding depletes the system of hemoglobin, and cyanosis is not observed. A fever may be present if the respiratory distress or failure is the result of an infectious process.

Auscultation may reveal expiratory grunting or wheezing and inspiratory strider. Upper airway problems usually involve a barking cough or strider, whereas wheezing and grunting breath sounds are associated with lower airway disease or obstruction. Diminished breath sounds may be present even in the face of a nontraumatic event.

Examination of the traumatized child may yield findings similar to those previously discussed. However, palpation, percussion, and a high index of suspicion are necessary for a thorough examination. The chest wall and mediastinal structures are more mobile in children than in adults. Children can withstand severe blunt chest trauma without sustaining rib fractures, but the heart and lungs may be severely contused. Likewise, the child with a tension pneumothorax may have a shift of the mediastinal structures much faster than an adult would. Interventions for the child with chest trauma are discussed subsequently. The transport team must recognize that any sign or symptom of respiratory compromise warrants aggressive airway management in children.

INTERVENTION

BASIC LIFE SUPPORT AIRWAY INTERVENTIONS

In the patient with a history of trauma, all airway interventions must be performed with protection of the cervical spine. The airway should be opened, all blood or emesis suctioned, and foreign bodies removed. The need for ready access to a working suction machine throughout transport cannot be overemphasized. The tongue may be displaced from the oropharynx through placement of an airway adjunct or use of a modified jaw thrust. If the patient's mandible is not intact, the tongue can be protracted directly with traction with a towel clip, suture, or clamp. When properly positioned, an oropharyngeal airway rests in the lower posterior pharynx. The oropharyngeal airway should be inserted with a tongue depressor. Proper position must be confirmed with assessment of airflow and efficacy of ventilation. An incorrectly placed oropharyngeal airway may worsen airflow or create an airway obstruction where none existed, created by the tongue being pushed posteriorly against the pharyngeal wall or the epiglottis being pushed against the laryngeal opening. The use of an oropharyngeal airway may induce vomiting in conscious patients; therefore, it should be used only in unconscious patients (Figure 11-6).

Nasopharyngeal airways may be used in patients with marginal stupor or coma who need assistance in maintaining an open airway. However, nasopharyngeal airways should be avoided for any patient with suspected head or facial trauma. Like that of the oral airway, the nasal airway's tip lies in the posterior pharynx behind the tongue. Selection of the appropriate size of nasal airway is important because traumatic insertion may cause severe epistaxis or adenoid bleeding, especially in children. Lubricant use facilitates its insertion. The airway is inserted with the beveled edge along the nasal septum. When the left nostril is used, the nasopharyngeal airway must be inserted upside down to maintain the beveled edge against the septum and then rotated once the airway tip is in the posterior pharynx. If significant resistance is met, the other nostril should be tried. The appropriate size for both oral and nasal airways is obtained by means of comparison of the length of the airway device to the distance from the nares or mouth to the angle of the mandible (Figure 11-7).

In patients with intact airway reflexes, placement of either device may precipitate vomiting, gagging, or laryngospasm. Breath sounds must be assessed after placement to ensure airway patency has not been compromised, and likewise, head position must be optimized to ensure obstruction has not occurred. Where indicated, the cervical spine must be protected. The addition of a simple mechanical adjunct can maintain the patient's airway and free the provider to perform other activities.

Ventilatory assistance must be initiated immediately for the patient with apnea and for the patient with severe hypoventilation. In preparation for intubation, respirations can be assisted with a bag-valve-mask device. Supplemental oxygen can be delivered through this device. The bag-valve-mask device with

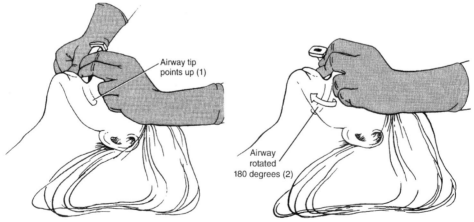

Airway tip
points up (1)

Airway
rotated
180 degrees (2)

FIGURE 11-6   **Insertion of oropharyhgeal airway.** (From Lynn-McHale D, Carlson K, editors: *AACN procedure manual for critical care,* ed 4, Philadelphia, 2001, Saunders.)

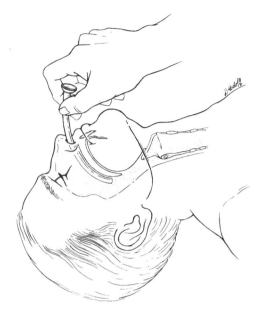

FIGURE 11-7   Correct placement of nasopharyngeal airway. (From Proehl J: *Emergency nursing procedures,* ed 4, Philadelphia, 2009, Saunders.)

a reservoir can deliver a fractional concentration of oxygen in inspired gas (Fio_2) of 90% to 100% at flow rates of 10 to 15 L/min. For emesis to be immediately identified, all masks should be transparent, the airway should be promptly suctioned, and assisted ventilations should be resumed.

BAG-MASK VENTILATION

Good bag-valve-mask skills are an essential competency for the transport nurse. Delivered tidal volumes vary with bag type, hand size, and patient body characteristics. The transport team must evaluate the effectiveness of bag-valve-mask ventilations, particularly single provider ventilations, and proceed to two-person bag-valve-mask technique if doubt exists as to the effectiveness of manual ventilations. The addition of an oral or nasal airway improves the effectiveness of manual ventilation, and placement should be considered a mandatory step in the process of using a bag-valve-mask on any patient in whom use is not contraindicated.

Important considerations in bag-mask ventilations are the quality of the mask seal and a patent airway. Patients with beards or who are edentulous present unique challenges to mask ventilations. The use of a water-soluble lubricant liberally applied to the mask area in contact with the beard surprisingly gives a much better seal in these patients. In patients who are edentulous, leaving the teeth in place to give the cheeks structure and then removing them just before intubation often aids ventilations. Lastly, the use of an oral airway should not be seen as a sign of weakness. It is an essential part of good masking skills and should be encouraged in patients who are deeply obtunded.

Often in obese patients, good valve-bag-mask skills are a team effort with one or two people maintaining a proper mask seal while another squeezes the bag reservoir.

In patients with hyperdynamic conditions, with high oxygen demands or poor oxygen delivery capabilities, hypoxia develops more quickly. Children normally have twice the metabolic demand for oxygen as do adults and have a smaller reserve capacity; desaturation can occur quickly, as with pregnant women and obese patients. Initially, evidence of good masking technique includes adequate chest rise. Pulse oximetry should be available to aid in oxygen desaturation detection, and if end-tidal CO_2 capnography is available, a regular waveform with exhalation should be noted.

The ability to perform advanced airway maneuvers must begin with knowledge of normal anatomy. Knowledge of the anatomic structures is especially important when structures are only partially visible or are displaced as a result of injury. Familiarity with the anatomic differences between the adult and child is equally important.

AIRWAY MANAGEMENT TECHNIQUES

THE LARYNX

Endotracheal intubation entails manipulation of the anatomy to allow passage of an endotracheal tube (ETT) through the larynx, either blindly or through direct visualization with a laryngoscope. An understanding of the relationship of the cartilages of the larynx and their relative positions helps with faster and more confident intubation.

The larynx, or voice box, is an intricate arrangement of nine cartilages, three single and six paired, connected by membranes and ligaments and moved by nine muscles. From above, it attaches to the hyoid bone and opens into the laryngopharynx, and on the inside, it is continuous with the trachea. In an adult, it extends from the level of the fourth to the sixth cervical vertebrae.

The three single cartilages form the basic boxlike structure of the larynx and provide the major external landmarks. The thyroid cartilage, commonly known as the Adam's apple, is formed by the fusion of two curving cartilage plates and is typically larger in men than in women because of the growth-stimulating influence of male sex hormones during puberty. Manipulation of the thyroid cartilage can displace the vocal cords posteriorly and improve laryngeal visualization during laryngoscopy. The ring-shaped cricoid cartilage is sandwiched between the thyroid cartilage above the first tracheal ring. Because the cricoid cartilage is a complete ring, the tracheal diameter does not narrow during cricoid pressure. Pressure on the cricoid from the anterior neck, known as the Sellick maneuver, compresses the esophagus and may prevent passive regurgitation of stomach contents during laryngoscopy. The cricoid cartilage is connected to the thyroid cartilage by the cricothyroid membrane and is the desired location for a cricothyrotomy. The upper free edge of the cricothyroid membrane forms the vocal cords. Because of the attachment of the vocal cords to the cricoid ring, downward pressure on the cricoid ring may help to bring the vocal cords into view when they are hidden behind the tongue (the Sellick maneuver). The third single cartilage is the epiglottis, a spoon-shaped structure that lies directly over the glottic opening and prevents anything other than air from entering the tracheal inlet. The epiglottis is the major visual landmark for performance of tracheal intubation (Figures 11-8 and 11-9).

The most important paired cartilages of the larynx are the arytenoids. The arytenoids are pyramid-shaped and anchor the vocal cords in the larynx. The vocal cords look pearly white because of their avascular nature. At rest, the vocal cords lie partially separated or abducted. Excessive secretions or aspiration stimulate the airway and activate the defense reflexes. Laryngospasm, or spasmodic closure of the vocal cords, is the most severe form of airway closure and can totally

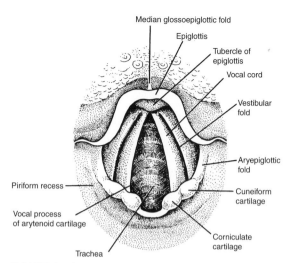

FIGURE 11-8   Laryngoscopic view of airway. (From Rosen P, et al: *Emergency medicine: concepts and clinical practice,* vol 1, ed 3, St Louis, 1992, Mosby.)

prevent ventilation and the passage of an ETT. If a tube is forced through the cords with excessive pressure, an arytenoid can be dislocated and permanent hoarseness can result. The remaining two pairs of cartilages, the cuneiform and corniculate, form the posterior wall of the larynx. Committing these structures to memory assists the laryngoscopist in quickly identifying the glottic opening; when the opening is obscured from view, the ETT can be steered into position with the structures in view as reference points.

TRACHEAL INTUBATION

Intubation of the trachea is considered the gold standard for artificial airway support. Tracheal intubation provides protection against aspiration, allows for controlled and precise ventilation, and provides a method of drug administration. In addition, intubation protects the airway in situations of progressive airway closure caused by epiglottitis, inhalation burns, soft tissue trauma or infections, and other obstructive conditions. In the broader world of medicine, endotracheal intubation is generally successful, with failure occurring in as few as one of 2000 elective general anesthesia cases.[5] Success rates in the emergency department are lower but still well over 97%.[8,41,45,71,81]

Complications of oral and nasal endotracheal intubation can be both significant and disastrous

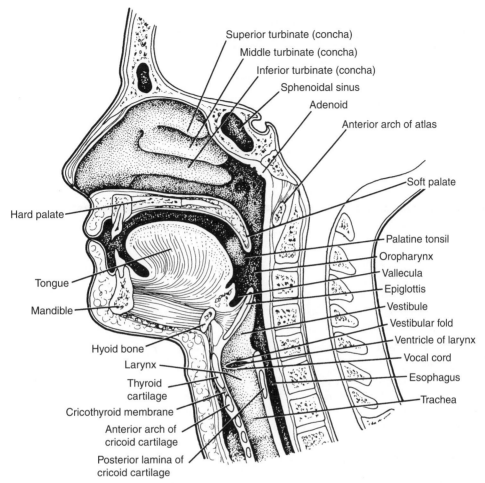

Superior turbinate (concha)
Middle turbinate (concha)
Inferior turbinate (concha)
Sphenoidal sinus
Adenoid
Anterior arch of atlas

Soft palate

Hard palate

Palatine tonsil
Oropharynx
Vallecula
Epiglottis
Vestibule
Vestibular fold
Ventricle of larynx
Vocal cord
Esophagus
Trachea

Tongue

Mandible

Hyoid bone
Larynx
Thyroid cartilage
Cricothyroid membrane
Anterior arch of cricoid cartilage
Posterior lamina of cricoid cartilage

FIGURE 11-9   **Sagittal view of airway.** (From Rosen P, et al: *Emergency medicine: concepts and clinical practice,* vol 1, ed 3, St Louis, 1992, Mosby.)

(see Box 11-1). Unsuccessful intubation or a missed inadvertent esophageal intubation may lead to prolonged hypoxia and result in long-term injury or death. If the patient cannot be intubated, other means of oxygenation and ventilation must be substituted. Pulse oximetry during intubation can help prevent oxygen desaturation during multiple intubation attempts and should always be available. Intubation predisposes the patient to a number of harmful physiologic responses, including laryngospasm, bronchospasm caused by airway irritability or aspirated secretions, hypertension, and dysrhythmias unrelated to hypoxia.[8] In addition, the process of intubation increases the patient's ICP.[40]

Unrecognized right mainstem bronchus intubation is a complication that may lead to inadequate ventilation and left lung atelectasis.

Orotracheal Intubation

Orotracheal intubation is the most common method of airway management for all age groups. In children, orotracheal intubation is used almost exclusively. It is a safe procedure that involves psychomotor skills that are easily mastered. Few, if any, true contraindications to orotracheal intubation exist in the emergency setting. However, during circumstances in which major facial and neck trauma prevents recognition of landmarks or during isolated mandibular

---

BOX 11-1   ## Complications of Intubation

Early Complications That Occur During the Intubation Procedure

1. **Neck**
   Cervical strain: subluxation/dislocation, fracture, and neurologic injury
2. **Mouth**
   Soft tissue injury that results in abrasion and hemorrhage involving lips, tongue, buccal mucosa, and pharynx
   Temporomandibular joint subluxation/dislocation
   Dental injury
3. **Airway/respiratory**
   Arytenoid: dislocation and avulsion
   Vocal cord: spasm, avulsion, and laceration
   Pyriform sinus perforation that results in pneumothorax and pneumomediastinum
   Tracheal and bronchial rupture
   Right mainstem bronchus intubation, with atelectasis and respiratory compromise
   Bronchospasm
4. **Gastrointestinal**
   Esophageal: intubation and perforation
   Vomiting and aspiration
5. **Cardiovascular**
   Hypertension, tachycardia, bradycardia, and dysrhythmias
   Cardiac arrest and interruption of CPR

Late Complications That Occur After Tube Is in Place

1. **Airway/respiratory**
   Tube obstruction: secretions, blood, and kinking
   Accidental extubation and endobronchial intubation
   Vocal cords: ulceration
   Trachea: ulceration, ischemic necrosis, and paralysis
   Pneumothorax and pneumomediastinum
   Aspiration and atelectasis
   Cough that results in increased intrathoracic, intracranial, and intraocular pressures
2. **Gastrointestinal**
   Esophageal intubation
   Tracheoesophageal fistula
3. **Cardiovascular**
   Tracheoinnominate artery fistula
4. **Infections**
   Sinusitis, pneumonia, tracheobronchitis, mediastinitis, and abscess
5. **Tube dislodgment**

From Walls R, editor: *Emergency airway management,* Philadelphia, 2000, Lippincott Williams & Wilkins; and Dauphinee K: Orotracheal intubation; nasotracheal intubation, *Emerg Med Clin North Am* 6(4):7110, 1988.

---

trauma in which the temporomandibular joint may be immobile, the orotracheal route becomes much more difficult and may necessitate a surgical airway. Other conditions that might dictate a surgical airway include circumstances in which significant bleed-ing is found in the oral pharynx or supraglottic area and patients with epiglottitis in whom landmarks are obscured or passage of a tube is impossible. Again, these conditions are considered relative, not absolute, contraindications.

At one time, laryngoscopy was considered contraindicated in patients with known or suspected cervical spine injury. The safety of inline immobilization of the cervical spine performed by an assistant combined with a gentle laryngoscopy is well established. Intubation of such patients has been greatly aided with pharmacologic agents, which improve the ease of intubation and make it much safer for the patient. Trauma to the teeth, soft tissues of the mouth, posterior pharynx, or vocal cords caused by improper use of the laryngoscope blade or by forcing an endotracheal is a complication of oral intubation.

In the adult, the narrowest portion of the airway is the glottic opening, the space between the true vocal cords. In children, the narrowest portion is at the cricoid cartilage below the vocal cords. The larynx of the child is therefore considered to be cone shaped. Because of this cone shape, it is possible to see the tube pass through the vocal cords but be unable to pass the tube through the cricoid ring. If this situation occurs, the tube should withdrawn and a smaller tube chosen; an ETT should never be forced down a child's airway.

Cormack and Lehane[22] quantified the ability to visualize the glottic opening during laryngoscopy (Figure 11-10). In the Cormack Lehane scale, grade I is visualization of the entire glottic opening, grade II is just the arytenoids cartilages or posterior glottic opening, and grade III is only the epiglottis; with grade IV, only the tongue is visible. Grade I and II views are associated with high intubation success rates, and grade III and IV views are linked with lower success rates. Other operators simply describe the percent of glottic opening (POGO) that is visible during the laryngoscopy.[22,65]

The choice of blade, straight or curved, is left to the personal preference of the person performing the intubation. Blades come in curved shapes, such as the MacIntosh, or straight shapes, such as the Miller, Phillips, or Wisconsin. Generally speaking, the wide flange of the curved blade aids in controlling the tongue, considered the primary obstacle to intubation, better than the straight blade. The ability of the flanged curved blade to control the tongue also leaves more room on the right side of the mouth to manipulate the endotracheal blade into place. In addition,

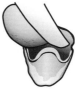

Grade I — Glottis, including anterior and posterior commissures, can be fully exposed.

A

Grade II — Glottis can be partly exposed (anterior commissure not visualized).

B

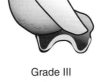
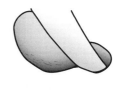

Grade III — Glottis cannot be exposed (only corniculate cartilages visualized).

C

Grade IV — Glottis, including corniculate cartilages, cannot be exposed.

D

FIGURE 11-10   **Cormack Lehane scale for visualizing glottic opening during laryngoscopy. A,** Grade I. **B,** Grade II. **C,** Grade III. **D,** Grade IV. (From Duchynski R, Brauer K, Jones S, et al: The quick look airway classification, *Air Med J* 17(2): 46-50, 1998.)

the curved blade follows the natural curvature of the anatomy better than the straight blade, which often must be inserted in a stepwise fashion of lifting, relaxing, and advancing. The straight blade, although more difficult for control of the tongue, has an advantage in viewing the glottic opening of patients who are considered to have an anterior positioned larynx. Such is the case in pediatric patients, patients with receding chins, and patients with short muscular necks. In these patients, the larynx is located more forward, and curved blades often do not provide an adequate view. The difficulty with use of the straight blade is that the rounded barrel shape of the blade is less optimal at controlling the tongue. If the laryngoscopist secures a good view of the cords without totally maintaining the tongue to the left of the blade, the tongue may lap over the blade and prevent manipulation of the tube through the cords. The laryngoscopist's attention may be so focused on the cords as to not notice that the tongue is thwarting efforts at the level of the mouth.

The adult-size blade is a no. 3 or 4. The curved tip of the MacIntosh is inserted into the vallecula, the space between the base of the tongue and the pharyngeal surface of the epiglottis. Lifting the blade lifts the epiglottic ligament and indirectly lifts the epiglottis to expose the larynx. The straight Miller blade is passed so that the tip lies beneath the laryngeal surface of the epiglottis. The epiglottis is then directly lifted to expose the vocal cords. Steps for orotracheal intubation are included in Box 11-2.

Selection of the appropriately sized tube is an important consideration in patient intubation. In general, the largest tube possible should be selected to minimize airway resistance, assist in suctioning, and minimize the need for excessive inflation of the tube cuff, which can cause mucosal damage. The cuff pressure should be at minimal occluding volume. At pressures greater than 25 mm Hg, mucosal ischemia starts to occur. A persistent air leak in the balloon is often caused by a faulty valve at the pilot balloon. To correct this condition without reintubation, the transport team member should attach a stopcock to the balloon, reinflate the balloon, and close the stopcock.[1] The average adult female airway can accommodate a 7-mm to 8-mm tube (the size refers to the inside diameter of the tube), and the average male airway, an 8-mm to 9-mm tube. The pilot balloon should be tested for leaks before insertion.

Preoxygenation is an important step that is frequently terminated prematurely. In the patient who is spontaneously breathing, the procedure requires an adequate seal on the face mask and use of a bag-valve-mask device with reservoir to deliver the highest FIO_2 for 3 to 5 minutes. If done correctly, preoxygenation washes out the nitrogen in the patients lungs and supersaturates them with oxygen, which allows for as much as 5 to 8 minutes of apnea. Another method of preoxygenation involves placement of a high flow mask on a breathing patient for, again, a period of 3 to 5 minutes. In the patient who needs ventilatory assistance, avoidance of peak airway pressures greater than 20 to 25 mm Hg aids in minimizing gastric distention, which increases the risk of vomiting leading to aspiration and hypoxia.

The BURP method is an additional maneuver to improve visualization of the glottis during intubation. The *BURP method* (Backward, Upward, Rightward, Pressure) involves pressure on the thyroid cartilage. When the laryngoscopic view is suboptimal, the assistant performing cricoid pressure

---

BOX 11-2   Steps for Orotracheal Intubation

1. Position the patient. Nontrauma patient: Flex the neck forward and extend the head backward, creating a sniffing position. Trauma patient: Maintain in-line traction.
2. Preoxygenate the patient.
3. Hold the laryngoscope in the left hand, and open the patient's mouth with the right hand.
4. Insert the blade into the right side of the mouth, sweep the tongue to the left, and advance to the appropriate landmarks. The Miller (straight) blade tip goes beyond the epiglottis; the MacIntosh (curved) blade tip enters the vallecula.
5. Pull the laryngoscope blade at a 45-degree angle; avoid twisting the laryngoscope handle. Visualize the epiglottis and vocal cords. Apply cricoid pressure.
6. Insert the ETT from the right corner of the mouth, and watch the tube pass through the vocal cords. Use the largest tube possible. Remove the stylet.
7. Inflate the tube cuff with 5 to 10 mL of air or to minimal occluding volume. (Minimal occluding volume is determined by placing the hand over the mouth and noting cessation of air leak with ventilation.) Capillary flow pressure in the tracheal mucosa is approximately 25 mm Hg, so cuff pressure should be less than that.
8. Confirm tube placement by auscultating bilateral breath sounds over the chest and axilla and by noting a lack of gurgling over the epigastrium. Observe for symmetry of chest wall motion. For a child, observe the cardiac monitor for the maintenance of an appropriate pulse rate and improvement in the patient's color.
9. Secure the tube in place.

may apply firm backward, upward, and rightward pressure on the thyroid cartilage to bring the glottic opening into view; or the laryngoscopist may perform the movement with a free right hand and, when the view is optimal, ask the assistant to hold the new found position. In this manner, the assistant performs both cricoid pressure and BURP maneuver to improve the view of the laryngoscopist and aid in prevention of stomach insufflation and regurgitation. When the laryngoscopist uses a hand to improve laryngeal visualization, the method is also referred to as *external laryngeal manipulation* (ELM) or *optimal external laryngeal manipulation* (OELM).[84]

Gastric emptying ceases with significant trauma, and patients are considered to have a full stomach if they have eaten within 6 hours of trauma or anesthesia. The Sellick maneuver (digital pressure over the cricoid cartilage exerted posteriorly to compress the esophagus against the underlying vertebral body) is applied to prevent the regurgitation of gastric contents into the pharynx and subsequent aspiration into the pulmonary tree and is considered an integral part of rapid sequence tracheal intubation during emergency airway management.[30] Occasionally, cricoid pressure may improve visualization of the glottic opening by pressing the larynx downward and perhaps into the field of view. That cricoid pressure may worsen laryngeal view and reduce airway patency is also clearly understood.[30]

If cricoid pressure is too great, or the pressure is over the thyroid cartilage and not the cricoid ring, it may prevent the passage of an endotracheal tube. This case is especially true in the pediatric patient because of the child's pliable airway structures. If difficulty is encountered, the assistant should release part or all of the pressure. If the patient actively vomits, the assistant should immediately release the cricoid pressure and actively suction the patient's airway.

Insertion of the tube through the relaxed cords should continue until the cuff is just past the cords. To ensure the tip of the tube is above the carina, the tube is placed so that the teeth are approximately at the 21-cm mark on the tube for women and at the 24-cm mark for men. A quick way to facilitate tube depth is to place the tube to a depth equal to three times the tube size. This formula works as well with pediatric tubes, provided the correct tube size is chosen. With completion of the intubation, the laryngoscope is gently withdrawn, the cuff is inflated with 5 to 10 mL of air, and placement of the tube is confirmed. Tube placement confirmation begins with auscultation of breath sounds in the right and left chest areas and over the stomach. A number of adjuncts are available to assist in confirmation of tube placement and are discussed later in this chapter.

Once intubation and oxygenation are complete, patients who were previously hypoxic may have an increased level of consciousness and may become combative. A patient's first priority in this confusion is extubation. Soft restraints and a bite block may be in order. An oral airway may be used as a bite block to prevent the patient from biting down on the ETT. The bite block should be secured in place separately from the ETT. If the bite block and the ETT are secured together, the patient may inadvertently cause extubation by lodging the tongue behind the oral airway and pushing it and the ETT out.

Nasotracheal Intubation

Nasotracheal intubation is referred to as a blind procedure because the larynx is not visualized as in the orotracheal method. Once considered an ideal technique for intubation of the patient with suspected cervical spine injury, nasotracheal intubation technique has since been replaced with inline cervical immobilization together with rapid sequence intubation (RSI) and oral intubation. All blind techniques can produce airway trauma that includes laryngeal and glottic damage, esophageal intubation, and significant bleeding that leads to a "can't ventilate, can't intubate" situation.[18]

Today, the nasotracheal technique has few true indications. In patients with spontaneous respirations and limited oral access, such as angioedema or other obstructive oral processes, nasotracheal technique with a cooperative patient and an experienced provider is a reasonable alternative to a surgical airway.[73] Other patients who might potentially benefit from a nasotracheal intubation include patients with severe dyspnea who cannot tolerate lying supine, such as those with pulmonary edema, congestive heart failure, or chronic obstructive pulmonary disease (COPD) exacerbation. Patients with dyspnea often have breath sounds that are easily heard and a glottis that tends to remain open, making nasotracheal intubation relatively easy provided the patient is well prepared.

For successful performance of the blind method of tracheal intubation, the patient must have spontaneous respirations, although the use of a lighted stylet in an patient with apnea can facilitate the nasotracheal route. In addition to the patient having spontaneous respirations, the nasotracheal method also requires a relatively quiet environment, which could make a procedure at a noisy scene difficult. In general, the nasotracheal technique requires more time than the orotracheal technique but also offers some slight advantages over the orotracheal technique (Box 11-3).

In trauma cases, the procedure can be performed with no movement of the cervical spine and can be performed on a patient who is sitting. Therefore, the nasotracheal method can be a useful procedure in the trauma patient who needs airway management but is still entrapped upright in a vehicle. Also, the patient cannot bite the tube, and the tube is easily secured in place. A disadvantage of blind nasal intubation is that any upper airway bleeding induced by this technique can obscure visualization during subsequent attempts at direct laryngoscopy should the blind technique fail.

The only absolute contraindication to the standard blind nasotracheal technique of intubation is apnea or near apnea. Other contraindications to nasotracheal intubation are considered relative, and they include: (1) a suspected basilar skull fracture (may risk cranial intubation) or other closed head injury[58]; (2) acute epiglottitis; (3) severe nasal or maxillofacial fractures; (4) upper airway foreign body, abscess, or tumor; and (5) anticoagulation therapy or other blood-clotting abnormalities that cause epistaxis. The disadvantages that are not contraindications to the procedure should be noted. Nasotracheal intubation puts the patient at risk for the development of meningitis or encephalitis. Special consideration must also be given to the patient for whom bacteremia would be detrimental, such as the patient with an immunocompromised condition or the patient with a cardiac valve abnormality or prosthesis.

The most common complication of nasotracheal intubation is hemorrhage. Traumatic intubation may cause epistaxis through abrasion of the nasal mucosa or rupture of a nasal polyp. Bleeding can be minimized with use of a tube 1 mm smaller than would be used orally and with the use of a vasoconstrictive agent to the nasal mucosa, such as topical phenylephrine. Oxymetazoline may also be used. It provides equally good vasoconstriction and can be used liberally without development of excessive hypertension in sensitive cardiac patients from mucosal absorption of phenylephrine. In addition, one should lubricate the tube well and avoid excessive pressure to help prevent excessive bleeding. The nasal passage may be gently dilated with successfully larger nasopharyngeal airways with 2% lidocaine lubricant applied to each airway. Some practitioners dilate the nasal mucosa with a gloved small finger. In the patient who is awake, administration of nasopharyngeal anesthesia with lidocaine or Cetacaine is also advisable, and 2% lidocaine gel may also be used to lubricate the tube. In children, the relatively large size of the tonsils and adenoidal tissue may produce

---

BOX 11-3   Advantages of Nasotracheal Intubation Versus Orotracheal Technique

1. Tube is more easily secured and hence is less likely to be dislodged.
2. More comfort during awake intubation and on the patient awakening.
3. Easier insertion in a patient with impaired neck or jaw motion.
4. No danger of the patient biting the tube.
5. Facilitates surgery to the oral cavity.
6. Favored in patients in whom laryngoscopy is difficult or contraindicated.
7. Useful in patients in whom neuromuscular blockade is hazardous.

Modified from Walls R, et al: *Manual of emergency airway management,* Philadelphia, 2000, Lippincott Williams & Wilkins.

severe bleeding if ruptured. Perforation and dissection of the posterior pharyngeal wall have also been reported. For these reasons, nasotracheal intubation in the child should only be attempted by an experienced and skilled provider. Steps for nasotracheal intubation are included in Box 11-4.

The proper head position for the patient who undergoes nasotracheal intubation is the sniffing position with a bit less extension than when an oral intubation is performed. Extreme extension creates a more acute angle for the tube to pass through the larynx and makes the procedure more difficult. However, if cervical spine injury is suspected, the head and neck must be maintained in the neutral position. The beveled edge of the tube should be introduced against the nasal septum of the nostril chosen. The tube is advanced through the nose and into the pharynx with continuous forward pressure and gentle rotation. If the nasal passage appears to be obstructed, the other nostril may be used or the tube may be substituted with a smaller one. The tube must never be forced. The intubation specialist must listen and feel for air movement through the tube as the tube enters the pharynx and advances toward the glottis. Cricoid pressure may also be helpful. As the tube approaches the glottis, breath sounds are heard maximally. On inspiration, the tube is advanced through the cords. Tube position is then verified as described previously.

Several devices are available to aid placement of the nasotracheal tube. The Endotrol tube is specifically designed for nasotracheal intubation and for use in patients with an anterior larynx. The Endotrol tube has a ring on the upper portion that directs the tip anteriorly when traction is applied to the ring. Should cord spasm develop, a topical anesthetic may be sprayed onto the cords through the tube. Another device used to aid placement of the nasotracheal tube is the airway whistle or Beck Airway Airflow Monitor (BAAM).[18,19,31] The whistle is attached to the standard 15-mm endotracheal connector and amplifies the patient's breathing as the tube is advanced through the posterior nasopharynx. As the tube is advanced further, the sound increases in intensity. Deviation from the airflow tract results in a decrease or loss of the whistle sound, which indicates the need for tube redirection. Once intubation is complete, the airway whistle is removed.[51] An air medical program evaluated the BAAM airway whistle and found that it was easy to use even in the noisy in-flight environment and had the added advantage

---

BOX 11-4 **Steps for Nasotracheal Intubation**

1. Assess nasal patency. Alternately occlude each naris, listen to air passage, and ask the patient or family members about past medical problems.
2. Anesthetize the nasal passage with lidocaine and a vasoconstrictor such as phenylephrine. Cetacaine to the posterior pharynx may also be used.
3. Position the patient. Nontrauma patient: May sit upright or assume a sniffing position with a bit less extension than for oral intubation. Trauma patient: Maintain in-line traction.
4. Provide supplemental oxygen.
5. Lubricate the tube liberally.
6. Introduce the tube perpendicular to the floor for the supine patient or to the bed for the upright patient.
7. Point the bevel of the tube toward the nasal septum. (If the left naris is used, the tube is inserted backward.)
8. Gently pass the tube and listen to breath sounds through the end of the tube as it is advanced. Occlusion of the opposite naris may make the breath sounds louder.
9. Just proximal to the glottis, the breath sounds become maximal. Take care not to touch the cords prematurely so as not to induce laryngospasm and cough.
10. Quickly advance the tube on inspiration into the trachea. An assistant should apply the Sellick maneuver (cricoid pressure) to help align the glottic opening.
11. Confirm the tube position by auscultating breath sounds and observing symmetric chest wall motion, and ensure that the patient is unable to speak.
12. Secure the tube in place.

of protecting the intubation specialist against contact with blood, vomitus, and sputum during the intubation procedure. A technique for use of the BAAM airway whistle combined with the controllable-tip ETT during blind oral intubation and digital intubation has also been described.

Digital Intubation

Digital intubation, or tactile orotracheal intubation, is another blind intubation technique that was the original method of intubation beginning in the mid 1700s.[2] With the invention of the laryngoscope, the technique became obsolete and is of limited usefulness in clinical practice. However, digital intubation can be helpful when other conventional methods have failed or in the prehospital setting where limited equipment, lighting, or space is problematic. The technique is useful in comatose patients with head and neck trauma, in obese patients or those with short muscular necks, and in patients with severe bleeding or excessive secretions that prevent direct visualization via laryngoscopy. The digital technique may also be useful in cramped spaces, such as ground or air ambulances in which space is limited, or in situations in which equipment such as a laryngoscope or suction apparatus is lacking or has failed.

Digital intubation requires that the patient be completely unconscious and that the mouth be opened widely without fear of the patient biting.

This technique has been used with remarkable success in children and neonates, despite their small mouth openings.[3] It relies on the ability of the intubation specialist to guide the tip of the tube through the glottic opening with the middle and index fingers of the nondominant hand (Box 11-5). The primary limitation of this technique is the length of the intubation specialist's fingers in relation to the patient's oral and upper airway anatomy.

AIRWAY RESCUE DEVICES

ENDOTRACHEAL TUBE INTRODUCER

MacIntosh, the British anesthesiologist who developed the MacIntosh blade, is credited with developing the *endotracheal tube introducer* (ETI) in the 1940s.[4] Later, it became known as the Eschmann Tracheal Tube Introducer, which remains available. And recently, a plastic disposable ETI became commercially available. Many anesthesia care providers consider the ETI the first choice in conditions where only the posterior arytenoids or the epiglottis are visualized during the intubation attempt.

The ETI is 60 cm long and is curved at a 35-degree at the end. The tip permits it to be steered behind the epiglottis and into the glottic opening. To use the ETI, perform laryngoscopy in the usual manner.

BOX 11-5   **Steps for Digital Oral Intubation**

1. Position the patient. Nontrauma patient: Flex the neck forward and extend the head backward, creating a sniffing position. Trauma patient: Maintain in-line traction.
2. Preoxygenate the patient.
3. Select the appropriately sized ETT in the usual manner. Insert an intubation stylet and bend the tube stylet in an open J configuration. Lubricate the tube.
4. Kneels or stand on either side of the patient at the level of the shoulders, facing the patient.
5. With gloved hands, insert the fingers of the nondominant hand along the patient's tongue, pull the tongue forward, and walk the fingers down to palpate the epiglottis with the middle finger. If the epiglottis is not palpated, pull forward on the tongue.
6. The tube stylet is then slid along the left side of the mouth, with the medial aspect of the middle finger and the volar aspect of the index finger used to guide the tube tip in the direction of the epiglottis. Keep the index finger above the tube and the tube tip in contact with the middle finger.
7. Hold the tube against the epiglottis with the index finger, and slip the tube distally toward the glottic opening.
8. As the tube enters the glottic opening, resistance increases. At this point, hold the tube firmly and withdraw the stylet slightly. Advance the tube through the cords and then completely remove the stylet.
9. Confirm proper tube placement in the usual manner.

Hold the ETI in the right hand and advance it toward the epiglottis, or where the cords are presumed. If the introducer goes blindly down the trachea, the laryngoscopist receives confirmation by way of feeling "clicks" as the curved tip of the introducer slides over the tracheal rings or "hold up" where the introducer reaches the carina or the right or left mainstem bronchus and cannot be further advanced. If the introducer is advanced without clicks or hold up, it has likely gone down the esophagus. This route is confirmed when the laryngoscopist literally realizes that the entire introducer has been inserted with only a few centimeters left in the hand. In this situation, pull back on the introducer until the curved tip is seen again and redirect it.[6]

If hold up is noted, which may or may not be accompanied with clicks, it is nearly 100% confirmation that the introducer is in the trachea. Clicks are confirmed in 90% of tracheal intubations with the ETI.[4,5] Hold up may possibly occur in a patient with esophageal stenosis with a false-positive result or with cricoid pressure.

Once the intubation specialist is confident the ETI has entered the trachea, with positive hold up, click, or both signs, an assistant places a lubricated endotracheal tube over the introducer. The intubation specialist then advances the tube, similar to the Seldinger technique, over the introducer while holding the laryngoscope in the left hand. Maintaining the laryngoscope in place facilitates sliding the tube over the introducer. The assistant can stabilize the introducer by holding the free end above the endotracheal tube as the intubation specialist advances the endotracheal tube. At times, the endotracheal tube may resist passing through the cords. If this should occur, back the tube out slightly and rotate the tube 90 degrees to the left (the Murphy eye is now in the upright position), then advance. If this maneuver is unsuccessful, rotate the tube to the right 90 degrees and advance. In rare situations, the tube may need to be rotated 180 degrees to pass through the cords. Once the endotracheal tube passes through the cords, remove the introducer and confirm placement in the usual manner.

Although not extensively studied in the prehospital setting, a number of good studies suggest the ETI is a safe, inexpensive, and effective rescue device for the difficult intubation situation.[54,67,68]

LIGHTED STYLET

An optional method of endotracheal intubation is the use of the *lighted stylet*. Referred to as the *transillumination method*, it uses a rigid wire stylet with a light bulb at the distal end and is powered by a small battery source in the proximal end. The technique relies on the transillumination of the neck tissue to guide the placement of the ETT. The lighted stylet was originally designed to aid in the blind nasotracheal method of intubation; however, design modifications have now been made to allow use in both orotracheal and nasotracheal methods and for pediatric use as well. The brighter transilluminated glow from the trachea is easily distinguished from the dull or absent glow should the esophagus be intubated. Medical personnel can also use the lighted stylet to accurately position the ETT of a patient with intubation by adjusting the stylet so that the transilluminated glow is at the level of the sternal notch. The tube is then slid to align proximally with a point that also aligns the light with the distal tip of the ETT (Box 11-6).

The lighted stylet is most commonly used as a rescue tool where other more traditional airway management techniques have failed. An added advantage with the lighted stylet is that is does not require extension of the neck for proper placement. A number of studies indicate that learning to use the intubation stylet is easy when compared with direct laryngoscopy and associated with few complications.[28]

SUPRAGLOTTIC AIRWAY DEVICES

The past 15 years have seen propagation in airway devices that are designed to be inserted blindly, in circumstances of failed intubation, or in "can't intubate, can't ventilate" situations. All of these devices can trace their development to the late 1960s with the marketing of the *esophageal obturator airway* (EOA). The original EOA was a two-part device, a mask and tube, that required one person to maintain tight seal on the mask and a second person to provide ventilations. Eventually, the EOA was replaced by the *esophageal tracheal combitube* which remains an effective intermediate airway used primarily in the prehospital setting. Transport teams may encounter the Combitube, or any number of supraglottic devices in areas where medical personnel are not

| BOX 11-6 | **Steps for Use of the Lighted Stylet** |

1. Position the patient. Nontrauma patient: Flex the neck forward and extend the head backward, creating the sniffing position. Trauma patient: Maintain in-line traction.
2. Preoxygenate the patient.
3. The lighted stylet should be checked to ensure its light is bright enough by directly looking at the light. If the light is not uncomfortable to the eyes, it should be discarded and a new one used.
4. The lubricated stylet is inserted into a transparent ETT, and the light is positioned at the tip of the ETT, but not beyond.
5. The distal end of the ETT is then bent at a slightly greater than 90-degree angle.
6. The intubator kneels or stands on either side of the patient at the level of the shoulders, facing the patient.
7. For the oral technique, lift the tongue or the tongue and jaw, pulling the epiglottis anteriorly and clearing the supraglottic area for introduction of the tube stylet. Slide the tube down along the tongue, and lift the glottis in a "soup ladle" motion. For the nasal technique, use the lighted stylet with a directional tip tube such as the Endotrol tube. The tube stylet is inserted with the beveled edge against the septum after application of a topical anesthetic and phenylephrine.
8. As the tube stylet is advanced, observe for the transilluminated glow in the midline. If the tip is off midline, a dim glow is observed. If the glow is extremely dim or cannot be seen, the epiglottis has not been elevated and is probably covering the glottic opening. Correct by lifting forward on the jaw, tongue, or both.
9. When a bright midline glow is observed, the tube stylet is advanced until the glow is located at the sternal notch.
10. Carefully remove the stylet without dislodging the tube. Secure the tube.
11. Confirm proper tube placement in the usual manner.

trained in endotracheal intubation techniques or when attempts at intubation are not successful. In addition, one of the following devices may likely be part of the transport team's algorithm for failed intubation. Following is a review of some of the supraglottic airway devices in use today. Most of these numerous devices are fairly new and awaiting critical review.[34,76]

Combitube

The *Combitube* is a double-lumen system that, when inserted blindly, allows for either tracheal or esophageal intubation without ventilatory compromise. During blind placement, the distal tube enters the esophagus approximately 98% of the time. Bending the Combitube at the pharyngeal portion between the cuffs for a few seconds, known as the Lipp maneuver, enhances the preformed curvature and eases insertion.[13] The Combitube incorporates a dual-cuff system that serves as airway seals. The distal balloon, which holds 12 to 20 mL of air, seals the esophagus and prevents gastric regurgitation or, in the event of tracheal intubation, aspiration. The proximal or oropharyngeal balloon is a high-volume cuff designed to be positioned between

the base of the tongue and the soft palate so that the mouth and nasopharynx are sealed off and the escape of air through the mouth is prevented. The pharyngeal balloon may also tamponade oral bleeding and prevent aspiration of blood into the trachea. Tube 1 is always ventilated first, in confirmation of placement of the tube. The presence of breath sounds during lung auscultation and absence of gastric insufflation confirm esophageal position of the Combitube and ventilation should continue through the esophageal lumen. Use of a colorimetric end-tidal CO_2 detector can also aid in determination of which tube to ventilate. The stomach may occasionally harbor residual carbon dioxide from esophageal ventilation of expired air into the stomach during bag-valve-mask ventilations. For this reason, ventilation between 6 and 12 times is recommended before relying on a colorimetric CO_2 detector or electronic CO_2 detector to confirm proper ventilations.[6] If placement of Combitube results in failed ventilation, the most likely cause is that the perforated pharyngeal section has been placed too deep and is positioned in the esophagus. Pulling the Combitube back 3 to 4 cm usually corrects the situation.

The oropharyngeal balloon does not prevent aspiration of teeth or other oral debris, and the oropharyngeal balloon can migrate out of the mouth anteriorly, partially dislodging the airway. If blind insertion results in tracheal placement, the Combitube can be used as an endotracheal tube.[69,70]

Esophageal tubes are contraindicated in patients who are awake and semiobtunded, in infants, in children, and in patients less than 120 cm in height. They cannot be used in patients with known esophageal injury or in situations of caustic ingestion. A criticism of the design is its potential complexity and confusion in use; however, numerous studies published since its introduction have indicated that the Combitube deserves strong consideration as a rescue airway and as a primary airway in certain clinical situations.[69,70] Figure 11-11 illustrates insertion of the Combitube.

Classic Laryngeal Mask Airway

The *classic laryngeal mask airway* (cLMA) developed by a British anesthesiologist Archie Brain and introduced in 1988 was the first of the modern day supraglottic airway devices. The less expensive and disposable model of the cLMA is the *laryngeal mask*

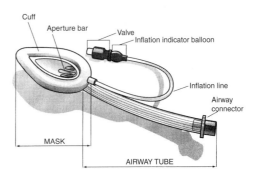

FIGURE 11-12   **Laryngeal tracheal mask.** (Courtesy LMA North America, Inc.)

airway (LMA) unique. The device is designed to surround and cover the supraglottic area in appropriate sizes for all patients, including neonates to large adults. The LMA consists of an airway tube, a mask, and a mask inflation tube (Figure 11-12). The LMA provides for ventilation by forming a seal over the larynx above the cords. Two rubber bars cross the tube opening at the mask end to prevent herniation of the epiglottis into the LMA tube. The tip of the LMA rests in the top of the esophagus. The LMA is an excellent bridge device that allows ventilations in situations where mask ventilations are difficult, ineffective, or impossible. Typical first-time insertion success rates

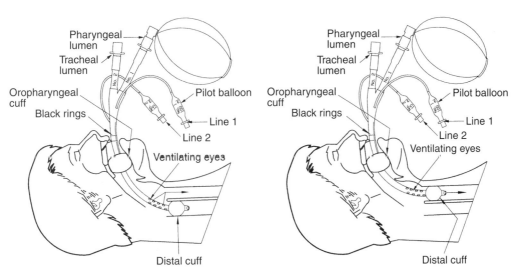

FIGURE 11-11   **Insertion of combitube.** (From Proehl J: *Emergency nursing procedures,* ed 4, Philadelphia, 2009, Saunders.)

range between 90% and 95% if time for proper insertion is approximately 30 seconds.[11,60,91,99] The major disadvantage of the classic and unique LMAs is that they do not offer defense against regurgitation and aspiration and therefore the airway remains unprotected. Insertion of the LMA is shown in Figure 11-13. A concern for air transport teams is that a properly inserted and inflated LMA may undergo expansion of the cuff at altitude and result in overinflation unless properly monitored and corrected.[98]

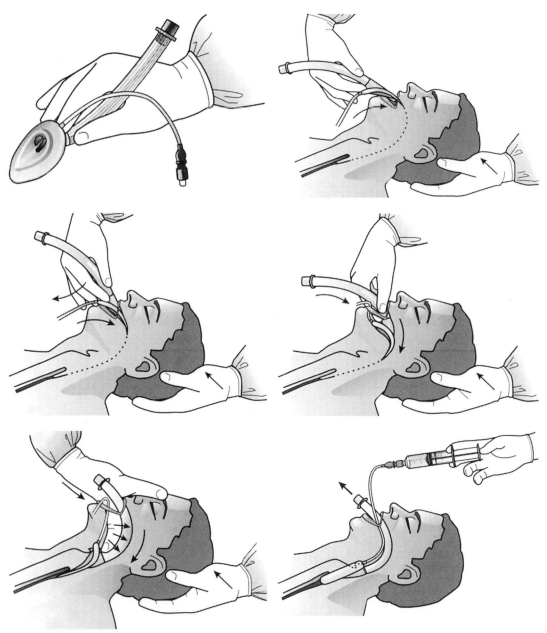

FIGURE 11-13   **Insertion of laryngeal mask airway.** (Courtesy LMA North America, Inc.)

Laryngeal Mask Airway ProSeal

The LMA is available in several variations. The *ProSeal LMA* (PLMA) incorporates a bite block built into the airway tube, a softer larger bowl, and a drainage tube that permits the insertion of an oro-gastric tube for decompression and venting of air. The addition of the drain tube allows for decompression of the stomach in a patient who has been mask ventilated with a result of abdominal distention and pulmonary compromise. In addition, the PLMA is known to have an improved seal pressure, up to 40 cm H_2O, compared with the classic LMA. The improved seal pressure is the result of an improved dorsal cuff, designed to push the cuff deeper into the periglottic tissues.[8,20] Improved seal pressures allow higher peak airway pressures, useful in ventilation of patients with reductions in airway compliance, such as the obese individual. The major disadvantage of the ProSeal LMA is that it is slightly more difficult to place than the LMA classic or unique. Although reports are found in which the Proseal LMA was successfully used as a rescue airway, these reports come primarily from the anesthesia literature and occurred in the operating room with providers skilled with its use. At present, no prehospital reports of its use exist. The future value of the ProSeal LMA as a prehospital rescue airway adjunct is yet to be determined.

Laryngeal Mask Airway–Fastrach

The intubating LMA or *LMA-Fastrach* is an adaptation of the classic LMA that allows for ventilation and provides a conduit for blind passage of a specially designed endotracheal tube for intubation. The LMA-Fastrach is available in three sizes: no. 3, no. 4, and no. 5. The proper size is based on the patient's weight in kilograms, with a range starting at 30 kg for a no. 3 to 70 kg and greater for a no. 5. Generally speaking, a 10-year-old to 12-year-old child and small adult need a no. 3, larger women and small men need a no. 4, and large men need a no. 5.

The LMA-Fastrach has a long history of successful use in the management of the difficult airway both in and out of the hospital.[7] The intubating LMA provides an alternative solution for the unexpected difficult airway, especially when inline cervical stabilization is necessary, because the device does not require extension of the neck. As a result of its rigid metal conduit, large metal handle, and curved shape that anatomically follows the natural curvature of the mouth and hypopharynx, a lubricated LMA-Fastrach may be easier to place than the LMA classic or the LMA unique. It is reported to be faster to insert with a greater degree of success than the LMA classic in inexperienced users.[16] The intubating LMA is of particular usefulness to the prehospital provider given its ability to be inserted from the front, side, or back of the patient who might be entrapped in a vehicle making laryngoscopy difficult or impossible.[55,87,88] The curved metal tube of the LMA-Fastrach allows for the specially designed flexible endotracheal tube to be guided through it, but other airway tools may also passed through the conduit as well. The lighted stylet, the Eschmann endotracheal tube introducer, and flexible fiberoptic scopes have been used in conjunction with the LMA-Fastrach for endotracheal tube intubation. Box 11-7 and Figures 11-14 and 11-15 contain the steps for insertion of the LMA-Fastrach.

Laryngeal Mask Airway CTrach

The *LMA CTrach* is the latest version of the LMA and one of the first of a new type of self-contained intubation tools that relies on fiberoptics to allow viewing of the larynx and tracheal intubation on a detachable liquid crystal display. The LMA CTrach is built on the success of the LMA-Fastrach and is indicated for use in the anticipated and the unexpected difficult intubation. The LMA CTrach is a relatively new intubation tool that has received some investigation in the operating room (OR) in fasted patients. It has not at this time been tested in any significant studies outside the OR or in the prehospital setting. The usefulness of such a tool in the management of the difficult airway outside the OR or outside the hospital remains unclear at this time. However, the idea of clearly viewing, on a small screen, the laryngeal structures and using the view to successfully intubate any patient, particularly one who could not be intubated conventionally, is intriguing. Perhaps these first generation optical or video laryngoscopes, discussed subsequently, will someday result in oral tracheal intubation as practiced today being relegated to a rescue technique.

| BOX 11-7 | **Steps for Insertion of the Fastrach** |

1. Completely deflate the mask of the LMA-Fastrach.
2. Lubricate the posterior surface with a water-based lubricant.
3. Hold the LMA-Fastrach in the dominant hand by the metal handle while opening the mouth with the other hand.
4. Insert the LMA-Fastrach in a circular motion, maintaining firm pressure against the hard and soft palate, and advance it until meets resistance, with only the metal tube protruding from the mouth. Use the metal handle and lift in a frying pan motion to properly seat the LMA in position.
5. Inflate the cuff of the LMA and ventilate the patient. Note adequate chest rise and and assess pulse oximetry to verify adequacy of the airway. Fully oxygenate the patient in preparation of intubation.
6. Disconnect the ambu bag and pass the specially designed silicone-tipped endotracheal tube through the LMA-Fastrach. Ensure that the ETT has been well lubricated with a water-soluble lubricant. The black vertical line on the endotracheal tube indicates proper orientation for the tip to pass through the glottic opening. Insert the ETT to the depth of the horizontal black ring encircling the ETT. The black ring indicates that the tube is positioned just behind the epiglottic elevating bar and is about to emerge from the bowl of the LMA.
7. Advance the ETT while lifting up on the metal handle. The user may feel a loss of resistance that indicates the tube passed through the cords. Inflate the pilot cuff of the ETT, connect a CO_2 detector, and ventilate. If CO_2 is noted, the tube is in proper placement. If CO_2 is not confirmed, release the air from the pilot cuff, pull the ETT back to the horizontal ring, readjust the LMA-Fastach with fine adjustments with the metal handle, and again attempt to advance the ETT. With each pass, confirm end tidal CO_2 as previously noted.
8. At this time, the LMA-Fastrach may be left in place or the decision to remove the LMA-Fastrach with the specially designed push rod may be made.
9. To remove the LMA-Fastrach, remove the 15-mm endotracheal tube connector from the ETT. Leaving it attached to the ambu bag ensures that it is not misplaced. Deflate the mask cuff and then deflate the ETT pilot balloon. This keeps the pilot balloon from being caught in the metal tube and possibly damaging the balloon. Use the push rod and push the ETT down through the LMA; at the same time, withdraw the LMA-Fastrach over the tube. As the LMA-Fastrach is withdrawn, grasp the ETT with the nondominate hand and secure it with the thumb and index finger. Remove the push rod, and continue to withdraw the LMA-Fastrach, allowing the ETT pilot cuff to come through the LMA-Fastrach while continuing to secure the ET tube with the other hand.
10. The LMA-Fastrach is now out of the mouth. Position the ETT at the proper depth, inflate the pilot balloon, and reconnect the ambu bag with the ETT connector already in place. As previously described, reconfirm end tidal CO_2.

The LMA CTrach looks similar to the LMA-Fastrach except it has a detachable high-resolution color display viewer that, when attached to the airway portion of the CTrach, aligns with the built-in fiberoptic channels to project light down one channel while projecting the image up to the viewer through a second channel. The viewer, in addition to providing the light source, has adjustments for brightness, color, and focus. It is powered by a rechargeable battery and is both water and shock resistant. In 2005, the manufacture redesigned the unit to improve the quality of the transmitted image. Like the LMA-Fastrach, the CTrach may be left in place to maintain an airway if intubation fails. At this time, studies to evaluate the LMA CTrach suggest that the success of obtaining a view and the quality of the laryngeal images were unpredictable.[56,89]

King Laryngeal Tube

A recently developed subpraglottic device, the *King Laryngeal Tube* is similar in design to the Combitube in that it incorporates a high-volume low-pressure oropharyngeal and esophageal cuff. The difference in the King Laryngeal Tube (King LT) is that its S-shaped design decreases the likelihood of tracheal intubation and no tube exists beyond the distal cuff. The distal cuff is designed to seal off the esophagus, and the proximal cuff seals the oropharyngeal area, which allows ventilation to take place via airway orifices that lie between the cuffs. Another difference in the King LT is that the two cuffed balloons are inflated by one port. Because of its single lumen and S-shaped design, the King LT may be less technically difficult to use and determine correct placement.[39]

Early evaluations of the King LT indicated the device was easy to insert but was associated with a high incidence rate of airway obstruction.[39] As a result, the King LT underwent design changes with improved performance.[39] The King LT is available for neonates to adults in sizes 0 to 5.

The I-Gel

The I-gel supraglottic airway is the newest supraglottic airway device that, unlike previous devices, does not use inflatable cuffs to achieve a seal of the esophagus and pharyngeal structures. The I-gel is produced from an entirely synthetic medical-grade thermoplastic (styrene ethylene butadine styrene), which gives it a gel-like feel.[35,53] It incorporates into its design a bite block and a gastric channel that allows for passage of a size 12F to 14F gauge suction catheter. The I-gel is an anatomically designed device that effectively fits snugly into the perilaryngeal structures, essentially mirroring the supralaryngeal anatomy. Current available sizes allow use in patients who weigh from 65 to 200 lbs, with additional pediatric sizes under development. In a review of 100 patients in the OR, the I-gel was positioned in 98 of the patients on the first or second attempt, and peak airway pressures of greater than 30 mm Hg were achievable, which allowed for positive pressure ventilations. The study found that as the device warmed to body temperature, the sealing properties of the I-gel improved as a result of the thermoplastic properties of the gel cuff.[53] A supraglottic device that can easily be inserted, has no inflatable cuff to risk tissue compression or distortion, and seals effectively to allow for positive pressure ventilations while keeping aspiration risks to a minimum seems to be the ideal rescue device in a failed intubation situation. The I-gel, although promising, has not yet undergone extensive study, and the future value of the I-gel as a prehospital rescue airway adjunct is yet to be determined.

VIDEO-ASSISTED LARYNGOSCOPY

Video-assisted laryngoscopy transmits, via a camera element located on the laryngoscope blade, an image to a monitor. The views obtained with the video-assisted laryngoscope can be enhanced via

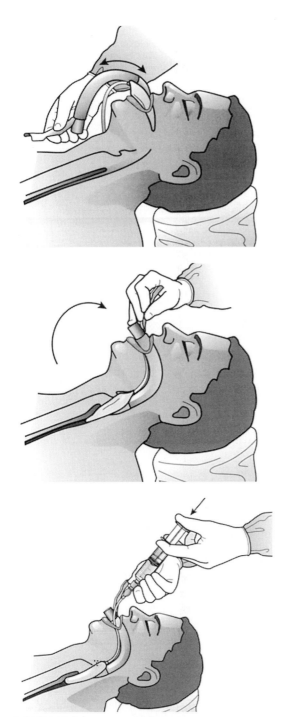

FIGURE 11-14 **Insertion of intubating laryngeal mask airway.** (Courtesy LMA North America, Inc.)

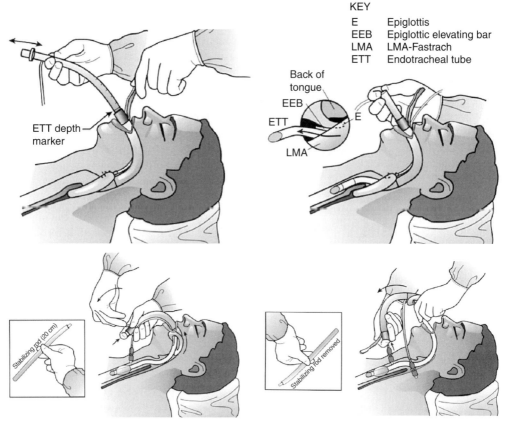

FIGURE 11-15   **Insertion of LMA-Fastrach endotracheal tube and removal of LMA-Fastrach.** (Courtesy LMA North America, Inc.)

magnification and wide-angle view. The video laryngoscope addresses some of the shortcomings of rigid laryngoscopes such as the Bullard, WuScope, and Upsherscope, all of which required maintenance of a skill level with the complexity of the technique and equipment, and the inability of rigid laryngoscopes to visualize the larynx because of blood, emesis, or secretions. Videolaryngoscopy is becoming a widely accepted airway management technique in anesthesia. Advantages over direct laryngoscopy include a better view of the larynx with no need for head extension in patients with limited cervical spine motion and reduced intubation time.

As video laryngoscopes and techniques improve, they are finding their way to the emergency departments and eventually will become tools used by critical care transport providers for airway management. The role of such devices as first-line techniques, or as rescue tools, is unclear at this time. The topic requires training and controlled trials to determine the utility of these new tools and their role in emergency airway management.

The *GlideScope* is a recently developed video laryngoscope designed for management of the difficult airway. The GlideScope use a MacIntosh-like blade coupled with a digital camera with a wide angle lens and an anti-fogging device built into the blade. The 60-degree anteriorly directed viewing angle allows for a panoramic view of the glottic opening without manipulation of the neck. The camera view is displayed in black or white or, in the newer models, on a 7-inch color screen. Newer models of the GlideScope include the Cobalt, which incorporates a disposable plastic blade into a video baton. Most recently, the GlideScope Ranger was released. Specifically designed for out-of-hospital airway management, the GlideScope Ranger features rugged construction, a nonglare monitor for use in bright light conditions, and the same viewing features as the original GlideScope. Advantages of the GlideScope include ease of use, the ability to intubate with the head in neutral position, and simultaneous viewing by numerous providers to assist in confirmation of tube placement and in teaching.[21] The design of the GlideScope, with the camera located back from the tip, and the antifogging technology gives an excellent view of the glottis that is not obscured by blood, emesis, or secretions, and the user maintains a safe distance from the patient's mouth to avoid potential infectious secretions. Failed intubations with the GlideScope result from the inability to pass the tube through the larynx, despite a good laryngeal and glottic view.[21] To enable easier passage of the endotracheal tube, use a stylet and angle the tip upwards to match the angulation of the blade. If resistance at passing the stylet tube is encountered, back the stylet out 3 to 4 cm and also withdraw the blade 1 to 2 cm.[21] As the tip and cuff of the tube enters the glottic opening, have an assistant remove the stylet before advancing the tube. Although rare, complications associated with the use of the GlideScope have been reported, most recently pharyngeal injury.[21]

McGrath Videolaryngoscope

The *McGrath videolaryngoscope,* newly released in January 2006, is a device that is completely portable and looks much like a standard laryngoscope. Mounted on top of the laryngoscope handle is a color liquid display that swivels and tilts to allow for optimal viewing by the operator. The battery, stored in the handle, powers two hyperbright light-emitting diodes and a small color camera located at the distal end of the blade and the viewing screen.[49,78,79] An innovative blade design allows for the blade to be adjusted to multiple lengths. Although no large studies support the use of the McGrath laryngoscope, preliminary evidence suggests that it is a compact, portable, and easy-to-use alternative to direct laryngoscopy and can be valuable in circumstances

of difficult or failed tracheal intubation.[78,79] As with the GlideScope, advancing the tube through the cords is enabled with the use of a stylet angled 60 to 70 degrees upwards at the tip.

PEDIATRIC MANAGEMENT

Successful management of the pediatric airway begins with the knowledge that anatomic differences in children require adaptations to the techniques described earlier for proper care to be provided. In addition to the obvious anatomic differences in children are many physiologic differences that are not as easily appreciated. Fortunately, the differences slowly diminish as a child ages. Not only should the clinician be familiar with anatomic and physiologic differences, but the clinician should also be aware that the child's fear or apprehension can complicate treatment efforts. Even the routine act of supplemental oxygenation with a nasal cannula or mask can become a challenge in a child who is awake because of the child's fear of having something in the nose or wrapped around the face. The child should be prepared with conversation and with comfort as much as possible. This step is important to the child and to the adult.

Indications for intubation in children are parallel to those of the adult. They include respiratory failure, failure to protect the airway because of altered mental status, and airway obstruction. Complications are also similar in both populations. The most common complications of orotracheal intubation for all age groups include dental trauma and esophageal and right mainstem bronchus intubations that go unrecognized.

The role of prehospital tracheal intubation has become controversial since the 2000 publication that examined survival and neurologic outcome in pediatric patients intubated in the prehospital setting.[36] The study, done in two large urban rapid-transport emergency medical systems (EMS) systems staffed with paramedics, compared the survival and neurologic outcomes of 830 pediatric patients treated with bag-valve-mask ventilations with those of patients treated with bag-valve-mask ventilations followed by endotracheal intubation. All patients entered in this study underwent intubation without the use of sedatives or paralytic agents. Results of the study found no significant difference in survival rates between the two groups. The study also revealed scene times were prolonged and fatal complications related to tracheal intubation were frequent. This management plan may be the best option for providers primarily trained in caring for adults. A common cause of unsuccessful pediatric intubation is operator inexperience.

ANATOMIC DIFFERENCES IN CHILDREN[37]

The pediatric airway differs from the adult until about the age of 8 years when the larynx resembles that of the adult in structure and position. The greatest differences exist in the child who is 2 years or less, and patients between the years of 2 and 8 represent a transitional period.

An infant's head is much larger in proportion to the rest of the body and results in a natural sniffing position. As a result, neck flexion is not necessary to attain the sniffing position and bag-mask ventilations. In infants and some young children, the sniffing position is too pronounced, and the transport team provider may need to place a towel under the infant's shoulders to raise the rest of the body and straighten the airway, thereby improving airflow.

The infant is also an obligate nose breather, and secretions or edema in this area can cause airway compromise more easily than in adults. Infants and small children have tongues that are large in relation to the size of the oropharynges, which makes the tongue, as it is in the adult, the most common cause of airway obstruction. The relatively small size of children's mouths also makes intubation more difficult. Because of the small size of the pediatric airway, minimal edema can create a life-threatening obstruction. An infant's airway, normally 4 mm in diameter, decreases to 2 mm with 1 mm of circumferential edema caused by secretions or trauma caused by intubation. In comparison, the adult airway, normally 8 mm in diameter, decreases to 6 mm with 1 mm of circumferential edema (Figure 11-16). The result is only a 25% decrease in diameter in the adult as compared with a 50% decrease in the infant with an equal amount of swelling.[62,75]

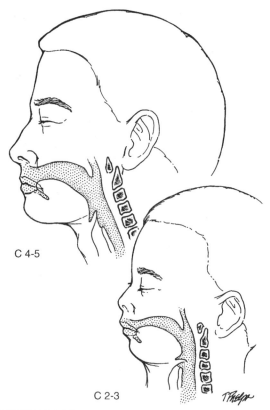

FIGURE 11-16   **Comparative anatomy of adult and infant airways.** (From Nichols DG, et al, editors: *Golden hour: the handbook of advanced pediatric life support,* ed 2, St Louis, 1996, Mosby.)

The vocal cords of a young child are more pliable than those of the adult and are easier to damage, resulting in potential obstruction. The presence of hypertrophied tonsils and adenoid tissues can cause rapid development of upper airway obstruction and is a significant source of bleeding when traumatized. In addition, the larynx is situated higher in relation to the cervical spines that in the adult. In the infant, the glottic opening is at C-1; as the child ages, the glottic opening moves down to the level of the adult at C-4 to C-5. The anterior position of the larynx in the infant and young child leads to more frequent intubations of the esophagus. In a situation in which the laryngoscopist recognizes no landmarks, a likely indication is that the laryngoscope blade has been passed to far and needs to be withdrawn until structures are recognized.

In addition to the anatomic differences noted, the critical care transport team members must be aware of the physiologic differences between children and adults. Of critical importance is the recognition that infants and children experience oxygen desaturation much quicker than adults. This faster desaturation time after apnea is the result of the higher metabolic oxygen consumption rate compared with the adult. The infant and child's oxygen consumption rate is twice that of the adults and the functional residual capacity (FRC) is significantly less.

Physiologic differences in infants and children influence drug administration and dosages. Children are known to have a relatively greater volume of water than adults. Water-soluble drugs, such as neuromuscular blockers, are therefore dissolved in a greater volume of water, which necessitates a greater bolus dose to achieve a given plasma level. Like all neuromuscular blockers, succinylcholine is water soluble. Therefore, the intravenous (IV) bolus dose needed in infants and young children (2 mg/kg) is larger than for older children and adults (1 mg/kg). Elimination clearance is likewise different in children. An intramuscular dose of 4 mg/kg provides a maximal onset of blockade in 3 to 4 minutes and lasts for 20 minutes. Its elimination clearance is more rapid in children, so its duration of effects is less than for adults.[75]

An indispensable tool in assisting with and reducing medication dosing errors is the use of the Broselow-Luten Resuscitation Tape system. The Broselow tape was initially designed to assist in the estimation of weight in cases of pediatric trauma. Since that time, information on equipment sizes and medications has been added, greatly reducing the anxiety of caregivers who primarily treat adult patients.[29]

Lungs can easily be overdistended, and barotrauma induced by overzealous positive pressure ventilation can develop. Ventilation should be limited to the amount of air needed to cause the chest to rise. Excessive volumes exacerbate gastric distention and increase the risk of pneumothorax. When possible, a self-inflating bag-valve ventilation system should be used, optimally with a pop-off valve. Resuscitation bags are available for neonates (delivering volumes of 500 to 600 mL) and adults (delivering volumes of 1.0 to 1.5 L). An oxygen reservoir should be used to enhance the oxygen concentration. Initial respiratory rates used for controlled ventilation should approximate normal spontaneous respiratory rates based on age.

The use of uncuffed endotracheal tubes has long been a practice in pediatric airway management. The practice is based on the belief that because the larynx is cone shaped and the subglottic cricoid ring is the narrowest portion of the pediatric airway, an adequately placed noncuffed tube provides protection from pulmonary aspiration and ensures sufficient ventilation. Uncuffed tubes are relatively smaller in external diameter than a cuffed tube of the same internal diameter. Therefore, a relatively larger sized internal diameter tube can be inserted comfortably. The larger tube offers less resistance to airflow, facilitates suctioning of secretions, and lessens the likelihood of development of subglottic stenosis. Subglottic stenosis is a serious airway complication that results from inflammation and scarring of the laryngeal mucosa, which leads to narrowing of the trachea. It can occur as a result of excessive intracuff pressures (greater that 30 cm H_2O) and lead to tracheal capillary ischemia. Currently, in many pediatric intensive care units (ICUs) and in anesthesia, the standard of care is to use cuffed tubes in patients as young as 2 years provided the tubes are carefully selected and cuff pressures are monitored.[46,64] A recent study of endotracheal intracuff pressures of adult patients in the emergency department (ED) and prehospital setting found that a substantial percentage of patients in this setting had cuff pressures that exceeded safe pressures.[17,46,82] Some authors have advocated the use of cuffed tubes in the prehospital setting, but at this time, no out-of-hospital research has been conducted on cuffed tubes in children. The 2005 American Heart Association guidelines for cardiopulmonary resuscitation and emergency care of pediatric and neonatal patients allows for the use of cuffed endotracheal tubes in infants, except newborns, and children in in-hospital settings provided cuff inflation pressure is maintained at less than 20 cm water pressure.[2] Uncuffed endotracheal tubes are generally used in children younger than 6 to 8 years.[2,32]

The proper ETT size can be determined in several ways. It can be approximated by the size of the child's little finger or nares. A more precise method to ensure proper ETT size is as follows:

Newborn: preterm, 3.0 mm;
             full-term, 3.5 mm.

Then:

$$\frac{[age(y) + 16]}{4} = \text{internal diameter of ETT (mm)}$$

ETT depth (cm) in orally intubated children
(or adults), tube measured at lip line
= tube size × 3

The anatomic differences between the pediatric and adult airways are illustrated in Figure 11-16. The anatomic differences can be summarized as follows:

1. A child's larynx lies more cephalad than an adult's.
2. A child's epiglottis is at an angle of 45 degrees to the anterior pharyngeal wall, whereas an adult's lies parallel to the base of the tongue.
3. A child's epiglottis is large, stiff, and U-shaped, whereas an adult's is flattened and more flexible.
4. The larger tongue of infants and children and the position of the hyoid bone depress the epiglottis.
5. The cricoid ring is the narrowest portion of a child's airway.

The use of a Miller (straight) blade permits easier cord visualization. A straight blade is inserted beyond the epiglottis, which is lifted up along with the tongue and jaw. If the blade is inserted too far and landmarks are not easily recognized, the blade should be gently backed out, and the glottic opening often pops into view. Inability to recognize the epiglottis increases the likelihood of tracheal intubation. Pediatric Miller blades range in size from 0 to 2. The 0 blade is used for the premature and small newborn, and the Miller 1 is used for the larger newborn to age 2 years. A Miller 2 or the MacIntosh 2 is used in children older than 2 years. For the child older than 12 years, the MacIntosh 3 is frequently used.

During intubation, assigning an assistant the task of observing the cardiac monitor for heart rate is beneficial. In young infants, the cardiac output is rate dependent, and bradycardia is universally associated with hypotension. A heart rate of less than 100 bpm in a neonate, less than 80 bpm in an infant, and less than 60 bpm in a child constitutes bradycardia. Should this be observed, the intubation attempt is aborted and oxygenation via bag-valve mask is initiated. Atropine should be administered to all children and adolescents receiving succinylcholine to block vagal stimulation.

Tube placement is confirmed via auscultation with observation, palpation, and the use of an endotracheal tube confirmation device such as an end-tidal CO_2 detector or capnography. Breath sounds are transmitted readily, although the child's thorax and abdomen make tube placement hard to judge. Therefore, along with auscultation, the transport team should observe the symmetric rise and fall of the chest wall, monitor for maintenance of heart rate, and check the patient's color for improvement. The chest wall should also be palpated for symmetry of movement.

The ETT depth is generally three times the inside diameter of the tube size. This rule of thumb applies to premature infants and to adults when the appropriately sized tube for the patient's age is in place. Once placed, the tube should be well secured with tape and tincture of benzoin. Tracheostomy tape should be avoided because it may kink the tube or reduce the tube's diameter if secured too tightly. Because the tube is cuffless and the child's trachea is so short, movement of the child's head may lead to a mainstem intubation or to extubation. As with the adult, assessment of tube placement should occur after each patient transfer (e.g., after the child is loaded into an aircraft or ground unit).

A part of airway management for children is the placement of a gastric tube. A child's stomach is relatively larger than an adult's and may contain food and a significant amount of air. Children tend to swallow air when crying (aerophagia). If full, the stomach may impinge on the diaphragm and decrease vital capacity. If a postintubation chest radiograph is available, the tip of the ETT should be at the T2 to T3 vertebral level or at the level of the lower edge of the medial aspect of the clavicle.

INVASIVE AIRWAY MANAGEMENT

Invasive airway management offers additional methods of management of a difficult or failed airway.

The likelihood is good that at some time these skills will be needed, particularly for the transport team who frequently care for trauma victims. Because of the relatively infrequent opportunity to gain experience, reluctance to attempt the procedure can occur even when the clinical situation clearly dictates the need for an invasive airway. This reluctance and the delay that results can add additional urgency to a situation that necessitates swift action. Transport team members must be knowledgeable in the techniques of invasive airway management: needle cricothyrotomy and surgical cricothyrotomy.

Cricothyroidotomy is a procedure used to gain airway control that necessitates a surgical incision through the cricothyroid space. It is performed when other forms of airway management have failed and the patient cannot be adequately ventilated and oxygenated with a bag and mask. Indications for the establishment of a surgical airway include: (1) the inability to gain airway access by other means (the failed airway); and (2) complete upper airway obstruction. Airway inaccessibility during orotracheal or nasotracheal intubation may be the result of trauma, which can cause abnormal anatomy or profuse bleeding and thereby obscure visualization of the glottic opening. Upper airway obstruction may be the result of a foreign body, mass lesion, or edema. Edema can be caused by infection, caustic ingestion, allergic reaction, or inhalation injury. Relative contraindications include: (1) the inability to locate the correct landmarks for puncture; (2) gross infection over the puncture site; (3) primary laryngeal injury; (4) coagulopathy; and (5) a patient younger than 12 years old.[92,93]

A *needle cricothyrotomy* (also called transtracheal jet ventilation and percutaneous transtracheal jet ventilation) is a method of airway control that uses a needle through the cricothyroid space and therefore requires less surgical skill than a cricothyroidotomy. Palpation and identification of landmarks of the neck are difficult in children, and identification of the cricothyroid membrane is nearly impossible in infants. An additional complicating factor is that the laryngeal prominence does not develop until late childhood and adolescence. Percutaneous transtracheal ventilation is generally accepted as the preferred surgical airway maneuver in children 12 years and younger. The goal is to avoid damage to the cricoid cartilage, which in children is the only circumferential structure that supports the larynx and upper trachea (Figure 11-17). In the future, the availability of alternative airway devices in the hands of trained personnel may reduce the significance of this airway management technique.

NEEDLE CRICOTHYROTOMY

Needle cricothyrotomy involves the insertion of an over-the-needle cannula through the cricothyroid membrane into the trachea. The needle cricothyrotomy

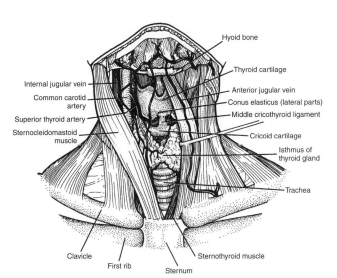

FIGURE 11-17 **Anterior aspect of neck with relative anatomic structures.** (From Rosen P, et al: *Emergency medicine: concepts and clinical practice,* vol 1, ed 2, St Louis, 1988, Mosby.)

Hyoid bone

Thyroid cartilage

Internal jugular vein

Common carotid artery

Superior thyroid artery

Sternocleidomastoid muscle

Anterior jugular vein

Conus elasticus (lateral parts)

Middle cricothyroid ligament

Cricoid cartilage

Isthmus of thyroid gland

Trachea

Clavicle

First rib

Sternum

Sternothyroid muscle

| BOX 11-8 | **Steps for Needle Cricothyrotomy** |

1. Stabilize the patient's head in a neutral position.
2. Identify the cricothyroid membrane and prepare the skin.
3. Stabilize the cricoid and thyroid cartilages with the nondominant hand.
4. Insert a 12-gauge or 14-gauge over-the-needle intravenous catheter into the membrane at a 45-degree angle caudally (toward the feet). On passage into the trachea, the needle is removed, and the cannula is advanced caudally.
5. The hub of the needle is connected, preferably to a jet ventilator capable of delivering oxygen at a pressure of 50 psi. Otherwise, the connector is removed from a 3.0-mm ETT and attached to the intravenous catheter. It is then connected to a bag-valve-mask device. This method is temporary until other means of airway securement can be achieved.

is quicker and easier to perform than a surgical cricothyrotomy and is an alternative technique for practitioners unable to perform a cricothyrotomy. Steps for this procedure are included in Box 11-8. The use of a kink-resistant catheter, 10-gauge, 14-gauge, or 16-gauge cannula, is recommended. The needle is removed, and the cannula is left in place. Commercially available cannulas are designed with side holes in addition to the distal port and incorporate a flange that aids securement of the catheter. The additional holes decrease pressure-related mucosal damage. When used in an adult, the cannula must then be connected to an oxygen-delivery device capable of delivering short bursts of oxygen from a high-pressure source of 50 psi. When used in pediatric patients, a pressure regulator set at a maximal pressure of 20 to 30 psi should be used to decrease the risk of barotrauma. This method of ventilation is known as *translaryngeal jet ventilation,* and it provides emergency oxygenation and ventilation by passive recoil of the chest wall and exhalation by way of the upper airway. In situations in which complete upper airway obstruction is suspected, a needle cricothyrotomy does not allow for exhalation and barotrauma results. In such a situation, a cricothyrotomy is the airway of choice.[93]

The ventilatory rate should be from 12 to 20 bpm with an insufflation time of about 1 to 2 seconds. In young children less than 5-years-old, an alternative method to the use of the jet ventilator allows for the connector from a no. 3 ETT to be connected to the cannula, which is then connected to a resuscitation bag. This technique meets oxygen requirements. However, ventilation is minimal at best, and respiratory acidosis quickly results. The respiratory

acidosis that results generally limits ventilation in this manner to approximately 30 minutes. The use of a resuscitation bag is at best a temporary measure, whereas jet ventilation is considered a true-positive pressure-ventilation technique.

SURGICAL CRICOTHYROTOMY

Surgical cricothyrotomy is an invasive procedure that should be governed by protocols. Steps for surgical cricothyrotomy are detailed in Box 11-9. In circumstances in which the anatomy of the neck is distorted, the trachea can be identified with slow advancement of a needle connected to a syringe through the skin and attempted aspiration of air. Once air has been aspirated, signaling entrance into the trachea, the needle and syringe should be left in place and cut down over the needle. If the incision is too small, identification of the structures is more difficult. A vertical incision over the midline is recommended for minimization of bleeding. The nondominant hand should be used for grasping and stabilization of the larynx until the tracheostomy hook can be inserted. If a tracheostomy hook is not available, one can be made with removal of the cannula from a 16-gauge or 14-gauge catheter and bending of the needle into a hook about 0.25 inches above the tip with a hemostat. After the skin incision has been made and the cricoid membrane identified, the membrane should be incised and the tracheostomy hook should be inserted through the membrane and used to stabilize the inferior border of the trachea. The diameter of the cricothyroid space is enlarged by insertion and spreading of a Trousseau dilator. Once the dilator is in place, the hook is removed to prevent puncture of the balloon of the tracheostomy

---

BOX 11-9	**Steps for Surgical Cricothyrotomy**

1. Stabilize the patient's head in a neutral position.
2. Identify the cricothyroid membrane and prepare the skin.
3. Stabilize the cricoid and thyroid cartilages with the nondominant hand.
4. Make a vertical incision 5 to 7 cm through the skin.
5. Identify the cricoid membrane, and insert the tracheal hook. Use the tracheal hook, now in the nondominant hand, to stabilize the thyroid. Apply upward traction (45-degree angle) on the inferior margin of the thyroid cartilage.
6. Use the tip of a no. 11 blade to create a horizontal incision through the cricoid membrane. Avoid insertion of the blade too deeply and injury of the posterior wall of the trachea or the esophagus.
7. Insert a Trousseau dilator and spread vertically to enlarge the diameter of the cricoid space. Mayo scissors may be used to help enlarge the space in the transverse direction.
8. Remove the tracheal hook.
9. Place a cuffed ETT or tracheostomy tube through the dilator.
10. Remove the dilator. Secure the tube, and verify proper position in the usual manner.

---

tube. A cuffed 6.0-mm ETT or a cuffed no. 4 Shiley tracheostomy tube is placed through the dilator, and the dilator is then removed. The balloon is inflated, and the tube is checked for correct position in the usual manner.

RAPID FOUR-STEP CRICOTHYROTOMY TECHNIQUE

The Rapid Four-Step Cricothyrotomy Technique was developed for use in the prehospital environment. This technique relies on palpation rather than direct visualization of the cricothyroid membrane, thus decreasing the need for suction and additional light (Figure 11-18). Studies suggest the rapid four-step technique aids in establishing an airway quicker than the traditional technique but may be associated with a higher complication rate. The steps for this procedure include[9,27,44]:

1. **Palpation** (Figure 11-18,A). To perform the procedure, one should position oneself at the patient's left shoulder and palpate the cricoid membrane with the index finger of the left hand, allowing the thumb and middle finger to palpate and stabilize the trachea.
2. **Incision** (Figure 11-18,B). With the right hand, a no. 20 scalpel is used to make a horizontal incision into the inferior aspect of the cricothyroid membrane. The scalpel is pushed through the membrane at a 60-degree angle to create a

2.5-cm horizontal incision. The scalpel is *not* removed but held in place.
3. **Traction** (Figure 11-18,C). A tracheal hook is held perpendicular to the longitudinal axis of the patient. With the left hand, the tracheal hook is placed flush against the caudal surface of the scalpel blade and slid down along the trachea. The tip of the hook is rotated 90 degrees in the inferior direction, and ventral/caudal traction is applied to the superior margin of the cricoid cartilage. The scalpel is then removed, and traction is maintained on the trachea by placing the left hand on the patient's sternum.
4. **Intubation** (Figure 11-18,D). This step is similar to orotracheal intubation. A cuffed endotracheal tube or tracheostomy tube is placed with the right hand. Tube placement is confirmed, and the hook is removed. If an endotracheal tube is used, the beveled side initially should be facing the cephalad during insertion to decrease advancement of the tube superior to the vocal cords.

CRICOTHYROTOMY: SELDINGER TECHNIQUE

The development of the *Seldinger technique* for insertion of catheters and other tubes has also provided an additional method of performing a cricothyrotomy. Commercial kits are available that contain all the components needed to perform this procedure. Steps include:

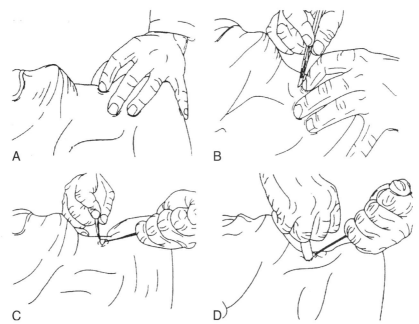

FIGURE 11-18   **Four-step cricothyrotomy. A,** Palpation. **B,** Incision. **C,** Traction. **D,** Intubation. (From Brofeldt BT, Osborn ML, Sakles JC, et al: Evaluation of the rapid four-step cricothyrotomy technique: an interim report, *Air Med J* 17(3):127, 1998.)

1. Position the patient and identify appropriate landmarks.
2. Insert a small locator needle into the cricothyroid membrane. Aspirate air to confirm needle placement into the trachea.
3. Pass a soft-tipped wire through the needle, and thread it into the trachea. Keep control of the wire at all times to prevent wire aspiration.
4. With a no. 11 blade, cut a small incision adjacent to the needle to facilitate passage of the airway device.
5. Place the airway tube with its internal dilator over the wire through the tissue into the trachea. If resistance is met, extend or deepen the skin incision. A gentle screwing motion may also facilitate passage.
6. Confirm tube placement.

PHARMACOLOGY OF ADVANCED AIRWAY MANAGEMENT

Since the 1980s, the use of sedation and neuromuscular blocking agents to facilitate advanced airway management before and during transport has evolved. Benefits of the use of sedation and neuromuscular blocking agents include rapid endotracheal intubation with improved oxygenation and ventilation, aspiration protection, spinal protection for those at risk, and facilitation of the transport of hemodynamically unstable, uncooperative, agitated patients who might otherwise put themselves and the transport team at an increased safety risk.

These agents were once used only by physicians in the hospital setting. Today, critical care transport teams consisting of physicians, nurses, and paramedics frequently use these agents; team members must possess a thorough understanding of their use, drug profile, and contraindications to use. Before sedation and neuromuscular blocking agents are used, each transport team member must develop strong clinical airway assessment and management skills that include training in airway management of patients who cannot be intubated and training in the use of backup rescue airway methods.[93] For the successful use of sedation and neuromuscular agents by a critical transport team, the team must possess strongly committed medical direction, a detailed training program that includes hands-on OR-based airway training, and the required use of continuous end-tidal CO_2 monitoring.[25,40]

RAPID-SEQUENCE INTUBATION

Rapid-sequence intubation has its roots in anesthesia where it is referred to as rapid sequence induction. Rapid sequence induction (RSI) of anesthesia was introduced for patients with a full stomach to protect the airway from potential aspiration of the gastric contents. The practice includes preoxygenation with 100% oxygen, administration of a predetermined induction dose (to induce unconsciousness), cricoid pressure, and the use of succinylcholine, followed by apnea and then tracheal intubation with a cuffed endotracheal tube. In the early 1980s, the technique of rapidly gaining control of the airway with the same drugs as in the OR became known as rapid sequence intubation when done in the ED. The practice is identical in both situations. Whether performed in the ED or outside the hospital, the procedure calls for preoxygenation of the patient with 100% oxygen and cautious avoidance, when possible, of positive-pressure ventilation, which results in gastric distention. Cricoid pressure and medication for sedation and analgesia, followed by a neuromuscular blocking agent (NMBA), typically succinylcholine, is then used to facilitate intubation. If the situation warrants, neuromuscular blockade may be maintained with administration of a longer-acting NMBA after confirming and securing the endotracheal tube. Before the use of NMBA, a brief neurologic assessment should be performed. This assessment must be performed and documented for comparison later. NMBAs can be classified in three ways: type of block produced (depolarizing versus nondepolarizing), duration of action (ultrashort, short, intermediate, or long), and structure (acetylcholine-like, benzylisoquinolinium compound, or aminosteroid compound).[10,12]

NEUROMUSCULAR BLOCKING AGENTS

All *NMBAs* work at the level of the neuromuscular end plate, disrupting neurotransmitter (acetylcholine) function and preventing effective contraction of skel-

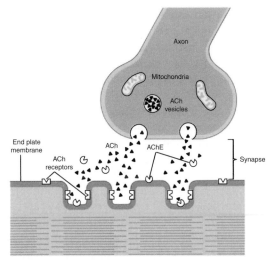

FIGURE 11-19   **Disruption of actylcholine function by neuromuscular blocking agents.** (From Clark JB, Queener SF, Karb VB: *Pharmacologic basis of nursing practice,* ed 4, St Louis, 1993, Mosby.)

etal muscle (Figure 11-19). These agents do not produce analgesia, anesthesia, or amnesia, and reports exist of patients with total recall and pain perception who received neuromuscular blocking agents without sufficient anesthesia during operations and procedures. Therefore, sedation of the patient is essential before and during extended periods of use of neuromuscular blocking agents.

The use of succinylcholine produces many side effects and clinical considerations. Because of succinylcholine's structural resemblance to acetylcholine, the primary parasympathetic neurotransmitter, it stimulates cholinergic receptors at other sites in addition to those at the neuromuscular junction. The stimulation of nicotinic receptors in the sympathetic and parasympathetic nervous system and muscarinic receptors in the sinoatrial node of the heart can produce bradycardia and lead to hypotension. Associated bradycardia is more pronounced in children and adults who receive repeated doses and is attenuated by the use of atropine as a pretreatment drug.

Fasciculations signal the onset of paralysis by succinylcholine. Fasciculations are the result of uncoordinated motor unit contractions and are clinically important in that they are associated with an increase in ICP, resulting in a decrease in cerebral perfusion, and as a result may increase secondary brain injury.[38]

Lidocaine is administered often as a pretreatment to attenuate the physiologic responses to laryngoscopy and intubation. To date, no evidence supports the use of lidocaine as a pretreatment for RSI in patients with head injury. However, studies of intubated patients in the OR and ICUs have shown success in blunting reflex increases in ICP from endotracheal suctioning and bronchoscopy and its use is still widely practiced.[10,12,72]

Succinylcholine-induced hyperkalemia is rare but continues to be reported in the literature and is associated with cardiovascular instability, hyperkalemic dysrhythmias, and death. Normal muscle releases enough potassium during succinylcholine-induced depolarization to raise serum potassium by 0.5 to 1.0 mEq/L. In denervation injuries, acetylcholine receptors develop outside the neuromuscular junction, referred to as up-regulation. These extrajunctional receptors allow succinylcholine to affect widespread depolarization and extensive potassium release. The higher the up-regulation is, the more profound is the hyperkalemia. The presence of two or more etiologic factors magnifies the up-regulation of acetylcholine receptors in muscle, which in turn can lead to an earlier and more profound hyperkalemic response to succinylcholine. The potential for severe hyperkalemia with succinylcholine can occur as early as 4 to 5 days of immobilization and can persist as long as the condition that induced it continues to present. Quadriplegics and paraplegics with persistent paralysis, therefore, could have the potential for succinylcholine hyperkalemia throughout life.[10,12]

Pathologic conditions with potential for hyperkalemia with succinylcholine include: upper or lower motor neuron defect; prolonged chemical denervation (muscle relaxants, magnesium, clostridial toxins); direct muscle trauma, tumor, or inflammation; thermal trauma; disuse atrophy; and severe infection.

Electrocardiographic (ECG) changes that include tall T waves greater than 5 mm, small absent P waves, atrioventricular dissociation, or ventricular tachycardia/fibrillation associated with succinylcholine and hyperkalemia occur within 2 to 5 minutes

and may be classified as mild, moderate, or severe. Treatment should include the IV administration of calcium gluconate (10 mL of 10% solution administered over 2 to 3 minutes), which restores the gap between the resting membrane potential and the threshold potential in the heart and prevents spontaneous depolarization. Other agents that promote the movement of potassium into the cell with a subsequent drop in serum potassium include insulin with glucose, catecholamines, and sodium bicarbonate. In most patients, the succinylcholine-induced hyperkalemia lasts less than 10 to 15 minutes, but in some, it may last longer.[10,12]

A long-held common belief among practitioners is that the use of succinylcholine for induction in patients with open globe injuries is relatively or absolutely contraindicated. Physiologically, succinylcholine is associated with an increase in intraocular pressure (IOP). However, when an open globe injury occurs, it is often associated with crying, forceful blinking, and rubbing of the eyes, all of which create a much larger rise in IOP than that associated with the use of succinylcholine. The belief that succinylcholine caused vitreous extrusion has been perpetuated for nearly 50 years and relied on anecdote rather than documented case reports. As of 2003, no well-documented case reports describe vitreous extrusion or blindness related to the use of succinylcholine.[10,12,15]

Succinylcholine is known to be a trigger for malignant hyperthermia (MH) in susceptible patients. Malignant hyperthermia is a hypermetabolic disorder of skeletal muscle. Classic signs include hyperthermia, tachycardia, increased carbon dioxide production, increased oxygen consumption, acidosis, muscle rigidity, and rhabdomyolysis. If untreated, the syndrome is fatal. Early detection is essential and relies on an observed increase in end-tidal carbon dioxide followed by laboratory confirmation of acidosis. The incidence of MH in adults is rare; however, children are known to be at higher risk, with more than 50% of all cases of MH appearing in children less than 15 years of age. MH is treated with dantrolene sodium administered in doses of 2.5 mg/kg bolus followed by additional doses up to 10 mg/kg. Further treatment is aimed at cooling of the patient, treatment of arrhythmias (avoid calcium channel blockers), aggressive fluid therapy to maintain urine output, and monitoring for coagulation abnormalities. Patients should be monitored for 48 to 72 hours after the initial event because as many as 25% of patients have a recurrence of symptoms.[10,12,74]

NONDEPOLARIZING AGENTS[10,12,47,52,66,77,80,83,95,96]

The South American arrow poisons known as curares were described by the explorers of the new world as early as the 16th and 17th centuries. Investigations into these poisons led to the development in 1943 of the first nondepolarizing drug tubocurarine, which was used as a muscle relaxant during surgical anesthesia. The unwanted side effects of tubocurarine led to the development and widespread use, beginning in the 1960s, of pancuronium, which continued until atracurium and vecuronium were released in the mid 1980s. In the 1990s mivacurium and rocuronium were introduced. With the release of newer agents, unwanted cardiovascular side effects have been eliminated and a predictable recovery profile established. A major advancement in the development of nondepolarizing agents was the release of atracurium, which spontaneously breaks down in the body to inactive compounds through Hofmann elimination. This self-destruct mechanism is independent of metabolism and excretion and therefore especially useful in patients with kidney, liver, or multiorgan failure. Cisatracurium is similar to atricurium but causes less tachycardia and is slightly more potent.[10,12]

Unlike succinylcholine, which binds to the muscle receptor and acts as an agonist, nondepolarizing muscle relaxants bind to the receptors and prevent depolarization with acetylcholine. Therefore, nondepolarizers are referred to as competitive antagonists. Nondepolarizing agents as a rule have a slower onset of action and maintain neuromuscular blockade longer than succinylcholine. Although succinylcholine is associated with numerous undesirable side effects, the nondepolarizers are not considered a substitute in rapid sequence intubation because of their slow onset of action and prolonged recovery time. The onset of action of these medications may be increased with a higher dose of the drug, but a greater risk exists of triggering cardiovascular side effects, such as tachycardia, and prolonging the duration of paralysis in a "can't intubate, can't ventilate" situation, which could have disastrous consequences.

The search for a nondepolarizing muscle relaxant with the onset of action equal to that of succinylcholine and with minimal side effects led to the development of rocuronium. Rocuronium is a steroidal nondepolarizing agent with intermediate duration. In patients who need rapid sequence intubation but in whom succinylcholine is contraindicated, rocuronium is the only currently available nondepolarizing agent that can provide relaxation and intubation conditions similar to succinylcholine (60 seconds) when dosed in the range of 1.0 to 1.2 mg/kg.[8] Sakles et al[77] found rocuronium to be safe and effective for RSI of selected ED patients in whom contraindication to succinylcholine existed.

Vecuronium has also been used as a substitute for succinylcholine; however, even when the normal intubation dose of 0.1 mg/kg is tripled, the speed of onset was only reduced to 90 seconds. With the slow onset of intubation conditions, the need to provide bag-valve-mask ventilations to prevent desaturation puts the patient at risk for gastric insufflation, which can increase the risk of vomiting an pulmonary aspiration.[9]

Indications for the use of neuromuscular blocking agents in the critical care transport environment include: facilitation of intubation, ventilation control, safety (management of an agitated patient), and improvement in oxygenation and treatment of pathologic muscle rigidity. Table 11-1 lists some of the NMBAs used in critical care transport.

Medications, disease processes, and physiologic conditions may interfere with the effectiveness of neuromuscular blocking agents. Neurologic diseases such as myasthenia gravis can prolong paralysis. Hyperthermia and hypothermia may have an impact on the pharmacology of selected neuromuscular blocking agents. Electrolyte imbalances such as hypermagnesia may also prolong paralysis. Table 11-2 contains some of the medications that may affect neuromuscular blocking agents. The transport team must be knowledgeable of medications that they administer and the management of potential adverse reactions that might occur.

TABLE 11-1	NMBAs			
NMBAs	**Intravenous dosage (mg/kg)**	**Onset (min)**	**Duration (min)**	**Comments**
Depolarizing				
Succinylcholine	Adult dose: 1.0-1.5 Pediatric dose: 1.5-2.0	1.5-2.0	4-6	Pretreat with atropine in children and adolescents; many adverse effects.
Nondepolarizing				
Pancuronium	00.04-0.01	3-5	60-100	Stimulate heart rate and cardiac output; no histamine release.
Atracurium	0.4-0.5	2-3	20-45	Metabolism independent of kidney or liver function; histamine release.
Rocuronium	0.5-1.0	1-2	20-40	Shortest onset of all nondepolarizing NMBAs; no histamine release.
Vecuronium	0.1	2-3	20-40	Minimal cardiovascular effects; no histamine release.
Mivacurium	0.15-0.25	2-3	12-20	Shortest duration of all nondepolarizing NMBAs; histamine release. No longer available in the United States.

TABLE 11-2	Medications That May Affect NMBAs
Medications	**Effects**
Aminoglycosides	Prolonged duration of relaxation
Lidocaine	Prolonged duration of relaxation
Local anesthetics	Prolonged duration of relaxation
Beta blockers	Prolonged relaxation
Magnesium	Prolonged relaxation
Procainamide	Prolonged relaxation
Quinidine	Prolonged relaxation
Potassium-depleting medications	Prolonged relaxation
Lithium	Prolonged relaxation
Digoxin	Prolonged relaxation
Corticosteroids	Prolonged relaxation

REVERSAL OF NEUROMUSCULAR BLOCKADE

On rare occasions, prolonged paralysis after the administration of NMBAs presents a problem in patient evaluation or treatment, and the need to reverse the agent arises. Pharmacologic reversal of these agents is possible. However, in most situations, normal drug metabolism and excretion to clear the neuromuscular agent are safer and easier. Succinylcholine has no known reversal agent. The patient's respirations must be supported during the duration of action time (4 to 6 minutes), after which the drug undergoes normal metabolism and muscle action returns.

Reversal of the nondepolarizing agents involves administration of drugs that inhibit acetylcholinesterase, which allows the local concentration of acetylcholine molecules to rise. The reversal agents include neostigmine, pyridostigmine, and edrophonium (Table 11-3).[10,12] The administration of these anticholinesterase-inhibiting drugs causes a strong parasympathetic response that consists of cardiovascular effects, bronchoconstriction, and increased glandular secretions. The cardiovascular effects are of greatest concern and include bradycardia, heart block, and cardiac arrest. These effects can be countered with administration of anticholinergic agents such as atropine or glycopyrrolate, given in conjunction with anticholinesterase inhibitors.

Sugammadex is the first of a new class of drugs called selective relaxant binding agents that are in use in Europe and undergoing final phase 3 studies

TABLE 11-3	**Drugs Used to Reverse NMBAs**
Drug	**Dosage**
First-line Drug Combination	
Neostigmine	0.05 mg/kg (not to exceed 5 mg) and atropine 0.015 mg/kg
Given via slow intravenous push	
Repeat dose not recommended	
Second-line Drug Combination	
Pyridostigmine	0.2 mg/kg and atropine 0.015 mg/kg
Given via slow intravenous push	
Repeat dose not recommended	
or	
Edrophonium	0.5 mg/kg and atropine 0.007 mg/kg
May repeat 10 min after initial dose (mixed thoroughly in same syringe)	

Data from Nissen D, editor: *2001 Mosby's GenRx*, ed 11, St Louis, 2001, Mosby.

in the United States. At this time, the release of sugammadex is awaiting approval from the US Food and Drug Administration. Sugammadex has shown to be highly effective in reversing the aminosteroid muscle relaxant rocuronium by encapsulating the unbound muscle relaxant molecules and removing them from the neuromuscular junction. In addition, sugammadex enhances the renal excretion of rocuronium.[97] Sugammadex allows for rapid reversal of rocuronium after high-dose administration when used as an alternative to succinylcholine. In theory, rocuronium administered in high doses could replace succinylcholine and sugammadex could be administered as a rescue in the "can't intubate, can't ventilate" scenario.[97] The future role of sugammadex in rapid sequence intubation requires further study.

MEDICATION-ASSISTED INTUBATION[10,12,47,52,65,66,77,80,83,95,96]

Overview

The use of neuromuscular blocking agents for endotracheal intubation was first reported in the emergency department in the early 1970s and spread widely in the 1990s. Rapid sequence intubation using muscle relaxants is now the cornerstone of emergency airway management. Some interest exists in the use of sedative medications to facilitate

intubation without the use of neuromuscular blocking agents. This process is generally described as medication-assisted intubation (MAI) or drug-assisted intubation (DAI).

Rapid sequence intubation (RSI) is effective with great success in the emergency department. A success rate over 95% is the accepted quality threshold for specialty critical care transport programs. Although MAI does avoid creating a situation in which a patient is paralyzed, and unable to be intubated, it also produces less optimal intubation conditions and less success rates than traditional RSI with neuromuscular blocking agents. The use of any MAI approach in the out-of-hospital environment must be done with the same caution, and implemented in the context of a well-supervised well-managed system that has rigorous education, monitoring, and performance improvement standards as a similar RSI program.

The use of medications to facilitate intubation is part of a process characterized by the following steps: planning, preparation, preoxygenation, premedication, paralysis after induction, placement of the endotracheal tube, and postprocedural monitoring.

Plan

The most important skill in airway management is critical thinking. The transport nurse should develop an airway management plan that includes consideration of patient history, history of present illness, current situation, and anticipated clinical course. In addition to a primary plan, there must be a backup plan in case of difficulty or failure. The backup plan is dictated by the situation, available equipment, as well as the skill of the airway specialist. Multiple intubation attempts are associated with increased likelihood of procedure-related complications. In the emergency situation, any progression past two attempts results in a significant increase in the frequency of complications: hypoxia is 5.9 times as likely, regurgitation is 11.6 times, bradycardia 13.1 times, aspiration 16.3 times, and arrest 157 times as likely.[93] Progression past three attempts offers little increased likelihood of overall procedure success.[57,93]

Individual providers should consider this in the development of their airway plans, and organizations should consider it in the development of their airway management standards.

Prepare

Before tracheal intubation is attempted, the patient should be evaluated for the likelihood of intubation difficulty. If difficult intubation is predicted, strong consideration must be given to use of an alternative approach. This consideration is particularly important if medications are going to be used to facilitate the process.

For evaluation of potential difficulty with laryngoscopy, a commonly suggested system is the LEMON Evaluation[93]:

- **L:** Look externally. Evaluate normal face and neck anatomy, face and neck pathology, face shape, sunken cheeks, protruding front teeth, and a receding mandible. Include an evaluation for a beard, which reduces the ability to get a seal for mask ventilation, and consider neck circumference. Increasing neck circumference is an independent predictor of intubation difficulty, the risk of which increases from about 5% with a 40-cm neck to 35% with a 60-cm neck.[51,52]
- **E:** Evaluate the 3-3-2 rule. Direct laryngoscopy requires the ability to line up oral,

pharyngeal, and laryngeal axes, and the 3-3-2 rule identifies patients in whom the ability to achieve that alignment is more likely to be difficult.[53] Patients should be able to place three of their own fingers between the upper and lower incisors of a fully opened mouth, three fingers along the mandible from the tip of the chin posteriorly, and two fingers from the laryngeal prominence to the floor of the mouth.
- **M:** Mallampati score. The *Mallampati score* describes the ability to see structures in the oropharynx.[54] Classically, the patient sits up, opens the mouth maximally, and protrudes the tongue maximally without phonating. In a class I airway, the soft palate, uvula, fauces, and tonsillar pillars are visible. In a class II airway, the tonsillar pillars disappear, but the soft palate, uvula, and fauces are visible. Intubation is typically not difficult in class I and class II airways. In a class III airway, only the base of the uvula and soft palate are visible; direct laryngoscopy is predicted to be moderately difficult. In a class IV airway, none of the soft palate is visible. Direct laryngoscopy is unlikely to be successful in these patients.
- **O:** Obstruction. Evaluate for potential mechanical obstruction from a foreign body, tumor, swelling, expanding hematoma, or abscess.
- **N:** Neck mobility. The neck should flex freely and the head should extend freely, so the patient can assume the classic sniffing position.

Preparation also involves gathering all necessary equipment.[85] The mnemonic ABCS may be helpful:

- **A:** Airway procedure equipment. All equipment for the primary, backup, and surgical airway should be readily accessible before the procedure begins.
- **B:** Breathing supplies. An oxygen mask, bag-valve-mask device, oral or nasal airways, and oxygen source.
- **C:** Cardiorespiratory monitors. Continuous ECG and pulse oximetry should be in place

throughout the procedure, and the immediate availability of postprocedure end-tidal carbon dioxide detection ensured.

- **S**: Suction supplies. The suction device should be assembled, tested, and turned on before the procedure begins.

Preoxygenate

Prior to receiving an induction medication, all patients must be preoxygenated. During the preoxygenation phase, nitrogen in air is exchanged for oxygen, allowing the patient to tolerate a period of apnea during intubation. The length of time to desaturation varies and is highly dependent on the patient's age, preexisting medical conditions, and body weight. Children and pregnant women desaturate quickly because their oxygen requirements on a mg/Kg basis is much greater. The obese patient has a restrictive ventilation defect that decreases the functional residual capacity, or reservoir of oxygen, which significantly decreases the time to desaturation. Preoxygenation with the head of the bed elevated is more effective, particularly in obese patients. Pre-existing pulmonary and cardiac disease also shortens desaturation times. Adequate preoxygenation is achieved by having the patient breathe 100% oxygen for 5 minutes, or taking four to eight vital capacity (the greatest volume breaths the patient can take) while receiving 100% oxygen. When possible, positive pressure ventilation should be avoided to minimize the chance of gastric insufflation and regurgitation.

Premedicate

The stimuli of direct laryngoscopy and endotracheal intubation produce a well-documented sympathetic response that increases mean arterial pressure, heart rate, and intracranial pressure. This sympathetic response may be particularly detrimental to patients with cardiovascular disease, and head injury patients. Pretreatment medications can be administered in situations where the sympathetic response to intubation must be controlled. The most commonly used pretreatment medications are lidocaine, fentanyl, atropine and nondepolarizing neuromuscular blocking agents.

The mechanism of action of lidocaine is unclear, but thought to be a combination of reflex suppression, peripheral receptor anesthesia, brainstem depression, decreased cerebral metabolism, and cell membrane stabilization. When administering lidocaine as a pretreatment, timing is important to aid in attenuating laryngoscopy effects. The optimal time between administration and laryngoscopy is 3 minutes, and the optimal dosage is generally considered 1.5 mg/Kg.

Opioids provide anesthesia and analgesia and decrease sympathetic tone. Compared with morphine, fentanyl has greater lipid solubility and causes less histamine release, which gives it a faster onset, shorter duration, and greater hemodynamic stability. Accordingly, it is preferred for use in induction. Doses of 5 mcg/kg effectively minimize the reflex sympathetic response to laryngoscopy but at an increased risk of premature apnea. More moderate doses of 2.5 to 3 mcg/kg decrease adverse effects while still blocking roughly half of the sympathetic response. Blood pressure moderation is more effective than heart rate control.

Fentanyl can cause a chest wall muscle rigidity that makes ventilation impossible. Muscle rigidity appears to be related to dose and to administration rate. The likelihood of chest wall rigidity is rare in doses of 5 mcg/kg or less in adults, but the risk, even at traditional doses, is real in neonatal and pediatric patients.

Atropine is used to counterbalance the cholinergic effects of succinylcholine, which can produce significant bradycardia especially in children, young adults, and in patients given a repeat dose of succinylcholine. Any child who is to receive succinylcholine should receive pretreatment with atropine due to the pronounced vagal effect from airway manipulation that occurs in this age group, combined with cholinergic effects of succinylcholine. Atropine also decreases oral secretions, which can be a benefit to the intubation specialist. The dose is 0.01 to 0.02 mg/Kg in children, to a maximum of the adult dose of 0.5 mg.

Muscle fasciculations occur from the administration of succinylcholine and are associated with a significant increase in intracranial pressure, as well as several less clinically significant side effects that include intraocular pressure increases, and increased intragastric pressure. Succinylcholine stimulates the nicotinic acetylcholine receptors in skeletal muscle producing generalized involuntary muscle fiber contractions. In head injury patients the rise in intracranial pressure associated with succinylcholine can be attenuated completely with pretreatment with a nondepolarizing muscle relaxant such as vecuronium or rocuronium. Administering a defasciculating dose of vecuronium or rocuronium is accomplished by giving 0.01 mg/Kg of vecuronium or 0.06 mg/Kg of rocuronium about 3 minutes prior to the administration of succinylcholine.

When administering a defasciculating dose of a nondepolarizing muscle relaxant the patient must be observed for muscle weakness, followed at times by apnea, which occurs during preoxygenation prior to administration of succinylcholine. This is particularly frightening to an awake or non-sedated patient. The intubation specialist must intervene to support ventilations.

Induction and Paralysis

Induction agents are given to render the patient unconscious during intubation. It is advisable to administer an induction agent to all patients, event those with apparent unconsciousness, unless the patient is in full arrest. Common induction agents in use today are etomidate, propofol, thiopental, and ketamine.

Etomidate is a barbiturate-like derivative without the adverse effects of the barbiturates. It acts rapidly, producing hypnosis in less than 30 seconds at a dose of 0.3 mg/Kg and recovery is prompt. Cardiovascular stability is characteristic of patients receiving etomidate, with little or no decreases in mean arterial pressure in normovolemic patients and in patients with limited cardiac reserve. Blood pressure changes are more likely to occur in hypovolemic patients. Etomidate decreases cerebral blood flow, cerebral metabolic oxygen demand, and intracranial pressure. Etomidate does not suppress the sympathetic response to laryngoscopy.[83]

Disadvantages of etomidate administration include pain during injection, involuntary skeletal muscle movements, and adrenocortical suppression. During this time the adrenal cortex is not responsive to adrenocorticotrophic hormone. This may be det-

rimental to patients on long-term steroid replacement therapy, or other forms of adrenal suppression, or patients in septic shock.

Propofol is a lipid soluble induction agent that combines rapid onset with rapid awakening. Unconsciousness and excellent amnesia occur within 30 seconds following a dose of 2-2.5 mg/Kg. The awakening from propofol is more rapid and complete than any other induction agent. Propofol however, is a significant cardiovascular depressant resulting in decreases in mean arterial pressure as well as cerebral perfusion pressure. These decreases are more exaggerated in the hypovolemic patient making propofol a less than optimal choice in trauma patient requiring RSI.

Thiopental is a short acting barbiturate, which depresses the reticular activating system or the "wakefulness" center of the brain. Barbiturates (including thiopental) also selectively decrease transmission of impulses through sympathetic nervous system ganglia, which likely contributes to the decrease in mean arterial pressure seen following an injection of thiopental. The blood pressure decreases are often attenuated by a baroreceptor-mediated increase in heart rate. Hypovolemic patients are less likely to compensate and are more likely to experience an exaggerated decrease in blood pressure related to thiopental. The advantage of thiopental and other barbiturates (except methohexital) is their cerebral protection properties. Thiopental is a potent cerebral vasoconstrictor, which produces decreases in cerebral blood flow, cerebral blood volume, cerebral metabolic oxygen demand, and intracranial pressure. The recommended dose of thiopental is 3-5 mg/Kg. Because thiopental releases histamine, it should be used with caution in patients with reactive airway disease. Accidental subcutaneous injection or extravasation of thiopental results in significant local tissue irritation. Since the introduction of etomidate, with its stable cardiovascular profile, thiopental and other barbiturates are used infrequently for RSI.

Ketamine is a phencyclidine (PCP) derivative that produces dissociative anesthesia. Induction in 60 seconds is achieved following a dose of 1-2 mg/Kg IV or within 2-4 minutes following an intramuscular dose of 5-10 mg/Kg. Anesthesia and analgesia come from dissociation between the thalamus and limbic system. Patients appear to be in cataleptic states in which the eyes remain open with a slow nystagmic gaze. Ketamine is unique among induction agents, in that it is the only induction agent that provides amnesia and analgesia. Skeletal muscle tone remains intact, which helps to maintain a patent upper airway however, the presence of protective upper airway reflexes should vomiting or regurgitation occur cannot be assumed. Ketamine increases sympathetic tone and produces potent cerebral vasodilation and cardiovascular stimulation from the direct stimulation of sympathetic nervous system outflow. Ketamine induced cardiac stimulation may adversely increase myocardial oxygen demands in patients with ischemic heart disease, and predictably increases ICP in head injured patients. Airway secretions are increased by ketamine and may precipitate laryngospasm, which can be attenuated with the use of an anticholinergic agent, such as atropine, as a premedication. Ideally, ketamine is useful for induction of patients who are hypotensive and hypovolemic but do not have an associated head injury with potential for increased ICP. Awakening from ketamine anesthesia may be associated with unpleasant visual, auditory, and proprioceptive illusions that may progress to delirium. Administration of benzodiazepines can decrease the incidence of emergence reactions associated with ketamine.

MONITORING AIRWAY MANAGEMENT AND VENTILATION DURING TRANSPORT

Evaluation of airway interventions occurs under less than optimal conditions during transport. Transport vehicles may be noisy and dimly lit. Traditional auscultation is extremely difficult, and poor vehicle lighting may interfere with the normal visual cues of assessment. Parameters used for evaluation include the level of consciousness, stability of vital signs, observation of the patient's color, and symmetric rise and fall of the chest wall. Several pieces of equipment may assist with evaluation and provide objective data. A more in-depth discussion about ventilation management during transport is contained in Chapter 12.[48]

END-TIDAL CARBON DIOXIDE DETECTION

End-tidal CO_2 detection is the most accurate and easily available method to monitor correct endotracheal tube position in patients who have adequate tissue perfusion. The disposable end-tidal CO_2 detector Easy Cap (Figure 11-20) assists proper ETT placement by incorporating a nontoxic pH-sensitive chemically treated indicator that changes color in the presence of carbon dioxide. When the indicator is removed from the sealed package, it is purple. After applying the monitor to an endotracheal tube and providing ventilations, the monitor either stays purple, which indicates no CO_2; changes to yellow, which indicates CO_2 concentrations greater than 2%; or becomes beige, which represents an intermediate concentration between 0.5% and 1.0%. A beige color usually represents a state of hypoperfusion that can occur in patients in cardiac arrest. False-negative results (color remains purple despite correct tracheal placement) can occur during cardiac arrest, severe airway obstruction, and pulmonary edema and in severely hypocarbic infants.

In low perfusion states, such as occur in cardiac arrest, the colorimetric end-tidal CO_2 can produce a detectable color change. In a study of 566 prehospital intubations of patients in cardiac arrest, a color change occurred in 95.6%, with only one

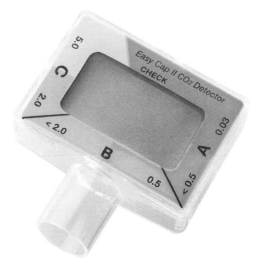

FIGURE 11-20   **Easy Cap end-tidal CO_2 detector.** (Courtesy Nellcor Puritan Bennett, Inc, Pleasonton, Calif.)

false-positive result.[24-26,50] In addition to verification of endotracheal placement after intubation, the Easy Cap device can also be used to monitor tube placement during transport. The device can reliably function for up to 2 hours and is not affected by environmental temperature extremes. If the indicator becomes contaminated with pulmonary secretions or comes in contact with medications administered through the ETT, the indicator no longer functions. The device may be removed from the ETT after administration of medications given through the ETT for at least six breaths, or until fluids are no longer visible, and then replaced with no loss of function. Pedi-Cap (Figure 11-21), a new smaller detector, is now available and is designed for neonates and children who weigh up to 15 kg. The adult model is not recommended in patients who weigh less than 15 kg because of the increased dead space of the device.

Capnography

Capnography is the measurement of end-tidal CO_2 volumes with each breath with use of infrared light absorption via placement of a sensor between the breathing circuit and the ETT. The instrument works by emitting an infrared light beam through a sensor located immediately distal to the ETT. As carbon dioxide is exhaled, the CO_2 molecules

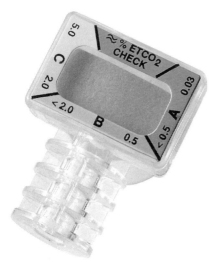

FIGURE 11-21   **Pedi-Cap pediatric end-tidal CO_2 detector.** (Courtesy Nellcor Puritan Bennett, Inc, Pleasonton, Calif.)

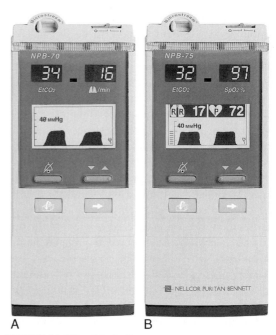

A   B

FIGURE 11-22   **CO_2 indicators. A,** NPB-70 handheld capnograph. **B,** NPB-75 combination handheld capnograph and pulse oximeter. (Courtesy Nellcor Puritan Bennett, Inc, Pleasonton, Calif.)

absorb the infrared light. The instrument then measures how much light was absorbed, thereby determining the concentration of CO_2. The data are then displayed in digital or waveform or both. Figure 11-22 shows two such instruments. The graphic waveform, called a capnogram, displays levels of CO_2 over time. Capnometry is the measurement of expired CO_2 and provides a numeric display of the CO_2 tension in torr (mm Hg) or CO_2. Normal end-tidal CO_2 volume is a close indicator of the arterial pressure of carbon dioxide, and the difference between these two parameters, known as the CO_2 gradient ($P\{a\text{-}ET\}CO_2$), has been reported to be less than 6 mm Hg in healthy patients.[24-26,33]

Capnography technology has been in use during the last decade in the operating room for assessment of the respiratory status of patients during surgery, for detection of hyperventilation or hypoventilation, and for detection of equipment problems. The value of capnography to the transport team is its ability to confirm proper ETT placement, to indicate situations in which the ETT has become displaced, and to detect disruption of the ventilator circuit.

Monitors that provide continuous waveforms can also assist the transport team in evaluating the clinical status of the patient. A sudden decrease in CO_2 to zero with no waveform indicates a dislodged endotracheal tube, a kinked or obstructed endotracheal tube, or a ventilator disconnect. An incremental decrease in CO_2 may indicate sudden and severe hypotension or cardiac arrest. An incremental increase in CO_2 can indicate hypoventilation or a partial endotracheal obstruction and can occur with sodium bicarbonate administration or rising body temperature. However, as with any piece of equipment, caution should be exercised when capnography is used to ensure the clinical picture matches the readings. Carbon dioxide present in the exhaled gas indicates that alveolar ventilation has transpired but does not necessarily mean that the ETT is in the trachea. A tube positioned in the pharynx also provides normal readings.

Continuous capnography has been used during blind nasotracheal intubation in spontaneously breathing patients. The posterior displacement of the tip of the tube to the larynx was recognized promptly with the use of continuous capnography. Likewise, when the tube was repositioned for entry into the trachea, the capnograph monitor displayed the presence of CO_2.

Recent advances in technology have allowed smaller more durable instruments for prehospital use. Although currently no national standard dictates the use of capnography during critical care transport, many transport programs use some type of monitoring during transport.

PULSE OXIMETRY

In the emergency department or critical care unit, healthcare providers rely on arterial blood gases or, more specifically, the partial pressure of oxygen tension (PaO_2) drawn on an intermittent basis to guide therapy. Pulse oximetry provides a reliable and continuous evaluation of oxygenation.

Oxygen in the blood is dissolved in the plasma or is bound to hemoglobin. The oxygen dissolved in the plasma is referred to as the partial pressure of oxygen (PO_2). The normal value of oxygen dissolved in the arterial blood (PaO_2) is measured in millimeters of mercury or torr. In children and adults, this value ranges from 80 to 100 mm Hg, with higher values expected in the pediatric population. The PO_2 accounts for 1% to 2% of the total oxygen content.

The portion of oxygen bound to hemoglobin is referred to as oxygen saturation (SO_2). In arterial blood, the normal value of oxygen saturation (SaO_2) ranges from 95% to 97.5%. The SO_2 accounts for 98% or more of the total oxygen content.

The relationship between the PaO_2 and SaO_2 is displayed in Figure 11-23, the oxyhemoglobin dissociation curve.[43] If one value is known, the other can be estimated. The relationship is not a linear one. The upper portion of the curve shows a compensatory mechanism of the body; in a healthy adult, more oxygen than necessary is carried. A drop in the PaO_2 from 100 to 80 mm Hg shows a minimal change in the SaO_2. The steep portion of the curve shows a rapid decline in SaO_2 with small decreases in PaO_2. When the SaO_2 falls to less than 90%, a rapid decline is seen in the oxygen content.

Pulse oximetry continuously monitors the SaO_2 value. A sensor device is placed across a pulsating arteriolar bed, such as the toe, nose, or finger. Figure 11-24 illustrates two types of pulse oximeters. The sensor houses a light source and photo detector device. The pulse oximeter processes the light

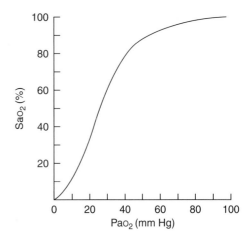

FIGURE 11-23 **Oxyhemoglobin dissociation curve.**

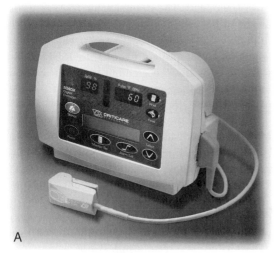

A

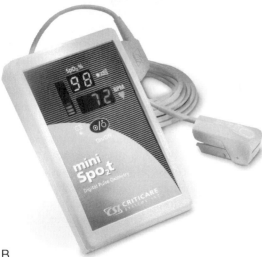

B

FIGURE 11-24   **Pulse oximeters. A,** 504DX portable pulse oximeter. **B,** 503DX miniSpO$_2$t handheld oximeter. (Courtesy Criticare Systems, Inc.)

absorption to determine SaO$_2$ values. The successful use of an oximetry device is dependent on proper placement of the sensor device. It should be positioned such that the light source and photo detector are in direct alignment. The patient's skin at the placement site should be clean and dry. The ability to obtain a pulse at the site of placement is also important. The accuracy of pulse oximetry may be affected by clinical conditions, such as hypotension or hypothermia, or during vasopressor therapy as a result of vasoconstriction.

The value of pulse oximetry to the transport team lies in its ability to act as an early warning system. A low SaO$_2$ value is detected much earlier than with clinical observation, permitting expeditious and aggressive interventions. Continuous pulse oximetry monitoring improves the recognition and management of hypoxemia during emergency endotracheal intubation, and during critical care transport, it offers visual reassurance to the team that airway management is having its intended effect. Pulse oximetry is valuable in the continuous monitoring of patients with unstable conditions; however, it is not a measure of ventilation.[61] If oxygen saturation measured with pulse oximetry suddenly changes, a repeat airway assessment should be performed to determine the cause and corrective action should be taken.

Pulse oximetry has also been found to be useful in determination of systolic blood pressure in the air medical setting with application of an appropriately sized blood pressure cuff on the same arm as the pulse oximetry probe. The cuff is inflated until the palatial display on the pulse oximeter is obliterated. The manometer reading at the point of obliteration is recorded as the systolic blood pressure.[61]

ESOPHAGEAL INTUBATION DETECTION[14,42,86,100]

Assessment of ETT placement is a routine maneuver after intubation. The potentially catastrophic consequences of an undetected esophageal intubation stress the importance of the ability to recognize and correct the situation should it occur. Observations such as chest movement, breath sounds, epigastric auscultation and observation, reservoir bag compliance, and tube condensation are some of the more commonly prescribed methods of tube position assessment. However, each of these methods at times may prove inaccurate.

The detection of CO$_2$ with capnometry or colorimetric devices is considered the gold standard for detection of tracheal intubation. However, in situations in which pulmonary blood flow is reduced, such as cardiac arrest, detection of end-tidal with such devices becomes problematic. The negative pressure test, with a specially designed syringe or a self-inflating bulb, is helpful in determination of endotracheal tube position. The detector consists of: 1, a 60-mL syringe fitted with a standard 15-mm ETT adaptor on the end of the syringe; or 2, a 75-mL self-inflating bulb with a standard 15-mm ETT adaptor. After intubation, either device is connected to the ETT, and the plunger is pulled back, in the case of the syringe, or the self-inflating bulb is compressed and then attached to the end of the ETT. Because of the rigid support provided by the cartilaginous rings, when the plunger of the syringe is pulled back, air is aspirated without resistance if the ETT is placed in the trachea. The easy aspiration of approximately 20 mL of air is a positive result for tracheal intubation. If resistance or negative pressure is encountered when the plunger is pulled back, the esophagus has been intubated. Likewise, if the compressed bulb reinflates, the ETT is assumed to be in the trachea. Inability to aspirate or aspiration that takes longer than 30 seconds is indicative of esophageal intubation; and if the bulb fails to self inflate, again, this indicates an esophageal intubation. The esophagus readily collapses when a negative pressure is applied because, unlike the trachea, it has no cartilaginous support. Initial studies done in the controlled environment of the OR or in animal studies concluded the device was near perfect at proper identification of ETT position. However, in follow-up studies, the device has shown to yield a 1% to 2% false-negative rate for tracheal intubation, although false-positive results for tracheal intubation appear to be extremely rare. Recent studies suggest that esophageal detection device failures are not uncommon and that these detectors be used in conjunction with other methods of detection, including end-tidal CO_2 and clinical assessment.

SUMMARY

Assessment and management of the patient's airway is the primary role of the transport team. Knowledge of when and how to perform basic and advanced airway management is critical in the transport environment. Good clinical judgment, skill, and familiarity with the pharmacology of airway management are necessary so that patients receive competent care and complications that can occur in the care of the critically ill or injured patient are prevented.

AIRWAY MANAGEMENT AND VENTILATION CASE STUDY

The transport team of a major regional trauma center was called by the local fire and EMS service of a small town 40 miles away for a motorcycle accident that involved two people. In 5 minutes, the BK-117 with a flight nurse and paramedic were en route for the 20-minute flight. The accident happened near the center of the small community within two blocks of the fire department, which was holding its monthly staff meeting when the call was received. On landing, the transport team was immediately met by the incident commander who told them that two motorcyclists without helmets were traveling an estimated 30 mph through an intersection when they were struck, T-bone fashion, by a pickup truck. The driver of the pickup was only slightly injured and refused treatment. The flight team was further told that a middle-aged man was the operator of the motorcycle and riding with him was a 20-year-old man recognized by EMS providers. They reported the young passenger had Down syndrome and many times had needed transport for a seizure disorder. The team was first directed to the middle-aged man. The initial assessment revealed the following information:

AIRWAY

The patient was awake, confused, and combative. He was lying supine on a backboard with a cervical collar in place. Oxygen was applied per nonrebreather mask, but he was attempting to remove it. No blood, vomitus, or other foreign material was obstructing the airway.

BREATHING

Respiratory rate was 28 bpm with bilateral equal chest expansion noted. The chest was palpated and found to have no subcutaneous air or crepitus.

CIRCULATION

Skin was pale, warm, and dry with 2+ radial pulses bilaterally. Capillary refill was 3 seconds.

DEFICITS

Movement was noted in all extremities. Pupils were midrange, round, and reactive bilaterally. The patient was screaming and was being physically restrained by numerous EMS personnel. He did not follow commands, and his speech was at times garbled. Upper extremity restraints were in place and secured to the back board. Glasgow Coma Scale (GCS) was 11 (E3, V3, M5).

EXTREMITIES

No upper extremity fractures were noted; however, he had an obvious open distal tibia-fibula fracture on the right. His pelvis appeared stable.

The transport team discussed options. Concern was found for the patient's mental status, and his uncooperative behavior presented a safety risk in flight. They decided to intubate the patient per RSI protocol. An intravenous line was started; the patient was preoxygenated and received lidocaine, an induction agent, and succinylcholine; and he was successfully intubated on the first attempt. The ETT was secured, and the patient then received a nondepolarizing paralytic agent and narcotic analgesic. While one team member finished up, the second team member went to evaluate the other victim.

The second victim, a 20-year-old man with Down syndrome, was lying supine on the pavement. No C-collar was in place, and the patient was being manually ventilated by two rescuers with an ambu bag. The emergency medical technician (EMT) in charge reported that the patient was found lying on his side in a head–chest position and was not breathing. His color was blue, and his pulse was slow and bounding. He was turned on his back, and bag-mask ventilations were started. One person was holding the mask, and another was squeezing the ambu bag. Numerous attempts to start an IV line were unsuccessful. The primary examination results were as follows:

AIRWAY

The airway was difficult to evaluate. The tongue was large, and it obstructed the view of the mouth. No obvious blood, vomitus, or foreign material was found in the mouth. The flight nurse inserted an oral airway, which immediately improved ventilatory exchange.

BREATHING

The patient had no spontaneous effort, and no subcutaneous air of crepitus was noted. Notable contusions were seen to the right anterior hemithorax. Adequate chest excursion seemed to exist with manual ventilations.

CIRCULATION

Color was ashen with slow bounding radial pulses bilaterally.

DEFICIT

No eye opening and no movement to pain on the left or right side was seen. The pupils were large, round, and minimally reactive. GCS was 3 (E1, V1, M1).

EXTREMITIES

Numerous abrasions and contusions were found but no obvious long bone fractures.

The transport team member was joined by the other, who was now finished packaging the first patient. The second patient also needed intubation, but IV access had still not been established. One team member attempted to start an IV line, while the other took over bag-mask ventilations. Despite multiple attempts, an IV line could not be established. The decision was made to attempt oral intubation. A cardiac and pulse oximeter were established. The heart rate was 68, and the pulse oximeter was 92%. The first attempt at intubation was made with a no. 4 MacIntosh blade, but the attempt was quickly abandoned because of the large tongue. A second and third attempt was made with a smaller no. 3 curved blade without success. Cricoid pressure with the BURP method was applied throughout each attempt. A decision was made that the second team member would attempt intubation. He chose to use a straight blade and on each attempt (3) was unsuccessful. He was unable to visualize any structures beyond the tongue. Between attempts, the oximetry reading dropped to the mid 80s. At this time, the flight crew elected to attempt intubation with their rescue device, the intubating laryngeal mask airway (ILMA or Fastrach). A no. 3-size ILMA was inserted into the mouth with the laryngeal surface down and pressed onto the hard palate. The device was advanced over the back of the tongue following the natural curvature of the oropharynx and hypopharynx to where it was seated over the larynx. The cuff was filled with approximately 20 mL of air. The patient was again ventilated, this time with the ILMA. In a few minutes, the saturations improved to 100%. Next, the silicone-tipped armored ETT was lubricated and inserted into the metal tube of the ILMA until the horizontal black line on the ETT was at the proximal entrance to the ILMA. Resistance was felt as the ETT advanced through the distal end of the ILMA. The metal handle was withdrawn slightly, and the ETT advanced without difficulty. The balloon of the ETT was inflated, and position was confirmed with a disposable end-tidal CO_2 detector. The ILMA cuff was then deflated and withdrawn over the ETT. The patient was quickly immobilized on a backboard; rolled towels were used to secure the head in neutral position. Both patients were loaded in the aircraft. While in flight, patient number one, the middle-aged man, remained hemodynamically stable with an oxygen saturation of 100%. Patient number two was hypotensive with a blood pressure of 80 mm Hg and a pulse of 60 to 70. His oxygen saturation remained 98% to 100% with significant improvement in color from the initial evaluation.

Patient number one's evaluation revealed a cerebral contusion and an open distal tibia-fibula fracture. He was taken to surgery for open reduction and internal fixation of the orthopedic injury and then admitted to the neurologic unit where he remained for 48 hours. At that time, he was extubated and moved to a regular floor. Four days later, he was discharged home with full neurologic recovery.

Patient number two was the son of patient one's girlfriend. The older man often gave the younger man rides on his motorcycle. The patient was found to have an atlantooccipital dislocation and a severe anoxic injury. He too was admitted to the neurologic intensive care unit (ICU) where, consistent with the family's wishes, he was removed from life support 36 hours after injury and died.

DISCUSSION

The transport team was faced a number of difficult patient management issues that were successfully negotiated. With a GCS of 11, the motorcycle operator needed intubation to facilitate safe transport more so than treatment of the neurologic compromise. The patient with Down syndrome displayed the usual airway characteristics of the abnormality. These include a short neck, irregular dentition, and a large tongue, which made the airway difficult to manage. In addition, he had a known seizure disorder. The congenital laxity of the ligaments of the neck most likely contributed to the atlantooccipital dislocation, and had the initial responders been delayed another minute, the patient would not have likely survived to be transported from the scene. The transport crew made several important decisions in caring for this patient. First, a properly sized oral airway is important as first-line management of a difficult airway. Secondly, after each intubation attempt, the patient was reoxygenated and ventilated. At the same time, the situation was reassessed and the team changed something. In this example, the size and type of laryngoscope blade was changed. After a failed intubation, good practice is to change something to improve the chances for success on the following attempt. The flight team also recognized that this was a "can't intubate, but can oxygenate" situation. Available options in this situation included lighted stylet intubation, retrograde intubation, digital intubation, the intubating laryngeal mask airway, and the esophageal tracheal combitube. The flight team recognized that because of the patient's short neck, a cricothyrotomy would have been extremely difficult and therefore chose to use the intubating laryngeal *mask airway (ILMA or Fastrach). This particular design differs from the original LMA in that the ILMA or Fastrach allows for the blind introduction of an ETT through it. The classic LMA does not constitute definitive airway management. The classic LMA does not protect against airway aspiration, ventilation pressures greater than 20 to 25 cm can dislodge the LMA, and the device is difficult to secure during patient transport. Patients must be significantly obtunded to allow insertion of the ILMA or the classic LMA. The combitube may actually be a better rescue device than the classic LMA because it allows for gastric decompression and aspiration of gastric contents by passing a suction catheter through the clear connecting tube into the stomach. In addition, it is more stable and less likely to become dislodged during transport. This case study underscores the importance of good airway skills and proper equipment, combined with sound judgment gained through practice and experience, in managing a difficult airway situation.*

REFERENCES

1. American College of Emergency Physicians: Drug assisted intubation in the prehospital setting, *Ann Emerg Med* 46(2):214, 2005.

2. American Heart Association: *2005 American Heart Association (AHA) guidelines for cardiopulmonary resuscitation (CPR) and emergency cardiovascular care,* Dallas, 2006, AHA.

3. Ardagh M, Moodie K: The esophageal detector device can give false positives for tracheal intubation, *J Emerg Med* 16(5):747-749, 1998.

4. Agro F, Barzoi G, Montecchia F: Tracheal intubation using a Macintosh laryngoscope or a glidescope in 15 patients with cervical spine immobilization, *Br J Anaesth* 90(5):705-706, 2003.

5. Asai T, Shingu K: The laryngeal tube, *Br J Anaesth* 95(6):729-736, 2005.

6. Bair A, Laurin E, Schmitt BJ: An assessment of a tracheal tube introducer as an endotracheal tube placement confirmation device, *Am J Emerg Med* 23(6):754-758, 2005.

7. Bhende MS, LaCovey C: End-tidal carbon dioxide monitoring in the prehospital setting, *Prehosp Emerg Care* 5(2):208-213, 2001.

8. Bowers R, Weaver JD: Compromised airway. In Stone K, et al, editors: *Current diagnosis and treatment: emergency medicine,* ed 6, New York, 2008, McGraw Hill.

9. Bracelet BT, Osborn ML, Sakles JC, et al: Evaluation of the rapid four-step cricothyrotomy technique: an interim report, *Air Med J* 17(3):127-130, 1998.

10. Brandom BW, Fine F: Neuromuscular blocking drugs in pediatric anesthesia, *Anesth Clin North Am* 20(1):45-58, 2002.

11. Brimacombe J: Analysis of 1500 laryngeal mask uses by one anaesthetist in adults undergoing routine anaesthesia, *Anaesthesia* 51(1):76-80, 1996.

12. Bowman WC: Neuromuscular block, *Br J Pharmacol* 147(Suppl 1):S277-S286, 2006.

13. Butler B, Little T, Drtil S: Combined use of the esophageal-tracheal Combitube with a colorimetric carbon dioxide detector for emergency intubation/ventilation, *J Clin Monitoring* 11(5):311-316, 1995.

14. Chew G, Vilke G, Davis D, et al: Toomey syringe aspiration may be inaccurate in detecting esophageal intubation after gastric insufflation, *J Emerg Med* 23(4):337-340, 2002.

15. Chidiac EJ, Raiskin O: Succinylcholine and the open eye, *Ophthalmol Clin North Am* 19(2):279-285, 2006.

16. Choyce A, Avidan MS, Patel C, et al: Comparison of laryngeal mask and intubating laryngeal mask insertion by the naïve intubatior, *Br J Anesth* 84:103-105, 2000.

17. Clements R, Steel A, Bates A, et al: Cuffed endotracheal tube use in paediatric prehospital intubation: challenging the doctrine? *Emerg Med J* 24(1):57-58, 2007.

18. Combes X, Soupizet F, Jabre P, et al: Out of hospital difficult intubation resolved with nasotracheal use of a gum elastic bougie, *Emerg Med J* 23(8):e46, 2006.

19. Cook RTJ, Stene J, Marcolina BJ: Use of a Beck Airway Airflow Monitor and controllable-tip endotracheal tube in two cases of nonlaryngoscopic oral intubation, *Am J Emerg Med* 13(2):180-183, 1995.

20. Cook TM, Hommers C: New airway for resuscitation? *Resuscitation* 69:371-387, 2006.

21. Cooper RM: Complications associated with the use of the glidescope videolaryngoscope, *Ca J Anaesth* 54(1):54-57, 2007.

22. Cormack RS, Lehane J: Difficult tracheal intubation in obstetrics, *Anesthesia* 39:1105-1111, 1984.

23. Danzl D, Vissers RJ: Tracheal intubation and mechanical ventilation: introduction. In Tintinalli J, et al, editors: *Tintinalli's emergency medicine: a comprehensive study guide,* ed 6, New York, 2004, McGraw-Hill.

24. Davis DP: Quantitative capnometry as a critical resuscitation tool, *J Trauma Nurs* 12(2):40-42, 2005.

25. Davis D, Dunford J, Ochs M, et al: The use of quantitative end-tidal capnometry to avoid inadvertent severe hyperventilation in patients with head injury after paramedic rapid sequence intubation, *J Trauma* 56(4):808-814, 2004.

26. Davis D, Dunford J, Ochs M, et al: The use of quantitative end-tidal capnometry to avoid inadvertent severe hyperventilation in patients with head injury after paramedic rapid sequence intubation, *J Trauma* 56(4):808-814, 2004.

27. Davis D, Bramwell K, Vilke G, et al: Cricothyrotomy technique: standard versus the Rapid Four-Step Technique, *J Emerg Med* 17(1):17-21, 1999.

28. Davis L, Cook-Sather S, Schreiner MS: Lighted stylet tracheal intubation: a review, *Anesth Analg* 90(3): 745-756, 2000.

29. Deboer S, Seaver M, Broselow J: Color coding to reduce errors, *Am J Nurs* 105(8):68-71, 2005.

30. Ellis D, Harris T, Zideman D: Cricoid pressure in emergency department rapid sequence tracheal intubations: a risk-benefit analysis, *Ann Emerg Med* 50(6):653-665, 2007.

31. Falk JL, Sayre R: Confirmation of airway placement, *Prehosp Emerg Care* 3(4):273-278, 1999.

32. Fine GF, Borland M: The future of the cuffed endotracheal tube, *Paediatr Anaesth* 14(1):38-42, 2004.

33. Frakes MA: Transport. In Gravenstein J, Jaffe M, Paulus E, editors: *Capnography: clinical aspects*, Cambridge, 2004, UK Press.

34. Frass M, Staudinger T, Losert H, et al: Airway management during cardiopulmonary resuscitation: a comparative study of bag-valve-mask, laryngeal mask airway and Combitube in a bench model, *Resuscitation* 43(1):80-81, 1999.

35. Gabbott DA, Beringer R: The iGEL supraglottic airway: a potential role for resuscitation? *Resuscitation* 73(1):161-162, 2007.

36. Gausche M, Lewis R, Stratton S, et al: Effect of out-of-hospital pediatric endotracheal intubation on survival and neurological outcome: a controlled clinical trial, *JAMA* 283(6):783-790, 2000.

37. Gilligan BP, Luten RC: Pediatric resuscitation. In Marx J, Hockberger R, Walls R, editors: *Rosen's emergency medicine: concepts and clinical practice*, ed 6, St Louis, 2006, Mosby.

38. Guidelines for the management of severe traumatic brain injury: XIV: hyperventilation, *J Neurotrauma* 24(Suppl 1):S87-S90, 2007.

39. Guyette F, Wang H, Cole JS: King airway use by air medical providers, *Prehosp Emerg Care* 11(4): 473-476, 2007.

40. Hayden S, Sciammarella J, Viccellio P, et al: Colorimetric end-tidal CO_2 detector for verification of endotracheal tube placement in out-of-hospital cardiac arrest, *Acad Emerg Med* 2(6):499-502, 1995.

41. Henderson JJ: Development of the 'gum-elastic bougie', *Anaesthesia* 58(1):103-104, 2003.

42. Hendey G, Shubert G, Shalit M, et al: The esophageal detector bulb in the aeromedical setting, *J Emerg Med* 23(1):51-55, 2002.

43. Hicks GH: Blood gas and acid-base management. In Dantzer D, et al, editors: *Comprehensive respiratory care*, ed 5, Philadelphia, 1995, Saunders.

44. Holmes J, Panacek E, Sakles J, et al: Comparison of 2 cricothyrotomy techniques: standard method versus rapid 4-step technique, *Ann Emerg Med* 32(4):442-446, 1998.

45. Jabre P, Combes X, Leroux B, et al: Use of gum elastic bougie for prehospital difficult intubation, *Am J Emerg Med* 23(4):552-555, 2005.

46. James I: Cuffed tubes in children, *Paediatr Anaesth* 11(3):259-263, 2001.

47. Jeevendra MJ, Richtsfeld M: Succinylcholine-induced hyperkalemia in acquired pathologic states, *Anesthesiology* 104:158-169, 2006.

48. Johannigman J: Prehospital respiratory care. In Dantzer D, et al, editors: *Comprehensive respiratory care*, ed 5, Philadelphia, 1995, Saunders.

49. Kaplan MB, Hagberg CA, Ward DS, et al: Comparison of direct and video-assisted views of the larynx during routine intubation, *J Clin Anesth* 18(5):357-362, 2006.

50. Katz SH, Falk JL: Misplaced endotracheal tubes by paramedics in an urban emergency medical services system, *Ann Emerg Med* 37(1):32-37, 2001.

51. Krishel S, Jackimczyk K, Balazs K: Endotracheal tube whistle: an adjunct to blind nasotracheal intubation, *Ann Emerg Med* 21(1):33-36, 1992.

52. Laurin E, Sakles J, Panacek E, et al: A comparison of succinylcholine and rocuronium for rapid-sequence intubation of emergency department patients, *Acad Emerg Med* 7(12):1362-1369, 2000.

53. Levitan RM, Kinkle C: Initial anatomic investigations of the I-gel airway: a novel supraglottic airway without inflatable cuff, *Anaesthesia* 60(10):1022-1026, 2005.

54. Lim Y, Yeo W: A comparison of the glidescope with the Macintosh laryngoscope for tracheal intubation in patients with simulated difficult airway, *Anaesth Intensive Care* 33(2):243-247, 2005.

55. Liu E, Goy R, Lim Y, et al: Success of tracheal intubation with intubating laryngeal mask airways: a randomized trial of the LMA Fastrach and LMA ctrach, *Anesthesiology* 108(4):621-626, 2008.

56. Liu EH, Goy L: The LMA Ctrach for unanticipated difficult intubation, *Anaesthesia* 61(10):1015, 2006.

57. Lowe L, Sagehorn K, Madsen R: The effect of a rapid sequence induction protocol on intubation success rate in an air medical program, *Air Med J* 17(3): 101-104, 1998.

58. Marlow T, Goltra DDJ, Schabel SI: Intracranial placement of a nasotracheal tube after facial fracture: a rare complication, *J Emerg Med* 15(2):187-191, 1997.

59. McGill J: Airway management in trauma: an update, *Emerg Med Clin North Am* 25(3):2007.

60. Miller D, Youkhana I, Pearce AC: The laryngeal mask and VBM laryngeal tube compared during spontaneous ventilation: a pilot study, *Eur J Anaesthesiol* 18(9):593-598, 2001.

61. Mohler J, Hart C: Use of a pulse oximeter for determination of systolic blood pressure in a helicopter air ambulance, *Air Med J* 13(11-12):479-482, 1994.

62. Moura JHS, da Silva P: Neonatal laryngoscope intubation and the digital method: a randomized controlled trial, *J Pediatr* 148(6):840-841, 2006.

63. Murphy MF, Walls RM: Identification of the difficult airway. In Walls RM, et al, editors: *Manual of emergency airway management*, Philadelphia, 2004, Lippincott William & Wilkins.

64. Newth CJ, Rachman B, Patel N, et al: The use of cuffed versus uncuffed endotracheal tubes in pediatric intensive care, *J Pediatr* 144(3):333-337, 2004.

65. Orhrocj EA, Hollander JE, Kush S, et al: Assessment of laryngeal view: percentage of glottis opening score vs. Cormack and Lehane grading, *Can J Anesth* 46(10):987-990, 1999.

66. Orebaugh SL: Succinylcholine: adverse effects and alternatives in emergency medicine, *Am J Emerg Med* 17(7):715-721, 1999.

67. Phelan MP: Use of the endotracheal bougie introducer for difficult intubations, *Am J Emerg Med* 22(6):479-482, 2004.

68. Phelan M, Moscati R, D'Aprix T, et al: Paramedic use of the endotracheal tube introducer in a difficult airway model, *Prehosp Emerg Care* 7(2):244-246, 2003.

69. Rich J, Mason A, Bey T, et al: The critical airway, rescue ventilation, and the combitube: part 1, *AANA J* 72(1):17-27, 2004.

70. Rich J, Mason A, Bey T, et al: The critical airway, rescue ventilation, and the combitube: part 2, *AANA J* 72(2):115-124, 2004.

71. Rich JA: editor: *Street level airway management*, Saddle River, 2007, Prentice Hall.

72. Robinson N, Clancy M: In patients with head injury undergoing rapid sequence intubation, does pretreatment with intravenous lignocaine/lidocaine lead to an improved neurological outcome? A review of the literature, *Emerg Med J* 18(6):453-457, 2001.

73. Roppolo LP, Vilke GM, Chan TC, et al: Nasotracheal intubation in the emergency department, revisited, *J Emerg Med* 17(5):791-799, 1999.

74. Rosenberg H, Davis M, James D, et al: Malignant hyperthermia, *Orphanet J Rare Dis* 2:21, 2007.

75. Rubin M, Sadovnikoff N: Normal pediatric airway anatomy. In Tintinalli J, et al, editors: *Tintinalli's emergency medicine: a comprehensive study guide*, ed 6, 2004, McGraw-Hill.

76. Russi C, Wilcox C, House HR: The laryngeal tube device: a simple and timely adjunct to airway management, *Am J Emerg Med* 25(3):263-267, 2007.

77. Sakles J, Laurin E, Rantapaa A, et al: Rocuronium for rapid sequence intubation of emergency department patients, *J Emerg Med* 17(4):611-616, 1999.

78. Shippey B, Ray D, McKeown D: Case series: the mcgrath videolaryngoscope: an initial clinical evaluation, *Can J Anaesth* 54(4):307-313, 2007.

79. Shippey B, Ray D, McKeown D: Use of the mcgrath videolaryngoscope in the management of difficult and failed tracheal intubation, *Br J Anaesth* 100(1):116-119, 2008.

80. Sparr H, Vermeyen K, Beaufort A, et al: Early reversal of profound rocuronium-induced neuromuscular blockade by sugammadex in a randomized multicenter study: efficacy, safety, and pharmacokinetics, *Anesthesiology* 106(5):935-943, 2007.

81. Steinfeldt J, Bey T, Rich JM: Use of a gum elastic bougie (GEB) in a zone II penetrating neck trauma: a case report, *J Emerg Med* 24(3):267-270, 2003.

82. Svenson J, Lindsay MB, O'Connor JE: Endotracheal intracuff pressures in the ED and prehospital setting: is there a problem? *Am J Emerg Med* 25(1):53-56, 2007.

83. Swanson ER: The use of etomidate for rapid-sequence intubation in the air medical setting, *Prehosp Emerg Care* 5(2):142-146, 2001.

84. Takahata O, Kubata M, Mamiya K: The efficiency of the "BURP" maneuver during a difficult laryngoscopy, *Anesth Analg* 84:419-421, 1997.

85. Takeda T, Tanigawa K, Tanaka H, et al: The assessment of three methods to verify tracheal tube placement in the emergency setting, *Resuscitation* 56(2):153-157, 2003.

86. Tanigawa K, Takeda T, Goto E, et al: Accuracy and reliability of the self-inflating bulb to verify tracheal intubation in out-of-hospital cardiac arrest patients, *Anesthesiology* 93(6):1432-1436, 2000.

87. Timmermann A, Russo S, Rosenblatt W, et al: Intubating laryngeal mask airway for difficult out-of-hospital airway management: a prospective evaluation, *Br J Anaesth* 99(2):286-291, 2007.

88. Timmermann A, Russo S, Crozier T, et al: Laryngoscopic versus intubating LMA guided tracheal intubation by novice users: a manikin study, *Resuscitation* 73(3):412-416, 2007.

89. Timmermann A, Russo S, Graf BM: Evaluation of the ctrach: an intubating LMA with integrated fiberoptic system, *Br J Anaesth* 96(4):516-521, 2006.

90. Velky T, et al: Early ventilation and outcome in patients with moderate to severe traumatic brain injury, *Crit Care Med* 34(4):1202-1208, 2006.

91. Verghese C, Brimacombe JR: Survey of laryngeal mask airway usage in 11,910 patients: safety and efficacy for conventional and nonconventional usage, *Anesth Analg* 82(1):129-133, 1996.

92. Vissers RJ, Bair AE: Surgical airway techniques. In Walls RM, et al, editors: *Manual of emergency airway management*, ed 2, Philadelphia, 2004, Lippincott William & Wilkins.

93. Walls R, editor: *Emergency airway management*, ed 2, Philadelphia, 2004, Lippincott William & Wilkins.

94. Walls RM: Airway. In Marx J, Hockberger R, Walls R, editors: *Rosen's emergency medicine*, ed 5, St Louis, 2004, Mosby.

95. Wang H, Davis D, Wayne M, et al: Prehospital rapid-sequence intubation: what does the evidence show? Proceedings from the 2004 National Association of EMS Physicians annual meeting, *Prehosp Emerg Care* 8(4):366-377, 2004.

96. Wang HE, Davis DP, O'Connor RE, et al: Drug assisted intubation in the prehospital setting, *Prehosp Emerg Care* 10(2):261-271, 2006.

97. Welliver M: New drug sugammadex: a selective relaxant binding agent, *AANA J* 74(5):357-363, 2006.

98. Wislon GD, Sittig S, Schears GJ: The laryngeal mask airway at altitude, *J Emerg Med* 34(2):171-174, 2008.

99. Young B: The intubating laryngeal mask airway may be an ideal device for airway control in the rural trauma patient, *Am J Emerg Med* (21):80-85, 2003.

100. Zaleski L, Abello D, Gold MI: The esophageal detector device: does it work? *Anesthesiology* 79(2):244-247, 1993.

CHAPTER

12

MECHANICAL VENTILATION

Carol Rhoades, Rose Linsler

The indications for endotracheal intubation are varied (Box 12-1). Once the airway is secured, the transport team must decide which method and mode of ventilation is most appropriate given the patient's clinical scenario.

Several advantages of mechanical ventilation over manual ventilation are found. Mechanical ventilation provides consistent and uninterrupted ventilation, which is of particular benefit in lengthy transports or in patients with minimal respiratory reserve in whom even a brief discontinuation of bag-mask ventilation may lead to desaturation and slow recovery. Ventilators also provide ventilatory parameter support that helps reduce lung injury and recruit alveoli in patients with acute lung injury (ALI) and acute respiratory distress syndrome (ARDS). In addition, patients with unstable conditions who need multiple interventions during transport are best served when all crewmembers are available to efficiently and quickly provide the care needed. The use of a ventilator eliminates the need for one crewmember to manually ventilate, thereby allowing all crewmembers to address other issues of care.

The advent of smaller, lighter, and more sophisticated ventilators extends the capability and flexibility available to the critical care transport provider.

The type of ventilator chosen and its capabilities depend on mission profile, weight and space restrictions, and population served. Whichever ventilator is selected, medical transport personnel are challenged to understand the terminology (Table 12-1), modes, strategies, and complications of ventilation to proficiently set parameters and troubleshoot ventilation problems. A thorough understanding of blood gas analysis is a prerequisite to monitoring and adjusting ventilation parameters.

TRANSPORT VENTILATOR SELECTION

Multiple resources are available to programs researching the purchase of a transport ventilator. In the United States, the Food and Drug Administration (FDA) is the regulatory agency that must approve all medical equipment, including transport ventilators, before utilization in practice. Transport teams can also look to the American Society of Testing and Materials (ASTM) for established minimal specifications for safety and performance requirements on ventilators.[30] In addition, programs should verify airworthiness testing, which analyzes equipment for electromagnetic disturbances (radio transmission) and for functionality with exposure to vibration and environmental extremes.

BOX 12-1   Indications for Endotracheal Intubation

Problem: Failure or Anticipated Failure to Protect the Airway
- Obtunded or comatose with loss of gag reflex
  - Traumatic brain injury
  - Overdose
  - Anoxia
  - Cerebral insults (cerebrovascular accident [CVA], aneurysms, etc)
- Obstruction
  - Edema related to trauma
  - Inhalation injury
  - Foreign body aspiration
  - Congenital anomaly
- Pharmacologic therapy: Profound sedation or analgesia used to treat or diagnose certain conditions, such as:
  - Status epilepticus
  - Increased intracranial pressures
  - Diagnostic procedures in combative patients
  - Elective procedures

Problem: Failure to Oxygenate
- Shunt ventilation: Alveoli are perfused but not ventilated
  - Pneumonia
  - Acute lung injury (ALI)
  - Pulmonary hemorrhage or contusion
  - Atelectasis
  - Congenital cardiac disease
- Dead space ventilation: Alveoli are ventilated but not perfused
  - Pulmonary embolus

- Hypotension
- Low cardiac output states
- Diffusion abnormalities: Obstruction or restriction of gas exchange across the capillary-alveolar membrane
  - Pulmonary edema
  - Pulmonary fibrosis
- Oxygen extraction: Inability to extract oxygen
  - Sepsis
  - Carbon monoxide poisoning
  - Cyanide poisoning

Problem: Failure to Ventilate
- Neurologic
  - Spinal cord injury or disease
  - Brain injury or disease
  - Overdose
  - Guillain-Barré syndrome
- Muscular
  - Myopathies
  - Myasthenia gravis
- Anatomic
  - Pleural effusions
  - Hemothorax or pneumothorax
  - Abdominal compartment syndrome
  - Bronchospasm, reactive airway disease
  - Congenital anomalies
- Infectious
  - Botulism
  - Respiratory syncytial virus (RSV)
  - Pertussis

Transport ventilators can be broadly classified as automatic resuscitators, simple, or sophisticated.[5] *Automatic resuscitators* are rudimentary devices with minimal or no monitoring and alarm capabilities. The fractional concentration of oxygen in inspired gas (FiO_2) is generally fixed, and set parameters are limited to rate and tidal volume. They are intended for the prehospital setting, to be used by medical personnel with limited exposure to ventilation management. Examples include Ambu Matic® (Ambu, Copenhagen), Vortran Automatic Resuscitators™ (VAR) Models RT and RC, (VORTRAN Medical Technologies, Sacramento,

CA) and Oxylator® EM-100, EMX, or FR-300 (CPR Medical Devices, Inc, Ontario, Canada). *Simple ventilators* offer greater choices in mode of ventilation, rate, volume, and FiO_2. They offer demand flow for spontaneously breathing patients, more alarm features, and minimal monitoring options. Examples of simple ventilators include AutoVent® 2000 and 3000 (Allied Healthcare Products Inc, St Louis, MO), Uni-Vent® 706 (Impact® Instrumentation, Inc., West Caldwell, NJ), and Pneupac® paraPAC (Smiths Medical PM, Inc., Waukesha, WI). These ventilators are also intended for use in the prehospital setting. *Sophisticated ventilators* supply multiple

TABLE 12-1	**Terminology Related to Ventilators**
Term	**Definition**
Acute Lung Injury (ALI)	Pulmonary condition characterized by acute hypoxemic respiratory failure, diffuse bilateral pulmonary infiltrates on CXR, pulmonary wedge pressure < 18 mm Hg, and PaO_2/FiO_2 ratio of < 300.
Adult respiratory distress syndrome (ARDS)	Severe form of ALI differentiated by a PaO_2/FiO_2 ratio < 200.
Asynchrony	Incongruity between patient's respiratory effort and ventilator breath delivery. Increases work of breathing.
Auto-PEEP	Gas trapped in alveoli at end of expiration caused by insufficient expiration time, bronchospasm, or mucous plugging. Causes dynamic alveolar hyperinflation and increases work of breathing. Also referred to as intrinsic PEEP.
Barotrauma	Damage to lung tissue from high airway pressures. Alveolar rupture may lead to pneumothorax, pulmonary interstitial edema, and pneumomediastinum.
Cyclic atelectasis	Repeated opening of alveoli on inspiration and collapsing on expiration.
Derecruitment	Collapse of open alveoli.
Dynamic alveolar hyperinflation	Increase in lung volume at end of expiration caused by incomplete exhalation.
Extrinsic PEEP	Mechanical application of PEEP. See *PEEP*.
Fraction of inspired oxygen (FiO_2)	Fraction of inspired oxygen ranges from 0.21 (21%) to 1.0 (100%). Normal ambient air FiO_2 is 0.21.
Functional residual capacity (FRC)	Volume of air remaining in lungs at end of normal expiration.
Ideal body weight (IBW)	Expected weight of person based on gender and height. Used to base targeted tidal volume in adult population.
Male	IBW = 50 kg + 2.3 kg for each inch over 5 ft.
Female	IBW = 45.5 kg + 2.3 kg for each inch over 5 ft.
I:E ratio	Ratio of inspiratory time to expiratory time. In normal conditions, expiratory phase is passive and twice as long as active inspiratory phase (1:2).
Inspiratory flow	Rate in which breath is delivered on ventilator. It is measured in liters per minute. The higher the flow, the faster the breath is delivered. Flow is equal to tidal volume divided by inspiratory time.
Inspiratory time (Ti)	Time over which tidal volume is delivered or pressure maintained (depending on mode). Set as I:E ratio or inspiratory flow.
Intrinsic PEEP	See *auto-PEEP*.
Mean Airway Pressure (P_{aw})	Average pressure to which lungs are exposed over one inspiratory/expiratory cycle.
Minute ventilation (VE; MV)	Volume of air that moves in and out of lungs in 1 minute. It is product of tidal volume and respiratory rate. VE = Vt × rate.
PaO_2/FiO_2 ratio	Calculation used to quantify to degree of hypoxemia and oxygenation abnormality in patients with acute respiratory failure. PaO_2 derived from arterial blood gas is divided by fraction of inspired oxygen. Normal is 500. Patients with ALI are at < 300, and patients with ARDS are at < 200. The lower the number, the greater the degree of pulmonary abnormality. For example, a patient on 60% FiO_2 has PaO_2 of 70 mm Hg: 70/0.6 = 115. By definition, this patient has ARDS.
Peak inspiratory pressure (PIP)	Measurement in lungs at peak of inspiration.

TABLE 12-1	**Terminology Related to Ventilators—cont'd**
Term	**Definition**
Permissive hypercapnia	Lung-protective ventilation strategy that uses low tidal volumes to reduce lung injury associated with high volumes and alveolar overdistention. Carbon dioxide is allowed to rise as consequence.
Positive end-expiratory pressure (PEEP)	Positive pressure maintained at end of expiration. Therapy used in mechanical ventilation to increase volume of gas remaining in lungs at end of expiration (FRC).
Plateau pressure	Pressure exerted on small airways and alveoli measured by holding inspiratory pause during ventilator delivered inspiration. Plateau pressures ≥ 30 mm Hg have been associated with alveolar overdistention lung injury.
Recruitment	Refers to opening of collapsed alveoli. Alveolar recruitment maneuvers refer to increasing PEEP, for short durations, to open collapsed alveoli and improve oxygenation. Level of PEEP, duration, and frequency of this maneuver is determined by clinician.
Tidal volume	Volume of gas inspired or expired in one breath.
Trigger-sensitivity	Measure of amount of negative pressure that must be generated by patient to trigger mechanical ventilator into inspiratory phase.
V/Q ratio	Ventilation (V) to perfusion (Q) ratio. High V/Q = deadspace ventilation. Alveoli are ventilated, but perfusion to lungs is impaired. Examples: pulmonary embolus, hypotension. Low V/Q = shunt ventilation. Alveoli are perfused, but there is impaired aeration. Examples: ARDS, pneumonia.
Volutrauma	Volume-related overdistention injury of alveoli inflicted by mechanical ventilation.

modes of ventilation, for example, continuous positive airway pressure (CPAP), synchronized intermittent mandatory ventilation (SIMV), continuous mandatory ventilation (CMV), and flow-by and pressure support, to list a few. These ventilators are equipped with a full complement of alarms and monitoring capabilities.[5] Trained medical personnel proficient in ventilation management use them for interfacility transports. Examples of these sophisticated ventilators include Crossvent 3 or 4 (Bio-Med Devices, Inc., Guilford, CT), Oxylog® 2000 or 3000 (Dräger Medical, Telford, PA), LTV® 1200 (Viasys® Healthcare, Minneapolis, MN) and Bird® Avian (Bird Products Corporation, Palm Springs, CA).

Choice of ventilator varies with program profile. Some factors that should be considered follow.

PROGRAM CONSIDERATIONS
Mission Type
Whether a program transports adult, pediatric, or neonatal patients influences ventilator choices. Pediatric patients need ventilators capable of delivering lower tidal volumes. For example, a 10-pound (4.5-kg) 2 month-old ventilated with a tidal volume of 6 mL/kg needs a ventilator to deliver volumes as low as 27 mL. If the program transports critically ill newborn patients, a ventilator with high-frequency ventilation mode may be necessary. Programs that transport the full spectrum of patients from neonates to adults often need more than one type of ventilator.

Critical care transport teams need a more sophisticated ventilator as opposed to programs whose primary mission is scene flights. Patients with severe adult respiratory distress syndrome are a challenge to oxygenate and ventilate, even with highly sophisticated ventilators, and attempts to bag ventilate are likely to be unsuccessful. Teams that cover a large geographic area want to look at oxygen consumption and battery life of the ventilator.

Budget
In addition to the outright cost of the ventilator, consideration of clinical engineering availability for preventative maintenance and repairs should be weighed.

Warranty coverage, loaner availability, manufacturer support, service record, and turnaround time for major repairs should also be explored.

Training

Mechanical ventilators require initial and on-going training. The more sophisticated the ventilator, the more training required. Highly sophisticated ventilators may require the addition of a respiratory therapist skilled in ventilation management. A transport program's quality assurance team should monitor the ability (or inability) to adequately ventilate patients during transport and address educational needs.

VENTILATOR CONSIDERATIONS
Guidelines

The American Association of Respiratory Care (AARC) has established a consensus statement on the essentials of mechanical ventilators.[1] Components are classified as either essential or recommended (Table 12-2). Manufactures of sophisticated transport ventilators are guided by these recommendations.

Durability and Safety

Transport ventilators should be compact, lightweight, and easy to secure; have proper electromagnetic shielding; and tolerate vibration and extremes of temperatures. Some monitor screens are difficult to see in the sunlight or dim lighting. Contrast adjustments should have a wide range. Alarms should have visual and loud audible alerts. Ventilator setting and alarm buttons or dials should not be easy to inadvertently reposition.

Oxygen Consumption

In addition to the patient-delivered gases, some ventilators use a gas source to drive the pneumatics, increasing the gas consumption of the ventilator during ventilation. A wide range of oxygen consumption exists between transport ventilators that should be compared with the transport range within a program.

Power

Battery life is of particular concern to programs that cover large geographic areas where transports occur over hours rather than minutes. Lithium ion

TABLE 12-2	**Transport Ventilator Guidelines**
Essential	**Recommended**
Set Parameters:	**Set Parameters:**
Positive pressure ventilation	Flow or I:E ratio
100% FiO_2	Spontaneous breath modes
PEEP	Triggering mechanism
Mandatory rate	
Monitoring Capabilities:	**Monitoring Capabilities:**
Peak airway pressure	Expired tidal volume
PEEP pressures	Expired spontaneous volume
	I:E ratio
	Mechanical rate
	Spontaneous rate

***Alarms: Level 1* (immediately life-threatening)**
Power failure
Loss of gas source
Absence of gas delivery (apnea)
Excessive gas delivery
Exhalation valve failure
Timing failure

***Alarms: Level 2* (potentially life-threatening)**
Battery power loss
Circuit leak
Blender failure
Circuit occlusion
Loss of or excessive PEEP
Auto-cycling

As outlined in the *Consensus Statement of the Essentials of Mechanical Ventilators* from the American Association for Respiratory Care.

batteries have one of the best energy-to-weight ratios and a longer shelf life as a result of a slower loss of charge when not in use and have no memory effect, which causes rechargeable batteries to lose charge capacity over time. They are also the most expensive. NiCad batteries are particularly susceptible to memory effect. Battery life on transport ventilators can range from less than 2 hours to 14 hours.

SELECTION PROCESS

An organized selection process should be used in the search for a transport ventilator. Following is one suggested evaluation tool:

1. With the mission profile in mind, have the members of the flight team list and rank desired ventilator criteria. Indicate required components versus "nice-to-haves." Is the team more comfortable with volume-controlled or pressure-controlled ventilators, or does the ventilator provide both options?
2. Recruit respiratory therapists and medical directors in the criteria listing process.
3. Gather a list of ventilators that best meet the criteria.
4. Rule out any ventilators on the list that do not meet airworthiness testing criteria or regulatory approval.
5. Search for published bench-testing reports.
6. Bring the ventilator into a clinical engineering bench test to verify that the ventilator functions as per published specifications. Some of the other considerations might be ease of use, safety, durability, portability, power usage, oxygen consumption, and functionality.
7. Use clinical engineering to assess for preventative maintenance, parts availability, and field repairs.
8. Use the ventilator on patients. If possible, trial it on patients in the hospital before field testing.
9. Review the data from steps 6, 7, and 8 against the criteria gathered in steps 1 and 2.
10. Rank the ventilators from most desired to least desired.
11. Use the program's budgetary process to assist with financial negotiations.
12. The evaluation team makes the final recommendation on the basis of the team criteria, clinical use, and financials.
13. Make a recommendation to management.

VENTILATOR-INDUCED LUNG INJURY

Ventilator-induced lung injury (VILI) is damage done to the lung as a direct result of mechanical ventilation. Patients with acute lung injury, ARDS, chronic obstructive lung disease (COPD), and asthma are particularly prone to VILI associated with high transpulmonary pressures, high tidal volumes, and cyclic atelectasis, which compounds the difficulty in ventilation management. *Transpulmonary pressure* is the pressure difference across the lung calculated by subtracting the pleural pressure from the alveolar pressure. Alveolar pressure is most closely approximated in ventilated patients by the end-inspiratory plateau pressure (Pplat). The Pplat is believed to be a better indicator of alveolar overdistention than the peak inspiratory pressure (Ppk) because it is not influenced by upper airway resistance or ventilator equipment.[26] The crew measures the Pplat by pressing the inspiratory pause button for 0.5 to 1 second and taking a pressure reading.

BAROTRAUMA

Barotrauma is the damage to lung tissue that causes alveolar rupture and migration of air into the extrapulmonary space. Historically, this has been attributed to high airway pressure. Barotrauma may lead to pneumothorax, tension pneumothorax, pneumomediastinum, air embolus (rare), and subcutaneous emphysema. Whether high Ppks are a direct cause of barotrauma or just a marker of severe lung disease is not clear.[16,34] In a retrospective study of patients enrolled in the ARDS Network trial of low-tidal volume ventilation, mean airway pressure and plateau pressure were not predictive indicators of barotrauma.[10]

VOLUTRAUMA

More recently, attention has been placed on ventilator-induced injury caused by high volumes and *alveolar overdistention,* also referred to as *dynamic hyperinflation.* The stretch of alveoli causes microvascular injury, high permeability pulmonary edema, accumulation of fluid in the interstitial and alveolar space, disruption of surfactant function, and alveolar collapse.[9,22,24] Monitoring and controlling the Pplat is one strategy used to prevent or minimize the excessive alveolar stretch associated with VILI. The ARDS Network study demonstrated that maintenance of the Pplat at ≤30 cm H_2O was associated with a statistically significant decrease in ventilator days and improved mortality rates.[4] The Network ventilation protocols set a goal plateau pressure of ≤30 cm H_2O and recommend it be checked after each change in positive end-expiratory pressure (PEEP) or tidal volume. Some controversy exists regarding the need to reduce tidal volume if the Pplat is ≤30 cm H_2O; however, a secondary analysis of the ARDS trial suggested that a beneficial effect was seen in tidal volume reduction from 12 mL/kg ideal body weight (IBW) to 6 mL/kg regardless of the Pplat before the tidal volume was reduced.[17]

Not only patients with ARDS/ALI are at risk for VILI with high volume ventilation. In a retrospective cohort study of 332 patients, 24% who did not have ALI at the initiation of mechanical ventilation developed injury within 5 days.[15] One of the primary risk factors for the development of ALI was high tidal volume (>9 mL/kg IBW) ventilation, which suggests that high tidal volumes may lead to the development of ALI in patients at risk.

Overdistention injury is not only associated with high tidal volumes. A normal tidal volume delivered to a diseased lung with large areas of low compliance can cause overdistention of available alveoli. Large segments of alveoli may be closed in patients with ARDS/ALI, leaving a small portion of the lung to receive the full tidal volume, which results in high pulmonary pressures and increasing susceptibility to volutrauma.[14]

CYCLIC ATELECTASIS

Cyclic atelectasis is the opening of alveoli on inspiration and collapsing on expiration. Animal models have shown that this repeated opening and closing causes the release of cytokines and development of local and systemic inflammatory response,[40] further extending lung injury. PEEP is used to curtail the collapsing of lung units on expiration, particularly in low tidal volume strategies.

OXYGEN TOXICITY

High levels of oxygen over a prolonged period of time have been shown to produce cytotoxic effects, presumably as the result of free radical production.[13] How this relates to the clinical care of patients with acute respiratory failure is unclear. Generally, transport times are of short enough duration not to produce the consequences of high oxygen levels in the adult or pediatric population. Administration of 100% oxygen to patients is reasonable during emergencies and resuscitation and for the duration of transport. Life-threatening hypoxia should always be treated with 100% oxygen delivered via facemask, endotracheal tube, or tracheotomy.

Some patients may be more susceptible to high levels of oxygen, for example, preterm neonates at risk for long-term retinal damage and bronchopulmonary dysplasia (BPD). Also susceptible are children with congenital cyanotic and partially repaired cyanotic-heart lesions who are at risk of hemodynamic instability as a result of oxygen-induced excess pulmonary blood flow.[38,43]

CLASSIFICATION OF POSITIVE PRESSURE VENTILATION

No universal consensus exists on classification of ventilators or ventilation modes, and descriptions vary with the literature. The elements in classification that are most pertinent to transport teams are volume-targeted or pressure-targeted positive pressure ventilation and continuous positive airway pressure. No research exists to suggest improved outcomes between volume-controlled and pressure-controlled ventilation strategies. Within these categories, ventilation modes can be described as mandatory, assisted, or spontaneous, depending on the dynamic necessary to initiate an inspiratory breath.

- *Mandatory:* Mandatory breaths are initiated, controlled (volume or pressure), and terminated by the ventilator. No synchronizing of the ventilator breaths occurs with patient-initiated breaths. Example: CMV.
- *Assisted:* Spontaneous breaths are initiated by the patient but controlled and ended (assisted) by the ventilator. Examples: Assist-control and pressure support.
- *Spontaneous:* Spontaneous breaths are initiated, controlled, and terminated by the patient. Example: CPAP.

VOLUME-TARGETED VENTILATION

Volume-controlled pressure-variable ventilation is the most common mode of ventilation used on transport ventilators. The tidal volume is preset and delivered during the set inspiratory time of the ventilatory cycle. Once that tidal volume is reached, inspiration ends and exhalation begins. The inspiratory pressure varies depending on the compliance and resistance of the lung, with higher pressures associated with greater lung resistance or low compliance. The advantage of this form of ventilation is the guarantee of minute ventilation (tidal volume multiplied by rate). On the other hand, the potential for lung injury exists when high pressures are required to deliver the set tidal volume in patients with low lung compliance. To mitigate against ventilator-induced barotrauma or lung injury, pressure limits are set. If the limit is reached during the delivery of the set tidal volume, the inspiration is terminated, even if the targeted tidal volume has not been achieved. Modes of volume-cycled ventilation include CMV, assist-control (AC), and SIMV.

Continuous Mandatory Ventilation

Continuous mandatory ventilation (CMV) is a volume-cycled mode of ventilation in which the tidal volume and ventilatory rate are set. Spontaneous respiratory effort by the patient is ignored, and no patient triggering is possible. This method of ventilation is uncomfortable and is primarily used in sedated or chemically paralyzed patients who make no spontaneous respiratory effort. *CMV-assist* is a term used by some ventilator manufacturers to refer to assist-control ventilation.

Assist-Control Ventilation

With *assist-control ventilation* (AC), the clinician sets a base ventilatory rate; however, the patient is allowed to breathe faster than the set rate. Every breath, whether patient or ventilator initiated, receives the full set tidal volume. This mode of ventilation requires minimal work from the patient and is often used during the early hours and days after intubation to allow the patient to rest while the underlying cause of respiratory failure is addressed.

Assist-control can be either *volume-controlled* (ACV) or *pressure-controlled* (PCV). In volume-targeted assist-control, both the ventilatory rate and tidal volume are set parameters. Parameters also set by the clinician on more sophisticated transport ventilators include inspiratory flow, waveform, and trigger sensitivity. Patient hyperventilation may occur in this mode; therefore, minute ventilation should be monitored. Auto-PEEP can occur when respiratory rates are rapid and expiration is incomplete. The use of pop-off valves and pressure limit alarms prevents excessive peak inspiratory pressures in such cases, but the tidal volume delivered is diminished.

Some ventilators use the CMV term in referring to assist-control mode. With setting of a trigger sensitivity in CMV mode, the ventilator assists spontaneous respiratory efforts in the same manner described previously.

Synchronized Intermittent Mandatory Ventilation

Synchronized intermittent mandatory ventilation (SIMV) is a volume-controlled mode of ventilation. The primary distinction between SIMV and assist-control ventilation is how the ventilator contributes to spontaneous respiratory effort. Similar to AC, SIMV mode provides breaths at a set rate and set tidal volume. Unlike AC, spontaneous respiratory efforts do not receive an assisted tidal volume. Most modern ventilators synchronize a patient's spontaneous efforts with the ventilator-delivered breath, preventing the delivery of a breath when the patient is already maximally inhaling or forcefully exhaling.

In SIMV, the tidal volume and ventilator rate are set. Some transport ventilators allow the clinician to set the inspiratory flow, waveform, and sensitivity.

PRESSURE-TARGETED VENTILATION

Pressure-controlled volume-variable ventilation involves the delivery of an inspiratory breath until a preset pressure limit is reached. Once the pressure is reached, inspiration is discontinued and the expiration phase begins. The tidal volume delivered varies depending on the compliance and resistance of the lung. For example, smaller volumes are delivered in patients with low pulmonary compliance or high airway resistance. The advantage of this mode of ventilation is that it limits the distending pressure of the lung, reducing the risk of ventilator-induced lung injury. The disadvantage of this mode is the absence of guaranteed minute ventilation with the potential for hypoventilation or hyperventilation. Modes of pressure-cycled ventilation include pressure-control and pressure support.

Pressure-Controlled Ventilation

Pressure-controlled ventilation (PC) delivers an inspiratory breath to a preset pressure limit. The inspiratory cycle is terminated when the inspiratory pressure limit is reached. In pressure-controlled ventilation, the clinician sets the base ventilatory rate, the inspiratory pressure, and the inspiratory time. The patient's spontaneous respiratory efforts are recognized (adjusted through the sensitivity setting), and breaths are assisted by the ventilator to reach the set inspiratory pressure. As lung compliance and resistance changes, so does the tidal volume. No guaranteed minute ventilation is used. Vigilant and continuous monitoring for hypoventilation and hyperventilation is necessary.

Pressure-Support Ventilation

Pressure-support ventilation (PSV) is an assisted mode of ventilation in which the patient initiates a breath, triggering the ventilator to deliver a preset level of inspiratory pressure. The patient determines the respiratory rate, inspiratory time, and tidal volume.[18] Because the patient triggers all breaths, this mode is only effective in the spontaneously breathing patient. The higher the pressure support is set, the less ventilatory workload for the patient. PSV can be combined with other modes of ventilation, such as SIMV and CPAP. It is also used in weaning patients from the ventilator by progressively decreasing the degree of pressure support. A minimal amount of PSV should be provided to overcome the resistance to the endotracheal tube and ventilatory circuit. If the intent is to provide complete ventilatory support, then PSV should be set relatively high. Minute ventilation should be closely monitored when used in patients with susceptibility toward respiratory depression.

Invasive Continuous Positive Airway Pressure

Continuous positive airway pressure (CPAP) is neither volume-controlled nor pressure-controlled ventilation. Patients breathe spontaneously at their own rate and tidal volume via an artificial airway with a continuous level of set pressure. This has the same effect as PEEP in opening collapsed alveoli and increasing functional residual capacity. This mode is primarily used to assess the patient's ability to ventilate and oxygenate before extubation. It is also used in patients without oxygenation or ventilation abnormalities who need only airway protection (e.g., patients who are alert and awake but have laryngeal edema or airway compression). This mode should be used with caution in patients who have potential to decompensate neurologically or hemodynamically.

NONINVASIVE POSITIVE PRESSURE VENTILATION

Noninvasive positive pressure ventilation (NPPV) refers to mechanical respiratory support provided without an endotracheal or tracheostomy tube. It is applied with a face or nasal mask, mouthpiece, and high flow nasal cannula or nasal prongs, although generally it is used with a snug fitting nasal or facial mask.[32] This method is useful in both chronic and acute disorders and is discussed here as it relates to acute respiratory failure or acute exacerbation of a chronic respiratory condition.

When successful, NPPV can eliminate the need for intubation and its complications, while preserving the ability to speak, cough, and swallow. NPPV decreases the work of breathing, increases alveolar ventilation, rests respiratory musculature, and improves gas exchange. The strongest evidence of support for the successful use of NPPV is in patients with acute exacerbation of COPD and in patients with acute cardiogenic pulmonary edema.[28,29] It may also be used in patients who refuse intubation. NPPV is contraindicated for patients who need emergent intubation because of cardiac or respiratory arrest and for patients with hemodynamic instability, inability to control the airway (high risk for aspiration), upper airway obstruction, facial trauma or deformity, unstable arrhythmia, or organ failure unrelated to respiratory failure.[18] Patients who have difficulty breathing in the supine position, especially when related to obesity, should be carefully considered before transport via NPPV. Lowering the head to load or for take-off and landing can turn a tenuous situation into an emergent one.

Noninvasive positive pressure ventilation can be delivered via CPAP, volume-cycled, or pressure-limited modes. CPAP delivers a constant positive pressure during inspiration and expiration. Volume-cycled ventilators are often not well tolerated because mask leaks result in high inspiratory pressures to achieve the preset tidal volume. Pressure-limited modes include pressure support, pressure-control, and bilevel positive airway pressure (BiPAP). BiPAP ventilation delivers both inspiratory positive airway pressure (IPAP) and expiratory positive airway pressure (EPAP; similar to CPAP and PEEP). The patient triggers each breath. In the event of apnea, alarms and back-up rates should be set. Skilled clinicians can perform manual NPPV with a facemask with a tight face seal and a flow-inflating device (anesthesia bag) or a self-inflating bag with a PEEP valve.

Success of NPPV is associated with user expertise, familiarity of equipment, and patient selection.[11,25,36,39] In initiation of NPPV, a properly fitting mask must be selected. Applying the mask gently until the patient is comfortable and in sync with the ventilator before securing the straps improves patient comfort. CPAP, as opposed to PSV or BiPAP, may be selected when hypoxemia from cardiogenic pulmonary edema or upper airway obstruction from underlying obstructive sleep apnea is contributing to respiratory failure. PSV or BiPAP modes are chosen when ventilatory failure is a component and positive pressure ventilation is needed to support failing respiratory muscles, such as in COPD exacerbation or neuromuscular disease. When using CPAP, start at a CPAP of 5 cm H_2O and gradually increase by increments of 2 cm of water until adequate oxygenation is achieved. Alternately, if using pressure-limited mode, increase the inspiratory pressures starting at 10 cm water, with 5 cm H_2O of expiratory pressure, while monitoring exhaled tidal volume. Depending on urgency of transport and degree of respiratory failure, if improvement is not noted within a short period, endotracheal intubation should be considered.

The efficacy of NPPV in the transport setting has not been clearly defined. Programs should develop specific criteria that involve not only proper patient selection but also the practicality of use in the medical transport environment. The use of NPPV in acute hospital and home settings is steadily increasing. Requests to transport patients already successfully managed on NPPV are on the rise. Compliance with protocols regarding electromagnetic interference must be maintained when considering use of a patient's personal NPPV device in an aircraft.

ADVANCED VENTILATORY MODES

HIGH FREQUENCY VENTILATION

High frequency ventilation (HFV) modes provide alveolar ventilation with tidal volumes that are less than or equal to dead space volume by delivering them at supraphysiologic frequency. The goal of HFV therapy is to produce adequate alveolar ventilation at low tidal volume with preservation of end-expiratory lung volume to minimize volutrauma and barotrauma. This form of ventilation is more commonly used for newborn and pediatric patients than adults. In practice, the high frequency devices most often used are high frequency oscillatory ventilation (HFOV) and high frequency jet ventilation (HFJV).

Indications for HFV include disease states such as bronchopleural fistulas and airway injuries and patients at risk for pulmonary barotrauma (i.e., those with mean airway pressure [P_{aw}], >18-20; plateau pressure, >35); and with diffuse alveolar disease (i.e., acute lung injury and ARDS), in which a major therapeutic goal is to preserve end expiratory lung volume while limiting end-inspiratory lung overdistention.

High Frequency Jet Ventilation

High frequency jet ventilation (HFJV) delivers inspiratory gas through a jet injector, near the carina, at high velocity. This is accomplished with a specific endotracheal tube (ETT) with a jet injector or an in-line jet injector adapter that is added to the existing ETT. HFJV is most often used simultaneously with a conventional ventilator that is able to provide PEEP and tidal volume breaths (10 mL/kg) to the patient to preserve end-expiratory lung volume.

- Rates of 100 to 600 bpm are delivered with a tidal volume of 3 to 5 mL/kg.
- Risks include airway injury from the jet flow of gas positioned near the carina and air trapping.

- Expiration is passive.
- HFJV is generally limited to patients less than 8 years of age because of limitations in minute ventilation support.

High Frequency Oscillatory Ventilation

High frequency oscillatory ventilation (HFOV) is the most widely used HFV technique in clinical practice today. High frequency oscillatory ventilators maintain lung recruitment by delivering a relatively high distending pressure (i.e., P_{aw}) while providing ventilation through superimposed piston-generated sinusoidal pressure oscillations (ΔP) at a frequency of 3 to 15 hertz. Adequate oscillatory pressure (ΔP) generally produces visible chest vibration ("wiggle") from the clavicles to the lower abdomen or pelvis.

High frequency oscillatory ventilation uses a relatively high P_{aw} to improve oxygenation. When transitioning to HFOV, the initial P_{aw} is generally set 3 to 5 cm H_2O above the P_{aw} on conventional ventilation immediately before transition. After the transition, the clinician should titrate the P_{aw} in 1 to 2 cm H_2O increments until oxygenation improves enough to allow a reduction in FiO_2 below 0.6 and global lung recruitment to a level at which both hemidiaphragms project at the level of the eighth to 10th posterior ribs on chest x-ray (CXR).[41,42]

- Ventilation is primarily determined with oscillatory pressure amplitude (ΔP). Increase the ΔP in 2 to 3 cm H_2O increments to improve CO_2 clearance. The chest wiggle is attained by adjusting the delta P (ΔP) on the ventilator.
- Ventilation is also influenced by the oscillation frequency, as frequency is inversely related to delivered tidal volume in HFOV. Although ventilation at higher frequencies generally delivers tidal volumes of 1 to 3 mL/kg, physiologic tidal volumes that approach those used in typical conventional ventilation strategies can be produced at the low end of the frequency spectrum.[35]
- HFOV is the only mode of mechanical ventilation in which expiration is active, rather than passive.

INHALED NITRIC OXIDE

Inhaled nitric oxide (iNO) is a naturally occurring vasodilator administered as an inhaled gas for selective pulmonary vasodilation, without associated systemic hypotension. As iNO diffuses across the alveolar-capillary membrane, the smooth muscle cells in the adjacent pulmonary vessels relax, which decreases pulmonary vascular resistance (PVR). Oxygenation improves as vessels that perfuse ventilated alveoli are dilated, redistributing blood flow and reducing intrapulmonary shunting. iNO in the bloodstream is bound to hemoglobin and is rapidly deactivated, thus causing little effect on systemic vascular resistance and blood pressure.

Therapy indications include pulmonary hypertension and isolated right heart failure. iNO can be administered through a nasal cannula or ventilator circuit at a dose of 5 to 40 ppm. Once therapy is started, do not abruptly discontinue or disconnect a patient from iNO without specific medical orders from a physician. PVR could significantly increase and cause acute hypoxia and right ventricular (RV) dysfunction.

Methemoglobinemia and alveolar cytotoxicity are rare adverse reactions reported with iNO therapy. Monitor methemoglobinemia levels with blood gas samples if available.

HELIUM-OXYGEN MIXTURE

Helium-oxygen mixture (Heliox) is a biologically inert gas with a much lower density than oxygen-nitrogen. With inhalation, resistance to airflow is reduced and areas of turbulent flow through obstructions may be converted to a streamlined nonturbulent (laminar) flow, thereby improving the work of breathing.

Clinical indications for heliox include upper airway obstruction associated with edema (postextubation stridor, croup), obstruction from compression, respiratory processes with high airway resistance or obstructive pathology (bronchiolitis, status asthmaticus), or respiratory distress syndrome. Heliox may also be used for children with bronchopulmonary dysplasia (to decrease the work of breathing), for augmentation in the delivery of nebulized bronchodilators to obstructed lower airways, and to allow time for the onset of therapeutic medications or the resolution of the disease process. If successful, it may negate the need for intubation. The benefits are usually evident in several minutes. Administration consideration includes:

- Usually administered with 30% oxygen through a tight-fitting mask.
- Commercially available in helium:oxygen concentrations of 80:20 or 70:30.
- Do not administer pure helium; always administer with oxygen. If manually blending helium and oxygen, place an in-line oxygen concentration device to ensure adequate oxygen mix.

Positive improvement has been reported in the adult population in patients treated for upper airway obstructions as a result of thyroid masses, radiation injury, lymphoma, cancer, or angioedema.[12]

VENTILATOR SETTINGS

Selection of ventilator mode and settings are determined by clinical assessment, degree of alteration in oxygenation or ventilation, disease pathophysiology, institutional or physician preference, and capabilities of the transport ventilator.

TIDAL VOLUME

Tidal volume (Vt) is set in volume-controlled ventilation modes. To reduce the likelihood of alveolar overdistention and high airway pressures, the tidal volume should be based on ideal body weight (IBW) rather than actual body weight in adult patients. Traditionally, high tidal volumes of 10 to 15 mL/kg have been used to maintain normocapnia and pH and to prevent atelectasis-related hypoxemia. However, adverse effects of barotrauma and volutrauma have led to recommendations for lower tidal volumes. The benefit of a low tidal volume ventilation strategy was shown in the landmark ARDS Network's randomized controlled multicenter trial of 861 patients that compared the use of low tidal volume (4 to 6 mL/kg IBW and plateau pressure $\leq$ 30 cm H_2O) with traditional tidal volume (12 mL/kg IBW and plateau pressure $\leq$ 50 cm H_2O) in ARDS. The trial was stopped early after interim

analysis results showed a 23% reduction in mortality rate in the low tidal volume group.[4]

In light of the study outcomes, tidal volume should be initiated at 6 mL/kg IBW in patients with ARDS/ALI. Adjust the respiratory rate to achieve the desired partial pressure of carbon dioxide in arterial blood ($PaCO_2$) or pH. Low tidal volume ventilation often requires acceptance of a degree of respiratory acidosis and is discussed in ventilation strategies (permissive hypercapnia).

Patients with obstructive disease such as COPD and asthma benefit from lower tidal volumes of 6 to 7 mL/kg IBW to reduce lung inflation and give the patient longer exhalation time.[27] In most other patients, use of a tidal volume greater than 8 mL/kg is rarely necessary, and a starting volume of 6 to 7 mL/kg with ventilator adjustments to meet pH and $PaCO_2$ targets is reasonable.

PEAK INSPIRATORY PRESSURE

Peak inspiratory pressure (PIP) is set in the pressure-targeted modes. When initiating pressure-control ventilation, the target pressure should initially be set to give the patient a measured tidal volume of 6 to 7 mL/kg IBW. As stated previously, tidal volume and minute ventilation are not static but change dynamically with lung compliance, which warrants close monitoring.

In volume-cycled modes, peak inspiratory pressure (Ppk) is a dynamic value reflective of a combination of patient and ventilator variables. Tidal volume, PEEP, and inspiratory time (Ti) are ventilator settings that contribute to inspiratory pressures. On some ventilators, inspiratory time is not a set parameter but is determined by the set respiratory rate and ratio of inspiratory time to expiratory time (I:E ratio). Ppk increases or decreases as lung compliance worsens or improves.

RATE, BREATHS PER MINUTE, AND FREQUENCY

In initial selection of the rate, consider the patient's age (pediatric, newborn, adult), minute ventilation, and tidal volume. *Minute ventilation,* or minute volume, is equal to the respiratory rate multiplied by the tidal volume; the normal parameters are 5 to 8 L/min. Adjustments to the rate depend on the clinical goal and disease process to meet the desired pH or

$PaCO_2$ range. Generally, increasing the rate decreases the $PaCO_2$ and increases the pH. Alternately, decreasing the rate increases the $PaCO_2$ and decreases the pH. With assisted ventilation modes in spontaneously breathing patients, care must be taken to monitor for hyperventilation and auto-PEEP.

FRACTIONAL CONCENTRATION OF OXYGEN IN INSPIRED GAS

If the partial pressure of oxygen in arterial blood (PaO_2) is unknown, the *fractional concentration of oxygen in inspired gas* (FiO_2) is typically set at 100% on initiation of mechanical ventilation and reduced as tolerated by PaO_2 or pulse oximetry. FiO_2 is used in combination with PEEP to maintain the PaO_2 or peripheral oxygen saturation (SpO_2) above the minimum threshold. The oxygenation goals set by the ARDS Network for patients with ALI/ARDS are PaO_2 of 55 to 80 mm Hg or SpO_2 of 88% to 95%.[4] The Brain Trauma Foundation recommends that PaO_2 be maintained at more than 60 mm Hg or SpO_2 at more than 90% in patients with traumatic brain injury.[7] The American Heart Association advises that oxygen saturations be maintained at or above 90% for patients with cardiac compromise.[2] If high levels of FiO_2 do not reverse hypoxia, then PEEP can be added incrementally to achieve oxygenation goals (see subsequent discussion).

The FiO_2 selections may be limited by the transport ventilator's blending or air entrainment capabilities.

POSITIVE END-EXPIRATORY PRESSURE

Positive end-expiratory pressure (PEEP) exerts pressure in the patient's airway above atmospheric level throughout the respiratory cycle, increasing the functional residual capacity (FRC) by opening collapsed alveoli. The FRC is the air that remains in the lungs at the end of passive expiration; it is reduced with loss of chest wall mobility (obesity) or lung compliance.[31] The increase in FRC through the addition of PEEP is referred to as *recruitment* and decreases intrapulmonary shunting of blood through lung regions with collapsed alveoli, improving ventilation to perfusion ratio (V/Q) matching. The ideal PEEP setting prevents cyclic atelectasis and

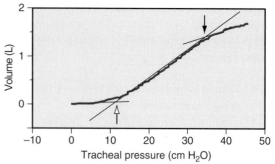

FIGURE 12-1   Volume-pressure (V-P) curve of respiratory system obtained on zero end-expiratory pressure by low-inflation constant-flow technique in representative acute respiratory disease syndrome patient, showing typical sigmoid shape. Three regions could be identified from this curve. First part of V-P curve at low lung volume is flat. This is followed by abrupt increase in compliance, heralding a linear part of V-P curve. Finally, near total lung capacity, compliance falls. The slope of the linear part of V-P curve amounts to 56 mL/cm H_2O. Intersection of first and second parts of V-P curve defines lower inflection point *(open arrow)*, coordinates of which are 30 mL and 12 cm H_2O. Intersection between second and third parts of V-P curve yielded upper inflection point *(closed arrow)*, whose coordinates are 1360 mL and 35 cm H_2O. (From Guerin C, Tantucci C: Respiratory mechanics in intensive care units. *Eur Respir Monogr* 4:255-278, 1999.)

overdistention injury while optimizing oxygenation. Intensive care clinicians may use the pressure-volume curve to balance the benefit of alveolar recruitment against the risk of hyperinflation by finding the ideal PEEP between the upper and lower inflection points on the curve (Figure 12-1). When possible, the overall goal should be to use the lowest PEEP setting necessary to acquire an acceptable PaO_2 with a FiO_2 of less than 0.60. Most patients benefit from the addition of 5 cm H_2O PEEP to overcome the decrease in FRC as a result of the airway resistance caused by the endotracheal tube.

In several circumstances, PEEP should be used with caution. PEEP increases intrathoracic pressure, thereby reducing venous return and preload. In patients with reduced circulatory volume, this reduction can cause or exacerbate hypotension. PEEP should be increased incrementally with close monitoring of blood pressure. By the same principle, mean arterial blood pressures should be monitored in patients with intracranial abnormalities when PEEP is increased to maintain cerebral perfusion pressure (CPP). Hypotension has been shown to increase mortality rates in patients with traumatic brain injured, and the Brain Trauma Foundation advises that the systolic blood pressure not drop below 90 mm Hg.[7] Blood pressure should, therefore, be monitored closely when increasing PEEP. Of note, one study of patients with severe traumatic brain injury showed that an increase in PEEP to as high as 15 mm Hg to optimize oxygenation did not compromise cerebral perfusion or oxygen transport.[21]

In patients with unilateral lung disease, preferential distribution of minute ventilation and PEEP may be directed to areas of healthy lung (least resistance) and do little for the injured or diseased lung. This can cause alveolar overdistention injury of healthy alveoli and compress the vasculature surrounding the alveoli, worsening the shunt. When possible, placement of patients in a lateral position with the good lung in the dependent position may help to improve blood flow and gas exchange to healthy tissue.

Auto-PEEP, also termed *intrinsic PEEP,* refers to air trapped in the alveoli at end expiration. Causes include high minute ventilation, mechanical expiratory flow limitation (foreign body obstruction, mucus plug), and physiologic expiratory resistance (asthma, COPD). Large tidal volumes or high respiratory rates increase the minute ventilation and reduce exhalation time. A new breath is delivered before full exhalation and traps air in the alveoli. Similarly, patient-generated rapid respiratory rates in assisted ventilator modes caused by agitation, patient-ventilator asynchrony, or low sensitivity thresholds can lead to subsequent incomplete exhalation and auto-PEEP. Patients with obstructive lung disease are particularly vulnerable to air trapping as a result of airway collapse or narrowing.

INSPIRATORY-TO-EXPIRATORY TIME RATIO AND FLOW RATE

The normal *inspiratory-to-expiratory time ratio* (I:E) is 1:2 or 1:3. The inspiratory time is calculated by dividing the tidal volume by the flow rate. An increase in the flow rate, or how fast a breath is given, causes a decrease in the inspiratory time,

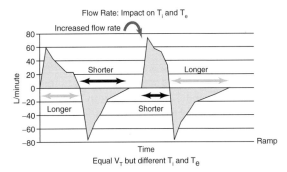

FIGURE 12-2   Effect of flow rate on inspiratory and expiratory times. Note that as flow rate changes, corresponding alterations are seen in effective time for inspiration and exhalation. Deflections above X-axis (time) indicate inspiration, and those below indicate exhalation. Delivered tidal volume for each cycle is the same, but inspiratory and expiratory times are different. (From Roberts and Hedges, editors: *Clinical procedures in emergency medicine,* ed 4, Philadelphia, 2008, Saunders.)

which allows for a longer period of expiration (Figure 12-2). The I:E ratio may be adjusted for disease pathology. Patients with reactive airway disease or asthma benefit from a longer expiratory time of 1:4 or more. Patients with hypoxia may benefit from a longer inspiratory time, reflective of an I:E time of 1:2. In some cases, I:E ratios of 1:1 can be attempted; however, these ratios may lead to hemodynamic compromise from auto-PEEP and contribute to volutrauma.

Although, for adults, flow rates of 60 L/min are usually adequate, higher flow is often needed to produce adequate ventilation, particularly in patients with obstructive lung disease.[6] Some transport ventilators are not equipped with the ability to adjust flow, and longer expiratory times are adjusted through the I:E ratio setting. The flow limitations of some transport ventilators, however, do limit extending of the expiration time and shortening of the inspiration time. In this situation, an inadequate time for expiration in patients with obstructive disease may lead to high plateau pressures, overdistention, and barotrauma. Clinicians can overcome this to some extent by decreasing the tidal volume or respiratory rate. This decrease may require some degree of respiratory acidosis to prevent lung overdistention from air trapping.

FLOW PATTERN

Some transport ventilators allow the clinician to select flow patterns, which dictate how an inspiratory flow is distributed. The primary waveforms available on transport ventilators are square (rectangular), sinusoidal (sine), and ramp (Figure 12-3). Flow pattern advantage depends on the patient's lung compliance, chest wall elasticity, airway resistance, and transport ventilator capability. Determination of which pattern optimizes ventilation-perfusion is not always predictable and is often an exercise of trial and error.[27]

Changing waveforms may require adjustments to the inspiratory flow or inspiratory time. Parameters should be checked after any change in flow pattern. In a review of studies during the past 40 years, the following conclusions can be drawn[23]:

- Mean airway pressure is higher with decelerating flow patterns than with accelerating patterns.
- Peak airway pressure is lower with decelerating patterns and higher with accelerating patterns.
- Gas distribution is improved with decelerating patterns.

TRIGGER-SENSITIVITY

An assisted breath (ACV, PCV, or PSV) can be triggered by either pressure or flow. *Pressure triggering* requires a demand valve that senses a negative airway pressure generated by the patient during initiation of a spontaneous respiratory effort. The demand valve sensitivity is set at a level that allows the patient to easily take a breath but not so sensitive that it interprets artifact, such as patient movement, air leak, or water in the ventilator circuit, as an attempted breath. This

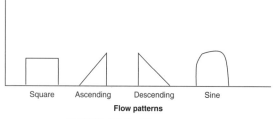

Square   Ascending   Descending   Sine

Flow patterns

FIGURE 12-3   **Flow patterns**.

could cause unintended hyperventilation, respiratory alkalosis, and auto-PEEP. If the sensitivity is set too high, the ventilator does not trigger a breath when the patient makes a spontaneous effort and increases the patient's work of breathing. The usual threshold is set at −1 to −3 cm H_2O.

Flow triggering detects a change in the flow of gas with spontaneous effort. A base flow continually moves past the patient. When the patient makes an inspiratory effort, the ventilator detects a deviation in the flow and is triggered to deliver a supported breath. A base flow of 10 L/min is often used with a trigger sensitivity threshold of 2 L/min.[19]

Changing of one ventilator parameter may affect other ventilator variables and should be reassessed after adjustments are made. For example, inspiratory time is equal to Vt divided by flow (Ti = Vt/flow), so when one of these parameters is changed, so are the others. Likewise, alteration in the FiO_2 may change the flow enough to alter the delivered tidal volume. Clinicians should be familiar with ventilator capabilities and limitations. Know the parameters that are automatically adjusted by the ventilator to compensate for changes made by the user.

VENTILATION STRATEGIES

PERMISSIVE HYPERCAPNEA

Normalizing pH and $PaCO_2$ in patients with obstructive lung disease or reduced pulmonary compliance often requires high tidal volumes and fast ventilatory rates that result in high peak inspiratory pressures and alveolar overdistention. *Permissive hypercapnea* is a lung protective strategy aimed at decreasing alveolar ventilation to prevent lung injury. The use of small tidal volumes produces higher $PaCO_2$ and lower pH. In permissive hypercapnea strategy, acidemia is tolerated to a pH of 7.20 to 7.25 mm Hg or lower. Hypercapnea and acidemia are not the goal of this approach, but rather the tolerated consequence. Acidosis at this level is generally well tolerated when achieved gradually.[20] The small tidal volumes associated with permissive hypercapnea may be uncomfortable and often requires sedation or paralysis to offset the increased respiratory drive and agitation associated with discomfort. The high $PaCO_2$ in permissive hypercapnea causes cerebral vasodilation and increased intracranial pressure. It is contraindicated in patients with head injuries or cerebral hemorrhage.

RECRUITMENT MANEUVERS

Recruitment maneuvers are an oxygenation strategy, for patients who need lung-protective ventilation management, that are aimed at reexpansion of atelectatic alveoli followed by the maintenance of optimal PEEP to prevent subsequent derecruitment. This technique may be most helpful in patients with significant alveolar atelectasis and derecruitment as a result of absent or insufficient level of PEEP delivery (e.g., after periods of endotracheal suctioning). Recruitment maneuvers refer to the application of elevated continuous airway pressure for variable duration, magnitude, and frequency to recruit collapsed alveoli and improve oxygenation. One technique studied in the ARDS Network trial is use of the CPAP mechanical ventilator mode with the CPAP set to 35 cm H_2O for 30 seconds.[8] The PEEP level after the recruitment maneuver can be set at the previous levels or higher for a period of time until oxygenation improves and is stabilized. To perform manually, hold a set continuous pressure generally less than 40 cm H_2O with a flow-inflating device for a defined period of time, generally less than 40 seconds. No consensus exists on the optimal alveolar recruitment strategy or whether this technique provides long-term improvements in oxygenation. The risks of this maneuver include alveolar overdistention, pneumothorax or pneumomediastinum, and hemodynamic compromise. Recruitment maneuvers are not suggested for the routine support of mechanically ventilated patients.

TROUBLESHOOTING

MONITORING

Patients on mechanical ventilation need vigilant and continuous monitoring of ventilator parameters and clinical assessment. Oxygen saturations and end-tidal carbon dioxide ($ETCO_2$) should be monitored, and their limitations in clinical use well understood. Pulse oximetry does not detect saturations below 83% with

the same degree of precision or accuracy as it does at higher saturations, nor does it perform well in low perfusion states. Many errors made in pulse oximetry readings are related to artifact. Pulse oximetry pulse reading should be compared with patient heart rate to ascertain accurate readings.

End-tidal carbon dioxide monitors have been shown to be accurate in hospital settings with healthy patients. However, prediction of $PaCO_2$ via $ETCO_2$ is not reliable in hypoperfusion states (hypovolemia, hypotension, reduced cardiac output) or in patients with ventilation-perfusion abnormalities. In normal conditions, the $ETCO_2$ reads 3 to 5 mm Hg lower than the $PaCO_2$. Changes in dead space or perfusion states related to treatment or worsening condition widen this gradient. Ventilation decisions made in these conditions may result in inappropriate patient management.

A baseline minute ventilation should be determined before a patient is transferred from a referring facility ventilator to a transport ventilator, particularly when ventilation modes are changed, to help guide adequacy in matching ventilation. Monitoring of minute ventilation also assists in the detection of hyperventilation or hypoventilation and reevaluation of treatment, ventilation mode, and ventilator settings.

VENTILATOR ALARMS

Alarm limits should be set to warn transport crew of mechanical and physiologic problems. Silencing alarms or changing limits without carefully considering the cause can be deleterious to the patient. Because peak inspiratory and plateau pressures are associated with VILI, alarm limits should be tightly controlled and assessed. Increased peak inspiratory pressure without change in plateau pressure is indicative of increased airway resistance, such as kinked endotracheal tube, secretions, bronchospasm or obstruction. Elevated peak *and* plateau pressures are associated with decreased compliance, such as pulmonary edema, pneumothorax, pleural effusions, or abdominal distension and auto-PEEP and asynchronous breathing.

Ventilator alarms are difficult to hear in the transport setting. They should be turned to maximal volume, and the machine should be positioned so that flashing alarm lights can be visualized. Airway status should be evaluated immediately with any patient deterioration. The DOPE acronym (*D,* displaced endotracheal tube; *O,* obstructed endotracheal tube; *P,* pneumothorax; *E,* equipment [ventilator] failure)[3] is a useful tool to remember possible causes of airway compromise (Box 12-2). If any question exists as to the cause of deterioration, the patient should be disconnected from the ventilator and manually ventilated until all possibilities are considered. Common ventilator alarms are listed in Table 12-3.

VENTILATOR ASYNCHRONY

Ventilator asynchrony occurs when disparity is found between patient respiratory effort and ventilator delivery, often described as "fighting the ventilator." Ideally, to unload the work of breathing and reduce respiratory distress, the ventilator should cycle with the patient's intrinsic respiratory rhythm.[6] Anxiety and discomfort are often associated with mechanical ventilation. Undersedation should be treated and reassessed. Initial ventilator settings can be adjusted after connecting the patient to the ventilator and assessing the patient's breathing pattern and demand. Generally speaking, spontaneous modes are more comfortable than control modes, and normal I:E ratios (1:2 or 1:3) are more comfortable than longer or inversed ratios.

TABLE 12-3	**Troubleshooting Ventilator Alarms**

Initial assessment:
- *Airway:* Is the endotracheal tube (ETT) in correct position? Check ETT insertion depth, check end tidal CO_2, check breath sounds.
- *Breathing:* Check breath sounds, look for chest excursion, check pulse oximetry, check patient color.
- *Circulation:* Check the pulse, electrocardiogram (ECG), and blood pressure.

Remove patient from the ventilator and manually use a resuscitation bag if any compromise is found.

Alarm	Cause	Management
Apnea	Insufficient spontaneous breathing by patient in CPAP or pressure-support mode.	Switch ventilator mode to one that provides set rate.
High airway pressure	ETT obstruction: sputum, kink, biting.	Suction airway.
	Decreased compliance or increased resistance.	Treat cause of resistance.
	Circumferential burns.	Adjust mode or settings.
	Bronchospasm, lung collapse, pneumothorax, endobronchial intubation, worsening of lung process.	Rule out hypoxia before treating agitation. CXR analysis.
	Anxiety/fear/pain/fighting of ventilator.	Change ventilator mode to one that is better tolerated or provides sedation/analgesia.
Low airway pressure	Ventilator disconnect.	Ensure that all connections are intact and tight.
	Leak in ventilator system.	
	Cuff leak.	Troubleshoot ETT cuff.
	Inadvertent extubation.	Bag-valve-mask if ETT was dislodged.
Oxygen pressure low	Oxygen cylinder is empty.	Check wall and cylinder connections.
	Cylinder valve is closed.	Bag-mask-ventilate until resolved.
	Unit not connected to wall terminal.	
	Aircraft/ambulance oxygen flow in off position.	

The patient's respiratory effort and triggering sensitivity should be assessed in assisted and spontaneous modes of ventilation, whether volume-limited or pressure-limited. If the sensitivity threshold is set too high, the patient's respiratory efforts are not recognized and the ventilator is not triggered to provide a breath. Alternately, if set too low, the ventilator auto-triggers or delivers breaths in response to extrinsic stimuli, such as patient movement or water in the circuit.

One problem related to volume-limited ventilators is inadequate flow of gas, which causes patients to feel that they are not getting enough air with attempts to extract more gas out of the ventilator.[33] This situation is uncomfortable for patients, and many transport ventilators only have the option of adjusting inspiratory time or I:E ratio and not flow. Patients with poor lung compliance or obstructive disease need high inspiratory flow rates to receive full tidal volume support during the set inspiratory time. Lengthening the inspiratory time compromises the long expiratory time needed by these patients who are already prone to air trapping and auto-PEEP.

Patient oxygenation and ventilation requirements may exceed the capabilities of some transport ventilators and may require deep sedation or neuromuscular blockade to complete the transport. This strategy should be undertaken after careful consideration of the cause of asynchrony, the ventilator capabilities, and alternative means of transport. More sophisticated transport ventilators and ventilation strategies often require the skill and knowledge of a respiratory therapist and the larger berth of an ambulance or fixed wing aircraft.

SUMMARY

Mechanical ventilation in the transport environment is challenging. The transport team must be familiar with indications for mechanical ventilation, pulmonary physiology, and the equipment that is used in the transport environment. This chapter provided an overview of these concepts. Transport team members must be skilled in this important transport concept.

MECHANICAL VENTILATION CASE STUDY 1

A 39-year-old 185-lb (84-kg) woman was seen at a rural Emergency Department with acute exacerbation of asthma. After medical interventions failed to reverse inadequate oxygenation and ventilation, she was paralyzed and sedated, intubated, and placed on a ventilator. On transport team arrival, the ventilator settings were: FiO$_2$, 100%; Vt, 850mL; assist-control rate, 35 breaths per minute; PEEP, 5mmHg. The corresponding arterial blood gas (ABG) results were: pH, 7.32; PaCO$_2$, 65; PaO$_2$, 60; oxygen saturation in arterial blood (SaO$_2$), 88%. The referring facility explained that they had increased tidal volume and rate three times in an attempt to decrease the PaCO$_2$; however, it continued to rise with each change. Other pertinent data: Ppk, 50 cm H$_2$O; blood pressure (BP), 88/62; heart rate (HR), 130; CXR showed overinflation and flattened diaphragms; breath sounds were diminished throughout. Initially, the transport team disconnected the patient from the ventilator and allowed her to completely exhale for almost 60 seconds. This maneuver improved BP to 125/82 and HR to 102. The ideal body weight for the 5'4" female was 50 kg. The initial settings on the transport ventilator were: FiO$_2$, 100%; Vt, 400 (8 mL/kg IBW); SIMV, 12; PEEP, 5mmHg; I:E, 1:3. The peak inspiratory pressures were elevated, so the team decreased the Vt to 300mL (6 mL/kg) and increased the respiratory rate to 16. The Ppk was reduced to 42. Continuous bronchodilator treatments were administered during transport and the patient was sedated and allowed to wake from the paralytic.

DISCUSSION

Patients with asthma are subject to airflow obstruction as a result of bronchospasm, airway inflammation, mucous plugging, and airway edema.[37] This obstruction limits the ability to completely exhale unless sufficient expiratory time is allowed. If left unchecked, hyperinflation, or auto-PEEP, can lead to increased intrathoracic pressures, decreased venous return, and cardiovascular collapse. In addition, the initial Vt of 850 mL set by the referring facility is 17 mL/kg of IBW (50 kg). With removal from the ventilator and full exhalation of trapped gas, the patient's hemodynamic state improved.

Mechanical ventilation strategies in patients with asthma are based on limiting gas trapping. Along with pharmacologic therapies to reduce obstruction, this can be accomplished with the ventilator through use of low tidal volumes (less gas to expire), lower respiratory rates (more time to exhale), and reduction of inspiratory time (longer expiration).[37] The ventilator used on this transport was limited to an I:E ratio of 1:3 and had no ability to directly adjust the inspiratory flow. Therefore, the team elected to reduce the tidal volume to lessen airway distention and high airway pressures. Permissive hypercapnia is an established strategy to control hyperinflation and reduce the potential of further lung injury in asthma. If, after these strategies are used, the pH remains less than 7.2, further sedation and chemical paralysis should be considered to reduce carbon dioxide production. No studies have shown any benefit in the use of sodium bicarbonate to treat pH of less than 7.2 in these patients.

MECHANICAL VENTILATION CASE STUDY 2

A previously healthy 11-year-old 50-kg child was admitted to the pediatric department of a community hospital with a diagnosis of respiratory distress and tracheitis from influenza B. He had a 7-day history of sore throat, lethargy, and fever. On admission, he had a room air saturation of 71%, increased work of breathing, and normal CXR results. Broad-spectrum antibiotics were started. The patient's oxygen saturation improved with a 15-L nonrebreather facemask. However, the patient's work of breathing continued to increase as evidenced by tachypnea, use of accessory respiratory muscles, and grunting, despite nebulized treatments of racemic epinephrine and albuterol. He was placed on facemask BiPAP of 16 IPAP and 10 EPAP. The child tolerated this method well but, despite this, showed signs of ongoing respiratory compromise and was referred for a higher level of care. The transport team arrived to find the patient sleeping, in a high Fowler's position, on BiPAP with 100% O_2. He woke quickly to verbal stimulation with appropriate mentation; although when he was not actively stimulated, he was unable to remain awake. Hemodynamics were stable with normal peripheral pulses, BP, and perfusion. The patient had a labored respiratory rate of 42 and was only able to speak in one-word to two-word sentences. Breath sounds were noted to be clear on the right and absent on the left, with an absence of wheezing. Recent ABG results showed a pH of 7.34, a $PaCO_2$ of 44, and a PaO_2 of 63. A discussion ensued among the flight team, referring staff, and medical control on the optimal airway support options for transport, which included continuing facemask BiPAP or proceeding with endotracheal intubation. Given the concerns of ongoing respiratory distress and signs of fatigue despite BiPAP, the patient underwent intubation to provide invasive oxygenation and ventilation support. During the laryngoscopy, purulent copious secretions were suctioned from the supraglottic area, which were sent for culture. After successful intubation, confirmed with end-tidal CO_2, the oxygen saturation decreased to 75%. To aid oxygenation, the patient was sedated and long-acting paralytic was administered. Breath sounds remained absent on the left, with the patient now exhibiting a visibly depressed left hemithorax. Postintubation CXR results showed the endotracheal tube 2 cm above the carina and a near whiteout over the left lung field with volume loss, suggestive of significant atelectasis. In an attempt to recruit collapsed alveoli and thereby improve oxygenation, the PEEP was increased to 10 mm Hg and the patient's oxygen saturation increased to 84%. The initial transport ventilator settings were as follows: SIMV rate, 20; Vt, 300 (6 mL/kg); FiO_2, 1.0; PEEP, 10; Ti, 0.8; I:E, 1:2.7, and pressure-limit, 40.

During the 25-minute flight, capillary blood gas (CBG) results showed a pH of 7.21, $PaCO_2$ of 60, and PaO_2 of 60. No ventilator changes were made. En route, the saturations decreased to 78%, and in response, the PEEP was increased to 13 cm H_2O and Ti adjusted to provide an I:E of 1:2, with a corresponding increase in oxygen saturation to 82%. On arrival, CXR results showed reexpansion of the left lung and no further visual discrepancy was noted between the right and left hemithorax.

In the intensive care unit (ICU), the patient continued to have difficulty with oxygenation and ventilation and was placed on HFOV with the following settings: delta P, 94; P_{aw}, 36; and Hertz, 7. Vasoactive drugs and fluid boluses were required for hemodynamic instability. The supraglottic culture was positive for group A Streptococcus and methicillin-sensitive Staphylococcus aureus. On day 5 in pediatric ICU, the patient was weaned to conventional pressure support with SIMV, and on day 6 was extubated after a spontaneous breathing trial. The child was discharged to home 5 days later.

REFERENCES

1. American Association of Respiratory Care: Consensus statement on the essentials of mechanical ventilators, *Respir Care* 37(9):1000-1008, 1992.
2. American Heart Association: *Advanced cardiac life support provider manual*, Dallas, 2006, American Heart Association.
3. American Heart Association: *Pediatric advanced life support provider manual*, Dallas, 2006, American Heart Association.
4. Adult Respiratory Distress Syndrome Network: Ventilation with lower tidal volumes for acute lung injury and the acute respiratory distress syndrome, *N Engl J Med* 342(18):1301-1308, 2000.
5. Austin, PN, Campbell RS, Johannigman JA, et al: Transport ventilators, *Respir Care Clin* 8:119-150, 2002.
6. Bhan U, Hyzy RC: Conventional mechanical ventilation. In Parsons, editor: UptoDate, Waltham, MA, 2008, UpToDate® Inc.
7. Brain Trauma Foundation: Guidelines for the management of severe brain injury third edition, *J Neurotrauma* 24(1):S1-S105, 2007.
8. Brower RG, Morris A, MacIntyre N: Effects of recruitment maneuvers in patients with acute lung injury and acute respiratory distress syndrome ventilated with high positive end-expiratory pressure, *Crit Care Med* 31(11):2592-2597, 2004.
9. Dreyfuss D, Basset G, Soler P, et al: Intermittent positive-pressure hyperventilation with high inflation pressures produces pulmonary microvascular injury in rats, *Am Rev Respir Dis* 132(4): 880-884, 1985.
10. Eisner MD, Thompson BT, Schoenfeld D, et al: Airway pressures and early barotrauma in patients with acute lung injury and acute respiratory distress syndrome, *Am J Respir Crit Care Med* 165(7):978-982, 2002.
11. Evans TW, Albert RK, Angus DC, et al: International consensus conferences in intensive care medicine: noninvasive positive pressure ventilation in acute respiratory failure, *Am J Crit Care Med* 163(1):283-291, 2001.
12. Feller-Kopman D, O'Donnell C: Physiology and clinical use of heliox. In Bochner BS, editor: UptoDate, Waltham, MA, 2007, UpToDate®, Inc.
13. Fisher AB, Forman HJ, Glass M: Mechanisms of pulmonary oxygen toxicity, *Lung* 162(1):255-259, 1984.
14. Fuhrman BP: Avoidance of ventilator induced lung injury, *Pharmacologica Sinica* 23:S44-47, 2002.
15. Gajic O, Dara SI, Mendez JL, et al: Ventilator-associated lung injury in patients without acute lung injury at the onset of mechanical ventilation, *Crit Care Med* 32(9):1817–1824, 2004.
16. Gammon RB, Shin MS, Groves RH, et al: Clinical risk factors for pulmonary: barotrauma a multivariate analysis, *Am J Respir Crit Care Med* 152(4):1235-1240, 1995.
17. Hager DN, Krishnan JA, Hayden DL, et al: Tidal volume reduction in patients with acute lung injury when plateau pressures are not high, *Am J Respir Crit Care Med* 172:1241-1245, 2005.
18. Hess DR, Kacmarek RM: *Essentials of mechanical ventilation*, San Francisco, 1996, McGraw-Hill.
19. Hill LL, Pearl RG: Flow triggering, pressure triggering, and autotriggering during mechanical ventilation, *Crit Care Med* 28(2):579-581, 2000.
20. Hivela E: Advances in the management of acute respiratory distress syndrome, *Arch Surg* 135(2):126-135, 2000.
21. Huynh T, Messer M, Sing RF, et al: Positive end-expiratory pressure alters intracranial and cerebral perfusion pressure in severe traumatic brain injury, *J Trauma-Injury Infect Crit Care* 53(3):488-493, 2002.
22. Ito Y, Veldhuizen RAW, Yao L, et al: Ventilation strategies affect surfactant aggregate conversion in acute lung injury, *Am J Respir Crit Care Med* 155(2):493-499, 1997.
23. Kacmarek RM, Chipman D: Basic principles of ventilator machinery. In Tobin MJ, editor: *Principles and practice of mechanical ventilation*, ed 2, San Francisco, 2006, McGraw-Hill.
24. Kolobow T, Moretti MP, Fumagali R, et al: Severe impairment in lung function induced by high peak airway pressure during mechanical ventilation: an experimental study, *Am Rev Respir Dis* 135(2):312-315, 1987.
25. Kramer N, Meyer TJ, Meharg J, et al: Randomized prospective trial of noninvasive positive pressure ventilation in acute respiratory failure, *Am J Respir Crit Care Med* 151(6):1799-1806, 1995.
26. Kratzert B, Minokadeh A: Plateau or mean pressure as a more accurate assessment of barotrauma than peak pressure. In Marcucci LA, Martinez EA, Haut ER, et al, editors: *Avoiding common ICU errors*, Philadelphia, PA, 2006, Lippincott Williams & Wilkins.
27. MacIntyre NR: Principles of mechanical ventilation. In Mason RJ, Murray JF, Broaddus VC, et al, editors: *Murray and Nadel's textbook of respiratory medicine*, ed 4, Philadelphia, 2005, Elsevier Saunders.
28. Martin TJ, Hovis JD, Costantino JP, et al: A randomized, prospective evaluation of noninvasive ventilation

for acute respiratory failure, *Am J Respir Crit Care Med* 161(3):807-813, 2000.

29. Nava S, Ambrosina N, Clini E, et al: Noninvasive mechanical ventilation in the weaning of patients with respiratory failure due to chronic obstructive pulmonary disease a randomized, controlled trial, *Ann Internal Med* 128(9):721-728, 1998.

30. Passini L: Trustworthy transport ventilators, *AirMed* 4(3):22-24, 1998.

31. Pelosi P, Croci M, Ravagnan I, et al: Total respiratory system, lung, and chest wall mechanics in sedated-paralyzed postoperative morbidly obese patients, *Chest* 109(1):144-151, 1996.

32. Phillips K, Hyzy RC: Noninvasive positive pressure ventilation in acute respiratory failure. In Parsons PE, editor: UptoDate, Waltham, MA, 2007, UpToDate®, Inc.

33. Sassoon CS, Foster GT: Patient-ventilator asynchrony, *Curr Opin Crit Care* 7(1):28-33, 2001.

34. Schnapp LM, Chin DP, Szaflarski N, et al: Frequency and importance of barotrauma in 100 patients with acute lung injury, *Crit Care Med* 23(2):272-278, 1995.

35. Sedeek KA, Takeuchi, M, Suchodolski, K, et al: Determinants of tidal volume during high-frequency oscillation, *Crit Care Med* 31(1):227-231, 2003.

36. Sinuff T, Keenan SP: Clinical practice guideline for the use of noninvasive positive pressure ventilation in COPD patients with acute respiratory failure, *J Crit Care* 19(2):82-91, 2004.

37. Stather DR, Stewart TE: Clinical review: mechanical ventilation in severe asthma, *Crit Care Online J* 9: 581-587 (DOI 10.1186/cc3733), 2005.

38. Sola A, Rogido MR, Deulofeut R: Oxygen as a neonatal health hazard: call for détente in clinical practice, *ACTA Paediatrics* 96(6):801-812, 1992.

39. Soo Hoo GW, Santiago S, Williams A: Nasal mechanical ventilation for hypercapnic respiratory failure in chronic obstructive pulmonary disease: determinants of success and failure, *Crit Care Med* 22(8):1253-1261, 1994.

40. Sugiura M, McMulloch PR, Wren S, et al: Ventilator pattern influences neutrophil influx and activation in atelectasis-prone rabbit lung, *J Applied Physiol* 77(3):1355-1365, 1994.

41. Ventre KM, Arnold JF: High frequency oscillatory ventilation. In Wheeler, Wong, Shanley, editors: *Pediatric critical care medicine: basic science and clinical evidence*, New York, NY, 2008, Springer-Verlag.

42. Ventre KM, Arnold JH: High frequency oscillatory ventilation in acute respiratory failure, *Paediatr Respir Rev* 5(4):323-332, 2004.

43. Welty S, Hansen TN, Corbet A: Respiratory distress in the preterm infant. In Taeusch HW, Ballard RA, Gleason CA, et al, editors: *Avery's diseases of the newborn*, ed 8, Philadelphia, 2004, Elsevier Saunders.

TECHNOLOGY IN TRANSPORT

Wesley Chasteen, Scott R. Singel

COMPETENCIES

1. Identify the use of new technologies in both air and ground communication systems.
2. Describe some of the new technologies that may be used for patient care.
3. Identify equipment that can be used for safe medical transport operations.

The pace of technologic advances over the past several decades has been dramatic. Concurrently, the healthcare industry has revolutionized its technology, with it becoming smaller, faster, more efficient, and more sophisticated. This technology not only includes equipment used during transport, such as satellite tracking, but also the equipment used to maintain and sustain a patient's life.

This chapter provides an overview of technology currently used in the transport environment and a review of communication devices, patient care, and documentation systems. It ends with information about technology that can improve safe operations, particularly in the air medical transport environment.

The chapter is not a comprehensive approach to all technology that may be available in air and ground transport, but it is an attempt to concentrate on some common pieces of equipment that

may be encountered in the transport environment. Technology continues to evolve and challenge those who must move critically ill and injured patients, and transport teams must be familiar with and ready to adopt this technology as needed to improve patient care and make the environment in which they operate as safe as possible.

COMMUNICATIONS

SATELLITE PHONE SYSTEMS

Communications in the air medical industry has acted as a lifeline for providers since its start. Most services use two standard types of radio communication: *very high frequency* (VHF) and *ultra high frequency* (UHF). VHF is a communication option that uses ranges from 30 Mhz to 300 Mhz. VHF is commonly referred to as "line of sight" communication and is ideal for the relaying of information over short terrestrial distances. Not commonly affected by atmosphere or electrical equipment, VHF frequencies are a reliable source of communications for the air medical industry. UHF is another commonly used frequency option in the prehospital environment. Unlike VHF, UHF frequencies use a spectrum of 300 Mhz to 3 Ghz, the same spectrum that modern cellular phones use. These frequencies are useful for longer range communications when used in concurrence with local repeaters to relay signals. Both UHF and VHF frequencies are still currently in use, but newer technology has surfaced to increase the reliability and range of air medical communications.[10]

The use of satellite-based devices has been a mainstay in aviation for many years. *Global positioning systems* (GPS) rely on satellite up links to provide aviators and ground crews with real-time position updates and directional assistance. The use of satellite technology has now found its way into other aspects of medical transport. Most air and ground emergency medical service (EMS) units have relied on complex radio hardware, which uses repeater systems to communicate with other units and the communications base. These systems are reliable but can pose problems when communication is initiated from low outlying areas. The introduction of the satellite phone messaging system (SATphone) has solved many of these issues.[10]

The *SATphone* operates by sending messages to satellites of the vendor for processing. The message then is routed to its destination via a landline or cellular network. Verbal communication is made through headsets on the internal communication system inside the aircraft. This technology prevents limitations during communications and allows access from virtually anywhere and in any type of meteorologic condition.[10]

Twelve-Lead Electrocardiographic Transmissions

Prehospital *12-lead electrocardiographic* (ECG) interpretations have become an invaluable tool in the diagnosis and proper treatment of acute myocardial infarction (AMI). The use of cellular telephone services has now given the field practitioner the ability to transmit these tracings to the receiving facility to facilitate treatment. Research has shown dramatic decreases in patient morbidity rates with use of this system. Many varieties of monitor defibrillators possess the ability to transmit ECGs with the placement of the appropriate upgrades by the particular vendor. Among these is the Rosetta-Lt model 7100 data translator for the LifePack 12 (Figure 13-1). This upgrade allows transmission over UHF, VHF, cellular, and landlines during continued transport in a moving vehicle. Fully formatted 12-lead ECGs can be transmitted in less than 1 minute. Once the transmission has been initiated, the tracing is received at the facility of choice at a stationary central computer with printing capabilities. Recent studies have shown a marked decrease in "door-to-drug" times and in diversion of EMS crews to appropriate facilities capable of performing cardiac catheterization. Currently, research is being performed to assess the effectiveness of the same transmission relayed to a specific cardiologist's handheld personal data device.[5]

Digital Patient Charting Systems

Patient care reports (PCR) are an essential tool for the relaying of information from prehospital providers

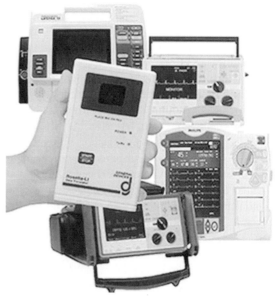

FIGURE 13-1   **Rosetta-Lt model 7100 data translator for LifePack 12**. (Courtesy General Devices, Inc, Ridgefield, NJ.)

to receiving hospitals.[3,8] Significant upgrades in this field have allowed for more efficient tracking and documentation of patient encounters. The practice of paper charting and patient flow sheets has been replaced with the introduction of digital charting through the use of portable computer tablets for prehospital personnel.

Many products are available on the market, such as Panasonic's Tough book, Toshiba's Tablet PC, and Golden Hour software; these products are increasing in popularity among air medical and ground EMS personnel. These charting devices are wireless and portable for easy mobility. They are encased in a shock-mounted carrier, which makes them extremely durable and well suited to meet the demands of both air and ground transport teams. Keyboards on the units are sealed to prevent contamination from bodily fluids encountered during transport. Some key benefits of digital charting are the ability to transfer precise patient information to receiving facilities and the ability to perform research and trends in patient care. The computerized format also allows for a more accurate approach to quality assurance and improvement.

TRACKING SYSTEMS

Satellite Tracking

To ensure the safety of both crew members and on-board patients, air medical transport units must be constantly tracked by communication officers. The Federal Aviation Administration (FAA) and individual flight programs set requirements for current position reports on all aircraft. When aircraft fail to meet the time requirements for these reports, emergency procedures are put into action.

Currently, with the introduction of satellite tracking systems, communication officers have the ability to constantly track and monitor aircraft location without the need for radio reports. Vendors such as Skyconnect offer these advanced services.[9] The global satellite tracking system uses 66 Low Earth Orbiting (LEO) satellites to maintain constant monitoring of inbound and outbound aircraft. The fleet can be equipped with a mission management unit (Figure 13-2), which is implanted into the cockpit control panel. The program director then has the ability to

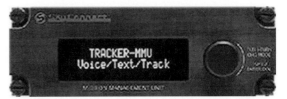

FIGURE 13-2 **Example of Mission Management Unit (MMU).** (Courtesy SkyConnect, Inc, Tacoma Park, Md.)

set the rate at which position reports are recorded. The tracking system is equipped with audio interface to dial direct numbers or send status reports via push button technology. The system is also compatible with other software to provide weather overlays, flight restrictions, and logging of events during flight. The system allows flight plan documentation for FAA auditing purposes.

Traffic Alert Systems

Air medical transport has been the subject of scrutiny because of numerous accidents in previous years. Satellite technology has contributed to a great decrease in these incidents. The *Traffic Collision Avoidance System* (TCAS) was created by the FAA to address the topic of mid-air collisions.[7] The TCAS operates freely of the ground-based Air Traffic Control (ATC) system. Currently, two types of TCAS are in use. *Type I* is for general aviation (GA) aircraft. The system sends advisories to pilots to assist in visual acquisition of aircraft that invade their flight path. *Type II* is a more sophisticated model in which, on identification of incoming traffic in the area, the program analyzes possible flight paths of the approaching aircraft. Along with path analysis, the issuance of resolution advisories (RAs) to operators provides a plan of action for avoidance of approaching aircraft.

Infrared Technology

The military has contributed a great amount of technology that is currently being adopted by civilian aviation agencies. Among these is the use of forward-looking infrared systems (FLIR). Infrared systems allow air crews to scan ahead of, and side to side of, their flight plan for tracking of approaching aircraft. Incoming images can be displayed on screens mounted in the control panel of the cockpit. FLIR technology is beneficial to EMS helicopter programs that perform search and rescue and for the tracking of downed aircraft. In addition to these specific uses, it is also used as an automated tracking device and landing assistance for night time operations and in severe meteorologic conditions. This specific system combines pinpoint tracking capabilities with aircraft collision avoidance technology. DRS Technologies is a leading vendor in this field and provides service to all branches of the Department of Defense (DOD).

AVIATION SYSTEMS

WIDE AREA AUGMENTATION SYSTEM

The global positioning system uses 24 satellites placed approximately 26,560 km above the center of the earth. These satellites broadcast continuous ranging signals that allow the GPS receiver to calculate its position relative to four or more satellites.

The *wide area augmentation system* (WAAS) augments this system by increasing the accuracy of the ranging signals. First, ranging signals are broadcast by communications satellites to increase the number of available reference points. Second, a nationwide ground network is used with fixed calibration points to evaluate the quality of the satellite ranging signals. Corrections are calculated for use by the GPS receiver, or the system advises that a ranging signal will not be used. These services address what are called integrity errors, which occur when the signal data are poor but, without a reference, cannot be detected. This correction improves the accuracy of the system from approximately 100 m to 8 m, a significant improvement in landings that are adjacent to multistory hospitals.[6]

NIGHT VISION GOGGLES

In a study done at the air medical transport conference (AMTC) in 2005, 94% of participants agreed that landing at a night scene was the most hazardous component of the mission. Survey participants also believed that the ground personnel on site did not adequately identify hazards at a scene. *Night vision goggles* address this problem by amplifying ambient light and giving the flight crew a clear view of the terrain features and obstacles. Although support for night vision goggles was not unanimous, 95% of participants from programs that operated in mountainous terrain supported use of night vision goggles.[2]

REAL-TIME WEATHER

Because weather significantly influences the safety of any transport, all pilots check weather reports before departure. However, weather is dynamic and can change rapidly; therefore, a system that presents real-time weather information during the flight contributes to safety. In 2003, WSI Corporation, a subsidiary of Landmark Communications, introduced a cockpit weather system that continuously broadcasts weather information directly to the cockpit via a satellite service.[3]

ACTIVE NOISE SUPPRESSION

One of the most irritating components of helicopter interior noise comes from high frequency structure-borne gear-mesh tones generated within the transmission. Passive noise suppression is traditional but adds volume and mass. Sikorsky Aircraft Corporation is engaged in a program to actively suppress gear mesh noise in the S-76. Structural actuation surrounding the gearbox mounts is used to cancel the gear-mesh vibration before it impacts the airframe (Figure 13-3). In the initial flight test in 1995, the primary gear-mesh tone (~800 Hz) was reduced by 7 to 12 dB. Follow-up flight tests in 1996 and 1997 achieved a 10 to 20 dB reduction.

To appreciate the extent of the noise suppression, consider that the decibel is a logarithmic unit that describes a ratio. Reduction of the sound level by half generates a decibel reduction of 3.

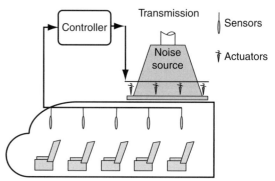

FIGURE 13-3   **Schematic of gear-mesh ANC architecture.** (From Millott TA, Welsh WA, Yoerkie CA Jr, et al: *Flight test of active gear-mesh noise control on the S-76 aircraft,* Proceedings of the 54th AHS Annual Forum, Washington, DC, May 1998.)

CABIN AIRFLOW

In transport of patients with airborne infectious diseases, such as severe acute respiratory syndrome (SARS), cabin airflow should be considered. Aircraft with a forward-to-aft cabin air flow and a separate cockpit cabin have reduced exposure of flight deck personnel. Aircraft that recirculate cabin and flight-deck air should have high efficiency particulate arresting (HEPA) filtration. In aircraft with uncontrolled interior air flow, such as helicopters, all personnel should wear disposable N-95 or higher respirators during transport of these patients.[4]

FUTURE SYSTEMS

TILT ROTOR

Many longer transports are done more efficiently via fixed wing. Currently, rotor-wing programs must refer the flight; even then, the flight needs to be airport to airport. Soon, a hybrid aircraft will be available to the civilian market and will allow direct transfer of these patients. Bell/Augusta Aerospace Company is introducing the BA 609 tilt-rotor aircraft. With a maximum cruise speed of 275 knots and a range of up to 1000 nautical miles, this aircraft may be ideal for many programs when the economies of scale bring the cost within reach.[1]

EMERGENCY CARE PRACTITIONER

The *emergency care practitioner* (ECP) is a paramedic with extensive additional training that includes diagnostics and pharmacology. In a pilot program in Essex, 12 paramedics received 24 months of full-time training that enabled them to administer 30 medications, including antibiotics, on the basis of patient group directions (PGDs). The ECPs see, treat, discharge, and refer patients in the out-of-hospital environment.[8]

SUMMARY

This chapter has addressed some of the technology that can be used for communications, patient care, and documentation in addition to technology that makes operations within transport easier and safer. The chapter concluded with some future possibilities so that medical transport can continue to meet the challenges of the 21st century.

REFERENCES

1. Bell/Agusta Aerospace Company: *The BA609: the world's first civilian tiltrotor,* available at http://www.bellagusta.com/air_ba_main.cfm, accessed January 2008.
2. Boonatra T, National EMS Pilots Association: NVG conclusions, *J Emerg Med Sys Pilots* 1-2, 1999, available at http://nemspa.org/nvgconclusions.html, accessed January 2008.
3. Boston Business Journal: *WSI cockpit weather system get FAA nod, Boston Business J* available at http://bostonbizjournals.com/boston/stories/2003/07/28/daily3.html?t=printable, accessed July 2003.
4. Centers for Disease Control: *Guidance on air medical transport for SARS patients,* available at http://www.cdc.gov?ncidod/sars/airtransport-sarspatients.htm, accessed January 2008.
5. Clemmensen P, Sejersten M, Sillesen M, et al: Diversion of ST-elevation myocardial infarction patients for primary angioplasty based on wireless prehospital 12 lead electrocardiographic transmission directly to the cardiologist's handheld computer: a progress report, *J Electrocardiol* 38:194-198, 2005, available at http://www.sciencedirect.com/science?_ob=ArticleURL&-udi=B6WJ4–4H9P5BT-3B&user=709071, accessed October 2008.
6. Enge P, Walter T, Pullen S, et al: Wide area augmentation of the global positioning system, *Proceedings IEEE* 8(8):1-8, 1996.
7. Federal Aviation Administration: *TCAS logic system,* available at http://adsb.tc.faa.gov/TCAS.htm, accessed January 2008.
8. Marsh A: *Emergency care practitioners,* available at http://216.109.125.130/search/cache?ei=UTF8&p=Emergency+Care+Practitioner&fr=yfp-t338-s&u=w, accessed February 2008.
9. SkyConnect: *EagleMed: saving lives, a case study,* available at http://www2.skyconnect.aero/1060.xml, accessed January 2008.
10. Strong R: *How do satellite phones work?* available at http://www.redsofts.com/articles/read/190/18959/How_Do_Satellite_Phones_Work.html, accessed January 2008.

SHOCK MANAGEMENT

Reneé Semonin Holleran

Shock has been described as the "rude unhinging of the machinery of life or a momentary pause in the act of death."[52] The pathophysiology of shock causes inadequate tissue perfusion, which results in the body's inability to meet its demands. This inability causes an alteration in cellular metabolism, which triggers the release of inflammatory mediators that promote a process that leads to coagulation disorders, continued hyperinflammatory response, organ damage, and death.[78] Despite the technologies and treatments available today, the mortality rate from shock remains high. Mortality and morbidity related to shock are best managed through prevention, early recognition, and rapid transport to definitive care.[2,16,26,28,33-35,51]

Shock is divided into three major phases: a compensatory stage, a progressive stage, and an irreversible stage. Shock can result from alterations in circulating volume, cardiac pump function, and peripheral vascular resistance. It causes a myriad of physiologic changes in the nervous, respiratory, renal, and gastrointestinal systems. Alteration in circulating volume, particularly hemorrhage, is one of the most common causes of shock and one that is frequently encountered by transport teams.

A complication of hemorrhage is the development of coagulopathy, which can be caused by dilutional effects of massive transfusions, continued bleeding, and hypothermia.[7,23,29,44] Disseminated intravascular coagulation (DIC) is a potential secondary complication of shock. DIC may be found in critically ill patients when transport has been delayed.[2]

This chapter discusses the etiology, pathophysiology, and initial management of shock. It also includes a discussion about coagulopathies that may challenge the care of patients in transport.

ETIOLOGY

Some of the causes of shock are summarized in Box 14-1. Although multiple causes have been identified as contributing to shock, the pathophysiology is essentially the same.

PATHOPHYSIOLOGY

The research on shock during the past 20 years has focused on the role of the immune system and the multisystem effects of clinical insult. The initial systemic inflammatory response that occurs after clinical insult is actually a protective mechanism. However, with prolonged inadequate tissue perfusion and consequential tissue oxygen debt, the body actually goes into a hyperinflammatory state that triggers a variety of systemic responses.

The immune system reacts with the activation of a complement cascade, which causes the release of cytokines such as tissue necrosis factor (TNF) and interleukin-1 (IN-1). In addition to cytokines, nitric oxide, reactive oxygen species, and growth factors are stimulated, which results in the triggering of polymorphonuclear neutrophils (PMNs),

endothelium macrophages, and lymphocytes.[53] These substances lead to bronchoconstriction, platelet aggregation, capillary permeability, and resultant vasoconstriction and vasodilation.[60] Specific products used for shock resuscitation can also contribute to an inflammatory response.[53] Recent research has shown a decrease in multiple organ failure complications after shock when a decrease occurred in the amount of blood transfusions used during resuscitation.[27] This research may also affirm the role of the immune and inflammatory responses in shock.

Even when shock or inadequate perfusion has been recognized, the resultant tissue ischemia and cell death continues to incite an inflammatory response. This process is known as reperfusion and inflammatory injury.[43]

Ischemic tissue in vulnerable organs converts xanthine dehydrogenase found in the vascular endothelium to xanthine oxidase (XO). Even when oxygen becomes available to ischemic tissues, the XO creates a burst of reactive oxygen metabolites that actually cause additional tissue injury.[60] Tissue injury stimulates more PMNs and the inflammatory process continues to contribute to multiple organ failure.[43]

SYSTEMIC INFLAMMATORY RESPONSE SYNDROME

In 1977, Eisman, Beart, and Norton[36] introduced a term called *multiple organ failure*. These authors described a man-made syndrome that involved principally the failure of the at least two major organ systems (i.e., pulmonary, renal, gastrointestinal, or

---

BOX 14-1 | **Etiology of Shock**

Hemorrhagic: Acute blood loss from an internal or external vascular injury.

External: Penetrating trauma, amputation, and open fractures.

Internal: Injury (splenic, liver); fractures, particularly pelvic; body tissue injury; bleeding from other internal source such as GI tract; and esophageal varices.

Hypovolemia: Fluid loss such as from third spacing, burn injury, vomiting, diarrhea, diabetes mellitus, diabetes insipidus, and diuresis.

Neurogenic: Spinal cord injury; alteration in vascular tone from drugs, food, plants, and venom.

Anaphylaxis: Allergic reaction to a foreign substance including drugs, food, plants, and venom.

Obstructive: Obstruction of blood flow (e.g., from a tension pneumothorax or cardiac tamponade).

Cardiac: Pump failure that may result from a myocardial infarction, valvular malfunction, septal defect, right-sided infarct, or direct injury to the heart such as a myocardial contusion.

Sepsis: Infectious agent that compromises the host defense mechanism.

hematologic). The authors tied it into an infectious process.[36]

The mechanism by which bacteria destroys so many remote organs remains unknown. Various toxins have been suspected but not universally proven.

Another interesting point raised in this paper was the expense and the ethics involved in keeping these patients alive.[36]

In the 1980s, several endogenous mediators were discovered that mimic a septic shock response in animal models. Multiple insults were also found to trigger these responses.[87] Soon, similar cascades were observed in patients, and reports began to appear in the literature to offer potential explanations as to why not all patients could be successfully resuscitated from an uncompensated or irreversible shock state.[59] However, many patients in whom septic shock, and eventually multiple organ failure and death, developed were discovered to not be infected at all.

In 1991, a consensus conference introduced the concept of *systemic inflammatory response syndrome* (SIRS) and the criteria to describe where patients fall on the continuum of shock.[15] These definitions are summarized in Box 14-2. This is the inflammatory model of shock or, as stated by Gross, "the rude unhinging of the machinery of life."[19]

BOX 14-2   Definitions

Sepsis Syndrome

Clinical evidence of infection
Rectal temperature, >38.3°C or <35.6°C
Tachycardia (>90 beats per minute)
Tachypnea (>20 breaths per minute)
At least one of the manifestations of inadequate tissue function/perfusion:
- Alteration in mental status
- Hypoxemia (PaO_2 < 72 mm Hg at FiO_2 0.21; overt pulmonary disease not the direct cause of hypoxemia)
- Elevated plasma lactate level
- Oliguria (urine output, 30 mL or 0.5 mL/kg for at least 1 h)

Systemic Inflammatory Response Syndrome

Two or more of the following conditions:
- Temperature, >38°C or <36°C
- Heart rate, >90 beats per minute
- Respiratory rate, >20 breaths per minute or PaO_2 < 32 mm Hg
- White blood cell count, >12.10^9 /L, <4.10^9 /L, or >10% immature (band) forms

Sepsis

The systemic response to infection manifested by two or more of the conditions mentioned under SIRS (SIRS related to infection).

Severe Sepsis

Sepsis associated with organ dysfunction, hypoperfusion, or hypotension. Hypoperfusion and perfusion abnormalities may include, but are not limited to, lactic acidosis, oliguria, or acute alteration in mental status.

Septic Shock

Sepsis-induced hypotension despite adequate fluid resuscitation along with the presence of perfusion abnormalities that may include, but are not limited to, lactic acidosis, oliguria, or acute alteration in mental state. Patients who are receiving inotropic or vasopressor agents may not be hypotensive at the time that perfusion abnormalities are measured.

Multiple Organ Dysfunction Syndrome

The presence of altered organ function in an acutely ill patient such that homeostasis cannot be maintained without intervention.

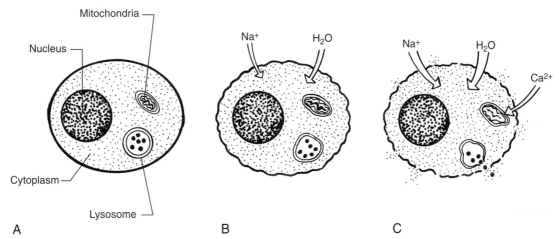

FIGURE 14-1 **A,** Normal cell. **B,** Massive amounts of water and sodium enter cytoplasm, causing blebs to develop. **C,** Calcium changes in mitochondria cause destruction; lysosomes rupture, spilling proteolytic enzymes into cytoplasm; cell wall loses integrity, and cell dies. (Modified from Kitt S, et al: *Emergency nursing,* Philadelphia, 1995, Saunders.)

Multiple Organ Dysfunction Syndrome

Bone[15] has described *multiple organ dysfunction syndrome* (MODS) as a clinical syndrome characterized by the development of potentially reversible physiologic dysfunction in two or more organ systems.[15,33] This pathology can be caused by a variety of acute insults, including trauma, sepsis, and poison. Research has shown that little consensus exists on what exactly constitutes MODS. However, most experts agree that the following seven systems are generally included in the definition: cardiovascular, central nervous, gastrointestinal, hematologic, hepatic, renal, and respiratory systems.

The patient with MODS is generally transported after a referring center can no longer provide care.[2] These patients present a unique challenge because they are more likely to have multiple invasive lines, treatment with many medications, and complex ventilator settings. Chapter 12 discusses the ventilatory management of these cases.

Cellular Response

A reduction in the amount of available oxygen causes an alteration in cellular metabolism, resulting in a cascade of significant cellular changes and leading to injury and death if interventions prove ineffective or are too late. Figures 14-1 and 14-2 illustrate the cellular and micropathophysiologic changes that occur during cellular ischemia.[20,38,59,61]

Body Systems Response

The transport team must always be cognizant of the causes of shock and the subtlety of its signs and symptoms in its early stages. They must also take into account comorbid risk factors that cause additional stress on the patient's body systems and that may increase a patient's risk of compromise, even with a moderate illness or injury. Some of these factors include a history of cardiovascular disease, pulmonary disease, or diabetes. Research continues to show that shock needs to be treated and reversed as soon as possible to prevent additional injury and eventual death.[5,9,77]

Regardless of the source of shock, if it is not quickly recognized, the concomitant changes that occur in blood pressure, blood flow, and volume and the alterations in oxygen transport that cause hypoxia lead to tissue hypoxia, organ dysfunction, multiple organ failure, and death.[1,23,49,60]

As previously discussed, the lack of available oxygen to the cell initiates a cellular response that results

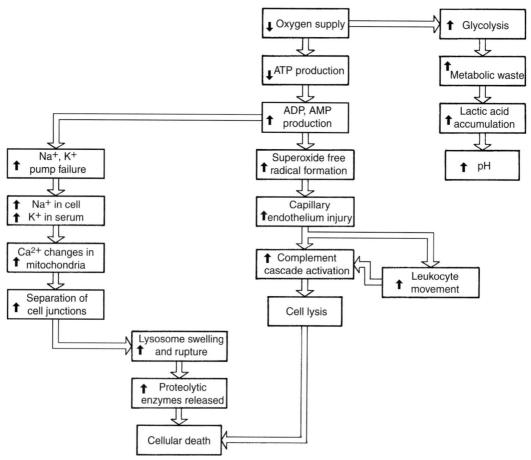

FIGURE 14-2   **Micropathophysiologic changes that occur during cellular ischemia.** *ATP,* Adenosine triphosphate; *ADP,* adenosine diphosphate; *AMP,* adenosine monophosphate; *Na⁺,* sodium ion; *K⁺,* potassium ion; *Ca2⁺,* calcium ion; *pH,* logarithm of reciprocal of hydrogen ion concentration. (Modified from Kitt S, et al: *Emergency nursing,* Philadelphia, 1995, Saunders.)

in body system changes. As shown in Figure 14-3, the immune system reacts with the activation of a complement cascade that eventually releases cytokines such as TNF and IN-1. These cytokines are key in the production of cellular toxins, such as arachidonic acid, thromboxane, and leukotrienes. These substances lead to bronchoconstriction, platelet aggregation, capillary permeability, and vasoconstriction or vasodilation.[1,39,41]

Figure 14-4 summarizes the other system changes associated with the hypoxia of shock that result in some of the classic signs and symptoms of shock. These signs and symptoms include altered mental status, changes in skin color and temperature, and a decrease in or absence of urinary output because of inadequate perfusion to the kidneys, which initiates a compensatory response to conserve water.[1,2,4,5]

STAGES

Shock has been divided into the following three specific stages: the compensatory stage, the progressive stage, and the irreversible stage. No matter what the origin of shock, a decrease in available oxygen triggers cellular responses, which in turn affect all body systems.[35]

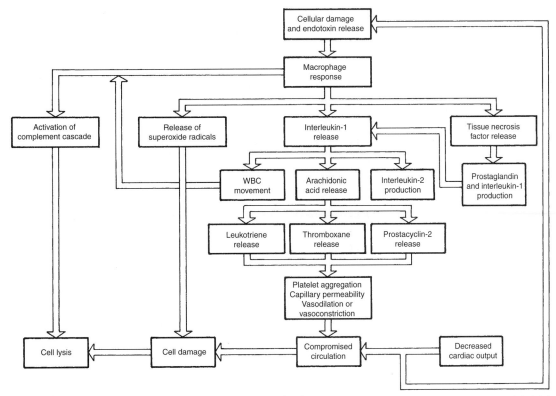

FIGURE 14-3 **Cascading response of immune system in shock.** (Modified from Kitt S, et al: *Emergency nursing,* Philadelphia, 1995, Saunders.)

COMPENSATORY

During the *compensatory phase* of shock, the body attempts to maintain perfusion in the face of illness or injury. Several compensatory mechanisms are stimulated so that the body may compensate and maintain end organ perfusion. The results of the triggering of these mechanisms, which include shifts of interstitial fluid, secretion of stress hormones, and increase in systemic vascular resistance, produce some of the classic signs and symptoms of shock. These signs and symptoms include tachycardia, tachypnea, pale skin, and diaphoresis. Figure 14-5 illustrates the compensatory mechanisms triggered in hypovolemic shock. This stage of shock is generally reversible.

PROGRESSIVE

If the presence of shock goes unrecognized or the cause of it is not managed, the shock cycle continues to progress. The initial insult that caused shock

continues to activate vicious cycles of compensatory mechanisms that, if not appropriately managed, lead to death. During this *progressive phase,* the effects of tissue hypoxia and anaerobic metabolism are experienced.[10-12] Cytokines such as TNF and the interleukins, especially 1 and 6, initiate the pathophysiologic changes that may eventually lead to multiple organ failure.

IRREVERSIBLE

In the *irreversible phase* of shock the body becomes refractory to treatment. In the final stages of shock, the patient may still be alive, but treatments such as fluid resuscitation, antibiotic administration, and ventilatory management become ineffective (Figure 14-6). The reason this occurs remains unknown but is probably related to the hyperinflammatory response of the body in shock as previously discussed.

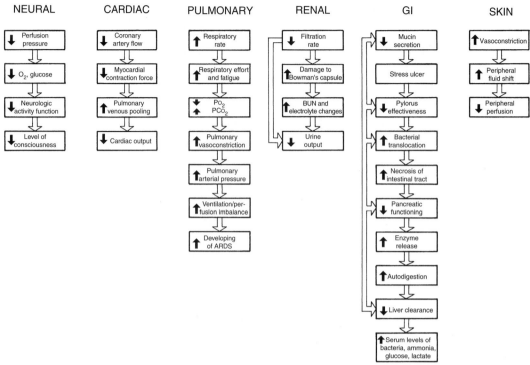

FIGURE 14-4 **Major organ system changes that occur from hypoxia associated with shock.** O_2, Oxygen; Po_2, partial pressure of oxygen; Pco_2, partial pressure of carbon dioxide; *ARDS*, adult respiratory distress syndrome; *BUN*, blood urea nitrogen. (Modified from Kitt S, et al: *Emergency nursing*, Philadelphia, 1995, Saunders.)

PATIENT ASSESSMENT AND SHOCK MANAGEMENT

The assessment and management of the patient in shock begins with the recognition that the patient is in shock. Early recognition of shock inversely affects the morbidity or mortality of the patient. Shock can be diagnosed on the basis of history and clinical signs.[2,37]

ASSESSMENT
Inspection
- Determine the patient's level of consciousness; restlessness, anxiety, and confusion may be indications of inadequate perfusion.
- Assess breathing effectiveness and respiratory rate; tachypnea occurs with increasing acidosis.
- Identify any source of uncontrolled bleeding. Inspect the chest, abdomen, and extremities.
- Assess the patient's skin color and presence of any moisture; the patient in shock may be pale, ashen, and diaphoretic.

Auscultation
- Obtain blood pressure; the patient's blood pressure may need to be palpated.
- Calculate the pulse pressure and monitor for trends in the blood pressure. A narrow pulse pressure indicates a fall in cardiac output and is an ominous sign.
- Listen to heart sounds; muffled heart tones may indicate a cardiac tamponade.
- Listen to breath sounds; absent breath sounds may indicate a pneumothorax or a hemothorax.
- Listen for bowel sounds; absent or hypoactive bowel sounds are common in shock.

Percussion
- Dullness in the chest may indicate blood in the thoracic cavity.
- Dullness in the abdomen may indicate blood in the peritoneal cavity.

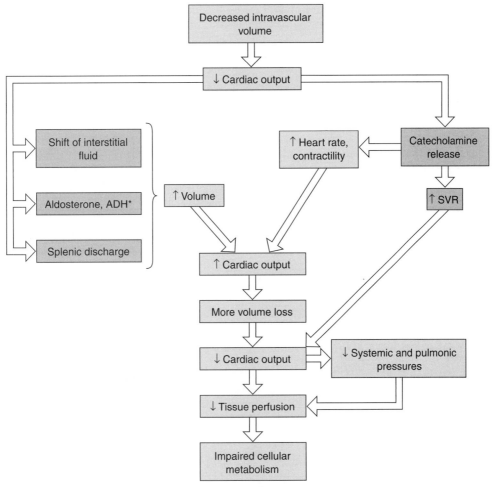

FIGURE 14-5   **Compensatory mechanisms triggered in hypovolemic shock.** (From McCance KL, Huether SE: *Pathophysiology: the biologic basis for disease in adults and children,* ed 5, St Louis, 2006, Mosby.)

Palpation
- Palpate central and peripheral pulses to assess adequate perfusion.
- Weak and thready pulse indicates decreased stroke volume as a result of hypovolemia.

Radiographic Studies
- Chest radiography is used to determine a pneumothorax or hemothorax.
- Computed tomographic (CT) scan of the chest is used to determine injury.
- Pelvic radiography is used to locate a fracture for a potential source of blood loss.

- Femur radiography.
- CT scan of the abdomen.

Other Studies
- Focus abdominal sonography for trauma (FAST).
- Diagnostic peritoneal examination (DPL).

Laboratory Studies
- Hemoglobin and hematocrit.
- Serum osmolarity.
- Electrolytes.

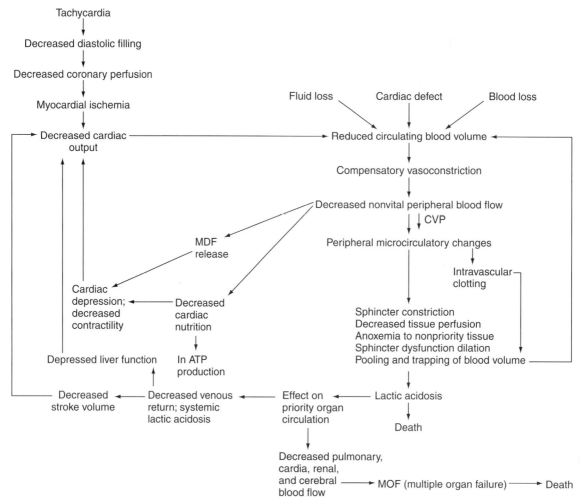

FIGURE 14-6   **Compounding factors in irreversible shock.**

- Blood urea nitrogen (BUN) and creatinine.
- Lactate level.
- Arterial blood gases (ABGs).
- Clotting studies.

MANAGEMENT

Simultaneous goals of therapy include the following[2,6,21,22,39,42,47,48]:

1. Correction of the initial insult.
2. Maintenance of adequate oxygen delivery.
3. Correction of secondary consequences such as acidosis, hypothermia, and coagulopathy.

4. Identification and management of preexisting disease.

A complete assessment and general therapy are accomplished almost simultaneously and should proceed as shown in Box 14-3.

Correction of Hypoxia

The goal for hypoxia during the initial resuscitation of the patient in shock is to correct the oxygen deficit that has occurred. The transport team should secure the patient's airway if indicated and provide oxygenation as soon as possible. This must always be

---

BOX 14-3 | **Steps in Initial Management of the Patient in Shock**

1. Assess airway patency, administer 100% oxygen, perform advanced airway management as indicated.
2. Assess breathing effectiveness, perform decompression if indicated.
3. Inspect for and control active bleeding.
4. Assess perfusion: peripheral and central pulses, capillary refill, skin temperature, color, jugular veins.
5. Initiate fluid resuscitation, closely monitoring patient during resuscitation.
6. Assess neurologic function: AVPU, GCS, pupillary function, motor and sensory response; immobilize patient if indicated.
7. Assess skin and skeleton; note abnormalities, deformities of skeleton, potential sources of blood, volume loss.
8. Keep patient warm.
9. Apply monitoring devices: cardiac, pulse oximeter, end-tidal.
10. Check invasive lines if in place.
11. Check urinary catheter if in place; monitor output.
12. Review laboratory studies before transport when available.
13. Review radiographic and diagnostic studies when available.

---

done with consideration for safety of both the patient and the team. Respiratory muscle effort is the major site of oxygen expenditure for the resting patient and may place undue metabolic demands on the heart. Assisted ventilation that provides maximal analgesia, sedation, and neuromuscular blockade may be necessary for the transport of a critically ill or injured patient. Mechanical ventilation of a critically ill or injured patient is discussed in Chapter 12.

Fluid Resuscitation

Fluid resuscitation has become one of the most controversial topics in shock management. Research has questioned some of the previously common methods used to manage shock in prehospital and transport environments.

The purpose of volume resuscitation is to restore oxygen transport and cellular uptake of needed oxygen, mitigate against the oxygen debt accumulation, repay a preresuscitation oxygen deficit, and prevent the complications of SIRS and the development of multiple organ failure. The prehospital and transport management of fluid resuscitation must pay careful attention to the long-term consequences of any intervention.[2,3,11,13,14,29,31,32,45,50,56,58,62,63,68,73,75,76,81,82,84,89,91,92]

Multiple fluids have been used for resuscitation, including lactated Ringer's, normal saline, hypertonic saline, Hetastarch, and Plasmanate. In hemorrhagic shock, blood and blood products are needed for resuscitation. Massive transfusion protocols have

been developed in multiple centers and should be used as a guideline in the use of blood and blood products in patient resuscitation. However, some transport programs do not carry blood or blood products. Regardless of which fluids are chosen for resuscitation, the patient needs to be monitored closely for the effectiveness of resuscitation and the potential complications that may occur.

Research has shown that hypotension may be a protective mechanism. Unless the source of bleeding can be adequately managed in the prehospital care environment, aggressive resuscitation may do more harm than good. Increasing a patient's blood pressure increases the risk of bleeding, may dislodge formed clots, and, depending on the resuscitation fluid, dilutes circulating volume and increases clotting time. Crystalloids and colloids do not carry oxygen, which is one of the primary survival needs for cells.[2,3,11,13,14,29,31,32,45,50,58,62,63,68,72,73,75,76,81,82,84,89,91,92]

The amount of fluid needed by patients in shock, particularly those in hemorrhagic or hypovolemic shock, depends on the amount of intravascular volume depletion. During resuscitation, the transport team needs to monitor the patient closely for sufficiency of volume replacement. The patient's blood pressure, pulse rate, level of consciousness, and urinary output (when available) provide parameters that can be monitored during transport. These parameters may also provide the transport team with indications of fluid overload.[2,22,37,70,71]

The complications of massive fluid resuscitation include hypothermia, coagulopathy, metabolic derangements such as hypocalcemia and hypokalemia, organ dysfunction, and extravascular fluid shifts. These complications may lead to the development of adult respiratory distress syndrome (ARDS), sepsis syndrome, acute renal failure, DIC, pneumonia, multiple organ failure, and death.[69,79,89,90]

Pneumatic Antishock Garment

One of the most common methods once used in the management of the injured patient in shock was the application of *pneumatic antishock garments* (PASG) or *military antishock trousers* (MAST). As the original name, MAST, suggests, this device was found to be of great use during the Vietnam War. However, little research had been done related to the effectiveness and potential complications that could occur once they were applied.[3,17,24,25,88,92]

Mattox et al[57] published a landmark study in 1989 that demonstrated several important points about the use of PASG. This study and other animal model studies proved that PASG did work but that their application in certain patient populations may actually increase patient morbidity and mortality rates.[57]

Currently, the International Trauma Life Support Course[22] recommends that the indications for the application of PASG in the prehospital environment include external hemorrhage that can be controlled (PASG possibly used initially until fluid replacement occurs), neurogenic shock without evidence of internal injuries, isolated fractures of legs without evidence of other internal injuries, and systolic blood pressure of less than 50 mm Hg (which still remains controversial).[22] Absolute contraindications to the use of PASG include pulmonary edema and bleeding that cannot be controlled. PASG must be used with caution in the woman who is pregnant, with pressure kept off the fetus.[22]

When PASG are used during transport, the transport team needs to weigh the advantages over the disadvantages and monitor the patient closely. Continued use of PASG can lead to the development of decubiti and other stasis injuries.[5,22]

Despite controversies, PASG are still used in some parts of the world to manage acute hemorrhage, particularly related to delivery. It might not be a bad idea to keep the PASG in a cool dry place and see what the future may bring.

Tourniquet Use

The use of tourniquets to control bleeding is not new. Recent information from the battlefields has shown a resurgence of the use of tourniquets. Tourniquets have been found to be of use in traumatic amputations related to battlefield injuries. Because of some successes, renewed interest has been seen in the use of tourniquets in civilian management of severe injuries with uncontrolled bleeding.

If tourniquets are used, the transport team must be familiar with their application and when they should be removed.[86]

Pharmacologic Management

The pharmacologic management of shock depends on the source of the shock. For example, usually little need exists for pharmacologic agents in traumatic hemorrhagic shock. The primary therapy is administration of fluids, blood, and blood products. However, once the primary therapy has been initiated, pharmacologic management may be indicated if the patient's condition does not improve.

Commonly used medications in the management of shock include inotropic agents, vasopressors, vasodilators, antibiotics, and steroids. Because dosages depend on age, size, and severity of the patient's condition, the transport team needs to be familiar with the indications, dosages, and side effects of the medications that may be used.[2,4,5,30,34,40,54]

Other Interventions

As summarized in Box 14-1, multiple causes of shock exist. When the blood flow is obstructed, as in cardiac tamponade and tension pneumothorax, the patient exhibits signs and symptoms of shock. Critical interventions in obstructive shock include pericardiocentesis and thoracic decompression. Although some disease states may induce a pericardial tamponade or tension pneumothorax and contribute to obstructive shock, the most common causes of these life-threatening maladies are blunt and penetrating thoracic trauma.[2,5,22]

Pericardiocentesis is indicated for the patient in shock when blunt or penetrating trauma to the chest (particularly the sternum) has occurred and the patient is hypotensive and has brady-cardia, distended neck veins, and muffled heart sounds.[2,5,22]

Needle decompression or chest tube insertion is indicated when the patient is in shock and has severe respiratory distress, hypotension, bradycardia, jugular vein distention, and tracheal deviation. When the patient is intubated, difficulty in ventilation should alert the transport team to the potential of a tension pneumothorax, once again in the patient with a history of blunt and penetrating trauma.[2,5,22]

Another source of a tension pneumothorax that should be considered by the transport team is barotrauma. Aggressive bagging or mechanical ventilation could cause a pneumothorax that contributes to a tension pneumothorax and obstructive shock. Chapter 12 discusses the potential complications related to the use of mechanical ventilation during transport.

Other interventions that may be used in the management of shock are the mechanical devices to assist circulation or increase tissue perfusion. Some of these devices include intraaortic balloon pumps (IAB), left ventricular assist devices (LVAD), and extracorporeal oxygenation devices (ECMO). The uses of these types of equipment require special skills and significant preparation. Chapter 23 contains a discussion about the indications and management of some of these devices.[74]

Clinical Monitoring

Depending on the time, location, and initiation of interventions, the patient in shock may not have clinical monitoring devices in place. Multiple methods may be used to monitor the patient in shock, including hemodynamic and venous oxygen saturation (SvO_2) monitors. Box 14-4 contains a summary of some of these clinical monitors.[4,55,83]

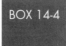

BOX 14-4	Cardiopulmonary and Metabolic Measurements in Shock

Arterial pressure
Left ventricular function (pulmonary artery catheter)
Cardiac output
Cardiac index
Mixed venous blood gases
Lactic level
Base deficit
Intramucosal pH

Central venous and pulmonary artery catheter pressures provide an index of the status of absolute and relative blood volume, the need for fluid replacement, and the effects of interventions. Accurate serial measurement of heart rate and rhythm, respiratory rate, cardiac filling pressure, cardiac output, tissue perfusion indices, and end organ function (mental state and urinary output) must be done when possible.[8,18,26]

Regardless of the types of clinical monitor used, the transport team needs to ensure that they can be used during transport. All ports, intravenous and invasive lines, and monitors need to be secured and accessible and protected from the possibility of contamination, particularly when invasive lines are in place.[4] If invasive monitors are used, the transport team should document an initial reading once equipment has been changed and according to transport protocols or as the patient's condition indicates during transport.[2]

SELECTED CAUSES OF SHOCK

HEMORRHAGE
Description

Circulation can be compromised in various ways. Failure of circulation occurs either locally or systemically and results in shock. Systemic circulation failure is caused by inadequate blood volume or a pump defect. The first of three types of inadequate volume is *hemorrhage,* or loss of plasma and red cell mass from the vascular system. Hemorrhage is either internal or external; the amount depends on the vessel, the extent of damage, and the ability to form and maintain a clot. The effect of hemorrhage depends on the preexisting state of the cardiovascular, respiratory, renal, and hematologic systems.[16,64]

Normal blood volume is approximately 7% of the ideal adult body weight (approximately 70 mL/kg) and 80 to 90 mL/kg in children.[5] In hemorrhage, a graded physiologic response is based on the percentage of blood volume lost acutely. The clinical symptoms progress as blood loss increases.

Changes in blood pressure at times may not be seen until 30% to 40% of the total blood volume is lost. Specific attention should be paid to pulse rate, respiratory rate, skin circulation, pulse pressure, and the patient's mental status.[5]

Intrathoracic and intraabdominal bleeding (cavitary hemorrhage) are well recognized as causes of hypovolemia in trauma. Significant losses from noncavitary causes (pelvic fracture, skin laceration, and multiple long bone fractures) may result in a 20% to 50% total blood loss, which places the patient in a severe shock state.

An isolated closed femur fracture can result in up to 2 L of blood lost in the fracture hematoma. In pelvic fractures, 40% to 50% of the total blood volume may be lost. The mortality rate in pelvic fracture is 6.4% to 15%; however, 42% to 70% of the deaths are attributed to blood loss. These patients need aggressive resuscitation.

Noncavitary blood losses contribute to additional loss of blood in 85.2% of patients with intraabdominal or intrathoracic hemorrhage. Blood losses occur 2 to 5 hours after the injury, so transport team members should be alert for delayed hypovolemia.[64]

Treatment requires tamponade of the bleeding and supporting and splinting fractures. Fluid management includes administration of crystalloid, blood, and blood products. Knowledge that severe volume losses can occur with noncavitary bleeding is essential for early recognition to ensure proper treatment and prevent wasted time in searching for cavitary hemorrhage.[2,3,11,13,14,29,31,32,45,50,58,62,63,68,72,73,75,76,80,81,82,84,89,91,92]

Indicators

A history of any of the following factors should lead to suspicion of hemorrhage:

> Trauma to the thorax, abdomen, pelvis, or an extremity.
> Melena or hematochezia.
> Hematemesis.
> Hemoptysis or epistaxis.
> Vaginal bleeding.
> Surgery.

Predisposing Conditions

The following conditions can predispose to hemorrhage:

> Anemia.
> Hemoglobinopathies.
> Thrombocytopenia.
> Liver disease.
> Any hemorrhagic diathesis, hemophilia, or DIC.
> Neoplastic disease.
> Peptic ulcer disease.
> Alcoholism.
> Atherosclerosis.
> Sepsis.
> Surgery.

Causes

Internal Hemorrhage

Pleural cavity hemorrhage: intrathoracic vessel trauma, leaking aortic aneurysm, aortic dissection, ruptured varices, fracture.

Peritoneal cavity hemorrhage: liver, spleen, or any artery trauma; abdominal aneurysm; tumor; arteritis; volvulus; strangulated ovarian cyst.

Retroperitoneal hemorrhage: tumor, trauma fracture, ectopic pregnancy; soft tissue extremity trauma, fracture, venipuncture; skin trauma, purpura.

Bladder hemorrhage: tumor, transurethral prostatectomy.

Cavity hemorrhage: complication of surgery.

External Hemorrhage

Gastrointestinal (GI) tract hemorrhage (associated with hematemesis): inflammatory gastritis, peptic ulcer disease (PUD), esophagitis, and tumor of esophagus, stomach.

Endotracheal hemorrhage: esophageal lacerations, foreign body ingestion, abdominal trauma.

Vascular hemorrhage: varices, aneurysms, mesenteric occlusion, and hematologic disease.

GI tract (associated with hematochezia): ulcerative colitis (inflammatory), shigellosis (infectious), amebiasis, tumor, vascular hemorrhoids, volvulus, mesenteric occlusion; Meckel's diverticulum (congenital).

Respiratory tract hemorrhage: trauma, inflammation, infection, vascular lesions, infarction of lung, bleeding in an abscess, ruptured aortic aneurysm, and bronchiectasis.

Vaginal hemorrhage: pregnancy, abortion, abruptio placentae, placenta previa, lacerations from delivery, cervical and endometrial cancer, dysfunctional uterine bleeding.

Fluid Loss
Description
The second of the three major types of inadequate volume is *fluid loss*. Fluid loss occurs in conditions with reduced blood volume and hemoconcentration because of water loss and unusually high solute loss. The usual modes of fluid loss are vomiting, diarrhea, excessive sweating (fever, heatstroke), excessive urination, and loss from body surface area of denuded skin. (The management of burns and burn shock is discussed in Chapter 20.)

Indicators
A history of the following indicates low blood volume from fluid loss:

Burns.
Diarrhea, vomiting, excessive urination, sweating.
Poorly controlled diabetes, lowered insulin usage with polyuria.
Exposure to environment for prolonged time with decreased food and water supply.
Fever.
Ascites.
Extensive surgery.
Diuretic use or abuse.

In addition, hematocrit levels and central venous pressure (CVP) values are good indicators of fluid loss.

Predisposing Conditions
A patient with any of the following conditions could be predisposed to low blood volume caused by fluid loss:

Age: very young or very old.
Surgery: GI resections, hyposectomy, and extensive resections.
Diabetes mellitus.
Adrenal insufficiency.
Drugs: diuretic therapy.
Hyperthyroidism.
Regional enteritis, ulcerative colitis.
Liver disease.
PUD.
Malnutrition, anemia.
Peritonitis, pelvic inflammatory disease.
Neoplasia.
Diabetes insipidus.

Abnormal Peripheral Distribution (Distributive Shock)
Description
Loss of blood volume can be caused by vasomotor dysfunction with sequestration of blood in the resistance circuit or venous capacitance bed. The absolute blood volume does not change, but an increase in vascular space results in a decrease of effective blood volume and tissue perfusion. Vasomotor dysfunction results in: (1) high or normal arterial resistance with expanded venous capacitance (pooling); or (2) low arterial resistance with arteriovenous shunting. This is sometimes referred to as *distributive shock*.[20]

Sepsis
Septic shock was a term used to describe the shock state associated with infection. In 1992, septic shock was reclassified and defined as sepsis-induced hypotension despite adequate fluid resuscitation with lactic acidosis, oliguria, and acute alteration in mental status.[15] *Sepsis* is described as a spectrum of clinical conditions caused by the immune response of a host to a clinical insult such as an injury or

illness and characterized by systemic inflammation and coagulation.[33] Each year thousands of people in the United States die of sepsis.[34]

The body responds to infection through an inflammatory response. Multiple proinflammatory mediators, such as tumor necrosis factor (TNF-a), interleukins 1 and 6, and platelet activating factor (PAF), are released. These mediators help the body repair and prevent further injury. The body also releases antiinflammatory mediators to balance the effects.[34]

In sepsis, an overwhelming inflammatory response occurs. TNF and interleukins cause tissue and capillary injury. One of these injuries is the activation of the coagulation system and depletion of endogenous anticoagulants, which results in diffuse microthrombus formation.[33] The primary cause of sepsis and septic shock is an event that interferes with local or systemic host defense mechanisms. These causes may include a primary infection (e.g., pneumonia) or an iatrogenic cause, such as the presence of a urinary catheter or pulmonary catheter. The increased indiscriminate use of broad-spectrum antibiotics has lead to a proliferation of antibiotic-resistant infections and increased the risk of sepsis.[33,85]

As with the management of any type of shock, prevention is primary in the treatment of sepsis. The transport team must use meticulous methods to decrease the risk of exposing patients to infection, particularly when transporting patients with invasive lines.

Indicators and risk factors for sepsis or septic shock include:

- Fever.
- Hypothermia.
- Obvious source of infection:
  - Urinary catheter.
  - Central venous access.
  - Invasive monitoring.
  - Open wounds.
  - Postsurgery conditions.
- Risk of infection:
  - Penetrating injury.
  - Open fractures.
- Hyperdynamic state:
  - Increased cardiac index.
  - Decreased vascular resistance.
- Hypoxia.

Neurogenic Shock

Neurogenic shock is a result of an injury or insult to the reticular activating system (RAS) and spinal cord. In the presence of major brain stem dysfunction or spinal cord injury, hypotension without tachycardia or cutaneous vasoconstriction may be a neurogenic cause. Vasoactive drugs should *not* be administered until volume is restored. Many times, if no blood loss has occurred, hypotension may be resolved by placing the patient flat or in a slight Trendelenburg's position if no injury to the cervical spine has occurred, as confirmed by medical personnel. Respiratory insufficiency is common, and ventilatory support should be implemented as necessary.[22,28,30,65]

The management of spinal shock includes appropriate immobilization for transport and initiation of pharmacologic management for hypotension. Vasoactive drugs may be needed to maintain peripheral vasoconstriction once any source of bleeding has been ruled out. High dose steroids were recommended in the past. However, research has challenged their use. High dose steroids should only be initiated after consultation with a neurosurgeon.[30]

The transport team must also ensure that the patient is kept warm because spinal cord injury leaves the patient poikilothermic. In addition, the team must be sure no pressure is exerted on the patient's skin that may cause further injury because the patient is insensitive to it.

Anaphylaxis

Anaphylaxis is an acute systemic allergic reaction that results from the release of chemical mediators after an antigen-antibody reaction. The reaction is mediated by immunoglobulin E (IgE), which rests on the surface of mast cells and basophils in the body, especially along the respiratory and GI tracts. When a reaction occurs, it results in the formation and release of histamine, the kinins, and the slow reactive substance of anaphylaxis, which cause three major effects: (1) vasodilation; (2) smooth muscle spasm; and (3) increased vascular permeability with edema formation (Figure 14-7).[2,37]

Anaphylactic reactions (not mediated by IgE) have identical signs and symptoms and are caused most often by drugs, such as iodinated radiograph

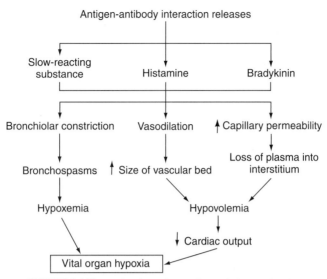

FIGURE 14-7   **Pathophysiology of anaphylactic shock.**

contrast, procaine compounds, and fluorescein. In either reaction, the sooner the onset, the more severe the reaction is likely to be.

Patients experience a sense of impending doom; pruritus, especially of the palms and feet; and sudden headache. Adverse reactions may occur quickly and affect all systems[37]:

Respiratory: upper airway edema; angioedema of hypopharynx, epiglottis, larynx, and trachea; asthma; stridulous breathing with supraclavicular, suprasternal, and intercostal retractions.

Cutaneous: flushing, pruritus, urticaria, and angioedema.

Cardiovascular: arrhythmias and electrocardiographic (ECG) abnormalities, probably caused by decreased coronary perfusion and oxygenation; vasodilation and hypotension, with or without other symptoms from venous pooling or increased capillary permeability and water loss into the interstitial space.

Neurologic: sudden loss of consciousness, seizures, cerebral anoxia from airway obstruction, and decreased blood pressure.

Gastrointestinal: rarely, GI spasm of smooth muscle that leads to cramps, diarrhea, sudden and explosive involuntary defecation, and vomiting with potential for aspiration.

Genitourinary: incontinence and labor-like pains in female uterus.

Death from upper airway obstruction, vomiting and aspiration, bronchospasm, and vascular collapse.

Management.   Treatment for anaphylaxis is as follows:

For some stings and bites, compression dressings may be applied to decrease the progress of the toxin. The Sawyer extractor may be used to remove the stinger.

Resuscitation should be initiated, depending on the severity of the reaction. The transport team must keep in mind that airway management may be more difficult because of swelling. Definitive airway management may need to be performed before transport, depending on the size of the transport vehicle and the length of the transport.

Epinephrine: Administration of 1:1000 epinephrine subcutaneously dilates bronchial smooth muscle, causes vasoconstriction, and decreases vascular permeability.

For severe reactions, a 1:10,000 epinephrine solution (5 mL) may be given intravenously and repeated every 5 to 10 minutes until reaction absolves and hemodynamics restored (recommendation of consultation with medical direction).

Antihistamine (diphenhydramine): An antihistamine competes with the binding sites.

Administration of steroids is also needed.

Unexpected anaphylaxis with a rapid clinical course may result in a swift recovery or death. Little time to act is available; early recognition is therefore essential.

Obstructive Shock

Description.   Circulation can be compromised and the patient can become hypotensive and hypoxic because of direct failure of the heart muscle or compression or obstruction of vessels that provide central circulation. The result of this pathophysiologic process may be a pericardial tamponade or tension pneumothorax.[22]

Cardiac tamponade and tension pneumothorax, once recognized, are easily reversible mechanical obstructions to cardiac output. *Cardiac tamponade* occurs when blood or effusion accumulates in the closed pericardial sac. The heart is unable to fill, the central venous pressure rises, blood pressure and pulse rate decrease, and heart sounds may be muffled (Beck's triad).[34] Needle pericardiocentesis is the treatment of choice.

Tension pneumothorax results in a complete collapse of one or both lungs with compression on mediastinal vessels and organs. Air under tension may be evacuated via needle or chest tube insertion.

Indicators.   A history of any of the following may indicate the potential for mechanical obstruction that results in hypotension and hypoxia:

Chest pain.
Dyspnea.
Syncope.
Trauma to the chest.

Signs and symptoms include:

Apprehension.
Shortness of breath.
Tracheal deviation.
Jugular vein distention.

Predisposing Conditions.   Predisposing conditions include the following:

Blunt or penetrating trauma.
Preexisting pulmonary disease, such as chronic obstructive pulmonary disease or asthma.
Cardiomyopathy.
Bacterial endocarditis.

Management should include:

Decompression of the obstruction via needle or chest tube for a tension pneumothorax.
Pericardiocentesis.
Transportation of the patient at lower altitudes.

COAGULOPATHIES

One of the common complications of shock is the development of coagulopathies and DIC, particularly as the result of massive blood loss and fluid resuscitation. In addition, the presence of a preexisting condition, such as hemophilia, or the patient's use of a medication such as warfarin that interferes with coagulation poses further challenges in patient care.

Most patients who are bleeding have normal clotting mechanisms (Figure 14-8), and when normal measures taken to control bleeding are not effective, a coagulopathy, or bleeding disorder, may be suspected. Diagnosis of a specific coagulopathy in the transport environment is difficult or impossible, but an index of suspicion should be raised in certain cases on the basis of assessment of the patient, available history, and evaluation of laboratory findings that may be available. Some patients have an established history of inherited coagulopathy, whereas others may be expected to have a bleeding disorder or tendency toward such a disorder on the basis of the current disease process. Confirmation of that suspicion requires more extensive laboratory testing than is available in most community hospitals and is best determined by consultation with a hematologist or an internist in a medical center with experience and facilities to properly evaluate and care for the patient.

A *coagulopathy* is defined as "any disorder of blood coagulation."[42,46,54,67] This is a broad categorization of a variety of disorders that interfere with the body's ability to control hemorrhage. Some coagulopathies are inherited disorders, whereas others are acquired and

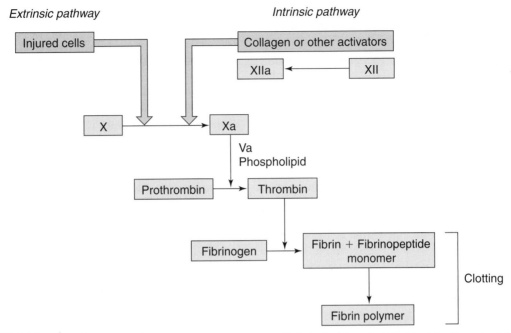

FIGURE 14-8   **Coagulation cascade.** (From McCance KL, Huether SE: *Pathophysiology: the biologic basis for disease in adults and children,* ed 5, St Louis, 2006, Mosby.)

unrelated to genetic tendencies. Coagulopathies can be either primary disorders or the result of an underlying disease. One of the 12 clotting factors (Box 14-5) may be deficient, or another stage of the clotting cascade may not function normally. Some coagulopathies are life threatening; others are so mild that they go undetected until late in life. Approximately 80,000 deaths in the United States occur each year from bleeding disorders of acquired or congenital origin.[54,67]

INCIDENCE

Some coagulopathies are hereditary in origin. The famous "bleeders" of history have had hemophilia. Any deficiency of one of the 12 clotting factors may cause a clotting disorder, but the most commonly seen hereditary coagulopathies are hemophilia A, hemophilia B, and von Willebrand's disease.[46]

HEREDITARY COAGULOPATHIES
Hemophilia A

Of all the hereditary coagulopathies, *hemophilia A,* sometimes called classic hemophilia, is the most common. About 70% to 90% of "hemophiliacs"

BOX 14-5	Common Names of Coagulation Factors
Factor I	Fibrinogen
Factor II	Prothrombin
Factor III	Tissue thromboplastin
Factor IV	Calcium
Factor V	Ac globulin
Factor VII	Proconvertin
Factor VIII	Antihemophilic factor (AHG)
Factor IX	Plasma thromboplastin component (PTC; Christmas factor)
Factor X	Stuart factor
Factor XI	Plasma thromboplastin antecedent (PTA)
Factor XII	Hageman factor
Factor XIII	Fibrin stabilizing factor

have hemophilia A. It is seen in 1 to 2 of every 10,000 people in the United States.[54] The gene is found on the X chromosome and is transmitted as a sex-linked recessive trait; therefore, nearly all its victims are male. Female carriers (heterozygotes) pass the gene to one half of their daughters, who then also become carriers, and to one half of their sons, who will have the disease. Males with the disease (hemizygotes) pass the gene to all of their daughters, who become asymptomatic carriers; sons are healthy. Of hemophilia patients, 30% have no family history of the disease.

Hemophilia B

Also called Christmas disease, *hemophilia B* is similar to hemophilia A. About 9% of those with inherited coagulation defects have this disease. It is 15% as frequent as hemophilia A and is found in approximately 1 of every 100,000 persons in the United States.[54] Like hemophilia A, it is found almost entirely in males as a sex-linked recessive trait.

von Willebrand's Disease

This form of hemophilia occurs in 5 to 10 of every 1,000,000 persons in the United States. *von Willebrand's disease* is found in both genders because it is inherited as an autosomal dominant trait.[46]

ACQUIRED DISORDERS

Coagulopathies may also be acquired rather than inherited. Acquired disorders occur much more commonly than inherited ones.[54] These bleeding disorders are the result of another disease process or therapy. Although many varieties exist, the types most likely to confront the transport team are described in the following sections.

Vitamin K Deficiency

Vitamin K must be present in the blood for clotting to occur. It is obtained by the body through the diet and produced by intestinal bacteria. In *vitamin K deficiency,* levels may be deficient because of poor diet or sterilization of the gut from antibiotic therapy. Patients at risk include the postoperative patient with oral intake who is on an extended course of antibiotic therapy.

Hepatic Coagulopathy

Liver disease is one of the most common risk factors for the development of coagulopathy. Because 11 of the 12 clotting factors are synthesized in the liver, patients with liver dysfunction, particularly those with severe cirrhosis, are deficient in those factors. In addition, vitamin K deficiency often contributes to the *hepatic coagulopathy* because patients with liver disease are unable to store vitamin K at optimal levels.

Disseminated Intravascular Coagulation

Disseminated intravascular coagulation (DIC) is a complex disease and is not uncommon in critically ill or injured patients. It is a secondary response to many diseases, including some infections, malignant diseases, and obstetric complications.[54,67] Box 14-6 lists many of the disease states for which DIC may be a further complication.

Disseminated intravascular coagulation appears to result from the entrance of substances into the blood that cause accelerated clotting, thus the variety of primary diseases (see Box 14-6) with which it has been associated.

Drug-Induced Coagulopathies

A variety of medications can either enhance or inhibit clotting. *Drug-induced coagulopathies* may be the most commonly seen cause of abnormal bleeding.[54] However, a few of these medications alone cause significant problems without accompanying platelet or clotting-factor deficiency.[54]

Massive Transfusions

Another cause of bleeding that can be encountered by transport team personnel is the coagulopathy associated with *massive transfusions*. Massive blood loss; the use of banked blood, which is deficient in clotting factors and platelets; and resuscitation with large amounts of crystalloids and colloids are significant contributing factors to the coagulopathy associated with massive transfusions. Those at risk include patients with major trauma, GI hemorrhage, or obstetric complications.[45,62,63,66]

NORMAL PHYSIOLOGY

Hemostasis, the arrest of bleeding, is an extremely complex process. The normal coagulation process is a balance between uncontrolled bleeding and generalized thrombosis or clotting. The transport team needs some understanding of the coagulative process

| BOX 14-6 | **Diseases That Precipitate DIC** |

Obstetric

Abruptio placentae
Amniotic fluid embolism
Toxemia of pregnancy
Hydatidiform mole
Retained dead fetus
Septic abortion

Infection

Bacterial: gram-negative or gram-positive septicemia
Rickettsial: Rocky Mountain spotted fever
Viral: varicella, rubella, arboviruses, influenza A
Parasitic: plasmodium falciparum malaria
Fungal: histoplasmosis

Trauma

Trauma with shock
Head injury
Burns
Anoxia
Heatstroke

Malignant Disease

Metastatic carcinoma: pancreas, lung, breast, stomach, prostate, colon
Acute promyelocytic leukemia

Shock States

Cardiac arrest

Miscellaneous

Aortic aneurysm
Snakebite
Transfusion reactions
Anaphylactic drug reactions
Prostatic surgery
Lung surgery
Extracorporeal circulation

to be adequately prepared for patients with actual or potential coagulopathies.

At least four components are necessary for normal clotting to take place: (1) blood vessels; (2) platelets; (3) clotting; and (4) fibrinolysis, or clot dissolution.[54] If any one of these components malfunctions or is deficient, a coagulopathy results. Nearly every conceivable aspect of these four components has been known to malfunction. A few disorders are

seen much more frequently than others; the remaining bleeding disorders are rather rare.

Blood vessels are composed of connective and smooth muscle tissue lined with endothelial cells. Vessel walls serve as an important protective barrier to contain and protect the circulating blood. If injured, the vessel constricts at the site of injury through a reflex nervous system response. This response decreases blood flow and slows bleeding. In addition, after blunt trauma, blood flowing into the injured tissue creates a hematoma, which decreases blood loss by mechanical pressure and tamponades the ruptured vessel.

The second and third components, platelets and clotting factors, interact to form the clot. Platelets, also known as thrombocytes, are actually cell fragments from larger cells called karyocytes, which are formed in the bone marrow. When a blood vessel is injured, collagen is exposed in the connective tissue. Collagen is oppositely charged to the circulating platelets, which causes platelets to be attracted to the injured site. The platelets adhere to exposed tissue and vessel walls, but they also stick or aggregate to one another, forming a platelet plug. Platelets then rupture as they plug the damaged vessel wall, releasing incomplete thromboplastin, also known as clotting factor III. Clotting factor III reacts with calcium, called factor IV, and several other blood factors to help form the permanent clot. The platelet plug is adequate to stop minor bleeding at least temporarily, but more severe bleeding also requires the interaction of coagulation factors to form a stable fibrin clot.

Collagen exposed at the injured site activates factor XII, which stimulates other reactions, eventually forming thrombin and enhancing the aggregation of platelets. Thrombin also converts fibrinogen, factor I, which is present in plasma, into fibrin, an insoluble protein of densely intertwined threads that catch erythrocytes and platelets.

After the clot has served its purpose in stopping the hemorrhage, the fibrin clot is dissolved by the fibrinolytic system. This process, known as fibrinolysis, begins within 24 hours after clot formation. Plasminogen, a serum globulin found in the clot, is activated by substances in the blood and becomes plasmin, a proteolytic enzyme that digests proteins, including fibrin, fibrinogen, and factors V and VIII. This prevents the permanent thrombosis of the injured blood vessel.

PATHOPHYSIOLOGY

HEREDITARY COAGULOPATHIES
Hemophilia A
The hemophilias are the most common hereditary bleeding disorders, and hemophilia A is the most prevalent of the hemophilias. The deficiency in this disease is factor VIII, also known as antihemophilic factor, with severity of symptoms closely related to the level of factor VIII in the blood. Platelet plug formation is normal; however, deficiency of factor VIII impairs the capacity to form a stable fibrin clot. The disease is almost always discovered by age 5 years, although mild cases may not be recognized until after trauma or surgery as an adult.[54]

Between acute episodes of bleeding, hemophiliacs may be without symptoms unless they are anemic from previous blood loss. Medical attention is sought for hemarthroses (bleeding into joints), hematuria, and epistaxis. Bleeding can also occur into deep tissues. Mucosal bleeding is unusual, as is GI bleeding, unless peptic ulcer disease is also present. Trauma is often the cause of bleeding, and that bleeding may occur or reoccur 8 hours or even 1 to 3 days after the injury and continue for days or weeks.

Bleeding is particularly dangerous when pressure is exerted on organs, vessels, or nerves. It can be life threatening when it is intracranial, lingual, laryngeal, retropharyngeal, pericardial, pleural, or simply exsanguinating. Central nervous system (CNS) hemorrhage is the leading cause of death of hemophiliacs and should be taken seriously.[54] CNS bleeding may occur spontaneously, unrelated to trauma or a specific lesion.

A long history of severe or poorly controlled hemophilia may leave the patient severely handicapped, with permanent joint damage from hemarthroses, which causes fibrous or bony ankylosis. Hemophiliacs may also have complications from the treatment process. Multiple blood product transfusions or factor-concentrate infusions can result in liver disease, hepatitis, and HIV.

Hemophilia B
Hemophilia B is similar to hemophilia A. It is a hereditary disorder with the same genetic pattern; males are primarily affected. Hemophilia B is caused by a deficiency of factor IX activity, which results in prolonged partial thromboplastin (PT) times. Clinical symptoms and bleeding are the same as in hemophilia A, as is the risk to the patient's life.

von Willebrand's Disease
von Willebrand's disease is a result of two defects: defective platelet adherence and decreased levels of factor VIII. Platelets occur in normal numbers but do not adhere to the subendothelial collagen of the capillary wall to form the platelet plug. Therefore, bleeding is prolonged. von Willebrand's disease is usually milder than hemophilia A or B. Bleeding is mostly from skin or mucous membranes rather than deep bleeding into tissue or joints. Easy bruising, epistaxis, dental bleeding, menorrhagia, and GI bleeding are the usual clinical manifestations.[46]

ACQUIRED COAGULOPATHIES
Bleeding disorders that are acquired are seen more often by the transport team than inherited coagulopathies.

Vitamin K Deficiency
Factors II, VII, IX, and X are vitamin K dependent and require the presence of vitamin K to function normally.[54] The body acquires vitamin K from leafy green vegetables in the diet and as a byproduct of intestinal bacteria. If these sources are not available to the body, a deficiency results in 2 to 4 weeks. Hemorrhage from vitamin K deficiency can occur in patients who undergo antibiotic therapy for extended periods while taking nothing by mouth because antibiotics may sterilize the gut, eliminating the bacterial source of vitamin K. Intestinal malabsorption and liver disease can cause bleeding from vitamin K deficiency. Hemorrhagic disease of the newborn is also a vitamin K deficiency, caused by a lack of vitamin K–producing intestinal flora and the immaturity of the liver.[54]

Hepatic Coagulopathy

Liver disease is a common cause of coagulopathy. It is most often seen in patients with severe hepatic cirrhosis but also occurs with other acute and chronic liver diseases. Any patient with severe liver dysfunction is at risk for hemorrhage. All coagulation factors except VIII are synthesized in the liver by hepatocytes. Therefore, patients with liver disease are deficient in those factors. However, before bleeding occurs, liver disease is usually advanced and easily recognized by other signs of the disease.

Other factors may contribute to bleeding tendencies in the patient with liver disease. A vitamin K deficiency may result from intestinal malabsorption, poor dietary habits, or the anorexia associated with liver disease. Further coagulopathy is often present because of low platelet count and platelet dysfunction. Finally, liver disease results in increased proteolytic activity in the blood, probably because the liver has a decreased ability to remove these proteolytic substances from circulation. The clinical picture is very close to that of DIC, which may also develop.

Disseminated Intravascular Coagulation

Disseminated intravascular coagulation has been called the most important coagulopathy in the emergency department.[2,54] This life-threatening disorder is actually a secondary complication of a broad spectrum of diseases (see Box 14-6). It may have a variety of causes, including the entry of foreign protein into circulation or massive vascular injury, as occurs in crushing trauma. Whatever the cause, the result is that the coagulation and fibrinolytic systems are out of control. Platelets and coagulation factors are consumed by this abnormal clotting. Thrombin formation overwhelms its inhibitor system and further accelerates clotting and activation of fibrinogen. Fibrin is deposited in the microvasculature of many organs, which results in poor tissue perfusion and eventual focal necrosis of tissue. Organ failure may result. Later the fibrinolytic system loses fibrin and impairs thrombin formation, and clots wash away. In summary, platelets, clotting factors, and fibrinogen are consumed so quickly that the body is unable to

replace them and maintain hemostatic levels. This creates a clinical picture of petechiae, peripheral cyanosis, GI bleeding, vaginal bleeding, prolonged bleeding, ecchymosis, hematomas, bleeding from surgical or invasive procedure sites, and signs of organ injury.

Drug-Induced Coagulopathies

Coumarin. The coumarin drugs, primarily dicoumarol and warfarin, are medications frequently prescribed. Coumarin interferes with the action of vitamin K, which causes a deficiency with resultant bleeding. Levels of prothrombin and factors VII and X are particularly decreased. Inappropriate dosage levels, the need for dosage adjustment, or intentional overdosage by the patient can be the cause of the coagulopathy.

Heparin. Heparin has several actions, the most important of which is the inactivation of thrombin.

With the inactivation of thrombin, fibrinogen is not converted to fibrin (insoluble protein threads that strengthen clots). Heparin also interferes in the action of factors IX, X, XI, and XII, which results in bleeding at single or multiple sites.

Other Medications. Aspirin affects platelet function and may cause bleeding. Aspirin blocks an enzyme called cyclooxygenase, which results in a decrease in platelet aggregation and decreased vasoconstriction. The clinical manifestations of aspirin-induced platelet dysfunction are minimal unless the patient also has an underlying coagulation defect such as von Willebrand's disease or other platelet or coagulation disorders.[54]

Fibrinolytic therapy is used in the management of acute myocardial infarction, pulmonary embolus, and stroke. A serious complication of this therapy is bleeding.

These medications work by causing clot dissolution with specific mechanisms, such as binding to fibrin and activating plasminogen to form plasmin, which in turn dissolves fibrin clots, fibrinogen, and other clotting factors. Although some drugs are clot specific, their action mechanisms leave the patient at risk for bleeding from puncture sites, from procedures such as intubation, and into specific places such as the brain or GI tract. Patients with histories of medical or surgical problems that can leave them at risk for bleeding are particularly vulnerable.[54] Other medications may interfere with platelet and clotting functions, but symptoms are generally mild and easily treated (Box 14-7).[54]

Massive Transfusions

Patients who receive large quantities of banked blood over a short period of time experience coagulopathies because of a dilutional effect. Banked blood becomes deficient in platelets and factors V and VII after storage at 4°C for 48 hours or longer. An estimated 10 to 12 units or more of blood given in a 24-hour period causes coagulopathies if platelets or fresh blood are not also given to increase platelet and clotting-factor levels.[2,91] The transport team must help prevent this type of coagulopathy from reaching clinically significant proportions.

BOX 14-7	**Drugs That Cause Decreased Platelet Number or Function**

Drug-Induced Thrombocytopenia

Alcohol
Antibiotics (sulfa, rifampin)
Aspirin
Cytotoxic agents
Digitoxin
Diphenylhydantoin
Estrogen
Gold salts
Heparin
Heroin
Nonsteroidal antiinflammatory drugs (NSAIDs)
Paraaminosalicylic acid
Phenylbutazone
Phenytoin
Quinidine, quinine
Streptokinase
Thiazides
Fibrinolytics

Drug-Induced Decreased Platelet Function

Aspirin
Clofibrate
Dextran
Dipyridamole
NSAIDs (indomethacin)
Sulfinpyrazone

ASSESSMENT

PHYSICAL ASSESSMENT

As with any other physical assessment, the transport team should first evaluate the airway, breathing, circulation, and disability (the ABCDEs). Once any necessary interventions have been undertaken to support those systems, attention can be given to a more detailed physical assessment.

Most bleeding, ecchymosis, and hematoma nearly always result from identifiable local trauma. However, as the transport team continues to assess the patient, certain observations indicate that a coagulopathy may be present. Some of these red flags include the following[2,37]:

1. Bleeding at multiple sites or in several body systems concurrently.
2. Spontaneous deep hematomas or hemarthroses.
3. Unusually prolonged bleeding after local injury.
4. Disproportionately large hemorrhage after a minor insult.
5. Late bleeding that follows a period of apparently normal hemostasis after surgery or trauma.
6. Inability to find an organic cause for hemorrhage in a specific area or organ system.

The transport team must be careful not to overlook the obvious. Many patients with previously diagnosed coagulopathies wear an identification tag such as the Medic-Alert tag as a necklace or bracelet, others carry a card that identifies the specific disorder, and some carry a treatment protocol at all times. This kind of documentation saves valuable time in directing patient assessment and care delivery.

During the assessment, the transport team should examine the skin and mucous membranes for signs of bleeding and note petechiae, purpura, ecchymosis, and hematomas. Oozing from intravenous (IV) sites or hematoma or ecchymosis around those sites may be significant. The patient should be observed for gingival or other mucous membrane bleeding; hematuria or GI bleeding may be part of the pattern that indicates coagulopathy. Joint deformities or stiffness may be present from previous hemarthroses. CNS bleeding is a life-threatening occurrence that is easily missed, and headache or other CNS signs should be aggressively pursued. The team should look for signs of liver, renal, or splenic disease or infection.

Any bleeding that is unusual or does not stop with direct pressure as expected should alert the team to suspect a coagulopathy is present. Identification of a specific coagulopathy on the basis of physical assessment, particularly in the transport environment, is almost impossible. However, characterization of the signs and symptoms of some of the major categories of coagulopathies is useful. Bleeding typical of a coagulation defect, such as the hemophilias, is large-vessel bleeding, often intramuscular, with large deep hematomas and hemarthrosis. Crippling joint deformities may be present from previous hemarthrosis.

In hemophilia, the platelet plug forms normally, but coagulation, which should follow, is defective. Therefore, the platelet plug may initially control bleeding. Later, delayed onset of bleeding may occur, or rebleeding may be seen after initial control of hemorrhage. In general, coagulation factor deficiencies are less responsive to local pressure than platelet abnormalities. Bleeding in DIC usually occurs at multiple sites, such as an oozing around IV or venipuncture sites or frank bleeding from mucosa. Purpura and ecchymosis may be present. The patient is often in shock.

Platelet defects, as in aspirin-induced bleeding or other types of thrombocytopenia, are manifested as small-vessel bleeding. Spontaneous bleeding occurs into the skin, such as petechiae, purpura, or numerous overlapping ecchymosis. Bleeding may be mucosal. Bleeding after trauma is more immediate than in clotting-factor deficiencies, and it usually stops with local pressure. Bleeding does not reoccur hours or days later, as does the pattern seen in clotting factor disorders.

HISTORY

A thorough history is extremely important in patients with suspected coagulopathies. The patient with a known coagulopathy may be more knowledgeable and expert about needed clinical management than the average nurse or physician. Family history of a coagulopathy may also guide in the assessment; however, this information should be substantiated by accompanying clinical signs and symptoms of the disease.

The patient's medical history may include unusual bleeding from the umbilical stump after birth and bleeding after dental extractions, trauma, or surgical procedures. A history of hemarthrosis, frequent epistaxis, or menorrhagia is significant. The flight nurse should question the patient about anticoagulants or other drugs that affect platelet function. A history of liver disease or other organ system failure is significant, as is evidence of infection or DIC-associated factors.

LABORATORY VALUES

Frequently, laboratory values are included in the patient's medical record received during an interfacility transport. These values should be referred to when the transport team undertakes the initial evaluation of the patient's condition (Box 14-8).

Table 14-1 lists possible diagnoses on the basis of results of the most readily available blood tests that evaluate coagulation and fibrinolysis. A definitive evaluation and diagnosis of the patient requires further laboratory testing at the receiving medical center.

In general, the intrinsic pathway is measured by the partial thromboplastin time (PTT). The extrinsic pathway is also evaluated by the PT (Figure 14-9).

A platelet count reveals thrombocytopenia but does not establish that platelet function is normal. Bleeding time, another widely available screening test, is increased in significant thrombocytopenia or platelet dysfunction disorders such as von Willebrand's disease. Fibrinogen concentration does not measure fibrinolysis directly but can suggest it when evaluated in conjunction with the other tests described.

BOX 14-8	**Normal Laboratory Values***

Bleeding time (Surgicutt)	1.5-8 min	
Fibrinogen concentration	195-365 mg/dL	
Hematocrit	Male:	42.0%-54.0%
	Female:	38.0%-46.0%
Hemoglobin	Male:	14.0-17.0 g/dL
	Female:	12.0-15.0 g/dL
Partial thromboplastin time (activated)	25-35 sec	
Prothrombin time	10.9-12.8 sec	
Platelet count		

Male:			
	6-11 y	235-534	$10^3/\mu L$
	12-16 y	184-485	$10^3/\mu L$
Female:	>16 y	184-370	$10^3/\mu L$
	6-11 y	227-539	$10^3/\mu L$
	12-16 y	200-390	$10^3/\mu L$
	>16 y	196-451	$10^3/\mu L$

*Normal values vary among laboratories depending on reagents used and method and instrumentation used.

TABLE 14-1	**Laboratory Evaluation of Coagulopathies**

Abnormal Tests	**Possible Diagnoses**
Plat or Plat BT	Idiopathic thrombocytopenic purpura, drug reaction, bone marrow depression
Plat, PT, PTT, Fib	DIC, liver disease
BT	Platelet dysfunction, mild von Willebrand's disease, salicylates, uremia
BT, PTT	von Willebrand's disease
PT	Factor VII deficiency (rare)
PTT	Hemophilia, heparin
PT, PTT	Vitamin K deficiency, coumarin drugs, liver disease, heparin, factor V, X, II, or I deficiency
Fib	Decreased fibrinogen (rare)
Fib, PT, ± PTT	DIC, primary fibrinolysis
All normal	Normal hemostasis, factor XII deficiency, allergic vasculitis, scurvy, dysproteinemia, etc

BT, Bleeding time; *Fib,* fibrinogen concentration; *Plat,* platelet count; *PT,* prothrombin time; *PTT,* partial thromboplastin time.

INTERVENTIONS AND TREATMENT

Diagnosis of a specific coagulopathy is difficult or impossible in the transport environment. Emergency interventions appropriate for patients with acute effects of coagulopathy are primarily supportive.

The first priority is airway management, which may be required if evidence is found of obstruction caused by bleeding or hematomas in the pharyngeal or laryngeal areas. Airway obstruction worsens as bleeding continues into the airway. An enlarging hematoma caused by bleeding into the soft tissues could completely obstruct the airway. Endotracheal intubation may be necessary to preserve the airway. Nasal intubation should be avoided because of a high likelihood of serious epistaxis. Supplemental oxygen should be delivered to the bleeding patient.

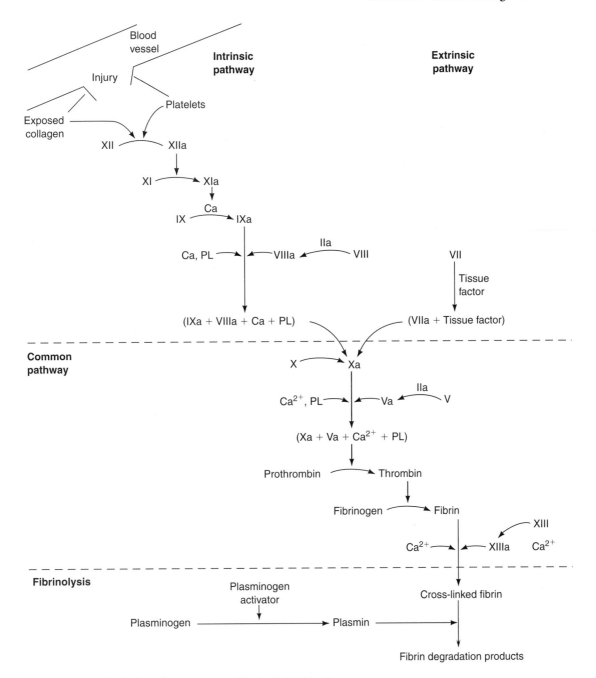

(1) Factors in the intrinsic pathway are present in circulating blood.
(2) The extrinsic pathway depends on the release of thromboplastin from damaged cells.
(3) "a" refers to the activated form of the designated factor.
(4) Ca = calcium. PL = phospholipid.

FIGURE 14-9 **Coagulation and fibrinolytic system.**

The next priority is to stop ongoing major hemorrhage. Patients who continue to hemorrhage should be treated in a similar way to any bleeding patients that the transport team may encounter. Direct pressure or pressure applied to appropriate pressure points helps control bleeding. Raising the bleeding part above the patient's heart decreases hydrostatic pressure and slows bleeding; however, pressure must be held for a much greater time than for the patient with normal coagulation mechanisms.

Volume replacement of shed blood is important. Fluids should be administered, and the patient's response closely monitored. If assessment indicates the need for additional volume replacement, blood products should be considered if available.

The patient should be protected from additional trauma during loading and unloading from the transport vehicle. The transport team should minimize needle sticks, and prolonged pressure should be applied to venipuncture sites. Intubation, catheterization, and other invasive procedures should be undertaken gently with good technique and only when indicated by the patient's condition.

Medications that depress platelet function should be withheld until medical consultation is available. Anticoagulants should also be withheld, with the exception of heparin in the case of DIC. This accepted therapy is appropriate in some situations to control the clotting system that is out of hemostatic balance.

Infusion of packed red blood cells, fresh frozen plasma, or platelets may be started at the referring hospital in an attempt to raise clotting factor or platelet levels. This therapy is useful but rather inexact when undertaken before complete laboratory evaluation. Only the specifically indicated blood component should be given because of the risk of autoimmunization and the possible transmission of infectious disease.[42,46,54,91]

Fresh frozen plasma can be infused to increase clotting factor levels in patients with deficiency. A unit of fresh frozen plasma raises any clotting factor level 2% to 3% in the average size adult. Fresh frozen plasma is not recommended if PT and PTT times are less than one and one-half times normal. Fresh frozen plasma is a useful method for correction of warfarin-induced hemorrhage when the seriousness of the patient's condition does not allow time for correction with simple discontinuation of warfarin therapy or administration of vitamin K.

Platelets can also be infused to correct bleeding caused by low platelet counts (thrombocytopenia) or deficiencies in platelet function. One unit of platelets should raise the platelet count by at least 5000 in the average adult. The decision to infuse platelets depends on clinical parameters in addition to platelet count. Patients with clinically stable conditions may need platelet counts for less than 10,000 to 20,000/μL. Patients undergoing invasive procedures generally should have a platelet count of 50,000/μL. However, patients with coagulation defects, hemorrhage, sepsis, or other unstable conditions may need higher platelet counts.

Specific treatment of certain disorders bears comment. Patients with hemophilia A should be treated early and aggressively for any bleeding episode. Standard treatment involves infusion of a factor VIII replacement. Cryoprecipitate is a frozen form of factor VIII concentrate. Most patients use factor VIII concentrate supplied in powder form. A single dose corrects minor bleeding, but severe hemorrhage may require continuous infusion for up to several weeks.

Hemophilia B is clinically indistinguishable from hemophilia A but requires treatment with either fresh frozen plasma or a concentrate enriched in the deficient factor IX. von Willebrand's disease is treated similarly to hemophilia A, often with cryoprecipitate.

Vitamin K deficiency should be treated with parenteral replacement. Administration of vitamin K intravenously is in a slow diluted infusion. An attempt should be made to correct the cause of the deficiency. Emergency treatment of hemorrhage with fresh frozen plasma should correct the clotting defect, at least temporarily.

Emergency treatment for hepatic coagulopathies includes administration of vitamin K. Fresh frozen plasma infusion replaces all known coagulation factors and is a safer and more complete therapy than prothrombin complex replacements. For patients with thrombosis, treatment with anticoagulation with heparin can be dangerous because heparin metabolism is unpredictable in cirrhosis and severe bleeding may result.

Disseminated intravascular coagulation is treated with identification and treatment of the underlying cause. Once this cause is eliminated, DIC resolves. Any significant bleeding or thrombosis requires immediate treatment. Fresh frozen plasma and cryoprecipitate are recommended to replace clotting factors. Platelet concentrates are given to increase the platelet count. Heparinization is a controversial treatment of the thrombosis seen in DIC. The clotting cascade is out of control in DIC, and clotting factors are rapidly consumed, which results in uncontrollable hemorrhage. Heparin reduces thrombin generation and prevents the further consumption of clotting factors. The risk is that heparin may cause further bleeding.

SUMMARY

The management of the patient who is in shock or may have complications of coagulopathy is based on early recognition, swift and appropriate treatment, and rapid transport. Regardless of the cause, uncontrolled shock leads to fatal derangement. The early diagnosis of shock requires consideration of the history of the precipitating incident, the patient's medical history, and the sometimes subtle signs exhibited by patients while compensatory mechanisms manage to maintain blood pressure and cardiac output.

An improved understanding of the pathophysiology of shock helps the transport team recognize patients in shock and potential or actual bleeding disorders. Although definitive diagnosis and treatment are generally not possible during transport, early recognition enhances the patient's chances for timely treatment. Supportive measures routinely practiced by transport teams help stabilize the patient in shock until further evaluation and treatment become available at the tertiary receiving facility.

SHOCK AND COAGULOPATHY CASE STUDY

A 23-year-old female restrained passenger of a motor vehicle was struck on her side of the car by a tractor-trailer. The car was driven into a ditch. On arrival of the transport team, they found a confused and combative patient in the back of an ambulance. The patient was on 100% oxygen via mask and was appropriately immobilized; one intravenous line of normal saline solution had been established.

Primary Survey

Spontaneous airway
Equal breath sounds
Pale, diaphoretic, cool skin
No palpable peripheral pulses; palpable femoral pulse
Monitor showed heart rate of 157, sinus tachycardia
Combative patient, Glasgow Coma Scale (GCS): 9
  Eye opening: 1
  Verbal: 3
  Motor: 5

Because of her signs of shock, the patient was intubated with rapid sequence induction (RSI) including amidate, lidocaine, and succinylcholine. She was intubated on the first attempt and ventilated with 100% oxygen. Initial color change on the end-tidal CO$_2$ was yellow.

A second line was established because the first line was tenuous. Additional sedation was given with the amidate, soft restraints were applied, and the patient was secured to the stretcher. During the 10-minute flight, 1500 mL of fluid was administered. The patient had a palpable pulse of 90 and a heart rate of 140, which decreased briefly to 110. Her ventilations were assisted with 100%, and she occasionally pulled against the restraints. Verbal assurance was given by the team.

On arrival at the trauma center, the patient was hot unloaded and taken to the Shock Resuscitation Unit. Her heart rate increased again to 150, and no blood pressure could be palpated. It was obtained with Doppler at 70 over palpation. A FAST examination was performed on arrival. A large amount of fluid was observed. Within minutes, she was taken directly to the operating room.

Blood and fluid resuscitation in the operating room (OR) returned a pressure of 90. The patient had sustained a severe splenic injury, and as repair began, her blood pressure dropped and she began to bleed profusely. A lacerated inferior vena cava was found.

Despite aggressive resuscitation and repair of the injury, the patient continued to bleed. Unfortunately, she died approximately 90 minutes after the accident.

This case illustrates the need for early recognition of shock (no palpable peripheral pulses, tachycardia, altered mental status), the initial critical interventions (intubation and oxygenation with 100% oxygen, fluid bolus), and rapid transport to an appropriate center for definitive care. However, it points out that even when all the pieces fall in place, the injury or illness that causes irreversible shock remains a challenge.

REFERENCES

1. Ackerman M: The systemic inflammatory response, sepsis, and multiple organ dysfunction, *Crit Care Nurs Clin North Am* 6:243, 1994.
2. Air and Surface Transport Nurses Association: *Transport nurse advanced trauma course (TNATC)*, ed 6, Denver, 2006, ASTNA.
3. Ali J, Qi W: Fluid and electrolyte deficit with prolonged pneumatic anti-shock garment application, *J Trauma* 38(4):612, 1994.
4. Alspach JG: *Core curriculum for critical care nursing*, ed 6, Philadelphia, 2007, Saunders.
5. American College of Surgeons Committee on Trauma: *Advanced trauma life support for doctors*, ed 8, Chicago, 2008, American College of Surgeons.
6. Anderson HL III, et al: Extracorporeal life support for respiratory failure after multiple trauma, *J Trauma* 37(2):266, 1994.
7. Angelica A, Todaro A: Action stat! Reversing acute dehydration, *Nursing* 23(6):33, 1993.
8. Barone J, Snyder A: Treatment strategies in shock: use of oxygen transport measures, *Heart Lung* 1:81, 1991.
9. Battistella F, Wisner D: Combined hemorrhagic shock and head injury: effects of hypertonic saline (7.5%) resuscitation, *J Trauma* 31(2):182, 1991.
10. Beere HM, Green DR: Stress management: heat shock protein–70 and the regulation of apoptosis, *Trends Cell Biol* 11(1):6, 2001.
11. Behrman S, et al: Microcirculatory flow changes after initial resuscitation of hemorrhagic shock with 7.5% hypertonic saline/6% dextran, *J Trauma* 31(5):589, 1991.
12. Berry R: Management of shock in trauma, *Anaesth Intens Care Med* 9(9):390-393, 2008.
13. Bickell W, et al: Immediate versus delayed fluid resuscitation for hypotensive patients with penetrating torso injuries, *N Engl J Med* 331(17):1105, 1994.
14. Bickell WH, et al: Resuscitation of canine hemorrhage hypotension with large volume isotonic crystalloid: impact on lung water, venous admixture, and systemic arterial oxygen saturation, *Am J Emerg Med* 12(1):36, 1994.
15. Bone R: Sepsis, sepsis syndrome, and the systemic inflammatory response syndrome (SIRS): Gullivar in Laputa, *JAMA* 273:155, 1995.
16. Boswell SA, Scalea TM: Initial management of traumatic shock, In McQuillan K, Makic MB, Whalen E, editors: *Trauma nursing: from resuscitation through rehabilitation*, ed 4, Philadelphia, 2009, Saunders.
17. Brees C, Hensleigh PA, Miller S, et al: A non-inflatable antishock garment for obstetric hemorrhage, *Int J Gyncol Obstet* 87:119-124, 2004.
18. Bridges EJ, Woods SL: Pulmonary artery pressure measurement: state of the art, *Heart Lung* 22(2):99, 1993.
19. Britt LW: Priorities in the management of profound shock, *Surg Clin North Am* 76(4):645-660, 1996.
20. Brown KK: Critical interventions in septic shock, *Am J Nurs* 94:21, 1994.
21. Brown KK: Septic shock: how to stop the deadly cascade, *Am J Nurs* 94:20, 1994.
22. Campbell JE: *International trauma life support, advanced prehospital care*, ed 6, Upper Saddle River, NJ, 2008, Pearson/Prentice Hall Health.
23. Carcello JA, Han K, Lin J, et al: Goal-directed management of pediatric shock in the emergency department, *Clin Pediatr Emerg Med* 8:165-175, 2007.
24. Cayten CG, et al: A study of pneumatic anti-shock garments in severely hypotensive trauma patients, *J Trauma* 34(5):728, 1993.
25. Chang FC, et al: PSAG: does it help in the management of traumatic shock? *J Trauma* 39(3):453, 1995.
26. Chikanori T, et al: Effects of mild Trendelenburg on central hemodynamics and internal jugular vein velocity, cross sectional area flow, *Am J Emerg Med* 13(3):255, 1995.
27. Ciesla DM: Multiple organ dysfunction during resuscitation is not postinjury multiple organ failure, *Arch Surg* 139(6):590-595, 2004.
28. Cocchi MN, Kimlin E, Walsh M, et al: Identification and resuscitation of the trauma patient in shock, *Emerg Med Clin North Am* 25:623-642, 2007.
29. Cohn SM, Farrell TJ: Diasprin cross-linked hemoglobin, resuscitation of hemorrhage: comparison of a

blood substitute with hypertonic saline and isotonic saline, *J Trauma* 39(2):210, 1995.

30. Consortium for Spinal Cord Medicine: *Early acute management in adults with spinal cord injury: a clinical practice guideline for health-care providers.* Washington, DC, 2008, Paralyzed Veterans of America.

31. Cross J, et al: Hypertonic saline fluid therapy following surgery: a prospective study, *J Trauma* 30(6):817, 1989.

32. Dabich MA, Wade CE: A review of the efficacy and safety of 7.5% nacl/6% dextran 70 in experimental animals and humans, *J Trauma* 36(3):323, 1994.

33. Darling GE: Multi-organ failure in critical patients, *Can J Surg* 31(3):172, 1988.

34. Dellinger RP, Levy MM, Carlet JM, et al: Surviving sepsis campaign: international guidelines for management of severe sepsis and septic shock, *Crit Care Med* 36(4):1394-1396, 2008.

35. Dutton RP: Current concepts in hemorrhagic shock, *Anesthesiol Clin* 25:23-34, 2007.

36. Eisman BB, Beart R, Norton L: Multiple organ failure, *Surg Gynecol Obstet* 144:323-326, 1977.

37. Emergency Nurses Association: *Trauma nursing core course,* Des Plaines, 2007, ENA.

38. Epstein CD, Herning RJP: Oxygen transport variables in the identification and treatment of tissue hypoxia, *Heart Lung* 22(4):328, 1993.

39. Ertel W, et al: Release of anti-inflammatory mediators after mechanical trauma correlates with severity of injury and clinical outcome, *J Trauma* 39(5):879, 1995.

40. Fisher J: *The plague makers,* New York, 1994, Simon and Schuster.

41. Frankel DA, Acosta JA, Anjaria DJ, et al: Physiologic responses to hemorrhagic shock depends on rate and means of hemorrhage, *J Surg Res* 143:276-280, 2008.

42. Gaedeke MK: Action stat! Disseminated intravascular coagulation, *Nursing* 24(7):53, 1994.

43. Hazinski MF: Shock, multiple organ dysfunction syndrome, and burns in children. In McCance KL, editor: *Pathophysiology: the biologic basis for disease in adults and children,* St Louis, 2006, Elsevier Mosby.

44. Jacobs L: Timing of fluid resuscitation in trauma, *N Engl J Med* 331(17):1153, 1994.

45. Johansson PI, Bochsen L, Stensballe J, et al: Transfusion packages for massively bleeding patients: the effect on clot formation and stability as evaluated by Thrombelastograph (TEG®), *Transfusion Apheresis Sci* 39:3-8, 2008.

46. Kasper C: *von Willebrand disease.* available at http://www.med.unc.edu/isth/publications/vwd_monograph/VWD_mon_2008.pdf, accessed September 2008.

47. Keenan A: Hematologic emergencies. In Kitt S, et al, editors: *Emergency nursing,* Philadelphia, 1995, Saunders.

48. Kirkpatric AW, Ball C, D'Amours Zygun D: Acute resuscitation of the unstable adult trauma patient: bedside diagnosis and therapy, *Can J Surg* 51(1):57-69, 2008.

49. Kokiki J: Septic shock: a review and update for the emergency department clinician, *J Emerg Nurs* 19(2):102, 1993.

50. Kowalenkno T, et al: Improved outcome with hypotensive resuscitation of uncontrolled hemorrhagic shock in a swine model, *J Trauma* 33(3):349, 1992.

51. Liberman M, Mulder D, Sampalis J: Advanced or basic life support for trauma: meta-analysis and critical review of the literature, *J Trauma* 49(4):584, 2000.

52. Maclean LD: Shock: a century of progress, *Ann Surg* 201(4):407, 1985.

53. Malkevich NV, Dong F, VanderMolen CA, et al: Innate immune response after resuscitation with hemoglobin-based oxygen carrier and recombinant factor VIIA in uncontrolled hemorrhagic shock in a swine model, *J Trauma* 64(6):1498-1510, 2008.

54. Mansen TJ, McCance KL: Alterations of leukocyte, lymphoid, and hemostatic function. In McCance KL, Huether S, editors: *Pathophysiology: the biologic basis for disease in adults and children,* St Louis, 2006, Elsevier Mosby.

55. Marthay MA, Chatterjee K: Bedside catheterization of the pulmonary artery: risks compared with benefits, *Ann Intern Med* 109(10):826, 1988.

56. Martin R, et al: Prospective evaluation of preoperative fluid resuscitation in hypotensive patients with penetrating truncal injury: a preliminary report, *J Trauma* 33(3):354, 1992.

57. Mattox K, et al: Prospective MAST study in 911 patients, *J Trauma* 30(8):1104, 1989.

58. Mazzoni M, et al: The efficiency of iso- and hyperosmotic fluids as volume expanders in fixed-volume and uncontrolled hemorrhage, *Ann Emerg Med* 19(4):350, 1990.

59. Moore E, et al: The post-ischemic gut serves as a priming bed for circulating neutrophils that provoke multiple organ failure, *J Trauma* 37:881, 1994.

60. Moore F, Moore E, Peterson V: Inflammatory models of multiple organ failure, *Trauma Q* 12(1):47, 1995.

61. Mountz J, et al: The role of programmed cell death as an emerging new concept for the pathogenesis of

autoimmune diseases, *Clin Immunol Immunopath* 80(3):S2, 1996.

62. Oman KS: Use of hematocrit changes as an indicator of blood loss in adult trauma patients who receive intravenous fluids, *J Emerg Nurs* 21(5):395, 1995.

63. Owens TS, et al: Limiting initial resuscitation of uncontrolled hemorrhage reduces internal bleeding and subsequent volume requirements, *J Trauma* 39(2):200, 1995.

64. Pedowitz RA, Shackford SR: Noncavitary hemorrhage producing shock in trauma patients: incidence and severity, *J Trauma* 29(2):219, 1989.

65. Pettijean ME, et al: Thoracic spinal trauma and associated injuries: should early decompression be considered? *J Trauma* 39(2):368, 1995.

66. Querin JJ, Dixon LS: Twelve simple sensible steps to successful blood transfusions, *Nursing* 20(10):68, 1990.

67. Rifkind R, et al: *Fundamentals of hematology*, ed 3, St Louis, 1986, Mosby.

68. Rottman S, Larmon B, Manix T: Rapid volume infusion in prehospital care, *Prehosp Disaster Med* 3:225, 1990.

69. Rueden K, Dunham CM: Sequelae of massive fluid resuscitation in trauma patients, *Crit Care Nurs Clin North Am* 6:463, 1994.

70. Ryan KL, Batchinsky A, McManus JG, et al: Changes in pulse character and mental status are late responders to central hypovolemia, *Prehosp Emerg Med* (12):192-198, 2008.

71. Samuels D, Bock H: *Air medical crew national standard curriculum*, Pasadena, CA, 1988, ASHBEAMS.

72. Sayre MR: What's new in the treatment of hemorrhagic shock, *J Air Med Transport* 10(5):20, 1991.

73. Schmoker JD, et al: Hypertonic fluid resuscitation improves cerebral oxygen delivery and reduces intracranial pressure after hemorrhagic shock, *J Trauma* 31(12):1607, 1991.

74. Schrieber TL, Miller DH, Zola B: Management of myocardial infarction shock: current status, *Am Heart J* 117(2):435, 1989.

75. Schultz SC, et al: The efficacy of diasprin cross-linked hemoglobin solution resuscitation in a model of uncontrolled hemorrhage, *J Trauma* 37(3):408, 1994.

76. Schultz SC, et al: Use of base deficit to compare resuscitation with lactated Ringer's solution, Hemaccel, whole blood, and diasprin cross-linked hemoglobin following hemorrhage in rats, *J Trauma* 35(4):619, 1993.

77. Schwartzberg S: Cytokines: experimental and clinical studies, *Trauma Q* 22(1):7, 1995.

78. Selfridge-Thomas J: Shock, In Kitt S, et al, editors: *Emergency nursing*, Philadelphia, 1995, Saunders.

79. Shatney CH: Initial resuscitation and assessment of patients with multisystem blunt trauma, *South Med J* 81(4):501, 1988.

80. Shekarriz B, Stoller ML: The use of fibrin sealant in urology, *J Urol* 167:1218-1225, 2002.

81. Shires GT, Browder LK, Steljes T, et al: The effect of shock resuscitation fluids on apoptosis, *Am J Surg* 189:85-101, 2005.

82. Sommers M: Rapid fluid resuscitation: how to correct dangerous deficits, *Nursing* 20(1):52, 1990.

83. Spearing-Bolgiano C: Administering oxygen therapy: what you need to know, *Nursing* 20(6):47, 1990.

84. Stern S, et al: Effect of blood pressure on hemorrhage volume and survival in a near-fetal hemorrhage model incorporating vascular injury, *Ann Emerg Med* 22(2):155, 1993.

85. Talan D: Recent developments in our understanding of sepsis: evaluation of antiendotoxin antibodies and biological modifiers, *Ann Emerg Med* 22:1871, 1993.

86. Tien HC, Jung V, Rizoli SB, et al: An evaluation of tactical combat casualty care interventions in a combat environment, *J Am Coll Surgeons* 207(2):174-178, 2008.

87. Thijs LG: Definitions and epidemilogy, In Dhainaut JT, editor: *Septic shock*, Philadelphia, 2000, Saunders.

88. Valedi MH: Pneumatic anti-shock garment associated compartment syndrome in uninjured lower extremities, *J Trauma* 38(4):616, 1995.

89. Vassar MJ, et al: Prehospital resuscitation of hypotensive trauma patient with 7.5% nacl vs 7.5% nacl with added dextran: a controlled trial, *J Trauma* 34(5):622, 1993.

90. Warren BL, et al: Kybersept trial study group, *JAMA* 286(1):1894, 2001.

91. Wilson M, Davis D, Coimbra R: Diagnosis and monitoring of hemorrhagic shock during initial resuscitation of multiple trauma patients: a review, *J Emerg Med* 24(4):413-422, 2003.

92. Zakaria ER, Matheson PJ, Flesner M, et al: Hemorrhagic shock and resuscitation-mediated tissue water distribution is normalized by adjunctive peritoneal resuscitation, *Am J Surg* 206(5):970-980, 2008.

UNIT IV
Trauma

CHAPTER

15

GENERAL PRINCIPLES OF TRAUMA MANAGEMENT

Reneé Semonin Holleran, Steven W. Neher

COMPETENCIES

1. Demonstrate the ability to perform scene safety and trauma triage.
2. Perform a primary and secondary assessment of the injury.
3. Initiate critical interventions for the injured patient before and during transport.

Trauma is defined as injury to human tissue and organs from the transfer of energy from the environment. Injuries are caused by some form of energy that is beyond the body's resilience to tolerate.[1,2] Regardless of gender, race, or economic status, unintentional injury is the fifth leading cause of death for all ages in the United States and the leading cause of death for those aged 1 to 44 years.[1,2] Approximately 164,112 deaths annually result from trauma.[3] Traumatic events are rarely accidental; most are actually preventable.[3] Thus, the term *accident* is no longer used in the trauma literature. Unintentional injuries are a major source of morbidity and mortality. For this reason, injury prevention has become a major public health goal.[24]

The cost of trauma-related injuries has exceeded $400 billion annually in the United States.[4] These costs are accounted for by lost wages, medical expenses, insurance administration costs, property damage, fire loss, employer costs, and indirect loss from work.[4]

INJURY DYNAMICS

The time elapsed from the actual injury to initiation of definitive care is key to patient survivability. One of the most important factors that has positively influenced morbidity and mortality rates of trauma is rapid transport; the addition of highly trained medical personnel has brought critical care management outside the trauma center to the rural hospital or the scene of the trauma.

The transport of the patient with multiple injuries requires in-depth knowledge and skills and expert prioritization and organization skills. A thorough understanding of the mechanisms of injury and the kinematics of trauma are essential for any transport team member caring for injured patients. Knowledge of these principles helps guide appropriate assessment and treatment.

HISTORY

One of the first steps in care of a patient with multiple injuries is a history of events preceding and following the traumatic event. With interfacility transfers, this information is most commonly obtained from other nurses, physicians, and family members. The history at a scene call generally comes from many individuals, including law enforcement, firefighters, and other emergency medical services (EMS) personnel and bystanders.[1]

When responding via rotor-wing aircraft at the scene of a trauma, an aerial view of the situation helps the transport team to begin data collection about the patient (Figure 15-1). The transport team has the advantage of evaluating the entire scene, the damage sustained to the vehicles or the buildings, the extent of impact, and the objects thrown or blown out of the central area of impact.

At the scene, life-threatening injuries are always top priority, and a detailed history may be impractical in certain cases. However, the importance of a thorough history is vital to direct the patient's care. Because time is a critical factor for survivability, the history should be obtained while gaining access to the patient or while simultaneously performing the primary assessment. If the patient has an altered level of consciousness, the only history obtained may be from the hospital or emergency personnel present, who may not be going to the receiving hospital.

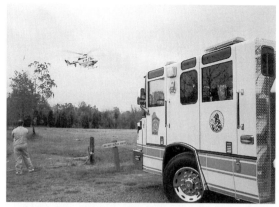

FIGURE 15-1   **When approaching a scene from the air, the transport team begins collecting information about the incident.**

The history should be elicited during concurrent patient assessment because the team may never get another chance to obtain needed information. When appropriate, the mnemonic *AMPLE* is used to elicit a history from the patient.

A: Allergies
M: Medications currently used
P: Past illness or Pregnancy
L: Last meal
E: Events or Environment related to the injury

Additional important information includes time of incident, mechanism of injury, any alteration in the patient's level of consciousness, and the patient's medical history, current medications, and allergies.

A further detailed history may be obtained from the patient during the secondary survey as time and patient condition allow and can be routinely performed in the transport vehicle.

MECHANISM OF INJURY

Injuries occur when external forces are applied to the body. The type and amount of injuring force and the tissue response to the force determine the extent of injury.[2] When the body's tissue cannot withstand any additional force, destruction occurs, as evidenced by common injuries seen in the patient with multiple injuries: fractures, lacerations, and ruptured internal organs. A complete understanding of a force and the way it is applied is necessary to predict potential injuries and thus adequately care for the injured patient.

Newton's first law of motion states that a body at rest tends to remain at rest and a body in motion tends to remain in motion until acted on by an outside force. When the body contacts an object, energy is transferred, and damage occurs (Figure 15-2).

Force is a result of energy transference, which can be explained by the laws of physics.

1. Energy can be neither created nor destroyed; it can only change form.
2. Kinetic energy (KE) = (Mass × Velocity²) / 2
3. Force = Mass × Acceleration

Because energy is neither created nor destroyed, it is transferred, and its transference is dependent on the mass of the object multiplied by the speed squared over a common denominator of 2. For example, an automobile that weighs 3000 lbs is traveling at 40 mph when it strikes a telephone pole.

$$KE = \frac{3000 \times 40^2}{2}$$

The kinetic energy transferred in this impact to both objects is 2,400,000 units.

The same force is applied to destruction of the body. Energy is transferred from the automobile to the human. Several factors determine the amount of energy the human absorbs, including the following:

1. The amount of energy absorbed by the objects that initially collide (e.g., the telephone pole and the automobile).
2. The amount absorbed by protective factors, such as seat belts, helmets, padded steering wheels, dashboards, and airbags.

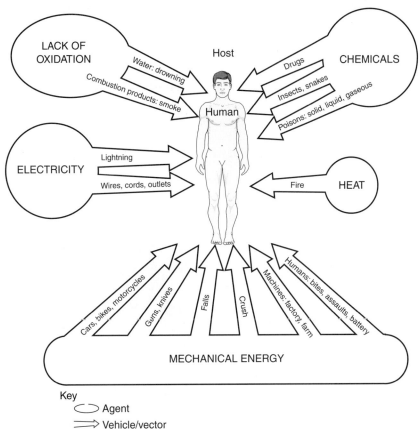

FIGURE 15-2 **Energy forces that can affect the human body.**

The forces involved in the impact cause varying degrees of destruction. The more slowly the force is applied, the less energy transference and the lower the degree of destruction. The extent of injury is also dependent on which body parts receive the impact.[19] For example; the skull can take more force before damage occurs than can the abdomen.

Force can be delivered via compression, acceleration, deceleration, or shearing.[19]

Compression: Direct pressure on a structure is the most common type of force applied. The amount of injury sustained is dependent on the length of time of compression and the area compressed.[19]

Acceleration/deceleration: Acceleration is the increase in the velocity of a moving object. Deceleration is the decrease in velocity of an object.[19] In an automobile crash, the body is thrown forward (accelerates) by the impact and decelerates as it comes in contact with the steering wheel, seatbelt, or dashboard. The internal organs initially also accelerate and decelerate as they come into contact with internal structures such as ribs, which causes destruction to the tissues and vasculature.

Shearing: Shearing forces occur when the tissues or organs or both are pushed ahead of underlying or overlying structures. The most common mechanism that causes a shearing injury occurs when a pedestrian is run over by a vehicle. As the vehicle grabs a part of the body, the area is pushed forward until it can no longer take the force, and it tears. Degloving routinely occurs from shearing forces.

The viscoelastic properties of tissues in the body help to absorb energy. When the energy delivered is below the limit of injury, the energy is absorbed and causes no damage. When the forces applied deliver more energy than the body can absorb, strains occur.[19] Strains may be classified as tensile, shearing, or compressive. Table 15-1 displays the characteristics and examples of each type of strain.

KINEMATICS OF TRAUMA

Patterns of injury have been identified with evaluation of the type of trauma that has occurred and the amount of force generated. Although all patients should be evaluated individually, certain injuries are common to certain forces. Prediction of these injuries is referred to as *kinematics*. Age, preventive

TABLE 15-1	**Characteristics of Strains**	
Type	**Reaction**	**Examples**
Tensile	Stretching	Bony fractures, aortic tears
Shearing	Movement of tissue in opposite directions	Brain injuries, lacerations/ avulsions
Compressive	Crushing force	Compartment syndrome, ruptures

measures taken, and velocity are factors in the alteration of injury patterns, and the caregiver should consider these factors in evaluation of a patient.[15]

BLUNT INJURIES
Motor Vehicle Crashes

Motor vehicle crashes account for most injuries and deaths in 70% of the 39 countries for which data are available (Figure 15-3).[4]

Head-on Collisions.   As an automobile collides with another automobile or with any object head on, energy is transferred to the vehicle. The front of the vehicle routinely stops less than one-half second after impact. The rear of the automobile continues to move forward until all the energy is dispersed. Although the front end of the car is destroyed, the rear of the

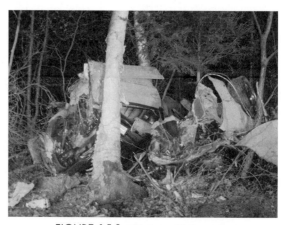

FIGURE 15-3   **Motor vehicle crash.**

vehicle causes the destruction by its continued forward movement. The same principle of injury occurs with the body during a head-on collision. The initial impact occurs in the front of the vehicle. The unrestrained driver hits the steering wheel with the thorax, the head may hit the windshield, and the knees contact the dashboard (Figure 15-4). Predictable injuries from initial impact are fractured ribs, pneumothorax, or hemopneumothorax; concussion; skull fractures; patella and femur fractures; dislocated hips; and acetabular fractures. The progression of injury proceeds, as does the automobile, and the person's internal organs are thrown from the rear forward until all energy is dispersed. Common injuries include ruptured spleens (direct compression from the steering wheel), lacerated livers (stretching of hilum until the tensile strength is exceeded), and ruptured thoracic aortas (heart and aorta are forcibly thrown forward, stretched, and then compressed against the ribs).

The restrained driver in a head-on collision has much of the energy absorbed by the seat belt and air bag, if present. The seat belt may impose a load 20 to 50 times as great as the body weight. The only portion of the human body capable of incurring this load is the pelvis. Unless the patient has the belt properly applied securely over the pelvis, direct compression of the abdomen may occur. The first indicator of these injuries is often the presence of abrasions over the abdomen from the seat belt. Other injuries associated with seat belt use include sternal fractures, breast injuries, and lumbar vertebral body fractures. As seen with abdominal seat belt injuries, abrasions or ecchymosis or both are important indicators. Lap belts should be worn with a diagonal shoulder strap to stop forward movement of the upper body. Diagonal straps worn alone can cause severe neck injuries, including decapitation. Air bags cushion forward motion only. They are effective in a first collision; but because they deflate immediately, they are not effective in multiple-impact collisions. When the air bag deploys, it can produce injury to the patient. The most common injuries seen are abrasions of the arms, chest, and face, which can include injuries caused by the patient's eyeglasses.[12,19,23]

Rear-end Collisions.   An automobile hit from behind rapidly accelerates, which causes the car to move forward under the patient. Predictable injuries are to the back (T12-L1 is the most common area of injury), legs (femur, tibia/fibula, and ankle fractures), and neck (cervical strain, cervical fractures caused by hyperextension), if the head restraint is not in the proper position. If the automobile undergoes a second collision by striking a car in front of it, the predictable head-on injuries also need to be evaluated.

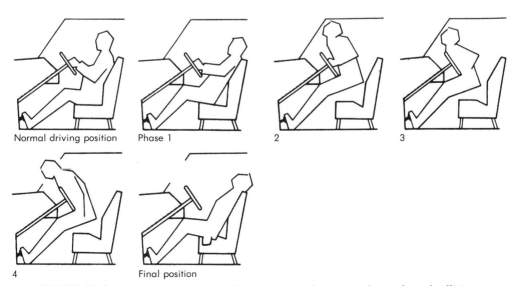

Normal driving position   Phase 1

2

3

4   Final position

FIGURE 15-4   **Phases of movement of the unrestrained occupant during frontal collision.**

Side Impact. An automobile hit on the side routinely causes lateral injuries to the patient. An unrestrained driver hit on the side can have initial injuries to the left clavicle, ribs, femur, and tibia/fibula. Abdominal injuries, such as ruptured spleens, are seen in these crashes, usually because of the fractured lower lateral ribs, but also because of direct compression on the abdomen.[19] Secondary injuries occur when the patient is propelled to the other side of the car, which causes injuries to the opposite side.

Rollovers. Predictable injuries caused by vehicle rollovers are more difficult to define (Figure 15-5). The unrestrained patient tumbles inside the vehicle, and injury occurs to the areas of the body that are hit. The caregiver should always care for these patients judiciously and realize the potential for multiple-system injuries.

Motorcycle Crashes

Because motorcycles offer minimal or no initial energy transference, energy is directly absorbed by the rider, and injuries are substantially more severe than with other motor vehicle crashes. The predicted injuries during a motorcycle crash, like those during other motor vehicle crashes, depend on the type of collision that occurs.

Head-on Collisions. For accurate prediction of injuries that involve the motorcycle rider, an understanding of the design of a motorcycle is helpful (Figure 15-6). The center of gravity is located

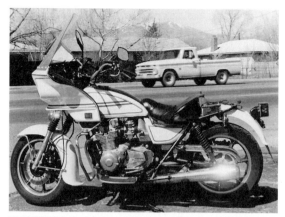

FIGURE 15-6   Construction of a motorcycle places the center of gravity in front of the driver's seat. Head-on collision causes the cycle to tip up and throw the occupant over the front.

in front of the driver's seat. As the cycle strikes an object head on, the rear (or lighter) portion tips upward from the weight under the handlebars, which prevents the driver, who is propelled over the handlebars, from total ejection. Associated injuries with this type of crash are fractured femurs, tibias, and fibulas (from the handlebars); chest and abdominal injuries (from direct compression against the handlebars or tire); and head and neck injuries (from impact with the tire or any object in front of the cycle). Any motorcycle crash can cause the rider to be ejected, but ejection is most common during head-on collisions. As with ejection from any vehicle, the head acts as the missile. Suspicion of and intervention for major head and cervical spine injuries are imperative with any ejected patient.

Side Impact. Injuries associated with a side-impact motorcycle crashes are related to the body parts crushed between the cycle and the second object. Most commonly seen injuries involve the leg and foot on the impact side. Open fractures of the femur, tibia/fibula, and malleolus are predictable.

Laying Down the Motorcycle. Motorcycle riders have learned the technique of laying down the bike and sliding off to the side before colliding with another object. The energy transference is a result

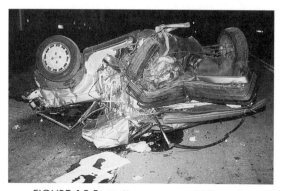

FIGURE 15-5   **Rollover motor vehicle crash.**

of sliding away from the bike. Commonly seen are abrasions on the affected side. Fractures may occur if the patient hits the road hard or comes in contact with another object. Preventive clothing, such as leather jackets, pants, and gloves, absorb more energy than average clothing; in this type of impact, they may prevent abrasions.

Falls

Falls from heights greater than 15 to 20 ft are associated with severe injuries. In predicting injuries associated with falls, caregivers should understand the following:

1. The average roof of a one-story house is approximately 15 ft off the ground; a two-story fall is approximately 30 ft.
2. With a fall greater than 15 ft, adults usually land on the feet. At less than 15 ft, adults land as they fall; that is, if they fall head first, they land on the head.
3. Because small children have proportionally larger heads, no matter what the distance, they tend to fall head first.

The caregiver must estimate the distance fallen. Second, what the patient landed on must be determined. A soft landing surface, such as dirt or sand, absorbs much more energy than a hard surface, such as concrete.

Three predictable injuries are seen in falls. The forces involved are deceleration and compression. The first injury, calcaneus fractures, is caused by compression of the feet on impact. Second, as the energy dissipates after impact and the top of the body pushes down toward the point of impact, compression fractures to T12-L1 are seen. Finally, as the body moves forward and the patient puts out both arms to complete the fall, bilateral wrist fractures occur.

PENETRATING TRAUMA

All objects that cause injury from penetration deliver the same two types of force: *crushing* and *stretching*.[13,1,4,16] Depending on the velocity of the penetrating object, the wound can be small or massive.

Stab Wounds

Stab wounds are considered low velocity and produce the major damage by crushing tissues as the penetrating object enters. An object that is narrow at the beginning and thicker at the end crushes the tissues as it enters and stretches them apart as the thicker part is inserted. The area of injury for stab wounds is typically localized to the area of insertion. The penetrating instrument might remain embedded in the patient or might have been removed; embedded penetrating objects should be stabilized with bandages for transport and not removed (Figure 15-7).

Firearm Injuries

Wounding from bullets can have four causes: (1) direct contact by the missile; (2) crushing force in the immediate vicinity of the missile; (3) temporary cavity formation; and (4) collapse of the temporary cavity.[10,14]

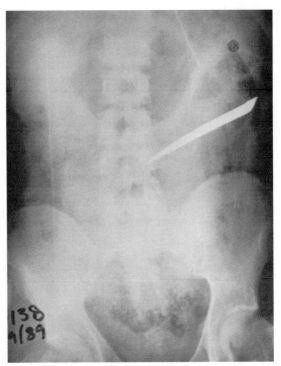

FIGURE 15-7 **Knife with the handle broken off embedded in a patient.** Object was discovered when the radiograph was taken.

The degree of wounding depends on the amount of energy transferred from the bullet to the body. The type of weapon used, the type of bullet, the distance from which the weapon was fired, and the body part penetrated are key factors in wound severity.

Firearms can be handguns, rifles, or shotguns. Handguns and some rifles are considered medium energy; assault rifles and hunting rifles are high energy. The greater the amount of gunpowder in the cartridge, the greater the speed of the bullet, and therefore, the kinetic energy increases.[19] The degree of deformation by the penetrating missile is influenced by the following factors.

Yaw and tumbling: Yaw is deviation of the bullet up to 90 degrees from a straight path, and tumbling is rotation of the bullet 360 degrees. Both cause increased tissue crush and stretching.

Deformation of a bullet when striking tissue: Certain missiles are constructed of soft lead and flatten on impact. Other bullets have hollow points that cause a mushrooming effect on impact; hollow-point bullets are also known as expanding bullets. The increased diameter of these bullets increases tissue destruction.

Fragmentation: Each fragmented portion of the missile causes damage in its path. Increased velocity increases the potential of fragmentation.

Explosive effect: Explosive bullets are intended to cause massive damage with a single shot. The bullet is composed of black powder and lead shot. On impact, detonation of the powder causes explosion and disintegration of the bullet casing, which further propels the lead shot.[19]

The closer to the target the bullet was fired, the greater the amount of kinetic energy transferred to the tissues. For that reason, firing distance is important to ascertain during the history taking.

Cavitation occurs with all penetrating objects. The permanent cavity is formed from the crushed tissue produced by the object. Temporary cavity formation occurs from transfer of kinetic energy from the missile to the tissue. The velocity, size, shape, and ballistic behavior of the missile and the biophysical properties of the tissue determine the extent of the temporary cavity. As a missile strikes tissue, temporary cavitation occurs forward of and lateral to the missile. Relatively elastic tissues, such as lung, bowel wall, and muscle, tolerate the stretch of the temporary cavity much better than the solid nonelastic organs, such as the liver and spleen.[15] The literature has estimated temporary cavity formation as large as 30 to 40 times the missile diameter.[5] Studies have indicated that temporary cavitation is usually no more than 10 to 20 times the missile diameter for high-velocity missiles (Figure 15-8).[15,18]

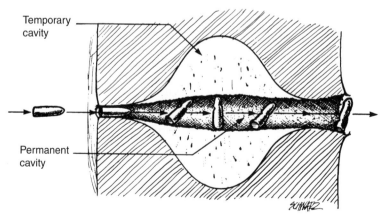

Temporary cavity

Permanent cavity

FIGURE 15-8   **Effects of yaw and temporary and permanent cavitation from a missile.** Permanent cavity is caused by necrotic muscle tissue. Temporary cavity is caused by stretching of soft tissue. (From Weiner SL, Barrett J: *Trauma management for civilian and military positions,* Philadelphia, 1986, Saunders.)

PATHOPHYSIOLOGIC FACTORS

Multiple trauma causes severe stress to the human body and is associated with a flux of hormones and physiologic reactions (Table 15-2). The degree of metabolic and hormonal changes depends on the severity of injury, the effectiveness of resuscitation, and the preinjury condition of the patient. The pathophysiologic analysis of traumatic injuries is discussed in detail in the chapters that individually discuss specific traumas. In general, metabolic response to shock from injury in the early stage differs from that in the late stage (Table 15-3).

In the early stage, the body responds to hypoperfusion as a stress to the body. Many of the changes that are mediated through the sympathetic nervous system occur rapidly. The overall effect is an increase in systemic vascular resistance. A response

is mediated through the renin-angiotensin system that occurs more slowly. The response is again to vasoconstrict and also to increase blood volume via retention.[8,21]

In the early stage, the compensatory mechanisms are beneficial in that the heart and brain receive adequate blood supply, but at the expense of the kidneys and other abdominal organs. If the underlying cause of shock is corrected, then the patient may do well. If it is not, the compensatory mechanisms are not able to continue to perfuse vital organs well enough, and the mechanisms themselves become deleterious to the body. The shock then progress to the late stage.[21]

During the late stage, as shock progresses, blood flow to all body tissues is impaired. Cell metabolism fails, and acidosis and energy deficiency result. Without enough energy, the cell functions fail, and

TABLE 15-2 Major Pathophysiologic Changes in Shock

Change	Effect
Early Stage (Compensatory/Nonprogressive)	
Increased epinephrine and norepinephrine	Increased cardiac output to increase blood flow to tissues
Alpha-adrenergic and beta-adrenergic receptors stimulated	
Alpha effects: skin and most viscera	Vasoconstriction and decreased blood supply
Beta effects: heart and skeletal muscles	Vasodilation and increased blood supply and heart rate
Renin-angiotensin response	Vasoconstriction and secretion of aldosterone; sodium and water retention, which supports intravascular volume; potassium loss
Increased glucocorticoids and mineralocorticoids	Sodium and water retention to increase intravascular volume; potassium loss
Hypoxemia	Hyperventilation and bronchodilation; provides more oxygen to tissues; may cause respiratory alkalosis
Decreased hydrostatic fluid pressure	Fluid shifts from interstitial space to intravascular space to increase vascular volume
Late Stage (Noncompensatory/Progressive)	
Decreased blood flow to heart	Impaired cardiac pumping ability (decreased cardiac output); blood pressure decreases
Anaerobic metabolism	Acidosis; decreased adenosine triphosphate; failure of cellular sodium-potassium pump (potassium leaves cell; sodium and water enter cell); cellular damage
Arteriolar dilation and venule constriction	Fluid shift from intravascular to interstitial space, reducing blood pressure
Decreased blood flow to kidneys with acute tubular necrosis	Decreased kidney function (oliguria or anuria, retention of nitrogenous waste products and potassium)
Decreased blood flow to pancreas	Production of myocardial depressant factor (MDF)

From Phipps WJ, Sands JK, Marek JF: *Medical-surgical nursing: concepts and clinical practice,* ed 6, St Louis, 1999, Mosby.

TABLE 15-3 Comparison of Signs and Symptoms in Early and Late Shock by Body System

	Early Shock	Late Shock
Respiratory system	Hyperventilation; ↑ minute volume; ↓ $PaCO_2$;* normal PaO_2; bronchodilation	Respirations shallow; breath sounds may suggest congestion; ≠↑ $PaCO_2$; ↓ PaO_2; pulmonary edema; ↓ pulse oximetry
Cardiovascular system	Blood pressure normal to slightly lowered; ↑ diastolic pressure; narrowed pulse pressure; tachycardia; cardiac output normal in hypovolemic shock, slightly decreased in cardiogenic shock, and increased in septic shock; mild vasoconstriction in hypovolemic and cardiogenic shock; vasodilation in septic shock	↓ Blood pressure; ↓ cardiac output; tachycardia continues; vasoconstriction worsens in hypovolemic, cardiogenic, and septic shock
Renal system	Decreased urine output; ↑ urine osmolarity; ↓ urine sodium concentration; hypokalemia	Oliguria or complete renal shutdown; hyperkalemia; buildup of waste products
Acid-base balance	Respiratory alkalosis	Metabolic acidosis; respiratory acidosis
Vascular compartment	Fluid shift from interstitial space to intravascular compartment; thirst	Fluid shift from intravascular to interstitial and intracellular spaces, causing edema
Skin	Minimal to no changes in hypovolemic and cardiogenic shock; warm flushed skin in septic shock	Cool clammy skin in hypovolemic, cardiogenic, and septic shock; cool mottled skin in neurogenic and vasogenic shock
Hematologic system	Release of RBCs from bone marrow to increase vascular volume; platelet aggregation	DIC; ↓ hematopoiesis leading to ↓ white blood cells, ↓ hemoglobin, ↓ hematocrit, ↓ platelets
Mental-neurologic system	Restless; alert; confused	Lethargy; unconsciousness
GI-hepatic system	No obvious changes	Perfusion decreases; bowel sounds diminished; gastric distention; nausea, vomiting

*GI, Gastrointestinal; *PaCO₂,* arterial carbon dioxide pressure; *PaO₂,* arterial oxygen pressure; *RBC,* red blood cell; *DIC,* disseminated intravascular coagulation.

From Phipps WJ, Sands JK, Marek JF: *Medical-surgical nursing: concepts and clinical practice,* ed 6, St Louis, 1999, Mosby.

lysosomes are damaged, spilling digestive enzymes into the rest of the cell and destroying it. As the enzymes come into contact with adjacent cells, these cells also are destroyed, and eventually, the cellular death results in organ death. Shock is a dynamic process; at some point, a cycle begins that cannot be stopped, and an irreversible stage of shock develops.

One syndrome is seen after a severe physiologic insult with initial successful resuscitation of the patient. The syndrome has been termed *multiple organ dysfunction;* the belief is that the local

injury from trauma and hypoperfusion causes a local inflammatory response. The response is probably a result of endothelial injury, platelet activation, the release of inflammatory mediators, and activation of the clotting cascade. This response leads to the development of a hyperinflammatory state and a hypermetabolic state, with increases in oxygen consumption and demand. The lung is usually the first organ to fail, with the kidneys, immune system, gastrointestinal tract, and liver following, resulting ultimately in sepsis, cardiovascular collapse, and death. Evidence suggests that the gastrointestinal tract plays a strong role in the initiation and continuation of the syndrome. Patients who are subjected to circulatory shock may sustain mild ischemia to the gut, which may lead to necrosis of the superficial mucosa, with loss of epithelial barrier function. Once the barrier function is lost, bacterial translocation is facilitated. This release of bacteria, endotoxin, and other luminal factors is thought to contribute to a systemic inflammatory response.[22]

These factors emphasize the importance of the amount of physiologic stress the patient receives and the need for rapid assessment and transport of the trauma patient to definitive care.

PRIMARY AND SECONDARY ASSESSMENT

In development of a systematic approach for assessment of trauma, caregivers must intervene in life-threatening injuries, discover occult injuries, and prioritize care. In the prehospital setting, scene evaluation is important and includes an assessment of safety. Every transport team member is responsible for recognizing all possible dangers and ensuring that none still exist. No one should become a victim. Caregivers should evaluate the scene and, if necessary, move the patient to a safe area before initiation of treatment. The transport team is challenged by many factors during attempts to perform a detailed assessment. Three of the most common factors are time, noise level, and the inability to fully disrobe a patient. The transport team is responsible for evaluating each patient situation individually to determine the best approach for assessment. For example, transport of a patient via helicopter from the scene of the accident may routinely require that the team performs the primary assessment on the scene, loads the patient, and performs the secondary assessment in the aircraft or ground vehicle, thus avoiding delay of definitive care. However, the auscultation of breath sounds and bowel sounds is not possible during rotor-wing transport and thus should be performed before liftoff and out of the normal assessment sequence.

PRIMARY ASSESSMENT

The focus of the primary assessment is evaluation and identification of life-threatening conditions (Figure 15-9). Problems identified during this portion of the evaluation are managed by the transport team immediately and simultaneouly. The mnemonic *ABCDE* is used to complete the primary assessment:[17,20]

A: Airway and cervical spine stabilization
B: Breathing and ventilation
C: Circulation with hemorrhage control
D: Disability (neurologic status)
E: Exposure (the patient is undressed)[3]

Airway

A secure patent airway is the first priority. The airway always is assessed immediately for patency, protective reflexes, foreign body, secretions, and injury. While the airway is assessed, the cervical spine should be protected simultaneously. Basic maneuvers should be instituted, including suctioning and opening of the airway with a chin-lift or jaw-thrust technique. A patient with a head injury or facial fractures risks losing the airway, and the transport team should always be prepared to manage the airway before it occludes. Frequent suctioning is often indicated, and the equipment should be at hand. Endotracheal intubation allows for optimal control of the airway. The transport team must be able to recognize the indications for airway management and perform the type of intervention (basic or advanced) that is optimal for the situation and clinical condition. Patients with a Glasgow Coma

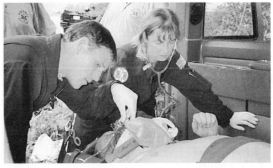

FIGURE 15-9 **Transport nurses performing a trauma assessment.**

Scale (GCS) of 8 or less are at risk for aspiration and hypoventilation. A definitive airway should be considered for patients with a GCS of 8 or less.

Breathing

Breathing is assessed with determining the patient's respiratory rate, depth, and effort of inspiration. Breath sounds should be auscultated bilaterally in all quadrants. Pulse oximetry and end-tidal carbon dioxide monitoring are the gold standard for monitoring the patient with intubation for transport. Most life-threatening injuries are in the chest and affect breathing (Box 15-1). Recognition of these injuries is imperative to effective management of ventilation. Once a patent airway is established, the caregiver must determine the effectiveness of air exchange. Observation of the rise and fall of the chest alone is not sufficient for the caregiver to determine the status of breathing. The caregiver should assess the rate of ventilation, use of accessory muscles, and presence of circumoral cyanosis. If spontaneous breathing is absent, the crew should initiate positive-pressure ventilation through a bag-valve device and appropriate airway adjunct. For patients who do not need a bag-valve mask, high-flow oxygen through a nonrebreather mask is effective to augment oxygenation. All patients with multisystem trauma should receive supplemental oxygen during transport, regardless of whether or not they are symptomatic.

Circulation

Evaluation of circulation is accomplished with assessment of the patient's mental status, skin color, temperature, and pulse. A quick palpation of radial pulses may be sufficient for the caregiver to determine effective circulation in the unconscious patient. If a radial, femoral, or carotid pulse is not palpated, then chest compressions should be initiated. As soon as possible, the patient should be placed on a cardiac monitor.

The crew who performs airway, breathing, and cervical spine control at the scene and gains vascular access en route may best treat patients who need immediate surgical intervention. This process allows minimal delay for the patient who needs immediate surgery. The concept that an intravenous line is supportive, rather than restorative, care to the patient is important to remember. Unlike intubation and ventilation of the patient, an intravenous line cannot correct a problem. It only provides supplemental fluid until the underlying condition is corrected. A patient in hypotensive shock may need immediate surgery, and extra time taken, especially at the scene, for lines to be initiated only adds to the delay of definitive care for that patient.

Vascular access may be needed to administer medications to secure the airway and to provide pain management during transport. Advanced training and technology has provided transport teams with a variety of new ways to gain vascular access. Intraosseous devices such as the EZ-IO have proven to be a simple quick way to gain vascular access in both the conscious and unconscious patient, pediatric and adult. External jugular venous, subclavian venous, and femoral venous catheterizations have been used by transport teams to gain vascular access. However, the transport team needs to carefully evaluate whether a delay may occur with multiple attempts in gaining vascular access on scene.

Choices of fluids for resuscitation may include crystalloid, colloid, and blood products. Initial fluids should be crystalloids such as normal saline solution or Ringer's lactate solution. Patients who do not respond to 1 to 2 L of crystalloid resuscitation or who appear to be in hypovolemic shock should be infused with type O uncross-matched blood. Rh factor is dependent on the gender or child-bearing status of the patient.[25]

BOX 15-1	**Indicators of Immediate Life-Threatening Chest Injury**

1. Open pneumothorax
2. Flail chest
3. Massive hemothorax
4. Tension pneumothorax
5. Cardiac tamponade
6. Penetrating cardiac wounds
7. Air embolus

Disability/Neurologic

A rapid neurologic examination establishes the patient's level of consciousness. The mnemonic *AVPU* (Alert; responds to Verbal stimuli; responds to Painful stimuli; or Unresponsive), the Glasgow Coma Scale Score and pupillary response and symmetry, the presence of extremity movements, and lateralizing motor findings can be used by the caregiver to assess disability. The GCS and the gross motor and sensory status of all four extremities should be determined and noted. The AVPU scale may also provide a quick assessment of the patient's level of consciousness and assist the transport team in determination of whether critical interventions, such as airway management, may be needed before transport.

Exposure/Environmental Control

The patient should be disrobed and evaluated for any life-threatening injuries. Environmental control involves assessment of the core body temperature and prevention of hypothermia. Exposure is particularly important in the patient with a traumatic mechanism of injury in which failure to identify a second or third injury may result in misassessment of the clinical picture.

Baring of the chest is essential for evaluation of life-threatening injuries, and exposure of the abdomen is crucial for proper examination; both should be done in all trauma patients. All restrictive clothing, such as belts or bras, should be removed or cut away. With exposure for assessment, attention must be given to keeping the patient warm; blankets should cover the body areas not being examined at the time.

Before the secondary assessment, the caregiver should judiciously check the patient for any uncontrolled hemorrhage. Active bleeding is controlled with direct pressure.

SECONDARY ASSESSMENT

The secondary survey is a complete assessment of the patient from head to toe. A more complete and traditional history and physical examination is performed.

The secondary assessment proceeds in a systematic fashion from head to toe to reveal all injuries the patient has sustained. During this assessment, the caregiver strictly adheres to assessment of the patient and does not intervene for specific injuries. To avoid missed injuries, the caregiver must develop a routine when performing the secondary assessment. Inspection, auscultation, palpation, and information the patient offers are the keys to performing this assessment. When proficient, the transport team should be able to perform the secondary assessment in approximately 60 seconds. Focus on obvious injuries is easy during this assessment, but the challenge is to discover occult injuries that may have an adverse affect on the patient's morbidity or mortality and cause major problems for both the patient and the team during transport.[9]

After completion of the secondary assessment, the caregiver can focus on the patient's specific injuries to determine their severity and to intervene when necessary, for example, by splinting an extremity. During the assessment and transport of the trauma patient, remember the importance of protection from hypothermia, which can be detrimental. Also, reporting all information regarding the patient to the receiving trauma team is important, especially any episodes of hypotension or loss of consciousness that the patient may have had. The mnemonic *FGH* can be used to complete the secondary assessment.

Full Set of Vital Signs, Focused Adjuncts, and Family Presence

The *F* in the FGH mnemonic stands for: Full set of vital signs, focused adjuncts, and family presence. A full set of vital signs should include blood pressure, pulse rate, respiratory rate, oxygen saturation, and temperature. This should be obtained before initiation of the head-to-toe assessment. Focused adjuncts can include attaching necessary equipment, placing indwelling urinary catheter, and inserting a gastric tube for the patient with intubation. Family presence can assist the transport team with language or cultural barriers.

Give Comfort Measures

The *G* of the FGH mnemonic is a reminder to the transport team to provide comfort measures. These measures may include reassuring the patient or pain management with the conscious or unconscious patient.

History

The *H* of the FGH mnemonic stands for history. This information obtained may be prehospital information from EMS caregivers or patient-generated information.

The primary and secondary assessments, along with the treatment of life-threatening injuries, are the most important aspects of trauma care the transport team can deliver. They direct the priorities of care during transport and for the staff at the receiving hospital and are the cornerstone for optimal outcome of the patient with multiple injuries.

Inspect the Posterior

Inspection of the posterior is generally not done in the transport process.

SCORING OF TRAUMA PATIENTS

Numeric scoring for determination of the severity of injuries is common practice. Scoring provides a potential outcome classification for trauma patients, through either single-system injuries, multisystem injuries, or the patient's physiologic condition. A variety of injury-severity scores exist; none are 100% accurate, and their questionable reliability should be considered with their use. Two common prehospital scoring systems and accepted retrospective scores are discussed in the following subsections.

PROSPECTIVE SCORING

A goal of emergency response personnel has long been to develop a numeric score to determine the severity of a patient's injuries at the accident scene. Use of such a score would mean rapid verification of trauma patients and appropriate triage to a trauma center; thus, appropriate resources could be used, and morbidity and mortality rates could be significantly improved. Numerous prehospital scoring indexes have been developed, and two have gained national support.

Trauma Score

The *Trauma Score* is a physiologic index that is composed of five categories: systolic blood pressure, respiratory rate, respiratory expansion, capillary refill rate, and score on the Glasgow Coma Scale (Figure 15-10). The score is a number between 1 and 15. Associated with each score is a probability of survival for that score. The lower scores are associated with higher mortality rates. To increase reliability of outcome predictions, the *Revised Trauma Score* has been developed. The Revised Trauma Score includes the Glasgow Coma Score, systolic blood pressure, and respiratory rate (Table 15-4), but both capillary refill rate and respiratory expansion have been removed because of subjectivity.[10] The major limitation to the Trauma Score remains the fact that it measures physiologic response; as long as the patient compensates, the score does not accurately reflect condition. The Trauma Score has a sensitivity rate of approximately 80%; therefore, 20% of patients with severe injuries are not identified with this score.[6]

RETROSPECTIVE SCORING

Attachment of a numeric score to each diagnosed injury is the concept of retrospective scoring.

Abbreviated Injury Scale

The *Abbreviated Injury Scale* (AIS), published by the American Association for Automotive Medicine, categorizes injuries into six body regions (head, neck, thorax, abdomen, spine, and extremity and external) and assigns an individual score to each injury (Box 15-2). Scores are integers from 1 to 6, according to severity. The lower the score, the less severe the injury.[11] The AIS method was designed to determine severity of motor vehicle injuries. In the 1985 revision of the AIS, penetrating injuries were addressed in all body regions, but the scale is still considered more sensitive to blunt injuries. The AIS allows determination of individual injury severity but does not take into account multisystem injuries.

Injury Severity Score

The *Injury Severity Score* (ISS) quantifies multisystem injury by use of the AIS scores. The ISS is determined by adding the squares of the highest AIS scores in the three most severely injured body systems. The ISS is a number between 1 and 75, with 1 being a minor injury and 75 being largely nonsurvivable. A patient

	Rate	Codes	Score
A. Respiratory rate	10-24	4	
Number of respirations in 15	25-35	3	
seconds: Multiply by 4	>35	2	
	<10	1	
	0	0	A. _____
B. Respiratory effort	Normal	1	
Retroactive: Use of accessory	Retractive	0	
muscles or intercostal retraction			B. _____
C. Systolic blood pressure	≥90	4	
Systolic cuff pressure: Either arm,	70-89	3	
auscultate or palpate	50-69	2	
	>50	1	
No carotid pulse	0	0	C. _____
D. Capillary refill			
Normal: Forehead or lip mucosa			
color refill in 2 seconds	Normal	2	
Delayed: More than 2 seconds			
capillary refill	Delayed	1	
None: No capillary refill	None	0	D. _____
E. Glasgow Coma Scale	Total GSC points	Score	
1. Eye opening			
Spontaneous _____ 4	14-15	5	
To voice _____ 3	11-13	4	
To pain _____ 2	8-10	3	
None _____ 1	5-7	2	
	3-4	1	E. _____
2. Verbal response			
Oriented _____ 5			
Confused _____ 4			
Inappropriate words _____ 3			
Incomprehensible			
sounds _____ 2			
None _____ 1			
3. Motor response			
Obeys commands _____ 6			
Purposeful move-			
ments (pain) _____ 5			
Withdraw (pain) _____ 4			
Flexion (pain) 3			
Extension (pain) _____ 2			
None _____ 1			
Total GCS points (1 + 2 + 3) _____		Trauma Score _____	
	(Total points A + B + C + D + E)		

FIGURE 15-10 **Components of the Trauma Score.**

TABLE 15-4	**Revised Trauma Score Variable Break Points**		
Glasgow Coma Scale Score	**Systolic Blood Pressure (mm Hg)**	**Respiratory Rate (breaths/min)**	**Coded Value**
13-15	> 89	10-29	4
9-12	76-89	> 29	3
6-8	50-75	6-9	2
4-5	1-49	1-5	1
3	0	0	0

BOX 15-2	**Abbreviated Injury Scale**

0. No injury
1. Minor
2. Moderate
3. Severe
4. Serious
5. Critical
6. Maximum; virtually unsurvivable

who receives a score of 6 in any AIS category is automatically scored as having an ISS of 75. Any patient with an ISS greater than 15 is widely considered to be a major trauma patient.

TRISS

The *TRISS* method ties together the Trauma Score, ISS, age, and type of injury to determine the probability of survival for the patient.[6,7]

With the focus on percent of mortality, the injury scoring systems have yet to address the probable morbidity associated with physiologic response and actual injuries.

FIELD TRIAGE

Use of triage to determine whether to take a patient to a trauma center is a necessary skill for caregivers in many parts of the United States today. Proper identification of patients who meet trauma center criteria is routinely based on physiologic criteria, such as blood pressure lower than 90 mm Hg; anatomic criteria, such as two long-bone fractures; and a field triage score, such as the Revised or Pediatric Trauma Score.[1] Figure 15-11 displays the standard field triage criteria for delivery of a patient to a trauma center.

TRIAGE PATIENT TRANSPORT

Care of the patient with multiple injuries during transport is aimed at maintaining adequate airway, breathing, and circulation; continued stabilization; and constant monitoring of the patient. The success of the transport depends on the caregiver's ability to anticipate the patient's progression and expect the unexpected (Figure 15-12).

SUMMARY

The members of the transport team provide a critical level of knowledge and expertise of care for the patient with multiple injuries in the prehospital setting. By understanding the kinematics of trauma, performing a thorough assessment, and delivering care in an organized manner, the transport team has a positive effect on decreasing morbidity and mortality rates of such patients.

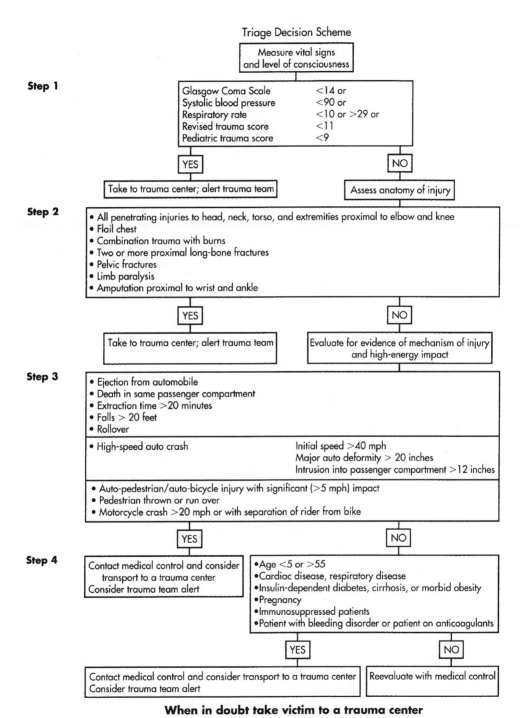

When in doubt take victim to a trauma center

FIGURE 15-11 **Trauma triage decision making.** (From Committee on Trauma, American College of Surgeons: *Resources for optimal care of the injured patient,* Chicago, 1993, American College of Surgeons.)

FIGURE 15-12   **Transport team performing field triage.**

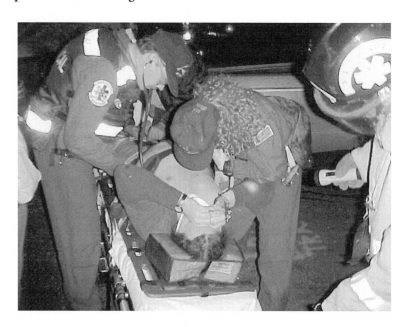

MULTIPLE TRAUMA CASE STUDY

The transport team was dispatched to a multiple-victim scene in a rural area, 30 minutes from the hospital. Reports were that two victims were dead and two others were severely injured. Initial responders performed the initial basic care practice. On arrival, the flight crew's aerial view of the scene revealed a single car that had been split in half. Rescuers were attending to two victims, and two bodies lying near the wreckage were covered with sheets.

On the basis of the report the transport team received before arrival, they began preparation to transport two victims in the aircraft. Both viable patients had been thrown from the vehicle over the guardrail. Patient 1 was a 15-year-old girl whose left leg had been amputated above the knee. Bleeding was controlled with a pressure dressing. She had multiple abrasions and lacerations on her face and chest. Her Glasgow Coma Scale score was 7 (eyes, 1; verbal, 1; motor, 5). She was pale and diaphoretic. She had a palpable femoral pulse of 130 bpm and a respiratory rate of 8 bpm. Patient 2 was a 16-year-old girl who was awake, screaming, and not following any commands. She had multiple abrasions and lacer-

ations to her face, head, and extremities. Her vital signs included a radial pulse of 100 bpm and a respiratory rate of 22 bpm. Both were immobilized on backboards with cervical collars and head blocks. Each had one intravenous line in place.

The transport team elected to intubate the first patient because of her low Glasgow Coma Scale score and her advanced level of shock. Rapid-sequence induction was initiated, and the patient was intubated without difficulty. During the intubation, a member of the rescue squad placed a second intravenous line. A palpable systolic pressure of 70 mm Hg was ascertained. Both patients were loaded into the aircraft and secured. The second patient was placed on oxygen at high flow per nonrebreather mask. Soft restraints were applied as a precaution.

During the 15-minute transport to the trauma center, the first patient's condition remained hypotensive and tachycardic. No additional neuromuscular blocking agent was administered. The second patient's condition remained stable. Both patients were admitted to the shock resuscitation unit, and a report was given to the resuscitation team.

REFERENCES

1. National Center for Health Statistics (NCHS): *Health, United States, 2005 with chartbooks on trends in the health Americans*, Hyattsville, MD, 2005, NCHS.
2. Anderson RN, Smith BL: Deaths: leading causes for 2002, *Natl Vital Stat Rep* 53(17):1-10, 2005.
3. Emergency Nurses Association: *Trauma nursing core course provider manual*, ed 6, Des Plaines, IL, 2007, Emergency Nurses Association.
4. American College of Surgeons: *Advanced trauma life support student manual*, Chicago, 2008, American College of Surgeons.
5. Barach E, Tomlanovich M, Nowak R: Ballistics: a pathophysiologic examination of the wounding mechanisms of firearms: part I, *J Trauma* 26(3):225, 1986.
6. Boyd CR, Tolson MA, Copes WS: Evaluating trauma care: the TRISS method, *J Trauma* 27(4):370, 1987.
7. Champion HR, et al: A new characterization of injury severity, *J Trauma* 30(5):539, 1990.
8. Chan L, Bartfield JM, Reilly KM: The significance of out-of-hospital hypotension in blunt trauma patients, *Acad Emerg Med* 4(8):785, 1997.
9. Chandler CF, Lane JS, Waxman KS: Seatbelt sign following blunt trauma is associated with increased incidence of abdominal injury, *Am Surg* 63(10):885, 1997.
10. Copes W: Major trauma outcome study: letter to MTOS participants, Aug 11, 1988, American College of Surgeons.
11. Copes WS, et al: The Injury Severity Score revisited, *J Trauma* 28(1):69, 1988.
12. Daffner RH, et al: Patterns of high-speed impact injuries in motor vehicle occupants, *J Trauma* 28(4):498, 1988.
13. Fackler ML, Bellamy RF, Malinowski JA: The wound profile: illustration of the missile-tissue interaction, *J Trauma* 28(2 Suppl):S21, 1988.
14. Fackler ML, Malinowski JA: The wound profile: a visual method quantifying gunshot wound components, *J Trauma* 26(6):522, 1985.
15. Jacobs B, Baker P: *Trauma nursing care course*, Park Ridge, IL, 1995, Emergency Nurses Association.
16. Janzon B: *High-energy missile trauma: a study of the mechanisms of wounding of muscle tissue*, Goteborg, Sweden, 1983, University of Goteborg.
17. Mackenzie C, Lippert FK: Emergency department management of trauma, *Anesthesiol Clin North Am* 17(1):45, 1999.
18. Mattox K, Moore EE, Feliciano DV, editors: *Trauma*, Norwalk, CT, 1996, Appleton & Lange.
19. National Association of Emergency Medical Technicians: *Prehospital trauma life support student manual*, ed 3, St Louis, 1994, Mosby.
20. Pepe P, Eckstein M: Reappraising the prehospital care of the patient with major trauma, *Emerg Med Clin North Am* 16(1):1, 1998.
21. Phipps W, Sands J, Marek J, editors: *Medical-surgical nursing concepts & clinical practice*, ed 6, St Louis, 1999, Mosby.
22. Reilly P, et al: *Reactive oxygen metabolites, Scientific American*, Chicago, IL, 1997, American College of Surgeons.
23. Sumchai A, Eliastam M, Werner P: Seatbelt cervical injury in an intersection type vehicular collision, *J Trauma* 28(4):498, 1988.
24. US Centers for Disease Control, Harvard School of Public Health: *U.S. burden of disease and injury study, Preliminary, unpublished results*, Atlanta, 2000, CDC.
25. Watts DD, et al: Hypothermic coagulopathy in trauma: effect of varying levels of hypothermia on enzyme speed, platelet function, and fibrinolytic activity, *J Trauma* 44:846, 1998.

NEUROLOGIC TRAUMA

Reneé Semonin Holleran, Katherine Logee

COMPETENCIES

1. Perform a neurologic assessment.
2. Provide critical interventions for the patient with neurologic trauma to achieve maximal potential for recovery.
3. Use guidelines in the management of traumatic brain or spinal cord injury during transport.

Traumatic neurologic emergencies involve disorders of both the central and the peripheral nervous systems. In one way or another, most of these disorders ultimately affect the respiratory system; thus, airway management is crucial. However, depending on the patient's condition, specific treatment may be instituted to lessen the impact of emergencies with which the transport team has to contend. The ultimate result of the disorders may be a progression to coma, often in association with increased intracranial pressure (ICP) or spinal injury. Therefore, the transport team must understand the causes of increased ICP and the neurologic syndromes discussed subsequently in this chapter.

TRAUMATIC BRAIN INJURY

Traumatic brain injury statistics are staggering. Traumatic brain injuries (TBI) are the leading cause of death related to trauma. Estimates are that both fatal and nonfatal traumatic brain injuries in the United States occur in 403 of 100,000 emergency department visits and in 85 of 100,000 that require hospital admission.[13] Two thirds of patients with head injuries are under the age of 30 years. During the past 18 years, United States involvement in the Middle East wars has shown the devastation of traumatic brain injury. The cost of care for people who survive neurologic injuries is in the millions of dollars.[1,2,5,9,13,17]

Head injury is the major cause of death related to motor vehicle crashes.[1,2,9] The primary solution to the death and devastation caused by neurologic trauma is prevention.

The outcome for a patient who has sustained a traumatic brain injury (TBI) may be determined by the severity of the injury and the time elapsed before the patient receives adequate medical attention; thus, the need is for rapid evaluation, assessment, and transfer of the patient to an appropriate-level care facility by the transport team. The transport team must possess a basic knowledge of the principles of pathophysiology of traumatic brain injury to apply appropriate diagnostic and therapeutic methods and perform a thorough and ongoing systemic evaluation of the patient.

When trauma to the head occurs, the hair and scalp provide some dampening effect on impact. However, the brunt of the blow is delivered to the skull, which has enough elasticity to be flattened or indented when struck with a blunt object. The maximal depression occurs instantly and is followed within a few milliseconds by several oscillations. A severe blow to the skull actually causes a generalized deformation by flattening in the direction of the impact, with a corresponding widening of the diameter at right angles to the impact line.[16]

The skull travels faster under impact than does the brain. Although the unbending skull often contuses the brain at the site of impact, severe brain injuries occur when the brain is hurled against the skull's rough bony prominence, the crista galli, the major sphenoid wings, or the petrous bones. It is not uncommon for the frontal and temporal poles to be injured. The undersurface of the temporal poles and, less often, the occipital poles are contused or pulped as a result of the unbending skull. Similar damage can also be caused by the edges of the relatively unyielding falx and tentorium. So-called coup lesions develop in opposite areas of the brain on impact.[16]

Damage may result from direct injury or from compression, tension, or shearing forces caused by the particular injury. In addition, secondary complications result from the traumatic brain injury. Ischemia and cerebral edema may ensue. An immediate increase in ICP seems to occur on impact; however, a secondary increase also occurs several minutes after the injury. The increase in ICP at the time of impact results from acceleration and deceleration of the head and deformation of the skull, the former being more significant than the latter.[13,14,16]

During impact, cerebral spinal fluid may offer some protection to the brain. However, this protective layer is insufficient in the subarachnoid space around the frontal and temporal lobes, the most frequent sites of contusion.[13,16]

TYPES OF TRAUMATIC INJURIES: PATHOLOGIC AND CLINICAL CONSIDERATIONS

Traumatic brain injury may exist in isolation; however, various combinations of injuries usually occur. Each component contributes in a different degree to the overall severity and outcome of the injury.[25,30]

Skull Fracture

The skull is composed of three layers: an outer layer, a middle cancellous layer, and an inner layer that is half as thick as the outer layer and contains grooves that have large vessels. Whether a fracture actually occurs in the area of impact depends on the type of injury. The more concentrated and focused the impact tends to be, the greater the likelihood of a fracture.

Most skull fractures are linear. A *linear skull fracture* produces a line that usually extends toward the base of the skull. Impact can produce a single linear fracture or multiple fractures, referred to as linear stellate fractures, that radiate from the compressed area. Although linear fractures may look benign, they can cause serious complications. One such complication is infection. If the fracture line is open a few millimeters at the time of impact, debris such as hair, dirt, and glass may travel into the cranial vault. Linear fractures may also lead to epidural hematoma if the fracture line crosses a groove in the layer of the skull that houses the middle meningeal artery. Another complication occurs when the dura, which is strongly attached to the skull, tears at the fracture site.

Diastatic and Basilar Skull Fractures. *Diastatic fracture* involves a separation of bones at a suture line or a marked separation of bone fragments; both are usually visible on computed tomographic (CT) scans. Facial fracture may also play a role in head injuries. A blow to the lower jaw when the jaw is closed can cause the mandibular condyles to displace upward and backward against the base of the skull, leading to a concussion or a basilar skull fracture. Another type of facial fracture, which may or may not involve the cranium, is an orbital blowout fracture, which usually involves the floor of the orbit and is caused by blunt impact to the orbit and its contents.

Basilar skull fractures can occur when the mandibular condyles perforate into the base of the skull, but they most often result from extension of fractures of the calvaria. Basilar fractures often produce Battle's sign (an oval-shaped bruise over the mastoid) or raccoon eyes (ecchymotic areas around the eyes).

Depressed Skull Fracture.

The presence of depressed elements of a fracture may warrant specific diagnostic and therapeutic measures. If the depressed fracture is closed, the rationale for surgical correction is to evacuate any local mass if present, repair any dural lacerations to prevent cerebral herniation through the defect, and correct any cosmetic disfigurement caused by the depression. In general, if the depression on the tangential view of the skull is greater than the thickness of the skull, the dura is probably lacerated, and surgery is recommended. Depressions of a lesser degree, unless over the forehead, rarely necessitate surgical exploration.

A compound depressed skull fracture usually requires surgical debridement. If the injury has been caused by a blow to a static head, the patient's level of consciousness is frequently well preserved, and no neurologic deficits may be seen. When a blow has been sustained to a moving head, consciousness is impaired.

Skull fractures can be the source of various complications, including intracranial infections, hematomas, air within the cranium, and meningeal and brain tissue damage. Traumatic pneumocephalus may occur if the frontal, ethmoid, or sphenoid sinuses or the mastoid processes are fractured. Air that has entered the skull locates in the epidural, subdural, subarachnoid, interventricular, or intercerebral space. Pneumocephalus seldom produces symptoms unless it is under tension and thus produces

compression of the underlying brain tissue. The incidence rate of pneumocephalus and cerebral spinal fluid rhinorrhea with sella turcica fractures is small, but a high incidence rate of infection exists if this condition is present. Associated palsies of the oculi motor, trochlear, trigeminal, or abducens nerves may also be seen.[32-34]

In general, temporal bone fractures can cause pneumocephalus if dural tearing occurs in conjunction with injury to the eustachian tube, the middle ear, or the mastoid process. The patient may have sensory neurologic hearing loss, otorrhagia, or cerebral spinal fluid rhinorrhea in the presence of a temporal bone fracture.

Hemorrhage

Subdural Hematoma.   *Subdural hematoma* is a collection of blood between the brain surface and the dura. It may occur as a result of a contusion or laceration of the brain with bleeding into the subdural space, tearing of the veins that bridge the subdural space, or an extension of an intercerebral hematoma through the brain surface into the subdural space. Subdural hematoma might be unassociated with skull fracture.[1,9,27,39]

Subdural hematomas are classified as acute, subacute, or chronic, depending on the time elapsed between the injury and the appearance of signs and symptoms of neurologic dysfunction. As with other types of traumatic brain injury, the time course of development and the degree and rate of neurologic dysfunction depend on many factors. As a general rule, if dysfunction occurs within 24 hours, the hematoma is acute; if it occurs between 2 and 10 days, it is subacute; and if it occurs after 2 weeks, the hematoma is chronic. This particular classification is partially pathologic. The location of the hematoma and the amount of mass effect play important roles in determination of the timing of surgical intervention.

Elderly patients may have larger subdural hematomas with slowly developing symptoms because they have larger potential subdural spaces as a result of cerebral atrophy. In contrast, symptoms may be displayed rapidly and marked increases in intercranial pressure may develop in a younger patient with a small subdural space.

Subdural hematomas generally occur in children under the age of 2 years. Signs and symptoms include a bulging fontanel and a large head (because of separation of the sutures) and retinal hemorrhages (because of increased ICP). In the infant patient, a shock-like state may also develop because a relatively large blood volume loss may be caused by a subdural hematoma.

Acute subdural hematomas are usually associated with high morbidity and mortality rates, which reflects the usually severe nature of the associated injuries and the not-infrequent association of rapidly rising ICP resulting from the mass effect and development of cerebral edema. Two separate related pathophysiologic problems are cerebral contusion and edema and the presence of blood in the subdural space. The CT scan is valuable in determination of whether surgical intervention may be indicated. If the major problem contributing to poor neurologic status is the mass effect, then surgical intervention may be necessary. If the major problem is the cerebral injury, then corrective treatment should be directed toward the increased ICP.

Epidural Hematoma.   An *epidural hematoma* is the collection of blood, usually arterial, between the skull and the dura. Epidural hematomas are classified as acute or subacute. An acute epidural hematoma that is arterial in origin generally produces symptoms within a few hours. Subacute epidural hematomas are venous in origin and take a longer time to produce symptoms. These hematomas are associated with linear skull fractures in 90% of patients, but they may also occur as a result of blunt injuries in which no evidence of fracture is seen.[9] The classic symptoms displayed with epidural hematoma are transient loss of consciousness, recovery with a lucid interval during which neurologic status returns to normal, and the secondary onset of headache and a decreasing level of consciousness. As a result of the initial injury, the middle meningeal artery may tear and cause traumatic unconsciousness. Spasm and clotting then occur in the middle meningeal artery, and the bleeding stops. During the next several hours, the artery gradually bleeds, and a hematoma is formed, stripping the dura from the inside of the skull. Once a headache with a decreasing level of consciousness becomes obvious, the secondary rise in ICP has already occurred, and distortion of the brain with significant mass effect occurs. Because compensatory mechanisms of the inner cranial space have already been exhausted, the patient's neurologic status rapidly deteriorates. The patient experiences a downhill course, usually with dilation of the ipsilateral pupil because of third-nerve compression by the herniating temporal structures, progressive unconsciousness with weakness or decerebration of either the contralateral extremities or the ipsilateral extremities, Cheyne-Stokes respirations, and, if no treatment is initiated, loss of pupillary reflexes, caloric responses, bradycardia, and death. Thus, identification of the epidural hematoma in the earliest possible stage, when a headache and drowsiness are the only symptoms, and transfer of the patient for immediate neurosurgical intervention are extremely important.[1,39] The classic history and clinical progression, however, is only seen in one third of patients with epidural hematomas. Another third are unconscious from the time of injury, and the final third are never unconscious. In children, bradycardia and early papilledema may be the only warning signs.[3,4]

Cerebral Contusion.   *Cerebral hemorrhagic contusions* frequently occur in patients, particularly adults, after traumatic brain injury. Of the patients who die of traumatic brain injury, 75% have contusions at autopsy. Hemorrhagic contusions are infrequently seen in children, but areas of localized decreased density on a CT scan may represent nonhemorrhagic contusions or possibly local ischemia.[1,9,14,16]

Generally, no surgical intervention is recommended for cerebral contusions because brain matter cannot be removed in areas of the brain that control motor, sensory, or visual functioning. If, however, the contusion occurs over the frontal or temporal lobes, with significant edema and shift, surgical removal of contused portions of the brain is feasible. When a temporal lobe contusion is present and signs of herniation are seen, surgical excision of the temporal lobe may be beneficial. Generally, patients with contusion are treated with medical control of elevated ICP.

Intracerebral Hematoma. Movement of one section of brain tissue over or against another section causes tears in blood vessels, which leads to contusions or *intracerebral hematomas*. Most intracerebral hematomas are found in the frontal and temporal lobes, usually very deep, and are associated with necrosis and hemorrhage. The anatomic relationship between these areas and irregularities of the skull has already been discussed. Intracerebral hematomas are readily identified on the CT scan. The clinical picture may vary from no neurologic defect to deep coma.

Traumatic Brain Injury: Diffuse Axonal Injuries

Diffuse axonal injury (DAI) occurs when the delicate axons of the brain are stretched and damaged as a result of rapid movement of the brain. Mechanisms of injury associated with the acceleration and deceleration that occurs with high-speed motor vehicle crashes or ejection from a vehicle can cause this type of diffuse brain injury. Because the axons have been damaged, interference with neuron transmission is seen, and multiple neurologic deficits can range from headache and amnesia to severe deficits that include deep coma, posturing, and respiratory compromise. Severe DAI is usually associated with a high mortality rate.[10,16]

Penetrating Injuries

Gunshot Wounds. When a person is shot at close range, evidence of smoke may be visible on the skin. When the muzzle of the gun is somewhat farther from the scalp but still close, evidence of powder burns may exist. A bullet striking the skull can cause great destruction of the underlying brain tissue.

Although some of the energy of impact may be dissipated by the shattering of bones and soft tissues, the impact on the brain after a bullet penetrates the skull is still great. The bullet's ability to destroy tissues is directly related to its kinetic energy at the moment of impact. The degree of damage to the brain depends primarily on the muzzle velocity of the bullet and the distance between the gun and its target.

A bullet that passes through the head produces a larger defect on the inner table of the skull than that produced on the outer table. High-velocity bullets cause extensive injury to the brain and cranium. The entrance wound is usually smaller than the exit wound, but a great deal of variation in size may be seen. Multiple linear fractures that radiate from either the entrance or exit wound are common. Some fractures may be far away from the trajectory of the bullet, particularly in thin bones. The transport team should describe the wounds but not attempt to determine whether they are entrance or exit wounds.

Injuries to the major cerebral arteries, veins, or venous sinuses can occur in any of the bullet's intracranial passages. Cerebral injuries cause an immediate but transitory increase in ICP. The eventual ICP depends on the degree of intracranial bleeding, which may be profuse even in the absence of injury to major vessels. Secondary cerebral edema causes a delayed increase in ICP. Damage to the hemisphere causes loss of autoregulation, falling cerebral blood flow, an increase in cerebral blood volume and ICP, and eventually, brain death.

Intracranial hematomas are frequently associated with penetrating wounds to the brain. If the bullet passes close to or transverses the ventricle, an intraventricular hematoma may result.

Infection is seen often in injuries caused by shell fragments because these fragments are more likely than bullets to carry dirt, hair, and bone fragments into the brain. Infections develop most often from retained bone fragments, improper closure of the scalp and dura, and delay of definitive surgery beyond 48 hours.

Whenever the skull has been penetrated, a risk of intracranial infection exists. The injury should be managed to minimize that risk. All patients with penetrating injuries should receive tetanus prophylaxis.

Most stab wounds are caused by assaults with sharp instruments such as knives, scissors, and screwdrivers or when the patient (often a child) falls on a stick or sharp toy. The best method is to transport the patient with a stab wound with the object immobilized, secured, and left in place.

If the penetrating object has been removed, determination of exactly where penetration of the skull occurred may be difficult, particularly if entry occurred at the eyelid or sclera. When the patient arrives at the hospital, the area of injury is explored and debrided, as with an open injury.

PHYSICAL ASSESSMENT: TRAUMATIC BRAIN INJURY

Examination of a patient who is unconscious requires integration of information from several systems: mental status, pupils, other cranial nerves, motor system, and respiratory function (Table 16-1).

Level of Consciousness

The best indicator of changes in intracranial pressure, especially from a mass lesion, is a patient's level of consciousness.[16,30] *Consciousness* is a mental state in which the person is stimulated by the environment and can react appropriately to it. A useful way of describing the conscious state is to divide it into alert, lethargic, or obtunded stages (Box 16-1).

The *alert* patient readily responds to the examiner, although, depending on the state of the central nervous system (CNS) injury, some confusion, speech disturbance, and motor deficits may be seen. The *lethargic* patient appears to be drowsy or asleep but can be aroused easily and can respond reasonably appropriately to the examiner's questions. However, if left alone, the patient slowly returns to an apparent sleep state or certainly lacks attentiveness. The *obtunded* patient is extremely drowsy, arouses with greater difficulty than a lethargic

BOX 16-1	Stages in Progression from Consciousness to Unconsciousness

Conscious State

Alert: Patient responds readily but may have some confusion, speech disturbance, or motor deficit.
Lethargic: Patient appears drowsy or sleepy but can be aroused to respond to questioning.
Obtunded: Patient is extremely drowsy, is difficult to arouse, and rarely answers in complete sentences; examiner may have to repeatedly stimulate to gain patient's attention.

Unconscious State

Stuporous: Patient does not verbalize appropriately or coherently; may moan and groan or utter monosyllables; responds to painful stimuli by moving extremities.
Comatose: Patient gives no evidence of awareness.

patient, rarely answers in complete sentences, and certainly does not volunteer information. In fact, during the active questioning period, the examiner may have to repeatedly stimulate the patient to gain attention.

TABLE 16-1	Physiologic Disturbance Correlated With Anatomic Level of Lesion					
Parameters	**Cerebral Cortex**	**Diencephalon**	**Thalamus**	**Midbrain**	**Pons**	**Medulla**
Mental status	Awake, alert, lethargic, obtunded	Light stupor	Deep stupor	Coma	Coma	Coma
Motor response	Appropriate	Focal response to pain	General response to pain	Decerebrate posturing, decorticate posturing	Flaccid	Flaccid
Pupil response	Normal size and reactivity	Small	Small	Midposition	Small	Small
Oculocephalic, oculovestibular reflex	Not testable	Normal response	Normal response	Abnormal	Abnormal	Abnormal*
Respiratory status	Variable	Variable	Cheyne-Stokes	Central neurogenic hyperventilation	Apneustic pattern	Apnea

*May be normal with isolated medullary injury.

Deterioration beyond the obtunded level results in the unconscious state. This state may be classified as either stupor or coma.

The *stuporous* patient does not verbalize appropriately or coherently. Two distinct levels of activity can characterize this state. The patient in a lightly stuporous state may moan and groan in response to stimulation or may utter an occasionally recognizable monosyllabic word, often a slang or curse word. The patient who is in a light stuporous condition responds to pain by moving all extremities, unless a primary motor system injury exists, and appears to crudely localize the site of the pain. However, a patient who is in a deeply stuporous state does not appear to localize and protect against pain. The patient who is in true *coma* may have decorticate posturing, decerebrate posturing, or flaccid motor response.

In examination of the pattern of motor response, the examiner must be aware of the possibility of primary motor system injury. For example, a left cortical lesion or a lesion in the left internal capsule may cause a contralateral hemiparesis that even in the awake patient may distort the motor response.

The comatose state roughly divides into three levels of reflex motor activity: decorticate posturing, decerebrate posturing, and flaccidity, to use clinically descriptive terms rather than more precise neurophysiologic descriptions. The patient in a *decorticate state* is unconscious and gives no evidence of awareness. Painful stimulation causes extensor rigidity in the lower extremities combined with a flexor posture of the upper extremities. Depending on the extent of the underlying damage to the motor system, this posturing may occur spontaneously or after painful stimulation and may be more prominent on one side than the other. *Decerebrate posturing* is exhibited by extensor rigidity in all four extremities. The patient who is *flaccid* has no motor response to painful stimulation.

For consciousness to be present, a stimulus must be presented to the CNS and must pass through the brain stem (with the exception of visual stimulation) to the diencephalon. From there, the stimulus must reach the cerebral cortex, where it is recorded. The patient must have sufficient cortical function so that the stimulus can excite associations through memory, which lets the patient acknowledge the presence of the stimulus and make use of that stimulus to relate appropriately to the external environment.

For example, when an intracranial mass lesion develops after head trauma and unconsciousness does not initially result, the patient may be expected, as the mass lesion increases, to progress systematically through the various levels and stages just described. The mass lesion may be a hematoma or a significant cerebral edema. A patient with a traumatic brain injury resulting in a primary upper brain stem lesion might be unconscious and may immediately evidence a comatose state without ever having had cortical or diencephalic deterioration. A person who survives a near drowning or delayed cardiopulmonary resuscitation may have severe bilateral cortical injury and may not progress significantly. A person with a spontaneous hemorrhage in the brain stem, particularly in the region of the pons or midbrain, is expected to become suddenly comatose with no evidence of an orderly progression through the stages noted previously.

Examination of the Pupils

The pupils are innervated by both the parasympathetic (third-nerve) and the sympathetic systems, with the former causing constriction and the latter causing dilation. The size of the pupil depends on the degree to which each system influences the pupil at the time of examination. The normal pupil constricts promptly to light. Examination of the pupils consists of assessment of the relative size of the two pupils and their reactivity to light. Injury to the parasympathetic system results in pupillary dilation.

Injury to the parasympathetic system may occur within the midbrain at the origin of the parasympathetic contribution to the third nerve, or it may occur outside the brain stem where the third nerve exits and proceeds forward beneath the brain into the region of the cavernous sinus. The sympathetic innervation begins in the posterior hypothalamus, descends the length of the brain stem and cervical cord, and exits in the lower cervical upper thoracic area, where it proceeds up the neck in the cervical sympathetic chain to the base of the skull and then out to the orbit where innervation occurs.

Injury to the sympathetic system results in pupillary constriction because of the actions of the unopposed third nerve. The sympathetic system can be injured within the CNS anywhere along its pathway and during its course through the chest and neck. Because of the relatively small size of the structures involved, lesions within the brain or brain stem are unlikely to affect either the parasympathetic or the sympathetic systems unilaterally. Therefore, we can assume that if bilateral pupil abnormalities are seen, a lesion in the brain or brain stem has affected the nerve supply to the pupils. For example, bilaterally small pupils may very well be caused by a lesion within the brain stem that affects both descending sympathetic tracts. On the other hand, a unilaterally affected pupil can be expected to be caused by a lesion of the tracts outside the brain or brain stem (extraaxial). A unilaterally dilated pupil may be caused by compression of the third nerve by a herniating temporal lobe after it has exited the midbrain and as it crosses the floor of the skull. A unilateral small pupil that results from sympathetic denervation reacts more sluggishly to light. Bilaterally dilated and fixed pupils are generally caused by global hypoxia or by bilateral temporal lobe herniation from central cerebral edema with bilateral third-nerve compression. Bilaterally constricted pupils may be caused by central herniation of the posterior hypothalamus at the site of origin of the sympathetic fibers through the tentorial notch or by bilateral involvement within the brain stem, such as from a pontine hemorrhage. Midbrain lesions that affect the parasympathetic bilaterally yield pupils that are in midposition and are nonreactive to light. Examination of other cranial nerves is helpful because they can reveal the competency of brain stem function including the III, IV, and VI nerves.

Brain Stem and Cranial Nerves

The integrity of the brain stem can be evaluated with examination of certain cranial nerves, especially those related to conjugate gaze. In the patient who is awake, conjugate gaze is controlled by visual input through the complex system that coordinates the function of the extraocular muscles by way of cranial nerves III, IV, and VI. In the patient who is unconscious, however, visual input gives way to vestibular input to control conjugate gaze. This is best evaluated with examination of the oculocephalic or oculovestibular reflexes.[16,37]

The oculocephalic reflex is demonstrated by stimulating the vestibular system through movement of the head in reference to the neck. While the patient lies supine on the ground, stretcher, or bed, the person performing the assessment opens the patient's eyelids. In normal circumstances, the eyes should stare at the sky or ceiling. The nurse then rotates the head briskly but gently to one side or the other. In normal circumstances, the eyes may momentarily remain in their position in the orbits but immediately track conjugately to the side opposite the direction of the movement so that the eyes are directed once again toward the sky or ceiling. If conjugate activity cannot be observed (e.g., if one eye tracks and the other one does not or if neither eye tracks), this signals an abnormality and suggests a disturbance of the brain stem. This maneuver should never be performed in a patient with a traumatic brain injury or multiple trauma until the cervical spine has been determined to be without injury.

The oculovestibular reflex is demonstrated by cold caloric stimulation, in which cold saline solution is irrigated into the external auditory canal. In a few seconds, the eyes conjugately deviate to the side of the irrigation and remain in that position from several seconds to several minutes. If this response is not seen, an abnormality is present in the brain stem involving the medial longitudinal fasciculus, the vestibular system, or both.

The midportion of the pons may be evaluated by the presence or absence of the corneal reflex. The corneal reflex can quickly be assessed by lightly touching the cornea with the corner of a soft gauze dressing and observing whether a blink reflex occurs.

Motor Examination

The motor system is best examined in conjunction with an examination of the patient's mental status or level of consciousness. The awake patient can be asked to perform certain motor tasks, such as moving the legs or gripping. If the patient is unconscious, motor activity in response to pain is a good way to determine the level of unconsciousness, as previously described.

Respiratory Pattern

Most patients with significant head injuries have hypoventilation early after the injury. Later, the respiratory pattern may vary, depending on the level of the lesion. Patients with decorticate posturing often have an accompanying Cheyne-Stokes pattern of respiration with a regular crescendo-decrescendo change in the volume of inspiration, with the rate remaining rather regular. The patient with decerebrate posturing may have central neurogenic hyperventilation. Patients with brain stem lesions may have varying rates and depths of respiration, and an ataxic element is often noted. With lower brain stem lesions, the rate becomes more irregular, more shallow, and less frequent, until medullary lesions

result in respiratory paralysis. Often the transport team needs to intubate the patient for respiratory control.

The Glasgow Coma Scale

The Glasgow Coma Scale (GCS), as shown in Table 16-2, is widely used to measure the severity of coma in patients and is therefore an indicator of prognosis. However, eye-opening response may not be accurately assessed in the patient with severe maxillofacial injuries whose airway is mechanically supported. In

TABLE 16-2	**The Glasgow Coma Scale**		
Circle the Appropriate Number and Compute the Total			
Best eye-opening response:	_____ **Right**	_____ **Left**	
	Never	1	
	To pain	2	
	To verbal stimuli	3	
	Spontaneously	4	
Best verbal response:			
	No response	1	
	Incomprehensible sounds	2	
	Inappropriate words	3	
	Disoriented and converses	4	
	Oriented and converses	5	
Best motor response:	_____ **Right**	_____ **Left**	
	No response	1	
	Extension abnormal (decerebrate rigidity)	2	
	Flexion abnormal (decorticate rigidity)	3	
	Flexion withdrawal	4	
	Localizes pain	5	
	Obeys commands	6	
	Total:_____ **3-15**		
Neurologic evaluation:	Record on Glasgow Coma Scale sheet		
	Repeat evaluation frequently. A score of 15 is normal; below 7 indicates coma; 3 signifies brain death.		
	Vital signs:		
	Level of consciousness		
	Glasgow Coma Scale		
	Pupillary size and reactivity		
	Right_____		
	Left_____		
	Focal weakness		
	Present_____		
	Absent_____		

addition, in a patient with a contralateral mass lesion, the best motor response may not depict progressing hemiparesis. When examining a patient, the GCS results are best recorded in the narrative record that goes to the receiving healthcare providers.

Reexamination

Successful acute management of the comatose patient depends on frequent examination of the patient to determine the level of neurologic function and rate of deterioration. The information provided in Table 16-2 can be helpful in this analysis.

When the transport team sees the injured patient for the first time, a baseline neurologic evaluation should be performed. Findings during subsequent examinations provide the transport team with an understanding of the intracranial injury. When a focal mass lesion such as a hematoma or focal contusion develops in a patient, the patient shows steady progression in depth of coma through the various levels depicted in Table 16-2. For example, when the initial examination of a patient results in findings compatible with a diencephalic level of coma, the coma is determined to have deteriorated to a midbrain level if the patient is subsequently found to have decerebrate posturing, midposition pupils, and central neurogenic hyperventilation. If the insult is unilateral, hemiparesis and an ipsilateral dilated pupil are seen before bilateral motor signs of herniation are seen. If the patient initially shows signs of coma resulting from a primary brain stem injury, a static lesion, a further deterioration in the level is not demonstrated within the next few hours, other than what is normally seen with a developing mass lesion.

INTERVENTIONS AND TREATMENT

The management of traumatic brain injury is based on both national and international guidelines that are now evidenced based (Box 16-2).[4,23] Each transport team should have developed protocols to manage these patients. The primary focus of the transport team should be to prevent hypoxia and hypotension.

| BOX 16-2 | **Summary of the Guidelines for the Management of Severe Traumatic Brain Injury That Affect Patient Transport[4,23]** |

Initial Resuscitation

Complete and rapid physiologic resuscitation is the first priority, and no treatment should be directed toward intracranial hypertension in the absence of indications of deterioration in neurologic status or signs of impending herniation. However, when signs of neurologic deterioration are present, aggressive management must be initiated and should include:
- Hyperventilation
- Administration of mannitol
  Sedation, analgesia, and neuromuscular blockade must be used in a discretionary manner.

Resuscitation of Blood Pressure and Oxygenation

Hypotension defined as a systolic blood pressure of less than 90 mm Hg must be avoided or aggressively managed. At PaO_2 < 60 mm Hg, apnea should be managed by securing the patient's airway and maintaining adequate ventilation.

Intracranial Pressure Treatment Threshold

Interpretation and treatment of ICP based on any threshold should be corroborated by frequent clinical examination and monitoring.

Hyperventilation

Avoid hyperventilation during the first 24 hours because reduced blood flow compromises cerebral perfusion.

Use of Mannitol

Administration of mannitol may occur before initiation of ICP monitoring with signs of transtentorial herniations or deterioration of neurologic status.

Management is based on the severity of the injury, which is usually measured by the patient's GCS. The following classification with the GCS has been suggested to identify the gravity of the patient's injury.[8,13,16,31,36,37]

- Mild   GCS 14-15
- Moderate   GCS 9-13
- Severe   GCS 3-8

Because the transport team may not always know the patient's primary diagnosis (i.e., subdural hematoma or epidural hematoma), management of patients based on GCS and the related physical examination results assists the team in providing the appropriate care to these patients.

The transport team's highest priority is establishing an adequate airway, providing oxygenation, and preventing or managing hypotension.[4,12,23,29] The awake patient should be placed on 100% oxygen. If the patient is unable to maintain the airway or the transport team anticipates the potential for deterioration during transport, the patient should be intubated. Care must be taken to maintain cervical spine protection while gaining access to the airway. A gastric tube should be inserted with care to prevent aspiration. Pulse oximetry and end-tidal CO_2 ($ETCO_2$) devices should be used throughout the transport process to monitor the patient's oxygenation and perfusion.[4,23]

If the patient is restless or agitated, hypoxia should be suspected until a specific cause can be found. Most patients with head injuries have sustained other injuries that cause pain. Even in the patient who is inattentive or stuporous, hypoxia rather than pain should be considered the cause of restlessness until this is proven otherwise.

The intubated patient who is restless or resists ventilatory support is increasing the ICP, which may be extremely critical. These patients should be managed with pharmacologically appropriate doses of sedation, analgesia, and neuromuscular blocking agents.[4,18,23] Because of the effects of analgesic and sedation agents on the patient's hemodynamic status, the effects of these medications must be closely monitored by the transport team. However, pain can be a powerful stimulus to increasing physiologic metabolism and oxygen consumption, and its effects must be considered on the patient's ICP.

In general, hypertension and bradycardia may develop in patients who have increased ICP. Hypotension and tachycardia are not signs of intracranial injury, except in a patient with herniation. However, small children may become hypovolemic from scalp lacerations associated with head injuries and should be monitored and treated accordingly with volume replacement.

Hypotension has been found to contribute to the mortality and morbidity of patients with head injuries.[23] Fluids and blood products should be administered to maintain blood pressure. Rapid transport for definitive surgical intervention may be the only management for some hemorrhagic hypotension.

Patients with head injuries may lose cerebral autoregulation (Figure 16-1). If this is the case, cerebral perfusion is directly related to mean systemic arterial pressure. Thus, hypotension may lead to underperfusion, and hypertension may lead to vascular congestion and mass effect. Both extremes should be avoided.

Seizures that develop during transport should be promptly treated because they produce hypoxia and cause increased ICP. Intravenous administration of benzodiazepines is indicated for initial seizure management. Prophylactic use of antiepileptic medications may also be considered, especially if the patient is receiving neuromuscular blocking agents.[23] Unconscious patients or those who have a depressed level of consciousness associated with seizure activities should be intubated for maximal

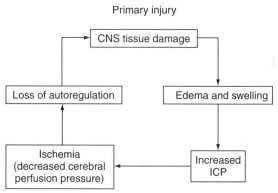

FIGURE 16-1   **Sequence of pathophysiologic events initiated by primary injury.**

control of the airway. Because an adequate airway is of paramount importance, the airway should be secured immediately.

Hyperthermia also increases ICP; thus, normal body temperatures should be maintained with the use of acetaminophen suppositories or cooling techniques. Shivering should be controlled because it increases ICP.

If neuromuscular blocking agents are used, close monitoring of the patient's temperature is important for the presence of hypothermia, because of the inability of the patient to shiver, or for evidence of malignant hyperthermia, particularly in children.

Routine hyperventilation is no longer recommended in the initial management of the patient with a traumatic brain injury. It may be indicated with any of the following signs.[4,16,19,20,22,23]

- Unilateral or bilateral pupillary dilation
- Asymmetric pupillary reactivity
- Motor examination results that show either extensor posturing or no response
- Other evidence of deterioration of the neurologic examination, such a known midline shift or impending herniation on the CT scan results

The patient's CO_2 level should be maintained between 30 to 35 mm Hg. End-tidal CO_2 monitoring aids the transport team in the appropriate ventilation of the patient with a traumatic brain injury. The transport team must pay careful attention when manually assisting an intubated patient with head injury. Aggressive bagging can potentially cause additional injury.[4,16,23]

Mannitol may be used to treat increasing intracranial pressure manifested by deterioration in the patient's neurologic status. Mannitol decreases the patient's ICP by enhancing cerebral blood flow because it can draw excess fluid into the vascular space and reduce blood viscosity. Mannitol should be administered through an intravenous filter.[4,16,23]

SPINAL CORD INJURY

All trauma patients, especially those with a head injury, are suspect for spine injury and should be treated accordingly.[6,7] The transport team should perform a baseline evaluation of the patient with a spine injury before transfer and should monitor the patient closely for changes in neurologic status during the transfer process. These patients should be transferred supine on a firm surface with the spine in good alignment. Studies suggest that log rolling of patients with spine injuries is destabilizing at the fracture site and should be avoided if possible. A scoop stretcher may be used to transfer the patient onto the rigid transport stretcher to avoid the torsion effects produced by the log-rolling maneuver.[11,15,24-26,28,38]

When appropriate and delineated by established guidelines, patients with cervical spine injury may be transported in traction. Proper equipment, such as a spring-loaded scale system, is necessary because use of hanging weights is inappropriate in the transport setting.

ETIOLOGY AND INCIDENCE RATE

The incidence rate of spinal cord injuries (SCIs) that result in paralysis or debilitating weakness as a consequence of trauma to the spinal cord has been analyzed statistically in many different ways in many different countries. An estimated 11,000 cases of spinal cord injuries occur per year in the United States.[7]

The age distribution of acute SCIs peaks in the 15-year-old to 24-year-old age group. Frequency decreases in the middle-age group, with a second peak occurring at about the age of 55 years.[7] The incidence rate in women is lower for all age groups. Traffic accidents continue to be the most frequent cause of SCIs in all age groups. Among children, most cases of SCI are caused by traffic accidents. Motorcycles and bicycles cause 10% to 12% of SCIs. Excessive consumption of alcohol is a factor in one third of cases involving accident victims with SCIs.[7,9]

More than half of work-related SCIs are caused by falls, and falls are the primary cause of SCIs in the home, particularly among the elderly, who fall down steps, from chairs, or off ladders.[7]

Approximately 7% of SCIs are caused by accidents that occur during sporting and recreational activities, and these SCIs most commonly occur as a result of diving into shallow water. The increasing number of women involved in sports is reflected in the rise of injuries for that group.[7]

INITIAL ASSESSMENT

Management of spine trauma begins with the realization that the patient may have an unstable spine. Whether at the accident scene or at a local referring hospital, the transport team should conduct a rapid thorough primary and secondary assessment of the patient with an SCI before transfer. This assessment provides a baseline for serial assessments and reveals additional injuries and commonly associated complications, such as aspiration, neurogenic shock (bradycardia and hypotension), and poikilothermy.[1,7,9]

Airway

The patient's airway should be checked for patency and cleared of foreign matter or secretions. With the spine protected, the upper airway in a patient with an altered mental status should be opened with use of the modified jaw-thrust maneuver to allow spontaneous or assisted ventilation.[1,2,5,9,17,26]

Breathing

Breathing may be absent or inadequate in patients with high cervical cord injury (C4 or above), which results in loss of both diaphragmatic and intercostal phrenic nerve intervention and paralysis of these respiratory muscles. In such cases, assisted ventilation with a bag-valve-mask and tracheal intubation with oxygen supplementation is indicated.[1,2,5,9,17,26] Rapid-sequence intubation with judicious spine immobilization may be necessary for airway and ventilation control.[1,2,5,9,17,26] Whatever method is chosen to manage the patient's airway, the transport team must ensure proper consistent protection of the entire spine.

Circulation

As with all critically injured patients, intravenous access is mandatory for patients with SCIs. Intravenous lines may be inserted on the scene or en route, depending on the patient's condition, distance of transfer, and existing protocols. Isotonic solutions such as lactated Ringer's solution or normal saline solution are preferred, with the rate and volume of infusion based on the patient's cardiovascular response. Neurogenic shock may be present in patients with cervical or high thoracic spine injury. Interruption of sympathetic outflow below the level of injury results in loss of autoregulation, a decrease in vascular tone, and the inability of the heart to increase its intrinsic rate. With passive vasodilation and a normal or bradycardic state, the patient becomes hypotensive.[1,2,5,9,17,26] The transport team should differentiate this shock state from hypovolemia and infuse crystalloids accordingly. In the absence of hypovolemia, the patient with an SCI can be considered normotensive, with a blood pressure of 80 to 90 mm Hg. If the patient's condition is hemodynamically unstable, administration of a vasoactive drug such as dopamine may be indicated. Hypovolemia must be ruled out before vasopressor therapy is begun.[1,2,5,9,17,26]

This sympathetic block or injury-induced sympathectomy produces poikilothermy. In this state, the patient loses the ability to vasodilate and sweat in hot environments and the ability to vasoconstrict and shiver in cold environments. Thus, the patient's core body temperature often reflects the environment and must be considered if warming or cooling techniques are withheld.[1,2,5,9,17,26]

Vasovagal reflex with tracheal suctioning must also be considered for these patients. Preoxygenation is important to prevent vagal stimulation and severe bradycardia, which could lead to cardiac arrest.[1,2,5,9,17,26]

SECONDARY ASSESSMENT

Once the primary survey has been completed, critical interventions have been initiated, and the patient's condition has been stabilized, the transport team can perform a secondary assessment, which includes performing a baseline neurologic evaluation; obtaining a history of the incident and of allergies, medications, previous illnesses or injuries, and the time of the patient's last meal; and completely exposing and examining the patient. Data about the mechanism and time of injury are valuable. To help expedite the transfer, this information can be obtained during the head-to-toe assessment.

Examination of the patient with an SCI should be performed with the patient maintained in a neutral position and the entire spine protected. A sensory and motor assessment helps the transport team determine the level and extent of injury. Autonomic function such as anal sphincter control can be assessed, and if sacral sparing is present, the injury should be considered incomplete.[1,21]

The transport team should visually inspect and carefully palpate the cervical spine area to determine the presence of deformity, crepitus, pain, and muscle spasm, which is frequently associated with cervical spine injury.[1] A second team member should maintain cervical spine immobilization while this is performed.

Lower Spine Injuries

The patient should be asked to wiggle the toes. If the patient can move the toes of both feet, the patient should be asked to raise each leg slightly, one at a time. The patient's legs should not be raised if the prior examination revealed no movement or association. If the patient shows any obvious weakness, injury to the spinal cord must be assumed.

Cervical Spine Injuries

The patient should be asked to wiggle the fingers. If the patient can do so, the patient should be asked to raise each arm, one at a time. Again, substantial active movement of the upper extremity should be avoided if evidence exists of obvious fractures of the spine or extremity. The transport team should ask the patient to squeeze the fingers with both hands. In addition, the transport team should ascertain the patient's dominant hand and cross over, matching the team member's dominant hand to the patient's dominant hand. The strength of the patient's grasp should be similar. If the patient cannot move the fingers and arms or has obvious weakness, SCI in the cervical region should be assumed.[1,2,5,9,17,26]

Sensory Examination

The presence of a sensory deficit confirms the suspicion of a cord or nerve-root injury. The transport team should test the patient's ankles and wrists and ask the patient if he or she can feel the touch. In the event that the patient cannot feel the touch in one or more places or reports numbness or tingling, SCI can be assumed.[1,2,5,9,17,26]

Neurologic Examination of the Unconscious Patient

The condition of an unconscious patient's spinal cord should be checked by pricking the skin lightly on the soles of the feet or ankles with a sharp object. If no spinal cord damage has occurred, the painful stimulus triggers an involuntary muscle reflex and the extremities move, unless the patient is in a profound coma. If the cord is damaged, no such reaction may be seen. The lack of response to pin pricks in the upper extremities indicates damage to the spinal cord in the cervical region. Failure of only the lower extremities to respond indicates SCI in the thoracic or lumbar regions.[1,2,5,9,17,26]

The degree of functional loss with sudden spinal cord transection depends on the level of the injury. The higher the injury, the more function lost. Complete sudden cord transection results in complete flaccid paralysis below the level of injury, areflexia (spinal shock) below the level of injury, urinary retention, and occasionally, in the male patient, priapism.

Incomplete sudden cord transection results in varying degrees of paralysis and sensory loss below the level of injury, areflexia (below the level of injury), and varying degrees of bladder or bowel paralysis. Box 16-3 may be used as a guide for evaluation of muscle strength and motor function.

INTERVENTIONS AND TREATMENT

The patient with SCI frequently has association trauma and therefore may have varying degrees of stability. Judicious airway assessment and management is needed for the patient with SCI when injuries are found in the cervical region. In the absence of hypovolemia, intravenous fluids should be monitored closely and maintained at a rate that prevents pulmonary overload. The transport team may initiate steroids if the injury is at L1 or above, time from injury is within 8 hours, and the team has received authorization to do so. Methylprednisone previously has been recommended as one of the methods of treatment for the patient with an isolated SCI. The Consortium for Spinal Cord Medicine Member Organizations[4] does not recommend routine use of high dose steroids in the prehospital care environment. The administration of high dose steroids should only be performed after consultation with a neurosurgeon. If the patient's potential spine injury has not been appropriately ruled out, the transport team must ensure that the patient remains immobilized until arrival at the receiving facility. However, particularly in a patient who cannot move and who may undergo a lengthy transport, assessment of the patient's skin for injury from a backboard should take place frequently. New methods of immobilization are being introduced that hopefully will decrease the risk of skin breakdown when a patient must remain immobilized for long transports.[1,2,5,9,17,26]

CLASSIFICATION OF CERVICAL SPINE INJURIES BY MECHANISM OF INJURY
Flexion Injuries

Anterior subluxation (Box 16-3) is a flexion lesion characterized by disruption of the posterior ligament complex (Figure 16-2). Because the anterior longitudinal ligament remains intact and the disk is not completely disrupted, this lesion is stable at the time of injury and is difficult to see radiographically.[1,2,5,9,17,26,35]

Physicians disagree on whether bilateral interfacetal dislocations result from hyperflexion or a combined flexion and rotary force. Unilateral and bilateral *interfacetal dislocations* involve soft-tissue injury of the posterior ligament complex, and tomographic scans frequently reveal an unstable injury with a high incidence rate of cord damage.[1,2,5,9,17,26]

The stability of a *simple wedge fracture* depends on associated posterior ligament disruption. This flexion injury usually results from a compressive force on the anterior portion of the vertebral body with stretching of the posterior ligament complex. These fractures are generally in the mid or lower cervical segments and are considered stable fractures because

of maintenance of posterior and anterior ligaments and the integrity of the interfacetal points.[1,2,5,9,17,26]

Teardrop hyperflexion fracture dislocations are seen as a result of diving or traffic accidents and falls. This type of fracture is extremely unstable because the vertebra is displaced posteriorly as the person strikes an object, and displacement disrupts the apophyseal joint capsule disk below. The anterior margin of the vertebra fractures in a teardrop-shaped fragment, and the fractured vertebra remains displaced posteriorly. Although often severe, the degree of neurologic deficit depends on the severity of hyperflexion compression. Patients who sustain teardrop flexion fractures frequently have acute anterior cervical cord syndrome. Immediate quadriplegia, loss of anterior cord senses (pain and temperature), and retention of posterior cord senses (position, motion, and vibration) result.[1,2,5,9,17,26]

Flexion-Rotation Injuries

Fractures that result from *flexion-rotation* are characterized by the displacement or fracture of one or more vertebrae. Fractured vertebrae may produce a unilateral facet dislocation with corresponding nerve-root compression. Severe distraction forces may cause an anterior displacement of the upper cervical body greater than 50%, which can result in bilateral locked facets and major cord injury, such as quadriplegia.[1,2,5,9,17,26]

Extension-Rotation Injuries

Pillar fractures, usually caused by motor vehicle accidents and falls, are the most common combined

---

BOX 16-3	**Muscles to be Tested for Evaluation of Motor Strength**

Actions to be Tested	Muscles	Cord Segment
Abduction of the arm	Deltoid	C5
Flexion of the forearm	Biceps	C5, C6
Extension of the forearm	Triceps	C7
Flexion of digits 2, 3, 4, and 5	Flexor digitorum and profundus	C8
Opposition of metacarpal of thumb	Opponens pollicis	C8, T1
Hip flexion	Iliopsoas	L12
Knee extension	Quadriceps femoris	L3-L4
Dorsiflexion of foot	Deep peroneal	L5
Dorsiflexion of big toe	Extensor hallucis longus	L5
Plantar flexion of foot and big toe	Gastrocnemius flexor	S1

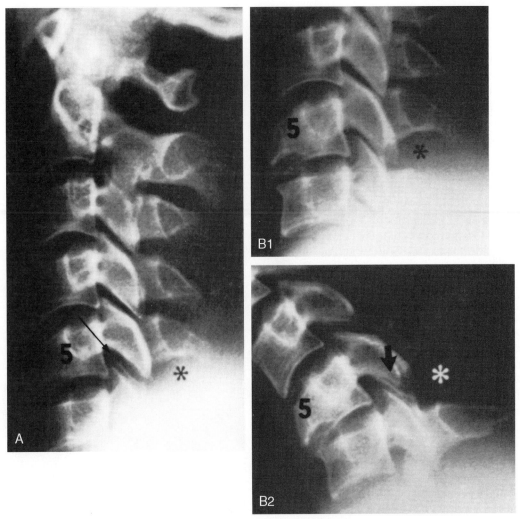

FIGURE 16-2   **Anterior subluxation of C5 on C6 associated with a wedge fracture of C5.** (From Harris JH Jr, Edeiken-Monroe B: *The radiology of acute cervical spine trauma,* Baltimore, 1987, Williams and Wilkins.)

injury of the cervical spine. The mechanism of injury results in force concentrated on the apophyseal joints of the mid and lower cervical segments and resultant vertical fractures of a lateral mass. A distraction of the fracture elements is probably caused by rebound flexion of the head and neck.[1,2,5,9,17,26]

Vertical Compression

Compression cervical spine injuries include the Jefferson fracture of the atlas and the bursting fracture of the lower cervical vertebrae. Compression fractures of the cervical spine are uncommon because the

injury must occur from force transmitted vertically through the skull and occipital condyles of the spine at the precise moment the spine is straight.[1,2,5,9,17,26]

Extension Injuries

Most *hyperextension* injuries result from contact with a windshield or other structure in the interior of an automobile. Extension injuries can be of three types. The *extension teardrop fracture* is a rare extension injury that involves the anterior corner of the axis. This type of fracture is usually associated with degenerative arthritis of the cervical spine.

The *hangman's fracture* is an unstable bilateral fracture of the pedicles of the axis. This fracture is often associated with dislocation of the C2 or C3 cord segment and prevertebral soft-tissue swelling.[1,2,5,9,17,26] *Hyperextension fracture-dislocation* injuries are associated with direct force backward or a backward and upward force without an axial loading force. The typical hyperextension-dislocation injury is accompanied by the following triad of signs: (1) midface skeletal or soft-tissue injury; (2) varying degrees of central cord syndrome; and (3) a lateral cervical spine radiograph that appears normal with the exception of diffuse prevertebral soft-tissue swelling (Figure 16-3).[17] This type of extension injury is believed to be responsible for the quadriplegia in the rare patient whose cervical spine films appear normal. The probable mechanism of injury is cord compression between the posterior vertebral body, lamina, and ligamentum flavum during extension.

Thoracic and Lumbar Spine Injuries

Injuries to the thoracic and lumbar spine vary in severity from muscle strains and ligamentous strain to fractures of the vertebral body, fractures of the dorsal elements, dislocation of the facets, and complex combination fracture dislocations. The spinal cord and the nerve roots may be injured by an encroachment into the spinal canal. Patients with stable compression fractures may sustain concomitant injury to the spinal cord, and patients with grossly unstable comminuted fractures may escape neurologic injury. In general, however, the more comminuted, displaced, and unstable the spine fracture, the greater the likelihood of severe cord damage.[1,2,5,9,17,26]

Direct injuries to the spine and the spinal cord may occur as a result of a direct blow, such as from a falling tree limb or other heavy object, a stab wound, or a gunshot wound. Most injuries are caused by indirect trauma to the vertebral column resulting from energy generated by forces applied to the head, shoulders, trunk, or pelvis. These forces may contain an axial load as the main force with varying degrees of lateral bending, flexion, extension, or torsion. The thoracic and lumbar spine are most commonly injured by the kinetic energy produced by the person's body traveling through space and a sudden deceleration of the shoulders, upper trunk, or buttocks against an

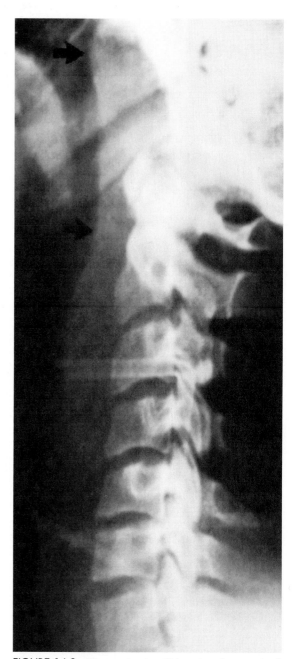

FIGURE 16-3 **Hyperextension dislocation characterized by intact cervical vertebrae and diffuse prevertebral soft tissue swelling *(arrows)* extending throughout the cervical region and into the nasopharynx.** (From Harris JH Jr, Edeiken-Monroe B: *The radiology of acute cervical spine trauma,* Baltimore, 1987, Williams and Wilkins.)

immovable object, with the vector of forces concentrated in an area of the thoracic or the lumbar spine. The most common area is that of the thoracolumbar junction, with specific patterns of vertebral body fractures and dorsal-element dislocation at T11 and T12, rotational-flexion fractures of both body and dorsal elements at T12 to L1, and bursting fractures of the body of L1. Fractures of the midthoracic spine usually occur at the T5 or T6 level.[1,2,5,9,17,26]

The most common site of lumbar fractures is L2 or L3. A specific type of flexion-distraction injury occurs when a person is restrained by a seat belt and experiences sudden deceleration, which causes sudden flexion and distraction centered at the midlumbar spine. Patients with these fractures often escape spinal cord cauda equina damage, and the fracture may be overlooked in the presence of traumatic brain injury or associated small intestinal injuries. Any person who has pain after being in an automobile accident in which a seat belt was worn must be examined specifically for the presence of a spinal fracture.

The thoracic spine is protected from injury by the rib cage, the sternum, and the chest wall. These bony structures permit little flexion and extension motion of the upper and midthoracic spine; however, a normal rotation motion does occur. The lumbar spine allows for more flexion, extension, and lateral motion because it lacks the previously mentioned supporting structures.[1,2,5,9,17,26]

Midthoracic spine injuries are usually caused by acute flexion, rotation, and axial load forces at the midthoracic region, resulting in either a simple compression fracture of the vertebral bodies or a complex fracture dislocation in which the vertebral body and the dorsal elements are fractured.

Most injuries at the thoracolumbar junction are caused by a combination of flexion, rotation, and axial load. An injury that is centered at T11 to T12 frequently causes a dislocation without fracture of the posterior facets and a slice fracture through the upper portion of the T12 vertebral body.

Rotational forces are commonly associated with fracture dislocations of T12 to L1 level. If the injury has more of an axial load than a rotational force, the body of L1 suffers a burst injury. In this type of injury, the posterior elements of the lamina, spinous process, and facet joints may be intact or may also be fractured.

SUMMARY

The management of all neurologic traumatic emergencies includes rapid assessment, airway management with spinal protection, and serial examinations throughout the assessment and transfer phases. On completion of the transfer, the receiving caregivers must be provided with a thorough report of events, including the time of the incident, the mechanism of injury or preceding events, care rendered by the referring facility and the transport team, response of the patient to care initiated, medical history of the patient, and observed changes in the patient's condition. This thorough report provides the receiving caregivers with information to guide their management and ensure continuity of care for the patient with the best possible chance for a positive outcome.

NEUROLOGIC TRAUMA CASE STUDY

A 22-year-old male unrestrained driver struck the back end of a parked car. He was thrown 25 ft from the vehicle. Because of the mechanism of injury, the local emergency medical services (EMS) agency called the transport team directly to the scene so that the patient could be transferred to a level I trauma center.

The transport team found on arrival that the patient was unresponsive with a GCS of 5. He had facial abrasions and swelling with palpable crepitus.

1. *Eye Opening: 1*
2. *Verbal Response: 1*
3. *Motor Response: 3*

He was being ventilated via bag-valve-mask (BVM) device, and his jaws were clenched. He was successfully intubated with rapid sequence intubation (RSI) on the first attempt. He had strong peripheral pulses, and the monitor showed a sinus tachycardia at a rate of 120 beats per minute. One intravenous line had been established before arrival, and the patient was appropriately immobilized and packaged for transport.

During transport, the patient's blood pressure was measured at 180/128 mmHg. His heart rate decreased to 48 beats per minute. His right pupil became fixed and dilated.

DISCUSSION

The patient's change in vital signs reflected increasing intracranial pressure. Based on his blood pressure, pulse rate, and fixed dilated pupil, the transport team initiated hyperventilation at a rate of 30 breaths per minute and administered 50 g of mannitol in route. These acute changes in the patient's neurologic status were clear indications for aggressive management to decrease the ICP.

On arrival at the receiving facility, the patient's blood pressure had decreased to 160/100 mmHg, and his heart rate had increased to 100 beats per minute. He was taken for emergent CT scan, which showed a large epidural hematoma with mass effect on the left. He was then taken to the operating room for decompression.

REFERENCES

1. Air and Surface Transport Nurses Association: *Transport nurse advanced trauma course*, Denver, 2006, ASTNA.
2. American College of Surgeons Committee on Trauma: *Advanced trauma life support course for physicians*, ed 8, Chicago, 2008, ACS.
3. Appleby I: Traumatic brain injury: initial resuscitation and transfer, *Anaesth Intensive Care Med* 9(5):193-196, 2008.
4. Brain Trauma Foundation Writing Team: Guidelines for traumatic brain injury, ed 2, *Prehosp Emerg Care* 12(1):S1-S53, 2007.
5. Campbell JE: *International trauma life support*, ed 6, Upper Saddle River, NJ, 2008, Pearson/Prentice Hall.
6. Chen FH, Fetzer JD: Complete cricotracheal separation and third cervical spinal cord transection following blunt neck trauma: a case report of one survivor, *J Trauma* 35(1):140, 1993.
7. Consortium for Spinal Cord Medicine Member Organizations: *Early acute management in adults with spinal cord injury: a clinical practice guideline for health care professionals*, Washington, DC, 2008, Paralyzed Veterans of America.
8. Dunn J, Smith M: Critical care management of head injury, *Anaesth Intensive Care Med* 9(5):197-201, 2008.
9. Emergency Nurses Association: *Trauma nursing core course*, ed 6, Des Plaines, IL, 2007, ENA.
10. Gennarelli TA, et al: Diffuse axonal injury and traumatic coma in the primate, *Ann Neurol* 12:564, 1982.
11. Geisler FH: Acute management of cervical spinal cord injury, *Trauma Q* 4(3):May, 1988.
12. Hastings RH, Wood PR: Head extension and laryngeal view during laryngoscopy with cervical spine immobilization maneuvers, *Anesthesiology* 80(4):825, 1994.
13. Maas A, Stocchetti N, Bullock R: Moderate and severe traumatic brain injury in adults, *Lancet Neurol* 7: 728-741, 2008.
14. Manifold S: Craniocerebral trauma: a review of primary and secondary injury and therapeutic modalities, *Focus Crit Care* 13:33, 1986.
15. McGuire RA, et al: Spine instability and logrolling maneuver, *J Trauma* 27:525, 1987.
16. McQuillan KA, Thurman PA: Traumatic brain injuries. In McQuillan KA, et al, editors: Trauma nursing: from resuscitation through rehabilitation, ed 4, Philadelphia, 2009, Saunders.
17. McSwain NE, Frame S, Salomone J: *Basic and advanced prehospital trauma life support*, St Louis, 2003, Mosby.
18. Miller JD: Traumatic brain injury and brain ischemia, *Br J Anesthesiol* 57:120, 1985.
19. Morris M, Kinkade S: The effect of capnometry on manual ventilation technique, *Air Med J* 14(2):79, 1995.
20. Muizelaar JP, Schroder ML: Overview of monitoring of cerebral blood flow and metabolism after severe traumatic brain injury, *Can J Neurol Sci* 21(3):S6, 1994.
21. Nikas D: Pathophysiology and nursing interventions in acute SCI, *Trauma Q* 4(3):May, 1988.
22. Norwood S, Myers MB, Butler TJ: The safety of emergency neuromuscular blockade and orotracheal intubation in the acutely injured trauma patient, *J Am Coll Surg* 179(6):646, 1994.
23. Povlishock JT: Guidelines for the management of severe traumatic brain injury, *J Neurotrauma* 24(S): 1-106, 2007.
24. Prolo DJ, Hanbery JW: Cervical stabilization-traction board, *J Am Med Assoc* 224(5):615, 1973.
25. Saboe LA, et al: Spine trauma and associated injuries, *J Trauma* 31(1):43, 1991.
26. Sanders M: *Mosby's paramedic textbook*, ed 3, St Louis, 2007, Mosby JEMS Elsevier.
27. Seeling JM, et al: Traumatic acute subdural hematoma: major mortality reduction in comatose patients treated within four hours, *N Engl J Med* 304:1511, 1981.
28. Smith M, Bourn S, Larmm B: Ties that bind: immobilizing the injury spine, *J Emerg Med Serv* 14(4):1989.

29. Stevens RD, Lazaridis C, Chalela J: The role of mechanical ventilation in acute brain injury, *Neurol Clin* 26: 543-563, 2008.

30. Sugerman RA: Structure and function of the neurogic system. In McCance K, Huether S, editors: Pathophysiology: the biologic basis for disease in adults and children, ed 5, St Louis, 2007, Elsevier Mosby.

31. Sullivan TE, et al: Closed traumatic brain injury assessment and research methodology, *J Neurosci Nurs* 26(1):24, 1994.

32. Tabaddor K: Nonoperative management of head trauma, *Contemp Neurosurg* 2(26):1, 1980.

33. Temkin NR, Dikem SS, Winn HR: Management of traumatic brain injury, posttraumatic seizures, *Neurosurg Clin North Am* 2(2):425, 1991.

34. Ward JD: Management of traumatic brain injury: prehospital care, *Neurosurg Clin North Am* 2(2):251, 1991.

35. Watts C: Trauma to the cervical spine, *Mod Med* 101, 1986.

36. Watts DD, Hanfling D, Waller M, et al: An evaluation of the use of guidelines in prehospital management of brain injury, *J Prehosp Emerg Care* 3(8):254-261, 2004.

37. White RJ, Likavec MJ: Current concepts: the diagnosis and initial management of traumatic brain injury, *N Engl J Med* 327(21):1507, 1992.

38. Whiteside TE Jr, Shah S: On management of unstable fractures of thoraco-lumbar spine, *Spine* 1:99, 1976.

39. York-Clark D, Stocking J, Johnson J: *Flight and ground transport nursing core curriculum*, Denver, 2006, ASTNA.

THORACIC TRAUMA

Reneé Semonin Holleran

COMPETENCIES

1. Identify clinical indications of thoracic injuries.
2. Recognize signs and symptoms of life-threatening thoracic injuries.
3. Perform appropriate critical interventions to manage a thoracic injury.

Thoracic injuries present a demanding challenge for patient transport. Thoracic injury remains second only to central nervous system injury as the leading cause of all trauma deaths.[1] In the pediatric population, with the exception of lung contusions, serious injuries to vital thoracic structures are associated with a mortality rate of more than 60%.[15] An understanding of the severity and mechanism of injury, management concerns of specific thoracic injuries, and special transport considerations aid the transport team in providing care.

Thoracic trauma is classified by either the mechanism of injury or the degree to which the injury is life threatening. Classification of thoracic trauma by mechanism of injury encompasses two categories: blunt and penetrating traumas. *Blunt trauma* is associated with motor vehicle crashes, compression injuries, falls, and assaults. *Penetrating trauma* occurs as a result of gunshot wounds, stab wounds, and impalement.

Thoracic injuries may also be categorized as life-threatening or potentially life-threatening conditions. *Life-threatening* thoracic conditions are airway obstruction, tension pneumothorax, massive hemothorax, open pneumothorax, flail chest, cardiac tamponade, aortic rupture, and myocardial rupture. *Potentially life-threatening* conditions are myocardial contusion, pulmonary contusion, aortic disruption, tracheobronchial disruption, esophageal rupture, and diaphragmatic disruption. Because many of the thoracic injuries are life threatening, rapid transport to a regional trauma center or tertiary care setting may be indicated.[5,13,18]

Special considerations for in-flight care of the patient with thoracic trauma relate to altitude changes and gas expansion. As previously discussed in transport physiology, gases expand with increasing altitude. Because of this expansion, a patient with an untreated pneumothorax or a nonfunctioning chest tube may be at great risk for development of a tension pneumothorax.[1,18,25] As part of the anticipatory planning and management of care during transport, the way changes in altitude may affect a patient with thoracic injuries must be considered.

The greatest threat in the management of a patient with a thoracic injury is hypoxia.[1,18,25] In addition to thoracic injury, the contributing causes of hypoxia may be decreased blood volume, failure to ventilate the lungs, ventilation-perfusion mismatches, or pressure changes within the intrapleural space. The ABCDEs of resuscitation serve as a framework for management of each injury. The ABCDE framework assists in quick detection of life-threatening injuries and implementation of rapid interventions.

LIFE-THREATENING THORACIC INJURIES

TENSION PNEUMOTHORAX

Etiologic Factors

Both blunt and penetrating thoracic traumas cause *tension pneumothorax*. A tension pneumothorax can also occur as a complication of the treatment of an open pneumothorax. Air progressively accumulates under pressure, and the flap of the injured lung acts as a one-way valve; air is allowed to enter the pleural space on inspiration but not allowed to escape on expiration.

Pathophysiologic Factors

Ventilation is inadequate because the air entering the pleural space increases the intrapleural pressure with each inspiration, which causes collapse of the ipsilateral lung and a mediastinal shift to the opposite side, leading to compression of the contralateral lung (Figure 17-1). Perfusion becomes inadequate because of decreased venous return to the heart as a result of the increased intrapleural pressure and shift of mediastinal structures.

Assessment

The mechanism of injury establishes a high index of suspicion. The patient with a tension pneumothorax

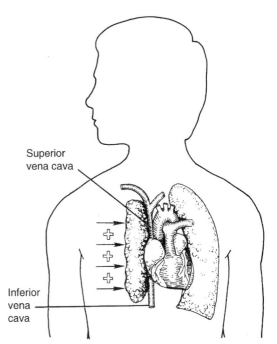

FIGURE 17-1   **Tension pneumothorax.** (From Sheehy SB: *Emergency nursing: principles and practice*, ed 4, St Louis, 1992, Mosby.)

has severe respiratory distress, dyspnea, and cyanosis. Agitation and anxiety are common.[1,11,16,19] Clinical evidence of shock may be present. Breath sounds are either decreased or absent over the involved hemithorax. The trachea should be assessed because a shift to the unaffected side occurs as intrapleural pressure increases. As air passes into the tissues, subcutaneous emphysema can be palpated, causing decreased preload into the heart. Jugular venous distention, a late sign, occurs because of the increased intrapleural pressure. Constant observation of the patient's chest excursion is important during transport because auscultation is next to impossible.

Interventions

The immediate life-saving intervention is rapid decompression of the pleural space. To release the intrapleural pressure, a large-bore needle should be placed into the pleural space, specifically into the second intercostal space, two-finger breadths lateral to the sternal border on the affected side. The needle should then be placed superior to the rib margin to avoid the intercostal artery. The anterior site is used for avoidance of the internal mammary vessels.[5,6,16,19] If a tension pneumothorax is present, a rush of air may be heard. This rush of air probably is not appreciated during transport. Instead, immediate improvement of the patient symptoms and a return to hemodynamic stability should be seen.

The needle thoracostomy must be converted to a tube thoracostomy as soon as possible. A single chest tube is acceptable for a pneumothorax, hemothorax, or hemopneumothorax.[7,16,21] In addition, intravenous access and fluid resuscitation should be initiated.

Evaluation

Constant reevaluation of the patient's cardiopulmonary status is warranted. If a chest tube is placed and a persistent air leak occurs, the presence of a tracheobronchial disruption must be considered.

MASSIVE HEMOTHORAX
Etiologic Factors

Massive hemothorax develops as a result of blunt or penetrating injuries of intrathoracic organs or laceration of an intercostal artery. The rapid and massive accumulation of blood and fluid in the pleural space can result in severe hemodynamic compromise.

Pathophysiologic Factors

The compliant lung offers little resistance to a large amount of blood becoming sequestered in the pleural space (Figure 17-2), and hypovolemic shock

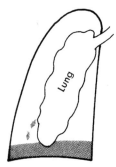

FIGURE 17-2   **Hemothorax.** (From Sheehy SB: *Emergency nursing: principles and practice*, ed 4, St Louis, 1992, Mosby.)

results. Compression of the ipsilateral lung occurs from the accumulation of blood, and a mediastinal shift can occur from compression of the contralateral lung. In this way, ventilation-perfusion mismatches happen.

Assessment

The mechanism of injury is vital to the initial assessment of a suspected massive hemothorax. Because of the decrease in blood volume, manifestations of hypovolemic shock may appear. Altered mentation, decrease in blood pressure, increase in heart rate, and signs of peripheral vasoconstriction are common. Breath sounds are decreased or absent over the involved hemothorax, and chest excursion on the affected side is decreased. Unlike the symptoms of cardiac tamponade, the trachea is generally in the midline, and the neck veins are flat unless a hemopneumothorax is present.[5,21]

Interventions

Restoration of lost blood volume is of primary importance, and an initial response is to achieve intravenous access with at least two large-bore catheters and to administer crystalloids or colloids. Supplemental oxygen should be administered. Endotracheal intubation may be necessary. Emergent management involves placement of a tube thoracostomy.

Fluid resuscitation must be carefully monitored. The transport team must also be cognizant that excessive fluid resuscitation, particularly in penetrating thoracic trauma, can be detrimental and lead to hypoxemia or worsening of hemothorax or cardiac tamponade.

In cases of massive hemothorax, the transport team may consider autotransfusion.[3,4] The use of autotransfusion in thoracic trauma has been greatly debated because of the potential effect of anticoagulants and abdominal contaminants.[2,12] Considerations related to autotransfusion are transport delay during supply setup and space limitation during transport. In situations of prolonged transport times, isolated chest trauma, conflicting religious beliefs, or cross-matching difficulty, autotransfusion may serve as a bridge until definitive care is provided.

Many transport programs today have access to blood and blood products that can be used when autotransfusion is not available, the wound is potentially contaminated, or time is an issue. In any resuscitation situation in which bleeding is actively occurring, the patient must be closely monitored to prevent additional bleeding. Resuscitation should occur cautiously until bleeding is controlled.[12] Rapid transport to definitive care should be one of the primary focuses of the team.[6]

The need for surgical intervention, a thoracotomy, is based not only on the initial amount of chest tube drainage, hemodynamic status, and fluid resuscitation amounts, but also on the location of chest-wall penetration or the rate of ongoing blood loss.[1,2,9,12,17,19]

Evaluation

Transport team members must constantly reassesses the ventilator neurologic and hemodynamic status of the patient and monitor the parameters of the patient's response to volume replacement.

OPEN PNEUMOTHORAX
Etiologic Factors

A penetrating object causes an *open pneumothorax*, or sucking chest wound. Air enters the pleural space through the opening or defect in the chest wall (Figure 17-3).

Pathophysiologic Factors

If the diameter of the chest-wall defect is greater than the diameter of the patient's trachea, air moves through the chest wound rather than through the trachea and airways. The defect in the thoracic wall leads to an equilibration of atmospheric and pleural pressure. The result is loss of the negative intrathoracic pressure, which leads to respiratory insufficiency. Air in the pleural space promotes collapse of the ipsilateral lung and a mediastinal shift to the unaffected side. The mediastinal shift and loss of normal negative intrathoracic pressure produce decreased venous return to the heart and cardiac insufficiency.

Assessment

A penetrating injury to the thorax should lead the transport team to closely assess the thorax to determine whether a sucking chest wound is present. The patient is in respiratory distress, with tachypnea and grunting, and as air enters and leaves the pleural space through the chest-wall defect, a sucking noise may be heard during respiration. Clinical manifestations of shock occur as a result of intermittent obstruction of venous return.[4-6,12,14,19,21]

Interventions

In the prehospital setting, the wound should be covered, but not sealed, with an occlusive dressing. A dressing taped on three sides creates a flutter-valve effect; air is prevented from entering the chest on inspiration but is not prevented from leaving the chest on expiration. If an occlusive dressing is used and a defect in the lung exists, a tension pneumothorax may develop because the air is not allowed to escape from the pleural space.

If a tension pneumothorax develops, the occlusive dressing should be immediately removed. The patient may need the placement of a chest tube to treat the underlying lung defect.[5,25] If the patient's ventilation and oxygenation continue to deteriorate, the team should immediately prepare to intubate. Maintenance of intravenous access is also imperative as a route for volume resuscitation and medication administration.

Evaluation

Evaluation must consist of continuous monitoring of the patient's cardiopulmonary status. Assessment parameters for expanding pneumothoraces are limited during transport because of the background

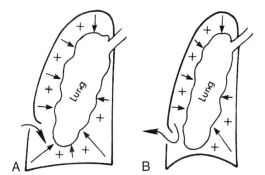

FIGURE 17-3 **Sucking chest wound. A,** Inspiration. **B,** Expiration. (From Sheehy SB: *Emergency nursing: principles and practice,* ed 4, St Louis, 1992, Mosby.)

noise levels. Astute evaluation of the patient's chest pain, tachycardia, increasing dyspnea, tracheal deviation, and development of subcutaneous emphysema and neurologic status prompts the transport nurse to begin hemodynamic compromise.[1,25]

FLAIL CHEST
Etiologic Factors
A *flail chest* usually occurs as a result of blunt thoracic trauma. Multiple rib fractures cause separation of a portion of the rib cage and loss of stability of the chest wall. The flail segment usually involves the anterior or lateral chest wall because heavy posterior muscles and the scapula protect the posterior chest wall.

Pathophysiologic Factors
Paradoxical chest movement interferes with the normal "bellows" function of the thoracic cage, causing inadequate gas exchange. The underlying pulmonary contusion causes progressive respiratory insufficiency. The instability of the chest wall and the pain from the fracture sites lead to hypoventilation and subsequent hypoxemia.

Assessment
Observation of chest excursion is important; however, the paradoxical movement may not be obvious except in cases of severe flail. The flail segment moves in the opposite direction from the rest of the thoracic cage during respiration, moving inward during inspiration and outward during expiration (Figure 17-4). Initially, the flail may not be obvious because of spasms of the muscles in the thoracic wall. The patient is also in respiratory distress, with cyanosis, grunting, and use of accessory muscles, and reports severe chest pain on the involved side.

Interventions
For the patient in severe distress, endotracheal intubation is needed to treat hypoxia. The patient should be manually ventilated if the transport ventilator does not have the appropriate settings to recognize the development of a tension pneumothorax. External stabilization techniques include application of gentle pressure over the flail segment with a pillow or a pad or placement of the patient with the

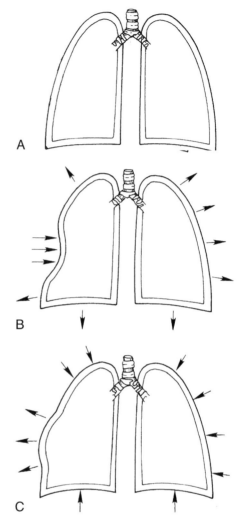

FIGURE 17-4   **Flail chest. A,** Normal lungs. **B,** Flail chest on inspiration. **C,** Flail chest on expiration. (From Sheehy SB: *Emergency nursing: principles and practice,* ed 4, St Louis, 1992, Mosby.)

injured side down, if the condition allows. Analgesia is warranted once the airway has been secured.

Evaluation
Constant reassessment of the patient's cardiopulmonary status is vital to treatment of the patient with a flail chest. Mentation, skin color, and Sao_2 measurements, in addition to vital signs, are parameters to monitor. Pain control cannot be accomplished until the patient's condition is fully evaluated but is warranted once stability is achieved.

ACUTE CARDIAC TAMPONADE
Etiologic Factors

Acute cardiac tamponade occurs when blood accumulates in the pericardial sac (Figure 17-5) as a result of blunt and penetrating cardiac trauma.

Pathophysiologic Factors

The hemodynamic effects of cardiac tamponade depend on how quickly fluid (blood) accumulates in the pericardial sac; rapid accumulation of blood (from 150 to 250 mL) may be fatal because the normal pericardial sac contains 20 to 50 mL of pericardial fluid. If the accumulation is slow, the fibrous pericardium stretches and may accommodate several liters of fluid without hemodynamic consequences. The main hemodynamic consequence is a decrease in diastolic filling because of increased intrapericardial pressure. Once the diastolic filling decreases, stroke volume and cardiac output fall. Central venous pressure increases as a result of increased intrapericardial pressure. However, because of the underlying pathophysiology, the patient may actually need fluid volume to maintain forward flow through the body's pump until definitive care is reached.[10]

Assessment

The patient with acute cardiac tamponade shows signs of decreased cardiac output, such as altered mental status, cool clammy skin, tachycardia, and a falling arterial blood pressure. Venous hypertension also occurs, as evidenced by marked neck-vein distention (unless the patient is hypovolemic) and rising central venous pressure. Distant muffled heart sounds may not be detectable in the field. *Pulsus paradoxus* is a fall in the systolic blood pressure greater than 15 mmHg during normal inspiration.[10] Collectively, the condition is known as Beck's triad (narrowed pulse pressure, increased central venous pressure [JVP], and distant/muffled heart sounds).

Interventions

The initial treatment of a patient with suspected cardiac tamponade is a rapid intravenous fluid bolus.[5,9,10] This measure improves filling pressures and temporarily improves cardiac output until pericardiocentesis can be performed. The emergent treatment of choice is pericardiocentesis (Figure 17-6).[19,25] A needle is placed into the pericardial sac and may withdraw as little as 15 to 20 mL of blood to improve the patient's condition. Pericardial blood generally does not clot because it has been defibrinated by heart motion. Pericardiocentesis may be extremely challenging to perform during

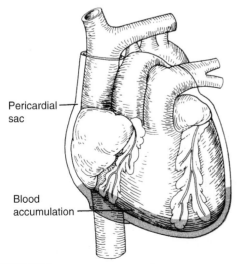

FIGURE 17-5   **Cardiac tamponade.** (From Sheehy SB: *Emergency nursing: principles and practice*, ed 4, St Louis, 1992, Mosby.)

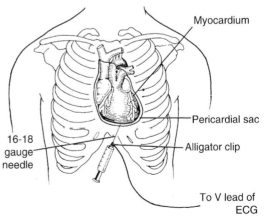

FIGURE 17-6   **Pericardiocentesis.** (From Sheehy SB: *Emergency nursing: principles and practice*, ed 4, St Louis, 1992, Mosby.)

flight because of the confined environment and air turbulence.

Because the long-term survival rate is less than 10%, aggressive interventions offer the best chance for patient survival. Failure to diagnose and repair aortic injuries within 24 hours of the patient's arrival results in mortality rates of 25% to 40%.[14] Transesophageal echocardiogram has been used as a rapid, accurate, and safe method of thoracic aortic transection identification.[5,8,18,20,22] However, aortography remains the gold standard for diagnosis of aortic injuries. Early recognition of this injury and rapid transport to definitive care is imperative.

Evaluation

When a trauma patient's condition continues to deteriorate even with aggressive management, the transport team should consider acute pericardial tamponade.

AORTIC RUPTURE
Etiologic and Pathophysiologic Factors

Aortic rupture occurs as a result of blunt or penetrating trauma, and death occurs immediately in 80% to 90% of patients. However, when the rupture or transection occurs in only the medial and intimal layers, the intact adventitia may prevent exsanguination temporarily.

Assessment

The patient may not show any external signs of chest trauma. Severe chest and midscapular pain is uncommon. If conscious, the patient may report dyspnea. Hypertension in the upper extremities is caused by a periaortic hematoma, partial aortic occlusion, or stretching of the cardiac plexus; a harsh systolic murmur can be auscultated along the precordium. If a radiograph of the chest (Figure 17-7) has been done (before interfacility transport), findings that promote a high index of suspicion on the part of the transport team are: (1) widening of the superior mediastinum; (2) loss of aortic knob shadow; (3) fracture of the first rib; (4) depression of the left main stem bronchus; (5) deviation of the trachea to the right; (6) pleural capping; and (7) deviation of the gastric tube in the esophagus.[5,18,25]

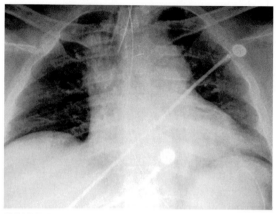

FIGURE 17-7 **Chest radiograph of an aortic aneurysm.** (From Mirvis SE: *Imaging in trauma and critical care*, ed 2, Philadelphia, 2003, Saunders.)

Interventions

Critical interventions and rapid transport to definitive care should be provided by the transport team. An immediate exploratory thoracostomy may be necessary.

MYOCARDIAL RUPTURE
Etiologic and Pathophysiologic Factors

Rupture of the heart, *myocardial rupture*, is the most lethal of blunt thoracic injuries.[1,25] Death occurs as a result of exsanguination. However, 61 cases of survival of nonpenetrating rupture of the myocardium have been reported; most cases were men who had been involved in motor vehicle accidents.[7,14]

Assessment and Interventions

Absent vital signs are key indicators that a fatal event has occurred. Resuscitation efforts are those used for any injured patient.

POTENTIALLY LIFE-THREATENING INJURIES

MYOCARDIAL CONTUSION
Etiologic Factors

Blunt trauma is the mechanism that produces *myocardial contusion*. The compression of the heart between the sternum and vertebrae occurs as a result of motor vehicle accidents, falls, or blows to the chest.

Pathophysiologic Factors

Lesions may vary in size from small areas of petechiae to large contusions and necrosis of the myocardium. Bleeding and edema occur at the site of injury.

Assessment

The patient should be suspected of having a myocardial contusion based on mechanism of injury (e.g., blunt trauma to the chest). The patient may be completely asymptomatic or may report chest pain that is characteristically identical to that of angina or acute myocardial infarction. Sinus tachycardia is common, and cardiac arrhythmias may occur. Patients at risk are those who have abnormal initial electrocardiogram findings with ST-T segment changes.[10] Use of cardiac enzymes as a diagnostic tool in patients with suspected myocardial contusions has been found to be of little value.[2]

Interventions

Management is similar to that for a patient who has sustained an acute myocardial infarction. Supplemental oxygen and intravenous access are part of the treatment regimen. If the patient has any dysrhythmias develop, advanced cardiac life support (ACLS) protocols should be used.

PULMONARY CONTUSION
Etiologic Factors

Pulmonary contusion occurs as a result of blunt thoracic trauma. Pulmonary contusion is not uncommonly associated with a flail chest or other blunt injuries to the chest.

Pathophysiologic Factors

Intraalveolar hemorrhage and edema occur as a result of blunt injury to the lung parenchyma. The alveolar-capillary integrity is lost, and interstitial hemorrhage and edema occur. Systemic hypoxemia is caused by decreased lung compliance and ventilation-perfusion mismatches.[15]

Assessment

The patient has a history of blunt thoracic trauma and usually has dyspnea and tachypnea. Tachycardia and anxiety, which may be caused by the stress of injury or hypoxemia, are also common. Rales and rhonchi are auscultated over the injured area. Lack of improvement in oxygen saturation during transport, despite oxygen therapy, may also indicate a pulmonary contusion. Maximum changes are seen in the chest radiograph from 48 to 72 hours after the injury.[1,25]

Interventions

Adequate ventilation with an aggressive pulmonary toilet is necessary. Supplemental oxygen should be administered. Endotracheal intubation is necessary when the Po_2 is lower than 60 mm Hg on room air or lower than 80 mm Hg with supplemental oxygen.

DIAPHRAGMATIC RUPTURE
Etiologic Factors

Herniation of abdominal viscera into the chest occurs with a traumatic defect in the diaphragm produced by blunt or penetrating trauma to the upper abdomen or lower thorax. If the injury occurred at the time the diaphragm was contracting strongly, a large avulsion tear results. Most *diaphragmatic ruptures* occur on the left side because the liver protects the right hemidiaphragm.[1,4,23]

Pathophysiologic Factors

Herniation of abdominal contents into the thoracic cavity causes compression of the ipsilateral lung and displacement of mediastinal structures. Cardiopulmonary insufficiency results, causing significantly reduced respiratory efficiency. The herniated viscera are compressed and cause gastric or intestinal obstruction or ischemia and gangrene.

Assessment

The patient may initially be asymptomatic or in severe distress. Abdominal or chest pain radiating to the shoulder may be present; dyspnea and cyanosis are also common signs. A paralytic ileus may accompany the injuries, so detection of bowel sounds may not be possible in the thorax cavity. Breath sounds are either decreased or absent on the side of the herniation. The abdomen is markedly scaphoid. A mediastinal shift is seen to the unaffected side.[1,4,5,24,25]

Interventions

Hypoxia should be treated, and ventilation must be maintained. The transport team should provide intravenous access and resuscitative measures. Immediate surgery for repair is indicated.

TRACHEOBRONCHIAL DISRUPTION
Etiologic Factors

Tracheobronchial disruption occurs most often from blunt trauma. Penetrating thoracic trauma is a less common cause.

Pathophysiologic Factors

Air passes through the tear into the pleural space or the mediastinum. In the pleural space, it produces a pneumothorax; in the mediastinum, it causes mediastinal emphysema. The patient's airway may be maintained initially because the tracheobronchial cartilage holds the lumen open.

Assessment

Hemoptysis, respiratory distress, and subcutaneous or mediastinal emphysema (or both) are present. A pneumothorax with a persistent air leak or failure of a lung to reexpand after tube thoracostomy should lead the transport team to suspect a tracheobronchial disruption. A tension pneumothorax may be the first visible sign of the problem.

Interventions

The transport team performs immediate endotracheal intubation with placement of the tube below the level of injury. Rapid transport for bronchoscopy and chest tube placement should be accomplished as soon as possible.[1,25]

ESOPHAGEAL PERFORATION
Etiologic Factors

The most common cause of *esophageal perforation* is iatrogenic traumatic instrumentation, although penetrating trauma, ingestion of a foreign body, and blunt trauma also can be causes.[17,24] A mortality rate of 10% is seen with early diagnosis; that mortality rate goes up to 50% with late diagnosis.[1]

Pathophysiologic Factors

Gastric contents and bacteria leaking into the mediastinum can lead not only to mediastinitis but also to fatal systemic toxicity. Perforation also results in massive fluid loss and can lead to hypovolemic shock.

Assessment

The location of the perforation determines the clinical signs and symptoms. Subcutaneous emphysema, dyspnea, dysphagia, fever, hematemesis, and shock are common observations.

Interventions

Intravenous access, gastric tube placement, antibiotic administration, and immediate surgery are the interventions of choice for esophageal perforation.

SUMMARY

The transport of a patient with a traumatic thoracic injury requires anticipatory planning to have all necessary equipment available. The transport team's prompt recognition and treatment of thoracic traumatic injuries, especially ensuring patency of the airway and performing specific measures for blunt or penetrating injuries, may reduce mortality and morbidity rates.

THORACIC TRAUMA CASE STUDY

The transport team was called to the scene of a high-speed single-car rollover motor vehicle crash. The patient was restrained, and because the car suffered extensive damage, he was trapped for more than 45 minutes. Patient extrication from the vehicle was in process when the air medical transport team arrived.

The primary survey completed and reported by the ground emergency medical service personnel revealed that the patient had an open airway, was having slightly labored breathing, and had a weak palpable pulse. No obvious bleeding was seen. His Glasgow Coma Scale (GCS) was 7 (E-1; V-1; M-5). The patient had multiple lacerations and abrasions on his face and upper extremities.

The secondary assessment, performed by the transport nurse on arrival at the scene of the accident, showed the following:

Vital signs: Blood pressure (BP): 164/110 mm Hg; heart rate (HR): 96 bpm; respiratory rate (RR): 45 bpm
Pupils: PERL
Airway: Patent

No obvious deformities of the head or face

GCS: 7

Chest expansion asymmetric; breath sounds could be heard over both sides, although they were decreased on the right

Minor abrasions to chest and back area

No other wounds or abnormalities noted

No abdominal wounds or distention noted

No obvious deformity to extremities

The transport team then initiated the following interventions.

The patient was immobilized on a long board with a cervical collar and head blocks.

Emergency medical service personnel initiated two large-bore peripheral intravenous lines, one in each arm. Because of the patient's GCS of 7, rapid sequence intubation (RSI) was used to intubate the patient on the first attempt with a no. 7.5 endotracheal tube. The patient was then hot loaded for transport to the trauma center.

During flight, patient ventilation became increasingly difficult. His heart rate dropped to 48 bpm. His oxygen saturation decreased to 88%. Because of the limited cabin size (Bell 407) and the inability to auscultate breath sounds, the transport nurse elected to perform a needle thoracostomy with a no. 10 gauge needle in the second intercostal space on the right side. Immediate improvement in ventilation was seen, and the patient's heart rate increased to 100 bpm.

The patient was hot off loaded and taken to the trauma bay for resuscitation.

OUTCOME

The patient was received in the emergency department of the area trauma center by the trauma team and was assessed by the trauma team. A chest tube was immediately inserted into the right chest. A FAST exam revealed fluid, and the patient was taken directly to the OR for further evaluation.

REFERENCES

1. Air and Surface Transport Nurses Association: *Transport nurse advanced trauma course*, ed 6, Denver, 2006, ASTNA.
2. American College of Surgeons Committee on Trauma: *Thoracic trauma: advanced trauma life support for doctors*, ed 8, Chicago, 2008, American College of Surgeons.
3. Blansfield J: Emergency autotransfusion in hypovolemia, *Crit Care Nurs Clin North Am* 2(2):196, 1990.
4. Bledsoe BE, Benner EW: *Critical care paramedic*, Upper Saddle River, NJ, 2006, Pearson Prentice Hall.
5. Brinkman W, Szeto W, Bavaria J: Overview of great vessel trauma, *Thorac Surg Clin* 17:96-108, 2007.
6. Campbell JE: *International trauma life support*, ed 6, Upper Saddle River, NJ, 2008, Pearson Prentice Hall.
7. Christensen MA, Sutton KR: Myocardial contusion: new concepts in diagnosis and management, *Am J Crit Care* 2(1):28, 1993.
8. Cohn SM, et al: Exclusion of aortic tear in the unstable trauma patient: the utility of transesophageal echocardiography, *J Trauma* 49(6):1087, 1995.
9. Cooper A: Thoracic injuries, *Semin Pediatr Surg* 4(2):109, 1995.
10. Daleiden A: Clinical manifestations of blunt cardiac injury: a challenge to the critical care nurse, *Crit Care Nurs Q* 17(2):14, 1994.
11. Emergency Nurses Association: *Trauma nursing core course*, ed 6, Des Plaines, IL, 2007, ENA.
12. Evans BJ, Hornick P: Penetrating injuries to the chest, *Surg* 24(11):406-409, 2005.
13. Feczko JD, et al: An autopsy case review of 142 non-penetrating (blunt) injuries of the aorta, *J Trauma* 44(1):846, 1992.
14. Fildes JJ, et al: Limiting cardiac evaluation in patients with suspected myocardial contusion, *Am Surg* 69(9):842, 1995.
15. Flagel BT, Luchette F, Reed T, et al: Half-a-dozen ribs: the breakpoint of mortality, *Surg* 148(4):717-726, 2005.
16. Herron H, Falcone RE: Prehospital decompression for suspected tension pneumothorax, *Air Med J* 14(2):69, 1995.
17. Klygis LM, et al: Esophageal perforations masked by steroids, *Abdom Imaging* 18(1):10, 1993.
18. Perez L, Chan G: Clinical decision making and management of blunt traumatic thoracic aortic injuries, *Air Med J* 27(4):139-144, 2008.
19. Proehl J: *Emergency nursing procedures*, ed 4, Philadelphia, 2009, Saunders Elsevier.
20. Saletta S, et al: Transesophageal echocardiography for the initial evaluation of the widened mediastinum in trauma patients, *J Trauma* 49(1):147, 1995.
21. Schrader KA: Penetrating chest trauma, *Crit Care Nurs Clin North Am* 6(4):687, 1993.
22. Shively BK: Transesophageal echocardiography in the diagnosis of aortic disease, *Semin Ultrasound CT MR* 14(2):106, 1993.
23. Sukul DM, Kats E, Johannes EJ: Sixty-three cases of traumatic injury of the diaphragm, *Injury* 22(4):404, 1991.
24. Tucker JG, Kim HH, Lucas GW: Esophageal perforation caused by coin ingestion, *South Med J* 87(2):269, 1994.
25. York Clark D, Stocking J, Johnson J: *Flight and ground transport core curriculum*, ed 2, Denver, 2006, ASTNA.

ABDOMINAL TRAUMA

Reneé Semonin Holleran

COMPETENCIES

1. Perform an organized and focused abdominal assessment.
2. Identify clinical indications of abdominal trauma.
3. Initiate critical interventions and provide appropriate treatment during transport for the patient with an abdominal injury.

Regionalized trauma care has drastically reduced the incidence rate of death after injury. However, despite improvements in prehospital, resuscitative, surgical, and critical care, unrecognized abdominal injury remains a preventable cause of death after injury.[2,3,15]

Exsanguination continues to be a common cause of death from traumatic injury. Because patients with abdominal trauma may have severe hemorrhage, rapid transport can significantly reduce the mortality and morbidity rates from both blunt and penetrating abdominal injuries. Four common causes of massive bleeding in trauma patients include external injury, massive hemothorax, retroperitoneal injury (e.g., pelvic fracture, renal laceration, or major vessel lesion), and intraperitoneal injury (e.g., liver, spleen, or major vessel laceration).[3,9,15,17] The likelihood of

significant intraabdominal injury is high when a patient has hypotension in the field, a major chest injury, or pelvic fracture.[14,35,42]

Patients with genitourinary injuries alone are not usually in danger of life-threatening hemorrhage. Although genitourinary trauma alone is not immediately life threatening, appropriate transport can significantly affect the recovery time and reduction of complications that result from these injuries. Many lower level facilities are not equipped to diagnose and treat specific genitourinary injuries. Air medical transport may be appropriate when a delay in ground time diminishes the chances of full recovery from renal, bladder, and genital injuries.

Shock and time elapsed between injury and arrival in the operating room are the major factors that affect survival of patients with abdominal injuries, and these factors can be ameliorated by intervention of trained transport personnel able to recognize life-threatening injuries, initiate treatment, and rapidly transport the patient to definitive care.

ABDOMINAL TRAUMA

ANATOMY OF THE ABDOMEN

The abdomen contains several major organs of the body responsible for digestion, nutrition, and elimination of toxins and waste from the body. Because the spleen filters aged red blood cells and one of the functions of the liver is to eliminate toxic waste from the bloodstream, both organs are vascular in nature. The spleen, liver, and vascular system of the abdomen are the primary sources of exsanguination during abdominal trauma.[1,2,11,18,19] Injuries to the hollow abdominal organs, such as the small and large intestine, can result in abscess formation, wound infection, and sepsis, especially if trauma to the intestine remains undiagnosed for a period of time. When injuries to the abdomen occur, they may have a large impact on morbidity and mortality.

The abdominal cavity includes all structures and organs between the respiratory diaphragm and the urogenital diaphragm. This space is divided into three compartments: the first, and largest, is the peritoneal cavity; the second is the space within the pelvic structure; and the third is the retroperitoneal space. The *peritoneal cavity* contains the diaphragm, spleen, liver, stomach, transverse colon, and most of the small intestine and mesentery.

The *bony structure of the pelvis* contains the rectum, bladder, iliac vessels, and female reproductive organs; the penis and scrotum are located outside the abdominal cavity below the urogenital diaphragm.

The *retroperitoneal space* is separated from the abdominal cavity by the posterior peritoneum and therefore is not always accessed with peritoneal lavage. Injuries in this area may be difficult to diagnose and are easily overlooked. The organs contained in this space are the aorta, vena cava, distal esophagus, kidneys, ureters, and portions of the duodenum, pancreas, colon, and rectum.

Knowledge of the basic anatomy of the abdomen and position of the organs is crucial because identification of organs possibly injured by blunt or penetrating trauma helps the transport team provide the treatment necessary for those injuries when preparing for or affecting the patient's transport.

CLASSIFICATION OF INJURIES

Abdominal trauma can be blunt or penetrating, depending on the mechanism of injury. *Blunt trauma* is caused by any type of force being exerted on the abdomen as the result of falls, motor vehicle accidents (MVCs), bicycle and motorcycle accidents, or any force striking the abdomen.[1,4,7,8,12,28] As the body receives an impact, the organs in the abdominal cavity continue moving forward; vessels and tissues tear away from their attachment points.

Patients have fewer fatal injuries with the increased use of seat belts, motorcycle and bicycle helmets, child restraint seats, and air bags and with enforcement of alcohol restraints. However, most blunt abdominal injuries (50% to 75%) are the result of MVCs.[1,7,11,13] The use of seat belts decreases the possibility of multisystem injuries, but improper placement across the abdomen rather than the pelvis, loose application, or use of only lap belts can result in visceral trauma. The abdominal organs most frequently injured by blunt trauma are the liver, spleen, and kidney, although hollow-organ (intestinal) injury can occur. Abdominal injuries among air bag–protected occupants occur less frequently than head, chest, and lower extremity injuries. However, abdominal injuries may be occult, and deformation of the steering wheel is an indicator of an increased likelihood of internal injury.[3,4,23,44-48]

Trauma is classified as *penetrating* when an object such as a knife or bullet enters the abdominal cavity; anything that has penetrated the abdomen and remains in place may be designated as an impaled object. Penetrating injuries of the abdomen are caused by gunshot wounds (GSWs) or stab wounds. The degree of injury of patients with GSWs depends on the caliber of the gun and its distance from the patient. High-velocity weapons and close-range shotguns cause more destruction to abdominal organs than do low-velocity weapons. However, bullets from low-velocity weapons can deflect off organs and bony prominences and create extensive injuries that are not easily recognized on initial examination. In stab wounds, the length of the knife or object, the depth of penetration, and the angle at which it was inserted determine the amount of injury. The major organs involved in penetrating injuries are the liver, small bowel, colon, stomach, and vascular structures. The large size and anterior position of the liver and bowel in the abdomen make them particularly vulnerable to penetrating trauma.[12,21-25]

Objects found impaled in the patient on arrival of the transport team should be left in place and stabilized for transport (Figure 18-1). Removal of the object may cause further injury or increase bleeding. If placing the patient into the transport vehicle is not possible because of the size and position of the object, it may have to be cut off while still in place within the abdominal cavity. The object should be moved as little as possible. In some instances, the trauma surgeon must be transported to the scene to assist in the shortening or removal of the object.[41]

PATIENT HISTORY

The history of the injury and the physical examination should be obtained before transport because the information is important to the transport team when they assess and stabilize a patient for transport. The trauma surgeon may use the information when deciding the degree of injury and whether surgery should be performed soon after arrival at the emergency center. When possible, a medical history, including medications, allergies, illnesses, and events leading up to injury, should be obtained from the

patient, family, or referring facility. Other helpful information is whether the patient has used alcohol or other substances, has a head or neck injury, has psychiatric problems, or has any underlying medical conditions (i.e., cardiovascular disease or coagulopathies).[1,10,15] Initial vital signs and level of consciousness, intake and output, and treatments done before the arrival of the transport team, and any changes or treatments in transport, should be reported to the trauma team at the receiving trauma center.

When a patient with blunt abdominal trauma is transported from a pedestrian accident or MVC, important information to obtain from the prehospital personnel at the site are the time of injury, probable speed of impact, damage to the vehicle (steering wheel, direction of impact on the vehicle), patient's position in the vehicle, and restraint devices used. When time permits, brief inspection of the damage to the vehicle by the transport team may provide more information on possible patient injuries. In patients injured from falls, the height of fall and position of impact help point to the type of injuries involved. The history of assault victims should include the type of instrument that struck them.[24,26]

Although internal bleeding is difficult to measure in penetrating injuries, the amount of blood lost at the scene should be noted for determination of the fluid replacement needed and indication of the degree of injury.

PHYSICAL EXAMINATION

The physical examination is one of the most important procedures for diagnosis of abdominal injury. It can be effective in determining the presence of blood in the peritoneal cavity or peritoneal irritation. Examination of the abdomen should be as thorough as possible. When a trauma patient who is in hemorrhagic shock is transported from a scene of accident or assault, the only assessment that time may permit is palpation for distention and tenderness. The abdominal assessment should include inspection, auscultation, and palpation before interfacility transport, especially when time and distance are great. Serial abdominal assessments should be done throughout transport because peritoneal irritation and accumulation of blood in the peritoneal cavity may not produce symptoms immediately.[1]

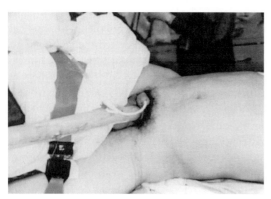

FIGURE 18-1   **Injury resulting from a logging accident.**

The abdomen should be fully exposed to allow the transport team to inspect for contusions, abrasions, deformity, hematoma formation, open wounds, and penetrating injuries. An ecchymotic discoloration around the umbilicus (Cullen's sign) can indicate intraabdominal or retroperitoneal hemorrhage. When examination of the patient's back is possible, the transport team should look for any obvious signs of trauma that indicate an abdominal or genitourinary injury. Flank bruising (also known as Grey-Turner's sign) may signify retroperitoneal hematoma formation from trauma to the kidneys, major blood vessels, or other organs contained in that space.

Auscultation should be done primarily in a quiet controlled area because bowel sounds are difficult to hear in the noisy transport environment. Absence of bowel sounds can be an important indicator of an ileus and abdominal injury, and assessment of bowel sounds before an interfacility transfer may alert the transport team to the possibility of abdominal injury. Absence of bowel sounds may indicate the need to consider the insertion of a gastric tube for patient comfort and to protect the airway from potential aspiration.

An abdomen that is tender and distended on palpation needs immediate attention, which generally requires rapid transport with continual observation of vital signs. The major causes of a distended abdomen are gastric dilation and rapid intraabdominal bleeding. Tenderness on palpation with involuntary guarding or rebound tenderness is indicative of peritoneal irritation.

Subjective reports of abdominal pain by a trauma patient should always be addressed. Because patients with head injury and a decreased level of consciousness are unable to identify abdominal pain, detection of a distended abdomen on palpation without any obvious signs of trauma may be the only indication of intraabdominal trauma.

The perineum should be visually inspected for any injuries to the genitals, urethra, or rectum. Peroneal hematoma formation can be caused by a retroperitoneal hematoma, pelvic fracture, or direct peritoneal trauma.

DIAGNOSTIC PROCEDURES

Three diagnostic studies are used to evaluate the injured abdomen. These studies are diagnostic peritoneal lavage (DPL), ultrasound scan (focused abdominal sonogram for trauma), and computerized axial tomographic (CT) scan.[1,7,19,20,30,34-38]

Diagnostic peritoneal lavage was the standard method used to evaluate abdominal trauma for decades. However, the advent of newer, more accurate, and less invasive technologies has made this procedure less commonly used than it once was. The American College of Surgeons Committee on Trauma recommends that a DPL be performed in a patient with an unstable condition if the abdominal examination results are suggestive of injury or unreliable.[1,2,19]

Focused abdominal sonogram for trauma (FAST) is generally used for torso evaluation of patients with multiple traumas.[28] The FAST examination is rapid and noninvasive but needs to be performed by qualified persons. It also can be distorted by bowel, gas, and subcutaneous air. It does not detect all abdominal injuries. Because intraabdominal injury cannot be totally ruled out with negative FAST results, especially in unstable conditions, a computed tomographic (CT) scan of the abdomen should be performed.[7,28]

Computed tomography of the abdomen for both adults and children offers both high specificity and sensitivity to the detection and location of abdominal injury. CT scan is effective in demonstrating solid viscous injuries such as spleen or liver lacerations, the presence and quantity of hemoperitoneum, and retroperitoneal injuries such as renal lacerations or hematomas associated with pelvic fractures. The CT scan has been helpful in decreasing the number of unnecessary laparotomies.[15,24,28]

Use of Ultrasound Scan Before and During Transport

In the past, several factors presented challenges to the use of ultrasound technology in the field. These factors included the size of the machine, the fragility of ultrasound probes, and the skills of those performing the tests. However, the availability of new technology has made it possible to use ultrasound in the transport environment.[30,36,38,43] Price, Wilson, and Murphy,[43] Mazur et al,[36] Melanson et al,[38] and Knobloch[30] have all looked at the advantages and disadvantages of performing a FAST examination before and during transport. Advantages include early identification of intraabdominal free fluid in the prehospital environment, which can contribute to rapid diagnosing of potentially life-threatening abdominal injuries and assure that the patient is transported to the most appropriate center for care. Another use of ultrasound scan in the prehospital environment is the evaluation of the ventricular situation before and after CPR, which could prevent the unnecessary transport of a dead patient.[30]

The disadvantages of the use of ultrasound scan in the transport environment have included the limited ability of transport team members to adequately perform the examination, the small size of the screen, the brightness of the screen, the cramped space within the aircraft and limited flight times, and the overall fragility of the equipment.[38] As technology continues to develop, a FAST examination before or during transport may become a useful assessment tool for the patient with abdominal trauma.

PATIENT ASSESSMENT, TREATMENT, AND TRANSPORT

In many cases, injury is not limited to the abdomen, particularly in patients with blunt abdominal trauma. Once the primary assessment is completed and critical interventions initiated, the secondary examination should be done for determination of any other injuries.

In addition to the usual airway and breathing assessment and management, signs and symptoms of cardiovascular system collapse, such as hypotension, delayed capillary refill, and decreased level of consciousness, are important indicators of abdominal injuries. Patients with visceral injuries have the potential for sudden onset of severe hypovolemic shock because of the vascular nature of many organs in the abdominal cavity and the space for occult blood accumulation. Rapid recognition of the possibility of major abdominal injury and rapid transport after the initiation of critical interventions should be the goal when a patient is in hemorrhagic shock or has impending exsanguination.

Patients in severe shock or near exsanguination exhibit a decreasing level of consciousness as hypoxia increases and pale to mottled skin that is cold, clammy, and possibly profusely diaphoretic (Box 18-1). Mucous

---

BOX 18-1   Symptoms of Shock

Decreasing consciousness
Pale-to-mottled skin that is cold, clammy, and possibly diaphoretic
Pasty white mucous membranes
Delayed or absent capillary refill
Distended and rigid abdomen with no bowel sounds
Potential shortness of breath and tachypnea
Tachycardia and hypotension
Unobtainable blood pressure reading
Blood pressure that does not respond to fluid administration
Reports of severe abdominal pain

---

membranes may be pasty white, and capillary refill is delayed or absent. When no obvious external bleeding is present, the transport nurse should examine the abdomen. If the abdomen is distended and rigid with no bowel sounds, the transport team member should suspect intraabdominal bleeding. The conscious patient reports severe abdominal pain. If the abdomen is tautly distended, pressure is exerted on the diaphragm, causing potential shortness of breath and tachypnea. The patient is tachycardic and hypotensive; a blood pressure reading may not be obtainable even with a weak brachial pulse. If the blood pressure does not respond to fluid administration, exsanguination is a real possibility. The survival of a patient who is exsanguinating may depend on the amount of time it takes for transport to definitive care. Not all patients with abdominal injuries display all the symptoms described previously. Varying degrees of these symptoms, such as abdominal tenderness without initial distention, decreased but not absent bowel sounds, and tachycardia without hypotension, should alert the transport team to the possibility of exsanguination.

Initial management at the scene when transport time should be short should consist of airway management, 100% oxygen delivery, and spinal protection. For the patient with an abdominal injury, fluid resuscitation should be initiated. This should be done while constantly monitoring the patient during transport. In addition to crystalloids, blood and blood products may need to be administered. The likelihood of significant intraabdominal injury is high when a patient has hypotension in the field, a major chest injury, or pelvic fracture.

Interfacility transfers may increase the patient transport time. Patient management should include all the treatment instituted for the short-scene-call transport. In addition, a gastric tube should be inserted for suspected intestinal injury, gastric distention, or aspiration. If massive external or internal hemorrhage is occurring, the referring hospital may have type-specific or O negative blood infusing or ready to send with the patient. If the report before transport indicates hypovolemic shock, the transport team should request that the referring hospital have blood ready for transport on the patient's arrival or obtain blood products for use during the transport. For some patients, blood transfusion before arrival at the level I trauma center can be the factor that decreases morbidity and mortality. Hypothermia caused by massive intravenous fluid resuscitation can have a negative influence on patient outcome; therefore, warming of intravenous fluids for the administration of many liters of fluid, or at least use of fluids from an emergency department instead of cold fluids in the transport vehicle, can be important. The goals of transport are initiation of critical interventions and rapid transport to the nearest facility capable of treating the injured patient.[5,6,14,29,32,40,45]

SPECIFIC ABDOMINAL ORGAN INJURIES

DIAPHRAGM
Incidence and Mechanism of Injury
Blunt injury to the diaphragm, resulting in rupture or partial tear, occurs when a tremendous force is applied to the abdomen. The left diaphragm is injured more often than the right because the liver absorbs the impact of the force on the right side. If a right-sided tear has occurred, liver injury will probably accompany it. Spleen injuries often occur with left-sided diaphragmatic trauma.[1,2,15,19,20] Diaphragmatic tears can occur without herniation of the bowel into the chest cavity. If an intestinal herniation into the pleural space does occur, intestinal strangulation may develop. A penetrating injury of the diaphragm should be suspected when a knife wound occurs at or below the nipple line anteriorly or at the inferior border of the scapula posteriorly.[2,50]

Assessment and Symptoms
The transport team may not be able to diagnose a diaphragmatic tear that has not resulted in bowel herniation. Further diagnostic procedures may be necessary to ascertain a diaphragmatic tear. Physical examination of the patient with a diaphragmatic hernia may reveal absent or reduced breath sounds on the affected side. Bowel sounds may be heard in the chest cavity when intestinal contents have herniated into the pleural space. Respiratory distress may accompany intestinal herniation. If stomach contents are returned when a needle thoracostomy is performed for a believed tension pneumothorax, diaphragmatic hernia should be suspected. Chest radiographic results may indicate intestinal herniation with the presence of stomach contents or a curled gastric tube in the chest cavity. Diaphragm injuries missed on diagnostic examination may result in intestinal incarceration or strangulation that occurs weeks to months later. Associated mortality rates are high.[2]

Treatment
Specific treatment for a known or suspected diaphragmatic tear with possible herniation should focus on airway management, oxygenation, and ventilation because of the potentially decreased lung capacity. Intubation and ventilation should be done when respiratory failure occurs. A gastric tube inserted for transport reduces the possibility of aspiration and gastric dilation, especially for patients with herniation.

LIVER AND SPLEEN
Incidence and Mechanism
The spleen is the most commonly injured organ in blunt abdominal trauma; the liver is second. These organs are frequently injured at the same time. In both spleen and liver trauma, early deaths are the result of hemorrhage or other injuries; late deaths result from infection. The mortality rate for liver injuries is 13%, with a higher percentage of deaths occurring from penetrating injury.[21,22] Penetrating injuries that occur below the nipple level of the thorax or in the upper abdominal cavities may involve the liver or spleen.

The mechanism of injury for liver trauma is direct trauma to the liver itself, which causes fractures in the organ, or deceleration forces that may avulse hepatic veins from the inferior vena cava and diaphragm attachments. Tears in the hepatic, arterial, and portal venous vessels from compressive or shearing forces can result in rapid bleeding. The biliary duct system and hepatic vasculature are injured more often in penetrating injuries of the liver than in blunt injuries.

Assessment and Symptoms

Patients with blunt and penetrating injuries can have symptoms that vary from slight tachycardia with abdominal guarding to profound shock and a distended taut abdomen when intraabdominal hemorrhage is occurring. A distended abdomen may indicate severe bleeding from either the liver or the spleen. When these patients are assessed, inspection and palpation of the abdomen should be done to locate contusions, abrasions, and pain. Other injuries, such as rib and scapula fractures, are associated with spleen and liver trauma. The amount of force involved in blunt abdominal injuries and the mechanism of injury and location of wounds in penetrating trauma are important indicators of spleen and liver injury.

Subjective symptoms of spleen injury may be localized tenderness in the left upper quadrant. Referred shoulder pain (Kehr's sign) from left hemidiaphragm irritation can also be present but is rarely seen. Localized abdominal pain from liver injuries occurs in the right upper quadrant.

Treatment

Because exsanguination may be the cause of death immediately after the accident in spleen and liver trauma, specific treatment should focus on hemodynamic status. Relay of information to the trauma center when obvious intraabdominal hemorrhage is present can prepare the trauma team for immediate care of the patient.

PANCREAS AND DUODENUM
Incidence and Mechanism

Both the pancreas and duodenum lie within the retroperitoneal space; they are in intimate proximity to each other and usually are injured together. Both are well protected and constitute less than 3% to 12%

of all abdominal injuries.[2] Mortality and morbidity from pancreatic and duodenal injuries occur more frequently from secondary complications of infection, pseudocyst or fistula formation, gastrointestinal tract malfunction, and chronic pancreatitis. Injury in blunt trauma should be suspected when direct force is applied to the left upper quadrant, as in steering wheel and bicycle handlebar impalement. Injury is caused by compression of these organs against the vertebral column. Injuries to both the pancreas and duodenum occur more frequently from penetrating than from blunt trauma.

Assessment and Symptoms

Symptoms of isolated blunt pancreatic and duodenal injuries may be difficult to observe. If duodenal digestive juices and blood are contained within the retroperitoneal space, the patient may not have many abdominal symptoms. Assessment of the patient usually shows tenderness over the area of the pancreas and the absence of bowel sounds. The patient's condition may be hemodynamically stable, with symptoms associated only with peritonitis (such as abdominal tenderness or guarding) or no symptoms at all. These injuries are difficult to diagnose, but careful history taking can assist in identification.

Treatment

The transport treatment for these patients includes a high index of suspicion for injury when the patient has vague abdominal symptoms after trauma. Treatment should include any procedures necessary for patient stabilization and supportive care if the patient's respiratory and cardiovascular status remains stable. If duodenal injury is suspected, gastric tube insertion reduces the gastric and duodenal juice infiltration of the peritoneal space. Outlying hospitals may transfer these patients several days after injury when isolated pancreatic and duodenal symptoms occur.

COLON AND SMALL INTESTINE
Incidence and Mechanism

Colon and small intestine damage occurs more frequently in penetrating than in blunt injuries, and in most cases, the liver, spleen, and other organs are also injured.[2,15,19] Colon injuries are caused by penetrating missiles such as bullets or stabbings 90% of the time. The small intestine is the most commonly injured organ in penetrating injuries, presumably because of the volume it occupies in the abdomen.[1] Blunt injury to the small intestine occurs with crushing of the bowel against the spinal column. Improper use of the seat belt, steering wheel impact, or a blunt object applied to the abdomen can produce this crushing effect. If a victim has a transverse bruise across the lower abdomen from a lap belt, rupture of the small intestine should be considered.[19] Bowel evisceration may occur with penetrating trauma, and bowel contents should be covered with sterile saline solution during transfer.

Assessment and Symptoms

The same thorough assessment for abdominal trauma should be done in suspected cases of intestinal injury. The transport team should inspect the location of all entrance and exit wounds with penetrating trauma. Examination of the back, buttocks, and perineum is important because wounds to these areas are easily overlooked. Documentation of the locations of wounds should be as accurate as possible. Evisceration of the bowel may be found with penetrating injuries; the color and size of protruding bowel should be noted on the initial examination.

Symptoms of isolated colon injury are associated with peritoneal irritation from blood or feces free in the peritoneum. Pain on palpation with guarding may be present, and symptoms of fever and leukocytosis may increase with time elapsed since injury. Fecal material may be present in the peritoneal lavage fluid when colon disruption has occurred. Abdominal radiographs may reveal free air in the peritoneum or a loss of the psoas shadow.

Symptoms of small bowel injury include tenderness, patient reluctance to change positions, rebound tenderness, and guarding. In small intestinal injuries, peritoneal lavage may show turbid or bile-stained fluid, an elevated white blood cell count, or presence of amylase. Radiographic films may reveal free air in the peritoneum or a small bowel ileus.

Treatment

Because most injuries of the intestine are associated with other more immediate life-threatening injuries, transport management should be prioritized accordingly. While airway and cardiovascular systems are being stabilized, saline solution dressings should be applied to any eviscerated bowel or dry dressings to any open wounds. The amount of blood loss at the scene should be noted. Most complications of bowel injuries occur later in the patient's course of recovery. The major factors related to morbidity and mortality are sepsis, abscess formation, wound infection, and intraabdominal peritonitis.

Gastric and Esophageal Trauma
Incidence and Mechanism

Gastric and esophageal injuries are uncommon because the esophagus and stomach are well protected within the upper abdominal cavity. The abdominal esophagus is 2 to 4 cm long and lies within the retroperitoneal space, anterior to the aorta. The pliability of the stomach reduces its chances of injury in blunt trauma, although a full stomach is more likely to rupture. Most esophageal and gastric injuries are caused by penetrating trauma.

Assessment and Symptoms

Symptoms of gastric and esophageal trauma are signs of peritoneal irritation, such as pain and guarding. Gastric tube drainage may show evidence of blood, which may indicate a gastric rupture in the absence of other obvious sources of bleeding, such as facial trauma, in which the patient may have swallowed blood. Review of the abdominal radiographs at the referring hospital may show free air in the peritoneum, indicating disruption of the intestinal tract, which may involve the esophagus, stomach, or both.

Treatment

Diagnosis of gastric and esophageal trauma injuries most likely is confirmed after arrival at the trauma center. Transport treatment of these patients is similar to that of any other trauma patient with life-threatening injuries. If a gastric rupture is suspected, a nasogastric tube should be carefully inserted for long transports. Time of last food consumption can be useful information to the trauma surgeon, especially in an unconscious patient.

ABDOMINAL VASCULAR INJURIES
Incidence and Mechanism

Injuries to the abdominal arterial and venous systems occur more frequently with penetrating trauma than with blunt trauma. A 5-year retrospective study of 530 MVC fatalities revealed that aortic injuries occurred in 18% of victims. The typical victim was a male driver with an elevated blood alcohol level who was involved in a head-on collision.[2,18,25,45,48,49] Compression or deceleration forces applied to the abdomen can result in avulsion of small vessels from the larger vessels from which they branch, and intimal tears within the vessel itself may occur. Intimal tears can result in thrombosis formation, whereas vessel avulsion tears can result in exsanguination. Penetrating injuries of vascular tissue cause lacerations and free bleeding. The major vessels frequently injured are the aorta; the inferior vena cava; and the renal, mesenteric, and iliac arteries and veins. Vascular system injury is the primary cause of death in patients with GSWs and stab wounds to the abdomen. Mortality rates are high, even when patients are not in shock at presentation.[18,25]

Assessment and Symptoms

A patient with no obvious active external bleeding source who has severe shock shortly after injury probably has arterial injury. Bleeding is profuse, and rapid fluid replacement may not maintain blood pressure and tissue perfusion when intraabdominal arterial lacerations are present. Patients with abdominal vascular injuries may present as or become the exsanguinating patient described previously, depending on the degree of intraabdominal bleeding and the time elapsed since injury occurred. With arterial injuries, the femoral pulse on the affected side may be absent. Major abdominal vein injuries can also produce profound shock, but shock may occur up to 30 minutes after the injury instead of immediately after. Bleeding from venous injuries may be controlled with direct pressure of the abdominal organs or abdominal pressure itself, limiting the possibility of early exsanguination.

Treatment

With abdominal vascular injuries, when exsanguination is imminent, rapid transport to a level I trauma center is critical to patient survival.

Complications after survival of the initial abdominal vascular injury include continued bleeding from vascular reconstruction areas or disseminated intravascular coagulation that develops from massive blood transfusions, liver ischemia, or profound shock. Thrombosis formation can occur and cause tissue ischemia to the kidneys or gastrointestinal tract. When renal or visceral veins are involved, pulmonary embolism can develop.

GENITOURINARY TRAUMA

Genitourinary trauma includes injuries to the kidney, bladder, ureters, urethra, and genitalia and is not usually immediately life threatening, as are the abdominal injuries previously discussed. Because of the position of the urinary and reproductive system within the abdominal cavity, a high index of suspicion for trauma in the genitourinary organs should be maintained when regions of the abdomen and back are injured.

RENAL AND URETER TRAUMA
Incidence and Mechanism

Renal trauma is frequently associated with abdominal injury; the kidney is the third most commonly injured abdominal organ.[1,8,16] Injuries sustained from blunt mechanisms such as MVCs, falls, contact sports, and assaults account for 70% to 80% of all renal trauma, and 5% of patients may eventually lose renal function.[19] Blunt injuries sustained from sudden acceleration or deceleration result in the stretching of the ureters and renal arteries and veins with the weight of the kidney. Contusions are generally from a direct blow to the flank. Of all renal and ureter blunt traumas, 85% are minor contusions; the remaining 15% consist of renal vascular injury, deep cortical lacerations, or shattered kidneys.[16,27]

Penetrating injuries are usually caused by GSWs or stabbings to the back or abdomen, with an 80% incidence rate of associated injury in other abdominal organs.[1,2,8,16] Low-velocity bullet injuries are more common than high-velocity bullet injuries (79% versus 8%); the damage is typically parenchymal laceration. Often, a high-velocity GSW injury results in nephrectomy because the kidney explodes from the impact or passage of the bullet.[1,16,35]

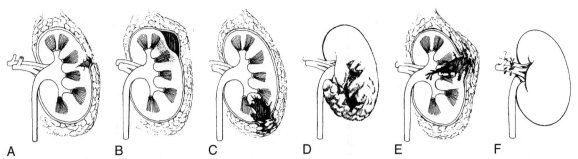

FIGURE 18-2   Renal injuries classified by severity. A and **B,** Minor injuries. **C, D, E,** and **F,** Major injuries. (Modified from Blaisdell W, Trunkey D, McAninch J: *Trauma management,* vol 2, New York, 1982, Thieme.)

Most renal injuries (80% to 85%) are minor and consist of contusions and minor lacerations; 10% are major and extend into the medulla, collecting system, or both, with the possible result of extravasation of urine (Figure 18-2). Vascular injuries occur in 1% to 3% of renal injuries, and retroperitoneal hematoma formation is likely.[8,39]

Ureteral injury, although rare, is generally a result of penetrating trauma such as GSWs or stab wounds. Rapid deceleration accidents may avulse the ureter from the renal pelvis.[2,31,33,46]

Assessment and Symptoms

On secondary assessment, any contusions, abrasions, or stab penetrations to the back and flank area should alert the transport nurse to the possibility of renal trauma. The patient may have flank pain. Kidney damage should always be suspected with gunshot injuries to the abdomen. Hematuria is a marker for both renal and extrarenal abdominal injuries after blunt trauma. All patients with gross hematuria should be evaluated after transfer for both renal and associated abdominal injuries. In addition, patients in shock or with a history of shock and microscopic hematuria after blunt trauma should also be suspected of abdominal injuries. Studies show that patients with microscopic hematuria but no shock do not have any major renal injury and are treated successfully without surgical intervention.[21]

Treatment

Because renal injuries are not immediately life threatening, the transport team should give supportive care and identify the patient's risk for kidney injury when other life-threatening injuries are absent. If a urinary catheter is in place, the transport team should transport with gravity drainage and monitor urine output. Ureter injury will probably not be diagnosed until full evaluation is completed at the trauma center; therefore, no specific intervention exists for air transport. At the receiving hospital, surgery may be indicated for major kidney injuries, ureteral tears, or renal vascular damage, although current literature indicates that the trend in treatment is toward nonsurgical management.[2,16]

BLADDER AND URETHRAL TRAUMA
Incidence and Mechanism

Blunt trauma to the bladder is most commonly associated with pelvic fractures (90% of cases of bladder rupture have associated pelvic fractures). Because the bladder lies within the pelvic girdle, bone fragments from the pelvis can penetrate the bladder. Rupture can also occur when a direct blow to the lower abdomen occurs with a distended bladder. Rupture can cause extravasation of urine into the peritoneal cavity. If diagnosis is not established immediately and the urine is sterile, no symptoms may be noted for several days; if the urine is infected, immediate peritonitis and acute abdominal pain develop.[16]

Urethral injuries are associated with bladder rupture and pelvic fractures and occur more often in men than in women. Shearing forces at the level of the prostate gland usually cause the most severe urethral damage during pelvic fracture; the urethra may be torn near the prostate gland. Straddle injuries caused by bicycle, horse-riding, or gymnastic accidents and direct penetrating trauma may cause injuries to the lower or more external urethra.

Assessment and Symptoms

Identification of patients at risk is the best way for the transport team to determine bladder and urethral injuries in the field. Subjective symptoms in common with both bladder and urethral injuries are lower abdominal pain, groin tenderness, and inability to void. Hematuria most likely is present with bladder trauma. Shock in these patients is usually associated with other visceral or vascular injuries. Blood at the urethral meatus is the single most important sign of urethral injury.

Treatment

Transport treatment of patients with bladder and urethral injuries should emphasize a high index of suspicion for their injuries; life-threatening injuries should take priority. A urinary catheter should not be inserted when blood is found in the urethral meatus. With a urethral tear, further damage can occur if a catheter is improperly inserted, although a prolonged transport time and a distended painful bladder are indications for careful controlled insertion of a urinary catheter in these patients. Autonomic hyperreflexia is a serious complication of a prolonged distended bladder that causes hypertension, bradycardia, and increased intracranial pressure.[19] The transport team should keep these symptoms in mind when transporting a patient with a diagnosed urethral tear and inability to void. When a ruptured bladder is suspected or diagnosed, transport should be accomplished without delay. The diagnosis is confirmed at the trauma center with retrograde cystography in bladder trauma or retrograde urethrography in the urethral injury.

GENITAL TRAUMA
Incidence and Mechanism

Genital trauma is more common in men than in women. The female reproductive tract is well protected within the pelvic bony structure; consequently, injuries are infrequent with either blunt or penetrating trauma. Bone fragments from a pelvic fracture may pierce the uterus, vagina, or other female organs. Injuries to the exterior female perineum from straddle accidents can result in hematoma formation. In men, penetrating trauma to the penis or scrotum is most often caused by a GSW. Urethral disruption may accompany these injuries. Other causes of blunt injury are MVCs, industrial accidents, and assault. Of scrotal injuries, 50% are caused by blunt trauma, and patients usually have contusions, hematomas, avulsions, lacerations, or testicular rupture at presentation.[16]

Assessment and Symptoms

Assessment of the patient with genital injuries includes a thorough history and a visual inspection. Respect for dignity should always be maintained. Reports of the event may be embarrassing for the patient, and the transport nurse must be careful to listen without judgment, although discrepancies between history and mechanism of injury should be noted. On physical examination, the transport team should visually inspect the perineal area for hematoma formation anywhere on the perineum, scrotum, or penis. If the scrotum is swollen and painful, ruptured testes should be suspected. Rectal injury can also be identified when the perineal area is examined, and the transport nurse should look for any obvious trauma and document any lacerations or avulsions, including the presence and amount of vaginal bleeding. Menstrual history is important for female patients if they are able to provide that information.

Treatment

Unless bleeding is profuse, injuries to the genitals are not immediately life threatening. Treatment for transport should consist of saline solution dressings to avulsions and lacerations, particularly those to the scrotum. Ice packs to both scrotum and penile hematomas help reduce swelling and pain; direct pressure should be applied to the areas of penile injury. In the case of penile or scrotum amputation, the parts should be transported in saline solution dressings on ice, and the transport team should ensure that the tissue is not in direct contact with the ice, which could cause further tissue damage.

Vaginal bleeding is difficult to control, and pressure dressings should be applied if possible. Exsanguination can occur with major vaginal tears because of the rich blood supply. When severe bleeding and shock are present, rapid transport to the nearest facility capable of treating gynecologic injuries should be the first priority. If objects are impaled in the genitalia, they should be left in place and immobilized.[19] The success rate of repair to genital injuries is high, and even penile reimplantation has been successful with microvascular surgery.[1,19,35]

SUMMARY

The initial treatment for all patients with suspected abdominal and genitourinary injuries from either blunt or penetrating trauma should include all procedures done for any injured patient.

Exsanguination, one of the major causes of death in trauma victims, can take place quickly with an abdominal injury because of the vascular nature of the abdominal organs and the large peritoneal space for blood accumulation. Calculation of the amount of lost blood is difficult in abdominal trauma patients because the abdomen can sequester large volumes of blood before signs of abdominal distention occur. The primary duties of the transport team when transporting patients with abdominal trauma should be recognizing and arresting profound shock and exsanguination by decreasing the blood loss from the intravascular space, replacing circulatory volume, and maintaining tissue perfusion.

Rapid transport reduces the time from injury to definitive treatment. Alerting the trauma center of the patient's condition through radio contact can provide the trauma team with valuable information, which also reduces delay of treatment of specific life-threatening injuries, thereby increasing the patient's chances of survival.

The primary role of the transport team in the management of the patient with abdominal trauma is to identify and manage any life-threatening conditions and to provide rapid transport to the appropriate facility where the patient will receive definitive care.

ABDOMINAL AND GENITOURINARY TRAUMA CASE STUDY

An air medical team was requested to respond to a rural county hospital for a farm tractor rollover; flight time was 20 minutes. En route, the faculty physician at the receiving facility relayed the following information to the transport team.

Mr. R. is a 75-year-old man who was found by his wife trapped under an overturned tractor for an unknown amount of time. She estimated the time to be approximately 6 hours based on when she had last seen him. Basic emergency medical services (EMS) responded to the scene, immobilized the patient, and transported him to the closest hospital, which was 10 minutes from the scene of the accident. The referring hospital reports that he has a patent airway and is on 100% oxygen via mask, with equal clear breath sounds, blood pressure (BP) of 100/70 mmHg, heart rate (HR) of 120 bpm, and respiratory rate (RR) of 28 bpm. He has severe abdominal pain.

On arrival at the referring hospital, the transport team performed an assessment and found the following:

AIRWAY

The airway was clear and patent. A nonrebreather mask was in place delivering 100% oxygen. A cervical collar with head blocks was in place.

BREATHING

Respirations were medium depth, equal expansion, and unlabored, with bilateral clear breath sounds and a respiratory rate of 28 bpm. Oxygen saturation of 95% was noted. No palpable deformities, crepitus, or subcutaneous air to the chest was found.

CIRCULATION

The patient's radial pulse was weak at a rate of 120 bpm, and he had a blood pressure of 80/64 mm Hg. His skin was pale, cool, and dry with a capillary refill of 2 seconds. The cardiac monitor showed sinus tachycardia.

NEUROLOGIC

Mental status remained unchanged with a Glasgow Coma Scale (GCS) of 15 and PERL; the patient was moving all extremities, although he had limited movement of his left leg. Patient denied any numbness or tingling.

SECONDARY ASSESSMENT

Abdomen

Abdomen was distended but soft. There was pain with palpation in the abdomen over both the right and left upper quadrants. Patient had severe pain with any movement of his pelvis. A large bluish area was found over the left flank area (Grey-Turner's sign). A urinary catheter had drained 25 mL of dark yellow urine, and a gastric tube was draining dark brown liquid. No bowel sounds were auscultated.

Extremities

Patient had left shoulder pain, but no deformities were palpated on either upper extremity. An open left tibia/fibula had been immobilized with a splint by the local EMS. Weak peripheral pulses were palpated in both lower extremities.

HISTORY

History of the Event

As previously described.

Medical History

Lopressor for treatment of angina.

DIAGNOSTIC INFORMATION

A second line was started, and a fluid bolus of 1 L of normal saline solution was begun.

Radiographs

C-spine visualized to C6.

Chest radiographic results reported as normal.

Pelvic radiographic results showed a left pelvic fracture with separation of the sacroiliac joint.

Left leg radiographic results showed a shattered tibia/fibula.

INTERVENTIONS

While preparing the patient for transport, a second intravenous line was started and a fluid bolus initiated. The patient was also allowed to see and talk with his family before leaving the emergency department.

TRANSPORT

During transport, Mr. R. lost his radial pulses and became agitated and confused. His skin was clammy. Despite receiving 2 L of crystalloids, his blood pressure dropped to 64/48 mm Hg. His heart rate continued at 120 bpm and above. His abdomen appeared more distended and became firm. Two units of O negative blood were infused, and the trauma center was notified of the patient's deteriorating condition.

On arrival at the trauma center, the patient was hot off loaded and taken directly to the Shock Resuscitation Unit. The trauma team performed a FAST examination that revealed fluid. The patient was taken to the operating room for immediate repair of his injuries, which included a lacerated spleen and liver, a pelvic fracture, and a left tibia/fibula fracture.

Recovery in the Surgical Intensive Care Unit (SICU) was tenuous with disseminated intravascular coagulation (DIC) and two episodes of angina occurring. After 3 weeks, he was transferred to the surgical step-down. After an additional uneventful 3 weeks in the hospital, Mr. R. was discharged home.

REFERENCES

1. Air and Surface Transport Nurses Association (ASTNA): *Transport nurse advanced trauma course (TNATC)*, Denver, 2006, ASTNA.
2. American College of Surgeons Committee on Trauma: *Advanced trauma life support program for doctors*, ed 8, Chicago, 2008, American College of Surgeons.
3. Anderson S, Day M, Chen M, et al: Traumatic aortic injuries in the pediatric population, *J Pediatr Surg* 43:1077-1081, 2008.

4. Augenstein JS, et al: Occult abdominal injuries to air-bag protected crash victims: a challenge to trauma systems, *J Trauma* 38:502, 1995.

5. Bicknell W, Pepe P, Bailey M, et al: Randomized trial of pneumatic antishock garments in the prehospital management of penetrating abdominal injuries, *Ann Emerg Med* 16(6):653-658, 1987.

6. Bickell W, et al: Immediate versus delayed fluid resuscitation for hypotensive patients with penetrating torso injuries, *N Engl J Med* 331(17):1105, 1994.

7. Bixby S, Callahan M, Taylor G: Imaging in pediatric blunt abdominal trauma, *Semin Roentgenol* 72-82, 2007.

8. Blaisdell W, Trunkey D, McAninch J: *Trauma management, urogenital trauma,* vol 2, New York, 1985, Thieme-Stratton, Thieme Verlag.

9. Blank-Reid C: A historical review of penetrating abdominal trauma, *Crit Care Nurs Clin North Am* 18:387-401, 2006.

10. Bourn M, Bourn S: Genitourinary emergencies: a prehospital perspective, *Emerg Med Clin North Am* 6:379, 1988.

11. Boyd CR, Tolson MA: Mechanisms of abdominal trauma: implications for initial care, *Emerg Care Q* 10:22, 1988.

12. Boyd CR, et al: Penetrating abdominal trauma and the basics of ballistics, *J Air Med Transport* 6:6, 1991.

13. Buckman RF, et al: Major bowel and diaphragmatic injuries associated with blunt spleen or liver rupture, *J Trauma* 28:1317, 1988.

14. Busani S, Cavazzuti C, Pasetto A, et al: Strategies to control massive abdominal bleeding, *Transplantation Proc* 40:1212-1215, 2008.

15. Campbell J: *International trauma life support,* ed 6, Upper Saddle River, NJ, 2008, Pearson/Prentice Hall.

16. Cutinha P: Genitourinary trauma, *Surg Med* 276-280. 2002.

17. Deree J, Shenvi E, Fortlage D, et al: Patient factors and operation room resuscitation predict mortality in traumatic aortic injury: a 20-year analysis, *J Vasc Surg* 45(3):493-497, 2007.

18. Eachempati S, Robb T, Inatury R, et al: Factors associated with mortality in patients with penetrating abdominal vascular trauma, *J Surg Res* 108:222-226, 2002.

19. Emergency Nurses Association: *Trauma nursing core course,* ed 7, Des Plaines, IL, 2007, ENA.

20. Eren S, Kantarci M, Okur A: Imaging of diaphragmatic rupture after trauma, *Clin Radiol* 61:467-477, 2006.

21. Feliciano DV, Marx JA, Sclafani SJA: Abdominal trauma, *Patient Care* 26:44, 1992.

22. Feliciano DV, Rozycki GS: The management of penetrating abdominal trauma, *Adv Surg* 28:1, 1995.

23. Fisher RB, Dearden CH: Improving care of patients with major trauma in the accident and emergency department, *BMJ* 300:1560, 1990.

24. Freshman SP, et al: Secondary survey following blunt trauma: a new role for CT scan, *J Trauma* 34:337, 1993.

25. Garner J: Blunt and penetrating trauma to the abdomen, *Emerg Surg* 223-228, 2005.

26. Goins WA, Anderson BB: Abdominal trauma revisited, *J Natl Med Assoc* 83:883, 1991.

27. Guerriero WG: Etiology, classification, and management of renal trauma, *Surg Clin North Am* 68:1071, 1988.

28. Isenhour J, Marx J: Advances in abdominal trauma, *Emerg Clin North Am* 25:713-733, 2007.

29. Jacobs L: Timing of fluid resuscitation in trauma, *N Engl J Med* 331(17):1153, 1994.

30. Knobloch K: Letter to the editor related to the use of ultrasound in the preclinical environment, *Air Med J* 27(4):152-153, 2008.

31. Knudson MM, et al: Hematuria, as a predictor of abdominal injury after blunt trauma, *Am J Surg* 164:482, 1992.

32. Leicht MJ, et al: Rural interhospital helicopter transport of motor vehicle trauma victims: causes for delays and recommendations, *Ann Emerg Med* 15:450, 1986.

33. Lowe MA, et al: Risk factors for urethral injuries in men with traumatic pelvic fractures, *J Urol* 140:506, 1988.

34. Lucciarini P, et al: Ultrasonography in the initial evaluation and follow-up of blunt abdominal injury, *Surgery* 114:506, 1993.

35. Maull KI, et al: Retroperitoneal injuries: pitfalls in diagnosis and management, *South Med J* 80:1111, 1987.

36. Mazur S, Pearce A, Alfred S, et al: The F.A.S.T.E.R. trial: focused assessment by sonography in trauma during emergency retrieval: a feasibility study, *Injury* 39: 512-518, 2008.

37. McKennay M, et al: Can ultrasound replace diagnostic peritoneal lavage in the assessment of blunt trauma? *J Trauma* 37:439, 1994.

38. Melanson S, McCarthy J, Stromski C, et al: Aeromedical trauma sonography by transport teams with a miniature ultrasound unit, *Prehosp Emerg Care* 5(4): 399-402, 2001.

39. Monstrey SJM, et al: Renal trauma and hypertension, *J Trauma* 29:65, 1989.

40. Moylan JA: Impact of helicopters on trauma care and clinical results, *Ann Surg* 28:139, 1988.

41. O'Connell KJ, et al: Comparison of low- and high-velocity ballistic trauma to genitourinary organs, *J Trauma* 28:139, 1988.

42. Phillips GR, Kauder DR, Schwab CW: Massive blood loss in trauma patients, *Postgrad Med* 95:61, 1994.

43. Price D, Wilson S, Murphy T: Trauma ultrasound feasibility during helicopter transport, *Air Med J* 19(4): 144-146, 2000.

44. Rutledge R, et al: The cost of not wearing seat belts: a comparison outcome in 3396 patients, *Ann Surg* 217:122, 1993.

45. Shorr RM, et al: Selective management of abdominal stab wounds: importance of the physical examination, *Arch Surg* 16:1141, 1988.

46. Spirnak JP: Pelvic fracture and injury to the lower urinary tract, *Surg Clin North Am* 68:1057, 1988.

47. Wachtel TL: Critical care concepts in the management of abdominal trauma, *Crit Care Nurs Q* 17:34, 1994.

48. Weesner CL, et al: Fatal childhood injury patterns in an urban setting, *Ann Emerg Med* 23:231, 1994.

49. Williams JS, et al: Aortic injury in vehicular trauma, *Ann Thorac Surg* 57:726, 1994.

50. Worthy SA, et al: Diaphragmatic rupture: CT findings in eleven patients, *Radiology* 194:885, 1995.

Reneé Semonin Holleran

COMPETENCIES

1. Perform an assessment of an injured extremity before and during transport.
2. Appropriately apply the immobilization device needed for patient transport.
3. Identify and treat potential complications related to musculoskeletal emergencies.

A simple fracture or dislocation can become a devastating injury and result in severe permanent disability. Even a moderate sprain, if inadequately treated, can result in an unnecessarily extended disability and can lead to recurrent injuries.

The hands of a pianist, the elbow of a pitcher, the legs of a dancer are all vital to each of these people. Although musculoskeletal injuries are rarely fatal, they often result in long-term disability that accounts for millions of dollars lost to the economy each year.[14] The first care provided to a patient with a fracture, dislocation, or severe sprain often determines the ultimate results that occur as a consequence of the injury.[8] The transport team can often prevent permanent disability with a prompt temporary measure, such as immobilization or splinting, especially in patients with multiple traumas when more definitive management must be postponed until life-threatening injuries have been taken care of adequately.

MUSCULOSKELETAL SYSTEM

A basic understanding of the composition and function of the musculoskeletal system is essential to proper management of orthopedic emergencies and ultimately to the welfare of the patient as a whole. The *musculoskeletal system* is composed of bones, ligaments, muscles, joints, tendons, blood vessels, and nerves. The function of the musculoskeletal system is to allow movement, provide support, and protect internal organs.[1-5]

Bone is a living structure with its own neurovascular innervation and capacity to heal. Bone is a specialized connective tissue with a calcified collagenous intercellular substance and is either cancellous or compact. The calcium content of bone depends on many factors such as parathyroid hormone and estrogen, dietary intake, and stress. An acid-base balance with a slight decrease in pH can cause bone demineralization.[1-5]

DEFINITION

An *orthopedic injury,* a trauma to the axial skeleton, is rarely considered an emergency. However, it does require urgent care. In terms of orthopedic involvement with underlying organs, emergencies can exist. An example is the fracture or dislocation of the knee or elbow. These are extremely painful injuries, and they also can cause permanent damage to nerves and vessels distal to the injury if not taken care of immediately. Table 19-1 lists various orthopedic injuries with possible complications.

CLASSIFICATION OF ORTHOPEDIC INJURIES

When force is applied to a limb, the energy of the impact dissipates to deform supporting structures. An excessive amount of force may damage more than one structure in the line of force.[6,11] This type of stress to the axial skeleton and its supporting structures can cause various types of injuries, including fractures, dislocations, sprains, tendon injuries, and strains.

FRACTURES

A *fracture* is defined as any break in the continuity of the bone or cartilage, and it may be either complete or incomplete, depending on the line of fracture through the bone.[1-5] Fractures generally are classified as closed or open. If the skin is unbroken, the fracture is technically *closed,* regardless of the number of fractures; if the skin is broken, the fracture is *open,* although it may be simple and minor in nature. Any broken skin in the area of a fracture must be included in the report. An open fracture is more serious because of the risk of infection. Figure 19-1 illustrates nine different types of fractures as defined by radiographic appearance.

Fractures of the long bone may produce steady slow bleeding and can result in 750 mL of blood loss from the humerus or tibia and 1500 mL of blood from each femur.[1-5] These patients must be watched closely for shock, and the long bone fracture should be immobilized for comfort. Another risk associated with fractures, even uncomplicated ones, is that of fat embolism, which can cause varying degrees of respiratory distress, including respiratory failure. Signs and symptoms of fat embolism are petechial rash, diffuse pulmonary infiltrates, hypoxemia, confusion, fever, tachycardia, and tachypnea. Patients at highest risk of fat embolism are those with long bone fractures of the lower extremity.[1-5]

DISLOCATIONS

A *dislocation* is the displacement of the normal articulating ends of two or more bones. A *complete dislocation* causes a tearing of the ligaments. A dislocation may also be described as *compound* when the joint is exposed to the outside air. Joints that are frequently dislocated are shoulders, elbows, fingers, hips, and ankles. Less frequently seen are dislocated wrists or knees. A dislocation is referred to as *subluxated* when the displacement is incomplete.

TABLE 19-1	**Urgent Complications of Orthopedic Injuries**
Injury	**Possible Complications**
Clavicle fractures	Brachial plexus compression or damage; pneumothorax or hemothorax
Humerus fractures	Injury to brachial artery or radial nerve
Pelvic fractures	Injury to bladder, urethra, rectum
Distal femoral shaft fractures	Femoral or popliteal vessel injury
Proximal tibia fractures	Compression of the anterior tibial compartment; tibial nerve injury
Clavicular head dislocation	Compression of trachea, subclavian, and carotid arteries
Posterior elbow dislocation	Compression of brachial artery
Posterior hip dislocation	Aseptic necrosis of the femoral head and sciatic nerve damage
Knee dislocation	Compression of the popliteal vessel
Ankle dislocation	Compression of the pedal artery

From Perdue P: Abdominal injuries and dangerous fractures, *RN* 44(7):35,84, 1981.

TYPE OF FRACTURE	DEFINITION
Transverse 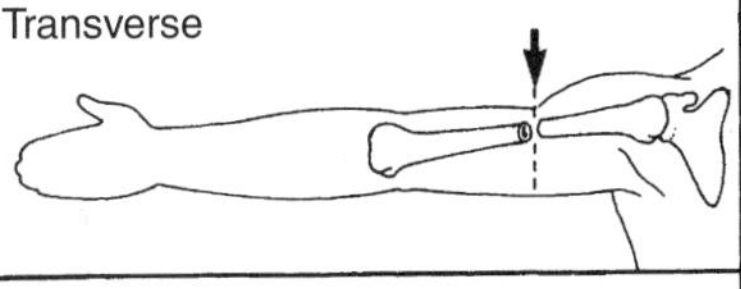	Usually produced by angulating force; once the fragments are aligned and immobilized, stability is ensured
Oblique 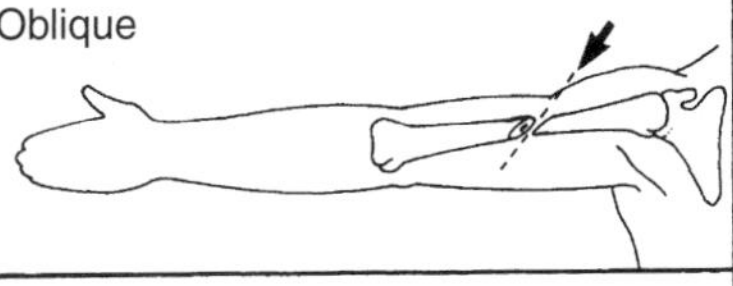	Fragments tend to slip by one another unless traction is maintained
Spiral 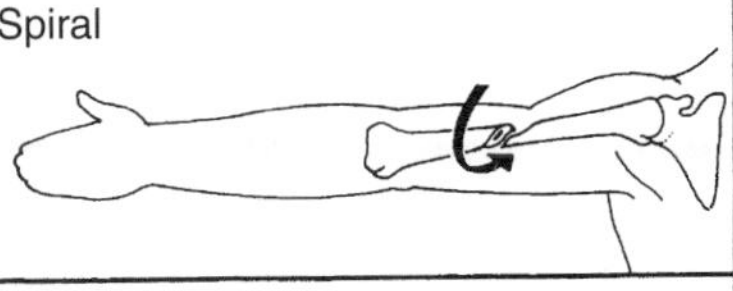	Produced by twisting or rotary force; reduction difficult to maintain
Greenstick 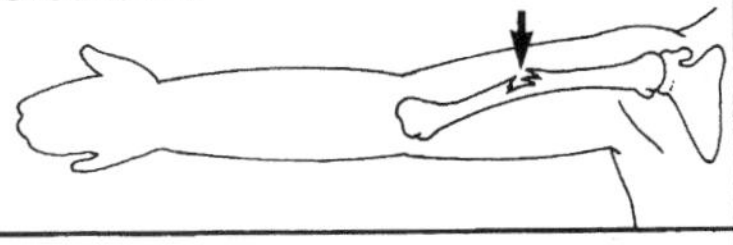	Caused by compression force in long axis of the bone; often seen in children under the age of 10
Compression 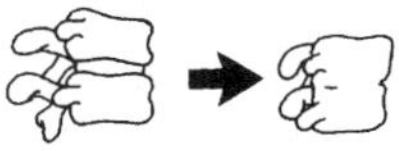	Usually produced by severe violence applied to cancellous bone, such as the spine
Comminuted 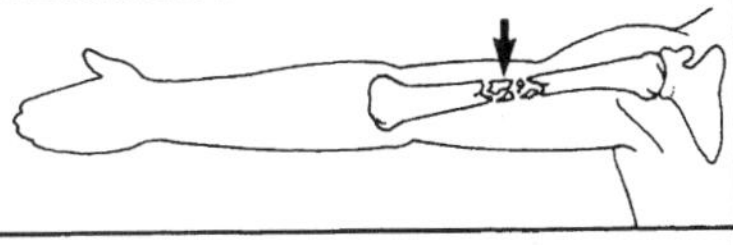	Always more than two fragments
Impacted 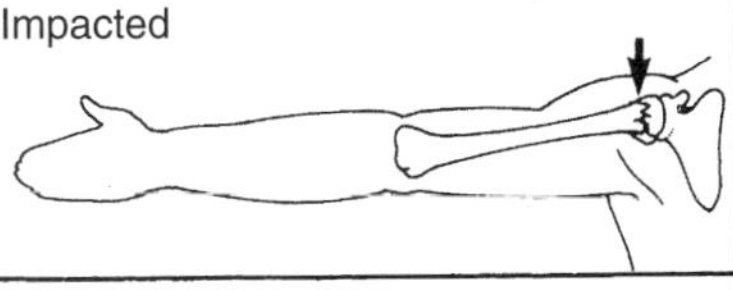	Produced by severe violence, driving bone fragments firmly together
Avulsion 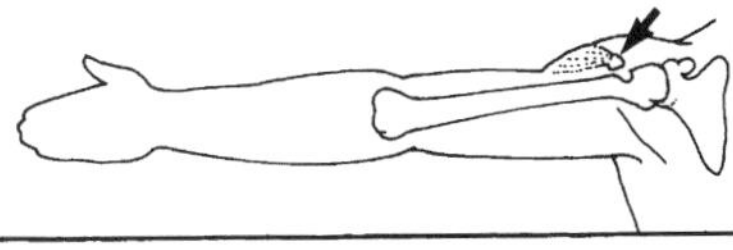	Produced by forcible contraction of a muscle, which pulls off a fragment of bone
Fracture dislocation 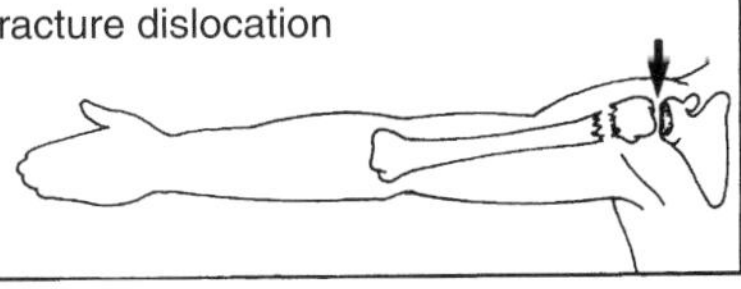	In addition to fracture there is a subluxation or dislocation of the joint

FIGURE 19-1   **Fractures according to radiographic appearance.**

MECHANISMS OF INJURY

Multiple mechanisms may cause injury to the musculoskeletal system, including motor vehicle collisions (one of the most common); falls, particularly to the elderly; sports, such as football and soccer; and routine activities, such as cleaning around the house. Either accelerating or decelerating forces may cause injury to bones, muscles, ligaments, and their surrounding nerves and blood vessels. An important point to remember is that when a force is applied to the musculoskeletal system and causes an injury, the surrounding tissue and organs may be injured along with the bones and muscles.[1,7,12,13]

ASSESSMENT OF AN ORTHOPEDIC INJURY

In patients with multiple trauma, musculoskeletal injuries are rarely life threatening. Thus, before assessing possible fractures, the nurse should evaluate for life-threatening injuries. The evaluation should begin with attention to airway, breathing, and circulation (the ABCDEs). Only when the patient has been fully evaluated and the condition is judged stable should an attempt be made to treat an injured limb. For adequate assessment data, a good history is important. This information can be obtained by talking to the first respondents on the scene or by reading the medical record. As previously discussed, an injury can often be anticipated by knowing the mechanism of injury and the circumstances under which it was sustained. To document a musculoskeletal assessment, certain orthopedic terms may be used. Box 19-1 lists common orthopedic terms.

Open fractures produce greater blood loss and risk of infection than closed fractures and so demand more immediate attention. However, closed fractures must be carefully monitored, too.[18] The examination for fractures should be organized by body areas, with observation first for obvious deformities. If conscious, the patient should be asked to try to move each extremity. If a fracture or dislocation exists, movement or attempted movement is almost always painful, or extremely limited with

---

BOX 19-1   **Common Orthopedic Terms**

Abduction: Movement of a body part away from the body's mid line.
Adduction: Movement of a body part toward the mid line.
Ankylosis: Decreased range of motion caused by stiffening of the joint.
Dorsiflexion: Movement of the hand or foot upward.
Eversion: Movement of the ankle outward.
Extension: Movement of the joint to open it or to maximally increase its angle.
External rotation: Outward rotation.
Flexion: Bending of the joint.
Hyperextension: Extension past neutral.
Internal rotation: Inward rotation.
Inversion: Movement of the ankle inward.
Kyphosis: Round back; increased flexion of the spine.
Lordosis: Sway back; increased hyperextension of the spine.
Plantar flexion: Movement of the foot downward.
Pronation: Movement of the forearm to place the palm downward.
Rotation: Movement of one bone turning on another.
Scoliosis: Lateral curvature of the spine.
Supination: Movement of the forearm to place the palm upward.
Torsion: Twisting of the bone on its axis.
Valgus: Deformity that causes an outward turning of the foot or toe (e.g., genu valgus or knock kneed).
Varus: Deformity that causes an inward turning of the foot or toe (e.g., genu varus or bow legged).

a dislocation. Range of motion, or lack of it, needs to be recorded. The extremities should be palpated proximally to distally, with evaluation for pain, displacement, crepitus, and decreased or absent pulses. The transport team should gently press laterally inward on the iliac crests and also press gently down on the symphysis pubis to assess for increased pain and to determine pelvic stability[6] and on the sternum and rib cage to determine stability of the ribs.

The classic signs of musculoskeletal trauma include deformity, localized swelling, pain, pallor, diminished or absent pulses, paresthesia, and paresis or paralysis.[6] If the patient is conscious, the transport team can ask about the patient's pain and its location. Peripheral pulses (especially those distal to the fracture site) should be checked bilaterally for presence and quality. Paresthesia should be checked in the conscious patient by touching or pinching the affected extremity and assessing for altered sensation. Always compare patient responses on each side.

Capillary refill should be monitored and skin temperature noted.[16,18] Paralysis at the time of the injury or ensuing paralysis on repeated examination may influence the transport location.

Joints above and below the fracture site or point of injury need to be evaluated. Neurovascular status assessments of the affected extremity should be done frequently, but especially before and after transport.

Children need special consideration in evaluation for musculoskeletal injuries. Because their bones are more flexible than those of adults, greater force is often necessary to cause a fracture. Therefore, a child who has sustained even minor rib fractures must be assumed to have sustained serious internal injuries. The transport team should suspect splenic or diaphragmatic injury in a child with low rib fractures. Injury to the flexible skeleton of the young child may cause different results than in the adult patient.[1-5]

MANAGEMENT OF ORTHOPEDIC INJURIES

Improper handling of a patient with an injury to the musculoskeletal system may convert a simple problem into a much more serious one. The closed wound may become an open one, a clean wound may become grossly contaminated, or blood vessels and nerves may be seriously injured. The five basic principles for management of fractures and dislocations are: (1) avoid unnecessary handling; (2) immobilize; (3) apply clean dressings to wounds; (4) control hemorrhage with direct pressure; and (5) check for the "5 Ps" distal to the injury—pain, pulselessness, paresthesia, pallor, and paralysis.[1,16-18]

WOUND MANAGEMENT

Local wound care is initiated by assessing the wound for evidence of severe hemorrhage or debris and the presence of bone ends protruding through the skin. These findings should be noted on the chart, and a dry sterile dressing should be applied. So that circulation is not further impaired, no attempt should be made at wound cleansing or pulling the bones back beneath the skin. Severe hemorrhage is generally controllable with direct pressure over the wound or over the arteries just proximal to the wound.[7] Good wound care is as important to a positive outcome as is good splinting. This technique should not be overlooked. Tetanus status should be noted at some point during patient care.

SPLINTING

Good emergency care rendered to a patient with any type of orthopedic injury decreases hospital stay, speeds recovery, and lessens the chance of serious complications. Because the extent of injury is difficult to assess initially, the best method is to assume a fracture is present and immobilize it until further evaluation can be made with radiography.

The primary objective of splinting is to prevent motion of fractured bone fragments or dislocated joints and thereby to prevent the following complications.[4,10,15,18]

1. Laceration of the skin by broken bones, which can increase the risk of contamination and infection.
2. Damage to local blood vessels, which can cause excessive bleeding into surrounding tissue, ischemia, and even tissue death.
3. Restriction of blood flow to an area as a result of pressure of bone ends on blood vessels.

4. Damage to nerves by inadvertent excessive traction, contusion, or laceration, which can result in possible permanent loss of sensation and paralysis.
5. Damage to muscles with possible subsequent necrosis, scarring, and permanent disability.
6. Increased pain associated with movement of bone ends.
7. Shock.
8. Delayed union or nonunion of fractured bones or dislocated joints.

Some basic principles of management for any type of orthopedic injury must be considered in splint application. These include[1,4,5]:

1. Visualize the injured area by cutting off all clothing in the surrounding area, which is especially important when the size of the transport vehicle may challenge one's ability to easily see all of the patient during transport.
2. Check and document neurovascular assessment before applying the splint. Marking the location of a palpated pulse makes consistent evaluation of the injured extremity easier.
3. If an extremity is extremely angulated and a distal pulse cannot be palpated, gentle traction may be applied to attempt to reduce the fracture. A fracture should never be forced.
4. All open wounds should be covered with a dry dressing.
5. A splint should be applied that to immobilize the joint above and below the fracture.
6. Padding should be placed in the splint to prevent pressure against bony areas and the risk of additional injury to the skin.
7. Bone ends should never be pushed back into a wound. Bone ends should be padded and covered. Keeping an open fracture clean may assist in decreasing infection.
8. Rapid transport of a patient with an unstable condition may override any attempts to splint fractures.
9. If a possible injury is suspected, apply a splint.
10. Reassess neurovascular status after the splint has been applied.

The transport team must address certain considerations, including the size of the transport vehicle, the transport vehicle's configuration, and altitude (if air splints are used) as it relates to the use of splints, when splinting a patient's injuries and preparing the patient for transport.

Soft Splint

A *soft splint* is one that has no inherent rigidity, such as a pillow or a rolled blanket. Both can provide considerable support when wrapped around an injured part and bandaged.

Rigid Splint

A *rigid splint* has inherent rigidity. It is placed along the side, front, or back of the injured extremity, and when used correctly, it immobilizes the fracture. Rigid splints are effective only when they are long enough to allow the entire fractured bone to be immobilized, are padded sufficiently, and are secured firmly to an uninjured part.[4,15,16]

Many items, such as rolled newspapers or pieces of wood, can be used to make a rigid splint. Whatever is used, however, must be long enough to immobilze the injured area one joint above and below the injured area, strong enough, and well padded enough to do the job (Box 19-2).

Traction Splint

Traction splints are also rigid splints. However, they are not used to reduce a fracture but rather to align it and immobilize the bone to prevent further damage during movement and transportation.[1,4,18] The traction splint immobilizes with a steady longitudinal traction pull exerted on the injured extremity. Traction splints should not be used on an injury to an upper extremity because of the danger of further damage or impeding circulation. Traction splints are contraindicated with possible fracture of the pelvis, fractured knee, fracture or serious wound to the tibia/fibula, and severe injury in which a wound and loss of bone continuity exists. Examples of traction splints are the Thomas half-ring, the Hare traction splint, Kendrick Traction Device, and the Sager splint.[4] Traction splints immobilize by pulling on the distal portion of the entire extremity below the fracture. The time necessary to apply a traction splint should be weighed against the need for rapid transport.

BOX 19-2	**General Principles of Splinting**

Expose and examine the injured extremity. Look for a wound, tenting of the skin, or obvious discoloration that may indicate the presence of or potential for an open fracture.

Support the body part.

Remove jewelry and constrictive items of clothing.

Assess and document sensory and circulatory status before immobilization. If no palpable distal pulse is found, medical control may recommend application of gentle traction along the long axis of the extremity (distal to the injury) until the distal pulse is palpable.

Immobilize the extremity so that the splint includes the joints above and below the fracture or the bones above and below the dislocation. Avoid excessive movement of the body part. (Movement may increase bleeding into the tissue space, increase the risk of fat embolism, or convert a closed fracture to an open fracture.)

Note: Immobilization requires a minimum of two rescuers.

When applying splints to the hand or foot, leave the fingers or toes exposed to provide for inspection and evaluation of neurovascular status.

Reevaluate and document sensory and circulatory status after immobilization. If a nerve or pulse deficit develops after splinting, remove the splint and place the extremity in its original position.

From Sanders MJ: *Mosby's paramedic textbook*, St Louis, 1994, Mosby.

Splinting Fractures of the Upper Extremities

Fractures of the clavicle usually occur at the middle and distal thirds of the bone from a blow to the shoulder. Pain, swelling, and deformity are generally evident. Supporting the arm in a sling and binding it against the chest with a swathe sufficiently immobilizes the fracture. However, injuries that occur in motor vehicle collisions may fracture the bone more medially, pushing it into the thoracic outlet and possibly injuring the long subclavian artery or vein or the brachioplexus.[4]

Fractures of the upper end of the humerus may or may not involve the shoulder joint. Pain and tenderness are seen, but severe angulation is less commonly observed. The goal in treatment of humeral fracture is to maintain shoulder function. This goal can best be achieved by treating the problem as a soft tissue injury that happens to involve bone.[4] If gross deformity is found at the fracture site, the arm should be splinted in the position in which it is found with padded boards and pillow splints. In most cases, however, little gross angulation occurs, and the arm may be splinted with a sling and swathe.[4,16]

Fractures of the mid shaft of the humerus endanger the radial nerve. The transport team can check for damage to the radial nerve by observing the patient's ability to spread the fingers. If damage has occurred, pain on movement and tenderness at the fracture site is seen. If angulation is present, a transport team member should use gentle constant traction, apply a sling, and, with traction still held, place a padded board along the outer border of the humerus. A swathe is applied around the sling, the padded board, and the injured arm, binding the arm to the chest. A fracture without angulation may be splinted in the same manner.

Fractures of the elbow endanger the radial, ulnar, and median nerves and the brachial artery. The transport team member should check for a pulse, movement, and sensation (Figure 19-2). The fracture should be splinted in the exact position found, with a rigid splint above and below the fracture. If possible, the arm should be bound to the side to offer additional support.

After gentle traction has been applied to any severe angulation of a fracture of the radius or the ulna, a rigid splint should be applied, immobilizing both the elbow and the wrist.

Fractures of the wrist without angulation should be splinted in the same manner as the radius and the ulna. Those fractures with severe angulation, however, should be splinted in the position found.

FIGURE 19-2   **Testing for neurologic function in the upper extremities.**

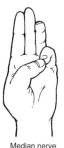
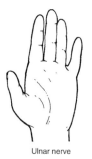
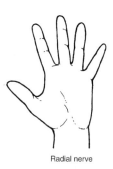

Median nerve   Ulnar nerve   Radial nerve

Severe hand injuries often involve both soft tissue and bone injury. In most cases, the hand should be splinted in the position of function, with the fingers slightly bent and a bulky fluff dressing in the palm of the hand. A rigid splint should also be used to immobilize the wrist.[4,16]

Splinting Dislocations of the Upper Extremities

When a shoulder is dislocated, the normal rounded appearance of the shoulder is flattened. The two basic types of shoulder dislocations are anterior and posterior. Most dislocations are anterior. In the anterior dislocation, the patient holds the arm away from the body, and a bony prominence is seen in the front of the shoulder.[11]

A pillow splint, and frequently the help of a second person to hold the arm, is used for maximal stability without changing the deformity. With a posterior dislocation, little deformity is evidenced, and the arm is held against the chest or abdomen. A sling and swathe are all that is necessary to maintain position. A rare inferior dislocation (the humerus is dislocated downward from the shoulder) may cause the patient to hold the arm above the head. The transport nurse splints it in the position found. These patients should be transported in a sitting position when possible.

A dislocated elbow may appear as a posterior or anterior dislocation. With a posterior dislocation, the more common, the arm is flexed. A long splint with the flexion maintained should be applied. A sling helps to maintain stability. This patient should also be transported in a sitting position if

possible. With an anterior dislocation, the arm is extended and the joint immovable because of pain. Again, the transport team splints the injury in the position found.

A dislocated wrist has an obvious deformity, and a well-padded splint should be used. The index finger is the most commonly dislocated finger, with the deformity being obvious and the fingertip slightly cyanotic and cold. A splint helps to control pain. Immobilization is all that is needed for both injuries.

Splinting Fractures of the Lower Extremities

Fractures of the hip and proximal femur are anatomically divided into two types: fractures of the neck of the femur (transcervical) and fractures through the trochanters (intertrochanteric). Both appear the same clinically, with pain and swelling around the hip, pain on hip motion, and various degrees of shortening and external rotation.[16] The fractured hip is best splinted with pillows in the position found. In assessment of hip injury, associated injuries to the knee, sciatic nerve injury, and ipsilateral femoral shaft fractures may be seen.

With fractures of the shaft of the femur, a strong contraction of the gluteus medius muscle occurs, with a tendency to pull the proximal fragment of the femur outward as the adduction causes bowing at the fracture point.[11,16] These fractures should be splinted immediately with a traction splint and kept in the splint until definitive orthopedic care is rendered. Femoral shaft fractures can cause extensive blood loss that can lead to hypovolemic shock, so these patients should be carefully monitored for early signs of shock.

Fractures of the knee should be splinted as they are found, with no attempt made to correct any angulation. Checking for and reporting changes in pulse, movement, and sensation is especially important with any type of knee injury. Fractures of the patella are recognizable as swelling of the anterior knee with little or no resistance to extension of the joint. A transport team member should splint this kind of fracture with a rigid splint and the patient's knee in extension.

Fractures of the tibia or fibula are managed with a rigid splint. The splint should immobilize both the ankle and knee joints and is best when carried as high as the groin. Great care must be taken with these fractures to prevent penetration of bone ends through the skin because the skin is thinner in this area of the leg.[4,18]

Severely angulated fractures of the ankle should be straightened with traction applied to the heel and forefoot. A rigid splint should then be applied to immobilize the foot and ankle. If any question of a sprain or fracture exists, the injury should be splinted until a diagnostic radiograph can be made. Another method that can be used to splint some injuries is the application of PASG. However, these are rarely available anymore. A PASG is effective in the splinting of both long bone and pelvic fractures and should not be overlooked by the transport team.

Splinting Dislocations of the Lower Extremities

Differentiating between a dislocated hip and a fractured hip is often impossible, although with a dislocated hip the patient's thigh is sometimes flexed to some extent and turned slightly inward. Treatment for either one is the same. The transport team should splint, with pillows or sheets and blankets, in the position found. Because of the close proximity of the sciatic and femoral nerves, an immediate neurologic assessment of the affected limb is of utmost importance (Figure 19-3).

Dislocations and fractures of the knee are treated the same. Any resistance to attempts to straighten an angulation indicates that it should be splinted in the position found, again paying heed to pulse, movement, and sensation. A rigid splint, preferably a padded board, should be used.

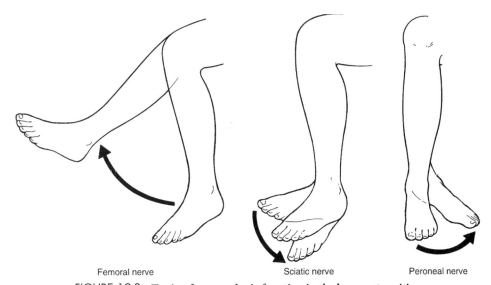

Femoral nerve   Sciatic nerve   Peroneal nerve

FIGURE 19-3 **Testing for neurologic function in the lower extremities.**

Ankle dislocations rarely occur without associated fractures and should be aligned and splinted exactly the same as ankle fractures. Dislocation of the foot is rare but generally involves more than one joint. It also should be treated the same as fracture of the foot. Toe dislocations are innately stable and need no splinting.[7]

Whenever possible after splinting a dislocation or a fracture, the transport team should elevate the affected extremity and apply ice to the injured part. This makes the patient more comfortable and can make the splinting of the extremity easier.

PELVIC FRACTURES

A pelvic fracture can be one of the most serious injuries that a patient can sustain. Arterial injuries occur in 20% of patients with pelvic fractures, and posterior fractures are more likely than anterior fractures to cause hemorrhage. The major cause of death is hemorrhage from arteries and veins torn by the fracture or dislocation.[1-5]

The most common form of pelvic fracture results from a severe external force applied directly on the pelvis or from an indirect force transmitted upward along the shaft of the femur. Minor fractures of the pelvis include breaks of individual bones without a break in the continuity of the pelvic ring. These fractures are relatively stable and rarely necessitate hospitalization. Major pelvic fractures are generally fractured in at least two separate places, and a separation of one or both sacroiliac joints may be found. These fractures are commonly seen in patients with multiple traumas.

Approximately 60% of pelvic fractures should be considered major injuries because of the complications of injury to the structures lying within the pelvis.[1-5] Besides the danger of damage to the major blood vessels within the pelvic girdle, fractures of the pubic ramus may lacerate the urethra, fractures of the brim of the pelvis may disrupt the ureters, and the bladder itself may rupture.[7] Open fractures of the pelvis occur with direct communication between fracture fragments and a laceration of the skin, vagina, or rectum. This uncommon fracture is caused by a high-velocity injury, and subsequent massive hemorrhage occurs with a 50% mortality rate. Even small amounts of blood on vaginal or rectal examination should indicate the possibility of an open fracture.[7]

Control of bleeding is a top priority.[1-5,7] Several devices may be used to immobilize the pelvis for transport, including PASG, slings made from sheets, and commercially available pelvic slings and belts.[4,16] Whichever device is chosen, transport team members need to be familiar with how the device is applied.

TRAUMATIC AMPUTATIONS

Complete *traumatic amputations* of extremities occur from time to time from various kinds of trauma, such as motor vehicle collisions, entanglements in farm or industrial machinery, or crushes caused by heavy objects or falls.

A primary assessment must first be made of the patient, and any life-threatening conditions must be addressed. Hemorrhage should be controlled with dry sterile pressure dressings, and the extremity should be elevated and immobilized. Recent research and field practice, especially in the Iraq and Afghanistan wars, may influence the management of massive bleeding from a traumatic amputation. The use of a tourniquet and the application of agents to stop bleeding may become a part of transport practice in the near future.[9,17] Transport team members should become familiar with these and their implications to prehospital and patient transport.

If bleeding is not a problem, then a transport team member should flush the wound with crystalloid solution depending on the local protocols, apply a dry sterile dressing and a mild pressure gauze wrap to the extremity, and immobilize and elevate the extremity. The transport team then should flush the amputated part with crystalloid solution, wrap it in a dry sterile gauze or towel (if unavailable, use a clean sheet), and place it in a plastic bag or container. Then, the severed part is put in another container and cooled with another plastic bag that contains ice. Dry ice should not be used because it increases necrosis. As with any acute vascular injury, the expediency with which the patient and amputated part reach definitive care directly correlates with the success of reimplantation.

FAT EMBOLISM

Fat embolism is a complication that may occur with large bone, pelvic, and rib fractures. It is generally not seen until 12 to 72 hours after injury. The transport team may encounter a patient with fat emboli, especially if it is a delayed transport.[1,18]

Clinical signs of fat emboli include respiratory failure, shock, and elevation in serum lipase levels. Thrombocytopenia can also occur, and patients may have multiple petechiae present. Low platelet count (<150,000) may be present also.

Long bone fractures should be appropriately immobilized. Patients should be closely monitored for respiratory distress, especially lack of improved oxygenation despite increasing the amount of FIO_2. If the patient in intubated, positive end expiratory pressure (PEEP) may be used to maintain an adequate PO_2 during transport.[1,18]

COMPARTMENT SYNDROME

Compartment syndrome develops with increased pressure within the compartment space of an extremity or other area of the body from bleeding, fluid accumulation (such as in a burn injury), or external sources such as splinting.[1,18] Fractures and crush injuries may put a patient at risk of compartment syndrome. Prolonged compression of an extremity in a splint can also cause compartment syndrome.

Clinical signs of compartment syndrome include progressive severe pain and decreased sensation and weakness in the involved extremity. Changes or absence in peripheral pulses and delayed capillary refill are late signs of compartment syndrome. Extreme pain with passive movement of the affected extremity is a hallmark symptom of compartment syndrome.

Removal of the constrictive device (splint or PASG) and elevation of the effected extremity to the level of the heart are some of the interventions the transport team may perform. If the compartment pressure is greater than 30 to 35 mm Hg, a fasciotomy may be indicated. Emergency fasciotomy must be done within 4 hours to prevent irreversible damage to muscles and nerves. However, the procedure should not be done without consultation with medical control.[1,18]

SUMMARY

In most cases, orthopedic and related vascular injuries are not life threatening; however, the long-term outcome for patients who sustain these injuries is greatly influenced by the initial care that they receive. The transport team should approach orthopedic and vascular emergencies with these goals in mind: (1) minimize the complications associated with fractures, both open and closed; (2) decrease complications of immobility caused by these injuries; (3) facilitate the general management of more definitive care; and (4) help to preserve and restore complete function of the affected extremity.[13]

ORTHOPEDIC VASCULAR TRAUMA CASE STUDY

A 25-year-old unrestrained intoxicated man was riding in the front seat of a car that struck the side of a hill. On arrival, the transport team found the patient in the back of an ambulance; the patient had severe right leg pain. The patient's ABCs were intact, but his right leg was lying beside his head. When the car had struck the hill, his leg had been crossed over on his knee. The impact of the collision caused dislocation of his right hip and multiple fractures of his leg, allowing it to assume this position.

No palpable pulse was found in the extremity. An intravenous line was inserted, and conscious sedation was administered with fentanyl and lorazepam. The flight physician then reduced the dislocated hip and splinted the fractures.

The patient was then transported without incident to the trauma center.

REFERENCES

1. Air and Surface Trauma Nurses Association (ASTNA): *Transport nurse advanced trauma course*, ed 4, Denver, 2006, ASTNA.
2. American College of Surgeons Committee on Trauma: *Advanced trauma life support course instructor manual*, ed 8, Chicago, 2008, ACS.
3. Blumen I, editor: *Principles and direction of air medical transport*, Salt Lake City, 2006, Air Medical Physician Association (AMPA).

4. Campbell J, editor: *International trauma life support for prehospital care providers*, ed 6, Upper Saddle River, NJ, 2008, Pearson Prentice Hall.

5. Emergency Nurses Association (ENA): *Trauma nursing core course*, ed 6, Des Plaines, IL, 2007, ENA.

6. Farrell J: The trauma patient with multiple fractures, *RN* 48(6):22, 1985.

7. Harrahill M: Open pelvic fracture: the lethal injury, *J Emerg Nurs* 20(3):243, 1994.

8. Heckman JD: Looking beyond the trees to the forest, *Consultant* 22(2):133, 1982.

9. Johansson P, Bochsen L, Stensballe J, et al: Transfusion packages for massively bleeding patients: the effect on clot formation and stability as evaluated by Thrombelastograph (TEG®), *Transfusion Apheresis Sci* 39:3-8, 2008.

10. Mabee JR: Compartment syndrome: a complication of acute extremity trauma, *J Emerg Med* 12(5):651, 1995.

11. Maher AB: Early assessment and management of musculoskeletal injuries, *Nurs Clin North Am* 21(4):717, 1986.

12. McSwain N: To manage multiple injury consider mechanisms, *Emerg Med* 16(4):56, 1984.

13. Pashley J, Wahlstrom NL: Polytrauma: the patient, the family, and the health team, *Nurs Clin North Am* 16(4):721, 1981.

14. Perdue P: Abdominal injuries and dangerous fractures, *RN* 44(7):35, 84, 1981.

15. Proehl J, editor: *Emergency nursing procedures*, ed 4, Philadelphia, 2009, Saunders Elsevier.

16. Sanders M: *Mosby's paramedic textbook*, ed 3, St Louis, 2007, Mosby JEMS Elsevier.

17. Tien H, Jung V, Rizoli S, et al: An evaluation of tactical combat casualty care interventions in a combat environment, *J Am Coll Surg* 207(2):174-178, 2008.

18. York D, Stocking J, Johnson J: *Flight and ground transport nursing core curriculum*, Denver, 2006, Air and Surface Transport Nurses Association.

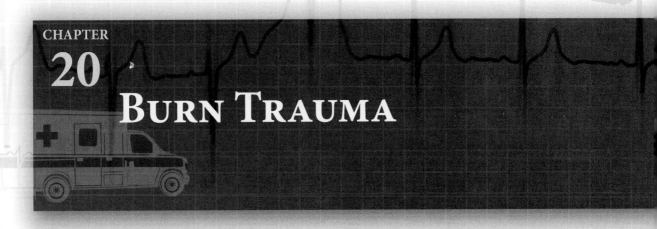

BURN TRAUMA

Heather McLellan

COMPETENCIES

1. Identify the pathophysiology of burn wounds.
2. Describe the initial assessment of the patient with burns.
3. Describe the management of the patient with burns during the transport process.

ETIOLOGY AND EPIDEMIOLOGY

A *burn wound* is an injury caused by the interaction of an energy form (thermal, chemical, electrical, or radiation) and biologic matter. Most burns are *thermal:* flame burns, scalds, or contacts with hot substances (Figure 20-1). Frostbite is often included in this category; however, no current statistics are available regarding its incidence rate.

Chemical injuries occur when the source of energy contacted is capable of causing tissue necrosis. Examples of necrosis-causing chemicals include strong acids, which cause coagulation necrosis from protein precipitation, and alkalis, which cause liquefaction necrosis.

Electrical burns occur when contact is made with a high-voltage current. The current itself is not considered to have any thermal properties while traveling through material of low resistance; however, the potential energy of the current is transferred into thermal energy when it meets resistance with biologic tissue and is dispersed throughout that tissue. This action is accomplished primarily by conduction.

Radiation injuries can be caused by both ionizing and nonionizing radiation. Radiation injuries make up a small percentage of burn injuries.

Approximately 700,000 individuals receive medical treatment for thermal burn injuries in the United States and Canada each year.[2,3] Of these, 40,000 need hospitalization, and 4000 die.[2,3,11] The World Health Organization estimates that 322,000 fire-related deaths occurred worldwide in 2002, with most of these in developing countries.[23] The survival rate from major burns has increased significantly and is now up to 94.4%.[2]

Estimates are that 500 deaths per year can be attributed to electrical and lightning injuries.[2,3]

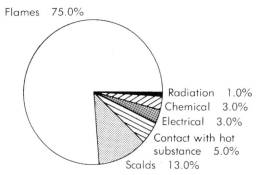

Flames 75.0%

Radiation 1.0%
Chemical 3.0%
Electrical 3.0%
Contact with hot
substance 5.0%
Scalds 13.0%

FIGURE 20-1   Causes of burn injuries.

Contact with electricity accounts for between 3% and 5% of all burns treated in the United States each year. All ages are affected, with the most common victims those who work with electricity professionally. The age group with the greatest electrical injury rate is infancy to 4 years of age.[2,3,11] These injuries are primarily caused by contact with exposed electrical cords and outlets. The second peak appears from ages 20 to 25 years. Those injuries occur predominately in the male population and are caused by work and industrial accidents. An estimated 150 people are killed by lightning each year in the United States. Most lightning injuries occur in the daytime hours of the summer and fall months. The outdoors enthusiast, athlete, camper, farmer, or golfer is more prone to lightning injury because of more frequent exposure to the elements.[2,3]

PATHOPHYSIOLOGY OF BURN WOUNDS

The causes of burns may vary, but the local and systemic responses are generally similar. The extent of the injury is influenced by three factors: (1) the intensity of the energy source; (2) the duration of exposure to the energy source; and (3) the conductance of the tissue exposed. The relationship between the duration of exposure to and intensity of the energy source is significant in determining the magnitude of the injury. Increased intensity with increased exposure causes increased amounts of tissue damage. Conductance can be affected by the presence of hair, water content of the tissues, and thickness and pigmentation of the skin. Significant

factors that determine severity of electrical injury are: (1) voltage and amperage; (2) resistance of internal body structure and tissue; (3) type and pathway of current; and (4) duration and intensity of contact.[8,24]

For a better understanding of the pathophysiology of burn wounds, one must know the anatomy and functions of the skin. Skin is composed of two layers: the epidermis and the dermis. The *epidermis*, the outer layer, consists of the basement layer of cells that migrate upward to become surface keratin. The inner layer, the *dermis*, consists of collagen and elastic fibers and contains hair follicles, sweat and sebaceous glands, nerve endings, and blood vessels. Beneath the cutaneous layers is a layer of subcutaneous tissue that consists primarily of connective tissue and fat deposits; this layer overlies muscle and bone.

The primary functions of skin include: (1) regulation of body temperature through dilation and constriction of the dermal and subcuticular vessels in response to environmental temperature; (2) protection against injury and bacterial invasion; (3) prevention of body fluid loss; and (4) sensory contact with the environment. A burn injury interrupts and compromises these functions.

THERMAL BURN INJURY

Responses of the body to thermal injury consist of varying degrees of tissue damage, cellular impairment, and fluid shifts. Locally, a brief initial decrease in blood flow to the area occurs, followed by a marked increase in arteriolar vasodilation. Release of toxic mediators of inflammation is activated with the burn, creating a complex circulatory dysfunction. These mediators include histamine, serotonin, kinins, oxygen free radicals, prostaglandins, thromboxanes, and interleukins. Although inflammatory activity is a necessary part of the healing process, excess production of mediators, especially oxidants and proteases, causes more capillary endothelial and skin cell damage.[10,13,17,20] This increases capillary permeability, particularly once the burned area reaches a size that is approximately 30% of the body surface area, which causes intravascular fluid loss and wound edema.

Hypoproteinemia that results from the increase in capillary permeability aggravates edema in the non-burned tissue. Myocardial contractility is thought to be decreased because of a release of tumor necrosis factor-alpha. Insensible fluid loss from the burn wound increases the basal metabolic rate and, along with fluid shift, leads to hypovolemia, hypotension, and inadequate end organ perfusion.[10,17]

The decrease in circulating plasma causes an increase in hematocrit, which in turn can cause hemoglobinuria when the hemoglobin is filtered through the kidneys and can contribute to renal failure. Increased peripheral vascular resistance leads to a decrease in venous return to the heart, decreased cardiac output, impaired tissue perfusion, and a decrease in renal perfusion, which can also contribute to renal failure.[10,13,18]

A decrease in splanchnic blood flow occurs, which increases the occurrence of mucosal hemorrhages in the stomach and duodenum. An increased risk of sepsis from bacterial translocation may also be seen as a result of diminished mucosal barrier function in the intestine. Patients with burns on more than 20% of the body surface area (BSA) can also have adynamic ileus, which can be of special concern for the patient transported by air at high altitudes.

Decreased immune response in both cell-mediated and humoral pathways increases the patient's susceptibility to infection.[10,17] Thus, the transport team must take extra precautions to prevent further injury to the burn victim through exposure to contaminated environments.

Thermal burns and pregnancy should be considered in any female of the reproductive age group. The outcome of the pregnancy is determined by the extent of the mother's burn injury. Spontaneous abortions can be anticipated with burns greater than or equal to 60% percent of BSA. The incidence rate of preterm labor or spontaneous abortion is reduced with adequate oxygenation, fluid resuscitation, and electrolyte imbalance correction.[2,3]

ELECTRICAL INJURY

Electrons flowing through the body produce injury by depolarizing muscles and nerves. They can also disrupt electrical rhythms in the brain and heart.

Electrical energy is also converted to thermal energy when it meets resistance from tissues. Resistance is described as the degree of hindrance to electron flow. Those tissues that contain the most electrolyte media, nerves, blood vessels, and muscles transmit current most easily because they have the least resistance. Tissues, tendons, and fat are most resistant and do not allow conduction, which causes burning and surrounding deep muscle damage. The intensity of the electrical current that passes through victims shows a direct correlation to the tissue damage produced.[10,18,24]

Voltage is defined as the force with which the electrical movement occurs. High-voltage injuries (>1000 V) and low-voltage injuries (<1000 V) are both common, and either type can cause death. High amounts of electrical voltage and amount cause more significant injury to the patient and result in tissue charring and extensive blistering. The type of current, alternating (AC) or direct (DC), can also determine the significance of injury.[10,18,24] Alternating current produces a tetanic contraction of muscles that "freezes" the victim to the source. This reaction is not seen with direct current; therefore, low-voltage AC exposure, such as to a household current of 110 V, can be more dangerous than a low-voltage direct current. The alternating current also has a greater potential to cause ventricular fibrillation from tetanic chest muscle contractions (Table 20-1).

The current pathway is critical because it may determine the severity of injury. Current passing through the head and thorax involves the respiratory center or heart and is likely to produce instant death. Current passing from hand to foot may not affect the respiratory center but may damage the heart. From the entry point, the electrical current follows the path of least resistance, causing one or more tracks of damage. The energy collects at the grounding point, causing significant tissue necrosis, and subsequently causing an explosive exit through the skin.[10,24] The mortality rate of hand-to-hand current passage is reported to be 60%; hand-to-foot current passage is 20%; and foot-to-foot current passage is 5%. Direct current has been noted to leave a discrete exit wound (Figure 20-2), whereas alternating current tends to be more explosive (Figure 20-3).

TABLE 20-1	Effects of Amperage by Household Currents (60-Hz AC)
mAmps	**Effect**
1-2	Tingling of skin
15-20	Muscle tetany: the "let go" current
50-90	Respiratory arrest (if directed through the medulla)
90-250	Ventricular fibrillation (if the myocardium is transversed)

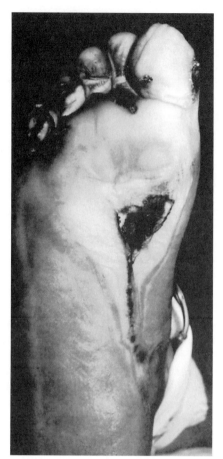

FIGURE 20-3   **Exit wound from alternating current.**

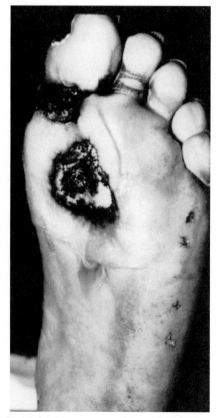

FIGURE 20-2   **Exit wound from direct current.**

With electrical injury, flame burns occur as the result of the ignition of clothing or other items by the current. These wounds could be severe when the victim is unconscious and has a long exposure to the flame. The ignition of clothing usually occurs

with high-voltage injuries that are greater than 350 to 1000 V. Frequently, high-voltage injuries cause combinations of all types of electrical burns, and determination of the proper course of therapy may become difficult.[10,17,18,24]

As electrical current passes through the body, severe dysrhythmia may occur. Ventricular fibrillation is frequently induced as a 60-cycle alternating current passes through the ventricles. Direct current injuries predominantly result in asystole by depolarizing the entire myocardium. In addition to those fatal rhythms, other dysrhythmia may occur, such as atrial fibrillation, sinus bradycardia, ventricular and atrial ectopy, supraventricular tachycardia, bundle branch block, and first-degree and second-degree block. Coronary artery spasm, coronary endarteritis, and direct myocardial injury are thought to be the cause of this dysrhythmia. Damage to the myocardium, including myocardial rupture, is also a result of an electrical injury. These injuries are believed to be caused by the heat generated by the current. Myocardial damage manifests itself in the same manner as the injury induced by ischemia.

The skull is a common entry point of electrical current; thus, the brain stem is often affected, which can lead to respiratory arrest and potential cerebral hemorrhage or edema.[8,24] Nervous system tissue is an excellent conductor of electrical current, so central nervous damage is not uncommon. Effects of electrical injury to the central nervous system are manifested by unconsciousness, seizures, disorientation, or amnesia. Other neurologic complications that have been identified are spinal cord injuries, particularly those associated with electrical current traversing a hand-to-hand or head-to-foot course, and local nerve damage with peripheral neuropathies. Incomplete spinal cord transection is a common delayed lesion caused by damage to the spinal cord by the heat of the electrical current or by blunt trauma from falls or severe tetanic contractions of the muscles surrounding the cord. Headaches, cerebellar dysfunction, optic atrophy, ascending paralysis, and transverse myelitis are neurological sequelae that are delayed.[8,24]

Extensive necrosis over vessels resulting from electrical injury may precipitate delayed hemorrhage from large blood vessels. Arterial thrombosis, deep vein thrombosis, and abdominal aortic aneurysms may also result. A major vessel that has been only partially damaged may cause difficulty with homeostasis in open or newly closed wounds. Injuries to the abdominal cavity commonly identified after electrocution are submucosal hemorrhages in the bowel, liver failure, pancreatitis, nausea and vomiting, paralytic ileus, and various forms and degrees of ulcerative disease.[8,24]

Long bone fractures and dislocations and vertebral fractures are caused by the rigorous tetanic muscle contractions that occur. Bilateral scapular fractures have been reported from exposure to a 440-V, 60-cycle current passing briefly through a person's upper extremities. Amputations have also

been the result of severe muscle contractions caused by high-voltage electrical injuries.[8,10,24]

Immediate burns to the eyes, optic atrophy, and the development of cataracts are not uncommon, particularly if the entrance or exit wounds appear on or around the head. Cataracts may develop unilaterally or bilaterally and occur as soon as 4 months or as late as 3 years after the injury.

For the pregnant patient, the hand-to-foot pathway of current invariably passes through the fetus. The amniotic fluid and abundant uteroplacental vascularity have a low resistance to current flow, and the fetus becomes an easy victim of electrical injuries. Regardless of how slight the injury may appear, the mother must be transported to a hospital in which extensive fetal monitoring can be done.

Acute renal failure is a complication that results from direct damage to the kidney by the electrical current or blunt trauma to the kidney or from myoglobinuria. Myoglobin is released as a result of extensive muscle necrosis, and myoglobinuria is proportionate to the amount of muscle damage incurred.[18]

ASSESSMENT

The assessment of the patient with burn injuries begins with the ABCDEs of the primary assessment. Burn wounds are often dramatic in appearance and can lure the transport team's attention away from more immediate life-threatening problems.

The subjective assessment includes as thorough a history as circumstances permit. The history should include the mechanism and time of the injury and a description of the surrounding environment, such as injuries incurred in an enclosed space, the presence of noxious chemicals, the possibility of smoke inhalation, and any related trauma. The time of the injury is especially important in the calculation of fluid resuscitation. Information regarding tetanus immunization status should also be obtained with the history.[12]

THERMAL BURNS

Assessment of a thermal burn includes estimating the burn size and depth, associated inhalation injuries, and calculation of fluid resuscitation needs. The size of a burn wound is most frequently estimated with the rule of nines[12] method, which divides the body into multiples of 9% (Figure 20-4). A more accurate assessment can be made of the burn injury, especially for pediatric patients, with a Lund and Browder chart,[12] which takes into account growth changes (Figure 20-5). For estimating scatter burns, a fairly accurate approximation can be made with the patient's entire palm size to represent 1% of the total BSA and visualization of that palm over the burned area. Use of electronic assessment tools is becoming popular because these tools not only increase the accuracy of assessment but also enhance continuity of care as they are easily transmitted to each level of caregiver.[15,25]

Primarily, the temperature of the burning agent, the duration of exposure, and the conductance of the tissue involved determine the depth of a thermal burn wound. Initially, the estimation of injury depth is difficult.

Burn wounds typically present in a bull's-eye pattern, with each ring representing a different zone of intensity. A *superficial partial-thickness* injury, formerly known as a first-degree burn, involves the epidermis and is represented by the outermost ring, the zone of hyperemia. This type of injury is usually red in appearance, is painful, and heals in 7 to 10 days.[10,12,17,20]

A *deep partial-thickness* injury, formerly known as a second-degree burn, involves both the epidermis and dermis. This burn is seen as the middle ring and is called the zone of stasis, which is potentially viable tissue, despite the heat injury. This wound is characterized by reddened skin that is wet or blistered, is painful, and generally heals in 14 to 21 days. However, these diagnostic signs can be misleading because a full-thickness burn is possible under a blister.[10,12,17,20]

Full-thickness injuries are the center ring, called the zone of coagulation. These injuries, formerly known as third-degree injuries, encompass wounds that consist of both dermal layers and extend into the subcutaneous tissue. Subdermal burns destroy both layers of tissue and extend into fat, tendon, muscle, and bone. Full-thickness injuries are charred and leathery in appearance or white and waxy, with thrombosed vessels that are easily visible under the surface.[10,12,17,20] They are painless because of destruction of sensory nerves, with no epithelial growth for healing. These wounds necessitate grafting.

Inhalation Injuries with Thermal Burns

The three types of identifiable inhalation injuries are: (1) asphyxiation from carbon monoxide poisoning; (2) supraglottic injury, which is primarily thermal in nature; and (3) infraglottic injury, which is primarily chemical. Inhalation injuries are the primary cause of death at the scene of a burn injury, and they contribute significantly to the overall morbidity and mortality rates of burn patients.[9,10,14,17]

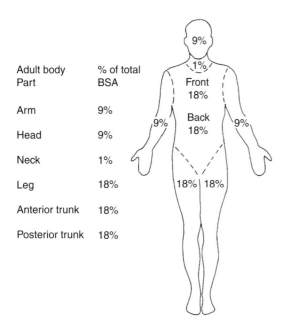

Adult body Part	% of total BSA
Arm	9%
Head	9%
Neck	1%
Leg	18%
Anterior trunk	18%
Posterior trunk	18%

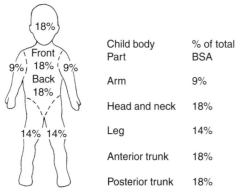

Child body Part	% of total BSA
Arm	9%
Head and neck	18%
Leg	14%
Anterior trunk	18%
Posterior trunk	18%

FIGURE 20-4   **Rule of nines.**

Age	0-1	1-4	5-9	1-14	15
A — ½ of head	9 ½ %	8 ½ %	6 ½ %	5 ½ %	4 ½ %
B — ½ of one thigh	2 ¾ %	3 ¼ %	4%	4 ¼ %	4 ½ %
C — ½ of one thigh	2 ½ %	2 ½ %	2 ¾ %	3%	3 ¼ %

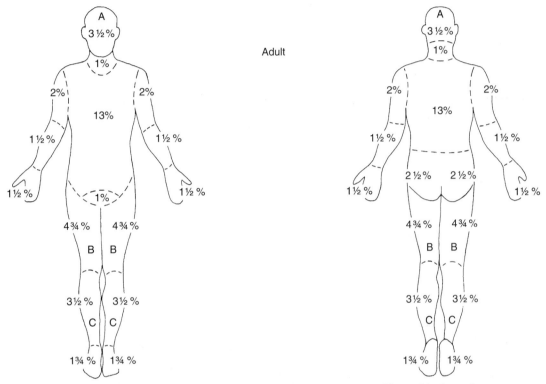

FIGURE 20-5 **Lund and Browder method for calculating percentage of burned body surface area.**

Carbon monoxide intoxication occurs because the affinity for carbon monoxide to hemoglobin is markedly greater than that of oxygen (approximately 12 times greater); therefore, the carbon monoxide displaces the oxygen and binds with the available hemoglobin to form carboxyhemoglobin, with resultant hypoxia. The signs and symptoms of carbon monoxide poisoning include pink to cherry-red skin, tachycardia, tachypnea, headache, dizziness, and nausea. Carboxyhemoglobin levels are helpful to determine the management approach for these patients. Levels of 0 to 15% rarely cause symptoms and may be normal, especially for a

heavy smoker. Levels of 15% to 40% cause varying amounts of central nervous system disturbances, such as confusion and headache. Levels greater than 40% can cause mental depression and coma. Any patient with suspected carbon monoxide injury should be given 100% oxygen.[9,10,14] The treatment of carbon monoxide poisoning is discussed in both Chapter 24, Pulmonary Emergencies, and Chapter 30, Toxicologic Emergencies.

Supraglottic injury should be suspected when facial burns, singed facial hair, or carbonaceous sputum are present. Other signs and symptoms of upper airway injury include presence of redness or blistering in the posterior pharynx, stridor, wheezing, bronchorrhea, or any other sign of respiratory difficulty. Absence of these signs and symptoms initially does not exclude the possibility of inhalation injury because upper airway edema may not be present until after the onset of fluid resuscitation.

Infraglottic injury is often more difficult to ascertain because the injury is progressive in nature. It is caused by the inhalation of the particulate byproducts of combustion. It is manifested by an increase in both pulmonary vascular resistance and pulmonary capillary permeability, which causes pulmonary edema. The primary symptom is hypoxemia that is resistant to oxygen therapy. Inhalation injuries are unpredictable in onset. Any patient with suspected inhalation injuries should be closely observed for 24 hours for onset of respiratory complications. Some experts advocate fiber optic bronchoscopy or xenon ventilation-perfusion scanning to identify inhalation injury earlier.[9,10,14,17]

ELECTRICAL INJURIES

If the patient actually becomes part of the circuit, they may incur direct contact burns. These wounds may appear devastating, and they frequently resemble a crush injury rather than a burn (Figure 20-6). The most common point of entry is the hand or skull, and the most common exit site is the feet. The sizes of these entrance and exit wounds are no real indicator of the amount of damage done to internal tissue. When the current leaves the body on its course to the ground, arc burns occur.[8,24] The arcing current produces extremely high energies, ranging from 3000 °C to 20,000 °C. Wounds are deeper because the heat intensity is closer to the body. Deep partial thickness and full thickness thermal burns may be indistinguishable when the heat source is more distant from the body.

Cutaneous injuries from electrical contact are frequently apparent because the skin is the first point of contact with the electrical current. Dry skin has a greater resistance than wet skin and thus produces greater generation of heat and subsequently a larger burn. Flexor crease burns are noted as the hallmark of the true conductive injury. Alternating current produces tetanic contractions of the flexor muscle of the upper extremities, causing the skin layers at the flexed joint to be more closely apposed. As the current path passes through the apposed skin layers, typical arc burns are produced at the wrist, elbow, and antecubital fossa.[8,24]

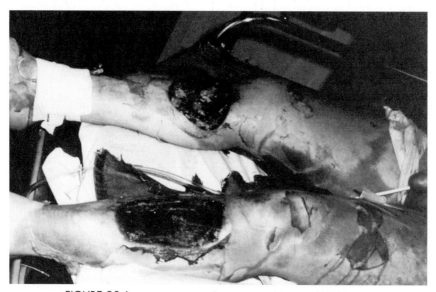

FIGURE 20-6   **Direct-contact burns resembling crush injuries.**

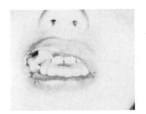 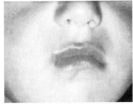

FIGURE 20-7　Oral commissure burns in a child less than age 2 years.

Oral commissure burns are commonly seen in children under the age of 2 years. These burns are typically caused by a child chewing or sucking on a low-tension (110-V) electrical cord. This type of burn is frequently localized but can cause associated injuries to the tongue, palate, and face (Figure 20-7).

LIGHTNING INJURIES

Lightning injuries are dissimilar to those caused by high-voltage contact; therefore, the effects and injuries differ. A lightning bolt may have a voltage of up to 1 billion V and induce currents greater than 200,000 A. Although the intensity of lightning is much greater than high-voltage electricity, the duration of exposure is much shorter, ranging from 1/100 to 1/1000 of a second. Because of this lesser duration, skin burns are less severe than those burns seen with high-voltage injuries.[8,24] Linear and punctate burns are frequently seen with lightning injuries, and feathering burns are pathognomonic to lightning injuries. With a lightning strike, the electrical current turns moisture on the skin to steam and frequently blows off or shreds clothing or shoes (Figure 20-8). Blunt trauma is frequently associated with lightning injuries and is caused when the victims are hurled to the ground by the current.[12] A victim may suffer a direct strike from a lightning bolt or may experience a splash injury. The splash injury occurs when lightning strikes an object and the stroke jumps to another object that acts as a better conductor. This mechanism causes multiple lightning strikes in people standing in close proximity to an object or to another individual who has been struck.

Patients with minor injuries usually are conscious; however, they may have lost consciousness transiently and are frequently confused and amnesic.

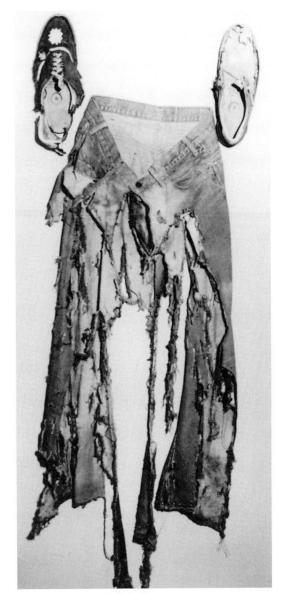

FIGURE 20-8　Clothing of a patient struck by lightning.

Patients with moderate lightning injuries show more obvious altered mentation and may be combative or comatose. They may have fallen or been thrown down forcibly from the current, which may have caused fractures and dislocations. Superficial and deep partial thickness burns may be apparent with a moderate lightning strike injury, as may tympanic membrane rupture caused by the explosive force of lightning strike. Difficulty in palpating peripheral pulses and a mottled appearance of the patient's lower extremities are caused by arterio-spasm and are frequently characteristic with a moderate injury. The condition usually clears in a few hours. Severe lightening injuries can be more dramatic. If lightning current passes through the brain, the direct current or blast effect caused by the strike may damage the brain. The patient is comatose and may possibly be undergoing a seizure. Closed head injury caused by a fall must also be considered in these cases.[8,24]

Cardiac arrest with ventricular fibrillation should be anticipated. The most common cause of death in lightning injuries is cardiopulmonary arrest. Lightning may cause paralysis to the medullary respiratory center, first causing respiratory arrest and then cardiac arrest. If immediate ventilation does not occur, a subsequent cardiac arrest follows, and brain death occurs from anoxia. Multiple arrhythmias are associated with lightning strikes, including ventricular tachycardia, PVCs, and atrial fibrillation. ST changes associated with ischemia are also common. Many ocular injuries have been reported, including detached retina, hyphema, direct thermal burn, corneal lesion, and cataract. As with electrical injuries, cataracts may appear as late as 2 years after the strike, but they are most commonly present in the first few days after the injury. Patients must be assessed for other signs of trauma caused by the impact of the strike and for life-threatening injuries.[8,24]

For the pregnant victim of a lightning strike, the fetus must be assessed with immediate use of fetal heart tones to determine viability. The prognosis of the unborn child is difficult to determine. Half of such pregnancies go on to normal delivery and produce no recognizable abnormality to the child, whereas the other half results in stillbirths.

CHEMICAL BURN INJURIES

Chemical burns differ from thermal burns in that the burning process continues until the agent is inactivated by reaction with the tissues, is neutralized, or is diluted with water. The degree of damage by a chemical agent depends on the concentration and quantity of the agent, its mechanism of action, and the duration of contact. Alkalis cause deeper and more significant wounds than acids.[10,17]

RADIATION BURN INJURIES

Dealing with radiation burns caused by ionizing radiation is a rare occurrence. Transport after a radiation accident is probably for more critical injuries than for radiation exposure itself.[10,17]

MANAGEMENT OF BURN INJURY

Transport of a burn patient requires an orderly prioritized approach. Equipment and supplies should be organized in advance when possible to expedite assessment and stabilization of the burn patient. Although supplies and equipment vary among transport programs, depending on protocols and primary service populations, little is needed beyond the standard emergency medical supplies to provide quality burn care. Sheets and blankets should be carried even in the summertime to prevent hypothermia during transport.

SCENE SAFETY

If transport of the burn patient involves scene response, the safety of all responders must be ensured. Safety precautions may include vigilance for toxic substances with the victim of a chemical burn, extinguishing sources of flame for the thermal burn, or use of special personnel and equipment for removal of electrical lines. Communication with ground personnel regarding the type of scene and landing zone is mandatory before approaching.

Removing the victim from any source of electrical current may place rescuers at risk. Wooden poles, rubber gloves, and ropes are not without risk and should be used only by those trained to work with electricity. The transport team must not assume that a downed wire is not dangerous because it is not producing sparks and because the surrounding areas are dark. Extrication is safe only when the power is turned off. If victims must be removed immediately because of injury, only trained individuals should attempt to do so. Management of the burn patient begins with the ABCDEs of the primary survey, including airway, breathing, and circulation, with a brief baseline neurologic examination. During assessments and interventions for life-threatening problems in the primary survey, the transport team should take precautions to maintain cervical spine immobilization if trauma is suspected. The transport team must be sure that the burning process has been stopped, which may require copious irrigation of the burn wound, as in the case of chemical burns, or simple removal of clothing and jewelry from the patient. The patient must be protected from further injury, and the safety of the transport team members must be ensured. The primary survey should then be performed.

AIRWAY/BREATHING/INHALATION INJURY MANAGEMENT

Intubation may need to be accomplished early because it could become impossible later with the onset of edema after the initiation of fluid replacement to manage the burned patient's airway. Assessment for dyspnea is more difficult during transport because of the noise and vibration, so the transport team should learn to rely on other parameters for assessment of respiratory status.[12,17,20] Securing an endotracheal tube may be difficult because tape, which is most often used, does not adhere to burned skin. Several alternatives are available, such as the use of cotton twill ties or suturing or stapling the tube to the nose or lip.

Inhalation injury is considered one of the most frequent causes of death in burn patients. Management includes careful assessment of the airway and rapid early intervention for signs of obstruction. Early intubation, before massive edema formation, is key for the patient with airway damage. Intervention for external sources of compression such as circumferential neck burns is also important.[12,16] Administration of humidified oxygen helps minimize inspissation of secretions, and frequent suctioning helps remove accumulated secretions. Use of bronchodilators is helpful for minimizing bronchospasm and encouraging mucociliary clearance.[12,14] Other medications that may be used include *N*-acetylcysteine alone as a mucolytic agent or in combination with heparin as scavengers for oxygen free radicals that are produced by activation of alveolar macrophages.[9]

CIRCULATION/FLUID RESUSCITATION

Two intravenous (IV) lines should be initiated peripherally with large-bore catheters. The fluid of choice for initial resuscitation is variable, but crystalloid is the most common. Ideally, lines should be placed in nonburned areas, but they may be placed through the burn if they are the only veins available for cannulation. Intravenous lines should be sutured in place if any danger of dislodgment exists because venous access may not be available peripherally after the onset of generalized edema. Blood should be obtained for initial laboratory studies when IV lines are initiated if that has not already been done.

The goal of initial fluid resuscitation is to restore and maintain adequate tissue perfusion and vital organ function, in addition to preserving heat-injured but viable tissue in the zone of stasis.[1,4,20] Fluid needs are based on the size of the patient and the extent of the burn. The two most common formulas for estimating fluid needs are the Parkland formula, which is 2 to 4 mL/kg/% total BSA (TBSA) burned. One half of the total amount should be given over the first 8 hours from the time of the injury, with the second half to be given over the following 16 hours.

Some controversy exists over the most appropriate fluid to be used in burn resuscitation. There are proponents of various combinations of hypertonic and isotonic solutions, crystalloid, and colloid. Choice of fluid largely is a matter of local opinion and current research. The transport team must consult with the physician or burn center that is accepting the patient to obtain orders for fluids and fluid resuscitation guidelines. A recent European survey noted that volume replacement remains almost exclusively crystalloids with a fixed formula.[5] An American study of fluid resuscitation during transport of burn patients indicated that fluid resuscitation was inappropriate in more than half of the patients transported, with the primary error overresuscitation.[21] These results were attributed largely to errors in documenting burn size and in monitoring IV flow rates.

Emphasis in pediatric fluid resuscitation is shifting to the minimum amount necessary to maintain vital organ function. Current research also suggests that children tolerate rapid initial volume infusion, with half the calculated volume given over 4 hours and the remainder given over 20 hours, a formula that differs somewhat from the adult regimen. The goal with pediatric fluid resuscitation is a urine output of 1 to 1.5 mL/kg/h.[7]

Burn Wound Management

Care of the burn wound includes covering the burned area with a dry clean dressing and, in the case of a large burn wound, placing the patient on one dry clean sheet and covering with blankets added over the sheets as needed. Wet dressings should not be used because they provide an open pathway for bacteria, cause additional tissue injury, and leave the patient at risk of hypothermia because of loss of skin integrity from the burn injury.[10,12,17,20]

With the exception of escharotomies, open chest wounds, and actively bleeding wounds, wound management in transport consists of simply placing the patient on and covering the patient with clean dry linen. Wet dressings are contraindicated because of the decreased thermoregulatory capacity of patients with large burns and the possibility of hypothermia. The burn patient should be covered with blankets to avoid hypothermia, and IV fluids should ideally be warmed. Some commercial wound care products are available. These should not be used without consulting a burn center.

Circumferential burns to the chest or extremities represent the more easily recognizable complications in burn care. Circumferential burns to the chest wall decrease chest wall compliance, creating respiratory insufficiency and hypoxia, especially in the pediatric population because chest walls are more pliable. This problem can be further aggravated by generalized edema.

Circumferential burns to the extremities or digits can be equally threatening to the circulatory stability of the affected limb, producing the "5 Ps" that represent the signs and symptoms of an arterial injury: pain, pallor, pulselessness, paresthesia, and paralysis. An ultrasonic Doppler scan device may be helpful in locating pulses in a particularly edematous area.

Escharotomies are the traditional way to deal with compression from circumferential burns (Figures 20-9 and 20-10). However, because this skill is difficult to teach and maintain, some recommendations are that a decompression technique should be used until a skilled provider is available.[6] Whichever method is used to relieve the compression, it should be performed before transport and should be performed only under the direction of the receiving physician. Several principles should be remembered

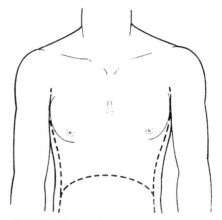

FIGURE 20-9   **Chest escharotomy sites.**

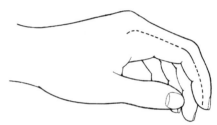

FIGURE 20-10   **Escharotomy site on the finger.**

in performing escharotomies. The procedures should be performed in as sterile an environment as possible to avoid seeding bacteria into already compromised tissue. The incisions should be made carefully and deep enough to penetrate the eschar and decompress the area without causing major bleeding in the zone of stasis because the tissue there is often too friable to maintain sutures.[12,17] When bleeding does occur, the appropriate treatment is direct pressure to the wound. The incisions should extend slightly beyond the constricted area for maximal effect. (See Box 20-1 for possible escharotomy sites.) Major vessels, nerves, tendons, ligaments, and joints should be avoided because future range of motion can be adversely affected. Results of the escharotomy should be carefully monitored. In most cases, relief of the constriction should be immediate.

Decompression is a more continual process with use of the least invasive methodology appropriate for the situation, including positioning, fluid management, ongoing clinical assessment, and incisions through eschar and superficial fascia only.[6]

BOX 20-1	**Possible Escharotomy Sites**

Chest

Anterior axillary incisions bilaterally joined with a
transverse incision along the costal margin (Figure
20-9).

Extremeties

Axially on medial or lateral aspect. If a single incision
is insufficient to relieve the constriction, then an
incision on both sides should be performed.

Elbow

Medial aspect anterior to the medial epicondyle.

Hand

Axially on the dorsum, between the tendons rather
than across them.

Fingers

Midlateral axial (Figure 20-10).

Ankle

Medial aspect anterior to medial malleolus.

Foot

Axially on the dorsum between the tendons rather
than across them.

For those burn patients who may not be transported until later in the disease process or those who may need long-distance transport to receive care, some debriding and dressings may be necessary. Mild soap and water may be used to clean simple burns. Blisters should be managed according to the burn center's wound care protocols.

When cleaning burns that are the result of contact with tar or asphalt, mixtures of cool water and mineral oil have been reported to be useful. The removal of these substances stops the burning process and helps decrease the patient's pain.[10,20]

PAIN MANAGEMENT

Burn pain varies depending on burn injury type and size. Factors that can affect burn pain include actual stimulation of nociceptors, fear of procedures, and anxiety regarding change in body image. Regardless of what types of medications are administered, they should all be given intravenously. The generalized edema during this time allows for only sporadic absorption of the medication if given intramuscularly. As fluid shifts reverse, a "dumping" and potential overdose of any medications that were given intramuscularly can occur.[12] The exception to this is a tetanus booster, which can be given intramuscularly.

For acute burn injury pain, opioids such as morphine are the analgesic of choice, particularly in conjunction with anxiolytic sedatives, such as benzodiazepines.[17,19,22] Adjunctive activity, such as diversion, guided imagery, and relaxation therapy, although of limited use during transport because of the distractions in transport vehicles, may be helpful during patient preparation.[19,22]

OTHER TRANSPORT CONSIDERATIONS

Electrocardiographic monitoring should be instituted on any patient with a large burn, an electrical injury, or preexisting heart disease.[8,10] Electrode patches may be a problem to place because the adhesive does not stick to burned skin. If alternate sites for placement cannot be found, an option for monitoring is to insert skin staples such as those used for wound closure and attach the monitor leads to them with alligator clips. This method provides a stable monitoring system, particularly for the agitated or restless patient who might displace needle electrodes. Burn electrodes that use needles attached to special cables for monitoring are available.

A urinary catheter with an urimeter should be placed to accurately monitor urinary output. As with intubation, the catheter should be inserted early, especially for the patient with perineal burns, because edema may make insertion impossible at a later time.

To combat the problem of adynamic ileus, the transport team should insert a gastric tube in all burn patients with significant burns to decompress the stomach. This process is especially important for the patient being transported at high altitudes.[10,12,17,20] Initial diagnostic studies should include hematocrit and electrolyte levels, urinalysis, chest radiograph, arterial blood gases with carboxyhemoglobin levels as indicated, and electrocardiography (ECG).

Accurate documentation of all treatment provided before and during transport of the burn patient is essential. This information provides the necessary history of the incident and its initial treatment to allow for consistent and quality planning of patient care at the receiving facility.

ELECTRICAL INJURY MANAGEMENT

As soon as the scene is secured and the patient is away from the current, primary and secondary assessment can proceed. Dysrhythmia should be treated with Advanced Cardiac Life Support (ACLS) algorithms or the transport program's individual protocols.

Cervical spine injury is of special concern for victims of electrical injury because of possible blunt trauma and because of severe tetanic contractions caused by the electrical current; therefore, the cervical spine must be immobilized.[8,10,20]

Initially, a minimum of two large-bore IVs with normal saline or lactated Ringer's solution should be started. Assessment of the area of surface burns is difficult because of the deep injury produced, and multiple liters of fluid may need to be infused.

Cervical and thoracic spine immobilization must be maintained. Adequate volume replacement, treatment of acidosis, and management of myoglobinuria must also be initiated. Fluid volume replacement formulae are not helpful with electrical injuries because of the deep tissue damage seen with the apparently mild cutaneous burns.

Higher rates of urinary output are essential to maintain because hemoglobinuria and myoglobinuria are common with electrical injuries.[8,10,18,20] The fluid resuscitation must be based on actual urine flow. A minimum of 50 to 100 mL/h of urine must be maintained; however, in the presence of urinary hemochromogen, the fluid volume must be of sufficient quantity to maintain a minimum output of 100 mL/h.[17,18]

Lactic acidosis is common because of the significant muscle damage caused by electrical injury. Sodium bicarbonate may be used to alkalinize the urine. Mannitol should be considered in the resuscitative phase to increase urinary output and to minimize acute tubular necrosis.[18]

LIGHTNING INJURY MANAGEMENT

Primary survey does not differ with the victim of a lightning strike. The patient's cardiopulmonary status must be assessed immediately, and CPR and intubation should be initiated on finding the patient in cardiac arrest. As with any unknown injury, the cervical spine must be immobilized before intubation and transport. The patient's cardiac status must be monitored continuously.[8,24]

Burns seen with lightning injuries are not as extensive as those seen with high-voltage injuries; therefore, massive amounts of fluids are not necessary unless the patient is in hypovolemic shock. Two IV lines should be established: one as a "keep open" line and one as a medication route. Observation and history taking must be performed with care to treat and transport these victims rapidly.[8,24]

CHEMICAL INJURY MANAGEMENT

Treatment of chemical injuries necessitates removal of all saturated clothing and a copious irrigation of the burn wound. In the patient with an otherwise stable condition, wound irrigation takes priority over transportation unless the irrigation can continue en route.[12] The transport team needs to ensure their safety and avoid placing a contaminated patient in a transport vehicle.

Dry chemicals such as lime should be brushed off before irrigation. Water and physiologic saline solution are the fluids of choice for wound irrigation. The time spent searching for a specific neutralizing agent may be more harmful than simply irrigation with water. The exogenous heat production by neutralization reaction can in itself cause further tissue destruction. In the treatment of chemical burns, the transport team must be aware of the possibility of exposure to the noxious agents and don appropriate protective gear before coming into contact with the patient or the patient's clothing.[10,20]

RADIATION INJURY MANAGEMENT

Radiation burns are treated like other kinds of burns. Any open wounds should be covered with gauze and fastened with an elastic bandage, never with adhesive. The focus beyond the lifesaving measures is to avoid contaminating the transport team and the transport vehicle. Gross contamination can be avoided with careful planning.[10,12,20]

EVALUATION

Evaluation of the burn patient consists primarily of assessment of the effectiveness of problem intervention and the recognition of future potential complications. Not all complications are, however, predictable or correctable.

Vital signs are not the most accurate method of monitoring a patient with a large burn because of the pathophysiologic changes that accompany such an injury. Blood pressure may be difficult to ascertain because of increasing generalized edema. An invasive monitoring device may not be accurate because of the peripheral vasoconstriction caused by release of vasoactive mediators such as catecholamines. Pulse may be somewhat more helpful in monitoring the appropriateness of fluid resuscitation.[4,10] Presence of more than a mild tachycardia or a persistent tachycardia is evidence of hypovolemia. However, even this can be confusing because tachycardia may be the result of pain and the stress response. The transport team should be careful not to overlook young, otherwise healthy adults whose normal resting heart rate may be in the 40-bpm to 60-bpm range or the elderly patient who may be taking medications, such as beta-blockers, that interfere with the normal physiologic responses. A heart rate of greater than 70 bpm may not indicate the underlying volume deficit for this type of patient.

A decrease in level of consciousness not associated with trauma may also be indicative of hypoxia or hypovolemia. This problem should be alleviated with appropriate adjustments in ventilatory and circulatory support. If the level of consciousness does not improve with increased hydration and oxygenation, other problem sources such as carbon monoxide poisoning or electrolyte imbalance should be suspected and investigated.[14,20]

Urinary output is perhaps the most accurate method of evaluation of the effectiveness of fluid replacement. Adults should have an hourly output of 30 to 50 mL.

The urinary output in children should be maintained at 1 to 1.5 mL/kg/h for children less than 30 kg. Oliguria is an indication of inadequate fluid volume and should be easily corrected by increasing the rate of fluid administration.[4,7,17] When this method is ineffective and fluid volume needs have been accurately assessed and administered, an osmotic diuretic such as mannitol can be given to avoid acute renal failure.

Myoglobinuria that occurs from the release of myoglobin after deep muscle damage can precipitate in the renal tubules and cause acute renal failure. This problem is especially common after electrical burns, and urine should be monitored in such cases for changes, such as to a dark tea color, that indicate the presence of myoglobin. Alkalinization of the urine through addition of bicarbonate to the IV fluids is done to prevent the myoglobin from progressing to its nephrotoxic metabolites. Diuresis through mannitol or loop diuretics also helps dilute the urine and flush the renal tubules.[18]

Pulmonary edema can occur from either overzealous fluid resuscitation or smoke inhalation, and the transport team should be careful to monitor respiratory function as fluid administration progresses. This problem is especially apparent when the transport of the burn patient has been delayed.[14]

Acidosis from the increased lactic acid production can occur and can be treated with sodium bicarbonate if increased fluid administration is ineffective.[17] Hyperkalemia from potassium released from the heat-damaged tissues can be reversed in several ways, including administration of sodium bicarbonate, glucose and insulin, or ion exchange resins. Hyponatremia from fluid replacement does not reflect a true sodium deficiency and seldom necessitates any type of treatment.[10] Hypoglycemia is a complication that frequently occurs with infants and young children because of their inability to maintain adequate glycogen stores. Blood glucose should be assessed frequently for pediatric patients. Intravenous fluids may be changed to lactated Ringer's solution with 5% dextrose if hypoglycemia becomes a problem.[7,10]

IMPACT OF TRANSPORT

For burn patients, two phases of transport usually occur. The first is the entry of the burn patient into the emergency medical services (EMS) system with transport from the scene of the incident to the initial care facility. The second phase is the interfacility transport of the stabilized patient from the initial care facility to a burn center or tertiary care center.

The increasing use of critical care ground and air medical services has had an impact on both phases of burn transport. In early transport, it has made a higher level of medical expertise more rapidly available to a larger service area, which has decreased the amount of time before assessment and resuscitation begins and enabled the critically injured patient to reach a definitive care facility quickly. In the second phase of transport, it has markedly decreased the amount of time spent out of a stable environment during transfer to a burn center.[2,21] A shift in the admission patterns for burn patients has been seen; increasingly, significant burn injuries are being transported to specialized burn care centers. These changes have had the combined effect of decreasing the morbidity and mortality rates of burn patients.[2,3,11]

The decision to transport to a burn center is made on the basis of the condition of the patient, the size of the burn, and, in the case of scene response, the distance to the burn center. Patients with concurrent traumatic injuries should first be evaluated at a trauma center if the traumatic injuries present the greatest immediate risk. If the burn injury is the greater risk to the patient and initial burn care can be facilitated en route, then transfer to a burn center may be appropriate. The American Burn Association has identified criteria for the transfer of burn patients to a burn center (Box 20-2).

SUMMARY

Burn and electrical injuries can present a major challenge to transport team members, but an orderly prioritized approach can greatly simplify

---

| BOX 20-2 | **Burn Unit Referral Criteria** |

1. Partial-thickness burns greater than 10% total body surface area (TBSA).
2. Burns that involve the face, hands, feet, genitalia, perineum, or major joints.
3. Third-degree burns in any age group.
4. Electrical burns, including lightning injury.
5. Chemical burns.
6. Inhalation injury.
7. Burn injury in patients with preexisting medical disorders that could complicate management, prolong recovery, or affect mortality.
8. Any patients with burns and concomitant trauma (such as fractures) in which the burn injury poses the greatest risk of morbidity or mortality. In such cases, if trauma poses the greater immediate risk, the patient may be stabilized initially in a trauma center transfer to a burn unit. Physician judgment is necessary in such situations and should be in concert with the regional medical control plan and triage protocols.
9. Burned children in hospitals without qualified personnel or equipment for the care of children.
10. Burn injury in patients who need special social, emotional, or long-term rehabilitative intervention.

Modified from American Burn Association: *Burn fact sheet, 2001*, available at www.Ameriburn.org/pub/factsheet.htm. Excerpted from Committee on Trauma, American College of Surgeons: *Guidelines for the operation of burn centers, resources for optimal care of the injured patient*, Chicago, 2006, ACS.

---

management. Patients may exhibit a wide spectrum of injuries from minor flesh burns to multiple traumas. Special burns such as chemical and electrical injuries have unique consequences that must be observed for early in management. The quality of treatment that the patient initially receives may determine the ultimate level of rehabilitation. A clear understanding of the pathophysiology of burn injuries is essential in providing quality burn care. Assessment and also underlying principles of intervention and resuscitation rely on this knowledge base. Transportation of these patients to an appropriate hospital and early involvement of a burn care specialist are invaluable.

CASE STUDY 1

15:00. Transport team received a request to respond to the scene of a minor methamphetamine laboratory explosion. EMS was assessing the patient while the local volunteer fire department (FD) was preparing the landing zone.

15:30. Contact was made with the landing zone (LZ) officer, and after checking for hazards, the aircraft landed safely near the scene of the explosion. The transport team was directed to the ambulance.

15:32. Report from EMS: A 23-year-old man was manipulating his methamphetamine laboratory apparatus when it exploded, causing burns to his upper body. The patient was found to have a large partial-thickness thermal burn injury covering his face, upper torso, arms, and legs. He was responding to painful stimuli only and had labored respirations. An acrid odor was on the patient's clothing, which was still in the ambulance. The patient was irrigated by EMS to avoid a risk of contamination with the anhydrous ammonia the patient had been working with, and he was covered with a clean dry sheet. Medical history included a long-standing history of IV substance abuse. Initial vital signs were pulse 132, respirations shallow at 40, and blood pressure (BP) 90/60 mmHg.

PRIMARY ASSESSMENT

Airway/Breathing

The patient had superficial partial-thickness burns on his face. His airway was moist and red, with blisters around his mouth. The transport team elected to intubate him because of his altered mental status and potential airway injury. His ventilations were assisted with 100% oxygen via bag-valve. Airway management was accomplished with c-spine immobilization in place.

Circulation

The patient had a rapid carotid pulse. His peripheral pulses were difficult to palpate because of his burn injury. The patient had one large-bore antecubital IV initiated.

Disability

After intubation and oxygenation, the patient was still responding only to painful stimuli. The transport team elected to load and go and complete the secondary assessment and additional interventions en route. The patient was covered with blanket during packaging to prevent hypothermia.

15:40. The patient was secured to the transport stretcher and was loaded in the aircraft for a 10-minute transport to the burn center.

15:44. En route, the transport team completed a brief secondary survey. The burn injury was estimated to be approximately 30% TBSA partial-thickness burns. Multiple small cuts from the shrapnel in the explosion were noted on the patient's face, arms, and torso. The patient weight was estimated at 65 kg. The transport team was unable to initiate a second IV line because of the poor state of the patient's veins. IV fluid resuscitation was managed through the existing IV.

Cardiac electrodes were applied to the patient's shoulders and waist to avoid the upper torso burns. Pulse oximetry was used, and the patient maintained saturations of 100% throughout the flight. Capnography was also used, and $EtCO_2$ levels were maintained between 30 and 34. Vital signs were pulse 112 and regular; and BP was 110/60. Morphine sulfate 10 mg was administered for pain.

15:48. Report was called to the burn center.

15:50. The patient was taken directly to the emergency department (ED) for assessment and treatment of both burn and soft-tissue injuries.

CASE STUDY 2

06:15. A 48-year-old man working at a rural pulp mill was walking across the crusted top of a lime slurry pit when the crust gave way and he was submerged in hot lime slurry to the hips; he incurred extensive thermal and chemical burns. Primary care given en route from the pulp mill included thorough irrigation of the lime slurry and administration of oxygen by the first responders. The transport team from the small regional facility was organized to transport the patient to the tertiary care center.

07:00. The transport team met the first responders at the regional treatment facility. Primary assessment revealed no problems with airway or breathing. Oxygen was administered at 15 LPM via NRB FM. Two large-bore IVs of NS were initiated in the patient's right arm. The patient was assessed as having approximately 50% BSA deep partial-thickness burns that were well irrigated. The patient had significant pain and was calling out during transfer to the transport stretcher. A Foley catheter was inserted to monitor urine output. No other injuries were noted.

07:20. The patient was loaded into the ground ambulance for the 1.5-hour journey to the tertiary care center and covered with a clean dry sheet and blankets to minimize heat loss during transport. En route, the transport team calculated burn size and fluid resuscitation requirements. The patient continued to have pain, and fentanyl and versed were ordered by the receiving physician for control of pain and anxiety. Urine output was monitored to evaluate effectiveness of end organ perfusion.

08:45. Report was called to the tertiary care facility, and the patient was delivered to the tertiary care center.

REFERENCES

1. Ahrns KS: Trends in burn resuscitation: shifting the focus from fluids to adequate endpoint monitoring, edema control, and adjuvant therapies, *Crit Care Nurs Clin North Am* 16(1):75-98, 2004.
2. American Burn Association: *Burn incidence and treatment in the US: 2007 fact sheet.* Available at http://www.ameriburn.org/resources_factsheet.php?PHPSESSID=4ac9a48b851c5293006c7ce6559aeb8c
3. American Burn Association: *National Burn Repository 2007 report dataset version 4.0.* Available at http://www.ameriburn.org/2007NBRAnnualReport.pdf
4. Arlati A, Storti E, Pradella V, et al: Decreased fluid volume to reduce organ damage: a new approach to burn shock resuscitation? A preliminary study, *Resuscitation* 72(3):371-378, 2007.
5. Boldt J, Papsdor M: Fluid management in burn patients: results from a European survey: more questions than answers, *Burns* doi:10.1016/j.burns.2007.09.005, 2008.
6. Burd A, Noronha FV, Ahmed K, et al: Decompression not escharotomy in acute burns, *Burns* doi:10.1016/j.burns.2005.11.017, 2006.
7. Carvajal HF: Fluid resuscitation of pediatric burn victims: a critical appraisal, *Pediatr Nephrol* 8(3):357-366, 1994.
8. Dega S, Gnaneswar SG, Rao PR, et al: Electrical burn injuries: some unusual clinical situations and management, *Burns* doi:10.1016/j.burns.2006/09.008, 2007.
9. Desai MH, Mlcak R, Richardson J, et al: Reduction in mortality in pediatric patients with inhalation injury with aerosolized heparin/N-acetylcystine therapy, *J Burn Care Rehabil* 19(3), 1998.
10. DeSanti L: Pathophysiology and current management of burn injury, *Adv Skin Wound Care* 18(6):323-332, 2005.
11. Edelman LS: Social and economic factors associated with the risk of burn injury, *Burns* 33(9):58-65, 2007.
12. Emergency Nurses Association: *Trauma nursing core course provider manual*, Park Ridge, IL, 2000, The Association.
13. Hettiaratchy S, Dziewulski P: Pathophysiology and types of burns, *Br Med J* 328:1427-1429, doi:10.1136/bmj.7453.1427, 2004.
14. Irrazabal CL, Capdevila AA, Revich L, et al: Early and late complications among 15 victims exposed to indoor fire and smoke inhalation, *Burns* doi:10.1016/j.burns.2007.06.025, 2008.
15. Malic CC, Karoo ROS, Austin O, et al: Resuscitation burn card: a useful tool for burn injury assessment, *Burns* 33:195-199, 2007.
16. Mlcak RP, Suman OE, Herndon DN: Respiratory management of inhalation injury, *Burns* doi:10.1015/j.burns.2006.07.007, 2008.
17. Newberry L: *Sheehy's emergency nursing: principles and practice*, ed 5, St Louis, 2003, Mosby.
18. Okafor UV: Lightning injuries and acute renal failure: a review, *Renal Failure* 27:129-134, doi:10.1081/JDI-200048216, 2005.
19. Patterson DR, Hoflund H, Espey K, et al: Pain management, *Burns* 30(8):A10-A15, doi:10.1016/j.burns.2004.08.004, 2004.
20. Regojo PS: Burn care basics, *Nursing* 33(3):50-53, 2003.

21. Shewakramani S: Adequacy of fluid resuscitation during transport of burn patients, *Ann Emerg Med* 48:4, 2006.

22. Summer GJ, Puntillo KA, Miaskowski C, et al: Burn injury pain: the continuing challenge, *J Pain* 8(7): 533-548, 2007.

23. World Health Organization: *International Society for Burns information sheet*. Available at http://www.ameriburn.org/WHO-ISBIBurnFactsheet.pdf

24. Wright RK: *Electrical burns*. Available at http://www.emedicine.com/EMERG/topic 162.htm

25. Yoshiro I, et al: Assessment of burn area: most objective method, *Burns* doi:19.1016/j.burns.2007.06.018, 2007.

Medical Problems

NEUROLOGIC EMERGENCIES

Katherine Logee

COMPETENCIES

1. Describe neurologic pathophysiology in terms of pressure-volume relationships and the components of the cerebral vault.
2. Perform a focused neurologic examination.
3. Describe common neurologic emergencies encountered in the transport environment in terms of pathology and management strategies.

Neurologic illness or injury is a common reason for air medical transport because of its potentially disabling or fatal consequences. The transport team is instrumental in assessing and determining the need for intervention on the basis of expert knowledge of the physiology of neurologic pathologies and how they relate to air medical transport. The two priorities of the air medical crew are effective management of those secondary injuries and rapid transport to an acute care facility.

NEUROLOGIC PATHOPHYSIOLOGY

A basic understanding of neuropathophysiology assists with the ability to critically think through management of patients with neurologic insults. We examine pressure-volume relationships and the volumetric components (cerebrospinal fluid [CSF], blood, and brain) of the neurologic system to gain an understanding of how changes in each of these components affect intracranial pressure (ICP), maintenance of ICP, alterations in ICP, and management of ICP changes.

PRESSURE-VOLUME RELATIONSHIPS

The main components of volume in the skull are the brain (1400 mL), blood (1400 mL), and CSF (150 mL). The latter two drain into the dural sinuses. In healthy individuals, venous pressure is the main determinant of ICP. However, any increase in the volume of one of these components without a corresponding decrease in the volume of the other two results in raised ICP.[20,27,33,39,45] Alteration in ICP is the prime concern in the care of patients with neurologic emergencies.[18,24,27,34,36]

How the volumes of CSF, blood, and brain maintain a relatively constant ICP is described by the *Monroe-Kellie hypothesis*. The Monroe-Kellie hypothesis states that the cranial compartment is incompressible and that the volume inside the cranium is a fixed volume. The cranium and its constituents (blood, CSF, and brain tissue) create a state of volume equilibrium such that any increase in volume of one of the cranial constituents must be compensated by a decrease in volume of another (Figure 21-1).

Because brain volume changes little (and when it does, it involves mainly interstitial water), most normal variations occur in the volumes of CSF and blood.[20,27,33,39]

The two principle factors that affect cerebral blood flow are the cerebral perfusion pressure (CPP) and the brain's autoregulatory system. *Cerebral perfusion pressure* is equal to the mean arterial pressure (MAP) minus the intercerebral pressure (ICP) or the central venous pressure, whichever is higher.

$$CPP = MAP - ICP$$

$$MAP = DBP + (SBP - DBP)/3$$

The *native autoregulatory system* refers to the brain's ability to keep the cerebral blood flow at a

$$K \sim V_{CSF} + V_{Blood} + V_{Brain}$$

FIGURE 21-1   **Modified Monroe-Kellie hypothesis.**

relatively constant level over a wide range of cerebral perfusion pressure, which is accomplished by varying the resistance in the precapillary arterioles.[36] A CPP greater than or equal to 70 mm Hg ensures adequate cerebral perfusion; ICP is normally 5 to 20 cm H_2O or 3 to 15 mm Hg. Constant cerebral blood flow is obtained with MAPs from 50 to 150 mm Hg, but these values may be higher in patients with chronic hypertension. At the low end of this curve (see Figure 21-2 and 21-3), CPP drops and cerebral hypoperfusion ensues; however, at the high end of the curve, cerebral hyperperfusion with cerebral edema occurs. In disease states, the curve becomes linear and the CPP approximates the CBF because of the loss of vessel autoregulation. Elevation of ICP or decrease in MAP results in cerebral hypoperfusion.[40,45]

To understand the ability of the intracranial components to compensate for the development of a mass (thinking of the combined volume of cerebral edema as mass is helpful), a look at the pressure-volume curve is useful (Figure 21-2).[20,27,39,41] As a change in volume of mass occurs, at first, no change in ICP occurs. This phenomenon is the result of compliance and is accomplished by reduction in volume

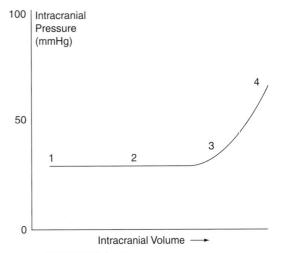

FIGURE 21-2   **Pressure-volume curve.**

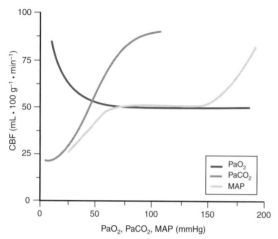

FIGURE 21-3   **Changes in cerebral blood flow (CBF) caused by independent alterations in PaCO$_2$, PaO$_2$, and mean arterial pressure (MAP).** (From Piyush M, Patel PM, Drummond JC: Cerebral physiology and the effects of anesthetics and techniques. In Miller RD: *Miller's anesthesia*, ed 6, Philadelphia, 2005, Churchill Livingstone.)

of CSF and blood. At some point, however, compliance is lost, and additional changes in volume result in great increases in ICP. In the acute state of cerebral edema, or a rapidly developing intracranial, the total shifts in volume amount to approximately 50 to 75 mL.[20,32,39,43,44,46]

Once the sutures and fontanelles close during childhood (by 18 months of age), the skull becomes a nondistensible structure. When a space-occupying lesion develops (whether that is a buildup of CSF, blood, or even a tumor), a reduction in the volumes of one or more compartments of the brain must occur for ICP to stay constant. The viscoelastic properties of the brain are such that if a mass, such as a growing tumor, exerts slowly increasing pressure, the brain may compensate through the slow loss of water or cellular elements through atrophy. However, with acute changes in the size of a mass, such as in an acute epidural hematoma, the brain is relatively noncompressible.

CEREBROSPINAL FLUID VOLUME

The volume of CSF is controlled by the rate of production and the rate of absorption of CSF. Production, except in the presence of very high ICP,

remains relatively constant in the adult at about 0.35 mL/min. CSF is actively secreted by the choroid plexus in the lateral, third, and fourth ventricles. CSF leaves the ventricular system, circulates throughout the subarachnoid space, and finally reaches the subarachnoid space overlying the cerebral convexities. Here, the CSF is absorbed passively by way of the arachnoid granulations located parasagittally along the sagittal sinus. The fluid passes through the structures of the granulation into the cerebral venous system and is carried away with venous blood.[26,34]

Absorption is pressure driven. The rate of CSF absorption is proportional to the ICP. CSF volume can be pathologically increased by an interference with absorption.[12,30,38] This increase can be caused by a mass or stricture in the ventricular system that prevents the CSF from exiting into the subarachnoid space. This accumulation of CSF is termed obstructive or *noncommunicating hydrocephalus*.[12,36]

Alternatively, after the CSF leaves the ventricular system, its circulation may be disturbed so that the fluid cannot reach the arachnoid granulation, resulting in *communicating* or *nonobstructive hydrocephalus*. Given that the subarachnoid space is so large, a focal lesion such as a tumor ordinarily does not produce this type of obstruction. Instead, a widespread disorder such as inflammation of the meninges or increased CSF protein results from such an obstruction.[35]

CEREBRAL BLOOD VOLUME

Cerebral blood volume comprises two relatively independent components: the arterial blood volume and the venous blood volume. Arterial blood volume accounts for approximately 25% of the total cerebral blood volume; venous blood volume accounts for the other 75%.[27,28,34]

Arterial cerebral blood flow (and volume) under normal circumstances remains relatively independent of systemic mean arterial blood volume and pressure through a process called *autoregulation*. Autoregulation is influenced by pressure and biochemical parameters.[2,3,23,27] As mean systemic arterial pressure increases, cerebral arterial blood vessels constrict, preventing the increase in blood volume and flow that normally occurs. If the mean systemic arterial blood pressure decreases, the cerebral arteries dilate, increasing cerebral blood flow. Alternatively stated, the blood flow is directly proportional to the perfusion pressure and inversely proportional to the total resistance of the system. Cerebral blood flow is maintained in a constant state between a mean systemic arterial pressure of approximately 60 and 140 mm Hg. Normal blood flow to the cerebral cortex averages 50 mL of blood flow/100 g of brain tissue (expressed as mL/100 g/min).[33] At perfusion less than 20 mL/100 g/min, neuronal cell membranes become impaired, which results in neurologic dysfunction. Despite this impairment, if the blood flow is restored, this damage is reversible. At perfusion flow less than 10 mL/100 g/min, the neuronal tissue rapidly becomes irreversibly damaged. In a no-flow state, cell death occurs within minutes.[33]

Arterial blood volume is also influenced by complex biochemical or metabolic action that can be summarized by the association of PaO_2, $PaCO_2$, and cerebral blood flow.

Increased $PaCO_2$ or decreased PaO_2 results in dilation of the blood vessel, presumably in response to greater cerebral metabolic needs.[27,29,46] As $PaCO_2$ decreases, blood volume and flow are reduced. Thus, this component of autoregulation may be influenced by respiratory control, with hyperventilation resulting in decreased cerebral blood flow and hypoventilation resulting in increased cerebral blood flow.[1,2,27] Venous blood volume is passively influenced by the delivery of blood from the arterial side and the ability of the cerebral venous system to drain from the head. This drainage depends on two influences: hydrostatic pressure and central venous pressure. Elevation of the head increases hydrostatic pressure on the venous side, permitting more rapid drainage from the cerebral venous system, mainly through the internal jugular veins bilaterally. Increased central venous pressure, whether caused by increased intrathoracic pressure or by right heart failure, decreases cerebral venous return.[2,13,27]

Respiratory management can greatly influence the volume of cerebral venous blood. If intrathoracic pressure is increasing because, for example, the patient is straining on an endotracheal tube that is blocked, a decrease in cerebral venous drainage (and thus an increase in cerebral venous blood volume) occurs.[27]

BRAIN VOLUME

Brain volume, except for a relatively insignificant alteration in interstitial water, does not change under ordinary circumstances. However, with injury, cerebral brain water may accumulate in the form of cerebral edema. An accumulation of water can be found in the intracellular space, extracellular space, or both. The three types of cerebral edema are: vasogenic, cytotoxic, and interstitial edema.

Vasogenic edema is an extracellular edema of the white matter that results from increased capillary permeability as a result of the widening of tight junctions and increases in pinocytotic vesicles at the level blood-brain barrier.[21] Vasogenic edema is seen locally around brain tumors, although it can develop around a cerebral infarct or a cerebral abscess as well. Generalized vasogenic edema occurs with cerebral trauma or meningitis.[16,21]

Cytotoxic edema is an increase in fluid in the neurons, glia, and endothelial cells as a result of ATP-dependent sodium-potassium pump failure so that fluid and sodium accumulate within the cell, leading to diffuse brain swelling. Development of cytotoxic edema is associated with a hypoxic or anoxic episode, such as a cardiac arrest or asphyxiation. It is also seen with hypoosmolarity conditions, such as water intoxication, hyponatremia, and the syndrome of inappropriate secretion of antidiuretic hormone.[21]

Interstitial edema occurs with hydrocephalus. The edema is found in the periventricular white matter when the intraventricular pressure is greater than the ability of the ependymal cells to contain the CSF within the ventricle.[21]

NEUROLOGIC EXAMINATION

A focused comprehensive neurologic assessment of the patient to be transported is important. After completion of a primary assessment, chief symptoms, history of present illness (including onset, duration, and sequence of symptoms), and medical history should be obtained. Box 21-1 contains a useful mnemonic for the differential diagnosis of an unconscious patient. Each of these items should be considered when identifying the etiology of an unconscious state. The examination itself should be conducted in a systematic, hierarchic, stepwise approach that

BOX 21-1	**Mnemonic for the Differential Diagnosis of Coma**

U Units of insulin
N Narcotics
C Convulsions
O Oxygen
N Nonorganic
S Stroke
C Cocktail
I ICP
O Organism
U Urea
S Shock

proceeds from the highest level of function (cerebral cortex) to the lowest level of function (reflexes). The cranial nerves, motor system, and reflexes should be assessed as well. In many cases, serial focused neurologic examinations are necessary for appropriate and timely interventions.

The focused neurologic assessment begins with obtaining vital signs and performing a general inspection of the patient. A rapid assessment of the patient's mental status should be made. Is the patient awake? Can the patient talk? Can the patient answer questions appropriately? Can the patient protect the airway? A complete mental status examination focuses on the following areas: awareness and mental function; and reception and interpretation of sensory stimuli, including an awareness and responsiveness to self, to the environment, and to the impressions made by the senses, and of cognitive function.[21]

There are 12 pairs of cranial nerves (a pair consists of a right and left nerve). Each nerve (right and left) must be evaluated separately to completely identify the extent of dysfunction that may be unilateral. Findings are compared for symmetry. As a brief review, cranial nerve (CN) I is the olfactory nerve. Testing of this nerve is often times deferred, unless an anterior fossa mass is suspected. CN II is the only nerve that can be examined directly. Testing encompasses an evaluation of visual acuity, visual fields, and an ophthalmoscopic examination.

An ophthalmoscopic examination is rarely completed in the transport environment because of the need to balance a comprehensive examination with a rapid transport and relatively short bedside time. CNs III, IV, and VI are all tested together because all three supply the extraocular eye muscles. CN V is composed of both sensory and motor components. Sensation on the face is tested here as is masseter and temporal muscle strength (clench/open jaw). CN VII is the facial nerve. This nerve also has both sensory and motor components. The sensory component includes the sense of taste on the anterior two thirds of the tongue. The motor component is tested by observing symmetry of the face at rest and during deliberate facial movements. CN VIII, also called the acoustic nerve, is a pure sensory nerve. Testing of this nerve involves the use of a tuning fork to test air and bone conduction. CNs IV and X are tested together because of their intimate association of function in the pharynx. Having the patient open the mouth and say "ah" allows visualization of the uvula for midline location and voice quality analysis and also allows for the testing for the presence of a gag reflex. CN XI is the spinal accessory nerve and is tested by having the patient shrug the shoulders against resistance and by having the patient turn the head to the side against resistance. Finally, CN XII is the hypoglossal nerve. Testing this nerve involves having the patient protrude the tongue and move it tongue from side to side. Clinical judgment must be used when deciding whether or not a judicious use of time involves performing a complete or partial cranial nerve assessment. This decision is based on the type of patient being transported and the agency's standing medical orders.

The next part of the neurologic examination is the motor system examination. The neck, upper limbs, trunk, and finally, the lower extremities should be examined (in that order). Generally speaking, muscle size, tone, and strength are examined.

The sensory system is examined next and is done with the patient's eyes closed. This portion of the examination is not generally included in a standard neurologic examination unless numbness, pain, trophic changes, or other sensory abnormalities are present.[21] Superficial, deep, and discriminative sensations are tested.[37]

The cerebellar system is tested by beginning with a finger-to-nose test. If this test is completed successfully, a further examination of upper extremity coordination is not necessary. Lower extremities are tested by having the patient draw a figure 8 on the opposite leg. Balance is also tested as part of the cerebellar assessment. This test is rarely indicated (or even advised) in the transport environment.

The final portion of the neurologic assessment involves the testing of reflexes. Knowledge of how to test reflexes in both the upper and the lower extremities is useful because many transport vehicles limit patient access to the lower extremities. Reflex testing involves muscle-stretch reflexes, superficial reflexes, and pathologic reflexes. Testing of reflexes is a routine part of the examination of a patient with acute spinal cord injury.

NEUROLOGIC EMERGENCIES

In treatment of a patient with a neurovascular emergency, maintaining a blood pressure adequate enough to perfuse the brain tissue, while ensuring that the pressure is not so high as to cause injury to the vascular beds in the brain, is imperative. Factors that must be considered when determining the target blood pressure include the type of neurovascular emergency, the level of hypertension that exists, the patient's blood pressure history, and the perceived condition of the patient's native autoregulatory system.[33] If the CPP is allowed to drop below the limits of autoregulation, ischemic damage may result. If the CPP is above the upper limit, then autoregulatory breakthrough occurs, leading to increased intracranial blood volume, increased intracranial pressure, and vasogenic edema. In addition, each type of neurologic emergency can have a significant impact on cerebral blood flow in its own unique way.

STROKE

The first type of neurologic emergency that we examine results from an interference with cerebral blood flow that causes ischemia of brain tissue. This interference of cerebral blood flow is also known as a *stroke* or *brain attack*. Atherosclerosis and hypertension lead to approximately half a million strokes annually; approximately 150,000 of those victims survive. According to the American Heart Association, stroke is the leading cause of permanent disability in adults. Approximately 700,000 individuals have a stroke each year in the United States.[10] The need to view stroke as a medical emergency is imperative to improving the outcome of stroke victims. A transport service, particularly air medical transport, is essential for providing rapid transport of the stroke patient to a tertiary care center where screening procedures such as computed tomographic (CT) scan, angiography, endovascular techniques, and intraarterial thrombolytic therapy are available as deemed necessary.[10,12,20]

Regardless of the underlying cause, a cerebrovascular episode that necessitates transport is frequently abrupt in onset and dynamic in progression. Treatment is directed at life-sustaining intervention, with an emphasis on prevention of extension of injury. Prognosis varies depending on the extent of involvement and the affected area of the brain. Recovery may be maximized by the prevention of additional cerebral insult through aggressive airway and cardiovascular support.[10,15,23,24,30]

A knowledge of normal cerebral circulation aids in the understanding of the pathophysiology of cerebrovascular disease. The importance of avoiding hypoxia has been discussed. Because the brain cannot store glucose, this substance must be constantly supplied in the blood flow. Critical reductions in glucose that result from hypoglycemia or decreased perfusion can cause irreversible cellular damage.

The brain receives its blood from two sets of vessels. Two common carotid arteries in the anterior neck bifurcate, each into an external carotid artery that supplies primarily facial tissue and the internal carotid arteries that provide most of the blood supply to the brain through its major subdivisions, the anterior cerebral and the middle cerebral arteries. In the posterior aspect of the neck on either side lie the vertebral arteries. These combine shortly after they pass through the foramen magnum into the single basilar artery, which mainly supplies the brain stem. The posterior cerebral arteries from the vertebral basilar system communicate through two posterior communicating arteries with the internal carotid arteries. A small anterior artery permits communication between the two anterior cerebral arteries.

Thus, at the base of the brain, a significant collateral circulation called the circle of Willis is formed where blood can flow as needed from one internal carotid system to the opposite internal carotid system, or to the vertebral basilar system, or to any combination of connections between the internal carotid systems and the vertebral basilar system.[2,17,26]

In addition, extensive collateral vessels may develop between the external carotid system and the internal carotid system. These collaterals are supplied mainly through facial anastomoses by way of the ophthalmic artery and through anastomoses between scalp vessels and vessels of the dura and arachnoid, called leptomeningeal vessels. Beyond this, however, in the depths of the brain, no collaterals assist deficient circulation. Therefore, occlusion of smaller vessels from the surface of the brain inward results in ischemia and infarction.[2]

The most common cause of vascular occlusion, resulting in the classic appearance of a stroke, is an embolus from some other part of the vascular system. Approximately one third of these emboli (especially in older persons) come from disease in the heart. Previous myocardial infarctions or valvular diseases may result in the development of mural thrombi, which are the source of emboli. In the great vessels a common location for thrombi formation is the bifurcation of the common carotid into the internal and external carotid. Disease at this location can often be detected with the auscultation of a bruit over the carotid bifurcation at the border of the involved sternocleidomastoid muscle just at the level of the angle of the mandible.[6,28] Auscultation must be performed carefully to prevent the dislodging of thrombi in the underlying vessel.

The next most common cause of cerebral ischemia is spontaneous intracerebral hemorrhage from cerebral aneurysms or arteriovenous malformations; that of accompanying hypertension is the most prevalent. As a result of this hemorrhage, the first vascular response is to contract and constrict to control hemorrhage in the region of the vascular injury. Second, as the hematoma develops in the brain tissue, the mass effect can place significant pressure on the distal arterioles, and capillary blood pressure becomes relatively low. Approximately 85% of hemorrhagic cases involve the cerebral hemispheres,

and only a relatively small number occurs in the cerebellum and brain stem as a result of involvement of the vertebral basilar system. In the case of hemorrhage in the cerebellum, the fourth ventricle may be acutely obstructed by the hematoma, resulting in sudden increase in ICP caused by impeded CSF flow. This increase is managed by the neurosurgeon with ventriculostomy drainage.[4,23,25,26]

In the extremely rare instance when a patient with such a condition is transferred, the neurosurgeon should be consulted on a case-by-case basis with regard to the care of the ventriculostomy or any other implanted device to monitor ICP before transport.[24,34]

A small subset of hemorrhagic cases involves the rupture of intracranial aneurysms into the subarachnoid space. This subarachnoid hemorrhage, besides causing primary brain injury, may result in cerebral ischemia caused by cerebral vasospasm. Little is found to distinguish this condition from other strokes except the symptom of severe, often focal, headache just before the hemorrhage.[5,7,9-11,33]

The use of crack cocaine has not only been implicated as a cause of intracranial hemorrhage but has been associated with acute intracranial arterial occlusive disease.[17]

Assessment

The transport team can be of help in the initial management of the patient who has had a stroke by performing a directed neurologic assessment once the patient's condition has been stabilized. Several stroke scales are available, including the Cincinnati Prehospital Stroke Scale, the Los Angeles Prehospital Stroke Scale, and the NIH Stroke Scale, that offer a framework for the evaluation of the stroke patient. These scales also assist in patient evaluation when specific therapies such as the administration of fibrinolytics have begun before transport.[10]

Plan and Implementation

A clear relationship between the duration of ischemia and the level of residual blood flow exists that differentiates tissue that is salvageable and that will die.[33] The American Stroke Association's most recent guidelines on the management of ischemic stroke state that the optimal management for the arterial hypertension seen after stroke has not yet been established.[33] Therefore, treatment decisions must be made on a case-by-case basis. Aggressive lowering of blood pressure in these patients has been shown to cause a reduction in the area of ischemia, which may expand the region of infarction.[33] Current recommendations support the lowering of blood pressure in patients with acute ischemic stroke who are candidates for fibrinolytic therapy, but even in this case, blood pressure lowering must be done cautiously. The agent of choice for lowering blood pressure must be easily titratable to avoid erratic or precipitous declines in blood pressure and ideally has a minimal vasodilatory effect on the cerebral vessels to avoid increasing ICP. Some examples of agents with these properties include nicardipine hydrochloride, labetalol, and esmolol.[33]

An intracerebral hemorrhage behaves like any mass lesion and causes an increase in ICP, thus decreasing CPP unless the MAP is also increased. Multiple studies of intracerebral hemorrhage (ICH) document a correlation between elevated blood pressure at presentation and poor outcomes.[33] Studies have also shown that hematoma growth in ICH may worsen outcomes.[33] Thus, if blood pressure is reduced, poor outcomes could be decreased. Little evidence directly supports this conclusion, however. In fact, one study found that the more rapid the decline in MAP over the first 24 hours, the higher the mortality rate.[33] Therefore, if blood pressure is lowered in patients with ICH, it must be done with extreme caution. Current guidelines suggest that MAPs in the setting of ICH should be maintained at or below 110 to 130 mm Hg. In all cases, the CPP should be maintained above 70 mm Hg.[33] Once the decision has been made to therapeutically lower blood pressure, agents that are used should be titratable and have minimal cardiovascular side effects (such as esmolol, labetalol, and nicardipine hydrochloride).

Current American College of Emergency Physicians (ACEP) guidelines do not support the use of nitroprusside for blood pressure control in patients with neurologic compromise with hypertension. Sodium nitroprusside is a potent vascular smooth muscle relaxant that makes the drug useful in lowering blood pressure. It is exactly this property, however, that makes the drug potentially less attractive for cases of hypertensive neurologic emergencies. Of great concern in this setting is the significant potential for this agent to not only reduce systemic blood pressure via relaxation of vascular smooth muscle but also to cause significant increases in intracranial pressure from dilation of the intracranial vasculature via the same mechanism.[33]

Evaluation

Evaluation of the success of interventions performed before transport may include assessment of a patient's neurologic status for either reperfusion or hemorrhage after fibrinolytic therapy. Evaluation of the effectiveness of interventions performed during transport include closely monitoring the neurologic status of the patient for changes in condition and performing the necessary interventions in a timely manner to minimize the neuronal injury and death for the patient.

SEIZURES

The annual incidence rate of *seizure* is estimated to be approximately 0.5% of the population (48 per 100,000) in the United States. The incidence rate is greater among males, particularly after the age of 20 years,[3,15,31] which may be to the result of a higher incidence rate of head injury with subsequent seizure activity. The highest incidence rate, however, is among children younger than 5 years (152 per 100,000 population annually). Overall, 650 per 100,000 of this population are affected by seizure activity in the United States. The prevalence rate is relatively constant between the ages of 10 and 60 years.[3,15,24]

The onset of epileptic seizures is associated with several types of generalized and focal brain lesions. The underlying neuropathophysiologic disturbances, however, are poorly understood. Although the belief is reasonable that an alteration exists in the neuronal pool or in the extracellular environment (both general theories have their advocates), neither laboratory investigations nor clinical experience with specific antiepileptic drugs have yielded a common therapy.[3,19]

Similar-appearing epileptic syndromes, however, are known to occur, caused by focal lesions such as brain tumors, arteriovenous malformations, stroke, and generalized states such as head trauma and viral or metabolic encephalopathies. In addition, in some idiopathic epilepsy syndromes, no obvious underlying cause is apparent. With more sophisticated recording techniques, several idiopathic epileptic syndromes are being associated with the presence of focal lesions, such as occult infarcts or sclerosis after birth trauma.[14,17,19]

Some patients present with *status epilepticus.* Traditionally, status epilepticus is defined as 30 minutes of continuous seizure activity or a series of seizures without return to full consciousness between the seizures. Many believe that a shorter period of seizure activity causes neuronal injury and that seizure self termination is unlikely after 5 minutes; some suggest times as brief as 5 minutes to define status epilepticus. In any case, these patients are considered to have true neurologic emergencies because of the neuronal injury that results.

Neuronal ischemic changes were once thought to be caused by decreased respiratory effort. They are theorized to occur in combination with ictal events and include a marked increase in metabolic rate and membrane changes that affect the transport of small ions at the neuronal level.[17,34]

Assessment

Several classification schemes for epilepsy have been proposed. The one with the most current widespread acceptance is from the International League Against Epilepsy,[3,32] which characterizes the syndromes as: (1) partial seizures that begin locally and may or may not spread generally; (2) generalized seizures that begin bilaterally and are symmetrical; (3) a large group of unclassified poorly understood syndromes; and (4) status epilepticus.

The same assessment criteria should be used regardless of the classification of seizure activity exhibited. The assessment criteria should include a thorough history, physical examination, and neurologic evaluation. The onset, type, and duration of seizure activity should be determined from the history. Additional pertinent information includes allergies, medications, cardiac problems, family history, recent illness, or injury.

In the physical examination, the airway is always of primary importance. The examiner must be alert to signs of trauma that may have occurred before or concurrent with the seizure activity. The physical assessment should then include motor, sensory, and psychomotor evaluation. The degree of involvement of these areas depends on the individual patient presentation. Involvement may range from isolated focal activity to generalized status involvement.[3,6,34]

Regardless of the level of involvement, motor activity during epileptic seizures is involuntary. Motor activity varies greatly depending on the type and neural focus of the seizure. In generalized tonic-clonic seizures, movement begins with the tonic phase, a continuous tense muscular state. This phase is followed by a hypertonic phase with hypertension and muscle rigidity. The clonic phase is characterized by rapidly alternating muscle rigidity and relaxation. During the clonic phase, sphincter control can be lost and the patient may be incontinent. Tachycardia, hyperventilation, and salivation result from autonomic discharge during seizure activity. Sensory assessment is subjective because the patient's symptoms may include visual, auditory, or proprioceptive phenomena. Psychomotor assessment is the determination of the level of consciousness, which may vary widely depending on the type of seizure activity and the time of evaluation. Other psychomotor observations include amnesia and repetitive behavioral patterns.[11,19,34] A few additional examples of seizure presentation include staring spells, a loss of motor control, blinking, lip smacking, and cycling extremity movements.

Plan and Implementation

A plan of care for the patient with seizure who needs transport includes rapid thorough assessment, appropriate interventions, and safe transfer to tertiary care.

Implementation of the plan involves management of the airway for prevention of hypoxia, support of the cardiovascular system, control of the seizure activity, and protection of the patient from physical injuries and additional complications associated with the seizure activity. Management of the underlying illness or injury that predisposed the patient to seizures may also be necessary.

Seizure management in the transport setting generally involves the use of a benzodiazepine (lorazepam or midazolam) and a longer acting anticonvulsant, such as phenytoin.

All patients with a generalized presentation of seizures characterized by bilateral tonic-clonic activity, altered level of consciousness, and possibly urinary or fecal incontinence should undergo aggressive treatment. Conditions can quickly become relatively hypoxic as a result of the seizure activity. Hypoxia tends to aggravate the seizure disorder and make treatment more difficult. The hypoxia occurs at two levels: generalized tissue hypoxia and cellular hypoxia. General tissue hypoxia occurs because the intense motor activity of the seizure interferes with adequate respiration. This aspect of the seizure disorder can be managed with the use of neuromuscular blocking agents in association with proper airway management. However, the intense neuronal activity characterized by sustained or rapidly intermittent bursts of neuronal discharge produces additional hypoxia at the cellular level. This hypoxia can result in a more long-term neuronal injury and is the reason for the aggressive use of an antiepileptic drug. The patient with a focal seizure (or partial seizure) characterized, for example, by facial twitching or motor activity limited to one extremity with no alteration of consciousness need not undergo aggressive management for short periods of time if attention must be paid to a more serious medical problem. However, a focal epileptic syndrome could become generalized fairly rapidly, so such a progression should be anticipated.[3,11]

Status epilepticus is the most dangerous syndrome. It is the most refractory to treatment, and the stress of the intense motor activity can cause not only respiratory insufficiency but also, in the elderly, myocardial strain that leads to myocardial injury.[8,34] Intense hypertension may also occur during status seizures, resulting in expected complications such as intracerebral hemorrhage.

Practically speaking, the acute management of a generalized seizure syndrome is simple and straightforward. An intravenous line should be placed for administration of the appropriate medication. However, some benzodiazepines are now available in a preparation that can be given rectally if intravenous access is not rapidly available.

Attention to the airway is most important, and intubation should be considered for any patient whose ability to control the airway is compromised.

Rapid sequence induction should precede any intubation attempts because of the neuroprotective benefits achieved with adequate sedation of the patient before intubation. Continued sedation is recommended. As mentioned previously, sedation with benzodiazepines serves to treat any additional seizure activity that might occur. The use of neuromuscular blockade is controversial primarily because it hinders the full neurologic examination of the patient by the receiving medical/neurology staff. Remember that antidotes to neuromuscular blockade do exist. The safety of the patient (including maintenance of an airway) is the primary concern in the transport setting.

Generalized epilepsy leading to status epilepticus is most often seen in the acute state in one of two situations: (1) with generalized encephalopathy, including that immediately following trauma; and (2) in patients who are known epileptics, who have reduced drug intake, and whose blood levels have fallen below therapeutic concentrations.[19,34]

Patients with recurrent seizures, whether they are experiencing seizures for the first time or have chronic epilepsy, may be given phenytoin in a relatively rapid loading dose of 18 mg/kg intravenously (IV; in normal saline solution) at a rate of 50 mg/min. Because this dose can precipitate supraventricular and ventricular arrhythmias, it is wise to observe the patient with a heart monitor. If arrhythmias are noted, administration of the drug should cease. If the cardiac rhythm returns to normal, especially if seizures continue, resumption of the administration of the phenytoin is appropriate at half the previously noted rate of administration.[11,34]

Evaluation

Obviously, patient outcome depends not only on the intervention but also on precipitating factors and any complications the patient might experience. The optimal goal in caring for the patient with seizures is prompt control of the seizure activity to minimize cerebral insult and prevent complications.

Evaluation data might include arterial blood gas values, chest radiographs, and laboratory results, including medication blood levels, and possibly CT scan or magnetic resonance imaging (MRI) to rule out cerebral pathology on the patient's admission to the receiving facility. In the trauma patient with seizure activity, radiographs of the skull and cervical spine are also evaluated.

Patients who present with seizure activity pose special problems. Most obvious is the safety of the uncontrolled seizure patient during transport. The patient, crew, and transport vehicle must be protected from the danger associated with the unpredictable motor responses of the seizure patient. Extra care should be taken in the application of protective patient restraints, and aggressive pharmacologic therapy should be instituted for all seizure patients.

Of particular note are visually induced seizures. The photosensitivity type is most prevalent. These seizures are induced by light flashes[8,11,17,22]; patients prone to these seizures may experience them in flight as a result of the strobe effect of aircraft lights. Pattern-induced seizures may occur in response to the light-dark pattern caused by a slowly rotating main rotor during start-up and shutdown.

NEUROLOGIC EMERGENCIES CASE STUDY

The transport team was called to transport a 12-month-old infant with febrile seizures.

HISTORY

The patient was an otherwise healthy 12-month-old infant who had a 3-day history of an upper respiratory type illness. The previous night, the patient had a fever of 101.4 °F (axillary). The mother witnessed the child having a 30-second full-body seizure. The seizure stopped on its own, but the patient was brought to the emergency department (ED) for further evaluation. On arrival to the ED, the patient had another seizure (never returning to baseline neurologic status between seizures). The patient was given benzodiazepines and dilantin in the ED. The patient was intubated. The transport team was called for rapid transport to the tertiary care Children's Hospital.

ASSESSMENT

On the transport team's arrival, the patient was found intubated but not sedated or paralyzed. She had one PIV in place with maintenance IV fluids running. Her vital signs were blood pressure 100/70 mm Hg, heart rate (HR) 160 bpm, respiratory rate (RR) 30 bpm, and temperature 101.4 °F rectal.

TRANSPORT

The patient was sedated with midazolam for transport. The patient did not exhibit any movements during the transport that necessitated the use of paralytics to either successfully ventilate or maintain endotracheal tube (ETT) security; therefore, the administration of paralytics was deferred to facilitate a full neurologic examination at the receiving facility. No seizure activity was noted during the transport. The patient was also given acetaminophen (rectally) as an antipyretic.

OUTCOME

The patient was transferred to the tertiary care Children's Hospital where she was diagnosed with febrile seizures. She was extubated the night she arrived and went home 2 days later.

REFERENCES

1. Albin MS, Babinski M: *Intensive life support of the neurosurgical patient: critical care of neurological and neurosurgical emergencies*, New York, 1980, Raven.
2. Bannister SR: *Brain and Bannisters' clinical neurology*, London, 1992, Oxford University Press.
3. Barker E: *Neuroscience nursing: a spectrum of care*, St Louis, 1994, Mosby.
4. Barnett HJM, et al, editors: *Stroke: pathophysiology, diagnosis and management*, New York, 1986, Churchill Livingstone.
5. Begley D, Newberry L: Neurologic emergencies. In Emergency Nurses Association, editors: *Sheehy's emergency nursing*, ed 5, St Louis, 2001, Mosby.
6. Bickley L, Hoekelman R: *Bate's guide to physical examination and history taking*, Philadelphia, 1999, Lippincott.
7. Biller J, et al: Spontaneous subarachnoid hemorrhage in young adults, *Neurosurgery* 21:664, 1987.

8. Bleck T: Seizures in the critically ill. In Ayers S, editor: *Textbook of critical care*, ed 3, Philadelphia, 2000, Saunders.

9. Bubb DI: Neurological problems. In *RN neurological problems: nursing assessment*, series 3, Oradell, NJ, 1984, Medical Economics Books.

10. Carrozzella J, Jauch E: Emergency stroke management: a new era, *Nursing Clin North Am* 37(1): 2002.

11. Clifford DB: The somatosensory system and pain. In Pearlman AL, Collins RC, editors: *Neurological pathophysiology*, ed 3, New York, 1984, Oxford University Press.

12. Daube JR, et al: *Medical neurosciences: an approach to anatomy, pathology, and physiology by systems and levels*, ed 4, Boston, 2001, Little, Brown.

13. Doczi T, et al: Blood-brain barrier damage during the acute stage of subarachnoid hemorrhage as exemplified by a new animal model, *Neurosurgery* 18:733, 1986.

14. Forster FM, Booker HE: The epilepsies and convulsive disorders. In Baker AB, editor: *Clinical neurology*, vol 3, Philadelphia, 1984, Harper & Row.

15. Garza M: Brain attack, *JEMS* 18(4):60, 1993.

16. Gelb LD: Infections. In Pearlman AL, Collins RC, editors: *Neurological pathophysiology*, ed 3, New York, 1984, Oxford University Press.

17. Gilroy J: *Basic neurology*, ed 3, New York, 2000, Pergamon.

18. Glaser GH: Convulsive disorders (epilepsy). In Merritt H, editor: *A textbook of neurology*, ed 6, Philadelphia, 1979, Lea & Febiger.

19. Greenberg M: Neurologic manifestations of AIDS. In Greenburg M, editor: *Handbook of neurosurgery*, ed 3, Lakeland, FL, 1994, Greenberg Graphics.

20. Guberman A: *Clinical neurology*, Boston, 1994, Little, Brown.

21. Hickey JV: *The clinical practice of neurological and neurosurgical nursing*, ed 5, Philadelphia, 2003, Lippincott Williams & Wilkins.

22. Holleran RS: *Prehospital nursing: a collaborative approach*, St Louis, 1994, Mosby.

23. Logee K: Neurologic transport. In York-Clark D, Stocking J, Johnson J, editors: *Flight and ground transport nursing core curriculum*, Denver, 2006, ASTNA.

24. Lothman EW, Collins RC: Seizures. In Pearlman AL, Collins RC, editors: *Neurological pathophysiology*, ed 3, New York, 1984, Oxford University Press.

25. Lynn-McHale DJ, Carlson KK: *AACN procedure manual for critical care*, Philadelphia, 2001, Saunders.

26. Macabasco AC, Hickman JL: Thrombolytic therapy for brain attack, *J Neurosci Nurs* 27:138, 1995.

27. McCance K, Huether S: *Pathophysiology: the biologic basis of disease in adults and children*, St Louis, 1998, Mosby.

28. McHenry LC Jr: *Cerebral circulation and strokes*, St Louis, 1978, Warren H Green.

29. Merritt H, Houston H: *A textbook of neurology*, ed 6, Philadelphia, 1979, Lea & Febiger.

30. Miller JD, Garabi J, Pichard JD: Induced changes of cerebrospinal fluid volume: effects during continuous monitoring of ventricular fluid pressure, *Arch Neurol* 28:265, 1973.

31. Millikan CH, McDowell F, Easton JD: *Stroke*, Philadelphia, 1987, Lea & Febiger.

32. Overbeeke JJ, et al: Higher cortical disorders: an unusual presentation of an arteriovenous malformation, *Neurosurgery* 21:839, 1987.

33. Pancioli AM: *Management of acute neurovascular emergencies*, Emergency Medicine Cardiac Research and Education Group Monograph, 2007 ACEP Scientific Assembly Satellite Symposia, 2008.

34. Plum F, Posner JB: *Diagnosis of stupor and coma*, ed 3, Philadelphia, 1983, FA Davis.

35. Powers WJ, Raichle ME: Stroke. In Pearlman AL, Collins RC, editors: *Neurological pathophysiology*, ed 3, New York, 1984, Oxford University Press.

36. Powers W: Acute hypertension after stroke: the scientific basis for treatment decisions, *Neurology* 43: 461-467, 1993.

37. Proehl J, editor: *Emergency nursing procedures*, ed 4, Philadelphia, 2009, Saunders.

38. Saper CB: Hypothalamus and brainstem. In Pearlman AL, Collins RC, editors: *Neurological pathophysiology*, ed 3, New York, 1984, Oxford University Press.

39. Schmidley JW: Cerebrospinal fluid, blood-brain barrier, and brain edema. In Pearlman AL, Collins RC, editors: *Neurological pathophysiology*, ed 3, New York, 1984, Oxford University Press.

40. Skinhoj E, Standgoard S: Pathogenesis of hypertensive encephalopathy, *Lancet* 1:461, 1973.

41. Toole JF: Vascular diseases of brain and spinal cord. In Merrit H, editor: *A textbook of neurology*, ed 6, Philadelphia, 1979, Lea & Febiger.

42. Treiman DM, Delgado-Escueta AV: Status epilepticus. In Thompson RA, Green JR, editors: *Critical care of neurological and neurosurgical emergencies*, New York, 1980, Raven Press.

43. Tsemetzis SA: Surgical management of intracerebral hematomas, *Neurosurgery* 16:562, 1985.

44. van Eijndhoven JHM, Avezaat CJ: Cerebrospinal fluid pulse pressure and the pulsatile variation in cerebral blood volume: an experimental study in dogs, *Neurosurgery* 19:507, 1986.

45. Weiner WJ, Goetz CG: *Neurology for the non-neurologist*, ed 4, Philadelphia, 1999, Lippincott Williams & Wilkins.

46. Williams FC, Spetzler RF: Hemodynamic management in the neurosurgical intensive care unit. In *Clinical neurosurgery*, Baltimore, 1987, Williams & Wilkins.

CARDIOVASCULAR EMERGENCIES

Christopher Manacci, Stephanie L. Steiner

COMPETENCIES

1. Perform a detailed cardiovascular assessment before, during, and after transport.
2. Recognize potential for lethal events, and institute appropriate interventions and therapeutic modalities.
3. Identify patients with acute cardiac events, including acute myocardial infarction, heart failure, cardiogenic shock, primary arrhythmias, and hemodynamic instability.
4. Use invasive monitoring during transport, as indicated, for the purpose of clinical management.
5. Provide treatment for patients with acute cardiac events and hemodynamic abnormalities.

One of the most challenging aspects for the transport team is the care of critically ill patients who need medical transport because of an acute cardiovascular event. The demand for medical transport of patients who are dependent on invasive devices and new sophisticated technology continues to increase.[33] This chapter describes advances in clinical care for patients with angina, acute myocardial infarction (AMI), congestive heart failure (CHF), aortic dissection, and other manifestations of cardiovascular disease, with a focus on assessment and management relative to the medical transport environment.

Cardiovascular disease is the leading cause of death in adults in the United States, accounting for about one third of all deaths in subjects over age 35 years.[49] In 2005, cardiovascular disease was responsible for approximately 4,036,000 emergency department visits. Cardiovascular disease is estimated to cost the healthcare system 448.5 billion dollars each year.[2] Recent data suggest that 13.7 million persons in the United States have coronary heart disease; half have myocardial infarctions (MIs), and half have angina.[49] Each day, 2400 deaths occur from cardiovascular disease alone, with one death every 37 seconds.[3] Cardiovascular disease, including hypertension, coronary artery disease (CAD), rheumatic heart disease, and stroke, affects more than 80 million Americans.[2,21]

A patient with an acute cardiac event, decompensated CHF, or an aortic dissection in a community-based limited-resource hospital often needs rapid critical care transfer to a tertiary care facility for further evaluation and emergent intervention. The transport of critically ill cardiovascular patients involves a number of issues, which include but are not limited to the potential effects of altitude and the difficulty associated with initiation of resuscitative interventions in a limited space in an uncontrolled environment.

Early research during the 1980s showed the safety and efficacy of interfacility air medical transport of patients with evolving MI who had undergone thrombolytic therapy under the care of a critical care clinician.[4,46] Current research has established the safe transport of patients who need advanced mechanical circulatory support. Interfacility transfer by air and surface critical care teams of patients dependent on intraaortic balloon pumps (IABPs), ventricular assist devices (VADs), and extracorporeal membrane oxygenation (ECMO) can now be accomplished.[23] Previous logistic restrictions, primarily because of the size of these devices and a lack of familiarity by crew members with this new technology, did not permit routine use of these circulatory support devices during transport.

ALTERATIONS OF CARDIOVASCULAR PHYSIOLOGY AT HIGH ALTITUDES

The potential for hypoxia poses one of the greatest risks to a patient with coronary artery disease. Decompensation of patients with acute cardiovascular disease during transport at high altitudes is generally caused by *hypoxic hypoxia,* which is defined as an oxygen deficiency in the body tissue sufficient to cause impaired function.[9,22] Individual patient tolerances vary, but the patient with cardiovascular compromise may be at risk if cabin pressure is above 6000 ft. For example, at an altitude of 10,000 ft, the barometric pressure decreases from 760 mm Hg at sea level to 523 mm Hg, which results in a lower partial pressure of oxygen. This reduction in the amount of oxygen in the blood decreases available oxygen to the tissues. As altitude increases, oxygen saturation decreases. If a patient has 98% saturation (PaO_2, 103) at sea level, they have 93% saturation (PaO_2, 68.9) at 8000 ft (the level at which commercial airlines routinely pressurize cabins).[9,22]

Healthy individuals can easily tolerate the effects of altitude without supplemental oxygen, but the patient with cardiovascular compromise can have clinical manifestations develop related to cellular hypoxia with even a change from 0 to 4000 ft. Compensatory mechanisms that occur to maintain adequate oxygen supply to the tissues include increases in respiratory rate, heart rate, and cardiac output. The increased workload on the heart increases myocardial oxygen consumption and necessitates increased blood flow to the heart muscle. In healthy people, cardiac reserve allows the body to compensate and meet the demand for increased blood flow to the tissues by altering heart rate, stroke volume, or both and increases blood flow to the heart muscle by dilating the coronary artery microvasculature. Cardiovascular heart disease and cardiac events limit the compensatory mechanisms available to increase cardiac output in response to increased myocardial oxygen demand. Patients with coronary artery disease may be unable to compensate for the increased workload imposed on the heart by the decreased oxygen tension experienced at high altitude. These patients may have development of chest pain, congestive heart failure, pulmonary edema, cardiac arrhythmias, or even cardiac arrest.[9,14,22]

Patients in cardiogenic shock on sodium nitroprusside therapy for afterload reduction and susceptible patients on nitroglycerin therapy can have development of *histotoxic hypoxia* because of the potential for cyanide toxicity. Carbon monoxide, cyanide, or alcohol intake can all cause histotoxic hypoxia, which results in the inability of the body to use available oxygen because of poisoning of the cytochrome oxidase enzyme system. Tissue hypoxia occurs because of the formation of methemoglobin (which has increased oxygen affinity when compared with normal hemoglobin); therefore, the ability for oxygen to be unloaded at the tissue level is decreased.

This situation can be made worse in the presence of a lower partial pressure of oxygen caused by high altitudes.[9,15,22,25] A patient with adequate available oxygen, who is profoundly anemic, may have such a low hemoglobin concentration that oxygen-carrying capability is reduced to the point that tissue hypoxia develops. This condition is referred to as *hypemic hypoxia,* which, again, can be aggravated by the low partial pressure of oxygen that can develop with increases in altitude. This situation is of special interest to the clinician transporting a patient with a recently placed VAD because of the potential for blood loss during surgical insertion. The hemoglobin concentration in these patients must be evaluated and transfused if necessary before departure from the referral institution.[9,22,25]

All patients with cardiovascular disease should receive supplemental oxygen when transported via air. The potential effects of altitude can be minimized if the aircraft is pressurized at or below 4000 ft and supplemental oxygen is delivered. In fixed-wing transport, limiting cabin altitude to a maximum of 6000 ft has been shown to eliminate problems for patients with cardiovascular disease. Cabin pressure is not a fixed variable and may need to be adjusted to accommodate patient condition. Cabin pressure can be adjusted to as low as sea level; however, a decrease in cabin pressure may come at the expense of travel at a lower altitude. Flights at decreased altitude may result in decreased speeds and therefore longer flights with an increased need for refueling stops during the trip.

Decisions regarding altitude restrictions or limitations must be based on patient history, current clinical condition, and pilot-in-command expertise and judgment. These decisions need to be evaluated throughout the mission and may need to be adjusted as a result of continued in-flight patient surveillance.[9,25]

SPECIAL CONSIDERATIONS FOR CARDIOPULMONARY RESUSCITATION IN THE TRANSPORT ENVIRONMENT

Cardiac arrest is of special concern to nurses involved in the transport of critical patients via either air or surface because CPR in the confined space of an aircraft cabin or ground transport vehicle often can be both difficult and challenging. The advanced cardiac life support (ACLS) guidelines are the standard of practice for resuscitation of the patient in cardiac arrest and should be used as such in the event of cardiac arrest in the transport environment. Transport team members are expected to have current verification in ACLS through the American Heart Association to participate in patient care within the transport environment.[24,25] Thorough pretransport assessment, planning, and intervention along with prompt correction of dysrhythmias, repletion of electrolytes, and continuous maintenance of adequate oxygenation may help to prevent the need for in-transport resuscitation.

However, the transport team must maintain a state of perpetual readiness for emergencies such as cardiac arrest. Preparation includes ensuring that resuscitation equipment and an adequate oxygen supply are easily accessible. ACLS drugs should be well labeled, not beyond the expiration date, and ready for quick administration. Generally, the number of crew members available to perform basic and advanced life support resuscitation is limited to only two medically trained personnel. For effective and rapid response in the event of an emergency, these team members must establish well-defined roles and responsibilities.

Special consideration should be given to transport vehicle configuration in anticipation of the potential need for CPR during admission. The position and height of the stretcher in relationship to the medical crew's ability to change positions is critical to facilitate proper hand and arm positioning in chest compressions. A well-designed configuration minimizes the need for crew members to extend or release restraint devices in administration of therapeutic interventions.[25]

DEFIBRILLATION DURING TRANSPORT

The most critical factor in determination of the success of a resuscitative effort is the time to restoration of effective spontaneous circulation. Immediate defibrillation is certainly the priority in the treatment of confirmed ventricular fibrillation and unstable ventricular tachycardia. The close quarters, metallic composition of transport vehicles, and proximity of vital electronic equipment, particularly in the rotor-wing environment, previously generated concern among transport personnel about safely defibrillation in this environment. Holleran[25] addressed the potential electrical risks of airborne defibrillation and showed that defibrillation with modern equipment in a medically equipped twin-engine helicopter is safe. Despite cramped quarters and sensitive electrical equipment, defibrillation can be carried out without hesitation, whether the aircraft is on the ground or in flight, provided that standard defibrillation precautions are observed. Air medical personnel should follow the ACLS defibrillation standards for selection of energy levels and use of self-adhesive monitor/defibrillation pads for the transport environment. The crew must inform the pilot before defibrillation and maintain clearance from the patient and stretcher when discharging the current.

CORONARY ARTERY DISEASE

DEFINITION AND PATHOPHYSIOLOGIC FACTORS

Coronary artery disease remains one of the most common health problems in Western civilization and is directly responsible for approximately 50% of all deaths annually in the United States.[2] Progressive atherosclerosis of the coronary arteries results in a reduction of blood flow to the myocardium. Risk factors for coronary artery disease (i.e., diabetes, hypertension, cigarette smoking, high levels of low-density lipoprotein [LDL], and low levels of high-density lipoprotein [HDL]) contribute to the formation of atherosclerotic plaques by injuring or interfering with the normal function of the vascular endothelium. The response-to-injury theory[8,15] of the development of atherosclerosis suggests injury to the endothelium and the subintimal accumulation of lipids. Chronic intimal injury encourages the deposit of lipids in the wall of the coronary artery, resulting in lipid-rich plaques with a fibrous cap.[8,15,31,40] The atherosclerotic plaque increases over time and at varying rates, depending on the degree of vascular injury

and risk factors present. An inflammatory process can be appreciated along the vessel wall with propagation of plaque formation and risk of shearing of the plaque. Acute coronary syndromes appear to be caused by rupture of an unstable coronary plaque that appears as a single lesion on angiography. However, increasing evidence shows that systemic effects, such as inflammation, are more widespread within the coronary circulation and lead to instability of multiple plaques. Significant obstruction to flow, as shown by coronary ischemia, occurs when the coronary arteries are narrowed by approximately 70%. At this point, myocardial oxygen blood supply may not be adequate to meet myocardial oxygen demand at times of stress, and ischemia of the myocardium develops.[10,15,31]

An area of the ventricular myocardium that becomes ischemic develops abnormal contractility almost immediately at the onset of ischemia, which results in decreased left ventricular function.[19] Although ischemic, the electrical homeostasis of the heart is altered, and life-threatening ventricular arrhythmias can occur.

PATHOPHYSIOLOGIC FACTORS OF CORONARY ISCHEMIA

Myocardial metabolism is an aerobic process in which the heart extracts about 70% of the available oxygen supplied by the coronary arteries. Increases in myocardial oxygen demand are normally met by increases in blood flow caused by dilation of the microcirculation system of the coronary arteries.

Angina pectoris or *angina* is a symptom of myocardial ischemia. It is caused by an imbalance between myocardial oxygen supply and demand. The end result is a buildup of metabolites in the ischemic tissue, which activates nerve endings and causes anginal pain.[15]

The myocardial oxygen supply and demand relationship is the basis for understanding both the causes of and the treatment for coronary ischemia. Myocardial oxygen supply is dependent primarily on patent coronary arteries and an adequate hemoglobin concentration to ensure adequate oxygen-carrying capacity. The major determinants of myocardial oxygen demand are heart rate, contractility, and wall stress. The imbalance between myocardial supply and demand can occur for a number of reasons:

1. Conditions that decrease supply:
   Decrease in the caliber of a coronary artery.
   Fixed (atherosclerosis).
   Transient (spasm).
   Severe anemia.
   Poor perfusion of the coronaries because of profound hypotension.
2. Conditions that increase demand:
   Tachycardia.
   Hypertension that results in increased left ventricular wall stress.
   Increased myocardial contractility caused by increased adrenergic stimuli, fever, or vasopressor agents.

Angina can be divided into several categories depending on the onset, severity, duration, and alleviation of symptoms. These categories include classic or stable angina, unstable angina, Prinzmetal's angina, or silent angina (more commonly termed silent ischemia).

Chronic Stable Angina

In the presence of a flow-limiting coronary artery atherosclerotic lesion, myocardial oxygen supply may be inadequate to meet periods of increased myocardial oxygen demand. When a patient with a significant atherosclerotic lesion undertakes an action that increases myocardial demand (such as walking on a treadmill), the patient begins to show signs of myocardial ischemia (angina with ST segment changes) when the myocardial oxygen demand begins to outstrip supply. This is the basis of the cardiac stress test to diagnose coronary artery disease.

Stable angina is usually precipitated by physical exertion or emotional stress. Chronic stable angina is predictable, given a measured work load. These symptoms usually last 1 to 5 minutes and are often abated with stopping the exertion activity or with the use of sublingual nitroglycerine (NTG).[10,26]

Unstable Angina

Unstable angina is a clinical syndrome and not a specific disease. Unstable angina is routinely classified with clinical descriptors, such as the presence of chest discomfort at rest.[13] The term unstable angina refers to an abrupt change in a patient's anginal symptoms. Unstable syndromes include angina with minimal exertion or angina with an exertion level that is much less than usual, new-onset angina, or angina at rest. The abrupt change in symptom pattern can occur as a result of any mechanism that suddenly increases myocardial oxygen demand (tachycardia from pain, fever, hypovolemia, profound hypertension, or thyrotoxicosis, or a sudden decrease in myocardial oxygen supply. This change includes a sudden decrease in the caliber of a coronary from progression of an atherosclerotic plaque or coronary spasm or anemia from acute bleeding. These symptoms and the ischemic electrocardiographic (ECG) changes that are associated with them are managed with treatment of the underlying problem.

The most common cause of a sudden decrease in myocardial perfusion is transient thrombus formation on the surface on a ruptured atherosclerotic plaque. Unstable angina, which is caused by an abrupt decrease in the caliber of a coronary artery, falls into the category of acute coronary syndromes, which are discussed extensively in a later section of this chapter.

Prinzmetal's angina, or variant angina, is a form of angina in which spontaneous chest discomfort with ST segment elevation occurs without relationship to exertion. Prinzmetal characterized it in 1959 as the result of temporary increased tone in a coronary artery resulting in a marked reduction in coronary blood flow. Evidence supports focal coronary spasm as the mechanism of transient ST segment elevation and concurrent symptoms.[27] Spasm is usually confined to a single epicardial vessel, but multivessel spasm can occur.[29] Spasm generally occurs in 1 centimeter of an atherosclerotic plaque in a mildly diseased vessel. Patients are generally young and often do not exhibit the classic atherosclerotic risk factors except for cigarette smoking. A circadian rhythm is often seen with anginal attacks, which are clustered in the early morning hours. During the period of time in which the coronary artery is in spasm, these patients are at risk for myocardial necrosis and the life-threatening arrhythmias that are associated with coronary ischemia. The pathophysiology of this disease appears to involve a combination of endothelial dysfunction and increased reactivity in response to vasoconstrictor substances. Treatment includes the use of vasodilator substances, such as NTG and calcium channel blockers, and risk factor modification.[10,29,43]

Silent Ischemia

Evidence of ischemia in the absence of symptoms occurs frequently. Upwards of 75% of ischemia in patients with stable angina is *silent,* or without clinical manifestations.[15] ST segment changes are often detected on ambulatory monitoring. Several explanations exist for the absence of anginal symptoms in patients with silent ischemia, including the observation that patients with this silent angina have less sensitivity to pain in general than do patients with more traditional angina.

Continuum of Acute Coronary Syndromes

An abrupt change in the caliber of a coronary artery can occur as a result of coronary blood vessel spasm or the abrupt worsening of an atherosclerotic plaque. Atherosclerotic plaques can suddenly become more narrowed because of the formation of atheroma in the wall of the vessel or the formation of a thrombus on the surface of a damaged plaque.[8]

Atherosclerotic lesions, which are rich in lipids, are susceptible to endothelial damage. Disruption of the protective endothelial lining, known as plaque rupture, leads to a cascade of processes, which are aimed at healing this damaged vessel. If these processes become overexuberant, a thrombus can form on the surface of the damaged endothelium, which results in the total occlusion of the blood vessel.[28,40]

Rupture of vulnerable plaques is responsible for 75% of all acute coronary syndromes and results in acute obstruction in blood flow to the myocardium normally served by the occluded coronary artery.[10] Acute coronary syndromes begin with a disruption of the endothelium overlying an atherosclerotic lesion. The lesions more likely to be involved in acute coronary syndromes are the mild to moderate lesions with thin fibrous tissue caps; larger lipid concentrations of the underlying coronary vessel wall causes both platelet activation and the stimulation of the clotting cascade to form thrombin. Thrombin

is a potent stimulant of platelet activation and is responsible for the conversion of fibrinogen in the bloodstream to fibrin. The newly formed fibrin is responsible for cross linking of platelets into a stable thrombus.

Platelets, once activated, bind to exposed areas of the vessel wall. More platelets are drawn to the area, and the activated platelets begin to bind to each other via receptors on their surface, known as glycoprotein IIb/IIIa receptors. These platelets eventually form a platelet plug. If large enough, they can completely occlude the relatively small (3-mm range) coronary arteries and occlude flow in the vessel. Platelet activation also leads to the secretion of vasoconstriction substances, which increases limited blood flow in the affected coronary artery.[18]

The degree to which a coronary artery is occluded and whether or not it remains occluded by this process subsequently determines in which part of the continuum of acute coronary syndromes an event is classified. For example:

1. Unstable angina caused by an acute change in the caliber of a coronary artery as a result of plaque rupture and thrombus formation. If transient occlusion of a coronary by activated platelets at the site of a ruptured plaque occurs with subsequent recanalization of the vessel, the patient may be symptomatic at rest (while the coronary is occluded) and have symptoms resolve spontaneously with recanalization of the vessel. Transient ECG changes may occur while the patient is symptomatic, but the episode is often too short to show either ECG changes or evidence of myocardial injury.
2. An event classified as a non–Q wave infarction begins in the same manner, but either occlusion of the coronary is prolonged (with myocardial necrosis) or distal embolization of small platelet clumps occurs, leading to occlusion of smaller distal coronary branches and therefore myocardial necrosis. Spontaneous recanalization may occur, but biochemical evidence of myocardial necrosis is found (troponin, CPKDMB).

In both of these instances, a significantly narrowed coronary artery (although recanalized) remains, and therapy is aimed at keeping the activated platelets present on its surface from progressing into a stable thrombus. In the patient with symptoms that resolve with therapy, the question of further management becomes less clear.[11] The data support the use of either of the following strategies:

1. Conservative management: Use of cardiac catheterization with subsequent revascularization only for patients with recurrent symptoms of angina or positive stress test results.
2. Invasive management: Performance of a cardiac catheterization with subsequent revascularization in all patients with documented acute coronary syndromes.

Acute MI represents the syndrome of acute plaque rupture, which continues to its ultimate end point, an organized thrombus made up of activated platelets with cross-linked fibrin, which results in a stable thrombus. These patients have continued chest pain and associated ST segment elevation because of injury caused by total occlusion of coronary blood flow. At this point, therapy must be aimed at immediate reperfusion.

Chronic Stable Angina: Assessment, Diagnosis, and Treatment. *Classic angina* is usually described as substernal chest discomfort, pressure, or heaviness that occurs with activity and is resolved with rest. The chest discomfort usually increases in intensity and often gradually self resolves. Occasionally, patients may report dyspnea, back, shoulder, arm, or jaw pain without the presence of chest pain. The location of the chest pain is most commonly in the middle or lower sternum or the left precordium. Patients may also have such symptoms as nausea, vomiting, diaphoresis, dyspnea, and fatigue, but in general, these symptoms are predictable and patients know their limitations. The patients usually stop exerting themselves or take NTG tablets before the symptoms become severe.

Physical examination results in patients with episodes of chronic stable angina are often normal, although patients could have an S4 because the ischemic area of the left ventricle is stiff.[15,19]

In stable angina, the ECG has limited diagnostic value. Transient ST depression may occur during exertion; it represents ischemia in the subendocardium, the inner surface of the myocardium. This area of the ventricular myocardium, just adjacent to the left ventricular cavity and farthest away from the oxygen rich blood supplied from the coronary arteries, is the most susceptible to ischemia. Cardiac arrhythmias, some potentially lethal, may occur with any episode of ischemia caused by alterations in the conductance of electrical activity through the myocardium at times of limited coronary blood flow.

The goal of treatment of chronic stable angina, as with all forms of angina, is identification of the imbalance in the myocardial oxygen supply and demand relationship and subsequent fix of the causative problem. Treatment involves strategies to either increase coronary blood supply or decrease myocardial oxygen demand, or both. This treatment may be accomplished through pharmacology, percutaneous angioplasty, or surgical interventions.[17]

Medical therapy for chronic stable angina is directed towards decreasing myocardial oxygen demand by controlling heart rate and blood pressure. Therapy includes beta-blockers, angiotensin-converting enzyme (ACE) inhibitors, transdermal or oral nitrates, and calcium channel blockers. Medical therapy is also aimed at risk factor modification, including smoking cessation and aggressive lipid lowering.

Nitroglycerin can be used in both short-acting and long-acting forms. Sublingual NTG is often used for the initial management of anginal pain and ischemia. It works by relaxing vascular smooth muscle, which leads to both arterial and venous vasodilation. Venodilation leads to a decrease in preload and therefore a decrease in ventricular wall tension. Arterial vasodilation leads to a decrease in systemic blood pressure. These actions both work to decrease myocardial oxygen consumption or demand. Coronary vasodilation, both epicardial and microvasculature, can help to increase myocardial oxygen supply. Patients who use long-acting nitrates should be warned of the tolerance effect with this medication and should have at least an 8-hour drug-free window to maintain drug efficacy. Patients often use sublingual NTG as prophylaxis before an activity that is known to precipitate an anginal attack.

Beta-blockers work by decreasing myocardial oxygen demand. These agents interrupt sympathetic impulses by competing with the neurotransmitter norepinephrine at the beta-sympathetic nerve endings. Beta-receptor inhibition results in decreased heart rate, myocardial contractility, and slowed impulse transmission through the cardiac conduction system. These effects lead to decreased myocardial oxygen consumption. In addition, beta-blockers decrease MI size and improve survival rates because of a decreased incidence of myocardial rupture and ventricular fibrillation.[17]

The calcium channel blockers verapamil and diltiazem slow heart rate, decrease blood pressure, and decrease myocardial contractility, with each of these contributing to a decrease in myocardial oxygen consumption. Although previously widely used for the management of angina, calcium channel antagonist use has decreased since controversial data were presented in 1995.

Beta-blockers should be used as first-line agents unless contraindicated, and calcium channel blocking agents can be added as an alternative or additional therapy if the maximal doses of beta-blockers have been achieved.[17,34]

All patients with coronary artery disease should take 81 mg of aspirin each day[34] and follow a lifestyle that promotes cardiovascular health. In patients with elevated cholesterol levels, a statin-type lipid-lowering agent should be used to achieve an LDL of less than 100 mg/dL.[34]

Percutaneous transluminal coronary angioplasty, with or without intracoronary stenting, can be performed in patients with symptomatic angina, which indicates ischemia in the territory of a significantly narrowed coronary artery. In patients with coronary artery disease that cannot be rescued with angioplasty, coronary artery bypass surgery may be needed to revascularize the entire myocardium. Again, aggressive risk factor modification in addition to interventional therapy is indicated.[41]

Patients with chronic stable angina often come into contact with transport personnel when they are faced with a sudden stressful situation not necessarily directly related to a cardiac event. Patients with significant coronary artery disease may be seen in the setting of a trauma, gastrointestinal bleed, or sepsis. The key to the evaluation and treatment of these patients is to ask the question "What is the underlying problem?" A patient with chest pain and ST segment changes in the setting of a broken pelvis and a hematocrit of 22% has symptoms caused by an increased myocardial oxygen demand, which therefore may provoke cardiac symptoms. This is again is from the increased demand on the myocardium and not necessarily a flow or supply issue. However, the true mechanism of what physiologically took place first is never truly known in this situation, and transport personnel should maintain a high suspicion. In the example used previously, no change has been seen in the caliber of the coronaries, therefore treatment should not be aimed at antiplatelet and anticoagulation therapy. The patient has stress caused by hypovolemia, anemia, and pain, which all lead to increased heart rate and therefore increased myocardial oxygen demand. The goal is correction of the underlying problem and accurate evaluation of the causes of the patient's clinical presentation, and therefore correction of the causative problem with transfusion, volume replacement, and pain control if indicated.

Acute Coronary Syndromes: Diagnosis, Assessment, and Treatment. The term *acute coronary syndrome* is applied to an abrupt change in anginal symptoms caused by the sequelae of a ruptured atherosclerotic plaque. The continuum of unstable angina, non–Q wave infarction, and AMIs is, in truth, a varying degree of the same underlying problem: a mild-to-moderate lipid-laden atherosclerotic plaque that suddenly ruptures exposing the underlying cholesterol gruel to the circulating blood and setting in place multiple mechanisms that are responsible for trying to repair the damaged vessel wall. Platelets cover the surface of the injured area and then attach to each other by receptors on their surfaces called GP IIb/IIIa receptors. The activation of platelets during this process releases regulatory substances, which cause further aggregation of platelets and vasoconstriction. At the same time, the clotting cascade becomes activated, which results in the formation of thrombin, a potent stimulator of platelets. Thrombin is also responsible for the formation of fibrin from fibrinogen in the blood.

As platelets accumulate in the area, a platelet plug forms, which itself can intermittently occlude flow in the coronary. As this mass of platelets becomes organized, fibrin interconnects the platelets into a stable blood clot, or thrombus.[28]

Once platelets have aggregated on the surface of ruptured plaque, the competition between antithrombotic and thrombotic processes in the body becomes intense. The vessel may reocclude at any time, or this area may heal without further symptoms, and the ruptured plaque/platelet plug may be incorporated into the atherosclerotic plaque, contributing to the progressive growth of atherosclerotic coronary artery disease. The goal of treatment in acute coronary syndromes is to augment the anticoagulant properties that the body possesses and interfere with the clot forming processes.

Acute coronary syndromes begin primarily as a process mediated by activated platelets; therefore, therapeutic strategies are primarily directed toward the inhibition of platelets and interference with platelet-to-platelet interactions.

Efforts aimed at decreasing myocardial oxygen demand, such as beta-blockers, pain control, and NTG, also help but do not address the primary problem of activated platelets on the surface of a ruptured plaque.

Aspirin is a potent inhibitor of thromboxane, a stimulated platelet aggregation. Many other pathways stimulate platelet aggregation and interactions. Aspirin has clearly been shown to decrease MI and death in patients who present to the hospital with unstable angina. All patients with symptoms consistent with unstable angina and without contraindications should receive at least 160 mg of aspirin.[1]

Ticlopidine and clopidogrel bisulfate inhibit platelet activation by inhibiting ADP-dependent platelet activation. This effect does not occur immediately; there is a risk of neutropenia with their use, and they should be used with caution. These drugs are primarily used in patients with true aspirin allergies and as an adjunct to anticoagulation therapy after intracoronary stent placement.

Heparin is a potent anticoagulant that augments the body's ability to reduce thrombin generation and fibrin formation. Heparin does not dissolve a clot that has already formed; however, it does halt the propagation of the clot or any new clots. Clinical evidence supports the use of heparin in acute coronary syndromes. The transport team should follow recommended protocols.

The glycoprotein IIb/IIIa receptors on the surface of platelets are responsible for the attachment of platelets to one another. Drugs that inhibit this process block the common final pathway of platelet aggregation and are therefore inhibitors of the formation of thrombus. The agents currently in use, such as abciximab, eptifibatide, and tirofiban, all have different mechanisms of actions, dosing strategies, and half-lives. A review of these drugs is not included here because it is beyond the intended scope of this chapter. These medications, which have become an important part of the treatment of patients with acute coronary syndromes, should be familiar to transport personnel. Current American Heart Association (AHA) guidelines recommend the use of GP IIb/IIIa inhibitors in addition to aspirin and heparin for patients with a non–ST segment elevation MI or refractory ischemia. In most patients, anticoagulation and antiplatelet therapies cause improvement of symptoms and signs of ischemia. For those patients with ongoing signs and symptoms of ischemia not relieved with medical therapy, cardiac catheterization with subsequent revascularization should be performed without delay. Depending on the patient's coronary anatomy, revascularization may include angioplasty with or without intracoronary stent placement or coronary artery bypass graft surgery.[1,34]

ACUTE MYOCARDIAL INFARCTION: ASSESSMENT, DIAGNOSIS, AND TREATMENT

An *acute myocardial infarction* occurs as a result of a coronary artery occluding from a thrombus forming on the surface of a ruptured atherosclerotic plaque. When flow no longer exists in the coronary artery, the entire distribution of that coronary artery is at risk for injury or myocardial cell death. Initially, that wall of the heart becomes stiff and then stops moving, which results in a loss of left ventricular ejection fraction and potentially leads to significant valvular dysfunction and ventricular arrhythmias. The longer the interruption to coronary flow, the more extensive the injury resulting in decrease of myocardial function.

As with the other acute coronary syndromes, an AMI begins as a platelet problem but evolves into a process that ends in the formation of a thrombus through the formation and infiltration of the platelet plug by fibrin cross-links. The initial treatment goals are therefore similar to those for other acute coronary syndromes. The use of aspirin, heparin, and GP IIb/IIIa inhibitors in addition to a definitive reperfusion strategy, such as emergent angioplasty, are the basic concepts of AMI therapy. Fibrinolytic therapy destroys fibrin in the intracoronary thrombus. In doing so, activated platelets are released from the thrombus. These activated platelets can reassemble and reocclude the vessel if adjunctive anticoagulation and antiplatelet strategies are not used. Agents such as beta-blockers, NTG, and morphine sulfate for pain control are important to decrease myocardial oxygen demand; reperfusion with definitive restoration of myocardial oxygen supply should be the primary goal.[12]

Diagnosis of Acute Myocardial Infarction

Patients who present with an AMI describe chest heaviness, discomfort, or pressure, often associated with shortness of breath, diaphoresis, or nausea. The discomfort may radiate to the neck, jaw, or arms. Ongoing angina associated with electrocardiographic results that show ST segment elevation in contiguous leads (leads that represent an area of the heart that is supplied by a single coronary), known as an acute injury pattern, together make the diagnosis of an AMI. ST segment elevation on the electrocardiogram represents ischemia, injury and subsequent myocardial cell necrosis in the area of the occluded coronary artery.[1,34]

The cardiac blood supply is made up of three principal coronary arteries. These vessels, the first branches off the aorta, originate from the coronary ostia at the level of the aortic valve cusps. The left main coronary artery divides into the left anterior descending (LAD) and the left circumflex arteries. The LAD supplies the anterior surface of the heart, the anterior two thirds of the septum, and part of the lateral wall. The LAD distribution is represented on the surface electrocardiogram in the V or chest leads. The circumflex coronary artery supplies branches to the lateral and posterior surfaces of the heart. The circumflex is not well represented on the standard electrocardiogram. Changes caused by ischemia or infarction in the circumflex coronary artery may be seen in the lateral (V5, V6, aVL, and I) leads or in the posterior wall by inference from changes in the V1 and V2 leads, which appear as ST segment depression that is actually elevation on the posterior surface of the heart.

In 85% of patients, the right coronary artery (RCA) is responsible for coronary blood flow to the inferior surface of the heart and to the posterior third of the interventricular septum by way of one of its branches, the posterior descending coronary artery. These areas of the heart are represented on the electrocardiogram as the inferior leads or leads II, III, and aVF. On the way to the inferior surface of the heart, the RCA is also responsible for supplying blood flow to the right ventricle.

Once the diagnosis of an AMI is clear, it should immediately prompt the decision of reperfusion therapy with rescue angioplasty and associated pharmacologic therapy. This decision must be made in a rapid fashion because for each minute the myocardium is devoid of blood flow, more injury occurs. The sooner an occluded coronary artery is reperfused, the less likely the patient is to die of an MI.[1]

Examination of the patient suspected of having an AMI should be focused and include evaluation for contraindications to therapy and a search for complications of the MI. Excessive sympathetic stimulation may result in an elevated blood pressure and an increased heart rate.

The patient should be evaluated for the presence of an S3, rales, or distended neck veins, which indicate the presence of congestive heart failure caused by either severe left ventricular failure from the AMI or flash pulmonary edema resulting from the acute onset of severe mitral regurgitation.[15]

Mitral regurgitation caused by the abrupt disruption of the mitral valve is often not audible on examination. It occurs as a consequence of occlusion of the blood supply to the lateral surface of the heart. Mitral regurgitation may also be related to a mechanical defect of the valve caused by untreated hypertension in some individuals. This may predispose the patient to acute onset of mitral regurgitation consequential to chordate rupture. Tachycardia and hypotension in association with the signs of congestive heart failure or pulmonary edema represent cardiogenic shock. These patients are best treated with emergent angioplasty, ideally after temporary placement of an intraaortic balloon pump. The intraaortic balloon pump is a counterpulsation therapy and assists in increasing both coronary perfusion and afterload reduction.[48]

These patients in cardiogenic shock must not receive beta-blockers; the tachycardia is a functional compensatory mechanism because of the severely limited stroke volume from an extensive MI.

Critical care transport personnel are involved in the transport of patients with cardiogenic shock to facilities that have the capabilities to perform emergency angioplasty. In patients transported before the placement of an intraaortic balloon pump, perfusion to the brain and vital organs must be maintained. The use of low-dose phenylephrine or norepinephrine to maintain blood pressure, albeit at a cost of increased myocardial oxygen demand, should be used. Dopamine is common; however, caution should be used because it not only increases myocardial depend but also the potential of tachyarrhythmias. These medications should be used at the lowest dose possible to maintain adequate perfusion of the vital organs, which can normally be achieved by a mean arterial pressure (MAP) of 65 to 70 mm Hg. Evidence of adequate perfusion includes not only adequate systolic blood pressure (SBP) but a patient who is conscious and making urine. However, ensuring an adequate preload status before initiating or increasing presser support is important.[19]

Profound bradycardia with complete heart block and hypotension can occur because of occlusion of the blood supply to the inferior surface of the heart. This generally responds to crystalloid infusion and administration of atropine. A patient with symptoms attributed to an inferior wall MI is extremely dependent on preload, and vigorous volume resuscitation is advised. A patient may need transcutaneous or transvenous pacing, and the transport personnel should be well versed in this use.

Hypotension with distended neck veins and clear lungs occurs in patients with right ventricular infarction as a result of occlusion of the proximal right coronary artery, which supplies blood to the right ventricle. Patients with right ventricular infarctions are extremely volume dependent because of inadequate preload to the left ventricle. Because the right and left ventricles work in circuit, a poorly functional right ventricle is unable to maintain adequate volume back to the left ventricle. The patient shows signs of poor cardiac output despite adequate left ventricular function. The basis of therapy for a right ventricular infarction is large volumes of intravenous fluid. Also, medication that reduces preload, such as nitrate and morphine, should be used with extreme caution if at all.

Therapy for Acute Myocardial Infarction

As with the previously described acute coronary syndromes, an AMI begins as a platelet problem; therefore, the same treatment, anticoagulation with antiplatelet therapies, is initiated.

Rescue angioplasty is angioplasty performed for the purpose of definitive reperfusion therapy and is considered the standard of care. The use of intracoronary stenting may result in decreased levels of restenosis in the future.

Critical care transport personnel are essential in the rapid transport of these patients to tertiary institutions with angioplasty facilities. Acknowledgment of the presence of an AMI at a referral institution should prompt the receiving institution to activate its cardiac catheterization laboratory staff. This process can be facilitated by transport personnel. Direct physician-to-physician contact and the timely fax of electrocardiographic results can avoid unnecessary delays in reperfusion therapy.

In patients with adequate blood pressure (SBP > 110 mm Hg) and the absence of posterior or inferior involvement, intravenous (IV) morphine sulfate (2 to 4 mg) and IV NTG therapy (goal is to decrease SBP by approximately 10% to 20%) can be used for pain control. Beta-blockers (metoprolol 5 mg IV q 5 min for three doses) can help decrease myocardial oxygen demand in the patient with no contraindication (i.e., severe congestive heart failure, bradycardia, or diffuse wheezing).

Emergency *coronary artery bypass surgery* (CABG) is performed in the setting of an AMI for patients with severe left main disease, failed angioplasty, and multivessel coronary artery disease not amenable to percutaneous revascularization. The time needed to activate a pump team and to place patients on bypass limits CABG as an initial strategy for reperfusion of an infarcting segment of myocardium.

Critical care transfer of these patients via air or ground is essential and should not be performed by basic or advance life support (ALS) units.

DYSRHYTHMIAS

Serious electrical abnormalities of the heart rate and rhythm are classified as *dysrhythmias.* They are described on ECGs as a deviation from the normal sinus rhythm in rate, too fast as in *tachycardia* or too slow as in *bradycardia;* in regularity, one or more beats occurring earlier or later than expected; or in a different pattern of activation of the cardiac muscle. Dysrhythmias can originate in any area of the heart. They are usually divided into arrhythmias that start in the atrium, that start in the atrioventricular (AV) node, and that start in the ventricle. Identification of the origin of the dysrhythmias is based on the following:

1. The relation between the P wave and the QRS complex.
2. The width and configuration of the P wave, which indicate how the atria are activated during the arrhythmia.
3. The width and configuration of the QRS complex, which indicate how the ventricles are activated during the arrhythmia.

Dysrhythmias are caused by a variation in the state of discharge of the sinoatrial (SA) node, ectopic impulses that compete with the SA node, or abnormal conduction of impulses from the SA node through the heart. The origin of a normal heartbeat is in the sinus node. The sinus node is located laterally near the junction of the superior vena cava and the right atrium. The sinus node is actually a region made up of groups of pacemaker cells, which automatically depolarize. The blood flow to this region is variable.

Dysrhythmias can be categorized as *tachyarrhythmias,* which include atrial tachycardia, supraventricular arrhythmias, and ventricular arrhythmias, and *bradyarrhythmias,* which include symptomatic bradycardia and conduction disturbances known as atrioventricular (AV) blocks.

PATHOPHYSIOLOGIC FACTORS

The cells that conduct the electrical current through the heart are known as the pacemaker or automatic cells. The pacemaker of the heart, the SA node, is located at the junction of the superior vena cava and the right atrium. An electric impulse is initiated at this node, and it travels through the internodal pathways to the AV node.

The AV node is located in the right atrium, directly above the tricuspid valve and anterior to the coronary sinus. The electrical impulse travels through the AV node and then moves through a common bundle of His, which divides almost immediately into the right and left bundles. The left bundle divides further to form two direct pathways to the anterior and posterior papillary muscle. The electrical impulse then permeates the many small fibers of the Purkinje network, beginning at the endocardium and ending in the ventricular myocardium.[19]

Dysrhythmias are the result of an irritable focus or foci in the electrical conduction system. Several mechanisms contribute to the development of dysrhythmias. The ischemic process and postnecrotic entities and underlying cardiac disease may enhance myocardial electrical instability. In addition, the development and treatment of myocardial failure result in mechanical dysfunction, metabolic changes, and electrolyte shifts and contribute to rhythm disturbances. Invasive cardiac instrumentation or pharmacologic therapies also have the potential to provoke serious dysrhythmias.

ASSESSMENT, DIAGNOSIS, AND TREATMENT
Tachyarrhythmias/Tachycardias

Atrial Tachycardia. *Atrial tachycardias* possess a regular rhythm; the impulse formation is in the atrium but outside the sinus node. P waves precede the QRS but are usually obscured because of the rapid heart rate, although AV conduction may be present.

The heart rates vary from 140 to 240 bpm. The incidence rate of atrial tachycardia seems to increase with age. Current classifications of atrial tachycardia are based on the three mechanisms responsible for the tachycardia.[19]

a. *Intraatrial reentry.* The characteristics of the reentrant circuit in atrial tachycardia are still not well understood. Many of these patients have other arrhythmias, specifically atrial fibrillation, or flutter.[19] Common symptoms are dyspnea, fatigue, and palpitation. Although the condition is symptomatic, usually no associated homodynamic compromise is seen. Catheter ablation is the primary therapy for reentrant atrial tachycardia with a suggested success rate of greater than 75%.

b. *Ectopic automaticity.* This is generated by a single or multiple atrial focus that clusters around the crista terminalis in the right atrium and around the base of the pulmonary veins in the left atrium. This condition has also been referred to as multiple atrial tachycardia (MAT). This is a descriptive entity that is characterized by an atrial rate of greater than 100 bpm with P wave morphology with varying AV intervals. It is easily confused with atrial fibrillation, and its mechanism is unknown. However, it is seen in patients with acute pulmonary disorders and accompanying hypoxia. Treatment is focused on the underlying cause. Patients with this mechanism are generally younger in age. This tachycardia does not respond to vagal maneuvers and is not terminated with atrial pacing. Treatment of precipitating causes is advisable. Also, amiodarone has been found to be useful.[19]

c. *Atrial flutter.* Atrial flutter presents as a series of rapid regular flutter waves, usually described as saw tooth or resembling a picket fence, with a rate from 220 to 350 bpm. Diagnosis is usually made in leads II, III, and AVF. Conduction through the AV node delays impulses and thus prevents rapid ventricular rates. The QRS complex during atrial flutter is usually the same as during sinus rhythm. Treatment methods are addressed in conjunction with fibrillation.

Atrial fibrillation. Atrial fibrillation represents chaotic atrial activity, with the atrial rate ranging from 300 to 700 bpm. Impulses are randomly conducted through the AV node to the ventricles, resulting in a typically irregular ventricular response that varies continuously in shape. Atrial fibrillation results in loss of effective atrial contraction, which reduces cardiac output and promotes mural thrombus development.

Treatment for patients with either atrial flutter or fibrillation is based on several clinical factors.

1. Is the patient's condition clinically stable or unstable?
2. Is impaired cardiac function associated with the flutter or fibrillation?
3. Is Wolff-Parkinson-White syndrome present?
4. Has the flutter or fibrillation been present for more or less than 48 hours?[40]

If the patient's condition is unstable, the patient should be appropriately treated immediately. The objectives of treatment are to control the rate, convert the rhythm, and use anticoagulation therapy when appropriate. Increased emphasis is placed on assessment of causes of the atrial fibrillation. Some underlying causes include hypoxemia, anemia, hypertension CHF, hypokalemia, and mitral regurgitation. The length of time of fibrillation or flutter is important because if such a rhythm continues for more than 48 hours, there is a risk of systemic embolization on conversion to a sinus rhythm if the patient does not undergo anticoagulation appropriately. If the condition in atrial fibrillation becomes unstable, cardioversion is recommended. If the patient is in atrial flutter, lower joules may be effective to convert the condition.

Supraventricular Arrhythmias.   *Supraventricular arrhythmias* originate above the ventricle and reflect atrial irritability. They can originate from the SA node, the AV node, the penetrating part of the bundle of His, or an accessory pathway.[28] These arrhythmias include premature atrial contractions, atrial tachycardia, atrial flutter, and atrial fibrillation.

Premature Atrial Contractions. *Premature atrial contractions* are an early atrial depolarization. They are predictors of impending supraventricular arrhythmias and do not necessitate intervention.

Sinus Tachycardia. *Sinus tachycardia* originates in the sinus node and is characterized by a heart rate greater than 100 bpm. It is a physiologic response to a demand for a higher cardiac output, and treatment is directed toward correcting the physiologic demand, as opposed to correcting the rapid heart rate. Causes can include infection, anemia, hypotension, and hyperthyroidism. IV or oral beta-blockers may be used when the tachycardia produces symptoms, as long as the underlying cause is corrected first.

Ventricular Arrhythmias. Ventricular ectopic activity is a common phenomenon in AMI, and *ventricular arrhythmias* are the major cause of sudden cardiac death in the United States. The most common cause of ventricular arrhythmia is ischemic coronary artery disease. Ventricular arrhythmias arise in the ventricles beyond the bifurcation of the bundle of His.

Death from a ventricular arrhythmia occurs through its interference with the cardiac pumping function. Several conditions that occur during the ventricular arrhythmia contribute to the decrease in cardiac output, which in turn can cause syncope and lead to arrest. The loss of the normal atrioventricular sequence is associated with a significant decrease in cardiac output. The rate of the ventricular arrhythmia also determines hemodynamic instability. A rate below 150 bpm does not usually cause hemodynamic compromise if the duration is short. If the ventricular tachycardia exceeds 200 bpm, significant symptoms are usually present and can include dyspnea, light-headedness, loss of vision, syncope, and cardiac arrest. Patients with ventricular tachyarrhythmias should be closely monitored because they have an increased risk of progression to ventricular fibrillation, especially with a history of compromised ejection fraction. In the absence of an independent licensed practitioner such as a physician or nurse practitioner or orders from online medical control, adhere to the American Heart Association's ACLS guidelines for specific algorithms for treatment of all arrhythmias or as indicated by prewritten orders.[11]

Premature Ventricular Complexes or Ventricular Premature Beats. *Premature ventricular complexes* (PVCs) or beats represent early ventricular depolarization that occurs before the next sinus beat. A wide bizarre configuration represents abnormal impulse conduction. PVCs or *ventricular premature beats* (VPBs) are fairly benign and are usually left untreated. They may, however, escalate to ventricular tachycardia or fibrillation, which necessitates careful observation of patients with VPBs. Assessment of these patients should include any underlying history of cardiac disease.

Paroxysmal Supraventricular Tachycardia. *Paroxysmal supraventricular tachycardia* (PSVT) is a regular tachycardia that exceeds the expected limits of sinus tachycardia at rest (>120 bpm) with or without discernible P waves. It usually has an abrupt onset and termination. It is supraventricular in origin and can be differentiated from atrial or junctional tachycardias by its abrupt onset and termination that the patient describes during assessment.[19] Current recommendations include the use of vagal maneuvers to resolve the PSVT. Adenosine IV is also still recommended. Be aware of some of the differing effects of adenosine in patients with asthma, in patients prone to bronchospasm caused by reactive airway disease, or in patients with preexisting cardiac disease. If the left ventricular (LV) function is preserved, additional options are amiodarone, calcium channel blockers, or digitalis. If evidence of cardiac compromise (ejection fraction, <40) is found, amiodarone should be considered first. Electric cardioversion should not be used in patients with PSVT who have impaired cardiac function.[11,34]

Ventricular Tachycardia. *Ventricular tachycardia* (VT) is three or more premature ventricular beats (PVCs) at an accelerated rate, usually greater than 100 bpm. The rhythm may be well tolerated or associated with hemodynamic compromise. Current emphasis related to treatment methods is still placed on whether the patient's condition is deemed stable or unstable. In assessment of the patient in ventricular tachycardia, instability is determined by symptoms displayed such as chest pain, hypotension, decreased level of consciousness, shock, shortness of breath, or pulmonary congestion that can be attributed to the rapid heart rate, usually greater than 150 bpm. If the patient's condition is determined to be unstable but pulses are detected, immediate synchronized electrical cardioversion is indicated at 100 to 200 J. If the patient is pulseless, immediate defibrillation should be instituted.[7,11]

If the patient is conscious and the condition is stable, assessment of type of VT is important for treatment decisions. With monomorphic VT, whether impaired cardiac function exists needs to be identified. When polymorphic VT is diagnosed, the QT baseline interval must be assessed. If the QT baseline interval is prolonged, which suggests torsades de pointes, medications used are magnesium, isoproterenol, phenytoin, or lidocaine with overdrive pacing. This type of VT is seen most often in patients with drug overdose. If the polymorphic VT has a normal baseline QT interval, the object is to treat the ischemia and to correct electrolytes. Medications recommended for use are beta-blockers, amiodarone, procainamide, sotalol, or lidocaine. In the absence of an independent licensed practitioner such as a physician or nurse practitioner or orders from online medical control, adhere to the American Heart Association's ACLS guidelines for specific algorithms for treatment of all arrhythmias.[7,11]

Ventricular Fibrillation.   *Ventricular fibrillation* (VF) is chaotic depolarization from multiple areas of the ventricle; no effective contraction occurs, which results in severe hemodynamic compromise. VF is the most common mechanism of cardiac arrest from myocardial ischemia or infarction and leads to sudden death if it is not converted to a more normal rhythm. The best treatment for VF is early defibrillation. Again, adherence to current ACLS guidelines regarding CPR, defibrillation, and pharmacotherapy is important. Pharmacologic therapy initiated can include epinephrine 1 mg IV push every 3 to 5 minutes or vasopressin 40 U IV as a one-time single

dose. Vasopressin is a natural-substance antidiuretic hormone that becomes a powerful vasoconstrictor when administered at much higher doses than found in the body. It has all the positive effects of epinephrine without the negative effects. Remember, AHA recommendations state that all antiarrhythmics can also behave as proarrhythmics that could generate VF/VT arrest.[7,11]

Accelerated Idioventricular Rhythm. *Accelerated idioventricular rhythm* (AIVR) is defined as a ventricular rhythm with a rate of 60 to 110 bpm. Most episodes are of short duration and terminate abruptly, slow gradually before stopping, or are overdriven by the basic cardiac rhythm. This rhythm is usually not treated but must be observed closely because of its propensity to degenerate into ventricular tachycardia or fibrillation.

Bradyarrhythmias

Bradycardia.   Absolute *bradycardia* is defined as a heart rate less than 60 bpm. It is a result of slowing of impulse formation by the sinus node and is most often associated with an inferior or posterior wall MI. It may also result from ischemic effects on the sinus node. The current treatment of choice for symptomatic bradycardia with the patient in a critical position or with no intravenous access is transcutaneous pacing. This can be accomplished with the application of an external pacemaker (which is preferable in the patient being considered for or receiving thrombolytic therapy). However, transcutaneous pacing is not as readily available as atropine (0.5 to 1.0 mg IV every 3 to 5 minutes to a total dose of 0.03 mg/kg for mildly symptomatic patients). For severe bradycardia, a maximum of 0.04 mg/kg is advisable. Atropine enhances sinus node automaticity and AV conduction. Patients with symptomatic bradycardia show signs of CHF, hypotension, shortness of breath (SOB), chest pain, or refractory ventricular ectopic activity. Dopamine at 2 to 5 mcg/kg/min can be given with accompanying hypotension. An epinephrine infusion of 2 to 10 mcg/min can be considered if pacing and atropine have failed. The use of lidocaine can be lethal to a patient with bradycardia when the bradycardia is a ventricular escape rhythm.[7,34]

External Pacing. An *external pacemaker,* or transcutaneous pacemaker (TCP), provides immediate pacing in an emergency without the risk of complications related to an invasive procedure. Pacing is accomplished with large electrodes that are placed over the precordium and on the posterior left side of the chest beneath the scapula. Standard electrodes provide the ECG tracing and allow demand-mode operation. The TCP operates asynchronously if the sensing electrodes are not in place.

Temporary Pacing. *Temporary pacing* is most commonly used for short-term management of symptomatic bradycardias, either as a bridge to permanent pacing or for self-limited bradycardias. Although the cause and reversibility of the bradyarrhythmia may not be known, prompt institution of external pacing may be crucial to maintain hemodynamic stability.[7] During transport, an external pacemaker may be used until a transvenous pacemaker can be inserted. External pacing is performed according to ACLS protocols. The catheters are inserted with aseptic technique, and the position of the electrode is validated with fluoroscopy. Ventricular pacing is used in most clinical situations, although atrial or AV sequential pacing may be indicated.

Some of the complications encountered with temporary cardiac pacing that may occur during critical care transport include sensing problems, failure to capture, myocardial penetration, and cardiac tamponade. Undersensing or failure to sense may be caused by malposition of the catheter, poor intracardiac signal quality, or generator malfunction. Undersensing is managed by turning the sensitivity setting of the pulse generator to full-demand position.[19] Oversensing, which results in pauses in paced rhythm, can result from sensing of atrial electrical activity if the pacing lead is positioned near the tricuspid valve, from sensing of T waves, or from sensing voltage transients that are the result of lead wire fracture, environmental influences, or signals from the generator. The problem of oversensing can be resolved by turning the sensitivity setting toward the asynchronous position until the unwanted signals are no longer sensed.[19]

Failure to capture can be related to malposition of the lead or to an increase in the myocardial stimulation threshold. To resolve this problem, the current output should be increased until consistent capture occurs. If electrolyte imbalance is the underlying problem, it should be corrected. The position of the lead should be checked and repositioned if necessary.

Myocardial penetration or perforation into the pericardial space is usually accompanied by a pericardial friction rub and often by a squeaking systolic sound or murmur. If the pacing has migrated, it should be repositioned. If cardiac tamponade occurs in association with perforation, immediate pericardiocentesis should be performed.

First-Degree Atrioventricular Block. *First-degree AV block* is characterized by prolongation of the PR interval beyond 0.20 seconds in adults and more than 0.18 seconds in children. A QRS complex with a constant prolonged interval follows each P wave. The usual range for the prolonged PR interval is 0.21 to 0.40 seconds, but the interval may extend to as long as 0.80 seconds. In this form of AV block, each atrial impulse is conducted to the ventricles. First-degree AV block has been associated with congenital structural heart disease such as endocardial cushion defects. It is rarely treated, but the cause should be determined and corrected.

Second-Degree Atrioventricular Block. *Mobitz type I* (Wenckebach AV block) is characterized by the progressive lengthening of the PR intervals until a single P wave is not followed by a QRS. The RR intervals become progressively shorter until the P wave is blocked, and a shortening of the PR interval postblock compared with the PR interval just precedes the blocked cycle. This type of arrhythmia has little clinical significance and is not treated.

Mobitz type II is recognized when the P waves are periodically blocked from conduction to the ventricles without a progressive prolongation of the PR interval or a progressive shortening of the RR interval. In this type of block, the PR interval of all conducted beats is constant, and the P-P intervals remain constant. Mobitz II is usually associated with bundle branch block or bifascicular block. Because Mobitz type II is usually a precursor of complete AV block and is generally irreversible, a permanent pacemaker is often necessary. Atropine is not indicated in type II blocks and third-degree blocks with widened QRS complexes.[11]

Third-Degree Atrioventricular Block or Complete Heart Block.

Third-degree AV block is a potentially lethal conduction abnormality that is characterized by separate and independent atrial and ventricular activity. Either sinus or ectopic atrial pacemakers control the atria, and a pacemaker that is distal to the AV block controls the ventricles. The ECG shows completely dissociated P waves and QRS complexes. The heart rate can be as low as 20 to 40 bpm with this type of block. Treatment almost always involves the use of a transcutaneous or external pacemaker or transvenous pacemaker, if available. Pharmacologic therapy with single agents can include atropine at 0.5 to 1.0 mg (although normally ineffective) or dopamine at 5 to 20 μg/kg/min. If atropine and pacing fail, epinephrine at 2 to 10 μg/min can be administered.

CARDIOGENIC SHOCK

Cardiogenic shock is defined as a decrease in cardiac output that results in a critical reduction in tissue perfusion, as evidenced by tissue hypoxia in the presence of adequate intravascular volume.[15,45] Cardiogenic shock is one of the most severe complications of AMI and is usually the result of extensive ischemic damage to more than 40% of the LV myocardium. Seven percent to 10% of patients with AMI have cardiogenic shock develop, with a mortality rate in medically treated patients between 50% and 70%. Although left ventricular failure is the most common cause of cardiogenic shock (78.5%), other common causes are the result of mechanical complications, including severe mitral regurgitation (6.9%), ventricular septal rupture (3.9%), isolated right ventricular shock (2.8%), and cardiac tamponade (1.4%). Myocarditis, end-stage cardiomyopathy, myocardial contusion, and septic shock with severe myocardial depression can also deteriorate into cardiogenic shock.[5,15,25,45] During the past two decades, the primary goal of therapy for the patient with AMI has been to manage or prevent pump failure. Because the amount of ventricular failure is directly related to

the extent of infarction, therapies aimed at limiting MI size and early revascularization are imperative in reducing the incidence and extent of pump failure. Prevention of the development of cardiogenic shock with early identification of the preshock state is the primary objective. Treatment should include relief or control of ischemia, prevention of arrhythmias, and inotropic hemodynamic support to support viable myocardial function. Thrombolysis and primary angioplasty have been shown to significantly reduce the incidence rate of cardiogenic shock.[34,48] Early intervention reduces the incidence rate of cardiogenic shock. Initiation of therapy for AMI following the AHA guidelines as soon as possible on presentation is important in the cycle of prevention of pump failure. However, the most extreme form of pump failure after an AMI remains cardiogenic shock.

Pathophysiologic Factors

Inadequate cardiac pumping present in cardiogenic shock results in a decreased cardiac output, hypoperfusion, and inadequate tissue perfusion. Both systolic and diastolic myocardial dysfunctions are characteristics of cardiogenic shock. Decreased compliance from ischemia results in hemodynamic changes that include a decrease in stroke volume (SV), which results in elevations in left ventricular end-diastolic pressure, left atrial pressure, and pulmonary capillary wedge pressure (PCWP). The concomitant hypotension causes a decrease in coronary artery perfusion, further contributing to myocardial depression. Elevation of left ventricular pressures can result in pulmonary edema and hypoxemia. Clinical cardiogenic shock constitutes the combination of hypotension and pulmonary edema. These changes eventually lead to complete circulatory failure.[45]

Assessment and Diagnosis

Patients in cardiogenic shock appear acutely ill and are in acute distress. Physical examination often reveals profound hypotension, signs of peripheral hypoperfusion, hypoxemia, acidosis, rales, and oliguria. They often have an ashen or cyanotic appearance, and the skin is cool and clammy with mottled extremities. Some patients have a depressed sensorium as a result of hypoxemia. Pulses may be irregular if arrhythmias are present, and peripheral pulses are faint and rapid. Jugular venous distention is usually present.

Hemodynamically, patients in cardiogenic shock manifest marked hypotension with SBP 80 to 85 mm Hg, low cardiac index 2.2 L/min/m^2, decreased urinary output (UO), elevated heart rates, and a pulmonary artery wedge pressure (PAWP) greater than 18 to 20 mm Hg. They also exhibit pulmonary congestion and arterial hypoxemia. Arrhythmias may occur as a result of hypoxemia, with chest radiographic results revealing pulmonary vascular congestion. However, the SHOCK Trial Registry[2] did indicate that 28% of the patients presented only with hypoperfusion and no congestion, whereas 64% of patients presented with the classic symptoms of congestion and hypoperfusion. Mortality rates for both groups were near the same (70% and 60%, respectively).[45]

MANAGEMENT

Specific issues to be addressed include correction of hypoxemia, correction of electrolyte levels and acid/base balance, maximization of volume status, treatment of sustained arrhythmias, inotropic/vasopressor support, early revascularization, and consideration of IABP/VAD support. Oxygenation and airway support are imperative, and correction of hypoxemia may include intubation and mechanical ventilation. Most patients need intubation with positive-end expiratory pressure (PEEP) if pulmonary congestion is severe. Electrolyte imbalances, such as hypokalemia and hypomagnesemia, create vulnerability to ventricular arrhythmias, whereas acidosis decreases contractility.

Maximization of volume status necessitates fluid resuscitation unless pulmonary edema is present. PAWP should be maintained at 18 to 20 mm Hg. Intake and output should be monitored carefully. Thirty percent of patients with inferior infarction have right ventricular infarction develop. The maintenance of right ventricular preload, with the administration of fluids, is the initial therapy for support of right ventricular infarction. Careful assessment of PCWP and cardiac output is essential. Antiarrhythmic drugs, cardioversion, and pacing should be used promptly as necessary to correct any arrhythmias or heart blocks that affect cardiac output. Inotropic agents and vasopressors should be initiated for cardiovascular support in the presence of inadequate tissue perfusion with adequate intravascular volume. Nitrates, beta-blockers, and ACE inhibitors, normally used to improve outcomes after AMI, can worsen hypotension and should be avoided in true cardiac shock. Although thrombolytic therapy has shown to reduce mortality rates in patients with AMI, no significant improvement in outcomes has been shown with established cardiogenic shock. However, even the possibility of saving a small number of lives advocates its use as a potential benefit in a certain high-risk group where both hypotension and tachycardia are present.[48] Aggressive use of vasopressors or IABP has been recommended to enhance the effect of thrombolysis.[16,48] Revascularization with percutaneous coronary angioplasty (PTCA) or coronary bypass surgery in 24 hours has been shown to significantly decrease mortality rates.[41] Other studies have shown that the placement of coronary stents provides better angiographic results and improves outcomes. Although CABG surgery shows favorable outcomes as well, the highly beneficial results of PTCA and the higher rates of surgical mortality and morbidity with CABG make the use of PTCA preferable.[46] Mechanical circulatory support, IABP, and VADs may be needed to stabilize patient conditions until coronary angioplasty and can be used as a bridge to surgical revascularization or heart transplantation. Early revascularization does significantly improve the outcome of patients in shock from MI. Patients in cardiogenic shock need frequent assessment of hemodynamic parameters, including blood pressure (BP), heart rate, and pulmonary artery pressures (if a pulmonary artery line is present). These patients should be kept in a supine position to improve cerebral blood flow and blood flow to the heart. They should be frequently assessed for peripheral perfusion, presence of edema, color and warmth of skin, blood gases, hemoglobin, and hematocrit to assess oxygen-carrying capacity and function.

Pharmacologic Therapy

Pharmacologic management includes the use of inotropic and vasopressor agents such as dopamine and dobutamine to improve cardiac output by increasing contractility. Dobutamine is the initial drug of choice when systolic pressure is greater than 80 mm Hg and is effective without a striking change in heart rate or systemic vascular resistance. Dobutamine can aggravate hypotension and precipitate tachyarrhythmias in some patients. Dopamine has both inotropic and vasopressor effects and is used when the systolic pressures are less than 80 mm Hg. Dopamine can result in tachycardia and an increase in peripheral vascular resistance, which exacerbates myocardial ischemia.

When dopamine and dobutamine are ineffective, norepinephrine, a catecholamine with potent alpha-adrenergic and beta-adrenergic effects, can be administered to improve coronary perfusion and to improve blood pressure. Norepinephrine should be carefully titrated because the combined increase in preload and afterload can threaten myocardial oxygen supply and demand, increasing the risk of ischemia and arrhythmia. It can also be used in conjunction with dopamine and dobutamine to allow for lower dosing. Vasodilators should be used with extreme caution because they can cause further hypotension and a decrease in coronary blood flow. Vasodilators are used to increase forward flow by reducing afterload; these drugs include sodium nitroprusside and NTG. Sodium nitroprusside reduces afterload by decreasing filling pressures and can also increase stroke volume. NTG reduces PCWP and left ventricular filling pressure and redistributes coronary blood flow to the ischemic area. Diuretic therapy is limited to treating pulmonary congestion and decreasing intravascular volume, thereby improving oxygenation.[34,48]

Intraaortic Balloon Counterpulsation

When pharmacologic support and adjunctive therapies fail to improve low cardiac output and poor perfusion associated with cardiogenic shock, alternative devices are often used, such as the IABP and VADs. IABPs have been used to treat cardiogenic shock for decades. Emergency revascularization in conjunction with *intraaortic balloon counterpulsation* (IABC) should be used in patients with AMI complicated by cardiogenic shock. Aggressive use of IABP has also been recommended to enhance the effect of thrombolysis. Stabilization with IABP and thrombolysis, followed by transfer to a tertiary care facility, is the treatment option for those facilities without direct angioplasty capability.[46] Air transport

of the patient with IABP has been done successfully for the past 25 years.[39]

A current IABP device such as Datascope has developed pumps specifically for transport. These machines can sense changes in balloon volume caused by the effect of altitude, reduced barometric pressure, and gas expansion and automatically adjust to these changes. These new balloon pump consoles are Federal Aviation Administration (FAA) approved. They are designed to withstand vibration and shock effects and are shielded from electromagnetic interference (EMI) and radio frequency interference (RFI). This design has eliminated previous concerns over IABP transports and the need to purge the pump to avoid overexpansion of the balloon. These devices and their use are explained in detail in Chapter 23.

Ventricular Assist Devices

For patients with AMI that develops to cardiogenic shock that necessitates a ventricular assist device, the prognosis is poor. Several circulatory assist devices are now available. Indications for these devices include postcardiotomy ventricular failure, myocarditis, cardiomyopathy idiopathic hypertrophic subaortic stenosis, cardiac transplant rejection, or as a bridge to transplant. These devices are explained in detail in Chapter 23.

The transport vehicle, rotor-wing, fixed-wing, or surface vehicles, must be capable of a team effort to ensure that the hemodynamic stability of the patient is not interrupted. This can be accomplished by organizing the transport team and efficiently using space aboard the aircraft to accommodate equipment and allow the nurse to adequately visualize the patient, monitors, and vasoactive medications.[52,56,67,89]

Fixed-wing considerations include the size of the aircraft and its medical configuration with a pressurized cabin.

The critical care transport nurse should have a diverse background in critical care and be well educated on the operation of the VAD and IABP pumps. It is highly recommended that three medical crew members accompany these specialty transports to accommodate the patient and equipment needs and the logistics of movement. The highest possible level of caregivers should be used for transport, with a minimum of two critical care trained nurses. Adequate oxygen and electrical power must be available during all facets of the transport process. To avoid catastrophic inadvertent disconnection of the devices during transport, all equipment must be well secured and the patient may need sedation.

CONGESTIVE HEART FAILURE

DEFINITION AND PATHOPHYSIOLOGIC FACTORS

Heart failure can be difficult to define, but generally it is recognized in the clinical setting. It is a complex clinical syndrome that can be brought on by any form of heart disease, resulting in ventricular failure that prevents adequate blood flow to meet tissue metabolic needs.[3,20] Heart failure has previously been defined as a circulatory disorder caused by left ventricular dysfunction. Recently, clinicians have recognized the need for a more encompassing definition of heart failure. Specifically, this definition highlights the process of left ventricular (LV) remodeling, the cellular events linked to the remodeling process, such as myocyte hypertrophy, interstitial fibrosis, myocyte dropout, and changes in the genetic expression of specific cardiac cell and subcellular proteins. Heart failure should not be defined solely on the presence or absence of congestion but should include a broad spectrum of characteristics such as acute or chronic, right-sided or left-sided failure, systolic or diastolic, and with or without compromised organ perfusion. The hallmark of acute heart failure is demonstrated by a decreased LV function that develops rapidly, canceling out the compensatory effect of the sympathetic nervous system. This is can be a result of exacerbation of a chronic condition or as an initial manifestation. When the ventricles cannot adequately deliver their preload, volume backs up in the left ventricle, then in the left atrium, and inevitably into the pulmonary circulation. An increase in preload, an increase in afterload, and a decrease in CO_2 are the hemodynamic outcomes of the body's response to myocardial dysfunction. The pathophysiologic processes of heart failure provide the basis for therapy that is directed at decreasing symptoms, promoting clinical stability, and decreasing the disease progression.[5,15]

ASSESSMENT AND DIAGNOSIS

A careful history usually reveals the cause of heart failure, such as MI, hypertension, or alcoholism. Left ventricular dysfunction from CAD and advanced age are the primary risk factors that contribute to the development of heart failure. Other risk factors include diabetes, angina, hypertension, history of cigarette smoking, obesity, elevated HDL, abnormally high or low hematocrit levels, proteinuria, and a history of CAD or previous MI. The patient has shortness of breath, which begins initially with exertion and progresses to shortness of breath at rest. In severe heart failure, the patient has orthopnea and must sit upright or lean over a table to breathe.

Physical examination reveals elevated central venous pressure, pulsus alternans, or a dicrotic pulse and pulmonary rales that do not clear with coughing and may extend to the lung apices. In right ventricular failure, an S3 and a holosystolic murmur of tricuspid regurgitation are often heard. Hepatomegaly is felt, and peripheral pitting edema without venous insufficiency is present. In left ventricular failure, the apical impulse is usually displaced laterally and downward and S1 is diminished. The S2 is sometimes paradoxically split, and an S3 gallop is present.[15]

Electrocardiographic monitoring may show the development of arrhythmias such as arterial fibrillation (AF), complete heart block (CHB), and rapid tachycardias that could exacerbate pump failure. Laboratory data are nonspecific, although arterial hypoxemia and metabolic acidosis are common and respiratory alkalosis may be present with significant tachypnea. Chest radiograph films can reveal cardiomegaly and may show pulmonary vascular congestion and interstitial edema. Because of an increase, invasive monitoring reveals an elevated PAWP, elevated systemic vascular resistance, and low cardiac output.[15,19]

Transport nurses must remain alert to factors that can aggravate underlying cardiac dysfunction. These factors may be an extension of active ischemia/infarction, uncontrolled hypertension, or heavy alcohol consumption. Viral infections and pneumonias frequently trigger the onset of symptoms and may necessitate weeks of close supervision for recovery, if recovery is even possible. Atrial fibrillation, which can cause or result from worsening failure, warrants the restoration of sinus rhythm to improve cardiac function. Obesity is both a primary cause and an aggravating factor for heart failure. Orthopnea is the most sensitive symptom of elevated filling pressures, and the degree of orthopnea parallels the amount of increased pressure. Jugular venous distention provides the most sensitive symptom of elevated resting filling pressures. Peripheral edema is present in only a few patients with chronic heart failure. Weight gain is another factor, which can indicate an impending episode of failure. Abdominal symptoms can result from hepatic congestion.

Once the patient is determined to be in failure, whether the patient is experiencing hypoperfusion must then be determined. Physical evidence of hypoperfusion includes low blood pressure, narrow pulse pressure, cool extremities, and occasionally altered mentation, with supporting evidence sometimes provided by decreased sodium levels and worsening renal function and lethargy.[15]

MANAGEMENT

Management of acute heart failure focuses on the reduction of preload for relief of pulmonary edema, reduction of afterload with vasodilators to enhance stroke volume, and enhancement of contractile function. Intravenous diuretics and nitrates are used for preload reduction. Afterload reducing agents and angiotensin-converting enzyme inhibitors are used in the chronic, as opposed to the acute, setting. Inotropic agents are rarely used to enhance contractility because of the increase in myocardial oxygen demand, unless shock is present.[15,34] Currently, beta-blockers are used to improve LV performance and improve survival.[6] Continuous ECG monitoring is necessary (potential ventricular arrhythmias may develop as a result of electrolyte imbalances), and strict intake and output measurements must be maintained and recorded.

CARDIOMYOPATHY

Cardiomyopathy is a general term used to describe disease that involves the muscle itself. The cardiomyopathies are unique because they are not the result of ischemic, hypertensive, congenital, valvular, or pericardial diseases.

Cardiomyopathies can be functionally classified into three categories: (1) dilated cardiomyopathy, which is characterized by ventricular dilation, contractile dysfunction, and symptoms of heart failure; (2) hypertrophic cardiomyopathy, which is marked by myocardial hypertrophy, with left and sometimes right ventricular hypertrophy, most commonly involving the interventricular septum; and (3) restrictive cardiomyopathy, characterized by excessively rigid ventricular walls that impede ventricular filling, with the impairment of diastolic filling.

DILATED CARDIOMYOPATHY

Dilated cardiomyopathy, formerly called congestive cardiomyopathy, is characterized by ventricular remodeling that produces dilated chambers, contractility dysfunction, and, in most cases, heart failure as a result of impairment of systolic pump function. Impaired systolic function can involve left, right, or both ventricles with ejection fraction of less than 40%. The total mass of the heart is increased, which results in dilation of the heart. This dilated cardiomyopathy is the end result of myocardial damage produced by a variety of toxic (e.g., cocaine), metabolic, or infectious agents and causes that can be familial, genetic, or idiopathic in origin. Secondary causes that may precipitate dilated cardiomyopathy include alcohol, hypertension, pregnancy, viruses, and hyperthyroidism.[10]

Pathophysiologic Factors

Myocardial hypertrophy results in dilation of the heart, and as the disease progresses, the altered hemodynamics of myocardial remodeling are characterized by diminished ejection fraction, decreased stroke volume, and elevated end-systolic volume caused by increased chamber pressure.[10,15] As a compensatory response, cardiac output initially rises but eventually declines in exercise or stress. Thrombus formation is enhanced because of the retention of blood in the cardiac chambers. The coronary arteries are usually normal. At the end stage of dilated cardiomyopathy, cardiac output declines and right-sided heart failure occurs, causing biventricular failure and symptoms of CHF.

Assessment and Diagnosis

Patients often have symptoms of low cardiac output or fluid overload. Congestion is not consistently present, especially in the milder stages. Chest pain is common even in the presence of healthy coronaries, and this may be associated with limited coronary vascular reserve or presence of ischemic heart disease. Severe ventricular dysfunction is frequently present with New York Heart Association class III or IV symptoms. Fatigue and weakness usually accompany these symptoms. Occasionally, patients have right-sided heart failure develop, with increased jugular venous distention (JVD), hepatomegaly, splenomegaly, ascites, and peripheral edema. Other clinical features include a persistent S3 gallop and symptomatic ventricular tachycardia. A reduction in pulse pressure and the presence of systolic murmurs may be seen. Patients may also have abdominal pain, a reflection of liver congestion, or gastrointestinal discomfort from mesenteric congestion. Fatigue and weakness are present because of decreased cardiac output. Arrhythmias and sudden death are not uncommon and may occur at any stage of the disease process.

On physical examination, the patient is breathless at rest or on exertion. The skin may be cool, pale, or cyanotic with peripheral edema. Palpation may reveal ascites, JVD, and pulsatile liver engorgement. An S3 and an S4 heart sound is often auscultated as a summation gallop in patients with rapid heart rates.[10,15]

Management

Treatment of dilated cardiomyopathy includes measures to improve the symptoms of heart failure and increase stroke volume. Pharmacologic therapy includes diuretics, digoxin, ACE inhibitors, inotropes, anticoagulants, antiarrhythmics, and beta-blockers. Inotropic agents such as amiodarone, dopamine, and dobutamine may be used for their positive inotropic effects to increase contractility and cardiac output. Diuretics decrease blood volume in heart failure, and anticoagulation therapy prevents systemic and pulmonary emboli. Beta-blocking agents may be used in patients with tachycardia at rest. Vasodilators can be used to decrease afterload and to improve cardiac output if intravascular volume is normal or high. Nitrates are most commonly used for this purpose. The aggressive use of ACE inhibitors and other therapies has resulted in improved outcomes.[34] Unfortunately, all forms of medical treatment are palliative rather than curative in the treatment of dilated cardiomyopathy. VADs may be used as a bridge to transplant to provide systemic support until cardiac transplant is available or other new surgical procedures can be initiated.

HYPERTROPHIC CARDIOMYOPATHY

Hypertrophic cardiomyopathy is characterized by disproportionate left and sometimes right ventricular hypertrophy. This most often involves the septum rather than the left ventricular free wall. Ventricular filling is impaired because of the abnormal stiffness of the ventricular septum. Hypertrophic cardiomyopathy is further characterized by disorganization of cardiac myocytes and myofibrils. The pathology of this disease leads to a gamut of abnormal processes that includes myocardial ischemia, diastolic dysfunction, ventricular and atrial arrhythmias, and congestive heart failure.[10,15]

Pathophysiologic Factors

Hypertrophic cardiomyopathy (HCM) is usually familial (up to 70%) with an autosomal dominant inheritance. Evidence exists that several genetic abnormalities might be associated with this disease. It is characterized by dynamic left ventricular outflow tract obstruction (LVOT) and increased left ventricular systolic performance. Most patients also have diastolic dysfunction as an effect of left ventricular relaxation and distensibility abnormalities. The high resistance to ventricular filling caused by diastolic dysfunction results in left atrial cavity size enlargement. Patients have shown reduced coronary blood flow that may result in myocardial ischemia, causing chest pain and dyspnea. Hemodynamically, patients with HCM have a high ejection fraction, which can result in increased myocardial oxygen consumption. The stiff ventricle requires high filling pressures, which often produce pulmonary hypertension. Poor outcomes are found when supraventricular and ventricular tachycardia are present.[10,15]

Assessment and Diagnosis

Patients with hypertrophic cardiomyopathy are usually young (in their second or third decade of life), active, and athletic, although idiopathic left ventricular hypertrophy is well described in patients over 60 years of age. The pattern of disease in this age group differs significantly. Patients with HCM typically are initially seen with a systolic murmur of late onset heard at the left sternal border and apex that radiates to the axilla. The murmur is increased by standing or during the Valsalva's maneuver. The arterial pulse is abrupt and has a jerky quality. Patients with significant left ventricular outflow gradients frequently have mitral regurgitation.

The most common symptom is dyspnea; other symptoms include angina as a result of oxygen demand exceeding supply and reduced coronary blood flow, syncope from inadequate cardiac output or arrhythmias, palpitations, fatigue, paroxysmal nocturnal dyspnea (PND), heart failure, and vertigo. Most of the symptoms are worsened with exertion. The ECG in hypertrophic cardiomyopathy reflects hypertrophy and atrial abnormality. Approximately 20% of these patients have atrial fibrillation.[15] Left ventricular hypertrophy (LVH) has been shown to be present 10 times more often in sudden death events than in those without LVH. Autopsy examination on apparently healthy young athletes with sudden death has revealed such cardiac diseases as hypertrophic cardiomyopathy. Even in those cases in which no apparent cause was found, physiologic LVH is noted to be present.

Management

Management of patients with hypertrophic cardiomyopathy consists of symptom relief and prevention of complications. Pharmacologic interventions that increase or maintain left ventricular end-diastolic volume and reduce ventricular contractility are usually used. Management currently includes beta-blockers, verapamil, dual-chamber pacing, and surgical myectomy. In patients with left ventricular outflow obstruction, beta-blockers to decrease myocardial oxygen consumption, decrease angina, and prevent increase in outflow obstruction with exercise are the first drug of choice. Verapamil can also be used for its negative inotropic effect, and often, in high doses, it may improve left ventricular relaxation and exercise tolerance in nonobstructive HCM. Dual-chamber pacing with a short program AV delay to maintain constant activation of the right ventricle

may improve symptoms in those patients with left ventricular outflow tract gradients. A myectomy to widen the left ventricular outflow tract should be considered in all patients with outflow obstruction of more than 50 mm Hg and symptoms nonresponsive to medical therapy. Percutaneous transluminal septal myocardial ablation (PTSMA) is a novel nonsurgical approach to ablate hypertrophied septal myocardium with injection of alcohol into the septal branches.[34] For long-term management, calcium channel blocking agents are used. The antiarrhythmic agent amiodarone is used for those patients with frequent ventricular ectopy or ventricular tachycardia. Prophylactic antibiotic therapy is indicated both before and after surgical procedures for protection from infective endocarditis.

RESTRICTIVE CARDIOMYOPATHY

Restrictive cardiomyopathy is the least common of the cardiomyopathies. It resembles constrictive pericarditis clinically and is characterized by a normal to slightly enlarged heart, decreased diastolic volumes, and, early in the disease process, a normal systolic function.

Pathophysiologic Factors

Diastolic function impairment results from excessively rigid ventricular walls that impede ventricular filling with the consequence of decreased ventricular compliance and filling. The walls of both ventricles are firm, noncompliant, and thickened. Mild cardiac enlargement may be seen with restrictive cardiomyopathy without significant ventricular dilation. The cause is usually unknown, but many specific pathologic processes may develop into restrictive cardiomyopathy, including myocardial fibrosis, hypertrophy, or infiltration.

Assessment and Diagnosis

Patients have signs and symptoms of myocardial failure with normal cardiac size. Most patients have chest pain, dyspnea on exertion, and fatigue. Often dyspnea on exertion is the only symptom in patients with early restrictive cardiomyopathy.[10,15] Because of the heart's inability to increase cardiac output, exercise tolerance is limited. Right-sided clinical presentation is frequently seen in advanced cases: increased jugular venous pressure, ascites, and peripheral edema. Mitral and tricuspid murmurs and S3 or S4 heart sounds are usually present. The ECG commonly reveals sinus tachycardia and atrial fibrillation with biventricular hypertrophy and decreased voltage.[10,15,34]

Management

Medical management of restrictive cardiomyopathy is similar to that for heart failure in that it is symptom limiting. The treatment focuses on fluid restriction, diuretic therapy, anticoagulation therapy, and administration of digitalis if atrial fibrillation is present. Surgical treatment consists of resection of thickened endocardial tissue. Valve replacement surgery is also done when necessary.

VALVULAR DYSFUNCTION

DEFINITION

Valvular dysfunction can result from either congenital or acquired causes that expose the valve to hemodynamic stress and may accelerate the degenerative changes that cause dysfunction. Changes that cause narrowing of the valve orifice are classified as *stenosis,* which may result in pressure overload. Changes that lead to valvular insufficiency because of improper closing of valves are classified as *regurgitation* and may result in volume overload.

MITRAL STENOSIS
Pathophysiologic Factors

Mitral stenosis most often is a result of rheumatic heart disease that usually occurs by the age of 12 years, with the associated murmur heard approximately 20 years later. Although rare, other diseases that result in mitral stenosis include but are not limited to congenital mitral stenosis and infective endocarditis. Mitral stenosis is a narrowing of the mitral orifice associated with abnormal flow patterns that result from valvulitis and develop into fibrosis and thickening of the mitral valve. The pathologic changes that occur in mitral stenosis are fusion of the commissures, fibrosis and thickening of the leaflets, shortening and fusion of the chordae and papillary muscles or both, and calcification of the leaflets. As the valve area is reduced, the gradient across the valve increases. Critical mitral stenosis occurs when the mitral valve opening is reduced to $1.0\,cm^2$; the normal mitral valve has an area of 4 to $6\,cm^2$. The stenosis leads to elevations in left atrial pressure that cause increased pulmonary venous and pulmonary artery wedge pressure.[7,19]

Assessment and Diagnosis

Symptoms develop gradually, with cardiac symptoms usually appearing in the fourth or fifth decade. The principal symptom of severe mitral stenosis is dyspnea with minimal exertion, pulmonary edema and hemoptysis that result from elevated left atrial, and pulmonary venous and pulmonary capillary pressure. Pulmonary edema develops when the pulmonary capillary pressure is greater 25 mm Hg. Hemoptysis results from ruptured pulmonary venules. AF is a frequently occurring arrhythmia as a result of atrial dilation and hypertrophy, which in return can cause further deterioration of the patient's clinical condition. Systemic embolization and thromboembolism may be a presenting symptom in the presence of atrial fibrillation. Fatigue is a common symptom, as are palpitations if AF has developed. Systemic venous hypertension with increased JVD develops when severe mitral stenosis leads to pulmonary vascular resistance and right-sided heart failure. Auscultation reveals an increased intensity of the first heart sound described as a snap and a low-pitched diastolic rumbling murmur that is best heard at the apex when the patient is in the left lateral decubitus position.[34]

Management

Medical management of mitral stenosis includes prevention of complications such as systemic embolism or bacterial endocarditis and treatment of AF. Symptomatic patients with dyspnea are treated with diuretics and short-acting or long-acting nitrate preparations. Those patients with AF should receive prophylactic anticoagulant therapy unless contraindicated. AF is treated with digitalis glycosides. Low-dose beta-blockers can be used to slow ventricular rates if necessary. The development of pulmonary edema from a rapid ventricular response necessitates urgent intervention with either cardioversion or intravenous procainamide. Prophylactic antibiotics are given before dental work, surgery, and other interventions that require instrumentation procedures to decrease the risk of development of infectious endocarditis. The best treatment for symptomatic mitral stenosis is relief of the valvular obstruction. Surgical management of mitral stenosis includes valvuloplasty or valve replacement, whereas nonsurgical treatment involves balloon valvuloplasty.[32]

Mitral Regurgitation
Pathophysiologic Factors
Acute *mitral regurgitation* (MR) is a result of severe mitral incompetence. The mitral valve fails to close completely. This allows blood to flow back into the atrium during ventricular systole. It involves abnormal loading conditions; a sudden volume overload is forced on an ill-equipped left ventricle and left atrium. Preload is elevated; afterload is initially decreased and then eventually increases as left ventricular function deteriorates. Although left ventricular stroke volume increases, a large amount of the flow is forwarded into the left atrium instead of the aorta. This results in an increase in pressure in the noncompliant nondilated left atrium and ventricle. Acute MR is a potentially fatal occurrence if the disease process includes mitral valve rupture. This valve disruption is caused by rupture of the base of a papillary muscle, usually from ischemic necrosis. Rupture of both valve leaflets is incompatible with life; however, if only one leaflet ruptures, resulting in an incompetent valve, prognosis is much better. From acute severe MR, pulmonary edema, left ventricular volume overload, and passive pulmonary hypertension develop. The pulmonary edema and hypertension are a result of left atrial hypertension from acute volume overload in a chamber of normal size and compliance.[6,32]

Assessment and Diagnosis
The symptoms of MR develop rapidly and are associated with left ventricular failure. Severe dyspnea at rest and angina result from increased left ventricular filling pressures. Tachycardia and tachypnea are common. The MR murmur is of variable intensity; it may be loud if normal left ventricular function is present and soft if left ventricular function is reduced.[32] If both leaflets are involved, the murmur is loud and widespread.

The ECG results may be normal or show evidence of an AMI. The rhythm is usually sinus rhythm; atrial fibrillation is indicative of chronic MR. Invasive monitoring discloses a prominent systolic regurgitant wave in the PAWP tracing.

Management
Surgical intervention (valvuloplasty or replacement) is almost always necessary, and medical management is used to stabilize the patient's condition before surgical treatment. Intravenous sodium nitroprusside therapy is given for vasodilator and afterload reducing affects. It lowers systemic vascular resistance, enhances stroke volume, and is effective in reducing pulmonary vascular congestion. Oral medical therapy includes ACE inhibitors, digoxin, and diuretics. Hypotension is usually treated with dopamine, and hemodynamic support with the IABP or VAD may be necessary.[6,32,42]

Aortic Stenosis
Pathophysiologic Factors
Aortic stenosis (AS) usually results from a congenital or degenerative origin. The most common cause of adult acquired AS is idiopathic degeneration and calcification of the aortic valve, with symptoms developing in the fifth and sixth decades of life. With rheumatic AS, which occurs in a small minority of patients, symptoms develop in the fourth decade. Congenital AS is diagnosed in childhood in the first decade, although occasionally some of these patients are seen for the first time as adults. The reduction in the valve orifice causes obstruction to the flow of blood from the left ventricle into the aorta during ventricular systole, which results in eventual ventricular wall thickening. Pressure overload and increased systolic wall stress contribute to the development of left ventricular hypertrophy, which acts as a compensatory mechanism. The progressive pressure overload, increased pressure gradient, and left ventricular hypertrophy can ultimately lead to total left ventricular failure.[10,15]

Assessment and Diagnosis
Both systolic and diastolic myocardial dysfunction may occur in AS, and patients have symptoms of heart failure. Angina develops because of myocardial

ischemia and abnormalities in oxygen supply and demand. Syncope is suspected of being caused either by an increase in intraventricular pressure during exercise that initiates a vasodepressor response or by supraventricular or ventricular arrhythmias. The presence of a systolic ejection murmur that radiates to the neck is frequently the first suspicion of the presence of AS; the murmur is loud early in the course of the disease and is associated with a systolic thrill. Later in the disease, the murmur is heard loudest at the end of systole and is heard over the aortic area and the apex. Palpation of the carotid arteries reveals a reduction in amplitude of the carotid upstroke. The palpation of a strong apical impulse in conjunction with the simultaneous weak and delayed carotid pulse is indicative of severe AS. ECG results may reveal left ventricular hypertrophy and left atrial abnormality, although a patient who is symptomatic can have fairly normal ECG readings.[34]

Management

Patients with asymptomatic AS have a nearly normal survival for long latency periods and most often do not need therapy at all other than antibiotic prophylaxis for the prevention of infective endocarditis. Patients with symptomatic AS have an average survival time of 2 to 3 years and need surgical intervention with aortic valve replacement (AVR). For those patients who are not surgical candidates, digitalis and diuretics may be used to treat CHF symptoms, and nitrates may be used with caution to treat angina.[34] Vasodilators and ACE inhibitors, widely used to treat CHF, are contraindicated in patients with AS. Vasodilators lower peripheral pressure and reduce preload, precipitating dangerous hypotension without increasing cardiac output.

AORTIC REGURGITATION
Pathophysiologic Factors

Acute *aortic regurgitation* (AR) results in a large volume overload at high pressure to the left ventricle, which cannot adapt acutely. The aortic valve fails to close completely, which allows the blood to flow back into the ventricle during ventricular diastole. Acute AR causes an early impairment in ejection, resulting in low forward stroke output, left atrial

hypertension, and pulmonary edema. The most common cause of AR is infective endocarditis; it is therefore common in younger patients with a history of intravenous drug use. Other causes include aortic dissection and nonpenetrating chest or upper abdominal trauma.[15]

Assessment and Diagnosis

The patient with acute AR is acutely ill with tachycardia, peripheral hypoperfusion, and congestive heart failure. Physical examination reveals a widened pulse pressure. S1 is diminished, and there is no S4. The diastolic murmur may be of variable intensity. The ECG results may be normal or show left ventricular hypertrophy if aortic dissection is present. Infective endocarditis is often mistaken for influenza. A high degree of suspicion should be present when a patient presents with the sudden development of high fever, malaise, and early symptoms of CHF with any prior history of an abnormal aortic valve or valve prosthesis.

Management

Medical management for patients with AR is a temporary measure until surgery can be performed. AVR is indicated for both survival and quality of life. Even if the patient is asymptomatic, AVR is indicated to prevent further deterioration into heart failure. Vasodilators may improve symptoms temporarily and assist in preparation for surgery. With endocarditis, broad-spectrum antibiotics should be started initially after blood cultures are drawn. Use of the IABP is contraindicated because it increases AR.[34]

ACUTE PERICARDITIS

Pericarditis refers to inflammation of the pericardium; it can have a number of causes. The most common conditions associated with the development of pericarditis include MI, infection, collagen vascular diseases, uremia, malignancy disease, drug therapy, and trauma.

The pericardium is a closed fibrous sac that envelops the heart. It consists of an inner serous membrane, the visceral pericardium, which closely adheres to the superficial myocardium and coronary vessels. The fibrous outer layer that surrounds the heart is the parietal pericardium. The space between the visceral and parietal layers normally contains between 10 to 20 mL of pericardial fluid that acts as a lubricant between the contracting surfaces. The exact role of the pericardium is not clear; however, it is believed to serve as a lubrication system, ensuring that cardiac motion is unimpaired by surrounding mediastinal structures. Because the pericardium resists stretching, it functions as a protective mechanism to prevent sudden dilation of the heart. The pericardium may also protect the heart from infection.

Pericarditis can be associated with AMI. It results from an extension of the infarction to the epicardial area and is associated with an inflammatory response localized to the pericardium bordering the infarction. It may also be a delayed response with a more generalized inflammatory response, such as in Dressler's syndrome.[10]

ASSESSMENT AND DIAGNOSIS

The presentation of pericardial heart disease depends on the pericardium's response to injury and subsequent effect on cardiac function. Diagnosis and recognition of acute pericarditis in the emergent situation are largely dependent on patient history of pleuritic chest pain. Typical chest pain is described as sharp, severe, and substernal and increases with inspiration or in the reclining position. Chest pain caused by acute pericarditis may further be aggravated by coughing or movement and may be relieved when the patient sits up and leans forward. Substernal pain may radiate to the neck, shoulder, and back. The physical examination may reveal a pericardial friction rub, which may be absent when effusion develops. ECG changes may show atypical T wave abnormalities. ST segment elevation is not common but may be present when pericarditis is more generalized. Diffuse ST segment elevation in conjunction with PR segment depression is the typical ECG presentation. Associated signs and symptoms of pericarditis include: (1) fever and leukocytosis; (2) dyspnea related to increased pain with inspiration; (3) dysphagia related to irritation of the esophagus by the posterior pericardium; and (4) sinus tachycardia.

Physical examination results show a pericardial friction rub that may be heard at various times and in various locations during the patient's course. The friction rub resembles a high-pitched grating or scratching sound. It is best heard with the diaphragm of the stethoscope placed at the lower left sternal border or apex with the patient sitting and leaning forward during held expiration. The presence of a friction rub does not exclude the presence of a large pericardial effusion or tamponade. A normal BP should be present without paradoxical pulse or venous distention. If the critical care nurse observes signs of restriction to ventricular filling, the presence of pericardial tamponade or effusion should be considered.

Dressler's syndrome appears later and may be related to an autoimmune reaction or may be related to activation of latent viral infections. Pathophysiology involves serosal inflammation and may involve the pleural or peritoneum.[15]

Purulent pericarditis is a rare syndrome with fever and hypotension frequently present. It is often mistaken for septic shock. Signs and symptoms associated with this syndrome are chest pain, pericardial friction rub, pulsus paradoxus, and elevation of jugular venous pressure. Patients only exhibit these classic descriptors 50% of the time, and a high index of suspicion is needed to diagnose this disorder.

MANAGEMENT

Evaluation and monitoring of acute pericarditis are important in the emergency setting to establish whether the pericarditis is associated with an underlying problem, such as MI or pericardial effusion, that necessitates specific therapy. The transport nurse should monitor for complications of pericarditis, such as signs of pericardial effusion that may accumulate rapidly and cause cardiac tamponade.

The chest pain of pericarditis may be managed with analgesics and antiinflammatory agents, such as aspirin and nonsteroidal antiinflammatory drugs (NSAIDs), such as ibuprofen. Because of the recurrent nature of Dressler's syndrome and the immunologic pathophysiology, steroids may be indicated for this condition.[34] The patient should be observed for atrial arrhythmias, such as beats and bursts of atrial tachycardia, which often accompany acute pericarditis.

CARDIAC EFFUSION AND TAMPONADE

Pericardial effusion refers to the development of fluid in the pericardial sac as a response to injury of the parietal pericardium or with all causes of acute pericarditis. *Cardiac tamponade* occurs with the accumulation of fluid and results in increased pressure and subsequent compression of the heart, to such an extent that cardiac output is significantly compromised. For emergency practitioners, cardiac tamponade is one of the most dramatic emergencies.

Pathophysiologic Factors

The hemodynamic effects of effusion are related to the speed of accumulation of the fluid. Rapid accumulation of 150 to 200 mL may produce acute cardiac tamponade; in contrast, large pericardial effusions, which develop slowly, can be totally asymptomatic. Under normal conditions, between 15 and 50 mL of fluid may be present in the pericardial space. The development of a larger volume of fluid may result from pericardial inflammation of any cause, heart failure, or traumatic injury to the heart, aortic dissection, or neoplasm. The presence of additional fluid causes the intrapericardial pressure to increase. When intrapericardial pressure is increased, diastolic filling of the ventricles is impeded, which results in a rise of ventricular pressure and decreased cardiac output. As the increased intrapericardial pressure reaches a critical level, a precipitous decrease in arterial pressure occurs.[7,19]

Assessment and Diagnosis

Mild to moderate pericardial effusion may not produce symptoms. If the fluid accumulates slowly, the fairly noncompliant pericardium stretches to accommodate the increasing volume with little or no rise in intrapericardial pressure until it reaches a size where it can no longer stretch. However, if the fluid accumulates rapidly, a small volume can be life threatening. Clinical symptoms of cardiac tamponade are related to systemic venous congestion, a reduction in cardiac stroke volume, and respiratory effects of impaired ventricular filling. Early tamponade manifests as tachycardia, tachypnea, edema, and elevated venous pressure. The classic signs, described as Beck's triad, include distended neck veins resulting from elevated central venous pressure (CVP), decreased BP, and muffled heart sounds. Pulsus paradoxus (abnormal fall in systolic pressure during inspiration caused by differential filling of the ventricles) may be present. Kussmaul's sign is a true paradoxical venous pressure abnormality associated with tamponade. It is manifested by a rise in venous pressure with inspiration when breathing spontaneously. If early signs of cardiac tamponade are not treated, rapid development of severe hypotension, right atrial and right ventricular collapse with profound circulatory failure, and shock result. Chest radiographic films may show a widening cardiac silhouette. Echocardiography is the recommended method for rapid and accurate diagnosis of tamponade.

Cardiac tamponade from trauma is usually the result of penetrating injuries, but blunt injury may also cause the pericardium to fill with blood from either injury to the heart itself or from the surrounding great vessels. Cardiac tamponade should be suspected in any trauma patient with electromechanical dissociation (EMD) or lack of response to volume resuscitation.[5]

Paradoxical Pulse

A finding of paradoxical pulse is elicited by measuring BP during quiet respiration. The technique involves pumping the blood pressure cuff above the systolic sounds and slowly deflating the cuff until the first systolic sound is heard. Normally, the systolic sound should disappear on inspiration. The critical care nurse should continue to deflate the cuff until all systolic sounds can be heard on inspiration and expiration. The paradox is the difference in millimeters of mercury between the pressure at which the systolic sound disappears and the pressure at which all systolic sounds are heard. A paradox of less than 10 mm Hg is a normal reflection of the inspiratory fall of aortic systolic pressure; however, it is exaggerated in the presence of cardiac tamponade. An inspiratory fall in systolic BP that exceeds 10 mm Hg indicates the presence of a paradoxical pulse.[5,47]

Management

Emergent evacuation of the pericardial fluid is definitive therapy in the presence of acute cardiac tamponade. Hemodynamic support during preparation of the patient for pericardiocentesis includes administration of blood, plasma, normal saline solution, or lactated Ringer's solution. Pericardiocentesis is accomplished with needle aspiration of pericardial fluid via the subxiphoid method. Removal of even small amounts of fluid with pericardiocentesis may have extremely beneficial effects and relieve symptoms temporarily. A positive pericardiocentesis caused by trauma necessitates an open thoracotomy for definitive treatment. Any trauma patient with EMD whose condition does not respond to volume resuscitation should indicate a high index of suspicion for cardiac tamponade.[5]

NONTRAUMATIC AORTIC DISSECTION

One of the most commonly seen life-threatening disorders of the aorta is dissection. *Aortic dissection* occurs when an intimal tear or separation develops in the aorta and results in hematoma formation in its medial layer. Dissections can originate anywhere along the length of the aorta and are classified according to location. The most common point of origin, and the most urgent clinically, is in the ascending aorta a few centimeters above the right or left sinus of Valsalva (65%). This condition can result in aortic valve insufficiency, compromise of a coronary artery, or rupture and cardiac tamponade or exsanguination. Other areas of common dissection include the proximal descending thoracic aorta just beyond the left subclavian artery origin (20%), the transverse aortic arch (10%), and the distal thoracic aorta or abdominal aorta (5%).[36,37]

The DeBakey system is the most widely used classification system for acute aortic dissection (Figure 22-1). In type I, the dissection originates in the ascending aorta and extends distally; in type II, the dissection is limited to the ascending aorta; and in type III, the dissection originates near and distally to the left subclavian artery and extends distally. Conditions associated with aortic dissection include systemic hypertension, congenital abnormalities of the aortic valve, advanced age, and heritable disorders of connective tissue such as Marfan's syndrome, a nonatherosclerotic disorder of connective tissue that involves massive degeneration of elastic fibers in the aortic media. Complications

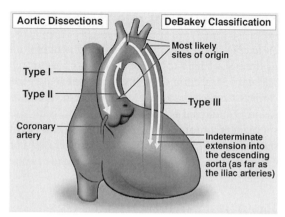

FIGURE 22-1   **Aortic dissections: DeBakey classification.** (Copyright 1995-2009, Challenger Corporation. Artist, Tom Rolain.)

of aortic dissection include compromise of flow to visceral organs and the extremities and neurologic deficits because of interruption of flow in branch vessels. Acute dissection of the ascending aorta that is untreated has a more than 90% mortality rate. Patients with distal dissection usually undergo medical management unless the dissection is complicated by rupture of the aorta or compromise of the blood supply to a vital organ. Surgery, emergent if necessary, is indicated for most patients with proximal dissection.[37,44]

ASSESSMENT AND DIAGNOSIS

The classic symptom of patients with aortic dissection is the sudden onset of pain, described as ripping, searing, and tearing, often originating in the back (interscapular) or substernal area and possibly extending down into the legs. The pain may be migratory and so changes in location as the dissection proceeds. Other signs result from obstruction of major vessels that originate from the aorta. Depending on the location of the dissection and the compromised vessels involved, the patient may have ischemia of various organ systems and signs and symptoms of cardiac disease. MI, cerebral insufficiency, cerebral vascular accident, hemiplegia or paraplegia, renal failure, and intestinal infarction may all result from dissection. Because of these diverse presentations and other less typical symptoms, a delay in diagnosis or misdiagnosis is common.

The patient with acute dissection is in severe distress and appears to be in shock with pallor, sweating, peripheral cyanosis, and restlessness. However, the BP may be normal or elevated, often as high as 200 mm Hg systolic, with a significant difference between both arms. Differential BP and pulses may indicate compromise of blood flow to one or both subclavian arteries. Absence of femoral pulses may indicate extension of the dissection into the aortic bifurcation, with compromising of circulation to one or both legs. Hypotension in aortic dissection is usually a result of rupture of the dissection into the pericardial space and may lead to cardiac tamponade. Rupture into the pleural space or mediastinum is more common with proximal dissection.[37,44]

Diagnosis of aortic dissection can often be made with physical examination alone. Transport of the acute case should not be delayed to obtain a chest radiograph. However, if a chest film is available on arrival of the transport team, it may be useful in conjunction with other diagnostic signs. Radiographic findings suggestive of an acute aortic dissection are: (1) mediastinal widening; (2) extension of the aortic shadow beyond a calcified aortic wall; (3) a localized bulge on the aortic arch; (4) tracheal deviation; and (5) left pleural effusion.[5]

MANAGEMENT

Prompt initiation of therapy and transport of patients with acute aortic dissection remains a challenge for transport nurses who often care for these patients during the brief interval between the onset of symptoms and the occurrence of life-threatening complications. Interventions are aimed at controlling pain and halting the progression of the dissecting force by reducing system blood pressure and the rate of change of pressure development. Blood pressure should be aggressively lowered to the lowest level compatible with adequate visceral, renal, and cerebral perfusion. Hypertension is treated with an intravenous beta-adrenergic blocking agent, given in conjunction with sodium nitroprusside. Beta-blockers must be given before afterload reduction to increase the force of left ventricular ejection, although it may aggravate the dissection. Labetalol can be given in place of a beta-blocker and sodium nitroprusside for short-term therapy for transport. For patients with

normotensive conditions, beta-blockers can be used alone. Infusions should be placed on the most accurate delivery pump available for transport, and doses should be titrated to BP response. Expert care and transport to definitive care requires pain relief and continuous ECG and BP monitoring. Pain may be managed with IV narcotic analgesia while the transport nurse constantly observes for signs of respiratory compromise. Decreasing the resistance to flow can reduce the pain. Type I and type II dissections necessitate emergent surgical repair with resection and Dacron replacement.[34,37]

Transport personnel should also be prepared to initiate intubation and assisted ventilation in the event that the patient's condition deteriorates. At least two large-bore IV access sites should be established for transport. Fluids should be kept to a minimum unless severe hypotension or rupture of the aorta occurs in flight. Blood should be available for transfusion during the flight if cardiac output becomes compromised. Inadequate pain or BP control and evidence of progressive dissection indicate an urgent need for surgical intervention. The transport team should not delay transfer to wait for laboratory results, blood products, or radiograph results. Coordination of efforts among transport personnel and the referring and receiving hospitals expedites admission to the surgical department for prompt intervention.

HYPERTENSIVE CRISIS

Hypertension is a common clinical condition that affects more than 60 million adult Americans. It is considered the most common risk factor for CAD. The prevalence rate of hypertension is expected to increase along with the aging population and increased life expectancy. Recent data from the Framingham Heart Study recognized the importance of elevated systolic blood pressure (SBP) and pulse pressure as significant risk factors for stroke and heart failure. Systolic hypertension and a widening pulse pressure are predominantly seen in the elderly.[10,15]

Hypertensive crisis is a potentially life-threatening complication of hypertension. Approximately 600,000 to 800,000 Americans have a hypertensive crisis develop. The presence of end-organ damage determines whether the crisis is defined as urgent or emergent. Hypertensive emergency with apparent end-organ damage necessitates an immediate reduction of blood pressure. The systolic blood pressure often exceeds 200 mm Hg, with a diastolic blood pressure greater than 120 to 130 mm Hg. No predetermined criteria exist for the level of BP necessary to produce a hypertensive emergency. The rate of rise of the blood pressure and the difference between the patient's usual level and that level present during crisis are the more important factors. A hypertensive crisis is a rapid progressive rise in BP sufficient to cause potential irreversible damage to vital organs. The major organs at risk are the brain, heart, and kidneys. the crisis may cause aortic dissection, cerebral hemorrhage, renal failure, and left-sided heart failure. Hypertensive crisis may occur in the clinical course of any patient with a persistent BP elevation, or it may occur as the initial presentation of a patient with hypertension. The evidence of organ dysfunction is the basis for diagnosis. Critical elevation of the blood pressure without end-organ damage is considered a hypertensive urgency, which can be treated with oral medication over the course of 24 to 48 hours.[10,15,25] Patients without prior hypertension may not tolerate BP levels as high as those patients with chronic hypertension.

ASSESSMENT AND DIAGNOSIS

The underlying pathologic process in accelerated hypertension and subsequent hypertensive crisis begins with arteriolar spasm and later leads to fibrinoid necrosis, release of vasoactive substances, continued vasoconstriction, and proliferation of the myointimal. Increased capillary permeability from cerebral arteriole dilation and increased cerebral blood flow or vessel wall damage are the effects of the pathophysiologic changes. The changes in the small arterioles are directly visible in the retina. The pathophysiology underlying specific target organ damage varies. Fluid leakage into the perivascular space from increased blood flow results in cerebral edema and hypertensive encephalopathy. The most devastating complication of hypertension is hypertensive encephalopathy. Hypertensive encephalopathy may be characterized by the presence of progressive central nervous systems signs and symptoms, including severe headache, nausea, vomiting, and visual difficulties. Focal neurologic findings can include blindness, seizures, aphasia, and hemiparesis. If left untreated, symptoms may progress to convulsions, stupor, coma, and death. Hypertensive emergencies are often caused by mismanagement or patient nonadherence. New onset of hypertension with no prior history of elevated blood pressure may be consistent with acute drug reactions.[34]

Accelerated hypertension without end-organ damage (hypertensive urgency) is more common than are hypertensive emergencies. Alterations in left ventricular performance from increased afterload are the primary mechanism by which an acute rise in pressure affects the cardiovascular system. Left ventricular failure, myocardial ischemia, or both can occur as a result of accelerated hypertension. Retinopathy, congestive heart failure, arrhythmias, or focal neurologic deficits may be present on clinical examination. Palpitations, angina, or congestive failure can present with cardiovascular decompensation. Signs and symptoms of left ventricular failure include chest pain, dyspnea, production of pink frothy sputum, rales, and bronchospasm. Neurologic symptoms may include headache, nausea, seizures, or obtundation.[15,19]

MANAGEMENT

The goal of therapy for patients with signs of hypertensive encephalopathy or malignant hypertension is to lower the BP in a controlled manner in 30 to 60 minutes to the baseline value (if known) for that patient. Systolic blood pressure reduction during the initial treatment is recommended to not exceed 25% to avoid the danger of cerebral hypoperfusion. Malignant hypertension may occur with or without associated diseases, such as intracerebral bleed, ischemic heart disease, pulmonary edema, pregnancy-induced toxemia, aortic dissection, renal failure, pheochromocytoma, and postoperative hypertension. Therapy should be based on each situation, critical organ involvement, and the desired time frame for lowering the blood pressure. For the transport nurse, the resolution of signs and symptoms should be used as a primary guide in the control of the pressure, in addition to the level of BP, frequent accurate BP readings may be difficult to obtain in transport. Monitoring the patient's cardiac rhythm and BP (by the most accurate means possible), observing the patient's level of consciousness, and assessing for signs of impending pulmonary edema or cardiac failure help the transport team evaluate whether the antihypertensive agents are effective. Either sodium nitroprusside or diazoxide may be used when immediate antihypertensive therapy is necessary. Both of these drugs have a controllable blood pressure reduction action. Other drug therapies should be based on the accompanying disease presenting with the malignant hypertension.[15,19,34]

Sodium nitroprusside acts by direct peripheral vasodilation with balanced effects on arterial and venous blood vessels. The antihypertensive effect of IV sodium nitroprusside is apparent in seconds and is dose dependent. Once the drug is discontinued, the pressure rises rapidly to the previous level in 1 to 10 minutes. Infusion rates must be closely monitored to avoid sudden fluctuations in BP.[35] Diazoxide exerts its hypotensive effect by reducing arteriolar vascular resistance through direct relaxation of arteriolar smooth muscle. When the drug decreases arterial pressure, baroreceptor reflexes are activated, leading to cardiac stimulation with increased heart rate, stroke volume, and cardiac output and resulting in mechanical stress on the aorta. For this reason, diazoxide should not be used for patients with dissection of the aorta and for patients with known CAD. Once the BP is controlled, the BP remains low and returns only gradually over 2 to 12 hours, which gives diazoxide an advantage over sodium nitroprusside in clinical situations in which monitoring the patient's condition closely for a long period of time is difficult.

HEMODYNAMIC MONITORING IN CARDIOVASCULAR ASSESSMENT

Accurate hemodynamic assessment is essential during the transport of the patient with cardiovascular compromise. Space limitations, noise levels, and vibration in the air medical environment may preclude the use of sophisticated invasive hemodynamic monitoring equipment during transport in some aircraft. The proficient transport nurse develops and refines the use of visual and tactile assessment skills for clinical patient evaluation. These skills should be used in conjunction with hemodynamic monitoring capabilities. Especially valuable are frequent examinations of mental status, skin color and temperature, pulse rate and quality, and urine output.

CARDIAC OUTPUT

The ultimate goal of monitoring and manipulation of hemodynamic parameters is to provide adequate perfusion of the body. This can be accomplished by directing and maintaining adequate cardiac output. Assessment of the cardiac output provides a useful measure of the pumping ability of the heart and is one of the major indicators of cardiac output. *Cardiac output* (CO) is defined as the multiplication of the heart rate and stroke volume (or amount of blood ejected from the left ventricle with each contraction). Changes in CO result from alterations in the rate of the heartbeat or the stroke volume. The major factors that influence stroke volume are contractility, preload (venous return or diastolic filling), and afterload (resistance imposed by normal aortic impedance). The normal range for CO is 4 to 8 L/min. CO is also used to calculate other parameters such as systemic vascular resistance (SVR) and stroke volume (SV; Figure 22-2).[7,19]

NONINVASIVE HEMODYNAMIC MONITORING

Noninvasive methods used to assess the hemodynamic status of the patient include the monitoring of the capillary refill, pulse rate and quality, BP, mentation, UO, and skin temperature. Mental status changes

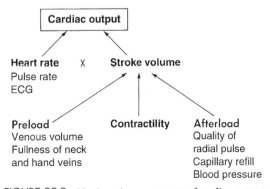

FIGURE 22-2 **Noninvasive assessment of cardiac output.**

are important in determination of the patient's overall condition. Significant changes in mentation occur in late shock when flow is compromised to the vital organs. Skin temperature and color, capillary refill, and UO in the absence of renal disease reflect tissue perfusion as it relates to cardiac output and intravascular volume. A combination of noninvasive methods such as capillary refill time, quality of the heart rate, and quality of the pulse or pulse contour should be used in conjunction with percutaneous monitoring and invasive hemodynamic monitoring to assess the adequacy of cardiac output during air medical transport of critically ill patients.

Blood pressure can be obtained noninvasively in the transport environment with the use of mechanical Doppler augmentation, automated BP devices, or palpation of the radial pulse with a sphygmomanometer and cuff. The cuff pressure measurements are usually adequate for a patient whose condition is hemodynamically stable; however, direct blood pressure monitoring via an arterial line is more accurate than indirect pressures specifically in the presence of hypertension, hypothermia, and shock. Transducer pressure measures systolic and diastolic BP from the same heartbeat. Cuff pressure measures systolic BP from one beat and diastolic from another. Indirect pressures are often difficult to hear in the presence of low CO and peripheral vasoconstriction. Although BP measuring devices can be useful to monitor trends in the patient's hemodynamic status, the patient's hemodynamic status should be evaluated with multiple methods rather than one specific parameter such as BP.[58]

Percutaneous Devices for Assessment of Oxygenation Status

The effects of altitude on the cardiovascular system are numerous. Adequate tissue oxygenation remains the highest priority in critically ill patients. The assessment of a patient's oxygenation and hemodynamic status can be augmented by various noninvasive transcutaneous devices that respond to physiologic changes in oxygenation and perfusion. Many monitors are available to monitor pulse oximetry during transport. Pulse oximetry provides continuous noninvasive monitoring of the percentage of oxygen saturation of arterial hemoglobin (SaO_2).

A probe or sensor can be placed on a patient's finger or ear lobe and detect a waveform from pulsatile blood with optical plethysmography. The probe contains red and infrared light emitters on one side and a photodetector on the opposite side. Red and infrared light not absorbed by the blood, bone, and tissue are measured by the photodetector and converted into a reading indicative of the arterial hemoglobin percentage.

A SaO_2 reading of 95% or higher at sea level is considered normal. This percentage decreases as altitude increases. However, a normal reading does not always mean adequate oxygenation. Some adverse events may not be detected until the event is totally or near irreversible. Several studies have shown pulse oximetry to be accurate and effective in identification of hypoxemia and other undesirable conditions associated with arterial desaturation. Continuous and routine pulse oximetry monitoring should result in fewer episodes of arterial desaturation and more rapid recognition of this event and thus may lower morbidity or mortality rates. The most common problem associated with the use of pulse oximetry is failure of signal detection. This can be related to motion, arrhythmia, hypothermia, hypotension or hypoperfusion, and vasoactive drugs. Some errors in detection can be easily resolved by changing or adjusting probe placement. Artifact from motion is more prevalent in the ground transport setting than in the air transport setting.[25]

Capnography measures carbon dioxide concentration or partial pressure on critically ill intubated patients and reflects the respiratory process. A normal waveform indicates carbon dioxide production, transport, and alveolar ventilation equilibrium. For critical care transport, capnometry can monitor $PaCO_2$, which is usually monitored through arterial blood gas (ABG) analysis. Changes in $EtCO_2$ levels can reflect airway complications or equipment problems and may reduce morbidity in the transport environment with early detection of airway and inadequate ventilation. Monitoring of end-tidal carbon dioxide in critically ill patients, such as those in cardiogenic shock, is recommended in the intensive care unit (ICU) environment and the prehospital environment when available.

INVASIVE HEMODYNAMIC MONITORING

The goal of transport for a patient who has been admitted to a coronary care unit is to provide a high level of care equal to that in the ICU. Often the patient has invasive intravascular catheters in place. Hemodynamic monitoring in a critically ill patient with intravascular catheters placed into a blood vessel or a chamber of the heart provides accurate information on initial and continuous cardiovascular status. Parameters assist with verifying diagnosis and guiding therapy and monitor clinical changes. For example, intraarterial pressure is more accurate than noninvasive sphygmomanometry in patients who are obese, hypotensive, peripherally vasoconstricted, or severely hypertensive.

Hemodynamic monitoring is an extremely valuable aid in assessment of patients who need specific interventions, such as volume, preload, and afterload reducing or inotropic agents, and of patients on IABP. Pulmonary artery (PA) catheters can provide information on both right and left heart pressures. PAWP and PA pressures reflect pressures in the left atrium and left ventricular end-diastolic pressure (LVEDP). These parameters can be used for assessment of left ventricular preload. The CVP is measured independently through a central venous catheter or through the proximal port of a PA catheter. CVP is reduced when preload, or the volume of blood returning to the heart, is reduced. A low CVP may be seen with bleeding, dehydration, drug-induced vasodilation, or overzealous diuresis. An elevated CVP may be seen with fluid overload (overtransfusion, overhydration), right ventricular failure, cardiac tamponade, tricuspid stenosis or insufficiency, or vasoconstrictive states. These parameters can help the transport nurse guide therapy. However, caution should be used not to concentrate on one cardiodynamic variable without a full evaluation of all physiologic information available, such as heart rate, capillary refill, pulse contour, BP, and UO.[58] Before transport, interpretation of intravascular hemodynamic parameters and trends provides the transport nurse with valuable information regarding the cardiovascular status of the patient. For safe practice, transport nurses who care for patients who need invasive hemodynamic monitoring must have knowledge of normal hemodynamic values, understand the significance of changes in these values over time, and demonstrate competency with hemodynamic equipment.

Preparation for transport of patients with existing intravascular monitoring lines varies from program to program; however, attention to detail and careful handling of the intravascular line are essential to avoid potential complications. When preparing a patient with intravascular monitoring lines for transport, the transport nurse must label all lines clearly, secure all connections, place sterile caps over all exposed ports, and maintain a heparin flush system during transport. For years, biomedical equipment designed for use in the hospital setting has been used in the transport environment with little research available to substantiate the accuracy of these invasive measures of hemodynamic status during air medical transport. Current biomedical devices developed and marketed for transport systems with features such as compactness, lightness, durability, and screen lighting conducive to this environment have not all been tested specifically for the air medical industry. The stresses of flight, such as the effect of vibration on biomedical equipment and electromagnetic interference, has not totally been defined.[15,24] Thus, the transport nurse must use a combination of invasive and noninvasive assessment methods to evaluate patient status throughout the transfer process.

CRITICAL CARE TRANSPORT OF THE CARDIOVASCULAR PATIENT

The level of care during medical transport should be at the level of the receiving hospital. The goal for critical care transport is to provide equal degrees of monitoring and support as in the hospital ICU. Proper patient preparation, stabilization, and resuscitation need to be completed to minimize any risk associated with transport. To efficiently organize the care and transport of critically ill patients, the transport nurse's performance must be consistent with the skills and knowledge as performed in an ICU.[15] Cognitive knowledge of the nursing process as it relates to the unique air medical environment is imperative. The nursing process helps the transport nurse formulate goals and a plan of action for the care of complex patient cases. The nursing process, assessment, planning, intervention, and evaluation, discussed next is related to air medical transport.

ASSESSMENT

Assessment of the cardiovascular patient begins with the initial information elicited from the referring agency by dispatch personnel. This information can be invaluable for evaluating the best vehicle for patient transport and is helpful for air transport (especially when flying in an aircraft with limited space and weight restrictions), for anticipating in-flight emergencies and preparing the receiving agency for the patient. Time en route to the referring agency can be spent developing a preliminary database and plan of care based on initial information obtained from dispatch and the referring agency.

For the cardiovascular patient, assessment and preparation for transport are directed toward recognition, prevention, and correction of hypoxia and maintenance of adequate tissue perfusion and cardiac output. The amount of time spent on assessment of the cardiovascular patient depends on the severity of the illness and the need for rapid intervention. The transport nurse should ascertain as much information as possible in the most efficient way possible to provide safe and efficient transport to a definitive care institution and to ensure continuity of care.

A brief history of the event may be elicited from the patient, family members, or referring agency personnel. A general appraisal of the patient can be made while approaching the bedside and observing, at that time, skin color, diaphoresis, activity or position of comfort, and respiratory distress. The transport nurse should also observe whether IV infusions have been initiated and are running wide open, vasoactive drugs are infusing, and oxygen is being delivered; inspect all invasive catheters; and note what rhythm is on the cardiac monitor. An initial perception of the situation helps to organize and direct management of the patient for efficient and safe transport.[25]

Physical examination is often abbreviated to the situation with skill and judgment used to determine what is vital and appropriate to evaluate under the circumstances. Hands-on assessment of the patient

includes confirmation of vital signs and hemodynamic readings and the identification of implications for continued emergency care. Initial evaluation of airway, breathing, and circulation is done in accordance with basic cardiac life support guidelines.[40] If the patient is not in immediate need of cardiopulmonary resuscitation, the overall cardiovascular status should be evaluated. Any necessary procedures should be performed at this time, such as intubation, central line insertion, chest thoracostomy tube insertion, or additional therapeutic interventions (initiation or adjustment of medications). Stabilization and management by an appropriate critical care trained medical team take precedence over speed of transport, unless the illness necessitates immediate access to the receiving facility (e.g., abdominal aortic aneurysm [AAA] with pending rupture that needs operative intervention).[25]

PLANNING AND INTERVENTION

Adequate management and preparation of the patient for transport can greatly reduce the need for resuscitative measures en route to receiving facilities. Planning care for transport of the critical cardiovascular patient includes anticipating complications that may occur as a result of the disease process and preventing the predictable. This requires a strong critical care knowledge base, orientation, and ongoing competency that encompass the principles and practice of transport nursing and meet the standards of the Air and Surface Transport Nurses Association.

EVALUATION

Throughout the transport process, the transport nurse systematically evaluates the patient's progress, analyzes data, and modifies the plan of care based on the patient's response to therapy. In the transport environment, continual assessment and monitoring of the patient provide data regarding the success or failure of each intervention.

SUMMARY

Technologic advancement is driving the medical industry, which in turn affects air medical transportation programs. The critical care transportation industry must adapt to and be proficient in the ever-changing technology that patients and their families are using in their communities. Chapter 23 contains a thorough explanation of the current methods used for mechanical management of the patient with cardiovascular disease. One day these patients will inevitably need emergent transportation, and critical care transport programs must be educated and prepared to properly care for them.

REFERENCES

1. Antman EA: *ACC/AHA guidelines for the management of patients with ST elevation myocardial infarction,* available at www.acc.org/qualityandscien, accessed November 2008.
2. Association AH: *AHA heart disease and stroke statistics update 2008,* 2008, Available at www.americanheart.org/statistics, accessed November 2008.
3. Braunwald EB: Congestive heart failure: fifty years of progress, *Circulation* 102:14IV, 2000.
4. Braxton C, Reilly P, Schwab C: The traveling intensive care unit patient, *Surg Clin North Am* 80(3):949, 2000.
5. Bursi FE: Heart failure and death after myocardial infarction in the community; the emerging role of of mitral regurgitation, *Circulation* 111:295-301, 2005.
6. Capomolla S, et al: Beta blockade therapy in chronic heart failure: diastolic function and mitral regurgitation improvement by carvedilol, *Am Heart J* 193(4):596, 2000.
7. Chulay MB: *AACN essentials of critical care nursing handbook,* New York, 2005, McGraw-Hill.
8. Corti RH: Evolving concepts in the triad of atherosclerosis, inflammation, and thromboses, *J Thrombolysis* 17(1):35-44, 2004.
9. Damergis JA: Physiological parameter changes of high altitude and their correlation with acute mountain sickness, *Ann Emerg Med* 51(4):536, 2008.
10. Cooper DK: *The Washington manual of medical therapeutics,* Philadelphia, 2007, Wolters Kluwer/Lippincott Williams & Wilkins.
11. Diamond L: Cardiopulmonary resuscitation and acute cardiovascular life support: a protocol review of the updated guidelines, *Crit Care Clin* 23(4):873-880, 2007.
12. Dugliano R: Antiplatelet therapy in early management of non-ST segment elevation acute coronary syndrome: the 2002 and 2007 guidelines from North America and Europe, *J Cardiovasc Pharmacol* 51(5):425-433, 2008.
13. Eid FB: The evolving role of medical therapy for chronic stable angina, *Curr Cardiol Rep* 10(4):263-271, 2008.
14. Erdmann JS: Effects of exposure to altitude on men with coronary artery disease and impaired left ventricular function, *Am J Cardiol* 81(3):266-270, 1998.
15. Fauci AE: *Harrison's principles of internal medicine,* New York, 2008, McGraw-Hill Medical.
16. Ferguson JE: The current practice of intraaortic balloon counterpulsation: results from the Benchmark Registry, *J Am Coll Cardiol* 38(5):1456-1462, 2001.
17. Fraker TE: 2007 Chronic angina focused update of the ACC/AHA 2002 guidelines for the management of patients with chronic stable angina, *J Am Coll Cardiol* 50(23): 2264-2274, 2007.
18. Freedman JL: *The role of platelets in coronary disease,* available at www.UpToDate.com, accessed November 2008.
19. Froelicher ES: *Cardiac nursing,* 2004, Lippincott Williams & Wilkins.
20. Grady K, et al: Team management of patients with heart failure: a statement for healthcare professionals from the cardiovascular nursing council of the American Heart Association, *Circulation* 102:2443, 2000.
21. Guidelines 2005 for cardiopulmonary resuscitation and emerging cardiovascular cardiovascular care, *Circulation* 112:57, 2005.
22. Hainsworth RD: Cardiovascular adjustments for life at high altitude, *Respir Physiol Neurobiol* 158(2-3):204-211, 2007.
23. Hatlestad DV: Air transport of the IABP patient, *Air Med J* 21(5):42-48, 2002.
24. Hickman BM: Stress and the effects of air transport on flight crews, *Air Med J* 20(6):6-9, 2001.
25. Holleran R: *Flight nursing: principles and practice,* ed 2, St Louis, 2003, Mosby.
26. Jackson G: Chronic stable angina: revised guidelines from the ACA/AHA, *Int J Clin Pract* 62(3):353, 2008.
27. Keller K: Prinzmetal's angina, *Am J Crit Care* 13(4):350-354, 2004.
28. Klein L: Clinical implications and mechanisms of plaque rupture in acute coronary syndromes, *Am Heart Hosp* 33(4):249-255, 2005.
29. Lanza GE: Current clinical features, diagnostic assessment and prognostic determinants of patients with variant angina, *Int J Cardiol* 118(1):41-47, 2007.
30. Lev EE: Effect of clopidogrel pretreatment on angiographic and clinical outcomes in patients undergoing primary percutaneous coronary intervention for ST elevation acute myocardial infarction, *Am J Cardiol* 101(4):435-439, 2008.
31. Libby PM: Inflammation and atherosclerosis, *Circulation* 105: 1135-1143, 2002.

32. Maogin SE: The clinical and hemodynamic results of mitral balloon valvuloplasty for patients with mitral stenosis complicated by severe pulmonary hypertension, *Eur J Intern Med* 16(6):413-418, 2005.

33. McBride LE: Transfer of patients receiving advanced mechanical circulatory support, *J Thoracic Cardiovasc Surg* 119(5):1015, 2000.

34. McPhee SJ: *CURRENT medical diagnosis and treatment*, New York, 2008, McGraw-Hill.

35. Nichols KW: Flight orientation curriculum for emergency medicine resident physicians, *Air Med J* 22(2):26-29, 2003.

36. Pagani F: Extracorpeal life support to left ventricular assist device bridge to heart transplant: a strategy to optimize survival and resource utilization, *Circulation* 99(2):206, 1999.

37. Patel PA: Pathophysiology, diagnosis, and management of aortic dissection, *Ther Adv Cardiovasc Dis* 2(6):439-468, 2008.

38. Pilmanis AS: Physiologic hazards of flight at high altitude, *Lancet* 362: 16-17, 2003.

39. Santa-Cruz RC: Aortic counterpulsation: a review of the hemodynamic effects and indications for use, *Catheter Cardiovasc Intervent* 67(1):68-77, 2006.

40. Shah P: Molecular mechanisms of plaque instability, *Curr Opin Lipidol* 18(5):492-499, 2007.

41. Silber S: Guidelines for percutaneous coronary interventions: the task force for percutaneous coronary interventions of the European Society of Cardiology, *Eur Heart J* 26(8):804-847, 2005.

42. Srichai MC: Cardiac tamponade masking clinical presentation and hemodynamic effects of papillary muscle rupture after myocardial infarction, *J Am Soc Echocardiogram* 15(9):1000-1003, 2002.

43. Sun HM: Coronary microvascular spasm causes myocardial ischemia in patients with vasospastic angina, *J Am Coll Cardiol* 39(5):847-851, 2002.

44. Theroux PW: Progress in the treatment of acute coronary syndromes: a 50 year perspective, *Circulation* 101(1):102, 2000.

45. Topalian SG: Cardiogenic shock, *Crit Care Med* 36(1):S66-S74, 2008.

46. *White paper on air medical transport. air medicine, accessing the future of healthcare*, available at www.fareonline.org: http://www.fareonline.org/english.pdf, accessed November 2008.

47. White R: 2005 American Heart Association Guidelines for cardiopulmonary resusciation: physiologic and educational rationale for changes, *Mayo Clinic Proc* 81(6):736-740, 2006.

48. Williams SW: Management of cardiogenic shock complicating acute myocardial infarction towards evidence based practice, *Heart* 83(6):621-626, 2000.

49. Wilson P: *UpToDate*, available at www.UpToDate.com, accessed November 2008.

23 MECHANICAL CIRCULATORY SUPPORT DEVICES IN TRANSPORT

Leslie C. Sweet, Allen C. Wolfe, Jr.

COMPETENCIES

1. Identify the indications for the use of a mechanical circulatory support device.
2. Perform an assessment of the patient with a mechanical circulatory support device.
3. Manage specific mechanical circulatory support devices before, during, and after the transport process.

The pace of technologic advances over the past several decades has been dramatic. Concurrently, the healthcare industry has revolutionized its technology, becoming smaller, faster, more efficient, and more sophisticated. The continued improvements in patient outcomes and the public's expectation for state-of-the-art medical care continue to propel healthcare technology into the 21st century. The rapid explosion of research in healthcare technology has hastened patient recovery and return to the community. In earlier decades, the prehospital healthcare providers' primary concerns with technology were automatic implantable cardioverter defibrillators (AICD) and insulin or vasoactive medication pumps. In regards to heart failure, cardiac assist devices have dominated the first decade of the 21st century, similar to how the cholesterol-lowering drugs, statins, dominated the 1990s. Although the

devices were in development for many decades, the evolution of cardiac assist devices seemed slow. With new technologic advancements and clinical understanding of engineering designs, the field of mechanical circulatory support has exploded.

HISTORIC PERSPECTIVE

In 1966, Dr Michael DeBakey implanted the first successful cardiac assist device in a female patient in her mid-thirties who had failure to wean from cardiopulmonary bypass (CPB). The patient was successfully supported by the device for a total of 10 days[12]; the device was then explanted, and the patient was ultimately discharged home. This landmark success fueled the race for widespread use of mechanical circulatory support devices for severe end-stage heart failure. Subsequently, the primary focus of researchers and physicians turned to total replacement of the injured myocardium with the use of a total artificial heart (TAH). In 1969, Dr Denton Cooley implanted a TAH, the Liotta Heart, in a patient with failure to wean from CPB. The patient was supported for 64 hours before undergoing cardiac transplant. The groundbreaking use of this device perpetuated further advances in the use of TAH and assist device technology. Additional modifications and clinical use continued into the 1980s with the first permanent implantation of a TAH in 1982 into an elderly dentist, Dr Barney Clark, at the University of Utah by Dr William Devries. The device, the Jarvik-7 TAH, was designed by Dr Robert Jarvik and associates for total cardiac replacement. Although Dr Clark ultimately died of multiple complications, he was fully supported for an unprecedented 112 days by a TAH without any native ventricles in place.[8,12] This mechanical circulatory support of a human for nearly 4 months was a pivotal achievement for the field of artificial organs. The Jarvik-7 has undergone further advances and is currently known as the CardioWest temporary TAH (SynCardia Systems, Inc, Tucson, Ariz). Limitations of the earlier technology, however, did prompt scientists and physicians to rethink whether assisting the heart, versus replacing it, may be more appropriate when feasible.[12]

In the 1980s, while heart transplantation gained prominence in the cardiac surgery arena, many end-stage heart failure patients died awaiting transplant due to an insufficient number of donor organs comparable to the profoundly increasing number of waiting transplant candidates.[1] In light of this skewed supply-demand ratio, medical researchers and engineers were tasked with developing a mechanical circulatory support device readily available and capable of sustaining patients as a bridge to transplant until a suitable donor organ became available and capable of providing lifetime support to patients with chronic heart failure deemed ineligible for heart transplant. The mid 1980s brought significant progress in the successful uses of ventricular assist devices (VADs) in patients awaiting heart transplant. Dr Phillip Oyer at Stanford University Hospital implanted a Novacor left ventricular assist system (LVAS; WorldHeart, Inc, Audubon, Pa).[17] This was followed in the early 1990s by other successful uses of VADs, including

Dr Robert Kormos and colleagues at the University of Pittsburgh who developed a program to allow the discharge of patients with VADs into the community.[12] These significant and successful uses with VADs as a bridge to transplant lead to the groundbreaking Randomized Evaluation of Mechanical Assistance for the Treatment of Congestive Heart Failure (REMATCH) trial to evaluate the use of the HeartMate VE LVAS for long-term cardiac support. Approved by the US Food and Drug Administration (FDA), the REMATCH trial was a multicenter clinical trial designed to compare optimal medical management (OMM) with long-term HeartMate VE LVAS support in patients with severe, medically refractory, end-stage heart failure deemed ineligible for cardiac transplant. The trial showed that the VE LVAS significantly improved long-term survival and quality of life in this very ill patient cohort. Although the VE LVAS outperformed the OMM strategies in the REMATCH Trial, the trial results still raised doubts with critics regarding the durability and infection-related complications of the left ventricular assist device (LVAD).[12,19] With the increased cost of LVAD patient management within the hospital setting, caregivers began to look to the management of these patients in the community. The goal of successful discharge of patients into the community was profound improvement of patient quality of life and survival with proper support, education, and training.

Concurrently, the development of the intraaortic balloon pump support began in 1958 when Dr Dwight Harken described a method to treat left ventricular failure with counterpulsation. His recommendation was removal of a certain amount of blood volume from the femoral artery during systole and rapid replacement of this volume during diastole.[15] Complications arose because of the need for bilateral arteriotomies of both femoral arteries and hemolysis of cells in the pumping apparatus.[15] This procedure necessitated surgical insertion and surgical removal, which increased the potential for postoperative complications. Later, at the Cleveland Clinic, a researcher in the 1960s named Dr Spiro Moulopolous, developed a form of treatment for left ventricular failure that expanded significantly in the years that followed.[4] With the concepts of his predecessors, he used what is today known as the intraaortic balloon pump (IABP) in three patients with cardiogenic shock. He made the simple, effective, and affordable circulatory assist device to support this challenging patient population.[9] The groundbreaking research gave rise to other great work at that time. Dr Adrian Kantrowitz in 1968 continued to work with counterpulsation and showed 27 patients with cardiogenic shock with both hemodynamic and clinical improvement. The cardiogenic shock was able to be reversed.[4] The evolution of all of these mechanical circulatory support devices (MCSDs) has created a more sophisticated set of treatment strategies to offer today's complicated patient cohort that is supported with both air and surface transport.

THE BASICS

Mechanical circulatory support devices (MCSDs) are mechanical devices or pumps designed to support the pumping function of a failing heart, whether attributable to acute cardiogenic shock or severe chronic cardiomyopathy. These devices may be separated into two major categories: total artificial hearts (TAHs) and ventricular assist devices (VADs). A *TAH* is a device that completely *replaces* the native heart physically, not just functionally. Implantation of a TAH involves removal of the native heart similarly to cardiac transplantation. Typically, the great vessels of the heart remain intact as does the atria, with complete excision of the remaining heart muscle. The TAH is then attached to the remaining atrial cuffs and great vessels. A caveat of a TAH is that if the device should fail no "back-up" native heart exists for compensation. In addition, because of the inherent size of a TAH, the patient must have adequate thoracic space to accommodate the pump. Total artificial hearts are most ideally suited for patients with biventricular heart failure (BVF), with both the left and the right ventricles having severe medically refractory end-stage heart failure.

Conversely, *VADs* are designed to *assist* the native heart in pumping adequate blood to vital body organs. The native heart remains intact, and the VAD is attached to the appropriate great vessels or heart chambers, typically with inflow and outflow cannulae. The extent of pumping support by the VAD varies depending on the design of the VAD and the capabilities of the native heart. With some devices, the native heart may serve primarily as a "funnel" or conduit through which the circulating blood is delivered to the artificial pump, which then provides complete cardiac output for that side of the heart.

Ventricular assist devices may be categorized by the side of the heart they support and the design of the pump itself. VADs that support the right side of the heart are *right ventricular assist devices* (RVADs), and VADs that support the left side of the heart are *left ventricular assist devices* (LVADs). When the technology is used to support both sides of the heart, it is a *biventricular assist device* (BVAD or BiVAD). Use of two different devices from two different manufacturers to provide BVAD support is feasible.[20] With BVAD support, another possibility is for the native heart to not contribute at all to the cardiac output. In this scenario, the native heart could develop clinically insignificant ventricular fibrillation with a fully coherent patient because the fully supporting BVAD sustains adequate circulatory support.

The specific indications for MCSDs include: 1, bridge to recovery; 2, bridge to more definitive therapy; 3, bridge to transplant; and 4, lifetime or destination therapy. Bridge to recovery (BTR) is indicated with suspicion that, given the opportunity to "rest" on a MCSD, the native heart function may be able to sufficiently recover and support native circulation, allowing for explantation of the device. Although initially this indication was thought to be limited to acute cardiogenic shock devices only, clinical experience shows that myocardial recovery may be achieved with the longer support duration provided by the long-term devices.[9,23]

Bridge to more definitive therapy describes the use of a short-term device to temporarily support the failing heart through an acute event. With time to stabilize the patient's condition, the cardiac function may be more thoroughly evaluated to better determine whether the insult is reversible or whether a more definitive long-term therapy is indicated and whether the patient is eligible for such therapy. Definitive therapy strategies may include more conventional percutaneous coronary interventions (PCIs) and coronary artery bypass graft surgery (CABG) or may expand to cardiac transplantation or permanent MCSD.

Bridge to cardiac transplantation (BTT) is the use of a MCSD to support a transplant candidate whose heart has become refractory to conventional pharmacologic support and for whom a suitable donor heart has not been identified. Current data from the United Network of Organ Sharing (UNOS) Registry continue to show that there are twice as many transplant candidates as there are recipients, which confirms the ongoing shortage of available donor organs. Historically, approximately 30% of transplant candidates die while awaiting a suitable donor heart. More recently, the mortality rate is down to 10% to 15%.[14,22] This reduction in mortality rates in the pretransplant cohort is attributable to multiple factors, including the use of ventricular assist devices to bridge these patients sooner rather than later, as shown by the increase of LVAD BTT cases from 3% in 1990 to more than 28% in 2004, as reported by Kirklin and Holman.[13] The use of MCSD to support these patients is intended to provide adequate circulatory support until a donor heart becomes available. At the time of transplant, the MCSD is removed along with the native heart.

Lifetime or *destination therapy* (DT) describes the use of MCSD to sustain circulatory support in patients with medically refractory end-stage heart failure who are also deemed ineligible for cardiac transplant because of other comorbidities. Historically, these patients would be sent home, if possible, with hospice care for the duration of their lives. With the advent of more permanent devices, these patients can feasibly be sufficiently sustained on MCSD and still be active members of their families and communities.

Further categorization of VADs includes the intended length of support and the design of the device. *Acute VADs* are usually those devices implanted for short-term use, typically 7 to 10 or up to 30 days. *Chronic* or *long-term VADs* are devices that are implanted for more long-term support, typically with the intent to discharge the patient into the community. Some indications exist for implanting devices for a duration of support between these two time lines and involve the use of devices that are otherwise specifically considered short-term or long-term devices.

With regards to the design of VADs, the technology has evolved significantly over recent years. The earliest designs of mechanical circulatory support included roller pumps for cardiopulmonary bypass and the intraaortic blood pump (IABP) for cardiogenic shock. Although the use of IABP for acute cardiogenic shock may increase the cardiac output by 10% to 15%, a significant mortality rate remains with shock patients. Both CPB and IABP are limited in the duration of support that they can provide. The goal of advancing VAD support is to provide even higher blood flow than the more conventional IABP, with potentially longer more tolerable support to assist in improving both acute and long-term outcomes.

The different devices developed in recent years may therefore be categorized per device design, regardless of indication for short-term or long-term use. *First-generation pumps* are devices that are described as *fill-to-empty* or *volume-displacement pumps*. These devices typically have a blood sac or chamber where blood collects, similarly to the native heart, before being ejected into the circulation. Like the diastolic phase of the human heart, the volume-displacement pump pauses for the blood chamber to fill optimally within a maximum time period before ejecting the blood into the appropriate artery of the supported ventricle. The rate at which these devices pump is often dependent on filling of the blood chambers and does not necessarily correlate with the patient's native heartbeat. Unlike an IABP with electrocardiogram (ECG) tracing capabilities, any apparent synchrony of pumping rates between these VADs and the native heart is coincidental.

Ejection of a first-generation pump may be pneumatically driven (i.e., air is compressed on a collapsible blood sac to exert sufficient pressure to cause forward blood flow from the blood chamber to the blood vessel; Figure 23-1) or mechanically driven (i.e., a metal plate is compressed against the collapsible blood sac or blood chamber to again cause forward blood flow, as previously described; Figure 23-2). Typically, these devices have inflow and outflow valves to ensure unidirectional blood flow through the pump. Examples of these types of devices are the Abiomed Circulatory Support System (CSS) composed of both the BVS Blood Pump and

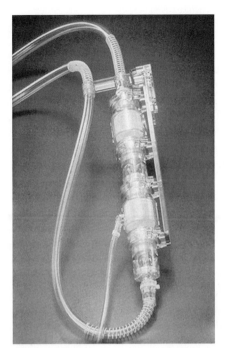

FIGURE 23-1   **Pneumatically driven Abiomed BVS Blood Pump.** (Courtesy ABIOMED, Inc, Danvers, Mass.)

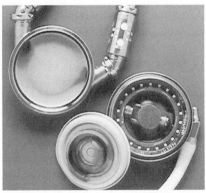

FIGURE 23-2   **Mechanically driven Thoratec HeartMate XVE LVAS.** (Courtesy Thoratec Corporation, Pleasanton Calif.)

the AB5000 Ventricle (ABIOMED, Inc, Danvers, Mass), the Thoratec Paracoporeal and Implantable VADs (Thoratec Corporation, Pleasanton, Calif), the HeartMate XVE LVAS (Thoratec Corporation), and the Novacor LVAS (WorldHeart Inc).

Rotary blood pumps, contrary to the volume-displacement pumps, draw blood continuously

from the supported heart. Rotary blood pumps do not have a blood collecting chamber or unidirectional valves and do not pause for optimal filling. They do have inflow and outflow cannulae, similar to the first-generation pumps, but instead of the blood chamber, they contain a high speed impeller. The impeller is likened to a turbine engine or propeller. Because rotary pumps draw blood continuously from the supported ventricle, pulsatility of the affected side may be dampened significantly. If the VAD is supporting the left side of the heart, for example, a peripheral pulse may be difficult to palpate, necessitating use of a Doppler flow probe to auscultate and confirm blood flow. Basic assessment skills of adequate circulation (e.g., capillary bed refill, adequate mentation, urine output, etc) have heightened importance in these patients.

Rotary blood pumps further differentiate into the second-generation and third-generation pumps. The rotary pump impeller uses rotational energy to propel the blood through the pump. It may be cylindrical or disc-shaped and uses blades or vanes to direct the blood flow forward. The *second-generation rotary blood pumps* are axial flow devices in which the blood path across the cylindrical impeller is linear, relying on circumferential energy (Figure 23-3). The rotational speed of an axial flow device is typically 8000 to 15,000 rpm. Examples of axial flow pumps available in the United States include the HeartMate II LVAS (Thoratec Corporation), the Jarvik 2000 (Jarvik Heart, Inc, New York), and the DeBakey LVAD (MicroMed Cardiovascular Inc, Houston).

The *third-generation rotary pumps* are centrifugal flow devices in which the blood path through the disc impeller involves a 90-degree turn via the perpendicular inflow and outflow ports, combining both centrifugal and circumferential energy to propel the blood forward (Figure 23-4). The rotational

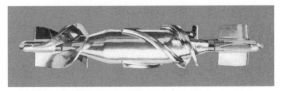

FIGURE 23-3   **Thoratec HeartMate II LVAS impeller.** (Courtesy Thoratec Corporation, Pleasanton, Calif.)

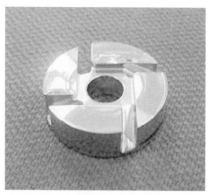

FIGURE 23-4   **HeartWare LVAS impeller.** (Courtesy HeartWare, Inc, Framingham, Mass.)

speed of the centrifugal pump is typically 2000 to 4000 rpm. In addition, the centrifugal blood pump impeller is magnetically or hydrodynamically (because of the flow of blood through the pump) suspended, which eliminates the amount of contacting mechanical surfaces that otherwise wear with time.[2,16] Consequently, third-generation pumps are often referred to as "wearless" pumps. As the technology advances through these generations, fewer and fewer contacting moving parts are used. The devices, inherent to their design, have also become smaller and more energy efficient. The benefits of these advances are that the pumps will likely last longer and can be implanted in a wider range of body sizes, which makes the technology more accessible to more patients. Examples of temporary external centrifugal pumps currently available in the United States include the TandemHeart System (CardiacAssist Inc, Pittsburgh) and the CentriMag VAD (Thoratec Corporation). The implantable centrifugal pumps currently or imminently available in the United States include the VentrAssist LVAD (Ventracor, Inc, Budd Lake, NJ), the DuraHeart LVAS (Terumo Heart, Inc, Ann Arbor, Mich), and the HeartWare LVAS (HeartWare, Inc, Framingham, Mass).

Of the six second-generation devices previously described, only the HeartMate II LVAS has FDA approval to date, specifically for bridge to transplant therapy only. The remaining axial and centrifugal pumps are in clinical trials in the United States for bridge to transplant, and destination therapy in some cases.

ACUTE CARDIOGENIC SHOCK DEVICES

As previously described, VADs used for acute cardiogenic shock are those devices indicated for immediate stabilization of the patient's condition with an average projected support time of 7 to 10 days. Common indications for these devices include acute cardiogenic shock associated with myocardial infarction, postcardiotomy shock, viral myocarditis, and temporary right ventricular failure (RVF) associated with implantation of a permanent LVAD. The advantage of these short-term devices is that they allow the clinical team the opportunity to stabilize the patient's condition for a more clear understanding of the clinical pathology and etiology of the cardiogenic shock and the most appropriate course for further therapy. Strategies at this time include the addition of pharmacologic therapies to maximize the potential for recovery and permanent removal of the VAD versus maximizing the pharmacologic therapy to determine whether weaning of the VAD is not feasible. In the latter case, the next strategies to consider are patient eligibility for cardiac transplant versus the need and appropriateness of lifetime VAD therapy. In extreme cases, withdrawal of pharmacologic and mechanical support may be warranted and requested by next of kin.

Typical acute cardiogenic shock devices that may necessitate medical transport are the intraaortic balloon pump (IABP), the extracorporeal membrane oxygenator (ECMO), the Abiomed BVS Blood Pump or AB5000 Ventricle (ABIOMED, Inc), the TandemHeart PTVA System (CardiacAssist Inc), the CentriMag VAD (Thoratec Corporation), and the Thoratec Paracorporeal or Implantable VADs (Thoratec Corporation). The major components of these blood pumps typically include cannulae that are attached to the appropriate anatomic part of the native circulation (i.e., blood vessels versus chambers of the heart) and then to the blood pump; the blood pump itself, which may either connect directly to the cannulae or require blood tubing to connect to the cannulae; and the console that runs the pump and provides power to the system, whether with electrical plug connections when stationary or with internal batteries for transportation of the patient while on support.

All of these devices currently require systemic anticoagulation therapy to minimize the potential for thrombus formation and occlusion and also minimize the potential for excessive bleeding and its associated complications, including multiple blood transfusions and subsequent right heart failure. Heparin is used most commonly, although an alternative agent such as argatroban may be needed if the patient has positive test results for heparin-induced thrombocytopenia (HIT). More long-term support of the AB5000 Ventricle and the Thoratec Implantable Ventricular Assist Device (IVAD) and Paracorporeal Ventricular Assist Device (PVAD) does allow for conversion of heparin to warfarin.

Intraaortic Balloon Pump

An *intraaortic balloon pump* (IABP) is a device whose primary purpose is to increase blood flow to the heart muscle through the coronary arteries with the assistance of diastole and to decrease the heart's workload through a process called counterpulsation. The secondary effects are the improvement of cardiac output (CO), stroke volume (SV), left ventricular emptying, and ejection fraction (EF). An increase in coronary perfusion pressure and systemic perfusion, with a decrease of heart rate, pulmonary capillary wedge pressure (PCWP), and systemic vascular resistance (SVR), also occurs.[11] This device is ideal for patients with poor cardiac output, chest pain unrelieved with medical therapy, and failed pharmacologic therapy associated with poor perfusion related to cardiogenic shock.

Placement of the IABP typically involves inserting a flexible catheter into the femoral artery and advancing it into the descending thoracic aorta (Figure 23-5). The placement of the catheter is confirmed with fluoroscopy or chest radiograph. As illustrated in Figure 23-5, proper location of the catheter is essential for ideal functioning. Poor placement of the IABP catheter can create other complications that are discussed subsequently in this section.

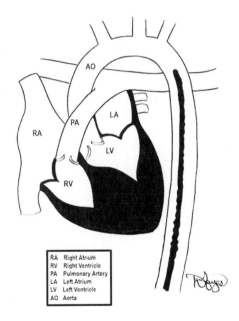

RA	Right Atrium
RV	Right Ventricle
PA	Pulmonary Artery
LA	Left Atrium
LV	Left Ventricle
AO	Aorta

The IABP is deflated during systole, as the heart contracts.

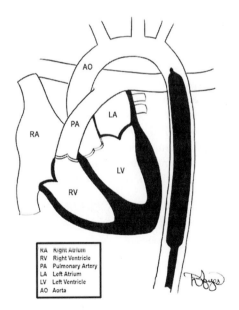

RA	Right Atrium
RV	Right Ventricle
PA	Pulmonary Artery
LA	Left Atrium
LV	Left Ventricle
AO	Aorta

The IABP is inflated during diastole as it improves coronary circulation.

FIGURE 23-5 **Placement of IABP balloon-tipped catheter.** The goal of inflation is to produce a rapid rise in aortic pressure optimizing diastolic augmentation, thereby increasing oxygen supply to the coronaries. During deflation, the reduction in end aortic diastolic pressure (afterload) causes improved cardiac performance. (Drawings courtesy of David Hayes.)

The newer generation intraaortic balloon pump offers operator flexibility, which allows the flight crew members the capability to care for a broad range of patients. These pumps are designed to work in conditions unique to the operating room, to the cardiac catheterization laboratory, to the intensive care unit (ICU), and to air and surface transport. The technology uses speed and quick algorithms, supplying support to patients with arrhythmias.[3] The balloon pumps have colorful display panels combined with pneumatic and electronic innovations. These balloon pumps possess cardiosynchronization capabilities, with auto select trigger selection and timing. The IABP adapts its deflation automatically while supporting ventricular ectopy or other arrhythmias.[20] If the timing is not correct, a number of physiologic changes can occur, as outlined in Table 23-1.

The automatic mode of the IABP uses the ECG trigger, but if the ECG trigger is lost, the pump searches for the next best trigger source and resets the time accordingly. A manual mode allows the transport team members to select and control all of the triggers and their timing even during changes in rhythm. This technology allows the flight team members to focus more on the patient and aviation safety rather than the pump.

Because of the large amount of background noise in air medical transport, the IABP console supports a large visual alarm display. The balloon is filled with a predetermined amount of helium. With use of the manual mode in the previous generation of these pumps (DataScope 97 and 98XT [Datascope, Corp., Fairfield NJ]), the pumps needed manual autofilling of the balloon catheter to compensate for the changes in balloon volume during air transport. This was done by the transport teams for every 2000 ft on ascent and 1000 ft on descent.[3] The newest generation IABP automatically refills the helium based on volume sensors, which detect changes in the volume of helium, prompting auto refill. This refilling also occurs every 2 hours automatically in manual or auto modes. In situations of very rapid descent, the pump refills many times, quickly causing a helium loss alarm.

The frequency of IABP counterpulsation is ordered by the physician. In most cases, it is 1:1; thus, for each contraction of the native ventricles and opening of the aortic valve, the IABP catheter is triggered to inflate during the subsequent diastolic phase timed to the dicrotic notch (Figure 23-6). The counterpulsation can be set for other frequency modes, such as 1:2 and 1:3, for which inflation of the balloon occurs on the dicrotic notch on every second or third beat, respectively. The balloon then deflates again at the onset of native ventricular systole. The most common IABPs used during transport are the Datascope CS 100 and 300 (Datascope, Corp., Fairfield, NJ), and the Arrow AutoCAT and AutoCAT WAVE 2 (Arrow International, Reading, PA). These types of balloon pumps have made significant changes in the past decade. The pumps are more operator-friendly, and their computerized monitoring systems allow for automatic timing of the inflation and deflation of the balloon catheter. The pumps also have transport designs that are more lightweight and safety conscious for air surface transport personnel.

TABLE 23-1	**IABP Timing Errors**
Timing Error	**Effect**
Early inflation	Premature closure of the aortic valve causing aortic regurgitation
Late inflation	Sub-optimal coronary perfusion
Early deflation	Retrograde coronary blood flow
Late deflation	Increases the resistance the balloon pumps against (afterload)

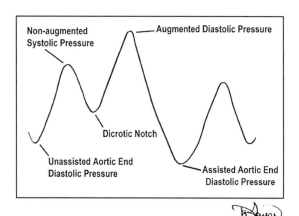

FIGURE 23-6   **IABP counterpulsation waveform.**
(Drawings courtesy of David Hayes.)

Patient Assessment

A complete assessment of the patient's hemodynamic status is vitally important before the transport of a patient with an IABP; however, the assessment should start with the primary survey. After the primary survey assessment and any interventions, a baseline neurologic examination is warranted. This examination is important because a highly placed IABP catheter can block blood flow to the subclavian and carotid artery.

The hemodynamic assessment should consist of evaluation of the patient's CO, cardiac index (CI), left ventricular stroke work index (LVSWI), SVR, pulmonary vascular resistance (PVR), and other pulmonary catheter data, if available. Assessment of heart sounds should be done with the IABP on standby so that the sounds are clearly heard, with a baseline assessment provided for monitoring the possible accumulation of an excessive amount of fluid around the pericardium (cardiac tamponade). In air transport, hearing capabilities are impaired; therefore, all the important sound-assessed information should be obtained before leaving the referring facility. The assessment of the IABP includes diastolic augmentation, pump timing, and any alarms.

Although the use of pulmonary artery catheters has decreased significantly in the past several years, standard practice in critical care transport of these devices is the continuous monitoring of the pulmonary artery (PA) catheter waveforms. Hence, transport teams should be properly trained in the management of PA catheters and waveform analysis. If the catheter migrates into the PA, a wedge waveform is visualized on the monitor. This displacement can result in occlusion or perforation of the pulmonary artery, which can cause pulmonary infarct and possibly death. In this situation, the caregiver needs to ensure that the balloon is deflated and then pull the catheter back until the PA waveform is visualized on the monitor. In instances in which the PA catheter slips into the right ventricle, the catheter should be withdrawn.

Physical assessment of the patient to assure proper positioning is important because of the anatomic positioning of the IABP. The patient may have specific clinical assessment deficits. If the patient's left brachial pulse is absent, the catheter may be positioned too high, causing occlusion of the subclavian artery and ultimately affecting blood flow to the left arm. A radiograph or fluoroscopy is best for identification of this misplacement. If the catheter is too low, the patient may have oliguria or anuria as a result of the catheter blocking the renal arteries, therefore decreasing renal blood flow.

Important laboratory values to review before transport include the most recent complete blood count (CBC), prothrombin time (PT), partial thromboplastin time (PTT), platelet counts, and basic metabolic panel. If oozing at the insertion site is present or occurs, use of a liter bag of intravenous (IV) fluids carefully placed over the exit site may be helpful. This placement applies light pressure without interfering with counterpulsation of the IABP. The oozing is most likely the result of the decrease in platelets caused by the counterpulsation of the IABP or anticoagulation effects from other medications. The head of the bed or stretcher (HOB) should be less than 30 degrees to prevent occlusion of the catheter. Light restraints or sedation may be helpful in securing the leg in which the catheter is inserted to prevent accidental IABP dislodgement or interference with balloon pump functioning. The diameter of the catheter varies from patient to patient; therefore, assessment for distal pulses is important to ensure perfusion of both extremities. An occlusion can cause ischemia of the affected extremity and result in clot formation, decreased circulation, and total arterial occlusion with possible amputation if the IABP is not adjusted or removed. The transport personnel must perform a thorough assessment and relay any complications from IABP therapy to the accepting physician with complete documentation in the flight chart.

Transport Considerations of the Patient with an Intraaortic Balloon Pump

1. In any vehicle, whether fixed or rotor-wing and ground, verify that the inverter can supply power to the IABP.
2. The two main manufactures of IABPs (Arrow and Datascope) both have adapters especially for transport personnel in the event the transport team's pump is different from the one at the referring facility. These adapters allow interfacing between the two different pumps.

3. A transport bag should accompany all IABP transports with auxiliary supplies for IABPs.
4. Assure that sufficient helium and a backup helium tank are provided.
5. All blood pressure readings should be taken from the IABP console, and not the noninvasive blood pressure cuff (NIBP) or manually. The highest pressure sensed or heard is the diastolic augmentation, not systolic. Therefore, documentation of the NIBP or manual pressures provides inaccurate information.
6. Positioning the patient with the head toward the front of the fixed aircraft decreases the patient's preload. The opposite occurs if the patient is positioned with the feet toward the front.
7. Ensure that the IABP console is plugged in whenever possible (e.g., in the transport vehicle and immediately on arrival at the bedside of the sending facility).

Management of Common Intraaortic Balloon Pump Emergency Procedures

In the transport environment, preparation for the worst case scenario in patient care and safety is a fact of life. Table 23-2 lists some emergencies that can occur with IABP therapy and their management.

Future Trends

As we have seen with IABP therapy in the past decade, balloon pumps have become smaller, smarter, and more user-friendly. Technologic advancement has switched focus from the pump console to the fiberoptic catheter. The fiber optic balloon pump catheter provides transport teams with two arterial waveform sources.[6] The traditional waveform is from the conventional transducer. The newer waveform is from the fiberoptic tip of the catheter inside the aorta. The traditional monitoring of arterial waveforms from transducers is delayed, whereas the fiberoptic waveform is in real time.[7] This real-time method provides more accurate timing. The transport considerations with these new catheters require the user to ensure it is properly zeroed and calibrated to the specifications of the manufacturer. At altitudes greater than 10,000 ft in an unpressurized cabin, the fiberoptic catheters may be altered and inoperable. They are more accurate below 10,000 ft.[3]

ABIOMED CIRCULATORY SUPPORT SYSTEMS: BVS BLOOD PUMP AND AB5000 VENTRICLE

The *Abiomed BVS Blood Pump* is a first-generation volume-displacement VAD. It received initial FDA approval in 1994 and is capable of providing RVAD, LVAD, or BVAD support. The BVS Blood Pump is a columnar blood pump that contains two blood sacs, an atrial and a ventricular chamber (see Figure 23-1 on page 439). The device-specific artificial trileaflet valves are located between the two bladders and distal to the ventricular bladder. A pneumatic (air-filled) flexible cable is attached to the blood pump at the level of the ventricular bladder at one end and to the external console at the other end.

TABLE 23-2	**IABP Emergency Interventions**
Problem	**Intervention**
Ventricular fibrillation (vfib) or pulseless ventricular tachycardia (VT) arrest	Follow Advanced Cardiac Life Support (ACLS) guidelines. Stopping the pump is not necessary. Pump is grounded and can accommodate electrical shocks.
Cardiopulmonary arrest: asystole or pulseless electrical activity (PEA)	Begin ACLS guidelines, and place pump on pressure mode during CPR. IABP pump will continue to pump with CPR as pressure is sensed.
Power failure	Attach 60-mL syringe to proximal stopcock and inflate IABP catheter once every 3-5 min to prevent clot formation on catheter.
Balloon rupture (evidenced by blood in the sheath, loss gas alarm, and rust-colored flecks)	Stop the pump immediately, clamp the catheter, and position patient in the left lateral position.

Compressed air trapped within the external console and pneumatic cable is then shunted between the console and the blood pump, which causes external pressure on the collapsible ventricular blood sac during the ejection phase of the pumping cycle, with subsequent release of that pressure during the filling phase. The pressure changes associated with filling and emptying of the ventricular bladder cause the proximal and distal valves to open and close, ensuring unidirectional flow of blood through the blood pump. Of note, the atrial bladder does not have a valve preceding it, so blood flows continuously into the atrial bladder, which is preload dependent. As with other volume-displacement first-generation pumps, the pump rate is dependent on the filling time of the ventricular chamber within a maximum period of time. Filling of the ventricular chamber is monitored by the console per the volume of displaced air through the pneumatic cable. Once the maximal amount of air is sensed by the console, the compressor shunts trapped air back, maintaining a minimum pump rate of 40 bpm.

To ensure adequate blood flow into the blood pump, the atrial bladder must be placed at a height relative to the patient's right atrium (Figure 23-7). The blood pump can be placed too high relative to the patient so that blood flow into the pump is limited. Conversely, if placement is too low, blood pump output may be limited.

The BVS blood pump is connected to the patient's circulation with device-specific cannulae. The inflow cannulae to the pump may be inserted into the native atria or ventricle, and the outflow cannulae are connected to the major artery attached to the side of the heart being supported. For RVAD support, typically the right atrium (RA) and pulmonary artery (PA) are the inflow and outflow cannulation sites, respectfully. For LVAD support, the left atrium (LA) or left ventricle (LV) may be used for the inflow cannula, and the aorta (Ao), typically the ascending portion, is used for outflow cannulation (Figure 23-8).

The *Abiomed AB5000 Ventricle* (ABV) received FDA approval through a postmarket approval (PMA) supplement in September 2003, with the longest support of a patient to date being greater than 300 days. The device consists of a single blood sac made of a special polyurethane material that is encased in a hard clear outer shell (Figure 23-9). Between the blood sac and outer case is a lubricant to protect blood sac integrity. Device-specific artificial valves are located in the inflow and outflow connectors (conduits) of the pump to ensure unidirectional blood flow through the pump. The pump casing has a similar flexible pneumatic cable that connects the blood pump to the external console.

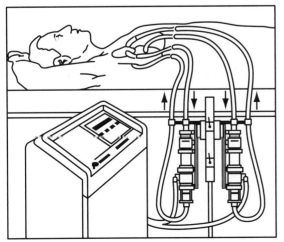

FIGURE 23-7 **Positioning of the Abiomed BVS Blood Pump.** (Courtesy ABIOMED, Inc, Danvers, Mass.)

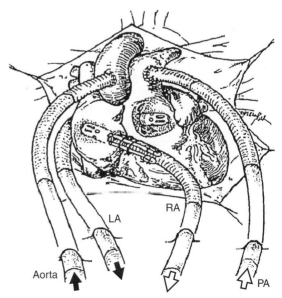

FIGURE 23-8 **Cannulation options for the Abiomed CSS.** (Courtesy ABIOMED, Inc, Danvers, Mass.)

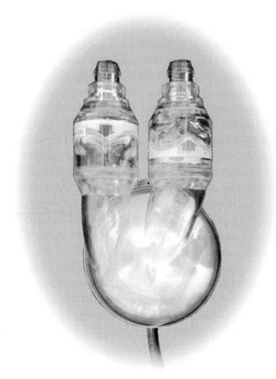

FIGURE 23-9   **Abiomed AB5000 Ventricle.** (Courtesy
ABIOMED, Inc, Danvers, Mass.)

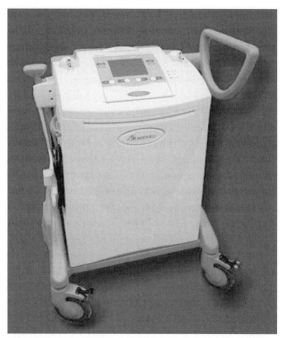

FIGURE 23-10   **Abiomed AB5000 console.** (Courtesy
ABIOMED, Inc, Danvers, Mass.)

Similarly, compressed air trapped within the external console and pneumatic cable is then shunted between the console and the blood pump, which causes external pressure on the blood sac during the ejection phase of the pumping cycle and release of that pressure during the filling phase. Unlike the BVS Blood Pump, the console does actively apply vacuum pressure to the AB5000 Ventricle to assist in filling the blood sac. The pressure changes associated with filling and emptying of the blood sac cause the proximal and distal valves to open and close to ensure unidirectional blood flow. The cannulae for attachment of the pump to the native circulation are the same as for the BVS Blood Pump, with similar cannulation sites as well. Both the BVS Blood Pump and the AB5000 Ventricle require open heart surgery for implantation.

ABIOMED has recently streamlined the technology so that the same external console, the AB5000 Console, may be used for both pumps, with one console for RVAD and LVAD support simultaneously if indicated (Figure 23-10). The distal ends of the pneumatic cables for the BVS Blood Pump and AB5000 Ventricle differ so that their connection to the console indicates to the console which device it is supporting. This differentiation is important because the amount of external pressure applied to the AB5000 Ventricle for adequate ejection is typically much higher than the BVS Blood Pump and more for an LVAD than an RVAD within each device type. In addition, a more measurable vacuum effect is used during filling of the AB5000 Ventricle than with the BVS Blood Pump. The console allows for manual adjustment of the amount of vacuum for the AB5000 Ventricle and for adjustment of alarm triggers for both devices. VAD flows for both devices range from 3 to 6 L per minute (lpm), with beat rates ranging from 40 to 60 bpm with normal automatic console function. The display screen provides information regarding pump beat rate, pump flow, alarm settings, vacuum pressure for the AB5000 Ventricle specifically, and alarm events with troubleshooting instructions. The console may also be programmed to a weaning mode that allows limitation of VAD support in an attempt to wean the native heart from the device. Should the VAD fail completely, a hand pump is attached to the console to support manual pumping of either device, whether univentricular or biventricular assist. The hand pump is directed with specific toggle buttons that must be manually preset to indicate which side of the heart is being supported and with which device (BVS versus ABV).

A discerning feature of the ABV from the BVS blood pump is that the ABV is capable of providing more long-term support with fewer bleeding and clotting issues. Unfortunately, the AB5000 Console is a hospital-based console with limited battery support of up to 1 hour. ABIOMED is in the midst of a clinical trial to evaluate the use of a portable driver for out-of-hospital support (Figure 23-11). Pending the results of this trial, in the future, patients who need prolonged Abiomed CSS support may be discharged into the community with the portable driver, allowing them improved quality of life while awaiting explantation of the device.

Frequent assessment of these pumps includes monitoring for adequate filling and emptying of the blood chambers and the presence of thrombus or fibrin layering. The most likely locations for fibrin or thrombus formation in the pumps are areas of low flow, specifically at the bases of the artificial valves, although they may also be identified on the surfaces of the bladders or blood sacs, or at the connections of the blood tubing. Initially, both blood pumps require full anticoagulation therapy with heparin, or argatroban if the patient is considered HIT positive. Anticoagulation goals may be altered if patient is coagulopathic or actively bleeding or if the device flow drops below 3 lpm. If prolonged support is necessary, which is most likely with the ABV, the intravenous anticoagulation therapy may be converted over to warfarin.

THORATEC PARACORPOREAL AND IMPLANTABLE VENTRICULAR ASSIST DEVICES

The *Thoratec Paracorporeal* and *Implantable Ventricular Assist Devices* (PVAD and IVAD, respectively) are also pneumatically driven VADs that are approved by the FDA for postcardiotomy shock and bridge to cardiac transplantation (Figure 23-12). Similar to the Abiomed CSS, the PVAD and IVAD are capable of providing RVAD, LVAD, and BVAD support. These may be used for short-term in-hospital acute recovery or for more long-term in-the-community BTT support. Community use of these devices is feasible because a portable driver is available. Patients may also be weaned from the PVAD and IVAD should native heart function recover. The longest duration of support for the PVAD is more than 1200 days, with more than 700 days for the IVAD.

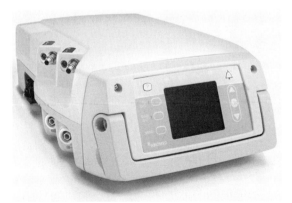

FIGURE 23-11 **Abiomed portable console.** (Courtesy ABIOMED, Inc, Danvers, Mass.)

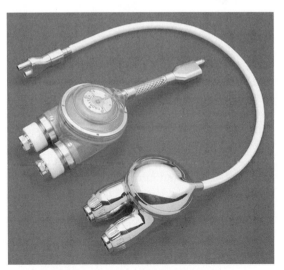

FIGURE 23-12 **Thoratec PVAD and IVAD.** (Courtesy Thoratec Corporation, Pleasanton, Calif.)

The three major components of the PVAD and IVAD are the blood pump, the cannula, and the consoles. The PVAD blood pump is composed of a flexible blood sac with a rigid clear case that houses a magnetic sensing device (Hall effect switch) to monitor filling of the blood sac. When the PVAD blood sac is full, the Hall effect switch is triggered to send a "full" signal to the console. The blood sac external surface is protected with a lubricant, which can be visualized through the protective rigid case. Two mechanical tilting disc valves are located in the inflow and outflow conduits to ensure unidirectional flow. A pneumatic cable with adjacent electronic cables connects the blood pump to the hospital-based dual-drive external console or the portable TLC-II driver. Air is shunted between the console or driver and the blood pump to actively facilitate emptying and filling of the blood sac, with application of direct air pressure for external compression of the pump and vacuum pressure to assist preload filling of the pump. The pump rate varies from 40 to 110 bpm, delivering a blood flow up to 7.1 lpm. The portable TLC-II pneumatic driver allows patients to ambulate more freely within the hospital and to be discharged into the community if appropriate.

The IVAD blood pump has the same blood sac and mechanical valves, but the case is made of titanium alloy with an optic sensor to monitor filling of the blood sac and to send the "full" signal to the console. The titanium alloy case allows the IVAD to be a fully implanted blood pump with a single percutaneous cable composed of both the pneumatic cable and optic sensors. As such, only the one percutaneous cable per VAD exits the body, instead of the two cannulae as with the externally placed PVAD. This percutaneous cable is wrapped in Dacron velour to encourage tissue ingrowth at the exit site as it is tunneled through the skin, to assist in stabilizing the exit site and minimizing the potential for infections. Filling and emptying of the IVAD blood pump is otherwise similar to the PVAD, with similar pump rates and volumes with either device console. A flashing green light on the console synchronizes with each pump beat, indicating complete emptying of the blood pump, which is otherwise observed directly with the PVAD.

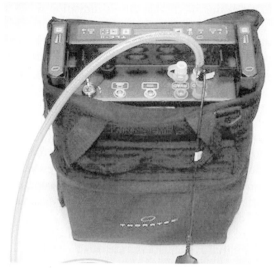

FIGURE 23-13   **Thoratec TLC II driver.** (Courtesy Thoratec Corporation, Pleasanton, Calif.)

The TLC-II driver is the portable driver for both the PVAD and IVAD and is capable of univentricular and biventricular support both in the hospital and in the community (Figure 23-13). It is powered with either electricity (AC power) or batteries and has a turn-key on the control panel to activate the driver. The AC adaptor allows for plugging the driver into an electric outlet to conserve battery power. The batteries provide 55 to 80 minutes of support, depending on whether the patient is receiving BVAD, LVAD, or RVAD support. Batteries are discharged individually, so when one battery is drained, its low battery alarm is triggered and the second battery begins support. The TLC-II driver also has its own internal battery for an added emergency back-up should all other power sources fail. A car power adaptor is available to serve as an alternate power source in the car. A functioning back-up battery in the TLC-II driver is needed with use of the car power adaptor. The car power adaptor does not recharge the batteries of the TLC-II driver.

The control panel of the TLC-II driver provides information about the VAD, including active power source type (electric versus battery), battery status, pump function (fixed or auto), type of pump (LVAD or RVAD), pump rate and calculated flow, fill signal per blood pump, alarm status, and a message that details how to correct it. The TLC-II driver offers a fixed or auto mode of pump function. With the fixed mode, the pump ejects at a predetermined rate regardless of filling of the blood sac, whereas the auto mode triggers ejection of the blood pump based on complete filling (positive fill signal) of the blood sac. The auto mode is more responsive to the patient's clinical condition. The vacuum regulator is located on the side of the console and is used to regulate the amount of vacuum necessary for maximal filling of the blood pump and subsequent activation of the fill signal. The eject pressure cannot be regulated through the TLC-II driver but rather through the hospital-based docking station and HeartTouch computer. Of note, immediately above the vacuum regulator is a grill that covers the air intake filter. This grill should be checked regularly for any obstructions or build up of dust and dirt. The control panel also has connection ports for both the pneumatic cable and the electric leads for both a LVAD and RVAD. The LVAD ports are colored red, and the RVAD ports are colored blue. For univentricular support, the unused ports should have the occluders in place to protect against loss of pneumatic pressure.

Surgical implantation of the PVAD is similar to the Abiomed CSS in that the heart and great vessels are cannulated and the cannulae exit the chest wall below the costal margin. The implantable IVAD may be placed in either a preperitoneal pocket or an intraabdominal pocket. The paracorporeal feature of the PVAD allows it to be implanted in pediatric patients; the primary size limitation is that of the cannulae. The IVAD, conversely, may only be implanted in patients with body surface area (BSA) of $1.3\,m^2$ or more. Surgical implantation of either device involves cannulation of the RA to the PA for RVAD support and the LA or LV to the aorta for LVAD support (Figure 23-14). With the paracorporeal approach of the PVAD, the cannulae exit the chest wall, which allows the pump to rest on the abdomen. Depending on which cannulation site is used, the pump may be flipped. The specific inflow cannulation site used for the LVAD also dictates where the LVAD sits relative to the RVAD. If the interatrial groove is used, then the LVAD sits to the right of the thoracic midline and to the right of the RVAD if BVAD support is indicated. Otherwise, the LVAD is typically located to the left of the abdominal midline. When patients

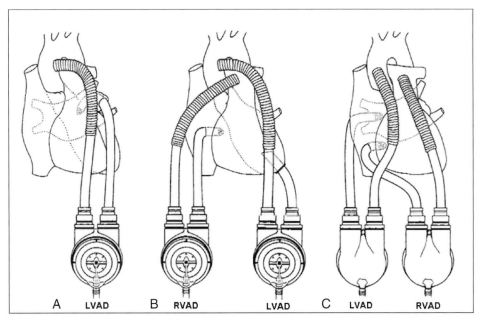

FIGURE 23-14 **Implantation approaches for Thoratec PVAD. A,** LVAD with LA cannulation. **B,** BVAD with apical cannulation of LVAD. **C,** BVAD with interatrial groove cannulation of LVAD. (Courtesy Thoratec Corporation, Pleasanton, Calif.)

become ambulatory, the pumps and the exit sites must be protected by providing a method to support the pumps without allowing them to dangle freely. Patients undergo full anticoagulation therapy with these pumps, initially with heparin or argatroban as indicated, with conversion to warfarin therapy in the patient with long-term support. Antiplatelet therapy may also be instituted. Patients need to have a minimum amount of equipment when discharged home, consisting of two TLC-II drivers, four hand pumps, at least eight fully charged batteries, AC and car power adaptors, a battery recharger, and a replacement pneumatic and electric lead.

Assessment of the PVAD blood pump includes observation for the "Flash Test." If the blood sac is ejecting adequately, a flashlight beam directed at the blood pump results in a flash of light beyond the blood pump at the end of the ejection cycle. Complete emptying of the IVAD is confirmed by the flashing green empty light on the signal processor after each VAD beat. As previously described, monitoring for the fill signal, two if the patient is on BVAD support, and the status of the power source is also important. If the device fails completely, hand pumping is possible with one hand pump per VAD at a pump rate of one pump per second. The hand pump is likened to a bulb syringe with an attachment port to allow for secure connection to the driver end of the pneumatic cable. The bulb is to be completely compressed with either hand pressure or foot pressure.

TANDEMHEART SYSTEM

The *TandemHeart System* (CardiacAssist, Inc) is an extracorporeal centrifugal pump also capable of providing RVAD, LVAD, and BVAD support. It can provide up to 5 lpm blood flow with a maximum speed of 7500 rpm. The pump is divided into two sections or chambers: the blood chamber or upper housing and the lower housing (Figure 23-15). The upper chamber contains the impeller, which propels the blood through the pump. The lower housing is filled with continuously flowing heparinized saline solution, which enters the pump housing and then passes into the blood chamber, providing a forward pressure that prevents detrimental backflow of blood into the lower chamber. The purpose of the heparinized infusate is to lubricate and cool

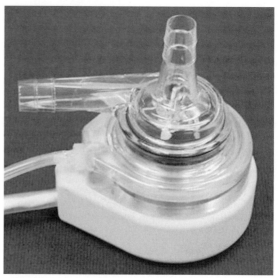

FIGURE 23-15   **CardiacAssist TandemHeart Pump.** (Courtesy CardiacAssist Inc, Pittsburgh)

the motor and to provide localized anticoagulation, which ultimately contributes to systemic anticoagulation as well. If the patient is suspected or deemed to be HIT positive, heparin is removed from the infusate and only injectable normal saline solution is used. Systemic anticoagulation therapy, however, may be achieved with an alternative peripheral anticoagulant such as argatroban. The infusate line is laced through an infusion pump in the external console to ensure adequate forward pressure of the infusate, delivering a fixed infusate rate of 10 mL/h. The electronic cable (the Communication line) attached to the pump is connected directly to the console or controller. CardiacAssist, Inc, has developed two types of consoles to run the TandemHeart System, the more recent design being targeted for medical transportation of patients with this pump (Figure 23-16). The console allows for adjustment of pump speed for maximal flow and houses a backup console as well. The display screen provides the pump speed and estimated flow, infusate diagnostics, and alarm messages. Weaning patients from support can be attempted by decreasing the speed of the pump slowly over time.

Implantation of the TandemHeart System may be performed surgically with an open chest or percutaneously. Special inflow and outflow cannulae are

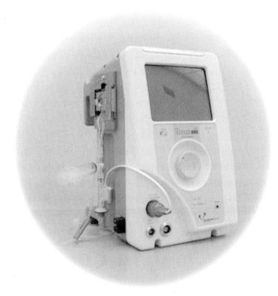

FIGURE 23-16   **CardiacAssist TandemHeart transport console.** (Courtesy CardiacAssist Inc, Pittsburgh)

used to connect the VAD to the native circulation, depending on which side of the heart is being supported. The inflow cannula is percutaneously placed in the right heart's venous system (inferior vena cava via the femoral vein). It is then passed into the right atrium (RA) for RVAD support or passed through the atrial septum into the left atrium (LA) for LVAD support (Figure 23-17). Percutaneous placement of the outflow graft for RVAD support is via the femoral vein or the right internal jugular vein into the PA, similar to pulmonary artery catheter placement. Outflow graft placement for the LVAD is performed percutaneously via the left femoral artery. Surgical placement with an open chest affords multiple options for direct surgical cannulation and percutaneous cannulation. Knowledge of the location of cannulae and the cannula stabilization techniques is imperative when caring for these patients because incidental movement of cannulae can be catastrophic, such as a percutaneous LVAD inflow cannula shifting from the LA into the RA or a femoral cannula receding out of the femoral artery. The TandemHeart transseptal inflow cannula has measurement markings on the cannula to assist in monitoring the stabilization of the cannula. The blood

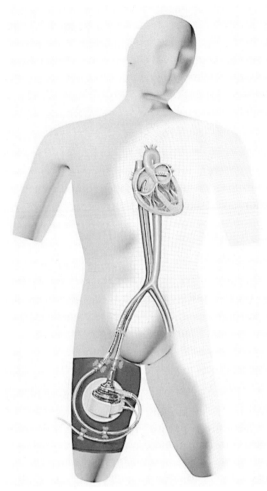

FIGURE 23-17   **Implantation approach for CardiacAssist transseptal TandemHeart LVAD.** (Courtesy CardiacAssist Inc, Pittsburgh)

pump itself may be anchored to the patient's leg with the TandemHeart Pump Holster with Velcro attachment to a thigh wrap.

Assessment of this device includes monitoring for signs of thrombus formation or fibrin layering, monitoring for signs of blood in the lower housing or infusate tubing, and monitoring for air bubbles in the infusate tubing. Unique to a continuous flow, centrifugal pump is the potential for suction of the inflow cannula as a result of inadequate blood volume to support the speed of the pump. Unlike the volume-displacement pumps that have intermittent filling of a blood chamber and therefore intermittent refilling of the native heart as well, a continuous flow device is continuously emptying blood from the heart chamber that it is supporting. If inadequate blood flow into the VAD occurs for any reason (e.g., inadequate filling of the native heart from tamponade, bleeding, hypovolemia, or obstruction of the inflow cannula, etc), the VAD may draw air into its system, which would in turn be delivered into the patient's arterial circulation. An indicator of this potential suction event is chattering (rapid bouncing or jerking) of the blood tubing. Such an occurrence needs immediate attention with either administration of volume or decrease in the pump speed.

CentriMag Blood Pump

The *CentriMag Blood Pump* (Thoratec Corporation) is a short-term extracorporeal magnetically levitated centrifugal blood pump capable of providing RVAD, LVAD, or BVAD support (Figure 23-18). The blood pump typically provides 4 to 5 lpm blood flow with normal pump speeds of 3000 to 4000 rpm. The CentriMag Blood Pump is approved for 6 hours of circulatory support, but an FDA-approved clinical trial is ongoing to evaluate its use for up to 30 days. The components of the CentriMag Blood Pump include the blood pump itself, which contains the magnetically suspended impeller; the motor, which encases the pump and drives the pump; the blood tubing, which is connected from the patient to the blood pump; an ultrasonic flow probe, which provides a direct measurement of the pump flows; and the console and back-up console, which are capable of supporting one blood pump per console.

With the ultrasonic flow probe placed directly onto the outflow blood tubing, the CentriMag Blood Pump has the unique ability to provide a direct measure of pump output, unlike the other acute devices in which flows are calculated. The flow probe can also detect retrograde flow and alarm accordingly. A minimum of 1000 rpm is suggested to ensure forward blood flow through the pump. The location of the flow probe should be changed regularly by approximately 1 cm. The CentriMag Blood Pump uses one of two consoles: the primary console or the back-up console (Figure 23-19). The display screen of the primary console provides the pump speed, pump flow, power source and status, and alarm messages. Console adjustments include the ability to adjust the speed ranges from 500 to 5000 rpm, along with low and high flow alarm triggers. The back-up console is designed to temporarily replace a failed primary console by providing support to the blood pump until a functioning primary console is available. The display screen of the back-up console provides limited information (pump speed, remaining battery time, and alarm messages), although it delivers the same speed and flow capabilities as the primary console.

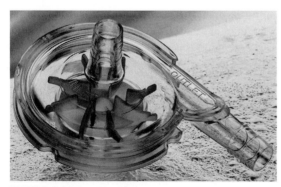

FIGURE 23-18   **Thoratec CentriMag Blood Pump.**
(Courtesy Thoratec Corporation, Pleasanton, Calif.)

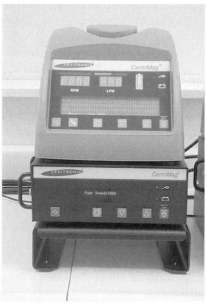

FIGURE 23-19   **Thoratec CentriMag primary and back-up consoles.** (Courtesy Thoratec Corporation, Pleasanton, Calif.)

Implantation of the CentriMag Blood Pump is most commonly performed intraoperatively via a sternotomy, with venous and arterial cannulation of the RA and PA, respectively, for RVAD support and similarly, the LA and aorta for LVAD support (Figure 23-20). Percutaneous placement may be performed with femoral venous and arterial access for inflow and outflow cannulation, respectively. The blood pump is locked into the pump motor, which in turn is mounted on a bracket attached to a bedside pole (Figure 23-21). Locking of the blood pump into the motor is critical to ensure proper function of the system. A motor cable attaches the motor and blood pump to the console, which is secured on a bedside stand. If a BVAD is implanted, two consoles and two pump motors are needed for the two blood pumps, with back-up consoles available for emergency support.

Assessment of the CentriMag Blood Pump includes monitoring patient hemodynamics, recognizing again that the continuous flow centrifugal pump may dampen arterial waveforms and minimize palpable pulses in the patient with LVAD

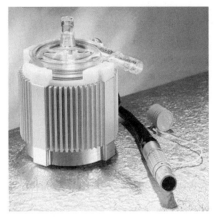

FIGURE 23-21 **Placement of Thoratec CentriMag Blood Pump within the motor.** (Courtesy Thoratec Corporation, Pleasanton, Calif.)

support, and monitoring for suction events as demonstrated by blood tubing chattering, presence of air in the tubing, and drops in pump flows. The blood tubing must be free of kinking and obstruction at all times, specifically on the inflow side, to help prevent air entering the arterial tubing. Prevention of suction is achieved with improving blood volume and decreasing pump speed. Full anticoagulation is required for the CentriMag Blood Pump, with systemic intravenous agents (e.g., heparin or argatroban if patient is HIT positive). Monitoring for thrombus formation or fibrin layering includes a focus on the tubing connections, which are frequently secured with tie-bands, and the blood pump. If the pump must be stopped at any time, a tubing clamp must be applied to the outflow graft before turning off the pump. An extra motor, console, and flow probe should be available at all times for the patient with CentriMag Blood Pump support.

Table 23-3 provides a brief overview of all of these acute cardiogenic shock devices.

TRANSPORT CONSIDERATION AND ASSESSMENT OF ACUTE VENTRICULAR ASSIST DEVICES FOR INTERFACILITY TRANSPORTS

The transport of acute ventricular assist devices requires a competent staff. The transport staff should have critical care experience and be trained on the

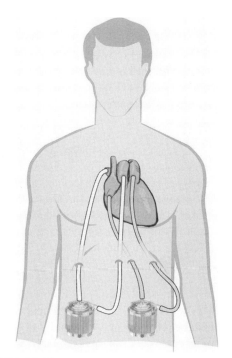

FIGURE 23-20 **Implantation approach for Thoratec CentriMag Blood Pump.** (Courtesy Thoratec Corporation, Pleasanton, Calif.)

TABLE 23-3	**Acute Cardiogenic Shock Devices: Characteristics and Features**					
Device name	BVS	ABV	PVAD	IVAD	Tandem-Heart	CentriMag
Type	Vol displ	Vol displ	Vol displ	Vol displ	Centrifugal	Centrifugal
Ventricle support	LVAD	LVAD	LVAD	LVAD	LVAD	LVAD
	RVAD	RVAD	RVAD	RVAD	RVAD	RVAD
	BVAD	BVAD	BVAD	BVAD	BVAD	BVAD
Rate/speed	40-60 bpm	40-60 bpm	20-110 bpm	20-110 bpm	3000-7500 rpm	1000-5500 rpm
Flow (lpm)	3-6	3-6	1.2-7.1	1.2-7.1	3-4, max 5	4-5, max 9.9
Flow probe	No	No	No	No	No	Yes
Internal back-up console	Yes, FR	Yes, FR	No	No	Yes	No
Console back-up battery (min)	60	60	55-80	55-80	60	Primary: 60 Back-up: 120
Manual pump	Hand pump	Hand pump	Bulb	Bulb	No	No
Defibrillation/ cardioversion	Yes, w/o disconnect	Yes, w/o disconnect	Yes, w/o disconnect	Yes, w/o disconnect	Yes, w/o disconnect	Yes, w/o disconnect
CPR	No	No	Per MD	Per MD	Per MD	Per MD
Anticoagulation	Heparin	Heparin Warfarin	Heparin Warfarin	Heparin Warfarin	Heparin	Heparin

Vol displ, Volume displacement; *max*, maximum; *FR*, fixed rate; *w/o*, without.

management of VADs or plan to transport a third rider who is considered the expert during the transport. Patient conditions are unstable from recent surgery. As more community hospitals implant VADs, the need for transport to more definitive centers for heart transplantation or more permanent devices is warranted. Before any transport on any device, an assessment for a properly working inverter is crucial. Consult the operational manual for specific information, which may vary with each device.

The physical assessment of the patient includes the primary and secondary survey with a review and analysis of laboratory values, advanced hemodynamics, adequate perfusion indicators, and adequate ventilation. In addition, auscultation of native heart sounds are recommended because peripheral pulses may be difficult to palpate if a centrifugal device is used. An assessment of device alarms and battery status should also be included, with review of the device display screen to obtain more specific information about device performance, including pump flow, rate, and speed. These data should be reviewed with a physician to assure specific device parameters are maintained.

The presence of "black specks" or clots or fibrin layering should be assessed in devices with external transparent outer cases, such as the BVS Blood Pump, the AB Ventricle, or the PVAD. If these clots or specks are noted, notify a physician immediately.

Patients have a stable (closed) or unstable (open) sternum. In either case, the sternum is weakened and a plan should be discussed on how to perform external compressions in the event of an emergency. The patients are typically sedated with IV medications. The Glasgow coma score is important to ascertain before the implant surgery to compare it with findings if the patient awakens during transport. Vasoactive medications, a PA catheter, intubation, a possible IABP, and systemic anticoagulation are common in all patients with acute devices. The higher than normal clotting time may be related to the earlier operating room procedure (VAD implantation). The activated clotting time should be greater than 200 seconds. All patients have some type of chest tube and should be watched carefully for increased bleeding. Epicardial pacing wires are available if temporary pacing is needed. If a patient has an AICD, the transport crews should assess whether it is activated or inoperable. If the patient has a continuous flow RVAD, extreme caution should be used when disconnecting any central vascular access device and exchanging IV bags. The continuous VADs could potentially pull air into the circulatory system if the lines are left uncapped. The most common postoperative issues facing acute patients with VADs are bleeding, arrhythmias, cardiac tamponade, hemodynamic instability, and sepsis. Other potential complications include acute respiratory distress syndrome (ARDS), pulmonary embolism (PE), and hypothermia related to heat loss from the external pump tubing, for which the BVS blood pump has a tubing cover.

Altitude considerations are important for all pneumatic driven pumps. Other devices without the ability to "vent" have an increase in air accumulation, which has operational effects on the device. The weight and space issues are important for rotor-wing and fixed-wing transports. Patients on the Abiomed CSS should be positioned with their feet toward the front of the aircraft to better maintain preload on takeoff and ascent.[5]

CHRONIC REFRACTORY SEVERE HEART FAILURE DEVICE

When a patient has development of severely decompensated heart failure, whether it is acute or chronic, that subsequently becomes refractory to conventional pharmacologic and mechanical means such that hospital discharge is not feasible, or frequent hospitalizations are needed to stabilize the patient's symptoms, the clinical team must direct treatment strategies to more definitive therapeutic options. The gold standard currently in patients with end-stage heart failure who are deemed eligible is cardiac transplantation, which offers a 50% survival rate at 10 years after transplant.[22] Alternatively, if VAD technology can be so perfected as to offer similar if not superior outcomes, without the delay for treatment (e.g., waiting for a suitable donor organ) and without the side effects attributable to immunosuppressive therapy for transplant patients, then VAD therapy may ultimately supersede heart transplant as the gold standard for this patient population. Hence, the competitive technologic race is to design mechanical support devices that are durable, applicable to multiple body sizes, easy to implant, and easy to manage technically, with minimal concurrent medication requirements including anticoagulation therapy and with applicability to all refractory heart failure indications. Following is an overview of the devices, both artificial hearts and VADs, that are currently striving to fulfill these needs.

ARTIFICIAL HEARTS

Two artificial hearts are currently clinically available in the United States. The *CardioWest temporary TAH* (SynCardia Systems, Inc) received FDA approval in October 2004 as a bridge to transplant in candidates at risk for imminent death (Figure 23-22). Although available for use in Europe, a portable driver that has been adapted for use with the CardioWest TAH is not yet available in the United States. Hence, US patients on CardioWest TAH support must remain hospitalized until a donor heart is available because the current console, named Big Blue, is not portable.

AbioCor Implantable Replacement Heart

The *AbioCor Implantable Replacement Heart System* (ABIOMED, Inc), the other clinically available artificial heart in the United States, is FDA approved as a life-saving measure when all other options have failed

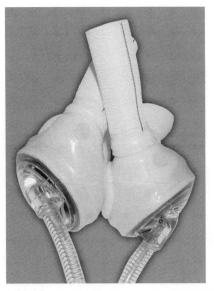

FIGURE 23-22 **SynCardia Systems CardioWest TAH.** (Courtesy SynCardia Systems, Inc, Tucson, Ariz.)

(Humanitarian Device Exemption approval) and does have portable power support, which makes it available for use in the community. It is intended for patients with irreversible end-stage biventricular heart failure, whose other major organs remain viable and who are not eligible for cardiac transplant. Patients evaluated for this technology are at risk of imminent death. The AbioCor System is composed of a totally implanted system with limited external components. The implanted components include (Figure 23-23):

- the thoracic unit, which is the blood pump composed of a right and left blood sac;
- the implanted controller and battery;
- the implanted cable, which connects the thoracic unit to the implanted controller and battery;
- and the internal transcutaneous energy transmission (TET), which communicates with the external power sources to recharge the internal battery and power the thoracic unit.

The external components of the AbioCor System include:

- the external TET;
- the AbioCor console and patient-carried electronics (PCE);
- the radio frequency module;
- and the handheld monitor.

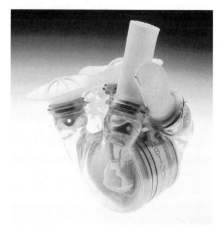

FIGURE 23-24   **Abiomed AbioCor thoracic unit.** (Courtesy ABIOMED, Inc, Danvers, Mass.)

The thoracic unit (Figure 23-24) essentially replaces the ventricles of the native heart and is attached to the remaining native atria. The outflow grafts of the AbioCor System are attached to the native PA and aorta (Figure 23-25). A chest computed tomography scan is performed before surgery to assist in evaluation of the feasibility of placement of the device. The thoracic unit has left and right blood sacs that are separated by the energy converter. The energy converter is designed to shunt hydraulic fluid back and forth between the two blood sacs, alternatively facilitating ejection and filling of the blood sacs. The frequency of this

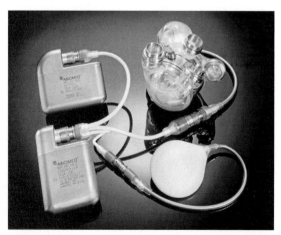

FIGURE 23-23   **Implanted components of Abiomed AbioCor System.** (Courtesy ABIOMED, Inc, Danvers, Mass.)

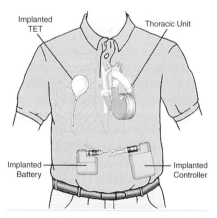

The AbioCor System has four main parts that are implanted inside the body.

FIGURE 23-25   **Implantation approach for the Abiomed AbioCor System.** (Courtesy ABIOMED, Inc, Danvers, Mass.)

shunting is the thoracic unit's beat rate and is manually controlled on the external console. The volume of hydraulic fluid shunted between the two blood sacs is determined by the balance setting on the console and affects the amount of blood pumped from each side. The implanted controller runs the thoracic unit, monitoring the system, controlling the system functions, and communicating to the external components the status and alarms of the system. The internal TET transmits energy from the external TET to the pump via conversion of transcutaneously transmitted radio waves into DC power. It also transmits alarm signals. The internal battery provides up to 45 minutes of battery power when the internal TET is not receiving power.

The external AbioCor Console provides electrical power to the external TET, which in turn transmits the energy to the internal TET. The external TET is anchored to the skin with a DuoDERM patch, placed directly over the internal TET. A TET status indicator on the console indicates how well the external TET is aligned (coupled) to the internal TET. The AbioCor console also communicates settings and information with the thoracic unit via the radio frequency communication module, which is most effective when held over the internal controller located in the patient's lower abdomen. The display screen on the console has two options, a clinical mode with intended use by trained clinicians and the home mode for use in the community. The display screen of the home mode provides information about the power status, pump rate and balance, radio frequency transmission status for the RF communication module, and alarm messages and responses. The patient-carried electronics (PCE) is a portable power transmission source for patients to use when active (Figure 23-26). It contains two sets of batteries, which when combined may provide up to 2 hours of power. The PCE control module is responsible for converting the battery or electrical power to be transmitted through the TET system. It may be powered by the portable batteries or through an AC power adaptor if an electrical socket is available. Patients are to travel with two PCEs, each with at least two fully charged batteries if the AbioCor Console is unavailable. The Handheld monitor is a personal digital assistant (PDA) that is

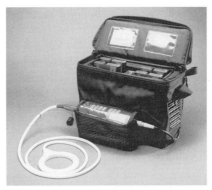

FIGURE 23-26 **PCE for the Abiomed AbioCor System.** (Courtesy ABIOMED, Inc, Danvers, Mass.)

able to provide pump information when the patient is connected to the PCE but cannot adjust AbioCor settings. The handheld monitor is battery operated and is set to recharge overnight while the patient is connected to the console.

In light of complete replacement of the native ventricles, ECG monitoring, pacing, defibrillation, inotropic or antiarrhythmic agents, and CPR are not indicated and, in the case of CPR, may be life threatening. Volume management of these patients is important relative to ensuring adequate atrial pressure to fill the artificial heart. Vasoconstrictors and vasodilators may be used to support blood pressure variances as needed. Patient conditions are also managed with antithrombin and antiplatelet therapy for the duration of support. A note of caution is that metal objects (e.g., the belt buckles of the stretcher straps) should be kept at least 3 inches away from the external TET to avoid a burn or fire hazard. In addition, patients should not be allowed to bend over at the waist to avoid affecting blood flow to the heart that may ultimately cause a loss of consciousness.

LONG-TERM VENTRICULAR ASSIST DEVICES

As previously described, and in contrast to artificial hearts, the *long-term VADs* are designed to support the native heart without removing it. Because of the evolution of the clinical trials to obtain FDA approval of these technologies for commercial use, an indication of BTT or DT had to be identified. In reality, as these devices enter the clinical arena after

FDA approval, the indication will more predominately be medically refractory severe end-stage heart failure. As described by Felker and Rogers,[10] the ultimate treatment goal of the therapy is driven by the patient's outcome after implant. To that end, the use of long-term VADs is becoming a more definitive treatment strategy in this very ill patient cohort while determining the treatment goal of BTT or DT.

Except for the Thoratec PVAD and IVAD, the remaining long-term VADs are intended for LVAD support only. Some of the smaller technologies are being evaluated in preclinical work for BVAD support,[18] but the current strategy is LVAD only. The HeartMate XVE LVAS (Thoratec Corporation) is the only long-term VAD with FDA approval for BTT and DT. The other devices remain in clinical trials for one or both indications. The major components of these devices are the blood pump, with an inflow cannula and an outflow graft; the controller, which runs the pump and provides device status and alarm indicators; and the power source. Not all of these devices use a bedside console, but they do provide interchangeable access to electricity and battery power. As LVADs, these devices cannulate the LV apex for the inflow access, with outflow anastomosis primarily to the ascending aorta. Interestingly, some European experience is found with descending thoracic aorta cannulation of rotary pumps.[21]

Unique to univentricular support, if the unsupported side is failing, it may not be able to deliver an adequate amount of blood to the supported ventricle, making adequate circulatory support difficult for the device to provide. Hence, adequate native right ventricular (RV) function must be ensured with these LVADs. The physiologic and subsequent geometric changes that occur with LV support commonly perpetuate otherwise benign RV failure, prompting the need for additional inotropic support if not temporary mechanical support for the RV. It is not unusual in this scenario, as previously described, to have the LVAD and RVAD be two totally different devices from two totally different manufacturers.[20] Typically, the RVAD is an acute device that is easily explanted after several days of RV myocardial rest. One of the added benefits of the continuous flow VADs over the volume-displacement devices is that the continuous flow devices may be more finely adjusted to provide sufficient LV unloading without compromising RV function. Unfortunately, the volume-displacement LVADs tend to provide all-or-nothing unloading of the failing LV. This maximal LV unloading tends to result in septal wall shifts into the LV chamber, with concurrent spherical reshaping of the RV and subsequent RV dysfunction. Manual adjustment of the speed of the continuous flow device allows significant influence over the alignment of the ventricular septum and the resultant RV function.

First-Generation Volume-Displacement Long-Term Ventricular Assist Devices

In review, the *first-generation VADs* are those VADs that contain a blood sac or chamber that allows for blood to collect before being ejected into the native circulation, either pneumatically or mechanically. Inflow and outflow valves, whether tissue or mechanical, ensure unidirectional blood flow. The PVAD and IVAD are first-generation pumps that may be used for short-term or long-term support. Because they have been discussed in detail previously, they are not revisited here. Suffice it to emphasize that patients supported with these technologies typically undergo conversion to warfarin therapy for full anticoagulation because of the prolonged support.

HeartMate XVE Left Ventricular Assist System. The *HeartMate XVE LVAS* (Thoratec Corporation) received FDA approval for BTT in an earlier version, the VE LVAD, in September 1998. The subsequent REMATCH Trial secured FDA approval for DT in November 2002. Although the REMATCH Trial showed a significantly increased survival and quality of life benefit with the HeartMate LVAD over OMM, the exposed limitations of the technology included limited device durability and significant sepsis events.[19] Many device improvements have since been incorporated to address these outcomes, although device durability remains limited as an inherent component of a volume displacement pump with many contacting mechanical parts that wear with time.

The titanium blood pump has tissue valves and textured surfaces throughout the pump blood path. These textured surfaces stimulate biologic deposition to create a pseudointimal layering that minimizes the potential for thrombus formation. The combination of the textured surfaces and tissue valves allows the HeartMate XVE LVAS to be adequately anticoagulated with antiplatelet therapy only. The blood pump may be placed in a preperitoneal pocket or intraabdominally and has a driveline that is tunneled subcutaneously across the abdomen to exit in the right upper quadrant (Figure 23-27). The Dacron velour-covered driveline is so designed to encourage tissue ingrowth over time as a barrier to bacterial infections that may contaminate down to the pump pocket. Because the XVE LVAS is a volume-displacement pump, the dead air space surrounding the internal motor must be shunted or displaced so that the flexible diaphragm of the blood chamber may move freely. Hence, the driveline contains an air tunnel that terminates externally through the vent port of the driveline beyond the exit site. A filter is attached at this port to prevent dirt particles from entering into the driveline and damaging the pump motor. The electronic wires of the pump are also contained within the driveline that then connects to the external system controller (Figure 23-28).

The system controller essentially runs the pump, monitors the system, provides alarm indicators and battery status, and provides a power conduit from the

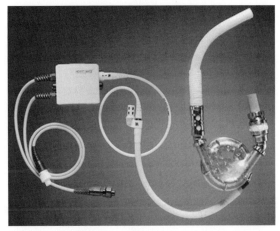

FIGURE 23-28 **Thoratec HeartMate XVE LVAS.** (Courtesy Thoratec Corporation, Pleasanton, Calif.)

power source to the pump. The controller has two power cables that connect either to a bedside electrical power base unit (PBU) or to portable batteries with battery clips. The display screen of the system controller has icons and buttons that allow for switching the modes from fixed to auto, for silencing alarms and checking battery power status, and for indicating active alarm situations. The PBU has either a system monitor or display module to provide a digital readout of pump parameters, including pump mode (fixed or auto), beat rate, stroke volume and flow, and current alarm messages. The PBU also recharges up to six batteries. Patients are instructed to connect themselves to the PBU whenever they sleep and then to batteries whenever they are awake and active. The PBU has an internal battery that is activated when electrical support to the PBU is interrupted. In addition to a minimum of six portable batteries, patients are also supplied with an Emergency Power Pak that provides prolonged battery support of up to 24 hours. In contrast to the rotary devices but similar to the PVAD and IVAD, the HeartMate XVE LVAS may be manually pumped should the device fail completely. A hand pump is attached to the vent port, following removal of the vent filter, converting the failed mechanical pump to a pneumatic pump. If device recovery is not feasible, the HeartMate XVE LVAS may be connected to the original device's pneumatic console for ongoing pneumatic support until the device can be repaired or replaced.

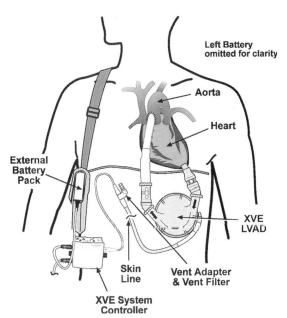

FIGURE 23-27 **Implantation approach of the Thoratec HeartMate XVE LVAS.** (Courtesy Thoratec Corporation, Pleasanton, Calif.)

Second-Generation Axial Flow Rotary Pumps

The *axial flow VADs* are continuous flow blood pumps with a linear blood path across the impeller. The three axial flow long-term blood pumps available in the United States are the HeartMate II LVAS (Thoratec Corporation), the Jarvik 2000 (Jarvik Heart, Inc), and the DeBakey LVAD (MicroMed Cardiovascular Inc). The HeartMate II LVAS (HMII) received FDA approval for BTT in April 2008 but remains involved in the investigational DT clinical trial. The DeBakey LVAD and the Jarvik 2000 are currently enrolling in their respective FDA investigational trials for BTT. In general, although the axial flow pumps have the advantage of finer control of LV unloading, they do not have the capability for manual drive should the device fail. This is applicable to the centrifugal flow devices as well. Manually pumping the HeartMate XVE LVAS (XVE) at 60 to 90 bpm is plausible, but attempting to manually drive the continuous flow devices at thousands of rotations per minute is not. Another feature of the continuous flow pumps is that they are valveless. Because these devices draw blood continuously through the system, valvular assurance of unidirectional blood flow is not needed. However, without the unidirectional valves and no mechanism for manually running the pump, pump failure and subsequent stoppage may potentially result in a significant retrograde blood flow (approximately 1-2 lpm) from the aorta back to the LV. Hence, efforts to prevent device failure have a heightened importance. Flow dynamics are dependent on the differential pressures at the inflow (LV) and outflow (aorta) cannulae, with sensitivity to preload and afterload. The higher differential pressure (higher aortic pressure relative to ventricular pressure) results in a lower pump outflow. Conversely, the lower differential pressure (increased ventricular pressure relative to aortic pressure) results in a higher pump outflow. Anticoagulation of these devices currently includes antiplatelet (usually aspirin) and antithrombin therapy (warfarin).

HeartMate II Left Ventricular Assist System. Except for the obvious engineering differences of the pump itself, the *HeartMate II LVAS* (Thoratec Corporation; Figure 23-29) has several similarities to the XVE LVAS. This valveless axial

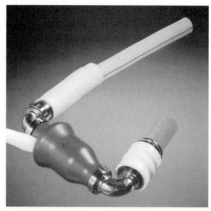

FIGURE 23-29   **Thoratec HeartMate II LVAS.** (Courtesy Thoratec Corporation, Pleasanton, Calif.)

flow VAD has an inflow cannula and an outflow graft that are attached to the LV apex and ascending aorta, respectively, with placement of the blood pump itself in a preperitoneal pocket, albeit a smaller pocket than the XVE (Figure 23-30). Of note, the inflow

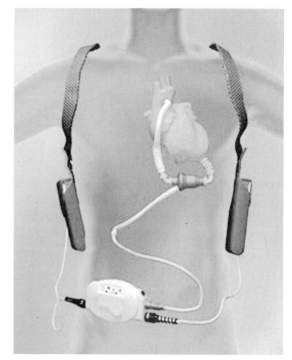

FIGURE 23-30   **Implantation approach of the Thoratec HeartMate II LVAS.** (Courtesy Thoratec Corporation, Pleasanton, Calif.)

cannula of the HMII has the same textured surface as found on all blood contacting surfaces of the XVE. The Dacron velour-covered driveline subcutaneously traverses the abdomen to exit in the right upper quadrant (RUQ) but is much smaller and more flexible than the XVE. The driveline is smaller because an air compensating tunnel is not needed, as it is with the volume-displacement pump. These changes in the driveline have shown to significantly reduce driveline-associated infections in comparison with the XVE. The HMII System Controller is larger and heavier than the XVE controller because of a fully functional back-up controller built in with the primary controller.

Because there is no mechanism to manually drive a rotary pump, a poised back-up controller provides additional reassurance. The icons on the controllers are slightly different as well. An important note is that the green light indicates two good power connections but does not reflect whether or not the pump is running, which may be confirmed with auscultation of the chest. Beyond the controller, all HeartMate accessories are interchangeable between the XVE and the HMII, as long as the display screens are programmed to handle either device. The portable battery sets provide 3 to 4 hours of power on average, and the Emergency Power Pak provides up to 12 hours of power.

Jarvik 2000. The *Jarvik 2000* (Jarvik Heart, Inc) axial flow pump (Figure 23-31) has a number of nuances that differentiate it from the other axial flow pumps. The inflow cannula contains the impeller, which is placed directly into the LV apex (Figure 23-32). The potential advantage of this intraventricular placement is that the pump pocket used by the other devices is obviated, as is the potential for pump pocket infections that still plague the other LVADs. The outflow graft similar to the other devices is anastomosed to the aorta. Similar to other LVAD controllers, the FlowMaker controller runs the pump, provides power to the pump, and monitors and triggers alarm statuses (Figure 23-33). In addition to these standard features, the FlowMaker controller uniquely allows the patient the ability to adjust the speed of the pump to accommodate the body's physiologic demands (e.g., lower speeds for rest, intermediate speeds for everyday activity, and

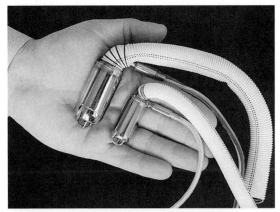

FIGURE 23-31 **Jarvik 2000 adult and child-size LVADs.**
(Courtesy Robert Jarvik, MD.)

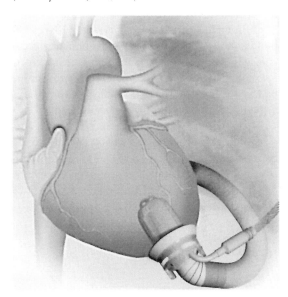

FIGURE 23-32 **Implantation approach for the Jarvik 2000 LVAD.** (Courtesy Robert Jarvik, MD.)

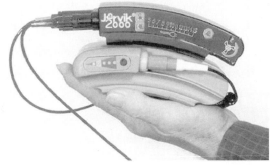

FIGURE 23-33 **Jarvik 2000 controller and battery.**
(Courtesy Robert Jarvik, MD.)

higher speeds for strenuous activity). The speed adjustment knob is located on the side of the controller next to the speed settings indicator. The speed settings are numbered 1 to 5, with 1000-rpm incremental speed rates per speed setting, ranging from 8000 rpm to 12,000 rpm. The speed rates correlate with a volume of augmented blood flow, not necessarily actual blood flow. Adequate filling of the blood pump affects the pump flow, as with any of the other devices. A setting of 1 provides an estimated augmented blood volume of 1 to 2 lpm, whereas a setting of 5 provides an estimated augmented blood volume of 5 to 7 lpm. The watts used to drive the pump are indicated on the controller providing a number range of 3 to 13. Normal watt range for the five speeds is 3 to 10. Of note, the watt lights blink rhythmically with the native heart beat. The cables that connect all of the external components of the system include an extension cable with a retractable coil that allows up to 6 additional feet from the patient to the controller. This is effective for various activities, including sleeping and showering.

The Jarvik 2000 is designed to be powered by battery sources only, and not electricity. The pump may be attached to the battery recharger for battery support, but it does not draw electricity even though the battery charger is plugged into a wall socket. The two types of battery sources for the Jarvik pump are the portable batteries that provide up to 7 to 12 hours of support per battery and the reserve batteries that provide up to 24 hours of support. All of the batteries recharge by being plugged into electricity.

DeBakey Left Ventricular Assist Device.

The *DeBakey LVAD* (MicroMed Cardiovascular Inc) evolved out of the experience of a National Aeronautics and Space Administration (NASA) engineer who needed LVAD support as a bridge to cardiac transplantation. Wanting to develop a small quiet fuel-efficient LVAD, a group of NASA engineers joined the clinical and research teams of Drs Michael DeBakey and George Noon to develop the DeBakey axial flow LVAD (Figure 23-34,A). The pump has undergone several engineering modifications since its initial clinical use to optimize clinical outcomes. It has received CE (Conformité Européene) mark approval, and is in the final stages of the US FDA–approved BTT clinical trial. The DeBakey VAD Child, intended for ages 5 to 16 years old as BTT, has also received CE Mark approval and an Human Device Exemption (HDE) approval by the FDA (Figure 23-34,B).

Pump components include the LVAD with a flow probe, the VAD controller (Figure 23-35) and

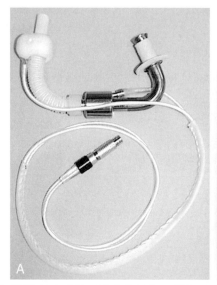
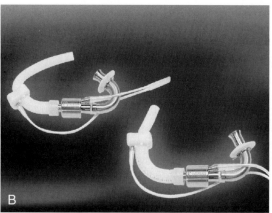

FIGURE 23-34 **A, MicroMed DeBakey VAD. B, MicroMed DeBakey VAD and VAD Child.** (Courtesy MicroMed Cardiovascular, Inc, Houston.)

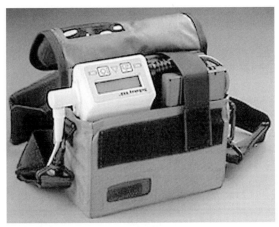

FIGURE 23-35   MicroMed DeBakey VADPAK. (Courtesy MicroMed Cardiovascular, Inc, Houston.)

VADPAK (carrying case), batteries, and the Patient Home Support System (PHSS). With implantation techniques similar to other LVADs, including inflow and outflow cannulae, a distinguishing feature of the DeBakey LVAD is that a flow probe is anchored to the outflow graft, providing a direct pump flow measure instead of the calculated pump flow of all other clinically available implantable LVADs (Figure 23-36). Pump parameters can only be changed by the hospital-based Clinical Data Acquisition System (CDAS) computer. The controller is programmed with a restart algorithm to allow for nine attempts to restart the pump if the device stops. The controller also contains a fail-safe mode that runs the pump at a fixed rate of 8500 rpm should the primary electronic system (Central Processing Unit, CPU) fail. The fail-safe dongle, which should be stored in the patient's VADPAK, can also activate the fail-safe mode by being inserted into one of the battery ports of the controller. Power sources include portable batteries and the Patient Home Support System (PHSS), which provides AC power with an emergency back up battery while recharging up to four portable batteries.

Third-Generation Centrifugal Flow Rotary Pumps

The *third-generation centrifugal blood pumps* are continuous flow pumps with disc impellers that are magnetically or hydrodynamically suspended. These pumps promise to have maximal durability because

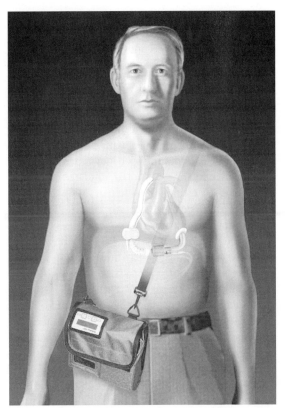

FIGURE 23-36   Implantation approach of the MicroMed Debakey VAD. (Courtesy MicroMed Cardiovascular, Inc, Houston.)

there are no contacting mechanical parts, which makes them "wearless" pumps. The disc impeller uses both centrifugal and circumferential energy to propel the blood through the blood path, which includes a perpendicular turn as the blood enters and exits the impeller. The third-generation pumps boast smaller drivelines, which should help minimize the arduous driveline infection issues of their predecessors. They also are more energy efficient to allow for the possibility of smaller and lighter batteries pending techno logic advancement. The three centrifugal flow pumps that are available for clinical trial evaluation in the United States are the VentrAssist LVAD (Ventracor, Inc), the DuraHeart LVAS (Terumo Heart, Inc), and the HeartWare LVAD (HeartWare, Inc). All three of these devices have received commercial approval (CE Mark) in Europe but are at various stages of the investigational trials in the United States. Their primary components, as with their predecessors, include the blood pump, the external controller, and the power source. Similar to the second-generation pumps, the pump flow dynamics of the centrifugal LVAD are sensitive to the differential pressure relationships of the inflow and outflow cannulae, and to preload and afterload. A unique characteristic of these pumps is that the patient's hematocrit value is entered into the controller and is combined with pump speed and watts to calculate pump blood flow. Incorrect entry of the patient's hematocrit or an outdated value may affect the flow estimate and trigger a flow alarm. In addition, these devices currently require both anti-thrombin and antiplatelet therapy.

VentrAssist Left Ventricular Assist Device.

The *VentrAssist LVAD* (Ventracor, Inc; Figure 23-37) is currently enrolling in both BTT and DT trials in the United States. The pump has inflow and outflow cannulae and is implanted in the left upper abdominal quadrant similar to many other devices (Figure 23-38). The controller provides the standard pump speed, power, and flow data and the pulsatility index and overpumping index, which reflect the amount of work being done by the device versus the heart and the potential for a suction event (Figure 23-39). Of note, the external cable or lead may actually be disconnected from the percutaneous lead of the LVAD and replaced if necessary. Replacement of the external lead should be done by two people and may warrant prophylactic intravenous anticoagulation therapy. Power source options include AC power and portable batteries that require recalibration monthly.

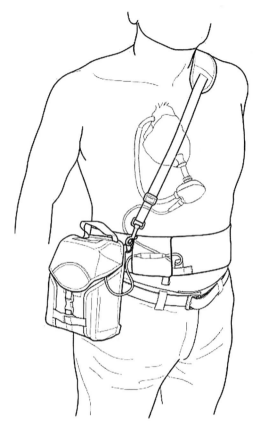

FIGURE 23-38   **Implantation approach of the Ventracor VentrAssist LVAS.** (Courtesy Ventracor, Inc, Budd Lake, NJ.)

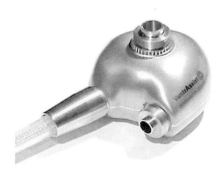

FIGURE 23-37   **Ventracor VentrAssist LVAS.** (Courtesy Ventracor, Inc, Budd Lake, NJ.)

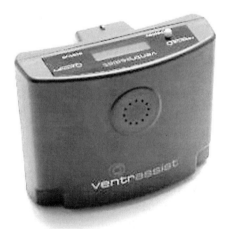

FIGURE 23-39   **Ventracor VentrAssist controller.** (Courtesy Ventracor, Inc, Budd Lake, NJ.)

DuraHeart Left Ventricular Assist System. The *DuraHeart LVAS* (Terumo Heart, Inc) has recently received conditional FDA approval to initiate its pivotal clinical trial in the United States for BTT. The DuraHeart LVAS is a fully magnetically levitated blood pump, with a special heparin-coating on all blood-contacting surfaces (Figure 23-40). The pump also has an implantation approach similar to the other pump pocket devices with inflow and outflow cannulae (Figure 23-41). The external controller includes a menu screen that displays alarm statuses and interventions to correct them. Power sources include portable batteries that are recharged by the portable battery charger, which can also provide AC power to the pump, and the emergency backup battery (EBB), which is used for extended power outages for a minimum of 15 hours. When hooked up to AC power through the battery charger, a fully charged battery must also be connected to serve as an emergency back-up should AC power failure occur. A hospital-based console may be used to provide electrical power for in-house patients.

HeartWare Left Ventricular Assist System. The *HeartWare LVAS* (HeartWare, Inc; Figure 23-42) has initiated its BTT trial in the United States.

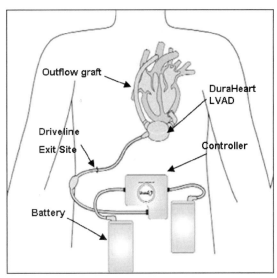

FIGURE 23-41 **Implantation approach of the Terumo DuraHeart LVAS.** (Courtesy Terumo Heart, Inc, Ann Arbor, Mich.)

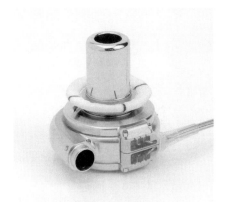

FIGURE 23-42 **HeartWare LVAS.** (Courtesy HeartWare, Inc, Framingham, Mass.)

Unlike the other centrifugal pumps, the HeartWare LVAS is implanted entirely in the pericardial space, with outflow graft anastomosis to the ascending aorta and subcutaneous driveline tunneling to the right upper quadrant of the abdomen (Figure 23-43). The driveline is significantly smaller than in its predecessors and is connected to the external controller (Figure 23-44), which is then connected to the appropriate power source. The controller provides the pump speed, flow, and watts parameters;

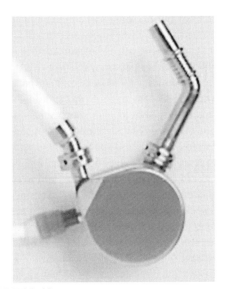

FIGURE 23-40 **Terumo Heart DuraHeart LVAS.** (Courtesy Terumo Heart, Inc, Ann Arbor, Mich.)

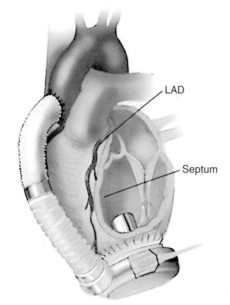

FIGURE 23-43   **Implantation approach of the HeartWare LVAS.** (Courtesy HeartWare, Inc, Framingham, Mass.)

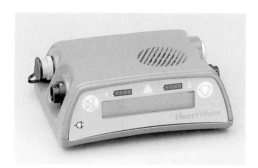

FIGURE 23-44   **HeartWare Controller.** (Courtesy HeartWare, Inc, Framingham, Mass.)

alarm messages and interventions; and power source and status. Power sources include external batteries, AC adaptor to an electrical outlet, and a DC adaptor to a car outlet. Portable batteries each provide 4 to 6 hours of support. A portable battery must be in place while using either the AC or DC adaptor to serve as a back-up should the other sources fail. The batteries are recharged by a portable battery charger.

Table 23-4 provides a brief overview of all of these chronic heart failure devices.

INTERFACILITY OR SCENE TRANSPORT CONSIDERATION OF LONG-TERM VENTRICULAR ASSIST DEVICES

The number of patients discharged in the community with VADs has increased in recent years. The likelihood that transport crews will come face to face with a device will increase because the FDA approved the HeartMate II in April 2008 as a bridge to transplant. These patients with chronic devices normally have stable conditions and are not immediately postoperative like their acute VAD counterparts. Some may have had their devices for weeks or months, and others for years. With the increased number of VAD options, transport crews are challenged to remain competent on all of them. Therefore, the educational leadership of these programs must ascertain which devices are in their area and develop training programs accordingly. The equipment necessary to safely transport these devices should include flashlights, clamps, and heparin. The patients are instructed to always carry a travel bag with all of the equipment needed to manage the device in an emergency. This bag should contain extra batteries, back-up controllers, and other specific equipment for the device. Also inside the travel kit is a reference card for the alarms and contact information for patient management. This equipment should always be transported with the patient. The patient is also instructed to be in the company of another person who is trained in emergency management of the device. If an emergency arises that renders the patient unconscious, the secondary caregiver should take over management of the pump. The secondary caregiver must also be transported if weight and space allow.

The assessment of a patient with a long-term VAD should consist of a primary and secondary survey. The assessment of pump functioning is done with auscultation of heart sounds. Each generation of devices presents different patient characteristics. For example, patients with volume-displacement devices have a pulse. Patients with either axial or centrifugal flow devices may be pulseless, depending on the function of the patient's native heart. In addition, with a continuous flow device, the patient's

TABLE 23-4 Chronic or Refractory Heart Failure Devices: Characteristics and Features

Device name	AbioCor	HM XVE	HMII	Jarvik	DeBakey	VentrAssist	DuraHeart	HeartWare
Type	Vo. displ	Vol displ	Axial	Axial	Axial	Centrifugal	Centrifugal	Centrifugal
Ventricle support	TAH	LVAD	LVAD	LVAD	LVAD	LVAD	LVAD	LVAD
Typical rate/Speed	85-150 bpm	50-120 bpm	8000-12,000 rpm	8000-12,000 rpm	7500-12,500 rpm	1900-2300 rpm	1500-1800 rpm	2400-3000 rpm
Flow (lpm)	4-8	2-10	4-6	Up to 8	Up to 10	4.5-6.5	4-6 (2.5-8)	2-10
Flow probe	No	No	No	No	Yes	No	No	No
Motor current	13-34 watts	–	6-8 watts	3-10 watts	0.3-2.0 amps	3.5-6.0 watts	0.4-0.7 amps	3.5-5.0 watts
Built-in back-up controller	No	No	Yes	No	No	Yes	No	No
Battery support (hours/battery set)	Int: ¾ TET: 2	4-6	3-4	7-12	6-8	4-8	3-7	8-12
Manual pump	No	Yes	No	No	No	No	No	No
Defibrillation/cardioversion	No	With disconnect	Yes	Yes	Yes, with PHSS disconnect	Yes	Yes	Yes
CPR	No	Per MD	Per MD	Per MD	Per MD	Per MD	Per MD	Per MD
Antithrombin	Yes	No	Yes	Yes	Yes	Yes	Yes	Yes
Antiplatelet	Yes	Yes	Yes	Yes	Yes	Yes	Yes	Yes

HM XVE: HeartMate XVE; *HMII:* HeartMate II; *vol disp:* volume displacement; *TAH:* total artificial heart; *LVAD:* left ventricular assist device; *rpm:* rotations per minute; *bpm:* beats per minute; *lpm:* liters per minute; *hrs:* hours; *int:* internal; *ext:* external; *defib/cardiovert:* defibrillation/cardioversion; *PHSS:* Patient Home Support System; *CPR:* cardiopulmonary resuscitation blood pressure should be assessed with mean arterial pressure (MAP) because a systolic or diastolic assessment is dependent on native function. A typical recommended MAP goal is 70 mm Hg. High blood pressures may limit pump outflow on most devices. These patients are on some type of blood thinning medications inclusive of antithrombin or antiplatelet therapy; therefore, examination of laboratory values is suggested. Assessment of the device function is completed with a thorough cardiac assessment and device data assessment with the display module if applicable. Management of arrhythmias should follow standard treatment algorithms, whether atrial or ventricular in origin. If the patient's condition becomes symptomatic or unstable, the arrhythmia should be treated, with consideration of device-specific issues (e.g., disconnecting the HeartMate XVE LVAS controller before defibrillation) before implementation of the therapy. Swift transport to the tertiary facility should be the goal.

The patients who return for readmission to the local hospital return for a number of reasons. Besides the device-related failure alarms unresolved by the patient, they may also return for non–device-specific issues, including altered mental status, falls, peripheral venous thrombosis (DVT), stroke or transient ischemic attacks, chest pain, sepsis, and nutritional and psychosocial issues.

SUMMARY

The use of VADs will only increase as the technology continues to evolve. The next frontier of MCSD projects to be smaller, more energy efficient, and possibly less invasively implanted. The potential for easier technology with easier implantation approaches allows the smaller hospitals the opportunity to implant these devices and potentially transport these patients to larger facilities. This progress will have a significant impact on the volume of critical care air and surface transports. As this occurs, transport teams must remain competent in transport and develop specific policies and guidelines related to the management and transport of this special patient population. Because the number of devices in this country is expanding,

---

BOX 23-1   Checklist Review for MCSD Transport

1. Can I do external CPR?
2. If not, is a hand pump or external device available for use?
3. If the device slows down (low flow state), what alarms are triggered?
4. How can I speed up the rate of the device?
5. Do I need to use heparinization for the patient if the device slows down?
6. Can the patient undergo defibrillation while connected to the device?
7. If the patient can undergo defibrillation, does anything need to be disconnected before defibrillation?
8. Does the patient have a pulse with this device?
9. What are acceptable vital sign parameters?
10. Can this patient be externally paced?

---

most prehospital personnel and transport personnel cannot remain comfortable and competent. Box 23-1 outlines a series of questions each transport team member can ask the patient, secondary caregiver, or knowledgeable physician to ensure safe and swift transport by the teams.

These questions provide the information needed to safely transport patients with MCSD during an interfacility or scene flight if a situation occurs where a patient presents with an unfamiliar device.

REFERENCES

1. American Heart Association: *Heart disease and stroke statistics: 2005 update*, Dallas, 2005, American Heart Association.
2. Antaki JF, Poirier V, Pagani F: Engineering concepts in the design of mechanical circulatory support. In Frazier OH, Kirklin JK, editors: *ISHLT monograph series mechanical circulatory support*, vol 1, Philadelphia, 2006, Elsevier, Inc.
3. Arrow International: *Counterpulsation applied: an introduction to intra aortic balloon pumping*, Reading, PA, 2007, Educational Materials Cardiac Assist.
4. Bolooki H: *Clinical application of the intra aortic balloon pump*, Armonk, NY, 1998, Futura Publishing Company, Inc.

5. ABIOMED: *Clinical reference manual: ABIOMED circulatory support systems*, Danvers, MA, 2003, ABIOMED, Inc.

6. *Datascope CS 100 educational materials: IABP counterpulsation*, Fairfield, NJ, 2008, Datascope Corporation.

7. *Datascope operators manual*, Fairfield, NJ, 2008, Datascope Corporation.

8. Devries W: The permanent artificial heart: four case reports, *JAMA* 259:849-859, 1988.

9. Farrar DJ, et al: Long-term follow-up of Thoratec ventricular assist device bridge-to-recovery patients successfully removed from support after recovery of ventricular function, *J Heart Lung Transplant* 21(5):516-521, 2002.

10. Felker GM, Rogers JG: Same bridge, new destination, *J Am Coll Cardiol* 47:930-932, 2006.

11. Gravelee GP, Davis RF, Stammers AH, et al: *Cardiopulmonary bypass: principles and practice*, ed 3, New York, 2008, Lippincott, Williams & Wilkins.

12. Kirklin JK, Frazier OH: Developmental history of mechanical circulatory support. In Frazier OH, Kirklin JK, editors: *ISHLT monograph series mechanical circulatory support*, vol 1, Philadelphia, 2006, Elsevier, Inc.

13. Kirklin JK, Holman WL: Mechanical circulatory support therapy as a bridge to transplant or recover (new advances), *Curr Opin Cardiol* 21:120-126, 2006.

14. Organ Procurement and Transplantation Network and the Scientific Registry of Transplant Recipients: *Transplant date 1997-2006, 2007 Annual Report of the US Organ Division of Transplantation*, Rockville, MD, 2007, Health Resources and Services Administration, Healthcare Systems Bureau.

15. Overwalder PF: Intraaortic balloon pump (IABP) counterpulsation, *Internet J Thoracic Cardovasc Surg* 2(2):1999, http://www.ispub.com/journals/UTCVS/Vol2N2/iabp.htm, retrieved 4/27/09.

16. Pagani FD, Aaronson KD: Mechanical circulatory support. In Mulholland MW, Lillemoe KD, et al, editors: *Greenfield's surgery: scientific principles and practice*, ed 4, New York, 2006, Lippincott Williams & Wilkins.

17. Portner P, Oyer P, McGregor C: First human use of an electrically powered implantable ventricular assist system, *Artif Organs* 9:36, 1985.

18. Radovancevic B, et al: Biventricular support with the Jarvik 2000 axial flow pump: a feasibility study, *ASAIO J* 49:604-607, 2003.

19. Rose EC, Gelijns AC, Maskowitz AJ, et al, for the REMATCH Study Group: Long-term use of a left ventricular assist device for end-stage heart failure, *N Engl J Med* 345(20):1435-1443, 2001.

20. Samuels LE, et al: Hybrid ventricular assist device: HeartMate XVE LVAD and Abiomed AB5000 RVAD, *ASAIO J* 54(3):332-334, 2008.

21. Siegenthaler MP, Martin J, Frazier OH, et al: Implantation of the permanent Jarvik-2000 left-ventricular-assist-device: surgical technique, *Eur J Cardiothorac Surg* 21(3):546-548, 2000.

22. Taylor DO, Edwards LB, et al: Registry of the International Society for Heart and Lung Transplantation: twenty-fourth official adult heart transplant report, *J Heart Lung Transplant* 26(8):769-781, 2007.

23. Wood C, et al: First successful bridge to myocardial recovery with a HeartWare HVAD, *J Heart Lung Transplant* 26:763-807, 2007.

REFERENCE MANUALS

ABIOMED: *AB5000 5000 operator's manual, ABIOMED circulatory support systems*, Danvers, MA, 2003, ABIOMED.

ABIOMED: *AbioCor clinician's guide to the AbioCor Implantable Replacement Heart System*, Danvers, MA, 2007, ABIOMED, Inc.

ABIOMED: *AbioCor Implantable Replacement Heart System patient and family guide*, Danvers, MA, 2007, ABIOMED, Inc.

ABIOMED: *AbioCor patient-carried electronics: mobile operation of the AbioCor System*, Danvers, MA, 2007, ABIOMED, Inc.

ABIOMED: *Clinical reference manual, ABIOMED circulatory support systems*, Danvers, Mass, 2003, ABIOMED, Inc.

Cardiac Assist: *TandemHeart PTVA System training manual*, Pittsburgh, 2006, Cardiac Assist, Inc.

HeartWare: *HeartWare Left Ventricular Assist Device (LVAD) System instructions for use* manual, Rev 07, Miramar, FL, 2008, HeartWare, Inc.

Jarvik: *Jarvik 2000 operator manual*, New York, 2005, Jarvik Heart, Inc.

Jarvik: *Jarvik 2000 patient handbook*, New York, 2005, Jarvik Heart, Inc.

MicroMed: *MicroMed DeBakey VAD operator's manual*, Houston, 2001, MicroMed Technology Inc.

MicroMed: *MicroMed DeBakery VAD patient user's manual*, Houston, 2001, MicroMed Technolgy, Inc.

Terumo Heart: *DuraHeart LVAD hospital guide-US*, Rev A, Ann Arbor, Mich, 2008, Terumo Heart, Inc.

Terumo Heart: *Patient and caregiver's guide-US, Rev A*, Ann Arbor, Mich, 2008, Terumo Heart, Inc.

Thoratec: *HeartMate II LVAS operating manual*, (103538B), Pleasanton, Calif, 2008, Thoratec Corporation.

Thoratec: *HeartMate XVE LVAS operating manual*, Pleasanton, Calif, 2007, Thoratec Corporation.

Thoratec: *Thoratec CentriMag Acute Circulatory Support Device training manual*, Pleasanton, Calif, 2007, Thoratec Corporation.

Thoratec: *Thoratec Ventricular Assist Device (VAD) & Implantable Ventricular Assist Device (IVAD) clinical operation & patient management*, Pleasanton, Calif, 2004, Thoratec Corporation.

Ventracor: *Clinical guidelines VentrAssist VA4 Left Ventricular Assist Device*, Budd Lake, NJ, 2007, Ventracor, Inc.

Ventracor: *Hospital quick reference guide VentrAssist VA4 Left Ventricular Assist Device*, Budd Lake, NJ, 2007, Ventracor, Inc.

Ventracor: *Patient and caregiver information VentrAssist VA4 Left Ventricular Assist Device*, Budd Lake, NJ, 2007, Ventracor, Inc.

24 PULMONARY EMERGENCIES

Reneé Semonin Holleran

COMPETENCIES

1. Perform a pretransport examination and evaluation of the patient's pulmonary function.
2. Demonstrate the management of a pulmonary emergency during transport.
3. Provide critical interventions during the transport process for selected pulmonary problems.

The transport of patients with medical disorders of the pulmonary system can be a significant concern. Oxygenation in many patients with pulmonary system disease is already compromised, and altitude or disconnection from set ventilators may have deleterious effects.[1] For the healthy person, alveolar oxygen tension (PaO_2) decreases to 65 mm Hg at 8000 ft with a decrease in arterial oxygen tension (PaO_2) to approximately 60 mm Hg.[4] Patients with significant pulmonary disease may show signs of hypoxemia at altitudes well below 8000 ft. Severe tissue hypoxia can occur with minimal obvious clinical signs. Thorough physical assessment and the use of pulse oximetry and capnography may help the transport team identify and intervene in impaired oxygenation situations.

ANATOMY AND PHYSIOLOGY OVERVIEW

ANATOMY
Airway

The upper airway consists of the nose, mouth, and pharynx. The pharynx extends from the nose to the larynx. The upper airway serves as a conducting system that warms, filters, and humidifies inspired air before it reaches the lungs. The pharynx branches into the larynx and the esophagus. The larynx contains the vocal apparatus, which includes the vocal cords, cartilage, and musculature. External landmarks of this area are the thyroid and cricoid cartilage, which can be palpated in the neck. The cricoid area is often the site for emergency surgical airway access. The epiglottis is a leaf-shaped flexible cartilage that covers the larynx during swallowing. Its primary function is to prevent food and liquids from entering the trachea and lungs. The lower airway consists of the trachea, the right and left mainstem bronchi, bronchioles, terminal bronchioles, respiratory bronchioles, alveolar ducts, and alveolar sacs.[3,6]

The trachea originates at the distal margin of the cricoid cartilage at the level of the sixth cervical vertebra. It continues distally to the bifurcation, the carina, which is at the level of the fifth thoracic vertebra. In adults, the length of the trachea is approximately 11 cm with an internal diameter of 12 mm. The trachea accounts for approximately 20% of anatomic dead space (approximately 30 mL).[3,6]

The mucosal surface of the trachea is made up of columnar epithelium and mucus-secreting cells. The carina branches into the left and right mainstem bronchi. The right mainstem bronchus is straighter and more in line with the trachea than the left mainstem, which may result in the endotracheal tube passing into the right mainstem rather than the left during intubation or suctioning.

The right and left mainstem bronchi branch into bronchioles. The bronchioles have some cartilage but consist of it less and less as the bronchioles progress distally. Further division gives rise to respiratory bronchioles that are the transitional zones between the bronchioles and the alveolar ducts. These zones are the transition between conducting airway and gas exchange areas. Alveolar sacs arise from the alveolar duct.[3,6]

The alveolar sac and pulmonary capillary are in close contact to facilitate gas exchange. The thin alveolar walls are made up of two types of epithelial cells: type I and type II. Type I cells are most abundant and are thin flat squamous cells across which gas exchange occurs. Type II cells secrete surfactant, a lipoprotein that coats the alveoli. Surfactant facilitates gas exchange by lowering surface tension of the fluids that line the internal surface of the alveoli, which prevents alveolar collapse during expiration.[3,6]

Thoracic Cage

The boundaries of the thoracic cavity are the sternum, ribs, and costal cartilage anteriorly and the ribs and thoracic vertebrae posteriorly. The clavicles and diaphragm establish the superior and inferior boundaries. Two layers of pleura line the thorax. The visceral pleura cover the outer surface of each lung. The parietal pleura lines the inner surface of the thoracic cavity. Between the two layers of pleural tissue is the pleural space, a potential space that contains a small amount of serous fluid. The fluid lubricates the two surfaces to facilitate ease of movement. It also creates a cohesive force that assists in maintaining the negative pressure that allows the lungs to remain inflated. Many organs are found within the thorax, including the heart, great vessels, trachea, esophagus, thymus gland, lymphatic vessels, and nerves.[13]

Muscles of Ventilation

Ventilation has two phases: *inspiration* and *expiration*. Inspiration is an active process. Contraction of the diaphragm and the external intercostal muscles increases the anterior posterior diameter of the thorax by raising the ribs and lowering the diaphragm. As chest cavity size increases, a negative pressure gradient is created, and air is inspired. The muscles then relax and cause passive expiration.

The accessory muscles used in respiratory distress include the scalene and sternocleidomastoid muscles, which assist with inhalation. The abdominal wall muscles and the internal intercostal muscles are used during active exhalation.[13,14]

Volumes and Capacities

For assessment of the events of pulmonary ventilation, the air in the lungs has been divided into four different volumes and four different capacities.[3] Volumes are distinct measurements (Table 24-1). *Total lung capacity* (TLC) is the sum of the volumes. Capacities are a combination of volumes (Table 24-2). Pulmonary volumes and capacities (Figure 24-1) are approximately 20% to 25% less in women than in men.[3]

PHYSIOLOGY

Effective ventilation depends on an intact thoracic cage, patent airway, integrity of the alveolar-capillary membrane, normal compliance, normal airway resistance, and adequate nutrition.

TABLE 24-1 Lung Volumes

Lung Volumes	Amount	Definition
Tidal volume	500 mL	Volume of air inspired or expired with normal breath
Inspiratory reserve volume	3000 mL	Extra air that can be inspired in excess of normal tidal volume
Expiratory reserve volume	1100 mL	Amount of air that can be expired by forceful expiration after normal tidal volume
Residual volume	1200 mL in a 70-kg patient	Volume of air remaining at end of maximal expiration

TABLE 24-2 Capacities

Capacities	Amount	Definition
Inspiratory capacity	3500 mL (~50 mL/kg)	Tidal volume plus inspiratory reserve volume: amount of air that can be breathed beginning at normal expiratory level and distending lungs to maximal capacity
Functional residual capacity	2300 mL	Expiratory reserve volume plus residual volume: amount of air remaining in lungs at end of normal exhalation
Vital capacity	4600 mL	Inspiratory reserve volume plus tidal volume: maximal amount of air that can be expelled from lungs after filling to maximum and expiring maximally
Total lung capacity	5800 mL	Maximal volume lung expansion with greatest inspiratory effort

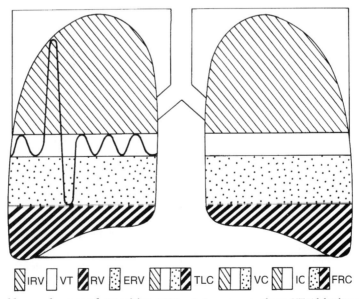

FIGURE 24-1 **Normal lung volumes and capacities.** *IRV,* Inspiratory reserve volume; *VT,* tidal volume; *RV,* residual volume; *ERV,* expiratory reserve volume; *TLC,* total lung capacity; *VC,* vital capacity; *IC,* inspiratory capacity; *FRC,* functional residual capacity. (From Des Jardins T, Burton CG: *Clinical manifestations and assessment of respiratory disease,* ed 4, St Louis, 2002, Mosby.)

Alveolar-Capillary Membrane

Gas exchange occurs in the alveolar-capillary membrane. Several structures are involved in this exchange (Box 24-1). Any change in these components alters gas movement across the respiratory capillary membrane.

The concepts integral to understanding gas exchange include diffusion, ventilation (V), perfusion (Q), ventilation-perfusion (V/Q) ratio, dead space, and shunts. *Diffusion* is the movement of gas from an area of higher pressure to an area of lower pressure—simply stated, from a greater concentration to a lesser concentration. Oxygen and carbon dioxide (CO_2) diffuse across the respiratory membrane.

Ventilation-Perfusion

Alveolar ventilation is the total volume of new air that enters the alveoli each minute. In the healthy adult male, alveolar ventilation is approximately 4 L/min.[3,6]

Perfusion is the amount of blood flow to the respiratory capillaries. Normally, the amount of blood that perfuses the alveoli is 5 L/min (i.e., cardiac output). In a perfect physiologic state, the ventilation of every alveolus is matched by an equivalent of perfusion, resulting in an equal V/Q ratio.

Various physiologic conditions alter the ventilation and perfusion relationship. When ventilation is less than perfusion, as occurs in atelectasis, more unoxygenated blood enters the systemic circulation. The condition that results in blood entering the system circulation without passing through a ventilated area of the lung is defined as *shunting*.[3,6] Anatomic shunting is the effect of blood that has not been oxygenated by the lungs traveling from the right to the left side of the heart, as with bronchial circulation.[5] Anatomic shunting normally occurs to less than 5% of cardiac output. Inspiration of 100% oxygen does not correct the shunt unit because all blood does not come in contact with functional alveoli. Shunting is the single cause of hypoxemia that cannot be rectified with delivery of 100% oxygen.[6]

When ventilation is greater than perfusion, a *ventilation-perfusion mismatch* occurs. A disease state that illustrates this situation is a pulmonary embolus. This physiologic occurrence is defined as a dead space unit.[6,16] *Dead space* is the inspired volume of air that does not come in contact with pulmonary capillary blood. Anatomic dead space is made up of the conducting airways and is normally 2 mL/kg of ideal body weight.[6]

In the setting of poorly ventilated arterioles, constriction occurs, thereby diverting the blood to better-ventilated areas. Similarly, poorly perfused alveoli collapse, which results in the diversion of airflow to more effectively perfused areas. This is termed a silent unit and helps to compensate for imbalanced V/Q ratios (Figure 24-2).

Transportation of Gases

Oxygen is transported in the blood as either bound to hemoglobin (97%) or dissolved in the plasma. The oxygen pressure (PO_2) reported on arterial blood gas analysis is a measure of dissolved oxygen only.

Oxygen-Hemoglobin Dissociation Curve

The *oxygen-hemoglobin dissociation curve* illustrates the relationship between hemoglobin saturation and PaO_2. This curve depicts the ability of hemoglobin to bind and release oxygen into the tissues. The relationship between oxygen content and the pressure of oxygen in the blood is not linear (Figure 24-3).

Various physiologic states change the relationship between hemoglobin saturation and PaO_2 (i.e., the oxygen-hemoglobin dissociation curve shifts in position).[3,6]

A shift to the left indicates an increase in the affinity of oxygen and hemoglobin. Physiologically, oxygen does not dissociate from the hemoglobin until tissue oxygen levels are very low because there must be a gradient. Situations that result in a left shift include alkalosis, hypocapnia, hypothermia,

---

BOX 24-1	**Structures Involved in Gas Exchange**

Surfactant
Alveolar membrane
Interstitial space
Capillary membrane
Plasma
Red blood cells

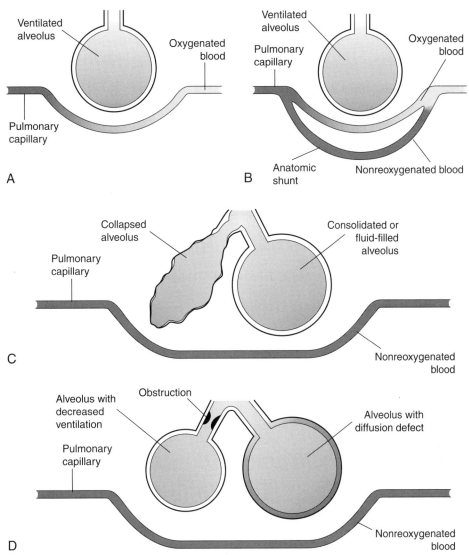

FIGURE 24-2 **Pulmonary shunting. A,** Normal alveolar-capillary unit. **B,** Anatomic shunt. **C,** Types of capillary shunts. **D,** Types of shunt-like effects. (Modified from Des Jardins T: *Cardiopulmonary anatomy and physiology: essentials for respiratory care,* ed 2, Albany, NY, 1993, Delmar.)

and decreased levels of 2,3-diphosphoglycerate (2,3-DPG). 2,3-DPG is an intermediate metabolite of glucose that assists in the dissociation of oxygen from hemoglobin at the tissue level. Levels of 2,3-DPG may be lower in patients who have received massive transfusions, related in part to the fact that stored blood is depleted of 2,3-DPG.[3]

The oxygen-hemoglobin curve shifts to the right in conditions that cause oxygen to dissociate more rapidly. In such cases, hemoglobin has a lessened

affinity for oxygen, which results in increased oxygen delivery at a cellular level. Physiologic conditions that result in a right shift include acidosis, hypercapnia, and hyperthermia (see Figure 24-3).

The understanding of this relationship is significant to the flight nurse to allow for the optimal intervention for patients. The amount of oxygen transported per minute is a product of oxygen content and cardiac output. This represents the quality of oxygen transported to the tissues per

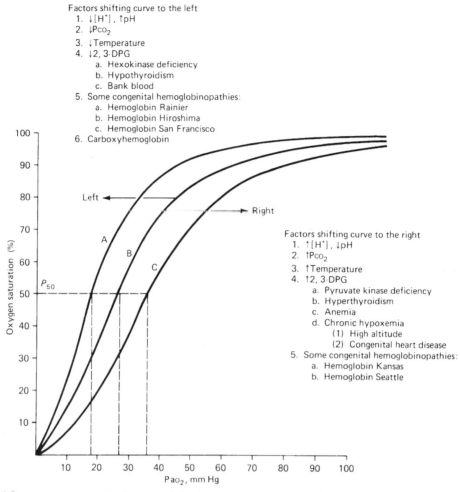

Factors shifting curve to the left
1. $\downarrow[H^+]$, $\uparrow pH$
2. $\downarrow Pco_2$
3. $\downarrow$ Temperature
4. $\downarrow 2, 3\text{-}DPG$
   a. Hexokinase deficiency
   b. Hypothyroidism
   c. Bank blood
5. Some congenital hemoglobinopathies:
   a. Hemoglobin Rainier
   b. Hemoglobin Hiroshima
   c. Hemoglobin San Francisco
6. Carboxyhemoglobin

Factors shifting curve to the right
1. $\uparrow[H^+]$, $\downarrow pH$
2. $\uparrow Pco_2$
3. $\uparrow$ Temperature
4. $\uparrow 2, 3\text{-}DPG$
   a. Pyruvate kinase deficiency
   b. Hyperthyroidism
   c. Anemia
   d. Chronic hypoxemia
     (1) High altitude
     (2) Congenital heart disease
5. Some congenital hemoglobinopathies:
   a. Hemoglobin Kansas
   b. Hemoglobin Seattle

FIGURE 24-3   *Curve B* is the standard oxyhemoglobin dissociation curve. *Curve A* shows the curve shifted to the left because of hemoglobin's increased affinity for oxygen. *Curve C* shows the curve shifted to the right because of hemoglobin's decreased affinity for oxygen. Factors responsible for shifting the curve are listed adjacent to curves A and C. (From Kinney MR, et al: *AACN's clinical reference for critical care nursing,* St Louis, 1988, Mosby.)

minute and is contingent on the interaction of the respiratory system, the circulatory system, and the erythropoietic system.[3] These relationships are defined in the formulas in Box 24-2.

Oxygen Consumption

The arterial-mixed venous difference in oxygen content is the difference between the arterial oxygen content and the mixed venous oxygen content. This difference indicates the actual sum of oxygen removed from the blood during circulation through the tissue. Normal oxygen transport is 1000 to 1200 mL/min.

In normal physiologic conditions, the tissues use 250 to 300 mL. Therefore, normal oxygen consumption is 250 to 300 mL. Mixed venous oxygen content values are determined from blood samples from pulmonary artery catheters.[3,6,9]

Carbon Dioxide

Carbon dioxide is transported in the blood by three mechanisms. CO_2 is dissolved in the plasma, which represents 10% of the CO_2 transported in the blood. Carbon dioxide also is moved by a chemical association with hemoglobin, carbaminohemoglobin.

BOX 24-2	**Oxygen Content Components**

Oxygen content = (Oxygen capacity × oxygen saturation) + (0.0031 × PaO_2)

Oxygen capacity = Maximal amount O_2 blood can carry	Stated as milliliters of O_2 per 100 mL of blood (vol%)	Multiply hemoglobin by 1.34
Oxygen saturation = % of hemoglobin saturated with oxygen	Stated as percent	SpO_2 or SvO_2

Systemic oxygen transport (mL/min) = Arterial oxygen content (mL/100 mL) × cardiac output × 10 (conversion factor) = 1000 to 1200 mL/min

This mechanism affects 30% of the CO_2 transported. It is a rapid system and can bind more CO_2 than oxyhemoglobin. The final and most significant mechanism is a conversion reaction as bicarbonate, which represents 70% of the CO_2 in the body. The bicarbonate reaction is slow in the plasma and rapid in the red blood cells.[3,6,9]

RESPIRATORY SYSTEM SUPPORT

OXYGEN THERAPY

Many critically ill and injured patients need oxygen therapy to augment the delivery of adequate tissue oxygenation. The most frequently used initial therapy for hypoxia is oxygen therapy.

Oxygen delivery systems are classified in two categories: high-flow systems and low-flow systems. *Low-flow systems* include a nasal cannula and simple oxygen face masks. These low-flow systems allow the patient to draw a supplemental amount of oxygen from the apparatus, and most of the inspired tidal volume comes from the room air within or around the apparatus. Therefore, the amount of oxygen that is inspired varies depending on the patient. The flow of oxygen from a cannula or simple mask is constant. The concentration of inspired oxygen is variable and depends on the patient's minute ventilation (Table 24-3).[3,6,9] For example, a cardiac patient with a high minute ventilation inspires less oxygen than a patient with a lower minute ventilation because the patient with high minute ventilation uses a greater amount of room air per minute.[9,10]

High-flow oxygen systems include nonrebreather masks. These devices result in the patient inspiring the total present fraction of inspired oxygen (FiO₂).

TABLE 24-3	**Low-Flow Oxygen Systems**	
Apparatus	**Oxygen Flow Rate (L/min)**	**FiO₂ (%)**
Nasal cannula	1-6	24-45
Simple face mask	4-6	35-45

Venturi masks operate by drawing oxygen through a narrow conduit that increases gas velocity and results in more room air being pulled into the mask. This high flow makes the concentration of inspired oxygen less dependent on the patient's ventilatory pattern. Venturi (air entrainment) masks can render precise low concentrations of oxygen between 24% and 50% (Figure 24-4).[3]

Nonrebreather masks have a reservoir bag that fills with 100% oxygen. These masks also use a one-way valve that allows inspiration from the reservoir and precludes inspiration of room air. The rebreather ensures that patients inhale basically 100% oxygen, regardless of inspiratory effort (Figure 24-5).[3,14]

VENTILATORY SUPPORT

Many patients with a pulmonary emergency need mechanical ventilation during transport. Chapter 12 contains extensive discussion about the use of ventilators during transport, including management of the machine and the patient.

RESPIRATORY MONITORING METHODS

Measurement of respiratory function during transport assists the team in assessment of acute changes in

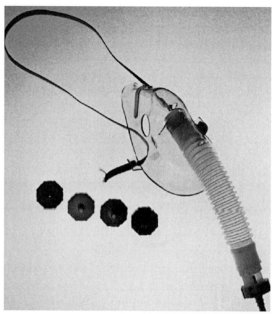

FIGURE 24-4   **Venturi mask and oxygen regulators.**
(Courtesy Richard Lazar, Stanford, CA.)

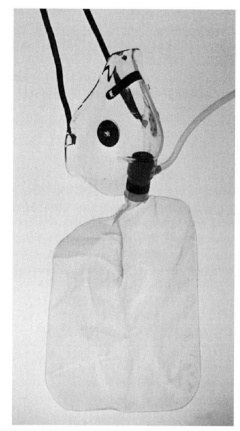

FIGURE 24-5   **Oxygen reservoir mask.** (Courtesy Richard Lazar, Stanford, CA.)

pulmonary function. Chapter 12 contains an in-depth discussion of current methods that can be used to monitor a patient's pulmonary status during transport.

ACUTE RESPIRATORY FAILURE

Acute respiratory failure can occur when chronic pulmonary disease or other factors affect the patient's ability to maintain adequate ventilation. Acute respiratory failure is defined as PO_2 less than 60 mm Hg and carbon dioxide pressure (PCO_2) greater than 45 to 50 mm Hg.[16] The transport team's initial concern is for adequate oxygenation and ventilation, followed by management of the underlying process that led to acute respiratory failure.

ACUTE RESPIRATORY DISTRESS SYNDROME

ETIOLOGY

Acute respiratory distress syndrome (ARDS) is a lung injury that has many causes (Figure 24-6). It may be a complication of other diseases or injuries,

with the most common severe sepsis with a pulmonary source of infection.[4] It is most commonly seen in patients with direct or indirect acute lung injury (ALS). Direct injuries may include gastric aspiration or inhalation injuries. Indirect injuries result in hypoperfusion of the lung and may be the result of severe hemorrhage, major burns, sepsis, multiple transfusions, multiple trauma, head injury associated with a change in mental status, pulmonary contusion, multiple fractures, and acute pancreatitis.[5,9]

PATHOPHYSIOLOGIC FACTORS

Acute respiratory distress syndrome results from a severe alteration in pulmonary vascular permeability, which leads to a change in lung structure and function. It is divided into two phases. Phase one is the

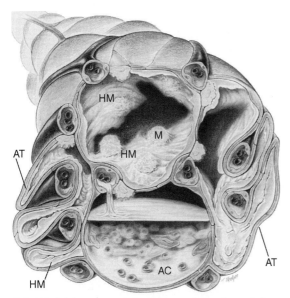

FIGURE 24-6 **Cross-sectional view of alveoli in adult respiratory distress syndrome.** *HM,* Hyaline membrane; *AT,* atelectasis; *AC,* alveolar consolidation; *M,* macrophage. (From Des Jardins T, Burton GG: *Clinical manifestations and assessment of respiratory disease,* ed 4, St Louis, 2002, Mosby.)

disease process that initiates an exudative state with an overwhelming expression of a proinflammatory response. This response results in damage to pulmonary endothelium and epithelium and in accumulation of fluid in the alveoli.[5] The second phase causes extensive pulmonary fibrosis and loss of normal alveolar structure.[5,6] The outstanding characteristic of ARDS is hypoxemia refractory to oxygen therapy. Because ARDS is a complication of other illnesses or injuries, the transport team must also consider the pathophysiology of the underlying problem.

ASSESSMENT

Assessment of the patient with ARDS includes the history of the present illness to determine the predisposing factors that led up to the diagnosis. Patients with ARDS report sudden onset of dyspnea; cyanosis occurs, and intubation with mechanical ventilation often becomes necessary. The patient appears in obvious acute distress. If the transport team is using mechanical ventilatory support for the underlying illness or injury, pulmonary compliance may decrease.[5,6]

Chest radiographs reveal widespread pulmonary infiltrates. Hypoxemia is present and may be severe. As the process worsens, accumulation of fluid in the alveoli significantly reduces pulmonary compliance. The patient's condition may progress to hypercapnia respiratory failure as the ability to maintain an effective minute ventilation is lost.[5]

INTERVENTION

Management of the patient with ARDS is a challenge. Positive end-expiratory pressure (PEEP) is added to mechanical ventilation in an attempt to improve arterial oxygenation. In addition, PEEP increases functional residual capacity (FRC). PEEP is measured in centimeters of water, and the lowest measurement possible should be used to restore FRC. As lung compliance decreases, higher levels of PEEP may be needed to maintain oxygenation levels. The management of the ventilated patient with ARDS is discussed in Chapter 12.[5,6,14,16]

Supplemental oxygen is necessary because hypoxemia is significant. Use of 100% supplemental oxygen may be necessary during transport. The oxygen delivery system used depends on the patient's condition.

The use of the pulse oximeter can help the transport team to monitor the patient's oxygen status. Changes in oxygen saturation (SpO_2) occur with ARDS, and subsequent changes may provide useful information for guiding other interventions. Ventilatory support with either a mechanical ventilator or a resuscitation bag is necessary for patients with endotracheal tubes in place. If a resuscitation bag is used, decreased lung compliance, decreased FRC, and impaired gas exchange may make adequate oxygenation difficult.

Capnography may also be used to monitor gas exchange and pulmonary ventilation. Figure 24-7 illustrates a normal capnogram. Both pulse oximetry and capnography assist in patient evaluation and management during transport.[5,6]

Fluids should be restricted unless shock is present. The impaired pulmonary capillary membrane allows fluids to leak into the alveoli. In the presence of shock, fluids must not be withheld. The main pulmonary system goal of air medical transport is to maintain adequate ventilation and oxygenation.

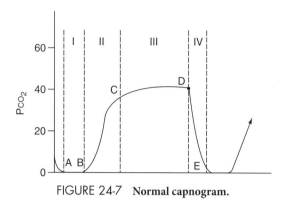

FIGURE 24-7 **Normal capnogram.**

CHRONIC OBSTRUCTIVE PULMONARY DISEASE

Chronic obstructive pulmonary disease (COPD) can be considered a continuum with asthma on one end, chronic bronchitis in the middle, and emphysema on the opposite end.[14] Emphysema and chronic bronchitis coexisting in varying degrees is not unusual. Although each entity is discussed separately, remember that different degrees of each can be present in the same patient.

One should not discount the effect of altitude on the patient with COPD because the ability to increase ventilation and cardiac output in response to stress is limited.[16]

ASTHMA
Etiology

Asthma is an obstructive pulmonary disorder caused by airway inflammation that results in restriction of airflow secondary to inflammation. The characteristics of asthma include: reversible airway obstruction, airway inflammation, and increased airway responsiveness to various stimuli.[8] Management of asthma now is directed at management of inflammation.

Pathophysiologic Factors

Various stimuli can trigger increased airway responsiveness. Once stimulation takes place, an inflammatory response occurs. Cellular infiltration and mucosal edema are seen (Figure 24-8). Airway hyperreactivity with smooth muscle contraction

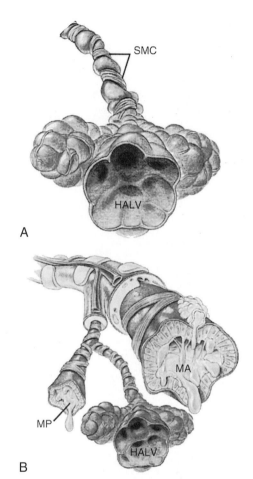

A

B

FIGURE 24-8 **Obstructive lung disorders. A,** Bronchial smooth muscle constriction *(SMC)* accompanied by air trapping. **B,** Tracheobronchial inflammation accompanied by mucous accumulation *(MA),* partial airway obstruction, and air trapping. *MP,* Mucus plug. (From Des Jardins T, Burton GG: *Clinical manifestations and assessment of respiratory disease,* ed 3, St Louis, 1995, Mosby.)

and additional mucus production and diminished secretion clearance also occurs and results in V/Q abnormalities, increased airway resistance, and hyperinflation of the lungs with an increase in residual volume. Status asthmaticus is a severe attack that is refractory to bronchodilator therapy.[6]

Assessment

The transport team should elicit a careful history to identify precipitating factors. For example, a viral illness may precede the acute exacerbation of asthma.

The patient may report a cough and dyspnea. A patient with a long history of asthma can usually rank the relative severity of the illness. A thorough medication history with regard to timing and dosage is helpful.

The physical examination reveals different degrees of respiratory distress based on the severity of the current episode. Tachypnea, wheezing, and a prolonged expiratory phase are not uncommon. If no wheezing is heard and the patient has difficulty talking, the transport team should consider the situation as emergent. Absence of wheezing may indicate that the patient is not able to ventilate sufficiently to produce breath sounds. Inspiratory retractions may be seen, as may the use of accessory muscles. The blood pressure is variable, and pulsus paradoxus may be present. Cyanosis and lethargy are late signs, and the presence of cyanosis or lethargy necessitates immediate attention.[6]

Diagnostic studies help determine the severity of the asthma. Resistance to airflow is measured with spirometry or a peak flow meter. Spirometric measurement of forced expiratory volume in 1 second (FEV1) is done before and after treatment to ascertain treatment success. Peak expiratory flow rate (PEFR) can be accomplished with a handheld meter and has been used to determine whether arterial blood gas (ABG) measurement is necessary.[8,15]

In addition to measurement of resistance to airflow, a chest radiograph may be done if other parameters are abnormal. Arterial blood gas measurement may be helpful in patients with severe asthma. Table 24-4 illustrates the stages of asthma with corresponding ABG results.

Intervention

Ensuring an adequate airway and providing supplemental oxygen are initial interventions. Asthma medications are divided into controller and rescue medications. Controller medications include orally inhaled corticosteroids (alone or in combination with β2-agonists), leukotrine modifiers, mast cell stabilizers, theophylline, omalizumab, and systemic corticosteroids. Rescue medications include short-acting β2-agonists and, in some cases, inhaled anticholinergics and short-acting theophylline. Intubation and mechanical ventilation are used only in severe cases. The indications for intubation and mechanical ventilation are listed in Box 24-3. Mortality rate increases for asthma patients who need intubation.[8]

Evaluation

The transport team should evaluate the patient's condition at regular intervals to ensure success of therapy. A decrease in dyspnea or in the degree of tachycardia and absence of accessory muscle use are parameters to evaluate success of treatment. Obvious improvement in FEV1 and PEFR measurements should occur. The patient should also be able to verbalize a subjective improvement in respiratory effort.

CHRONIC BRONCHITIS
Etiology

Chronic bronchitis is a chronic obstructive pulmonary disease that occurs most often as a result of cigarette smoking. Exposure to pollutants in the environment is also a contributor.

TABLE 24-4	**Stages of Asthma**			
Stage	pH	PO$_2$	PCO$_2$	Interpretation
I	↑	Normal	↓	Hyperventilation: ED treatment
II	↑	↓	↓	Hyperventilation; ED treatment consists of correcting hypoxemia
III	Normal	↓	Normal	Obstruction prevents hyperventilation; patient may need hospitalization
IV	↓	↓↓	↑	Severe; ICU admission; may necessitate mechanical support of respirations
V	↓	↓↓↓	↑↑	"Crossed" gases: PCO$_2$ > PCO$_2$; hospitalization and mechanical support of respirations after intubation necessary

From Hammond BB, Lee G: *Quick reference to emergency nursing,* Philadelphia, 1984, Lippincott.
ED, Emergency department; *ICU,* intensive care unit.

| BOX 24-3 | Seven Indications for Intubation and Mechanical Ventilation in the Patient with Asthma |

1. Decreased level of consciousness.
2. Progressive exhaustion.
3. Absent breath sounds or severe wheezing despite therapy.
4. pH 7.2.
5. $PCO_2 > 55$ mm Hg.
6. $PO_2 < 60$ mm Hg despite high-flow oxygen.
7. Vital capacity decreases to level of tidal volume.

Pathophysiologic Factors

The bronchi are the site of illness in the patient with chronic bronchitis. The mucus-secreting cells of the bronchial walls hypersecrete copious amounts of sputum, which prevents airflow into the alveoli. The alveolar gas exchange is normal, but the alveoli are underventilated because of the obstruction of airflow. Hypoventilation results in hypercapnia and hypoxemia. Figure 24-9 illustrates the pathophysiology of chronic bronchitis and emphysema.[6]

EMPHYSEMA
Etiology

Emphysema is a COPD that is defined anatomically as an irreversible increase in the size of air spaces distal to the terminal bronchioles. Most patients with emphysema are either current or past cigarette smokers. COPD develops in approximately 15% of smokers. Diantitrypsin may also play a role in the development of emphysema.[6]

Pathophysiologic Factors

Pathologic changes begin to occur years before the onset of obvious symptoms. The alveoli are destroyed, supporting structures fail to keep the alveoli open, and the air spaces beyond the terminal nonrespiratory bronchioles are increased in size. An increase occurs in the ratio of air to lung tissue in the alveoli. The alveolar capillary interface area is decreased, which results in a decrease in gas exchange. Air is trapped in the lungs and increases residual volume. The expiratory phase increases as the increased resistance to airflow continues. The patient's vital capacity is close to normal until the disease has progressed to a severe stage. Retention of CO_2 is also a late finding. Figure 24-9 illustrates the pathophysiology of emphysema.

Assessment of Chronic Bronchitis and Emphysema

Assessment of the patient with chronic bronchitis and emphysema is similar because the two entities often coexist in varying degrees. The history is important in determining the primary etiology of the disease. Exacerbations of stable states may occur with minor pulmonary infections, stress, changes in weather, or continued exposure to environmental pollutants (including smoking). The patient's subjective assessment of the condition is important to determine the usual status of the disease. The patient may report increased dyspnea, increased or a change in sputum production, or an increase in the malaise that may accompany the disease.

Physical examination of the patient may reveal rhonchi or expiratory wheezes. Rales may be present if the patient has an acute infection. The thorax is hyperresonant to percussion, and the anterior posterior diameter of the chest is increased. Observation of the patient's respiratory pattern reveals pursed lips and flaring nostrils. During acute exacerbations, every possible accessory muscle may be used because of the work of breathing. Patients with chronic bronchitis are frequently referred to as "blue bloaters" because they appear edematous and cyanotic. Conversely, emphysema patients are "pink puffers" because they are markedly dyspneic with a pink skin color. Tachycardia and the presence of dysrhythmias are also not uncommon. In the advanced

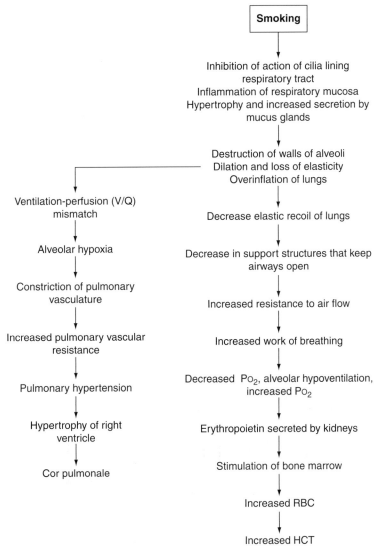

Smoking

Inhibition of action of cilia lining
respiratory tract
Inflammation of respiratory mucosa
Hypertrophy and increased secretion by
mucus glands

Destruction of walls of alveoli
Dilation and loss of elasticity
Overinflation of lungs

Ventilation-perfusion (V/Q)
mismatch

Decrease elastic recoil of lungs

Alveolar hypoxia

Decrease in support structures that keep
airways open

Constriction of pulmonary
vasculature

Increased resistance to air flow

Increased pulmonary vascular
resistance

Increased work of breathing

Pulmonary hypertension

Decreased Po_2, alveolar hypoventilation,
increased Po_2

Hypertrophy of right
ventricle

Erythropoietin secreted by kidneys

Cor pulmonale

Stimulation of bone marrow

Increased RBC

Increased HCT

FIGURE 24-9 **Basic pathophysiology of chronic obstructive pulmonary disease.**

stages of the disease, hemoptysis, fatigue, and weight loss may occur. Breath or heart sounds, or both, may be muffled because of the increased diameter of the patient's thoracic cavity. The patient frequently wants to sit and lean forward to better use accessory muscles.

The patient's mental status is an important component of the transport team's objective assessment of the patient. Retention of CO_2 occurs in the later stages of the disease process. Once the CO_2 level in the arterial circulation increases beyond the baseline level, one of the first signs is behavioral and emotional changes. The mental status changes may vary from confusion, irritability, and decrease in intellectual performance to obtundation.

Diagnostic studies include ABG measurement, chest radiograph, and electrocardiogram (ECG). The ABG results vary depending on the severity of the disease. A normal finding is for the patient with COPD to have a chronic respiratory acidosis compensated by metabolic alkalosis.[6] Chest radiograph reveals hyperinflation of the lungs, narrow and elongated heart shadow, increased anterior posterior diameter, and flattened hemidiaphragms in a lateral view.[6] The ECG findings are most often normal. However, some alterations that may exist include findings that show low voltage (again, because of the barrel chest), large peaked P waves in the inferior leads, and right-axis deviation as a result of elongation of the heart, respiratory volume strain, and signs of cor pulmonale. Atrial and ventricular arrhythmias are not uncommonly noted on the ECG. Pulmonary studies are vital capacity and FEV1. If either finding is less than 50% of normal for the patient, respiratory failure is present.

Intervention

Supplemental oxygen is given to attempt correction of the hypoxemia to the patient's baseline level. In the healthy person, CO_2 levels in the blood stimulate respirations. In the patient with COPD, the retention of CO_2 has rendered this reflex ineffective, and the drive for respiration becomes hypoxemia. Thus, administration of supplemental oxygen should be at low flow rates (≤ 2 L/min) unless the patient is being assisted with respirations by means of a mechanical ventilator or resuscitation bag.

The transport team may encounter some patients who have been placed on a noninvasive ventilation device. If the transport vehicle cannot accommodate the noninvasive device or the team is not familiar with the management of the device, a decision may need to be made to intubate the patient for safe transport. The team should always consult with the patient and family and the physician when this decision must be made.[16]

The patient may need assistance with removal of tracheobronchial secretions. Administration of intravenous (IV) fluids for rehydration may be necessary. IV fluids should be administered cautiously because there is usually some degree of right heart failure. Cardiac monitoring is necessary to detect dysrhythmias. Often treatment with pharmacologic agents may cause dysrhythmia. Life-threatening dysrhythmias should be treated according to standard advanced cardiac life support (ACLS) protocols.

Evaluation

Evaluation of the patient with COPD includes assessment of the patient's mental status for changes in baseline. Any alterations should be aggressively investigated. ABG results must be matched with the patient's clinical condition. Febrile illnesses are generally treated with antibiotics, and hospitalization may be necessary. If intubation and mechanical ventilation are necessary for respiratory failure in the patient with COPD, aggressive pulmonary toilet measures should be undertaken and evaluated for results.

SPONTANEOUS PNEUMOTHORAX

ETIOLOGY

A *pneumothorax* is defined as the accumulation of air or gas in the pleural space (Figure 24-10). *Spontaneous pneumothorax* most frequently occurs in young adult men, but it is not uncommon in older patients who have an underlying obstructive pulmonary disease.[6,14]

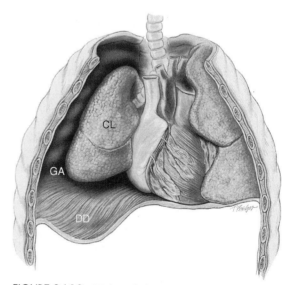

FIGURE 24-10   **Right-sided pneumothorax.** *GA,* Gas accumulation; *DD,* depressed diaphragm; *CL,* collapsed lung. (From Des Jardins T, Burton GG: *Clinical manifestations and assessment of respiratory disease,* ed 4, St Louis, 2002, Mosby.)

PATHOPHYSIOLOGIC FACTORS

Primary spontaneous pneumothorax most commonly occurs from the rupture of subpleural emphysematous blebs. The blebs are most often located in the apices of the lung.[6,14] The pathophysiology is similar to that of pneumothorax caused by thoracic trauma. The lung collapses in varying degrees, and hypoxemia may occur. If the pneumothorax is significant, a tension pneumothorax may occur when the air is trapped in the pleural space under pressure.

ASSESSMENT

Patients frequently have chest pain and dyspnea. The amount of pain may vary depending on the degree of lung collapse. In the patient with underlying COPD, the patient's condition deteriorates in spite of aggressive therapy. The breath sounds are decreased or absent on the affected side. In the patient with COPD, determination of any change in breath sounds may be difficult because of the increased anterior posterior diameter. If the hypoxemia becomes severe, changes in mental status can occur.

INTERVENTION

In patients who are asymptomatic with a small collapse of the lung, usually admission to the hospital for observation is all that is necessary. Symptomatic patients are usually treated with a tube thoracostomy. A chest tube is placed in the fourth intercostal space, with the anterior axillary line on the affected side.

The implications for transport, particularly air transport, are significant. Gases expand at high altitudes. The transport team should not transport a patient with a pneumothorax, even in a helicopter at low altitudes, without considering whether a chest tube should be inserted. If a chest tube is not inserted before transport, the equipment should be readily available to perform a needle thoracostomy in flight should a tension pneumothorax occur.[1] In transporting a patient with COPD, baseline parameters should be closely assessed before transport. If the patient's condition deteriorates during transport, in spite of aggressive management, the possibility of a pneumothorax should be investigated.

EVALUATION

The evaluation of a patient with a pneumothorax during transport includes reevaluation of mental status, observation of rise and fall of the thorax with respiratory movement, observation for changes in SpO$_2$, and ensuring patency of the chest tube (if present). Reports of chest pain and dyspnea should also be addressed and reevaluated. Sudden deterioration should lead to an evaluation of signs of tension pneumothorax (tracheal deviation, jugular venous distention, absent breath sounds, or chest movement on the affected side). Any interventions taken during transport should be constantly reassessed.

PULMONARY EMBOLISM

ETIOLOGY

Obstruction of pulmonary flow by emboli can result in alterations in lung tissue function, pulmonary circulation, and heart function. *Pulmonary emboli* contribute to the deaths of 50,000 to 100,000 patients annually and account for 5% to 10% of all the deaths in US hospitals.[2,6] The risk factors include heart disease, cancer, immobility, estrogen therapy, disorders in clotting and fibrinolysis, multiple trauma, obesity, and childbirth.

PATHOPHYSIOLOGIC FACTORS

Once the clot is produced, the lysing system is unable to compensate. The clot travels through the venous system to the right heart and on to the pulmonary vasculature. The obstruction of blood flow in the pulmonary vasculature may be small, massive, or complete. The results vary, depending on the location and size of the clot. Figure 24-11 illustrates the different types of emboli and the resulting symptoms and effects.

ASSESSMENT

Patients with pulmonary embolism report nonspecific and variable symptoms. Lower chest pain, dyspnea, cough, hemoptysis, anxiety, syncope, and diaphoresis are potential symptoms. The transport team should suspect pulmonary embolism in any patient when signs and symptoms of cardiorespiratory problems are not otherwise explained. A thorough history is necessary to determine risk factors.

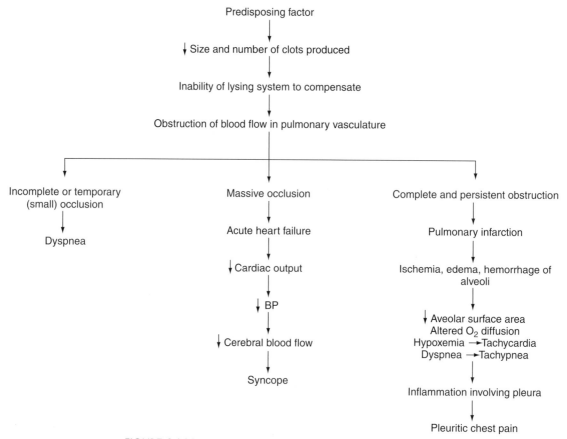

FIGURE 24-11   **Basic pathophysiology of pulmonary embolism.**

Physical examination may reveal fever, pleural friction rub, tachypnea, tachycardia, and anxiety. Although the patient exhibits signs of hyperventilation, ABG values reveal hypoxemia. The usual diagnostic tests are generally inconclusive in the patient with pulmonary embolism. The ventilation-perfusion scan (V/Q scan) is the test most often used in diagnosis of pulmonary embolism. To perform the scan, a small amount of radionuclide-labeled albumin is injected intravenously. After the injection, the labeled albumin particles attach to the pulmonary capillary bed. A pulmonary embolism reveals an area without radionuclide pickup, a perfusion deficit. The ventilation component of the scan assesses ventilatory function with the use of radioactive xenon. The perfusion and ventilation scans are compared, and a perfusion deficit without a correlation on the ventilation scan in the same area is supportive of a pulmonary embolism. With a low probability and a high index of clinical suspicion, or a high probability scan result, pulmonary angiography is done.

INTERVENTION

Supplemental oxygen should be administered during the diagnostic phase. Cardiac monitoring should be continuous because these patients are at risk of cardiac dysrhythmias. Anticoagulation therapy is started once the diagnosis has been determined; the standard anticoagulant used in treatment is heparin. Some studies of pulmonary emboli reveal thrombolytic therapy is associated with more rapid clot lysis when compared with heparin. As shown in one study, a trend toward a decreased death rate appeared when pulmonary embolism was treated with urokinase followed by heparin when compared with patients given heparin alone. However, many practitioners consider the benefits of thrombolytic therapy compared with heparin alone as yet unproven; therefore, many patients are treated with anticoagulation therapy alone (current oxygen saturation [SpO$_2$]). Some physicians use thrombolytic therapy in patients with hypotension and low cardiac output in spite of treatments such as streptokinase, urokinase, and recombinant tissue plasminogen activator that have been used to treat pulmonary embolism. In patients whose conditions cannot be managed with heparin, thrombolytics, or a combination of these two therapies because of the massive size of pulmonary embolism or contraindications to medications, surgical intervention may be necessary.[7] Intervention may include embolectomy or placement of an inferior vena caval umbrella filter.

EVALUATION

Evaluation of the patient transported with pulmonary embolism includes a thorough history of illness and any treatment started. Samples for baseline coagulation studies should be obtained before the initiation of anticoagulant or thrombolytic therapy. The transport team should assess the patient's cardiopulmonary status constantly during the transport to allow immediate intervention should deterioration occur.

PNEUMONIAS

ETIOLOGY

Pneumonia is an inflammation of the lung parenchyma, caused by either bacterium or viruses (Figure 24-12). Box 24-4 lists the different types of pneumonia with their causative organisms.

PATHOPHYSIOLOGIC FACTORS

Lobar pneumonia is an inflammatory process in which the affected alveoli are diffusely involved. Bacteria, neutrophils, and protein pass from one alveolus to another and produce compact infiltrates. The dense alveolar consolidations prohibit volume loss and produce air bronchograms on chest radiography. *Streptococcus pneumoniae* and *Klebsiella pneumoniae* are the most common organisms that produce lobar pneumonia.

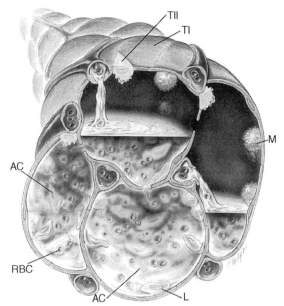

FIGURE 24-12 **Cross-sectional view of alveolar consolidation in pneumonia.** *TI,* Type I cell; *TII,* type II cell; *M,* macrophage; *AC,* alveolar consolidation; *L,* leukocyte; *RBC,* red blood cell. (From Des Jardins T, Burton GG: *Clinical manifestations and assessment of respiratory disease,* ed 4, St Louis, 2002, Mosby.)

Bronchopneumonias occur with areas of normal lung parenchyma interspersed with affected lung parenchyma. The condition is multilobar and bilateral, with areas of atelectasis. *Staphylococcus aureus* is the most common organism. *Interstitial pneumonia* is the result of an inflammatory process that affects the support structures of the lung.

ASSESSMENT

The history of the patient with suspected pneumonia includes fever and purulent sputum production. The specific signs and symptoms for different types of pneumonia are listed in Box 24-4. In addition to a careful history, a physical examination should include not only a thorough pulmonary assessment but also an assessment of the patient's overall health.

INTERVENTION

The type-specific interventions are summarized in Box 24-4.

BOX 24-4	Pneumonias

Streptococcus Pneumonia (Pneumococcal)
Organism
Streptococcus pneumoniae: Gram-positive, lancet-shaped *Diplococcus*; aerobe.
Risk Factors
Young, elderly, immunosuppression, alcoholism, COPD, cardiovascular disease, diabetes mellitus, hyposplenia; highest
   risk in winter months
Pathophysiology
Bacteria is normal inhabitant of upper respiratory tract; aspiration, inhalation, or hematogenous seeding are routes of
   entry; damage occurs from overwhelming growth, which impairs gas exchange
Clinical Manifestations
Malaise, sore throat, rhinorrhea, chills, fever, rust-colored sputum, pleuritic chest pain, nausea, vomiting, abdominal
   pain, tachycardia, tachypnea, dyspnea, decreased breath sounds, dullness, rales, pleural friction rub; in elderly
   patients, change in mental status or congestive heart failure possible presentation
Diagnostic Findings
Leukocytes up to 40,000 mL with left shift
Leukopenia
Liver function tests abnormal
Chest radiograph (CXR): Homogenous lobar or sublobular infiltrates
Treatment
Antibiotics
Fluids
Oxygen

Staphylococcus Aureus
Organism
Staphylococcus aureus pneumonia: Gram-positive nonmotile spherical organism
Risk Factors
Intravenous drug abuse, immunocompromise, and complication of influenza epidemic
Pathophysiology
Aspiration from upper respiratory tract leads to infections; growth occurs rapidly in the debilitated host;
   hematogenous seeding occurs with dialysis or IV drug use
Clinical Manifestations
Abrupt onset of fever, chills, cough, dyspnea, pleuritic chest pain; purulent sputum ranging from yellow to pink; frank
   hemoptysis common; toxic appearance; tachypnea, tachycardia, rales, rhonchi
Diagnostic Findings
White blood cell (WBC) > 150,000/mL
Positive blood cultures in 20% of cases
CXR: Bilateral lower lobe bronchopneumonia, early abscess formation or pleural effusion possible
Treatment
Antibiotics
Fluids
Oxygen

Klebsiella Pneumoniae
Organism
Klebsiella pneumoniae: Gram-negative, nonmotile, encapsulated rods
Risk Factors
Men, over 50 years of age, alcoholism, heart disease, diabetes mellitus, COPD, aspiration

BOX 24-4	Pneumonias—cont'd

Pathophysiology
Results in necrosis of alveolar walls, multiple abscesses, loss of lung volume, friable blood vessels

Clinical Manifestations
Fever, rigors, dyspnea, productive cough, hemoptysis, copious purulent sputum that is green or blood streaked

Diagnostic Findings
Leukopenia or leukocytosis
CXR: Lobar consolidation, typically of right upper lobe; rapid appearance of lung abscesses; pleural effusion common; bronchopneumonia in lower lobes

Treatment
Antibiotics
Fluids
Oxygen

Pseudomonas Aeruginosa

Organism
Pseudomonas aeruginosa: Gram-negative motile rod, not encapsulated

Risk Factor
Second most common nosocomial, decreased host defenses or antimicrobial therapy, alcoholism, diabetes mellitus

Pathophysiology
Aspiration, necrosis of alveolar walls, multiple abscesses, loss of lung volume, friable blood vessels

Clinical Manifestations
Same as those for *Klebsiella* infection

Diagnostic Findings
Leukocytosis with left shift
Arterial hypoxemia
Hypocapnia
Positive blood cultures in 33% to 50% of cases
CXR: Patchy infiltrates in lower lobes; cavitation, empyema

Treatment
Antibiotics
Fluids
Oxygen

Haemophilus Influenzae

Organism
Haemophilus influenzae: Gram-negative, pleomorphic motile rod; encapsulated and nonencapsulated strains

Risk Factors
50 years of age; >50% have alcoholism, COPD; upper respiratory infection (URI), 2 to 6 wk previously
Encapsulated strain: Alcoholism, diabetes mellitus, COPD, impaired immune system
Nonencapsulated strain: Exacerbation of bronchitis, nonbacteremic pneumonia

Pathophysiology
Bacterial infection that produces inflammation

Clinical Manifestations
Minimal elevations in temperature, pulse, and respiration (TPR), dyspnea, rales, rhonchi, pleuritic chest pain, nausea, vomiting

Diagnostic Findings
Leukocytosis
CXR: Bronchopneumonia, lower lobe and multilobular pleural effusions

Treatment
Antibiotics
Fluids
Oxygen

EVALUATION

Pulmonary status should be constantly reevaluated during transport of the patient with pneumonia. Mental status, SpO_2 readings, cardiac monitoring, and adequate V/Q parameters should be constantly assessed.

NEAR DROWNING

Each year, approximately 4000 people drown in the United States.[11,12] Most these victims are pediatric patients and under the age of five years. Drowning is the second-leading cause of injury-related death for children ages 1 through 14 years. However, any age group can be at risk for drowning or near drowning.

ETIOLOGY

Risk factors for the occurrence of a near drowning include inability to swim, seizures, head injury, hyperventilation, myocardial infarction, and stroke. Alcohol and substance abuse also are great risk factors. Alcohol use has been involved in one quarter of drownings.[11,12] Unfortunately, near drowning may also be an indication of child maltreatment or abuse.

PATHOPHYSIOLOGIC FACTORS

Persons who are submersed in a substance, most often water, panic and hold their breath. They may also hyperventilate, which can lead to aspiration and swallowing of water. Swallowed water may cause vomiting and further aspiration of fluid into the lungs, resulting in direct pulmonary injury and hypoxia.

The primary effect of drowning is generally pulmonary injury followed by hypoxia and cerebral edema. Whether the water aspirated into the lungs is fresh water or seawater, the end result is surfactant destruction, alveolitis, and destruction of pulmonary capillary membranes. This results in impaired gas exchange and hypoxia.[11]

ASSESSMENT

The assessment of the near-drowning victim begins with evaluation and management of the patient's airway, breathing, and circulation. The evaluation should include consideration of whether the patient may have sustained a cervical spine injury from falling or jumping into the water.

INTERVENTIONS

The management of a near-drowning victim includes removal of the victim from the water, basic and advanced life support with cervical spine immobilization, and rapid transport. Wet clothing should be removed and dry warm blankets applied to prevent hypothermia.

The primary intervention for near drowning is prevention. Box 24-5 contains a summary of interventions to prevent drowning. Teaching and assisting in implementing these prevention strategies should be an important role for transport team members.[16]

SUMMARY

The transport of the patient with a pulmonary medical emergency requires knowledge of the common disease pathophysiologic changes. The effect of even low altitude on oxygenation in the patient with a chronic pulmonary problem cannot be overemphasized. The transport team must combine the knowledge and skills to affect a safe expeditious transport of a pulmonary patient to the appropriate facility.

BOX 24-5   Drowning Prevention

When children are around water (swimming, bathing), they must be watched by an adult at all times.
Never swim alone.
Never drink alcohol or use drugs when swimming or boating.
People with backyard pools or ponds or who live near bodies of water should learn CPR.
Never use air-filled swimming devices (water wings) in place of life jackets or approved life preservers.
Know the local weather conditions to prevent being caught out on the water in a storm.
Follow beach warnings about dangerous tides, rip currents, or presence of danger in the water.

PULMONARY SYSTEM
CASE STUDY

HISTORY

The transport team was called to the scene of a near drowning. A 15-year-old boy was playing ice hockey with his friends on a farm pond. He suddenly fell through weak ice. He was pulled out by his friends, and CPR was begun.

On arrival of the transport team, the patient was found with a palpable pulse and a Glasgow coma scale (GCS) of 5 (E–1), (V–1), (M–5); pupils were 4 mm, and both were reacting equally. The patient's airway was secured with endotracheal intubation and rapid sequence intubation (RSI) after an intravenous access was obtained. His wet clothing was removed, and he was wrapped in a warm blanket. A cervical collar was applied, and the patient was placed on a backboard and prepared for transport to the trauma center.

During transport, lorazepam and fentanyl were administered for agitation. His vital signs were blood pressure (BP) 110/50 mm Hg, PR 130R, and assisted ventilations at 16. A pulse oximetry reading could not be obtained because of his cold extremities. His CO_2 level was measured at 30 on the end-tidal monitor.

OUTCOME

The patient was admitted to the critical care unit where his level of consciousness (LOC) continued to improve. However, pneumonia and sepsis developed, which were believed to be the result of aspiration of the water in the farm pond. Pseudomonas was cultured from his sputum. He needed a tracheostomy for ventilatory support. However, after several weeks, he was able to have the tracheostomy tube removed and eventually made a full recovery.

DISCUSSION

One important point this case makes is the success of basic life support (BLS) at the scene by this patient's friends. Mouth-to-mouth ventilation was started immediately once his friends pulled him out of the water, resulting in a limited amount of time that the patient was without ventilation. Some experts also believe that the water temperature may increase the chances of survivability.

REFERENCES

1. American College of Surgeons: *Advanced trauma life support-skills procedure, chest trauma management, needle thoracentesis (student manual)*, ed 7, Chicago, 2004, American College of Surgeons.
2. Anderson FA, Wheeler HB: Venous thromboembolism risk factors and prophylaxis, *Clin Chest Med* 16(2):235, 1995.
3. Brashers V: Structure and function of pulmonary system. In McCance KL, Huether SE, editors: *Pathophysiology: the biologic basis for disaese in adults and children*, ed 5, St Louis, 2006, Mosby Elsevier.
4. Cottrell JJ: Altitude exposures during aircraft flight, *Chest* 92:81, 1988.
5. Deal EN, Hollands JM, Schramm GE, et al: Role of corticosteroids in the management of acute respiratory distress syndrome, *Clin Therapeutics* 30(5): 787-799, 2008.
6. Ellstrom K: The pulmonary system. In Alspach G, editor: *Core curriculum for critical care nursing*, ed 6, Philadelphia, 2006, Saunders Elsevier.
7. Fields JM, Goyal M: Venothromboembolism, *Emerg Med Clin North Am* 26:649-683, 2008.
8. Krouse JH, Krouse HJ: Asthma: guidelines-based control and management, *Otolaryngol Clin North Am* 41:397-409, 2008.
9. Randhawa R, Bellingan G: Acute lung injury, *Anaesth Intens Care Med* 8(11):477-480, 2007.
10. Rozet I, Domino KB: Respiratory care, *Best Pract Res Clin Anaesthesiol* 21(4):465-482, 2007.
11. Sachdeva RC: Near drowning, *Environ Emerg* 15(2): 281-296, 1999.
12. Schoene RB, Nachat A, Gravatt A, et al: Submersion incidents drowing and near drowning. In Auerbach P, editor: *Wilderness medicine*, ed 5, St Louis, 2007, Mosby Elsevier.
13. Seidel H, Ball J, Dains J, et al: *Mosby's physical examination handbook*, St Louis, 2006, Mosby Elsevier.
14. Selfridge-Thomas J, Hoyt S: Respiratory emergencies. In Hoyt S, Selfridge-Thomas J, editors: *Emergency nursing core curriculum*, ed 6, Philadelphia, 2007, Saunders Elsevier.
15. Spahn JD, Covar R: Clinical assessment of asthma progression in children, *J Allergy Clin Immunol* 121(3):548-557, 2008.
16. York Clark D, Stocking J, Johnson J: *Flight and ground nursing transport core curriculum*, Denver, 2006, Air and Surface Transport Nurses Association.

ABDOMINAL EMERGENCIES

Reneé Semonin Holleran

COMPETENCIES

1. Perform a comprehensive assessment of the patient with an abdominal emergency.
2. Initiate the critical interventions for the management of an abdominal emergency during transport.
3. Identify the management of specific abdominal emergencies during transport.

Disorders encountered by transport teams may include esophageal obstruction and esophageal varices with rupture; stomach disorders, such as gastric or duodenal hemorrhage, ulceration, perforation, or pyloric obstruction; gallbladder and biliary tract disorders; liver disease; pancreatic disorders; and intestinal obstruction or rupture, ruptured diverticula, and acute appendicitis.

Transport via air may cause specific problems for the patient with an abdominal emergency.[11] The aerodynamics and biophysics that govern air medical care are especially important in relation to the gastrointestinal (GI) system, which encompasses 26 ft of liquid-producing and gas-producing viscous matter. Careful patient history, assessment, and pretransport planning are imperative for the patient transported via air.[1]

ESOPHAGUS

The esophagus is a hollow tube of striated and smooth muscle that is approximately 10 inches long in an adult. It lies posteriorly to the trachea, closely aligns the left mainstem bronchus, and exits the thoracic cavity at the diaphragmatic hiatus, or approximately at the T11 level. The esophagus provides the primary functions of peristaltic movement of food bolus, prevention of reflux with lower esophageal sphincter activity, and venting for gastric pressure changes.

Vascular supply to the esophagus is through branches of the descending thoracic aorta. Venous return from the esophagus is through the superior vena cava, azygos system, and portal vein system.

Neurologic intervention is initiated in the medulla and carried out by the vagus nerve.

Because the esophagus lies in the thoracic cavity, in normal atmospheric conditions, it maintains a subatmospheric pressure of –5 to –10 mm Hg, whereas the stomach, which is in the abdominal cavity, rests at an atmospheric pressure of +5 to +10 mm Hg. Acute esophageal occurrences are esophageal obstruction, esophageal varices, and esophageal rupture.

Esophageal Obstruction

Three areas in the esophagus are narrow and may be potential sites for obstruction and injury. These areas include the cricoid cartilage, the arch of aorta, and the point at which the esophagus passes through the diaphragm.[6]

Esophageal obstruction is fairly common. Strictures, webs, tumors, diverticula, foreign bodies, achalasia, and lower esophageal rings can all reduce or eliminate the venting property of the esophagus for the upper GI system. When air medical transport of a patient with obstruction is undertaken, intermittent exposure to variations in altitude is of great importance. Esophageal obstruction and an expanding gastrum can pose a serious threat if rapid decompression occurs at 35,000 ft. The venting property needs to be established before flight and depends on whether rotor-wing or fixed-wing transport is to be used.[11]

Assessment

The transport team should correlate careful physical assessment with interpretation of radiologic and laboratory data to anticipate any potential problems that may occur during the transport process.

Subjective Data.   The transport team should ascertain the patient's chief symptom and medical history. Included in these subjective data should be the patient's clinical course since the incident occurred. Medical history helps the transport team identify any other additional problems that may arise during transport.

Objective Data.   The flight nurse performs a physical examination that includes assessment of the following:

- The patient's ability to protect the airway.
- The patient's ability to clear secretions by swallowing.
- The presence and location of pain.

Diagnostic Tests

Radiographic studies of the obstruction should accompany the patient. If an esophagoscopy has been performed, a report should be provided to the transport team so they can prepare for any potential problems that may occur during transport.

Plan and Implementation

If the patient is being transported via air, the plan of care depends on the anticipated transport altitude. The transport team should carefully evaluate the patient's ability to maintain the airway. Even with aircraft pressurization, adequate gastric venting is extremely important if high altitude will be maintained. Pretransport medications and antiemetic therapy are often helpful not only for the antiemetic effect but also for the associated drowsiness. A gastric tube should be placed (if not contraindicated) and gastric contents emptied before and during transport. If the gastric tube is hooked to suction, its flow and contents should be closely monitored during transport. Continuous monitoring of respiratory status is also necessary.

Intervention

Caution must be exercised when a patient is placed on suction devices during transport; intermittent disconnection of suction from the gastric tube allows the pressures to equalize and prevents extreme suction against the gastric wall.

Children with a potential esophageal obstruction may benefit from an accompanying parent or other caregiver to decrease anxiety and prevent crying or other movement that may increase the risk of airway compromise.

Esophageal Varices

The most common cause of *esophageal varices* is hepatic congestion. Torturous, fragile, dilated esophageal veins can bleed from spontaneous rupture caused by increased portal hypertension or physical or chemical trauma. Esophageal varices are usually associated with cirrhosis. Varices occur frequently at the distal esophagus and hemorrhoidal plexus, and hemorrhagic shock from an esophageal bleed can occur rapidly. Bleeding occurs in 30% to 40% of patients who have esophageal varices.[10]

Assessment

Sequential history of the patient with esophageal varices helps the transport team anticipate probable needs during transport.

Subjective Data.   The transport team should obtain a history related to the cause of the esophageal varices, which can also provide information about other potential problems that could develop during transport. For example, the patient with severe liver disease also has bleeding and clotting problems. A patient with a history of alcoholism may be at risk for withdrawal, which may include seizures.

Objective Data.   Careful consideration of the patient's most recent pretransport laboratory data (hematocrit and hemoglobin levels, prothrombin time [PT]/partial thromboplastin time [PTT] or international normalized ratio [INR], and electrolyte profile) helps the transport team anticipate the patient's needs during transport.

If transport is between medical facilities, a transport team member should review radiologic findings and ensure that adequate interventions have occurred. If a patient has undergone angiography, the transport team must secure the cannulization site before any

patient movement and monitor the site frequently throughout transport.

Plan and Implementation

The transport team's primary priority is to ensure adequacy of the airway before transport. The transport team must consider what supplies are needed should an acute hemorrhagic episode occur during transport. Continuous gastric suction can produce large volumes of secretions, and a system to adequately dispose of secretions during transport needs to be ready, such as a supply of sealable bags or containers with tight seals.

An experienced transport member must maintain adequate care of any esophageal tubes, such as the Sengstaken-Blakemore, Linton, or Minnesota tubes. Although these devices are rarely used anymore, traction-dependent or specialized esophageal tubes can pose a problem for transport. Traction maintained with a football helmet can be used during transport (Figure 25-1). A plan of care must be predetermined in the event of airway loss.[5]

Airway loss from these particular types of tubes can be from either physiologic deterioration or tracheal obstruction. Saline solution, rather than air, can be used to inflate these cuffs to prevent further expansion during flight.

Intervention

If an acute hemorrhagic episode occurs, maintenance of airway and circulating volume is the first priority. Blood and blood product may be needed during

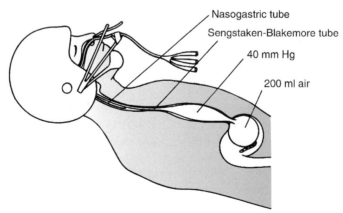

FIGURE 25-1   **Traction maintained with football helmet for Sengstaken-Blakemore tube.**

transport. Effective pretransport planning to prevent vomiting and ensure adequate venous access and volume resuscitation is crucial. Management of medications such as vasopressin and octreotide is necessary during transport.

Because these patients may have active bleeding during transport, the transport team should prepare with additional suction equipment, suction catheters, and bedding. "Preplanning" is a good idea; perhaps the patient can be placed in a transport bag to prevent leakage of blood or fluids.

Esophageal Rupture

Esophageal rupture commonly results from penetrating trauma but may also result from a blunt insult to the thorax. Rupture from invading lesions, tumors, or caustic exposure also occurs but to a lesser extent. If esophageal rupture has occurred, the venting properties and pathways have been altered. During transport, and with possible altitude changes, the distribution and displacement of gases are no longer circumvented by the appropriate course. Complications of gastric pneumonitis, hemopneumothorax, and alteration in gas exchange may all occur.

Assessment

The transport team ascertains the history of incidents that led to the current episode. Drugs known to have corrosive effects on the esophagus are doxycycline, tetracycline, acetylsalicylic acid, clindamycin, potassium chloride, quinidine, and ferrous sulfate. Caustic substances can quickly lead to burning or complete erosion of the tissue. Estimation of the degree and size of burns is extremely difficult and can quickly compromise respiratory status. If the rupture is caused by an extravasating tumor, hemorrhage and airway control can become quite difficult.

Plan and Implementation Priorities

The transport teams' priorities are as follows:

1. Ascertain adequacy of airway and oxygenation.
2. Maintain adequate venous access and volume support.
3. Place gastric tube with adequate suctioning if it is not contraindicated.

STOMACH

The stomach lies beneath the diaphragm and is secured in the peritoneum by the lesser omentum. The stomach is subject to alterations in intraabdominal pressure, unlike the esophagus, which has negative atmospheric pressure. The cardiac sphincter separates the esophagus from the stomach. Vascular supply is from the celiac artery branches, and venous return is through the superior mesenteric, splenic, and portal veins.

The stomach functions as a receptacle of ingested substances and attempts to provide chemical and mechanical breakdown. As the stomach expands, peristaltic action increases. The average time of gastric emptying is 1 to 8 hours. Chyme is then propelled through the pyloric sphincter into the duodenum. Decreased gastric motility and alterations in altitude can lead to complications.

Acute Gastric Occurrences

Acute gastric occurrences can take the form of gastric duodenal hemorrhage, gastric perforation from both mechanical and chemical means, pyloric obstruction, and gastric and duodenal ulceration.

Bleeding from peptic or duodenal ulceration occurs more frequently than does esophageal variceal bleeding. Several methods may be used to manage the bleeding, including insertion of gastric tubes, such as Linton or Minnesota tubes (rarely used anymore for the management of bleeding esophageal varices); pharmacologic management; endoscopy; thermal therapy; injection therapy, and if bleeding is massive and cannot be controlled, surgery. Anticipatory planning and thorough preparation can ensure a safe patient transport.[3]

Ulcerative lesions of the stomach or duodenum that lead to bleeding or perforation are in part caused by mucosal membrane erosion. The tissue beneath the mucosa is then subjected to general tissue corrosion. Ulcerations can lead to hemorrhage, perforation, or obstruction and may occur after an attempted repair.

Intervention

In the event of an acute hemorrhagic episode during transport, a transport team member should perform volume resuscitation, including administration of blood, blood products, and medications to manage the bleeding.[11] Complications may arise if the gastric tube becomes obstructed.[8] Gastric dilation and excessive hydrochloric acid can cause nausea and vomiting, which may mechanically induce hemorrhage. Maintenance of adequate gastric venting is imperative throughout any altitude changes when the patient is transported via air.

Movement can cause nausea whether via air or ground. The transport team should provide antiemetics and sedation to decrease the risk of vomiting, which may precipitate bleeding and potential airway compromise during transport.

GALLBLADDER AND BILIARY TRACT

The primary function of the gallbladder and biliary tract is to receive approximately 2 L of bile a day from the liver. Bile, which is stimulated not only by food ingestion but also by stress and acute illness, flows into the duodenum through the common bile duct. Fluid and electrolyte reabsorption takes place in the gallbladder before the bile enters the duodenum; therefore, with generalized volume deficit, an even more concentrated efficacious bile enters the duodenum.

Bile, which is composed of fatty acids, bile salts, phospholipid, cholesterol, conjugated bilirubin, and water, mixes with the chyme to aid digestion.

The ampulla of Vater and Oddi's sphincter are common sites of disease or injury that dramatically affect the entire tract. The gallbladder and biliary tracts are stimulated sympathetically by the splanchnic nerve and parasympathetically by the vagus. Vascular supply is provided by the hepatic artery and cystic vein.

Gallbladder and biliary disorders that necessitate acute air medical transport are infrequent. However, necrotic gangrenous cholecystitis can progress to septicemia, acute pancreatitis, or gallbladder rupture, hepatic failure, or both, because of obstruction of flow of bile production.

PLAN AND IMPLEMENTATION

Transport of patients with gallbladder and biliary tract disorders includes pretransport evaluation and determination of adequate drainage of gastric or tubes or both. Careful observation during transport is imperative for prevention of flow obstruction. As with any major abdominal disease or trauma, careful monitoring of oxygen tension and saturation should occur during transport.

LIVER

The incidence of liver disease and its associated illnesses is relatively frequent. Underlying disease processes, trauma, chemical abuse, or drug overdoses (especially acetaminophen) induce liver disease.[7]

An adult liver weighs approximately 3 lbs and is supplied by the hepatic artery and portal vein. The liver contains more than 50,000 lobules of hepatocyte.

The liver diseases most commonly encountered by transport personnel are cirrhosis, liver failure, or associated biliary atresia; also common are patients who are candidates for liver transplantation.

At times, the patient may have hepatic encephalopathy, which can present an unique challenge during transport. Hepatic encephalopathy can cause confusion, cognitive deficits, and coma. A confused and irritable patient could potentially become a safety threat. All other causes, such as electrolyte imbalance, must be ruled out and treated.[2]

PLAN AND IMPLEMENTATION

Hepatic encephalopathy, acid base imbalance, and electrolyte imbalances may make the patient confused and combative and can contribute to the challenge of transport, especially during flight.

When transporting a patient with liver disease, knowledge of what medications may not be effective because of liver dysfunction is important. For example, benzodiazepines that are used by many transport programs to decrease anxiety related to transport may not be as useful or may have to be administered in higher more frequent doses.[2,5]

Hepatic encephalopathy is often treated with medications such as lactulose that can cause diarrhea. The transport team needs to ensure that the patient is appropriately "padded" to prevent skin damage from the rectal output and possible contamination of equipment.[2]

PANCREAS

The pancreas, a gland approximately 8 inches long in an adult, is located behind the spleen. The pancreatic body is positioned horizontally across the abdomen. Its vascular supply is through celiac and mesenteric arteries. The pancreas consists of endocrine, alpha, beta, and delta cells. Pancreatic disorders include pancreatitis and hemorrhagic pancreatitis, cancer, and damage caused by trauma. Devastation of this organ leads to difficult care management of fluid and electrolyte balance, hemodynamic stability, and pain control.[11]

ASSESSMENT

A sound history is helpful in determination of the cause of the pancreatic disease process. The transport team should also ensure proper airway and venous access before transport. Careful evaluation of electrolyte balance may help the transport team determine additional treatment. A gastric tube must be in place before transport. If the patient has already undergone surgery and drains have been placed, the transport team must ensure proper venting for collection bulbs and surgical dressings. Pain management is an important transport intervention in the care of the patient with pancreatitis. An evaluation of what medications have been used to manage the patient's pain should be performed to ensure that the transport team has the appropriate medication to deal with the patient's pain during transport.[11]

INTESTINES

The small intestine (duodenum, jejunum, and ileum) is approximately 23 feet long. The primary functions of the intestines are absorption and digestion. The large intestine is composed of the cecum, ascending colon, transverse colon, descending colon, and sigmoid colon. This extensive, enclosed, gas-producing system can pose many difficulties for transport of a patient who has either direct intestinal disease or general acute illness.

The intestinal problems most frequently encountered by transport teams are obstructions, ruptures, ruptured diverticula, acute appendicitis, ischemic bowel, and mesenteric infarct.[6,11] Many of these patients have sepsis and septic shock.

ASSESSMENT

A careful history is necessary to determine whether the intestinal disease is a primary or secondary illness. A physical examination by the transport nurse should check specifically for abdominal distention, hyperactive high-pitched bowel sounds, and rectal blood, and the transport team should assess the patient for signs and symptoms of peritonitis or sepsis. The patient's temperature should be measured before transport.

PLAN AND IMPLEMENTATION

The transport team should evaluate venous access and volume needs before the transport. The patient in shock may need fluid resuscitation and vasopressors to support blood pressure. During transport, the team must ensure an adequate airway and provide oxygen, consider aircraft altitude or pressurization to reduce gas expansion, and ensure gastric tube patency. Continuous gastric tube suctioning is imperative throughout transport for a patient with an intestinal obstruction. Patients with stomas need adequate collection-bag venting.

If the patient has sepsis or septic shock, the transport team should direct care towards that management.

ABDOMINAL AORTIC EMERGENCIES

Patients with abdominal aortic injuries may require transport to definitive, specialized care.[9] The mortality rate from ruptured abdominal aortic aneurysms (RAAAs) is 75% to 90%.[4] Risk factors for *abdominal aortic aneurysms* (AAAs) include: increasing age, male gender, family history of abdominal aortic aneurysm, and smoking. Once the AAA has ruptured, operative intervention is necessary.

ASSESSMENT

Most patients with AAA or RAAA come from a referral center and have been diagnosed. Many are also in hemorrhagic shock. Because time is one of the most important factors for potential survival, the transport team's assessment should be focused on critical problems such as hypoxia, hypotension, and bleeding.

INTERVENTIONS

Rapid transport to an appropriate care facility is one of the most important interventions that can be provided by the team. Decreased time to the operating room has shown decreased mortality rates. A focused rapid assessment should be performed by the transport team. Blood and blood products are needed if a rupture has occurred and the patient is in hemorrhagic shock. However, the transport should not be delayed if at all possible for diagnostic data and such. A coordinated effort to decrease time but provide safe and competent care should begin with the initial call for transport.[2,9] The transport team needs to be prepared for cardiac arrest during transport and consider when possible allowing the family to see the patient before transfer or even accompany the patient because of the high mortality rate associated with RAAA.

SUMMARY

Careful planning by the transport team before transport, especially via air, helps provide effective safe care.

Because patient problems are difficult to predict, the transport team should plan for equipment and treatment methods that can be applied easily to all patients before transport. Gases that expand with altitude are ever present in the GI system; proper venting mechanisms should be placed before flight, and backup devices should be available on the aircraft. Calculation of flight time, ground time, and unanticipated diversions helps the transport team estimate the amount of volume, battery time, capacities, and therapeutic support needed for the entire transport time.

GASTROINTESTINAL MEDICAL EMERGENCIES CASE STUDY

The helicopter was called to transport an 82-year-old man with an upper GI bleed from a community hospital to a tertiary care center. Refractory massive hemorrhage had occurred during the previous 12 hours, and simple endoscopy by the local community hospital revealed what they believed to be a mass, greater than 13 cm, in the gastric pouch. Because of the size of the mass, clear visualization of the probable hemorrhagic sites was obstructed. This patient had a history of hospital admission 1 week before this occurrence for mild upper GI bleed brought on by food ingestion. A diagnosis of thrombocytopenia and hypertension was made at that time.

TRANSPORT TEAM EXAMINATION

The patient was a mildly obese man, who was pale and diaphoretic, in semi-Fowler's position on an emergency department stretcher. He was actively bleeding from a gastric tube and periodically vomiting large amounts of bright red blood and clots. The patient was visibly anxious and expressed fear of dying.

Cardiovascular: Skin was pale, cool, and diaphoretic, with petechiae over chest, abdomen, and thighs anteriorly.

Electrocardiogram (ECG): Global ischemia with occasional multifocal PVCs was noted. Two large-bore intravenous (IV) tubes were in upper extremities.

Respiratory: Nasal cannula delivered 4 L/min. Breath sounds revealed faint rales at bilateral bases. The chest radiograph revealed bilateral lower lobe infiltrates and a markedly distended gastrum elevating the left diaphragm. An approximately 13-cm mass with varying densities was seen.

GI-Genitourinary (GU): Normoactive bowel sounds were auscultated, and a large mass was palpated in the left upper quadrant. A urinary catheter was in place and draining clear yellow urine. A no. 18 Salem sump was in place and lying posteriorly to the gastric mass draining bright red blood. The emergency department staff was performing saline solution lavage.

Medications given before the flight crew's arrival were as follows:

Lasix 40 mg IV push (IVP)

Ativan 2 mg IVP

5 units of packed red blood cells

3200 mL of crystalloid

Laboratory data were as follows: Hematocrit (Hct) 27, PT 12.9, PTT 22.5; platelets 73,000; arterial blood gas (ABG) on 4 L/min nasal cannula O_2: pH 7.38, PO_2 68, PCO_2 32; vital signs: blood pressure 110/68 mm Hg; AP 108; respiration 30; temperature 96 °F, patient shivering.

Interventions

The transport team prepared the patient for transport and took iced saline solution in a cooler and four additional units of packed red blood cells. The stretcher was prepared with dry warmed linen and a space blanket. The oxygen was changed to 100% nonrebreather mask, and the patient was given safety orientation before flight.

The flight time to the tertiary facility was 20 minutes. Vital signs remained stable, and the saline solution lavage was continued throughout the flight, with noted clearing on landing. Units no. 6 and no. 7 of red packed blood cells were infusing. Patency of the gastric tube during air medical transport was crucial for this patient, and frequent manipulation of the tube was necessary to prevent occlusion.

Workup of this patient revealed that the gastric mass was a product of small bones, Styrofoam, hair, and paper products. The patient was taken to the operating room for removal of the foreign-body mass. It was noted at that time that the patient had no body hair.

DISCUSSION

Pretransport planning for the needs of the patient for the initial admission time and during the flight to the receiving facility is imperative.

This patient continued to receive colloid replacement during type-matching and cross-matching at the receiving facility.

The gastric bleeding was caused by mechanical lacerations from small bones. The patient underwent surgical repair and psychiatric evaluation after admission. In this extremely complicated case, a diagnosis of bezoar was made, and further psychologic evaluations were to follow.

REFERENCES

1. Air and Surface Transport Nurses Association: *Transport nurse advanced trauma course,* Denver, 2006, ASTNA.
2. Arora G, Keeffe EB: Management of chronic liver failure until liver transplantation, *Med Clin North Am* 92: 839-860, 2008.
3. Barnet J, Messmann H: Management of lower gastrointestinal tract bleeding, *Best Pract Res Clin Gastroenterol* 22(2):295-312, 2008.
4. Bounoua F, Schuster R, Grewal P, et al: Rupture abdominal aortic aneurysm: does trauma center designation affect outcome? *Ann Vasc Surg* 21(2):133-136, 2007.
5. Christensen T, Christensen M: The implementation of a guideline for patients with a Sengstaken-Blakemore tube in situ in a general intensive care unit using transitional change theory, *Intens Crit Care Nurs* 23:234-242, 2006.
6. Emergency Nurses Association: *Emergency nursing core curriculum,* ed 6, Des Plaines, IL, 2008, ENA.
7. Gunning EJ: Hepatic failure, *Anaesth Intens Care Med* 7(4):119-120, 2006.
8. Hearnshaw S, Travis S, Murphy M: The role of blood transfusion in the management of upper and lower intestinal tract bleeding, *Best Pract Res Clin Gastroenterol* 22(2):355-371, 2008.
9. Mitchel AD, Tallon JM: Air medical transport of suspected aortic emergencies, *Air Med J* 21(13):34-37, 2002.
10. Thabut D: Management of acute bleeding from portal hypertension, *Best Pract Res Clin Gastroenterol* 21(1):19-29, 2007.
11. York-Clark D, Stocking J, Johnson J: *Flight and ground transport nursing core curriculum,* Denver, 2006, Air and Surface Transport Nurses Association.

26 INFECTIOUS AND COMMUNICABLE DISEASES

Russell D. MacDonald

Transport personnel routinely encounter patients with infectious disease or suspected infectious disease. This encounter may be in the form of a sudden illness in the community setting or the transfer of a critically ill patient from one institution to a higher level of care. These emergencies put transport personnel at risk because the type, extent, and severity of these illnesses are not yet known. The Occupational Safety and Health Administration (OSHA) identifies more than 1.2 million community-based first-response personnel, including law enforcement, fire, and emergency medical service personnel, at risk for infectious exposure.[7] This large number highlights the need to protect these personnel against such exposures.

In the past, infectious and communicable disease preparation may not have been a priority. However, the 2003 severe acute respiratory syndrome (SARS) outbreaks made this preparation a priority. Medical personnel who cared for patients at the onset of the SARS outbreaks in Toronto[8] and Taipei[4] were exposed to or contracted SARS in significant numbers, and one paramedic died of SARS. More importantly, the loss of personnel from work because of exposure, illness, and quarantine impacted the ability to maintain staffing during the outbreak and highlighted the need to adequately prepare and protect the workforce from potential exposure.[3,5,9]

This chapter addresses communicable and infectious disease in a manner relevant to transport agencies and their personnel. The chapter is divided in two parts. The first is transport personnel and patient centered and describes the basics of communicable disease transmission and prevention, general approach to the patient with a suspected infectious or communicable disease, and specific disease conditions outlined by presenting symptom. The second is provider oriented and outlines occupational health and safety issues necessary to protect responding transport personnel.

TRANSPORT PERSONNEL AND THE PATIENT

COMMUNICABLE DISEASE TRANSMISSION AND PREVENTION

The Occupational Safety and Health Administration defines *occupational exposure* as "a reasonably anticipated skin, eye, mucous membrane, or parenteral contact with blood or other potentially infectious material that may result from the performance of the employee's duties."[7] Infection control practices are designed to prevent exposure to blood or potentially infectious material, including cerebrospinal fluid, synovial fluid, pleural fluid, pericardial fluid, amniotic fluid, peritoneal fluid, and any other body fluid, secretion, or tissue.

Universal precautions is the term formerly used to describe aspects of the methods used to prevent exposure, but this term is no longer used by healthcare workers. The more favored terms are *routine practices* and *additional precautions*. These terms indicate the same basic minimal level of precaution taken for all patients.

Infection is defined by the Association for Professionals in Infection Control and Epidemiology[1] as an invasion and multiplication of microorganisms in or on body tissue that causes cellular damage through the production of toxins, multiplication, or competition with host metabolism. Infectious agents capable of causing disease include bacteria, viruses, fungi and molds, parasites, and prions. These five types of microorganisms can be differentiated by their appearance on microscopic examination, reproductive cycle, chemical structure, growth requirements, and other detailed criteria. Although bacteria and viruses are the most common causes of illness in the developed world, parasites are more prevalent in other settings.

As shown in Figure 26-1, numerous factors are directly related to the ability of a microorganism to cause an infection. The dose is the amount of viable organism received during an exposure. Infection occurs with the presence of a large enough number to overwhelm the body's own defenses. *Virulence* refers to the ability of a microorganism to cause infection, and *pathogenicity* refers to the severity of infection. Additional factors determine the likelihood of transmission. Incubation and communicability peri-ods are the intervals between the organism entering the body and the appearance of symptoms and the time during which the infected individual can spread the disease to others, respectively. The host status and resistance refer to the host's ability to fight infection, which can be influenced by immune function and immunization status, nutritional state, and presence of comorbid illness.

An *infectious disease* results from the invasion of a host by disease-producing organisms, such as bacteria, viruses, fungi, or parasites. A *communicable* (or contagious) *disease* is one that can be transmitted from one person to another. Not all infectious diseases are communicable. For example, malaria is a serious infectious disease transmitted to the human bloodstream by a mosquito bite, but malaria is infectious, not communicable. On the other hand, chickenpox is an infectious disease that is also highly communicable because it can be easily transmitted from one person to another.

The *mode of transmission* is the mechanism by which an agent is transferred to the host. Modes of transmission include contact transmission (direct, indirect, droplet), airborne, vector-borne, or common vehicle (food, equipment). Contact transmission is the most common mode of transmission in the transport medicine setting and can be effectively prevented with routine practices. Table 26-1 contains a summary of disease transmission.

GENERAL APPROACH AND PATIENT ASSESSMENT

The risk of communicable disease is not as apparent as other physical risks, such as road traffic, power lines, firearms, or chemical agents. Transport personnel must use the same level of suspicion and precaution when approaching a patient before the risk of communicable disease is known. The use of routine practices, as a minimum, is necessary for every patient encounter to mitigate this risk.

The risk assessment begins with information from a dispatch or communication center, before patient contact is made. Call-taking procedures must include basic screening information to identify potential communicable disease threats and provide this information to all responding personnel. The screening information can identify patients

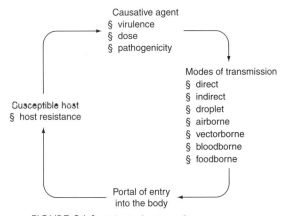

Causative agent
§ virulence
§ dose
§ pathogenicity

Modes of transmission
§ direct
§ indirect
§ droplet
§ airborne
§ vectorborne
§ bloodborne
§ foodborne

Susceptible host
§ host resistance

Portal of entry
into the body

FIGURE 26-1   **The infectious disease process.**

TABLE 26-1 Disease Transmission	
Type and Definition of Transmission	**Examples of Diseases Transmitted**
Contact transmission: *Direct* contact occurs between the infected colonized individual and a susceptible host. *Indirect* contact occurs with passive transfer of infections agents such as those left on a surface.	HIV Methicillin-resistant *S. aureus* (MRSA) Norwalk virus *C. difficile*
Droplet transmission: Large droplets generated from the respiratory tract of a patient when the patient sneezes or during invasive procedures such as suctioning.	Meningitis Influenza Rhinovirus Respiratory syncytial virus and SARS
Airborne transmission: Spread of disease via the airborne route.	Measles Varicella Tuberculosis
Vector-borne transmission: Disease is spread by means of an insect or animal (vector).	Rabies West Nile virus
Common vehicle transmission: Spread of an infectious agent by a single contaminated source to multiple hosts.	Water sources *(E. coli)* Contaminated food *(Salmonella)* Contaminated medical equipment

with symptoms of fever, chills, cough, shortness of breath, or diarrhea. The call-taking can also identify whether the patient location, such nursing home, group home, or other institutional setting, poses a potential risk to the responding personnel. This information helps responding personnel determine what precautions are necessary before they make contact.

When patient contact is made, personnel can identify the patient at risk for a communicable disease. A rapid history and physical examination can raise suspicion for a communicable disease. The following screening questions help assess whether the patient has a communicable disease:

- Do you have a new or worsening cough or shortness of breath?
- Do you have a fever?
- Have you had shakes or chills in the past 24 hours?
- Have you had an abnormal temperature (>38°C)?
- Have you taken medication for fever?

A screening physical examination also identifies obvious signs of a communicable disease. These signs may include any new symptom of infection (fever,

headache, muscle ache, cough, sputum, weight loss, and exposure history), rash, diarrhea, skin lesions, or draining wounds.

All personnel must take appropriate precautions when a patient has any signs or symptoms suspected to be the result of an infectious or communicable disease. All transport medicine agencies must provide appropriate training that enables personnel to identify at-risk patients and appropriate use of personal protective equipment (PPE). The levels of PPE needed based on perceived disease threat are addressed in detail in subsequent sections of this chapter.

SPECIFIC DISEASE CONDITIONS BY PRESENTING OR CHIEF SYMPTOM
Respiratory Infections
Respiratory infections may be suspected with symptoms that classically include any combination of cough, sneeze, shortness of breath, fever, chills or shakes. Infections above the epiglottis are classified as *upper respiratory tract infections,* and those below the epiglottis are classified as *lower respiratory tract infections.* Upper respiratory infections may be suspected when patients present with "cold" symptoms such as rhinorrhea, sneezing, lacrimation, or

coryza. More localized and possibly more serious upper respiratory infection may present with symptoms such as throat pain, fever, odynophagia, dysphagia, drooling, stridor, or muffled voice. Lower respiratory infections typically present with fever, shortness of breath, pleural pain, cough, sputum, or generalized symptoms such as chills, rigors, myalgia, arthralgia, malaise, and headache. More atypical symptoms of respiratory infection may be found in children, the elderly, and patients with immunocompromise. Children with respiratory infection may have gastrointestinal symptoms such as nausea, vomiting, abdominal pain, and diarrhea. The elderly and patients with immunocompromise may not have a fever with respiratory infection.

Respiratory infections are spread when people cough or sneeze and the aerosolized respiratory secretions directly come in contact with the mouth, nose, or eyes of another person. Because microorganisms in droplets can survive outside the body, indirect transmission can also occur when hands, objects, or surfaces become soiled with respiratory discharges. When respiratory infections are suspected in patients, providers should use droplet precautions and apply them to a patient.

Febrile Respiratory Illness. *Febrile respiratory illness* should be suspected when a patient has any combination of fever, new or worse cough, and shortness of breath. The elderly and patients with immunocompromise may not have a febrile response to a respiratory infection.

Cough

Pneumonia. In addition to cough, shortness of breath, and fever, patients with *pneumonia* may also have additional symptoms of tachypnea, increased work of breathing, chest or upper abdominal pain, and cough productive of phlegm, sputum, or blood. Generalized systemic symptoms such as myalgia, arthralgia, malaise, and headache may also be present. Gastrointestinal symptoms such as nausea, vomiting, and diarrhea may be associated with pneumonia.

Evidence indicates that the signs and symptoms traditionally associated with pneumonia are actually not predictive of pneumonia, whereas diarrhea, dry cough, and fever are more predictive of pneumonia. In elderly patients, the diagnosis of pneumonia is more difficult because both respiratory and nonrespiratory symptoms are less commonly reported by this patient group.

Infectious agents that typically cause pneumonia include *Streptococcus pneumoniae, Mycoplasma pneumoniae, Chlamydia trachomatis, Chlamydia pneumoniae, Pneumocystis carinii,* and *Haemophilus influenzae.* The incubation period from initial contact with the microorganism to development of symptoms is generally not well known for these organisms. For *S. pneumoniae,* it may be 1 to 3 days; *M. pneumoniae* may range from 6 to 32 days. *P. carinii* may appear 1 to 2 months after initial contact for those with immunosuppression. *S. pneumoniae* can be transmitted up to 48 hours after treatment is initiated. However, *M. pneumoniae* can be transmissible for up to 20 days, and the organism may remain in the respiratory tract for up to 13 weeks after treatment. For the other organisms, the time period for transmission is unknown.

Pertussis. *Pertussis* should be included in the differential diagnosis of a patient with chronic cough. Pertussis presents in three stages: first, a catarrhal stage that lasts 1 to 2 weeks; next, a paroxysmal stage that lasts 1 to 6 weeks; and finally, a convalescent stage that lasts 2 to 3 weeks. In the first stage, pertussis is virtually indistinguishable from any other respiratory illness; it is characterized by runny nose, sneezing, low-grade fever, and mild cough. The provider may suspect pertussis in the second, paroxysmal, stage when the patient has bursts of rapid coughs. The cough usually ends with a long high-pitched inspiratory effort described as a whoop, or it may end with vomiting. The third state is the period of recovery in which the cough becomes less paroxysmal. In adolescents, adults, and those who are vaccinated, pertussis is milder and thus may be indistinguishable from other respiratory illnesses, even in the paroxysmal stage.

Pertussis is caused by the *Bordetella pertussis* bacterium and transmitted via the respiratory route with airborne droplets. Thus, respiratory and contact precautions should be undertaken with known or suspected cases of pertussis.

Unfortunately, routine precautions are not always sufficient because pertussis is most infectious during the nonspecific catarrhal period and the first 2 weeks of the paroxysmal phase. The time from infection to the development of symptoms is usually 7 to 10 days.

Complications from pertussis most often occur in young infants. The major complication and most common cause of pertussis-related death is bacterial pneumonia.

With the introduction of routine pertussis vaccination, pertussis rates had declined from about 140 cases per 100,000 population in the 1940s to about 1 per 100,000 population in the 1980s. However, since the 1980s, pertussis rates have been steadily increasing. In 2002 in the United States, a rate of 3 cases per 100,000 population was seen. Most cases were in children under 6 months of age, the age group most at risk of pertussis-related complications.

Influenza. *Influenza* classically presents with the abrupt onset of fever (usually 38°C to 40°C), sore throat, nonproductive cough, myalgia, headache, and chills. Unfortunately, only about half of infected persons have the classic symptoms of influenza infection. From those classic symptoms, studies have attempted to identify the signs and symptoms most predictive of influenza. Unfortunately, these clinical decision rules are no better than clinician judgment alone.

Influenza is caused by a virus with three subtypes: influenza A, B, and C. *Influenza A* causes more severe disease and is mainly responsible for pandemics. Influenza A has different subtypes determined by surface antigens H (hemagglutinin) and N (neuraminidase). *Influenza B* causes more mild disease and mainly affects children. *Influenza C* rarely causes human illness and has not been associated with epidemics.

Influenza transmission occurs primarily through airborne spread when a person coughs or sneezes but may also occur through direct contact of surfaces contaminated with respiratory secretions. Hand washing and shielding of coughs and sneezes help prevent spread. Influenza is transmissible from 1 day before symptom onset to about 5 days after symptoms begin and may last up to 10 days in children.

Time from infection to development of symptoms is 1 to 4 days.

Individuals at high risk of influenza complications include young children, people over age 65 years, those with immunosuppression, and those with chronic medical conditions. Complications of influenza include pneumonia, either the more common secondary bacterial pneumonia or rare primary influenza viral pneumonia; Reye's syndrome in children taking aspirin; myocarditis; encephalitis; and death. Death occurs in about 1 per 1000 cases of influenza, mainly in persons older than age 65 years. Providers should be immunized annually, typically in October.

Four antiviral drugs are available for prevention and treatment of influenza in the United States. Amantadine and rimantadine belong to a class of drugs, adamantanes, which are active against influenza A; oseltamivir and zanamivir belong to the class of neuraminidase inhibitors, which are active against influenza A and B. When used for prevention of influenza, they can be 70% to 90% effective. When used for treatment, antiviral medications can reduce influenza illness duration by 1 day and attenuate the severity of illness. Antiviral agents should be used as an adjunct to vaccination but should not replace vaccination. The Centers for Disease Control (CDC) recommends influenza antiviral medications for individuals who have not as yet been vaccinated at the time of exposure or who have a contraindication to vaccination and are also at high risk of influenza complications. Also, if an influenza outbreak is caused by a variant strain of influenza not controlled with vaccination, chemoprophylaxis should be considered for healthcare providers who care for patients at high risk of influenza complications, regardless of vaccination status. Since the 2005 to 2006 influenza season, a high proportion of influenza A viruses are resistant to the adamantanes. As a result, the CDC has recently recommended against the use of adamantanes for treatment and prophylaxis of influenza. The neuraminidase inhibitors continue to be recommended as a second line of defense against influenza. For prophylaxis, the neuraminidase inhibitors should be taken daily until the exposure no longer exists or until immunity from vaccination develops, which can take about

2 weeks. For treatment, these antiviral medications should be started as soon as influenza symptoms develop, but no later than 48 hours after symptoms start, and treatment should continue for 5 days. In the setting of an influenza outbreak, transport agencies and systems may opt to restrict duties for providers who are not immunized or who have not yet received prophylactic antiviral therapy in attempt to prevent spread of the outbreak.

Avian Influenza. Influenza A virus infects humans and also can be found naturally in birds. Wild birds carry a type of influenza A virus, called *avian influenza virus,* in their intestines and usually do not get sick from them. However, avian influenza virus can make domesticated birds, including chickens, turkeys, and ducks, quite ill and can lead to death. The avian influenza virus is chiefly found in birds, but infection in humans from contact with infected poultry has been reported since 1996. A particular subtype of avian influenza A virus, H5N1, is highly contagious and deadly among birds. In 1997, in Hong Kong, an outbreak of avian influenza H5N1 occurred not only in poultry but also in 18 humans, six of whom died. In subsequent infections of avian influenza H5N1 in humans, more than half of those infected with the virus have died. In contrast to seasonal influenza, most cases of avian influenza H5N1 have occurred in young adults and healthy children who came in contact with poultry infected or surfaces contaminated with H5N1 virus. As of the end of 2007, 346 human infections with influenza H5N1 and 213 deaths (62%) were documented. Although transmission of avian influenza H5N1 from human to human is rare, inefficient, and unsustained, concern exists that the H5N1 virus could adapt and acquire the ability for sustained transmission in the human population. If the H5N1 virus gains the ability to transmit easily from person to person, a global influenza pandemic could occur. No vaccine for H5N1 current exists, but vaccine development is underway. The H5N1 virus is resistant to the adamantanes but likely sensitive to the neuraminidase inhibitors.

Tuberculosis. *Tuberculosis* (TB) is caused by the *Mycobacterium tuberculosis* complex. Most active TB is pulmonary (70%); the remainder is extrapulmonary (30%). Patients with active pulmonary TB typically have cough, scant amounts of nonpurulent sputum, and possibly hemoptysis. Systemic signs such as weight loss, loss of appetite, chills, night sweats, fever, and fatigue may also be present. Clinically, the provider is unable to distinguish pulmonary TB from other respiratory illness; however, certain risk factors may alert the provider to the possibility of tuberculosis. These risk factors are immigration from a country with a high prevalence rate, homelessness, exposure to active pulmonary TB, silicosis, HIV infection, chronic renal failure, cancer, transplantation, or any other state of immunosuppression.

Active pulmonary TB is transmitted via droplet nuclei from people with pulmonary tuberculosis during coughing, sneezing, speaking, or singing. Procedures such as intubation or bronchoscopy are high risk for the transmission of TB. Respiratory secretions on a surface lose the potential for infection. About 21% to 23% of individuals in close contact with persons with infectious TB become infected through inhalation of aerosolized bacilli. The probability of infection is related to duration of exposure, distance from the case, concentration if bacilli in droplets, ventilation in the room, and the susceptibility of the host exposed. Effective medical therapy eliminates communicability within 2 to 4 weeks of start of treatment.

If infected with TB, an individual may have development of active TB with symptoms or latent TB, which is asymptomatic. Time from infection to active symptoms or positive TB skin test results is about 2 to 10 weeks. The risk of development of active TB is greatest in the first 2 years after infection. Latent TB may last a lifetime, with the risk that it may later progress to active TB. About 10% of patients with latent TB have progression to active TB in their lifetime.

With transport of a patient who is known or suspected of having TB, respiratory precautions should be undertaken by the provider (in particular, a submicron mask). Patients should cover their mouth when coughing or sneezing or wear a surgical mask. In the event of suspected exposure to a patient with active pulmonary tuberculosis, the case and the exposure should be reported to the transport agency or public health authority. Close contacts should be monitored for the development of active TB symptoms. Two tuberculin skin tests should be performed, based on public health recommendations, on those closely exposed to patients with active TB. Because the incubation period after contact ranges from 2 to 10 weeks, the first test is typically done as soon as possible after exposure, and the second test is typically done 8 to 12 weeks after the exposure. If the provider or contact develops either active TB with symptoms or latent asymptomatic TB, as diagnosed with a new positive TB skin test, treatment should be sought.

Treatment for latent TB is typically isoniazid (INH) for 6 to 9 months. This single-drug regimen is 65% to 80% effective. For active TB, a four-drug regimen is typically used for 2 months: isoniazid, rifampin, pyrazinamide, and ethambutol. This regimen is followed by INH and rifampin for an additional 4 months. Several forms of multi–drug-resistant (MDR) TB and extensively drug-resistant (XDR) TB have been identified. These forms necessitate an aggressive multidrug regimen for prolonged periods of time and are dependent on the organism's patterns of drug sensitivity and resistance. In all cases, a physician skilled in management of TB must initiate and monitor treatment and provide suitable follow-up. Public health officials must also be notified.

Severe Acute Respiratory Syndrome. *Severe acute respiratory syndrome* (SARS) is difficult to distinguish from other respiratory infections because patients have symptoms that are similar to other febrile respiratory illnesses. On initial presentation, reliance on respiratory symptoms alone is not sufficient to distinguish SARS from non-SARS respiratory illness. Fever is the most common and earliest symptom of SARS and is often accompanied by headache, malaise, or myalgia. In patients with SARS, high fever, diarrhea, and vomiting were more common as compared with other patients with other respiratory illnesses. Cough occurred later in the course of disease, and patients were less likely to have rhinorrhea or sore throat as compared with other lower respiratory tract illness. Because clinical features alone cannot reliably distinguish SARS from other respiratory illnesses, knowledge

of contacts is essential. Contact with patients with known SARS, contact with SARS-affected areas, or linkage to a cluster of pneumonia cases should be obtained in the history.

Severe acute respiratory syndrome was first recognized in 2003 after outbreaks occurred in Toronto, Singapore, Vietnam, Taiwan, and China. The illness is caused by a coronavirus. The incubation period ranges from 3 to 10 days, with an average of 4 to 5 days from contact to symptom onset. About 11% of those with SARS eventually die, usually of respiratory failure. The risk of mortality is highly dependent on the patient's age and presence of comorbid illnesses. The case fatality rate is less than 1% for SARS patients less than age 24 years and up to 50% for those age 65 years and greater or those with comorbid illness.

The coronavirus is found in respiratory secretions, urine, and fecal matter. Transmission is via droplet spread from respiratory secretions, with high-risk transmission during intubation and procedures that aerosolize respiratory secretions. Transmission can also occur from fecal or urine contamination of surfaces. There have been no confirmed cases of transmission from asymptomatic cases. Preliminary studies show that transmission likely occurs after the development of symptoms, with the peak infectious period 7 to 10 days after symptom onset and a decline to a low level after day 23 from onset of symptoms.

If SARS is suspected, providers must use all routine practices and additional precautions. Transport agencies may also elect to limit or avoid any procedures that may increase risk to personnel, including tracheal intubation, deep suctioning, use of non-invasive ventilatory support (continuous positive airway pressure [CPAP], bilevel positive airway pressure [BiPAP]), administration of nebulizer medication, and any other procedure that may aerosolize respiratory secretions. During the SARS outbreaks in Toronto, emergency medical services (EMS) medical direction modified directives such that paramedics did not intubate patients or deliver nebulized therapy in the prehospital setting.[10] Finally, personnel and systems must also notify the receiving facility of a patient suspected of SARS, which permits staff to have appropriate PPE in place and a suitable isolation room prepared for the patient.

Rash

Methicillin-Resistant *Staphylococcal aureus.*

Skin infections with onset in the community or hospital may be caused *Staphylococcus aureus. S. aureus* is a bacterium that normally secretes beta-lactamases, rendering them normally resistant to antibiotics such as ampicillin and amoxicillin. Methicillin, a type of beta-lactam antibiotic, developed in 1959, was not broken down by these bacterial beta-lactamase enzymes. However, in the 1960s, infections of *S. aureus* were found to be resistant to methicillin and other beta-lactam antibiotics, resulting in the emergence of methicillin-resistant *Staphylococcal aureus* (MRSA).

In addition to skin and soft tissue infections, MRSA may less commonly cause severe and invasive infections such as necrotizing pneumonia, sepsis, and musculoskeletal infections, such as osteomyelitis and necrotizing fasciitis. MRSA skin infections typically present as necrotic skin lesions and are often confused with spider bites. The severity of MRSA skin infections may range from mild to severe. Unfortunately, no reliable clinical or risk factor criteria distinguish MRSA skin and soft tissue infections from those caused by other infectious agents.

Transmission of MRSA is mainly through hand contact from infected skin lesions, such as abscesses or boils. About 1% of the healthy population is also colonized with MRSA, mainly in the anterior nares but also in the pharynx, axilla, rectum, and perineum. Therefore, autoinfection may also be a route of infection. The transmissible period lasts as longs as skin lesions continue to drain or as long as the carrier state remains. Newborns, the elderly, and persons with immunosuppression are most susceptible.

Transmission of infection is prevented with routine precautions. Draining wounds should be covered with clean dry bandages. Contaminated surfaces should be cleaned with disinfectants effective against *S. aureus*, such as a solution of dilute bleach or quaternary ammonium compounds. One study has shown that ambulances may have a significant degree of MRSA contamination, highlighting the need for proper cleaning and decontamination of all equipment and the vehicle itself after every patient transport.

No data support the routine use of decolonization of MRSA with antiseptic agents or nasal mucopirocin. Decolonization may be considered in select circumstances, with multiple recurrent infections of MRSA or ongoing transmission in a well-defined group of close contacts. Little data are available on effective decolonization agents, but topical chlorhexidine gluconate or diluted bleach (3.4 g of bleach diluted in 3.8 L of water) is suggested.

With skin or soft tissue infections, any drainage should be cultured. Abscesses should be incised and drained. Antibiotic therapy may be considered with signs of cellulitis, systemic illness, associated immunosuppression, extremes of age, facial infection, or failure of initial incision and drainage. The choice of therapy should be dictated by local susceptibility patterns. Clindamycin, doxycycline, and trimethoprim-sulfamethosaxole (TMP-SMX) are considerations for treatment of CA-MRSA skin and soft-tissue infections. HA-MRSA may be resistant to many more classes of antibiotics, and vancomycin or linezolid may be necessary.

Measles. *Measles* is a viral disease that initially presents with a 2-day to 4-day prodrome of fever, cough, runny nose, and possibly conjunctivitis. In the prodrome stage, the provider is unable to clinically distinguish measles from any other viral upper respiratory illness. A measles rash follows, beginning on the hairline and then involving the face and neck, and over 3 days, proceeding downward and outward to the hands and feet. The rash produces discrete red maculopapular (flat and raised) lesions initially, which may become confluent. Initially, the lesions blanch and after 3 to 4 days become nonblanchable spots, which appear within 1 to 2 days before or after the maculopapular rash. Koplik spots, punctuate blue-white spots on the red buccal mucosa of the mouth, are pathognomonic for measles and alert the provider to the presence of measles.

Measles is transmitted via aerosol or droplet spread and is communicable from 4 days before appearance of the rash to 4 days after appearance. Providers likely encounter the patient in the transmissible stage and should use routine practices to prevent spread of disease.

The incubation period is approximately 10 days. Persons who have not been immunized or have never had measles (born after 1957) are susceptible to infection if exposed.

Rubella.   *Rubella* is a viral disease with a prodrome that precedes rash. Clinical diagnosis alone is unreliable. The prodrome, which consists of fever, upper respiratory symptoms, and prominent lymphadenopathy, lasts 1 to 5 days and mostly presents in older children and adults. During the prodrome, rubella is clinically indistinguishable from any other viral URTI. A maculopapular rash that appears 14 to 17 days after exposure and lasts 3 days typically follows the prodrome. Like measles, the rash starts on the face and progresses downward. In contrast to a measles rash, the rash from rubella is fainter, does not coalesce, and is more prominent after a hot shower or bath. Associated symptoms may include arthralgia or conjunctivitis. Confirmation of rubella infection is with laboratory diagnosis of virus or antibody.

Rubella is transmitted from respiratory secretions via airborne transmission or droplet spread, with an incubation period of 14 to 17 days. Although rubella is most contagious when the rash is present, it may transmitted by subclinical or asymptomatic cases of rubella, and 7 days before the onset of rash.

Life-threatening complications of rubella include encephalitis and hemorrhagic disease, but these are uncommon. The main objective of immunization is prevention of *congenital rubella syndrome* (CRS), the main complication of rubella. No specific treatment exists for rubella, only preventative vaccination. Rubella immunization is part of the routine childhood vaccinations, administered as a live vaccine along with measles and mumps as "MMR."

With exposure to patients later diagnosed with rubella, immunity of the contact should be assessed. Subsequent immunization of the nonimmunized contact does not prevent infection or illness. In adults, rubella is generally a mild febrile disease, and control measures are aimed at prevention of spread to nonimmunized pregnant women. In the case of spread, patients suspected of having rubella should be isolated with routine precautions in place.

Varicella.   Like measles and rubella, *varicella* starts with a prodrome that subsequently leads to a rash. In children, the prodrome of fever and malaise may be absent. Unlike measles and rubella, varicella infection, chickenpox, can be clinically diagnosed by the provider based on a more pathognomonic rash. The pruritic rash progresses from macules to papules and then to vesicles, which later crust over. The vesicles are unilocular and collapsible, in contrast to the multilocular and noncollapsible vesicles of smallpox. Lesions start on the scalp, progress to the trunk, and later move to the extremities.

Varicella virus infection that leads to chickenpox typically lasts 3 to 4 days, with an incubation period of 14 to 16 days. Transmission is via airborne droplets from the respiratory tract or via inhalation of aerosolized vesicular fluid from skin lesions. Chickenpox is transmissible 1 to 2 days before the onset of rash until all papules become crusted.

Complications in children include secondary bacterial skin infections, pneumonia, and dehydration. Nonimmunized adults may have more severe complications, including encephalitis, transverse myelitis, hemorrhagic varicella, and even death. In the United States, only 5% of the reported cases of varicella are from adults, but 35% of the mortality occurs in adults. The case fatality rate is 1 per 100,000 cases in children aged 1 to 14 years but 25.2 per 100,000 cases in adults aged 30 to 49 years.

Maternal varicella 5 days before to 48 hours after delivery may result in neonatal infection and subsequent mortality rates as high as 30%. Varicella infection in the mother at 20 weeks of gestation can lead to congenital varicella syndrome, which includes skin scarring, extremity atrophy, and eye and neurologic abnormalities.

Cases of chickenpox should be excluded from public places until the vesicles become dry. In the hospital, strict isolation measures should be undertaken to avoid contact with susceptible persons with immunocompromise. Articles soiled by discharges from the nose and throat should be disinfected.

If exposed to chickenpox, contacts should assess susceptibility based on immune status. If previously infected or vaccinated, contacts are immune. Susceptible nonimmune contacts have three choices to prevent infection: vaccination, varicella zoster immunoglobulin, or antiviral drugs. Varicella vaccine can prevent illness or attenuate severity if used within 3 days of contact. Vaccine is recommended in susceptible individuals. Varicella zoster immunoglobulin (VZIG) is recommended for newborns, persons with immunocompromise, and pregnant women and can also modify severity or prevent illness if given within 96 hours of exposure. Antiviral drugs such as acyclovir, if used within 24 hours of onset of rash, can reduce the severity of disease. These drugs are not recommended for routine postexposure prophylaxis but can be considered in persons over 13 years of age and those with immunocompromise.

Bites

Bites necessitate treatment for the physical injury itself and for the infectious disease exposure from the bite. Infection rates from bites mainly depend on the animal that has caused the bite and the site of injury. Cat bites can have an infection rate of up to 50%; about 10% of dog bites become infected. Bites on the face, scalp, hand, wrist, foot, or joints have the highest rate of infection. Hands are the most common site of human, dog, and cat bites. Bite infections may cause cellulitis, osteomyelitis, abscess, septic arthritis, or even septicemia. In addition to antibiotic therapy, bites may also necessitate treatment with rabies prophylaxis, tetanus prophylaxis, and HIV and hepatitis B prophylaxis. Prophylactic antibiotic treatment for bites depends on the specific infectious agents most commonly associated with the particular animal. Finally, personnel should also be aware of the risk of transmission of hepatitis C from human bites.

Animal Bites. Bites by dogs and cats account for 95% of animal bites. In up to 75% of infected cat bites and 50% of infected dog bites, the causal infectious agent is *Pasteurella* species. This bacterium can produce an infection in as short as 12 hours. *Pasteurella canis* is the most common organism in infected dog bites, and *Pasteurella multicoda* is the most common in cat bites. Other common organisms from infected cat and dog bites include *Streptococci, Staphylococci, Fusobacterium,* and *Bacterioides.*

Prevention of infection from bites should begin with copious high-pressure irrigation with sterile saline solution. Prophylactic antibiotics are advised for hand bites from cats or dogs and high-risk bites including any cat bite, deep dog bite punctures, and bites in individuals with immunocompromise Amoxicillin-clavulinic acid or cefuroxime, each for 5 days, provides appropriate broad-spectrum activity. In patients with allergies to penicillin, either azithromycin alone or clindamycin with levofloxacin can be given.

Human Bites. After dog and cat bites, humans are the next most common cause of bites. *Streptococci* species and *Eikenella corrodens* are the most common pathogens in infected human bites. Clenched-fist injuries, which result from a flexed knuckle of a fist striking human teeth, are common and serious causes of human bite injuries. This type of injury often leads to serious deep infections because the patient usually offers an alternative mechanism for the hand injury, resulting in delayed antibiotic therapy. Human bites can also transmit HIV and hepatitis B and hepatitis C.

Prophylactic antibiotics should be provided for all human bites that penetrate deeper than the epidermal layer and for bites to the hands, feet, or skin overlying joints or cartilaginous structures. Postexposure prophylaxis for HIV and hepatitis B should be considered for human bites according to a risk evaluation of the source. Patients should also be educated on the risk of transmission of hepatitis C.

Rabies. *Rabies* is caused by rabies virus, a rhabdovirus of the genus *Lyssavirus,* and may be transmitted by an animal bite. No treatment exists for rabies once it develops, and the mortality rate approaches 100%. The time from infection to development of disease is usually 3 to 8 weeks, and death is typically from respiratory paralysis. To determine the risk of rabies transmission, knowledge is needed on the type of animal that inflicted the bite, the geographic location of the incident, the vaccination status of the animal and person, whether the bite was provoked or unprovoked, and whether the animal can be captured and tested.

Patients with animal bites and suspicion of rabies should be given postexposure prophylaxis. For non-immune individuals, prophylaxis consists of 1 dose of human rabies immunoglobulin, half given into the bite site, accompanied by a 5-dose series of rabies vaccine on days 0, 3, 7, 14, and 28. Postexposure prophylaxis should always occur in consultation with local public health officials.

In the United States in 2006, of all cases of rabies from animal bites, 92% were related to wild animals and 8% to domestic animals. Among wild animals, rabies was most frequently found in raccoons, followed by bats, skunks, and foxes. Among domestic animals, cats were the most common cause of rabies, followed by dogs and cattle. Squirrels, guinea pigs, hamsters, chipmunks, gerbils, mice, rats, rabbits, and hares rarely have rabies. In the United States, two to three cases of human rabies have been seen each year for the last 10 years. Most were to the result of contact with bats, likely because bites from bats are superficial and not easily noticed. In the United States, Canada, and Western Europe, dogs account for less than 5% of animal rabies; in most developing countries, dogs account for more than 90% of cases of animal rabies.

Immunization against rabies is not routinely recommended for the general population in North America, unless the person is engaged in activities that place them at high risk of acquiring rabies. These persons include rabies laboratory workers and veterinarians. Most agencies recommend that domestic dogs, cats, ferrets, and livestock be vaccinated against rabies. Routine rabies immunization for personnel is not recommended.

Abnormal behavior in an animal or an unprovoked bite is more likely to indicate that a bite was from a rabid animal. This increases the risk of rabies transmission, and postexposure prophylaxis should be offered. If a dog, cat, or ferret that caused a bite can be captured, it should be confined and observed for 10 days for the development of rabies symptoms. If rabies develops, the bitten individual should receive rabies postexposure prophylaxis. For any bites with bats, raccoons, skunks, or foxes, postexposure prophylaxis should be offered regardless of whether the animal is captured or not.

Tetanus. Bites are at risk of being infected with *Clostridium tetani* because they are puncture wounds or are contaminated with saliva. Live *C. tetani* organisms are not present in the oral flora of humans or animals, but their resilient spores are ubiquitous and in the environment, soil, and feces. Crushed devitalized tissue produced by bites favors the production of tetanus.

Tetanus is an often fatal disease caused by the exotoxin of *C. tetani*. The incubation period ranges from 3 to 21 days, during which time the spores transform into live bacteria that then produce an exotoxin. Clinically, the exotoxin leads to convulsive spasms of the skeletal muscles and generalized rigidity, mainly involving the jaw and neck. Patients with any form of bites should receive prophylaxis with 0.5 mL of tetanus toxoid intramuscularly if they have not been immunized within the prior 5 years. Those who have not completed immunization series, are not up to date with the immunization, or have an unknown immunization history should also receive tetanus immunoglobulin.

Altered Mental Status, Neck Stiffness, Headache

Meningitis refers to inflammation of the meninges that cover the brain. It can be the result of infectious and noninfectious causes. Noninfectious causes include drugs, vaccines, systemic disease such as collagen vascular disorders, and malignancy disease. Infectious causes include viruses, bacteria, fungi, parasites, and rickettsiae.

Meningitis is typically classified as bacterial meningitis versus aseptic meningitis. *Aseptic meningitis* refers to meningitis with cerebrospinal fluid absent of microorganisms on gram stain or routine culture. The most common cause of aseptic meningitis is viral agents. *Viral meningitis* is generally more common and less severe and requires supportive measures with no specific treatment. *Bacterial meningitis,* on the other hand, has a case fatality rate of 13% to 37%, and as high as 80% in the elderly, despite appropriate antibiotic therapy. In addition, up to 20% of survivors of bacterial meningitis have permanent sequelae such as brain damage, hearing loss, or limb loss.

Bacterial meningitis should be suspected when the patient has at least two of the following four symptoms: headache, fever, neck stiffness, or altered mental status. However, the provider should be aware that only one of these symptoms may be present in the patient with bacterial meningitis. Focal neurologic symptoms such as extremity pain or temperature changes may be early signs. Although a petechial rash is classically associated with bacterial meningitis, only 11% to 23% of patients with bacterial meningitis actually have a rash. In the absence of diagnostic tests such as lumbar puncture, personnel are unable to use clinical signs and symptoms alone to distinguish bacterial from aseptic meningitis. Considering the rapid onset of symptoms and high morbidity and mortality rates with untreated bacterial meningitis, all patients with suspected meningitis should be treated as having bacterial meningitis until proven otherwise.

Neisseria meningitidis and *S. pneumoniae* currently account for 80% to 85% of adult community-acquired meningitis. *H. influenzae type b* was formerly a leading cause of meningitis, but introduction of routine childhood vaccination is making this bacterium less prevalent. Less common causes include staphylococci, group B streptococci, and *Listeria*. *S. pneumoniae* is a more common cause of meningitis, and the mortality rate is also higher (30%) as compared with the mortality rate of meningitis (7%) caused by *N. meningitides*. Since the introduction of routine childhood vaccination with *H. influenzae type b*, this is no longer a leading cause of meningitis.

Transmission is via droplet spread from respiratory secretions. Therefore, respiratory and contact precautions should be undertaken when transporting patients suspected of meningitis. The time from transmission to the development of symptoms is about 2 to 10 days for *N. meningitidis* and about 1 to 4 days for *S. pneumoniae*.

Empiric treatment of adult bacterial meningitis is vancomycin plus a third-generation cephalosporin, such as cefotaxime. In neonates, those over age 50 years, and those with altered immune status or alcoholism, ampicillin is added to cover *Listeria monocytogenes*. Treatment may last 14 to 21 days, depending on the infectious agent. In addition to treatment of the patient, personnel exposed or in close contact to patients with meningitis may need prophylactic therapy. This treatment is particularly important for personnel exposed to the patient's oral or respiratory secretions. Exposed personnel should contact the transport agency or local public health agency immediately. Public health will likely provide prophylactic treatment with ciprofloxacin, ceftriaxone, or rifampin to prevent infection from close contact.

Diarrhea

Diarrhea is practically defined by increased frequency, increased volume, and decreased consistency of stools. A strict definition is more than three stools in a 24-hour period, with the stools being liquid enough to adopt the shape of the container in which they are placed. *Acute diarrhea* lasts 2 to 3 weeks, with *chronic diarrhea* lasting longer. *Infectious diarrhea* is commonly associated with nausea, vomiting, fever, abdominal cramps, and intestinal gas-related symptoms. Diarrhea may be infectious or noninfectious in origin, and the provider should attempt to rule out noninfectious causes because most noninfectious causes are true diarrheal emergencies (mesenteric ischemia, gastrointestinal [GI] bleed, bowel obstruction).

Infectious diarrhea may be caused by viruses, bacteria, protozoa, or helminthes. The diarrhea may be caused by the organisms themselves or the toxins they produce. Gastrointestinal infections are typically spread via contaminated water, contaminated food, contaminated environments, direct contact among humans, and hand-to-mouth transmission. The differential diagnosis can be narrowed with selective testing of stool specimens for bacterial culture, ova, parasites, *Clostridium difficile* toxin, and viral enzyme-linked immunosorbent assay (ELISA) tests. These tests are not available in the prehospital setting, but history may identify prior testing results and the likely offending agent.

To prevent spread of infection, providers and systems must ensure routine practices and additional precautions are in place. In addition, equipment and transport vehicles must be thoroughly cleaned and decontaminated when transport involves a patient suspected of having infectious diarrhea.

Therapy that can be initiated by providers includes isotonic fluid replacement and management of hypovolemia and sepsis. Antibiotic therapy and antimotility therapy should only be considered once a thorough assessment has been conducted in the hospital setting because such therapy may be inappropriate in certain diarrheal conditions.

Acute infectious diarrhea may be bloody or watery, with bloody diarrhea signifying inflammatory destruction of the intestinal mucosa. Whether the diarrhea is watery or bloody provides clues as to the cause of the diarrhea and the consequent sequelae: in watery diarrhea, the main concern is dehydration, and in bloody diarrhea, the main concern is intestinal damage and sepsis.

The most common causes of diarrhea are viruses, which account for 50% to 75% of cases. As compared with bacterial diarrhea, viral diarrhea typically has less high fever and watery stools, whereas bacterial diarrhea typically has bloody stools with less severe abdominal pain. Among the viral causes of diarrhea, rotavirus and the noroviruses (Norwalk and Norwalk-like viruses) account for 50% of viral gastroenteritis. Adenoviruses are the second most common cause of acute viral gastroenteritis. Rotavirus diarrhea is the most common cause of viral diarrhea in children and usually occurs in children between 6 and 24 months of age (most individuals have antibodies by age 3 years). History and physical examination alone cannot clinically distinguish rotavirus from other enteric viral infections because rotavirus infection presents with watery diarrhea, vomiting, fever, and abdominal pain. It is usually diagnosed from rotavirus antigen in stools. In addition to transmission by the contact and the fecal-oral route, respiratory spread may also occur with rotavirus. The incubation period is 24 to 72 hours, with the period of communicability up to 8 days from the start of the watery diarrhea. Two rotavirus vaccines are available for children, RotaRix and Rotateq; Rotateq is licensed for use in the United States. In 1999, RotaShield was withdrawn from the market after being associated with intussusception.

Diarrhea by norovirus causes signs and symptoms clinically indistinguishable from rotavirus; nausea, vomiting, diarrhea, and abdominal pain also occur with norovirus infection. In children, vomiting is more prevalent, whereas in adults, diarrhea is more common. Diagnosis is made with nucleic acid hybridization assays and RT-PCR. The incubation period is 12 to 48 hours, and illness lasts for a shorter time than rotavirus diarrhea, 12 hours to 3 days. The period of communicability is unknown but lasts up to 7 days. Transmission routes are similar to rotavirus, including airborne transmission. No vaccine currently exists for norovirus infections.

Bacterial diarrhea typically includes bloody diarrhea, as opposed to watery diarrhea; however, not all bacterial diarrhea is bloody. Bloody diarrhea is often referred to as dysentery. Bloody diarrhea may not necessarily be the result of infectious causes, and other causes of bloody diarrhea should be considered, such as mesenteric ischemia or a gastrointestinal bleeding. Common causes of bacterial diarrhea are *Salmonella*, *Shigella*, *Yersinia*, *Escherichia coli*, and *Campylobacter*.

E. coli are classified by their O, H, and K antigens and also by their virulence properties. *E. coli* 0157:H7 is the main serotype that causes bloody diarrhea through secretion of a potent shiga-like cytotoxin. *E. coli* 0157:H7 is found in healthy cattle and is spread to humans from undercooked beef, raw milk, and produce. The incubation period is typically 3 to 4 days, and the period of communicability can be up to 3 weeks in children. Antibiotics and antimotility agents are not recommended for this infection. Treatment is directed at HUS, which may necessitate dialysis, steroids, or plasma therapy in the ICU setting.

C. difficile is a bacterium that can cause a spectrum of mild watery diarrhea to severe colitis, which may progress to perforation of the colon and sepsis. This infection is increasing in prevalence and is frequently associated with healthcare settings. More than 90% of cases occur after or during antibiotic therapy. *C. difficile* is also the most common cause of bacterial diarrhea in persons with HIV in the United States. The provider may only suspect *C. difficile*–associated diarrhea based on the risk factors because it is clinically indistinguishable from any other watery diarrhea based on signs and symptoms. Diagnosis is confirmed with enzyme immunoassays of stool samples. Providers should notify transfer and receiving facilities that a patient has

C. difficile–associated disease, if known. Treatment is cessation of existing antibiotic therapy if possible, rehydration, avoidance of antimotility agents, and therapy with metronidazole or vancomycin, orally, for 10 days.

Jaundice

Hepatitis A. *Hepatitis A* can cause acute disease or asymptomatic infection but not chronic infection. Although more than 70% of older children and adults are symptomatic, in children younger than 6 years, 70% of infections are asymptomatic. Symptomatic illness is characterized by fever, jaundice, and dark urine, in addition to malaise, anorexia, and nausea. Jaundice is the most common symptom. Unfortunately, the clinical signs and symptoms of hepatitis A are indistinguishable from other types of acute viral hepatitis. Diagnosis is usually with immunoglobulin (Ig) in blood, antihepatitis A immunoglobulin M in the acute phase, and antihepatitis A immunoglobulin G after 6 months.

Hepatitis A infection rarely progresses to fulminant hepatitis A, which can lead to death.

Hepatitis A is transmitted via the fecal-oral route from consumption of contaminated food or water. Rarely, hepatitis A can be transmitted via blood transfusion, particularly clotting factor concentrates. In the United States between 1990 and 2000, 45% of patients with hepatitis A could not identify a risk factor for infection. The time from infection to the presentation of symptoms, if any, is on average 28 days. Hepatitis A is most transmissible from feces 1 to 2 weeks before the onset of illness to about 1 week after the onset of jaundice.

If a provider comes in contact with a patient suspected of having hepatitis A, routine practices and additional precautions can prevent the spread of infection. Hepatitis A infection is prevented with vaccination administered in two doses 6 to 18 months apart. In 2005, the Advisory Committee on Immunization Practices (ACIP) recommended that all children aged 12 to 23 months of age receive the hepatitis A vaccination. International travelers, men who have sex with men, persons with clotting factor disorders, and those with chronic liver disease should also be immunized. Hepatitis A vaccination is not routinely recommended for healthcare workers.

Unvaccinated persons who have been exposed to hepatitis A may be candidates for postexposure antihepatitis A immunoglobulin, which has been shown to be 85% effective in prevention of hepatitis A infection if given within 2 weeks of exposure. Potential candidates include persons who have had household or sexual contact with a person with hepatitis A, persons who have shared illegal drugs with a person with hepatitis A, other food handlers working with another food handler diagnosed with hepatitis A, patrons of an infectious food handler if the food handler had diarrhea or poor hygiene, and staff and attendees at a child care center where a hepatitis A case was diagnosed. Vaccination should supplement immunoglobulin administration in postexposure prophylaxis but not replace it.

Hepatitis B. *Hepatitis B* infection can cause acute disease or chronic disease or be asymptomatic. Like hepatitis A, symptoms present more in adults than in children, and symptoms are not specific for hepatitis B. Even about 50% of adults with acute infection are asymptomatic. When symptoms occur, they are divided into phases: the prodromal, icteric, and convalescent phases. In the 3-day to 10-day prodromal phase, nonspecific symptoms of malaise, weakness, and anorexia are the most common symptoms, but low-grade fever, arthritis, rash, vague abdominal discomfort, nausea, and vomiting may also occur. The icteric phase lasts 1 to 3 weeks and is characterized by jaundice, with dark urine and light stools starting 1 to 2 days before the onset of jaundice. In convalescence, jaundice disappears but malaise and fatigue may persist for weeks. Definitive diagnosis of hepatitis B is with serologic testing.

Most acute hepatitis B infections result in complete recovery, but in 1% to 2% of patients fulminant hepatitis infection occurs, with a 63% to 93% case fatality rate. About 10% of acute infections progress to chronic infection, which leads to premature death from cirrhosis or liver cancer in 25% of cases. In the United States, an estimated 51,000 new hepatitis B infections occurred in 2005.

Hepatitis B is transmitted via percutaneous or mucosal exposure to infected blood or blood products. Transmission can also occur from saliva, semen, vaginal secretions, and cerebrospinal, pleural, peritoneal, pericardial, amniotic, or synovial fluid. Transmission to healthcare workers can occur not only from needle sticks or other sharp injuries but also through cutaneous scratches or abrasions. The hepatitis B virus can exist for at least 7 days outside the body on inanimate surfaces, and infection can occur with touching skin lesions or mucous membranes with any contaminated equipment. This is particularly important in the transport setting and emphasizes the need for adherence to routine practices and additional precautions and proper cleaning and decontamination of equipment and vehicle surfaces. If the hepatitis B HBs-antigen is present in the blood of a source, the source is communicable for hepatitis B. If infected, the incubation period is on average 60 to 90 days.

Hepatitis B vaccination is recommended for all infants at birth, at age 1 to 2 months, and at 6 to 18 months. For unvaccinated adults, a three-dose schedule is recommended for those at increased risk of hepatitis B infection, which includes healthcare workers.

If percutaneous or mucous membrane exposure occurs to blood that may contain hepatitis B, postexposure prophylaxis with hepatitis B immune globulin (HBIG) may be considered. Before this treatment, the vaccination status of the exposed person with hepatitis B should be assessed. If vaccinated, the exposed person should have an assessment of protective antibody levels to hepatitis B, as about 5% of vaccinated persons may not respond to the hepatitis B vaccine. If available, the source blood should also be assessed for the presence HBs-antigen, which signifies infection with hepatitis B and communicability. If an individual is exposed to HBsAg-positive fluid and is not immunized or lacks protective antibody levels, HBIG should be given within 24 hours and hepatitis B vaccination should also be started.

Hepatitis C.   About 60% to 80% of persons initially infected with *hepatitis C* are initially asymptomatic. Among the few 15% to 30% who become symptomatic, clinical signs and symptoms are similar to other acute viral hepatitis illnesses and include jaundice, fatigue, dark urine, abdominal pain, anorexia, and nausea. Diagnosis of hepatitis C is with serologic testing.

Unlike the other viral hepatitis infections, in up to 85% of hepatitis C infections, persistent infection develops. Among those with chronic infection, 70% have chronic liver disease develop, and 1% to 5% of those die prematurely of chronic liver disease. An estimated 20,000 new hepatitis C viral infections occurred in the United States in 2005, and 3.2 million Americans are chronically infected with hepatitis C.

Hepatitis C is transmitted via mucosal or percutaneous exposure to infectious blood or blood-derived body fluids. Sexual contact can lead to transmission but is a far less efficient route of transmission. The period of transmission may persist in infected persons indefinitely. If infected, the incubation period is on average 6 to 9 weeks, and 20 years may pass before the onset of liver disease.

No vaccine is available to prevent hepatitis C, and postexposure prophylaxis with hepatitis C immunoglobulin has not been shown to be effective. Providers must rely on routine practices and additional precautions to prevent occupational and nosocomial transmissions. Disposable injection equipment should not be reused and should be properly disposed of; reusable injection equipment should be appropriately sterilized.

Biologic Weapons

Anthrax.   The symptoms of *anthrax* are determined by the route of transmission of the bacterium which causes anthrax, *Bacillus anthracis*. The three forms of anthrax are: cutaneous, gastrointestinal, and inhalational.

Cutaneous anthrax presents as a small, painless, pruritic papule, which progresses to an enlarging vesicle in 1 to 2 days. The vesicle ruptures and erodes, leaving a necrotic ulcer that later is covered with a black painless eschar. Pathognomonic features of anthrax include the presence of an eschar, lack of pain, and edema out of proportion to the size of the lesion. Associated symptoms include swelling of adjacent lymph nodes, fever, malaise, and headache. Cutaneous anthrax is caused by *B. anthracis* entering a cut or abrasion in exposed areas of the body such as the face, neck, arms, and hands. The incubation period of cutaneous anthrax is 1 to 12 days. The case fatality rate can be as high as 20% without antibiotic therapy but 1% with therapy.

Gastrointestinal anthrax presents with more non-specific symptoms. The two forms are: oropharyngeal and intestinal. *Oropharyngeal anthrax* starts with edematous lesions at the base of the tongue or tonsils that progress to necrotic ulcers with a pseudomembrane. Sore throat, fever, cervical adenopathy, and profound oropharynx edema are associated symptoms. This form of anthrax initially presents with fever, nausea, vomiting, abdominal pain, and tenderness that may progress to hematemesis, bloody diarrhea, and abdominal swelling from hemorrhagic ascites. Gastrointestinal anthrax is caused by consumption of meat contaminated with anthrax. The incubation period for *intestinal anthrax* is believed to be 1 to 7 days. The case fatality rate of gastrointestinal anthrax is estimated to be 25% to 60%.

Inhalational anthrax initially causes nonspecific symptoms that mimic influenza. These early symptoms are low-grade fever, nonproductive cough, malaise, and myalgia. Two to 3 days later, the condition rapidly progresses to severe dyspnea, profuse sweating, high fever, cyanosis, and shock. Hemorrhagic meningitis occurs in up to half of patients. The provider must attempt to distinguish any influenza-like illness from anthrax because of the narrow window of opportunity for successful treatment. Nasal congestion and rhinorrhea are not common with inhalational anthrax but are more common with influenza-like illness. Further, shortness of breath is more common in inhalational anthrax and less common in influenza-like illness. Although not typically available to providers, the chest radiograph shows mediastinal widening or pleural effusion. These findings are the most accurate predictors of inhalational anthrax. Inhalational anthrax can be caused by inhalation of anthrax spores, commonly seen after intentional release of aerosolized anthrax, or by the processing of materials from infected animals, such as goat hair. The incubation period for inhalational anthrax is usually 1 to 7 days but can be as long as 43 days. Case fatality rates of inhalational anthrax can be as high as 97% without antibiotics and up to 75% with antibiotics.

Human-to-human transmission of any form of anthrax is rare. A vaccine for anthrax is licensed in the United States and is administered in a six-dose schedule with annual boosters thereafter. Vaccination is not currently recommended for emergency first responders or medical personnel; however, it may be indicated for certain military personnel. In cases of deliberate use of anthrax as a biologic weapon, first responders should wear a full face respirator with HEPA filters or a self-contained breathing apparatus, gloves, and splash protection. If clothing is contaminated, it should be removed and placed in plastic bags. Soap and copious amounts of water should be used to decontaminate skin, and bleach should be applied for 10 to 15 minutes in a 1:10 dilution if gross contamination occurs. If exposure to aerosolized anthrax occurs, postexposure prophylaxis with ciprofloxacin or doxycycline should begin and continue for 60 days. Vaccination given in three doses for postexposure prophylaxis should also be administered because of the persistence of anthrax spores in the lungs. Quarantine is not appropriate for persons exposed to anthrax because they are not contagious. Patients suspected of being infected with anthrax and needing hospitalization should be immediately started on intravenous (IV) antibiotics such as ciprofloxacin and one other active drug. Other active drugs include doxycycline, rifampin, vancomycin, penicillin, ampicillin, chloramphenicol, imipenem, clindamycin, and clindamycin. Treatment should continue for 60 days or longer.

Botulism.   *Botulism* is caused by a neurotoxin produced by *Clostridium botulinum*, which ultimately leads to a flaccid paralysis. The four forms of botulism are based on site of toxin production: food-borne, wound, intestinal, and inhalational.

In *food-borne botulism*, early symptoms are nonspecific gastrointestinal symptoms and include nausea, vomiting, and diarrhea. The condition may progress to blurred vision, double vision, dry mouth, and difficulty in swallowing, breathing, and speaking. Descending muscle paralysis occurs, starting with the shoulders and progressing to the upper arms, lower arms, thighs, then calves. Respiratory muscle paralysis ultimately leads to death. Food-borne botulism is caused by the ingestion of *C. botulinum* toxin present in contaminated food or by deliberate contamination as a biologic weapon. The incubation period is usually 12 to 36 hours. The case fatality rate in the United States is 5% to 10%.

Intestinal botulism is rare and occurs mainly in infants. It causes a striking loss of head control, constipation, loss of appetite, weakness, and an altered cry. Intestinal botulism occurs with ingestion of botulism spores, rather than ingestion of toxin. Spores, which may come from honey, food, and dust, germinate in the colon. The incubation period is unknown. It is estimated to cause 5% of deaths from sudden infant death syndrome. The case fatality rate of hospitalized cases is less than 1%.

Wound botulism causes the same symptoms as food-borne botulism. The incubation period is up to 2 weeks. This is also a rare disease, caused by spores entering an open wound from soil or gravel.

Inhalational botulism is the most common form in the case of use of botulinum toxin as a biologic weapon. Symptoms are the same as food-borne botulism, but the incubation period may be longer.

No reported cases exist of person-to-person transmission of botulism. Therefore, providers do not need any special equipment to manage a patient with suspected or known botulism infection. Supportive care is advised in all cases, including volume replacement. In the case of consumption of food suspected of being contaminated with botulism, treatment may include gastric lavage or whole bowel irrigation. In the case of suspected aerosol exposure to the toxin, clothing should be removed and placed in plastic bags, and the exposed person should shower thoroughly.

Antitoxin use should be considered and administered within 1 to 2 days of exposure. Treatment for botulism is botulinum antitoxin, given after blood is collected to determine the specific antitoxin. Patients should be transported immediately to a center with an intensive care unit. In intestinal botulism in infants, equine botulinum antitoxin should not be used. In the United States, an investigational human-derived botulinal immune globulin is available for infant intestinal botulism from the California Department of Health Services.

Plague.   *Plague* is caused by the bacterium *Yersinia pestis*. Initial signs and symptoms may be nonspecific and include fever, chills, sore throat, malaise, and headache. Tender, swollen, warm, and suppurative lymph nodes, mainly in the inguinal area, often follow. This swollen lymph node is called a bubo; hence, the term *bubonic plague*. Patients infected with the plague may then have progression to septicemia, meningitis, pneumonia, or shock. When plague progresses to the lungs, leading to *pneumonic plague*, person-to-person transfer may occur from infective respiratory droplets that are expelled with coughing. The exposed contact subsequently has development of primary plague pneumonia.

Untreated plague has a case fatality rate of 50% to 90%. With treatment, the death rate is 15%.

Plague is transmitted to humans via bites, scratches, respiratory droplets, or direct skin contact. Bites from infected rat fleas are the most frequent source of transmission, but bites or scratches from cats may also transmit plague. Airborne droplets from the respiratory tract of cats or humans infected with pneumonic plague are another source of transmission. In case of deliberate use as a biologic weapon, plague bacilli are transmitted via the aerosolized airborne droplets. Direct contact with tissue or body fluids of a plague-infected sick or dead animal can lead to transmission to humans through a break in the skin. The incubation period is 2 to 6 days for bubonic plague. For primary pneumonic plague, incubation period is shorter, typically 1 to 4 days.

Prevention of infection is with control of exposure to infected fleas. In addition, environmental flea and rodent control can be an effective means to prevent prevalence and subsequent transmission. A vaccine for bubonic plague exists, but a vaccine for pneumonic plague does not. The vaccine is administered in a three-dose schedule with booster doses every 6 months. Commercial plague vaccine is no longer available in the United States.

For patients with pneumonic plague, strict isolation is indicated with precautions against airborne spread until 48 hours after start of antibiotic therapy. Antibiotic therapy for bubonic or pneumonic plague is effective if started within 8 to 18 hours of onset of symptoms. First-line antibiotics are streptomycin or gentamycin. Chloramphenicol is used to treat plague meningitis.

Close contacts of patients infected with pneumonic plague should be provided with chemoprophylaxis with tetracycline or chloramphenicol for 1 week after exposure ends. Close contacts include any medical personnel, household contacts, and face-to-face contacts. Contacts should also be placed under surveillance for 7 days. If contacts refuse antibiotics, they should remain in strict isolation for 7 days. Articles soiled with sputum or purulent discharges should be disinfected.

Y. pestis could be used as a potential biologic weapon disseminated through aerosol spread and leading to pneumonic plague. Many patients with fever, cough, and particularly hemoptysis in a fulminant course with high case fatality should raise suspicions for deliberate use as a biologic weapon.

Smallpox.   The two clinical forms of *smallpox* are: variola major and variola minor. *Variola major* is the more severe form of disease with a case fatality rate of greater than 30%, and *variola minor* is the less severe form with a case fatality rate less than 1%. All smallpox begins with a prodrome that lasts 2 to 4 days. The prodrome starts abruptly and consists of fever, headache, nausea, vomiting, muscle pain, headache, and malaise.

Transmission of smallpox is via inhalation of the virus from airborne droplets or fine particle aerosols originating from the oral, pharyngeal, or nasal mucosa of an infected person. This transmission usually occurs from direct face-to-face contact within a distance of 6 ft. Transmission could also occur from physical contact with an infected person or with contaminated articles through skin inoculation. Transmission from dried skin crusts is uncommon. Smallpox is not transmissible during the incubation period but becomes infectious with the first appearance of rash until the disappearance of all scabs, which is about 3 weeks. The incubation period of smallpox is an average of 12 days, with a range from 7 to 19 days.

Personnel should be able to identify the smallpox rash and try to distinguish it from other less virulent diseases, particularly chicken pox. Identification of smallpox is important because its presence indicates a medical and public health emergency. Differentiation can be made through the prodrome and the rash. In smallpox, patients have a severe febrile prodrome, whereas in chickenpox, prodrome is short and mild or nonexistent. In smallpox, the rash consists of deep, hard, well-circumscribed lesions at the same stage of development; in chickenpox, the lesions are superficial, not well-circumscribed, and at different stages of development. In addition to chickenpox, other conditions may be confused with smallpox, such as herpes, impetigo, contact dermatitis, erythema multiforme, and scabies. Further information to differentiate these illnesses from smallpox is available from the CDC at http://www.bt.cdc.gov/agent/smallpox/.

Any new suspected cases of smallpox are a medical and public health emergency. Therefore, strict respiratory and contact isolation of confirmed or suspected smallpox cases must be undertaken. No antiviral drug is approved for the treatment of smallpox, but cidofovir may be useful as a therapeutic agent and could be used off-label under an investigational new drug protocol.

Contacts with suspect or confirmed smallpox cases should wear N95 fit-tested masks and use routine practices and additional precautions. All bedding and clothing should be autoclaved or laundered in hot water with bleach. Contacts include first responders, laundry handlers, housekeepers, and laboratory personnel.

Smallpox vaccine is administered as one dose, and success of vaccination is determined by a major reaction at the inoculation site, but its use as a childhood immunization was discontinued in 1972. In nonemergency situations, vaccination is recommended for public health, hospital, and other personnel who may need to respond to a smallpox case or outbreak. In an emergency situation, such as the intentional release of variola virus in a bioterrorist event, vaccination would be recommended for those exposed to initial release, contacts of confirmed or suspected cases, and those involved in direct care or transportation of confirmed or suspected cases. Some uncommon but serious adverse reactions, precautions, and contraindications to smallpox vaccine should be reviewed before administration at http://www.bt.cdc.gov/agent/smallpox/. Vaccinia immune globulin intravenous is available for the treatment of adverse reactions to smallpox vaccine. Smallpox vaccine can be used for postexposure prophylaxis in exposed contacts. If administered less than 7 days after exposure, contacts generally experience the mild modified type of smallpox.

Tularemia. *Tularemia,* caused by the bacterium *Francisella tularensis,* has various clinical manifestations related to the route of introduction. All forms have a sudden onset of nonspecific influenzalike symptoms, including high fever, cough, sore throat, chills, headache, and generalized body aches. Sometimes, nausea, vomiting, and diarrhea may also occur. All forms may lead to sepsis, pneumonia, and meningitis. The clinical forms include ulceroglandular, glandular, oculoglandular, septic, oropharyngeal, and pneumonic.

Ulceroglandular tularemia is the most common form. It begins at the skin site of the bite of a tick or fly. A papule appears that becomes pustular, later ulcerates, and finally develops into an eschar. Regional lymph nodes become swollen, painful, and tender and rarely suppurate and discharge purulent material. *Glandular tularemia* has no skin involvement, only regional lymphadenopathy similar to that which occurs with ulceroglandular disease. *Oculoglandular tularemia* is caused by the bacillus entering the eye; conjunctival ulceration occurs followed by regional lymphadenopathy of the cervical and preauricular nodes. *Septic tularemia* begins with nonspecific symptoms of fever, nausea, vomiting, and abdominal pain and eventual leads to confusion, coma, multisystem organ failure, and septic shock.

Oropharyngeal tularemia is caused by consumption of contaminated water or food that leads to exudative pharyngitis, which may be accompanied by oral ulceration. Abdominal pain, diarrhea, and vomiting may accompany this type. Regional lymphadenopathy again occurs and affects the cervical and retropharyngeal nodes.

Pneumonic tularemia may be caused by lung exposure to an infective aerosol from soil, grain, or hay or from deliberate use of an infective aerosol as a bioterrorist attack. The clinical presentation may be cough, pleuritic pain, and rarely, dyspnea. Chest radiographic findings show hilar lymphadenopathy, bronchopneumonia, and hilar lymphadenopathy. Despite the lungs being the primary route of entry, tularemic pneumonia can commonly present as nonspecific systemic signs without respiratory symptoms and often with normal chest radiographic results.

Tularemia is transmitted through the skin, mucous membranes, lungs, and gastrointestinal tract. The bacteria pass through the skin via bites, oropharyngeal mucosa, and conjunctiva by contaminated water or by contaminated blood or tissue during handling carcasses of infected animals. Through the gastrointestinal tract, it is transmitted via ingestion of insufficiently cooked meat of infected animals or via consumption of contaminated water. Finally, tularemia can be transmitted through the lungs via contaminated soil, handling of contaminated furs, or deliberate aerosolization of the bacterium as a biologic weapon. The incubation period is usually 3 to 5 days and can range from 1 to 14 days.

No documented person-to-person transmission of tularemia exists, including pneumonic tularemia. Routine precautions are adequate when transporting and caring for patients. The vehicle and equipment, however, must be thoroughly cleaned and decontaminated after patient transport.

Viral Hemorrhagic Fevers. *Viral hemorrhagic fevers* are caused by different distinct families of viruses and lead to similar clinical syndromes. In the case of bioterrorist attack, first responders must be able to recognize the illness associated with the intentional release of the biologic agent.

In hemorrhagic fever, the initial signs and symptoms are nonspecific and include high fever, headache, muscle aches, and severe fatigue. There may be associated gastrointestinal symptoms of nausea, vomiting, diarrhea, and abdominal pain. Respiratory symptoms of cough and sore throat may also occur. About 5 days after the onset of illness, a truncal maculopapular rash develops in most patients. As the disease progresses, bleeding occurs from internal organs, mouth, eyes, and ears, and from under the skin, which is seen as skin petechiae and skin ecchymosis. Shock, coma, seizures, and kidney failure may ensue in severe cases.

Transmission occurs when humans have direct contact with infected animals, mainly rodents, or are bitten by a mosquito or tick vector. Once a person has become infected, some viruses can be transmitted from person-to-person, mainly via close contact with infected people but also indirectly via objects contaminated with infected body fluids.

Transmission of viral hemorrhagic fever mainly occurs in the latter stage of illness when the patient has vomiting, diarrhea, shock, and hemorrhage. In the case of Ebola virus, reports are found of transmission within a few days of the onset of fever. The incubation period ranges from 2 days to 3 weeks, and no transmission has been documented during the incubation period.

No vaccine or established cure exists for viral hemorrhagic fevers, except for yellow fever and Argentine hemorrhagic fever. Ribavirin or plasma has been used for treatment with some success. Prevention is the best method of control. To prevent infection, contact with rodents and bites from ticks and mosquitoes should be prevented. Person-to-person transmission can be prevented with strict adherence to routine practices and additional precautions. In addition, patients with known or suspected viral hemorrhagic fever must be isolated. Although isolation is not possible in the setting, the transporting vehicle can serve to isolate the patient from the scene and while in transit.

If personnel are exposed to viral hemorrhagic fever, they should be placed under surveillance for fever. Surveillance should occur twice daily for at least 3 weeks after exposure. In case of development of temperature above 38.3 °C, patients should be hospitalized immediately with strict isolation.

OCCUPATIONAL HEALTH AND SAFETY

Immunization is a key and safe element in prevention and control of infectious diseases. In general, the following immunizations are recommended for personnel: tetanus-diphtheria, hepatitis B, polio, measles, mumps, rubella, varicella (if not already immune), and influenza. In addition, all personnel should be skin tested for tuberculosis exposure (TB or tuberculin skin test). Recommendations may also include immunization with polyvalent pneumococcal and meningitis vaccines and others that are more specific to local and regional requirements. Transport agencies should consult with regional or national public health authorities, such as the US Centers for Disease Control and Prevention (CDC), the Canadian National Advisory Committee on Immunizations (NACI), or similar agencies, to determine the appropriate immunization schedule and frequency of immunization for personnel.

Routine practices and *additional precautions* are a system of healthcare practices that combine the former universal precautions and body substance isolation into a new comprehensive standard of practice. The practice relies on recognition of signs and symptoms and modes of transmission of communicable disease instead of specific diagnoses. Routine practices assume all patients are potential reservoirs of organisms that may present a risk to healthcare providers and other patients. All healthcare providers should use routine practices at all times and in any healthcare setting, whether or not any evidence of a communicable or infectious disease is found.

Routine practices include patient assessment, hand hygiene, personal protective equipment, sharps safety, patient transport considerations, routine equipment cleaning, and routine vehicle cleaning and disinfection. Additional precautions are further methods of infection prevention and control based on the mode of transmission of the known or suspected infectious agents. Some additional precautions used to prevent spread of infection in a hospital setting, such as negative or positive pressure rooms, are not possible in the prehospital setting. Infection control practices must be simple, part of the routine work setting, and applied in all situations to be effective.

HAND HYGIENE

Hand washing is the single most important means of prevention of the spread of infection. Skin typically harbors two types of flora: resident and transient. The *resident flora* are normal bacteria found on skin that create an inhospitable environment for transient flora. *Transient flora* are recent contaminants on the skin acquired from colonized or infected patients or from contaminated objects in the environment. Transient flora on hands of healthcare workers are often the source of nosocomial infections. Proper and regular hand washing removes the dirt, organic material, and transient microorganisms that pose a risk of disease transmission.

Routine hand hygiene can prevent nosocomial infections and prevent contamination of patient care equipment and the environment.

Proper hand hygiene includes use of alcohol-based hand rubs, hand washing, and skin care. Care must be taken to ensure nonintact skin, especially on the hands, is adequately covered during patient care. Healthy intact skin is an effective barrier to infection. Use of soap and water and an alcohol-based hand rub are two effective hand hygiene methods.

Hand washing with soap and water for 10 to 15 seconds is preferred, but if soap and water is not available, an alcohol-based rub should be used. Waterless hand wash supplies should be available in all emergency response vehicles. When washing hands, remove all rings, bracelets, and watches before beginning. Obtain a moderate stream of comfortably warm water, and avoid splashing or letting water run from an unwashed part of the arm back down to the hands. Hands should be dried with paper towels, which are then disposed of, and a paper towel should be used to turn the tap off so as not to recontaminate the hands.

Hand chapping and dermatitis can be prevented or minimized by rinsing and drying skin completely, not using excessive amounts of soap, using hand creams, and alternating types of soaps. Personnel should avoid artificial nails or nail enhancements because microorganisms can accumulate under the nails and the nails are difficult to clean.

Alcohol-based or waterless hand wash solutions are not effective against spore-forming organisms such as *C. difficile*. Personnel must wash hands with soap and water (and not waterless hand wash solutions) when caring for patients with suspected spore-forming organisms.

Personnel must wash their hands:

- At the beginning and end of every shift.
- Before and after each patient contact, even if gloves were used.
- After handling potentially infectious materials, including body fluids, secretions, and excretions, or equipment potentially contaminated by infectious materials.
- After cleaning or decontaminating equipment.
- After using the bathroom.
- Before eating or drinking or smoking.
- Before and after handling or preparing food.

- Whenever the hands appear soiled.
- After removing PPE, such as masks, gloves, and gowns.

When hands are visibly soiled, they should ideally be washed with soap and water to remove the visible debris. If hand washing facilities are not available, visible soiling should be removed with a moistened towel or towelette, followed by use of an alcohol-based hand rub. All personnel should perform hand hygiene frequently and whenever indicated.

PERSONAL PROTECTIVE EQUIPMENT

Personal protective equipment (PPE) is specialized clothing or equipment that prevents blood or potentially infectious substances to pass through or reach personnel's clothing, skin, eyes, mouth, or other mucous membrane under normal conditions of use. The PPE acts to isolate personnel from exposure and can include items such as gloves, face mask, eye protection, face shields, and impervious gowns. These items should be available on all emergency response vehicles and should not be worn in the vehicle's driver compartment to prevent contamination of this area.

Personal protective equipment also includes disposable resuscitation and other equipment to protect providers against injury with potentially contaminated objects. These can include sharps containers, disposable bag-valve-masks, laryngoscopes, needleless intravenous delivery systems, and intravenous catheter insertion devices with retracting needles.

In general, regular surgical masks are considered adequate to prevent transmission of respiratory infections spread via large droplets. These masks may be used in cases where airborne transmission is not suspected. In the prehospital setting, however, personnel do not typically know the mode of transmission and cannot accurately determine whether the infection is spread via droplet or airborne means. In addition, personnel often perform procedures that generate aerosols, and the prehospital environment is typically uncontrolled and may have other particulate hazards. As a result, transport agencies and personnel may opt to use submicron particulate masks.

In cases of airborne respiratory infection, such as measles or tuberculosis, standard surgical masks are inadequate and submicron masks are necessary. The latter can filter in excess of 95% of airborne particles in a size range of 0.1 to 10 μm and provide a better facial seal than standard surgical masks. The masks, however, require fit testing and proper use to ensure maximal effectiveness.

All personnel should use an appropriate mask under the following circumstances:

- When caring for a patient with new onset cough or respiratory symptoms.
- When treating and transporting a patient with a known or suspected communicable disease transmitted via droplet or airborne route.
- When blood or body fluid splash is expected.
- When performing procedures, such as intubation or suctioning, that could result in aerosolization.
- When cleaning the vehicle and equipment after transport of a patient with known or suspected communicable disease transmitted via airborne or droplet route.

In addition to the indications for wearing a mask, the eyes and face should also be protected in any situation where splash contamination is possible. Specific eye protection should be used because regular or prescription glasses do not provide adequate protection against splash or spray. Face shields are an additional level of protection that may be used during invasive airway procedures. Personnel should not touch their face or eyes during patient care or before performing hand hygiene because of the risk of self contamination. Any eye or face protection worn must be carefully removed to prevent self contamination, followed by appropriate hand hygiene.

All personnel should use a new clean disposable pair of gloves that should be put on for each patient encounter. The gloves should be properly sized without any defects. If a gown is worn, the gloves must cover the gown's cuffs. Gloves must also be changed between patient care activities and procedures with the same patient when in contact with fluids or substances that may be highly contaminated with microorganisms, such as suctioning a tracheal tube or applying a dressing to an abscess. Personnel must perform hand hygiene immediately after removal of gloves and before touching one's eyes, nose, mouth, or another person. Gloves should never be worn in the vehicle's driver compartment.

Personnel should never perform hand hygiene while wearing gloves. Soap and alcohol-based agents break down the integrity of gloves and reduce their effectiveness. In addition, gloves should not be brought into a documentation or work room or worn while completing paperwork. This usage can result in transferring infectious agents to the work area or onto the paperwork. Finally, gloves are never a substitute for proper and adequate hand hygiene.

Long-sleeved impervious gowns are used to prevent the forearms and uniforms of responding personnel from becoming grossly contaminated with blood and body fluid. They should be used when large volumes of blood or body fluid are expected, such as treatment of an uncontrolled hemorrhage or during childbirth. Gowns should be impervious to fluids and completely cover the user, both front and back. The gown must also be removed and properly disposed of immediately after use and never worn in the vehicle's driver compartment.

Knowledge of when to use PPE is important; proper donning, removal, and disposal are equally important. The correct order to putting on PPE is gown or coverall first (if indicated), followed by mask, then eye protection, then gloves. Personnel should exercise care when removing PPE to avoid contamination of themselves or others or further contamination of the environment. If personnel are wearing a gown or coveralls, the gloves must be removed and disposed of first before gown removal. The gown is then removed, ensuring the outside of the gown is held away from the body and carefully rolled up inside out to avoid contaminating the wearer. The wearer should now perform hand hygiene, then remove face shield, eye protection, and mask without touching any potentially contaminated surfaces. Disposable items should be discarded in the appropriate waste receptacle. Personnel must repeat hand hygiene when all PPE has been removed. In summary, the proper PPE removal sequence is gloves, gown, hand hygiene, face and eye protection, mask, repeated hand hygiene.

Each transport service and agency must have in place both initial and recurrent training programs to ensure all personnel who provide patient care are appropriately trained in routine precautions and PPE use. Recurrent training is necessary because knowledge and skills decline with time,[11] which puts personnel at increased risk from incorrect use of routine precautions or PPE.

SHARPS SAFETY

The Association of Professional in Infection Control and the National Institute of Safety and Health (NIOSH)[6] report that the most frequent cause of blood-borne infection in healthcare settings is a needle-stick injury. Any healthcare worker, including emergency response personnel, is at risk of occupational exposure to blood-borne infectious agents. The risk of transmission of infection is variable, ranging from 0.5% risk of infection after a percutaneous exposure to HIV to up to a 30% risk after the same type of exposure to hepatitis B. Further details regarding specific infectious agents and postexposure prophylaxis are included elsewhere in this chapter and textbook.

All transport agencies must have a sharps handling system and mitigation strategy to decrease risk of transmission of blood-borne illness. Strategies must include proper containment and disposal systems, training of personnel in safe use of equipment, and adoption of safer systems, such as needleless drug and fluid administration systems and self-retracting IV catheter assemblies. All agencies must also have in place a reporting, treatment, and follow-up system in the event of an injury with a sharp object or of blood or body fluid exposure.

All personnel must also practice safe use of sharps at all times. This includes the following safe practices:

- Communication with other personnel regarding location of sharps (i.e., "sharp on floor", etc).
- Never leaving sharps for disposal by other personnel.
- Never passing exposed sharps to other personnel.
- Never carrying uncapped sharps in pocket.
- Never bending or recapping needles or other sharp objects.
- Immediate disposal of sharps in appropriate container.

- Disposal of sharps container when "full line" is reached.
- Immediate reporting of any injury involving a needle stick, other sharp object, or exposure to blood or body fluid.

PATIENT TRANSPORT ACCOMMODATION

Hospitals can isolate patients with an infectious disease in private or specialized rooms. Transport agencies and personnel do not have this ability. The transport vehicle becomes an isolation area while the patient is in transport. As a result, the vehicle itself must be treated in a manner similar to an isolation room in a hospital. To minimize further spread of disease, the ambulance's exhaust fan should be turned on to circulate air to the outdoors, and only essential personnel and patient escorts should accompany the patient to hospital. All personnel and escorts must wear appropriate PPE. Finally, the agency must notify the receiving hospital so they can prepare for patient arrival without further or unnecessary contamination of hospital personnel, other patients, or the surrounding patient care areas.

ROUTINE EQUIPMENT CLEANING AND DISINFECTION

Cleaning and disinfection are two distinct and separate processes. *Cleaning* is the removal of visible and invisible contamination from a surface using soap, detergent, or other physical means. *Disinfection* is a process that kills microorganisms on the surface, with the exception of spores that are resistant to disinfection. The three levels of disinfection are: low, intermediate, and high.

Sterilization is a third process that uses high-pressure steam, gas, or other harsh chemical process to destroy all microorganisms, including highly resistant spores. Sterilization is necessary for any equipment that penetrates a patient's sterile body cavity or vasculature. This includes surgical instruments, needles, catheters, and implanted devices. All sterile equipment used by personnel is for single patient use only and must be disposed of or resterilized after use.

Table 26-2 outlines the various levels of disinfection, and Table 26-3 describes which level is appropriate for

TABLE 26-2	Levels of Disinfection		
Level	**Effects**	**Uses**	**Methods**
Sterilization	Destroys all microorganisms, including highly resistant bacterial spores.	For instruments or devices that penetrate the skin or contact normally sterile areas of the body during invasive procedures. This is a rare occurrence in prehospital care.	Steam under pressure (autoclave). Gas process (ethylene oxide). Dry heat. Immersion in an approved chemical sterilizing agent for a prolonged period (according to manufacturer's instructions).
High-Level Disinfection	Destroys all forms of microorganisms, except bacterial spores.	For reusable equipment that comes into contact with mucous membranes, including: Airway bags. Laryngoscope blades. Suction bottles. Magill forceps.	Hot water pasteurization with placement of articles in water 176°F to 212°F (80°C to 100°C) for 30 min. Exposure to an approved chemical sterilizing agent for 10 to 45 min (or as directed by the manufacturer in accordance with manufacturer's instructions).
Intermediate-Level Disinfection	Destroys tuberculosis bacteria, vegetative bacteria, most viruses and fungi, but not bacterial spores.	For surfaces that only contact intact skin and have been visibly contaminated with body fluids. Surfaces must be precleaned of visible material before disinfection. Equipment that requires intermediate-level disinfection includes: Backboards and splints contaminated with blood. Suction tubing (tubing from collection unit to suction source).	Wiping with a hospital disinfectant/chemical germicide that has tuberculocidal activity. Wiping with a commercially available hard surface germicide or with a 1:100 chlorine bleach.
Low-Level Disinfection	Destroys most bacteria, some viruses and fungi, but not tuberculosis bacteria or bacterial spores.	For routine housekeeping or removal of soiling when no body fluids are visible. Equipment that requires low-level disinfection includes: Backboards and splints not contaminated with blood. Blood pressure cuffs. Stethoscope. Drug box. Monitoring equipment. Aircraft stretcher.	Wiping with a hospital disinfectant.

TABLE 26-3 **Level of Decontamination Required For Each Type of Equipment**	
Equipment	**Decontamination Procedure**
Airway bag (BVM)	High-level disinfection or disposal
Airways	
Nasopharyngeal	Disposal
Oropharyngeal	Disposal
Double lumen	Disposal
Bedpans	
Plastic	Disposal
Metal	High-level disinfection
Bite blocks	Disposal
Blood pressure cuffs	Low-level disinfection
Bulb syringe	Disposal
Cold packs	Disposal
Dressing	Disposal
Drug box	Low-level disinfection
Drug containers	Low-level disinfection
Tracheal tubes, stylets	Disposal
Head blocks	Low-level disinfection
Hot packs	Disposal
Intravenous poles	Low-level disinfection
K-basins	Disposal
Laryngoscopes	
Blades	High-level disinfection
Handle	Low-level disinfection
Magill forceps	High-level disinfection
Military anti-shock trousers (MAST)	High-level disinfection
Monitor, defibrillator paddles, includes patient cables and nondisposable lead wires	Low-level disinfection
Needles and syringes	Disposal in an impermeable container; do not break, bend, cut, or recap needles before disposal
Nitrous oxide delivery equipment	
Masks	High-level disinfection
Valve	High-level disinfection
Other electronic equipment (i.e., CO_2 monitors, glucometers, pulse oximeters)	Intermediate-level to low-level disinfection
Oxygen delivery equipment	
Nasal cannula	Disposal
Mask, non-rebreather	Disposal
Nebulizers	Disposal
Extension tubing	Disposal
Oxygen flow meter	Low-level disinfection
Oxygen regulators	Low-level disinfection
Oxygen tanks	Low-level disinfection

a particular purpose of piece of equipment. Cleaning must always be done before disinfection. Under no circumstances should equipment be reused, and transport agency or personnel should not return contaminated equipment to service without first properly cleaning, disinfecting, or sterilizing the equipment.

ROUTINE VEHICLE CLEANING AND DISINFECTION

The transport vehicle should be cleaned after every patient transport. Personnel cleaning the vehicle must use appropriate PPE when cleaning the vehicle. Good physical cleaning of all areas, including all equipment and surfaces, with the appropriate cleaning agent is necessary for effective cleaning. Although each agency should have a specific cleaning regime for each vehicle type, the following general method is suitable in most circumstances. All equipment must be removed from the vehicle storage locations before cleaning. All visible contaminants should be scrubbed and removed with soap and water, wiped or sprayed with an approved disinfecting solution, and then allowed to air dry. While the vehicle is drying, all equipment should be cleaned and disinfected as appropriate (see previous section). All items used in cleaning the vehicle (cloths, brushes, mops, etc) should be placed into an appropriate freshly prepared decontamination solution and allow to soak for 30 minutes or laundered. Once complete, all personnel performing the cleaning should remove PPE, perform hand hygiene, and ensure the vehicle has adequate infection control supplies and equipment to respond to multiple calls before returning to base.

Disposable equipment and other biohazardous waste generated during patient care or vehicle cleaning should be stored in suitable leak-proof biohazard containers. Transport agencies should have an agreement made with a local healthcare facility or suitable waste disposal company for disposal of biohazardous waste, including sharps containers.

ADDITIONAL PRECAUTIONS

Additional precautions supplement routine practices when spread of infectious disease is believed to occur via contact, droplet, or airborne routes. In the prehospital setting, the following situations mandate use of additional precautions.

Contact precautions are used in treatment of a patient with a communicable disease transmitted via direct contact. Examples include MRSA, VRE, or *C difficile*. In addition to routine precautions, personnel should use proper eye protection and not transport more than one patient in the same transport vehicle.

Airborne and droplet-spread diseases are not readily distinguished in the prehospital setting, so personnel should use the same precautions for both types of diseases. Recognition is the first step to taking appropriate additional precautions in this setting. Personnel must remain at least 3 ft from the patient while determining the need for additional precautions. The decision to use additional precautions must be made on the basis of patient history and presenting signs and symptoms. If a respiratory illness is suspected, the following additional precautions are indicated:

- Submicron particulate mask and eye protection worn at all times and removed when patient contact is complete.
- Surgical mask placed on the patient.
- If high-concentration oxygen is needed, use of a low-flow high-concentration mask fitted with submicron hydrophobic filter.
- Patient compartment exhaust system kept on and running during and after patient transport to ensure adequate air exchange.
- Transport of only one patient at a time.

SUMMARY

Although it is the provider's responsibility to use routine practices and additional precautions (where indicated), the services and agencies must provide the necessary infrastructure to promote safe working practices to mitigate the risk of disease. The Toronto SARS outbreaks showed that lack of adequate infection control implementation was a leading cause of infection among healthcare workers.[2] The workplace must provide the requisite administrative and work practice controls, including policies and procedures to ensure adherence to the safe working practices. An adequate amount of appropriate protective equipment and related supplies designed to prevent disease must also be provided.

REFERENCES

1. Association for Professionals in Infection Control and Epidemiology: *APIC text of infection control and epidemiology*, Washington, DC, 2002, APIC.
2. Centers for Disease Control and Prevention: Cluster of severe acute respiratory syndromes cases among protected healthcare workers–Toronto, Canada, April 2003, *MMWR* 52:433-436, 2003.
3. Dwosh H, Hong H, Austgarden D, et al: Identification and containment of an outbreak of SARS in a community hospital, *Can Med Assoc J* 168:1415-1420, 2003.
4. Ko PC-I, Chen W-J, Ha MH-M, et al: Emergency medical service utilization during an outbreak of severe acute respiratory syndrome (SARS) and the incidence of SARS-associated coronavirus infection among emergency medical technicians, *Acad Emerg Med* 11:903-911, 2004.
5. MacDonald RD, Farr B, Neill M, et al: An emergency medical services transfer authorization center in response to the Toronto severe acute respiratory syndrome outbreak, *Prehosp Emerg Care* 8:223-231, 2004.
6. National Institute of Occupational Health and Safety: *Preventing needlestick injuries in health care settings*, Atlanta, 1999, Centers for Disease Control.
7. United States Department of Labor: *Occupational exposure to blood-borne pathogens: precautions for emergency responders*, Washington, DC, 1992, OSHA.
8. Varia M, Wilson S, Sarwal S, et al: Investigation of nosocomial outbreak of severe acute respiratory syndrome (SARS) in Toronto, Canada, *CMAJ* 169(4):285-292, 2003.
9. Verbeek PR, McLelland IW, Silverman AC, et al: Loss of paramedic availability in an urban emergency medical services system during a severe acute respiratory syndrome outbreak, *Acad Emerg Med* 11:973-978, 2004.
10. Verbeek PR, Schwartz B, Burgess RJ: Should paramedics intubate patients with SARS-like symptoms? *CMAJ* 169(4):199-200, 2003.
11. Visentin LM: *Knowledge, attitudes, and behaviour of paramedics regarding personal protective equipment for communicable respiratory disease outbreaks*, MSc Thesis, Department of Community Health Sciences, University of Toronto, Toronto, Canada, June 2005.

UNIT VI
Environmental Emergencies

CHAPTER 27

COLD-RELATED EMERGENCIES

Reneé Semonin Holleran

COMPETENCIES

1. Describe thermoregulation and mechanisms of heat loss.
2. Define mild, moderation, and severe hypothermia.
3. Identify methods to prevent heat loss during patient transport.

Hannibal started over the Pyrenean Alps in 218 BC with an army of 46,000, but in 15 days, he lost more than 20,000 men to the cold.[8] Statistics have not significantly improved since Hannibal's time. US soldiers sustained 90,000 cold-related injuries in World War II, and Germany suffered 100,000. During two winter months in 1942, the Germans performed 15,000 cold-related amputations.[57] During the Korean War, the United States had a 10% cold-related casualty rate.[35,41,42]

Transport personnel must be aware of the risk of hypothermia regardless of the climate or terrain in which they practice. A hiker on a summer day in the Rocky Mountains, an older person in an unheated home in the Sun Belt, and a sailor stranded off the warm Florida coast are all at equal risk of hypothermia. Studies have shown that cold contributes to 16% of all recreational boating fatalities and 20% of all scuba diving fatalities.[33,34,36,52]

HYPOTHERMIA DEFINED

Hypothermia, defined as a core body temperature of less than 35°C, occurs because the body can no longer generate sufficient heat to maintain body functions.[7] *Accidental hypothermia,* in contrast to iatrogenic hypothermia, is the unintentional decrease in core temperature associated with trauma or exposure to the environment.[1,6,7,13,14,28] Core body temperature can be measured in the rectum, the esophagus, the tympanic membrane, or the bloodstream. Rectal thermometers provide the least reliable measurement of core body temperature. The esophageal and tympanic thermometers are more reliable. Table 27-1 lists thermometric equivalents for Fahrenheit and Celsius temperatures.[20]

TABLE 27-1 **Thermometric Equivalents (Celsius and Fahrenheit)**	
Degrees Celsius	**Degrees Fahrenheit**
15.0	59.0
16.0	60.8
17.0	62.6
18.0	64.4
19.0	66.2
20.0	68.0
21.0	69.8
22.0	71.6
23.0	73.4
24.0	75.2
25.0	77.0
26.0	78.8
27.0	80.6
28.0	82.4
29.0	84.2
30.0	86.0
31.0	87.8
32.0	89.6
33.0	91.4
34.0	93.2
35.0	95.0
36.0	96.8
37.0	98.6
38.0	100.4
39.0	102.2
40.0	104.0

CLASSIFICATION

Hypothermia can be both a clinical symptom and a disease.[8] It can be classified as *primary,* with simple environmental exposure in a healthy person, or *secondary,* with hypothermia as a part of a disease process or caused by a predisposing condition.[8] Multiple predisposing factors can place a person at risk of hypothermia. Age, diseases, medications, and type and length of exposure can all contribute to the development of hypothermia. The transport environment can especially place a patient at risk for hypothermia from loss of clothing, wet clothing, lack of protection from the environment, medications, diseases and injuries, and lack of environmental control within the transport vehicle itself.[14,22-25] Box 27-1 contains a summary of predisposing factors to hypothermia.

Hypothermia is classified into four stages. *Mild hypothermia* is defined as a core body temperature greater than 32°C and less than 35°C (90°F to 95°F) and is associated with low morbidity and mortality rates. The patient may display symptoms of ataxia, slurred speech, apathy, and even amnesia. Thermoregulatory mechanisms continue to operate.[16] *Moderate hypothermia* occurs when the core body temperature is greater than 28°C but less than 32°C (82°F to 90°F). Thermoregulatory actions

BOX 27-1	**Predisposing Factors for Hypothermia**

Diabetes
Malnutrition
Hemorrhagic shock
Stroke
Thermal injuries
Elderly
Infants
Emergency childbirth
Environmental exposure
Immersion in cold water
Fluid resuscitation with cold infusions
Aircraft frame
Failure to remove wet clothing
Lack of environmental control in the transport vehicle

Modified from Danzl D: Accidental hypothermia. In Auerbach P, editor: *Wilderness medicine,* ed 5, St Louis, 2007, Mosby.

such as shivering continue but begin to decrease and eventually fail. The patient's level of consciousness continues to decrease, and cardiac arrhythmia may develop. *Severe hypothermia* is defined as a core body temperature of 28°C (82°F) or less and is associated with a higher morbidity and mortality rates.[2,6,26,27] *Profound hypothermia* occurs at a temperature of 20.0°C to 9.0°C (68.0°F to 48.2°F). These zones and characteristics are summarized in Table 27-2.[7]

MORTALITY

Many factors influence the mortality from hypothermia, including degree and duration of hypothermia, age, poverty, predisposing disease, and complications. Hypothermia in a trauma patient can be deadly.[1,2] Most victims die of cardiac arrhythmia. The presence of a severe underlying disease is almost always associated with increased mortality. Rankin and Rae[47] noted no correlation between the severity of hypothermia or the rate of rewarming and the clinical outcome but did note, rather, that mortality was correlated with the presence or absence of severe underlying disease.

The old adage "the patient is not dead until they are warm and dead" still directs the medical management of the patient with hypothermia. Transport programs, particularly those that provide service in cold weather or rescue environments, must have policies and procedures that control when and how a patient with severe hypothermia is resuscitated and transported.

NORMAL TEMPERATURE REGULATION

Humans become uncomfortable with even a small deviation in core body temperature from 37.6°C. In *De Re Medicina*, Aurelius Cornelius Celsus described in 25 AD the universal discomfort of cold temperatures as "hurtful to an old or slender man, to a wound, to the precordia, intestines, bladder, ears, hips, shoulders, private parts, teeth, bones, nerves, womb and brain. It also renders the surface of the skin pale, dry, hard and black. From this proceed shudderings and tremors."[7,25] Normal body temperature is maintained in a narrow range by a delicate balance of heat loss and heat production regulated by a "thermostat" in the preoptic anterior hypothalamus. The hypothalamus is sensitive to temperature changes as small as 0.5°C.[4] Stimuli sent from the hypothalamus to the sympathetic nervous system increase heart rate and dilate muscle blood vessels to increase heat production. In addition, shivering generates heat by increasing muscle activity. At the same time, cutaneous vasoconstriction reduces heat loss by shunting blood from the periphery to the core.[50-56,58,61,65]

The ability to shiver is affected by hypoglycemia, hypoxia, fatigue, alcohol, and drugs. Shivering is the body's main mechanism of heat production and its strongest defense against hypothermia. However, shivering requires increased blood flow to peripheral muscles and consequently results in a 25% heat loss. Preshivering increases heat production by 50% to 100%. Visible shivering increases heat production by 500%. An average 70-kg person produces about 100 kcal/h of heat under basal conditions and up to 500 kcal/h when shivering.[7] This degree of heat production, however, cannot be sustained for long because the patient becomes fatigued once glycogen stores are depleted. Maximal shivering occurs at 35°C and stops below 32°C. Cessation of shivering is a sign that the patient has made the transition from mild to severe hypothermia.

Hypothermia results when the thermoregulation system becomes overwhelmed or damaged centrally at the hypothalamic level or systemically by a decrease in heat production or an increase in heat loss. Thermoregulation is disrupted at the hypothalamic level by head trauma, cerebral neoplasm, cerebrovascular accident, acute poisoning, acid-base imbalance, Parkinson's disease, and Wernicke's encephalopathy. Acute spinal injury can eliminate vasoconstrictive control by the hypothalamus. Heat production is decreased by malnutrition, hypothyroidism, hypopituitarism, and rheumatoid arthritis. Normally, 90% of the heat produced by the body is lost to the environment by way of conduction, convection, radiation, and evaporation.

METHODS OF HEAT LOSS[7]

Conduction together with convection each account for 15% of heat loss.[16] *Conduction* occurs when the body comes into direct contact with a heat conductor. Examples of good conductors are water, snow, metal, and damp ground. Normally, conduction plays a minor role in heat loss, but it is an important

TABLE 27-2	Physiologic Changes Related to Temperature	
Degrees Celsius	**Degrees Fahrenheit**	**Characteristics**
38.0	99.6	Normal rectal temperature
37.0	98.6	Normal oral temperature
Mild		
36.0	96.8	Increased basal metabolic rate in an attempt to balance heat loss, tachycardia, increased cardiac output
35.0	95.0	Shivering at the maximum, usually still responsive, but level of consciousness beginning to decrease, regulatory systems beginning to falter
34.0	93.2	Dysarthria, amnesia, blood pressure still normal, oxyhemoglobin curve begins to shift to the left
32.0	91.4	Heart rate decreases to 50 to 60 bpm, ataxia, poor coordination, apathy, lethargy
Moderate		
32.0	89.6	Vasoconstriction, level of consciousness progressively falls
31.0	87.8	Shivering stops, respirations and blood pressure may be difficult to obtain
30.0	86.0	Mental confusion, delirium, increased muscle rigidity; heart rate and cardiac output begin to decrease, arrhythmias begin to develop (atrial fibrillation)
29.0	84.2	Acidosis, hyperglycemia, metabolic rate decreased by 50%, decreased respirations, bradycardia, decreased stroke volume, decreased cardiac output, pupils dilated, paradoxical undressing
Severe		
28.0	82.4	Hypotension, loss of vasoconstrictive capabilities, ventricular fibrillation if patient handled roughly, increased myocardial irritability
27.0	80.6	Prolonged PR, QRS, and QT intervals; muscle flaccidity; no voluntary movement (appears dead); no pupillary reactions
26.0	78.8	Seldom conscious, areflexia
25.0	77.0	Stuporous, hypoventilation, ventricular fibrillation may appear spontaneously, cerebral blood flow one third of normal, cardiac output 45% of normal
24.0	75.2	Coma, pulmonary edema, respiratory arrest
23.0	73.4	No spontaneous movement, rigor mortis appearance, no corneal reflexes
22.0	71.6	Maximal risk of ventricular fibrillation, 75% decrease in oxygen consumption
21.0	69.8	Apnea
Profound		
20.0	68.0	Pulse is 20% of normal
18.0	64.4	Asystole
10.0	50.0	92% decrease in oxygen consumption

factor when the patient has been immersed in cold water, is lying in a snow bank, or is wandering without shoes for an extended period. Heat loss in water is approximately 24 times faster than heat loss in air of the same temperature.[17,19] Immersion in water in temperatures less than 10°C causes hypothermia in only a few minutes,[7] in contrast to more than an hour in air.[58]

Heat loss by *convection* occurs when either air or water moves over the patient or the patient moves through air or water. Heat loss is accelerated by increasing air movement (forced convection). The wind, the rotating blades of the helicopter, and the movement required to transport the patient to the transport vehicle all contribute to forced convective heat loss. Figure 27-1 lists temperature differences related to wind chill factors.

Body heat lost by radiation is 45%.[7,9] *Radiant heat transfer* occurs when a difference exists between body temperature and ambient temperature. The body absorbs heat when the ambient temperature is higher and emits heat when the ambient temperature is lower. Radiant heat loss, as convection, is directly related to dermal blood flow and percentage of skin surface exposed. Radiant heat loss is accelerated at night or when the sky is overcast.

Evaporation occurs when water on the body surface is converted from a liquid state to a gaseous state.[7,9] The body is cooled as the vapor moves off the body into the air. The evaporative process accounts for about 25% of heat loss[7,9] and occurs normally through the skin, lungs, and upper airway. Burns and various skin lesions expose more open moist surface area and thereby increase evaporative

Wind in m.p.h.	Local Temperature in Degrees Fahrenheit										
	32	23	14	5	−4	−13	−22	−31	−40	−49	−58
	Equivalent Temperature (Wind Plus Local Temperature)										
Calm	32	23	14	5	−4	−13	−22	−31	−40	−49	−58
5	29	20	10	1	−9	−18	−28	−37	−47	−56	−65
10	18	7	−4	−15	−26	−37	−48	−59	−70	−81	−92
15	13	−1	−13	−25	−37	−49	−61	−73	−88	−97	−109
20	7	−6	−19	−32	−44	−57	−70	−83	−98	−109	−121
25	3	−10	−24	−37	−50	−64	−77	−90	−104	−117	−130
30	1	−13	−27	−41	−54	−68	−82	−97	−109	−123	−137
35	−1	−15	−29	−43	−57	−71	−85	−99	−113	−127	−142
40	−3	−17	−31	−45	−59	−74	−87	−102	−116	−131	−145
45	−3	−18	−32	−46	−61	−75	−89	−104	−118	−132	−147
50	−4	−18	−33	−47	−62	−76	−91	−105	−120	−134	−148
	little danger for those properly clothed ▶		considerable danger ⟶			extreme danger ⟶						

FIGURE 27-1   **Chill factor: temperature plus wind.** (From Vaughn PB: Local cold injury-menace to military operations: a review *Milit Med* 5:307, 1980.)

losses. In addition, evaporation increases when the patient is wearing damp clothing or is covered with blood.

Heat loss is inversely proportional to body size and body fat. White fat insulates because it has less blood flow and consequently has less ability to vasodilate and lose heat. Consequently, large people conserve heat better than small people, obese people better than thin people, and adults better than children.

As newborns, about 5% of our body weight is made up of heat-producing brown fat cells, but as we age, the proportion of brown fat cells drops dramatically, giving way to more white fat cells. Brown fat cells are relatively abundant in races that are highly cold-adapted, such as the Inuit, and in most mammals, including humans as neonates.[50]

Brown (heat-producing) fat is typically located between the shoulder blades and wrapped around the internal organs close to the heart. People who live outdoors, such as the homeless or Inuit, have a lot more of this fat, and those people burn a lot of fat to keep warm. Urban humans who are usually reared in warm tightly temperature-controlled environments tend to have reduced populations of brown fat and hence reduced capacity for nonshivering thermogenesis, which has high survival value in cold environments. Long-term cold adaptation increases the amount of brown adipose tissue.[50]

Lipolysis with oxidation of fatty acids requires oxygen and can produce quite large amounts of heat. Brown fat cells are especially adapted to thermogenesis; it appears that they produce heat with little production of ATP. Norepinephrine release triggers lipolysis, oxidation of fatty acids, and heat production in both white and brown fat deposits. Nonshivering thermogenesis typically uses mitochondria in brown fat and is stimulated by the sympathetic nervous system, releasing norepinephrine. Mammals that acclimatize to cold temperatures build up brown fat stores mediated by the thyroid hormones.[50]

The transport team must carefully consider risk factors that may place the patient at risk for development of hypothermia. These risk factors include[2,4,16,22]:

Age: The pediatric patient has less fat, and shivering provides limited heat production. Elderly people may also have similar inabilities to generate heat.

Medications: Antidepressants, phenothiazines, narcotics, neuromuscular blocking agents, and nonsteroidal antiinflammatory drugs (NSAIDs) are only a few examples of the pharmacologic agents that may interfere with the patient's ability to maintain body heat.

Preexisting medical problems: Conditions such as Parkinson's disease, head injury, malnutrition, hypoglycemia, and shock place the patient at risk of hypothermia.

Prolonged exposure and weather conditions: Factors such as high humidity, brisk winds, and rain or snow may increase heat loss.

PHYSIOLOGIC RESPONSE TO HYPOTHERMIA[7,13,43,44,48,59,60,62,64]

METABOLIC DERANGEMENTS

Complications of hypothermia result mainly from the sequelae of *metabolic derangements*. Initially, metabolism increases to generate heat. Optimal metabolism begins to decrease at 35°C. Symptoms of mild hypothermia consequently include shivering, hypoglycemia, and increased respiratory rate, heart rate, and cardiac output. A dramatic decrease in metabolic rate occurs between 30°C and 33°C as the patient makes the transition from moderate to severe hypothermia. Every 10°C decrease in temperature decreases metabolism by half.[7] At 28°C, all thermoregulation ceases. The metabolic functions of the liver also begin to falter at temperatures below 33°C. The liver no longer efficiently metabolizes fats, proteins, and carbohydrates or drugs, alcohol, and lactic acid. Symptoms of severe hypothermia include absence of shivering, hyperglycemia, and decreased respiratory rate, heart rate, and cardiac output. Bowel sounds are decreased, if not absent, as a result of decreased gastric motility and gastric dilation.[27-29]

Hypoglycemia is associated with chronic mild hypothermia, whereas hyperglycemia is associated with acute severe hypothermia. Long-term shivering depletes glucose and glucose stored in the form of glycogen. Shivering can stop at temperatures greater than 33°C if glucose or glycogen stores are depleted or if insulin is no longer available. Shivering begins again when the core body temperature increases to 32°C if depleted glucose is replaced. Hyperglycemia occurs at temperatures below 30°C because insulin no longer promotes glucose transport into cells once metabolism significantly decreases.[9,23] Hyperglycemia does not occur if glucose and glycogen stores have been previously depleted but not replaced.

OXYGENATION AND ACID-BASE DISORDERS

Respiratory rate initially increases after sudden exposure to cold but then decreases as body temperature and metabolism decrease.[8] At temperatures above 32°C, ventilation is usually adequate. At 30°C, respirations are shallow and difficult to observe. Apnea and respiratory arrest commonly occur at temperatures between 21°C and 24°C. Although carbon dioxide production also decreases to about half the basal level with each 8°C drop in temperature,[25] the decreased respiratory rate is inadequate to effectively excrete CO_2 at a temperature below 33°C. Consequently, a respiratory acidosis develops in the hypothermia victim.

Cellular respiration is impaired by the decrease in metabolism, drop in cardiac output, and left shift on the oxyhemoglobin dissociation curve. Hypothermia decreases cardiac output by decreasing heart rate and circulating blood volume and by increasing blood viscosity and peripheral vascular resistance. Blood shifting to the core results in a perceived overhydration, and the body responds by removing the extra volume through diuresis. Prolonged hypothermia also causes plasma to leak from the capillaries, thereby increasing blood viscosity by 2% for every 1°C decline.[8,25]

Hypothermia begins to shift the oxyhemoglobin dissociation curve to the left at 34°C. Oxygen then binds tenaciously with hemoglobin, which results in reduced tissue oxygen delivery. In addition, Biddle has noted that oxygen consumption was half of normal at 27°C and, at 17°C, had fallen to one quarter the normal value.[8,10] Anaerobic metabolism and lactic acid production increase from the combination of decreased cardiac output, oxygen delivery, and oxygen consumption. The increase in lactic acid leads to cardiac arrhythmia and death.

The cardiovascular system is more sensitive to the effects of acid-base disturbances than any other body system. Acidosis is commonly associated with asystole, and alkalosis is associated with ventricular fibrillation.[8,9,39,41] Hypoventilation and lactic acid production lead to respiratory and metabolic acidosis. Acidosis usually corrects itself once the patient is rewarmed. Hyperkalemia is associated with metabolic acidosis and with muscle damage and kidney failure, which may all be present in the rewarmed hypothermic patient. Iatrogenic respiratory and metabolic alkalosis is difficult to treat and should be avoided.

CENTRAL NERVOUS SYSTEM

The central nervous system (CNS) displays some of the most impressive sequelae in the patient with hypothermia. Complete recovery is possible even after prolonged cardiac arrest. Hypothermia protects CNS integrity and may allow the brain to withstand long periods of anoxia.[15] Cerebral blood flow decreases 6% to 7% for every 1°C decline until 25°C is reached.[8,9] Cerebral oxygen requirements decrease to 50% of normal at 28°C, to 25% of normal at 22°C,[13,41] and to 12.5% of normal at 16°C.[52] Caroline[5] noted that the brain can survive without perfusion for about 10 minutes at 30°C, whereas it can survive for up to 25 to 30 minutes at 20°C.[52] Remarkably, Steinman[54] noted that at 16°C the brain can survive without oxygen for up to 32 to 48 minutes.[54,55]

Patients with mild hypothermia are clumsy, apathetic, withdrawn, and irritable. Reflexes are hyperactive at temperatures above 32°C. Level of consciousness begins to decrease markedly at 32°C, and patients become lethargic or disoriented and begin to hallucinate. Hypothermia victims even remove jackets, gloves, shoes, and other protective clothing. This reaction is known as *paradoxical undressing* and is often one of the first signs that patients are becoming severely hypothermic. Patients can no longer ascertain whether they are cold.

The cough reflex is absent at decreased temperatures, and aspiration of stomach contents can occur. Coma develops between 28°C and 30°C. At temperatures below 30°C, the pupils dilate and become nonreactive. In addition, corneal and deep-tendon reflexes may be absent. The patient with hypothermia must be carefully examined to rule out rigor mortis or death. At temperatures below 20°C, the electroencephalographic results, if they were available, would be flat.[54,55]

CARDIAC ARRHYTHMIA

The effects of hypothermia on heart rhythm were noted as early as 1912. Hyperthermia was found to produce bradycardia that progressed to asystole.[8-10] In 1923, subjects reportedly showed T-wave changes on electrocardiograms (ECGs) after drinking 600 mL of ice water.[45,46] Up to 90% of all patients with hypothermia are believed to have some electrocardiographic abnormality, including atrial fibrillation, sinus bradycardia, and junctional rhythms.[16,33-36,58,63]

The heart initially responds to mild hypothermia with an increase in heart rate as a result of sympathetic stimulation; this response is short lived. Heart rate then decreases to 50 to 60 bpm at 33°C and to 20 bpm at lower temperatures.[7,16] Atrial fibrillation with a slow ventricular rate is common at temperatures below 29°C. Okada, Nishimura, and Yoshiro[40] recently noted that atrial fibrillation was unusual in mild hypothermia (temperature greater than 32°C) and was often observed in moderate (32°C to 26°C) and moderately deep (less than 26°C) hypothermia. About half of the cases studied in moderately deep hypothermia remained in sinus, atrial, or junctional rhythm. Okada and colleagues[39,40] also noted that atrial fibrillation usually converted to sinus rhythm spontaneously after return to normothermia.

Changes in the conduction system begin at 27°C and may be observed as a widened QRS interval and prolonged PR and QT intervals. The Osborne, or J, wave is seen clearly at 25°C. The J wave is described as an extra deflection at the junction of the QRS and ST segments (Figure 27-2). The origin of the J wave is unknown. According to Okada, Nishimura, and Yoshiro,[40] the prolongation of the Q-T interval and the presence of J waves are directly related to the severity of the hypothermia. Large J waves

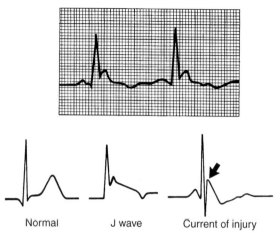

FIGURE 27-2   **ECG tracing showing the characteristic J, or Osborne, wave of hypothermia.**

(see Figure 27-2) are seen at temperatures of less than 30°C, whereas small J waves are seen at higher temperatures.

Several theories have been offered for the presence of J waves in hypothermia. The J wave may represent hypothermia-induced ion fluxes that cause delayed depolarization or early repolarization of the left ventricle. The J wave may also be a hypothalamic or neurogenic factor. J waves may also be seen in patients with central nervous system lesions or cardiac ischemia, in patients who are septic, or even in young healthy people.[21]

Ventricular irritability, which occurs at temperatures less than 30°C, is commonly associated with alkalosis and is the most lethal cardiovascular response to hypothermia. At 28°C, rough handling, careless intubation, or cardiac compressions can irritate the heart. Ventricular fibrillation can occur spontaneously at 25°C. Unfortunately, arrhythmia at temperatures below 30°C becomes increasingly refractory to drugs and defibrillation because of decreased perfusion and metabolic rate.

Asystole occurs at 20°C but has a surprisingly good prognosis if the patient is rewarmed quickly. Asystole is associated with acidosis and appears to be the primary arrhythmia in accidental hypothermia. Rankin and Rae[47] found that asystole was the terminal rhythm in all 22 patients they studied. Graham, McNaughton, and Wyatt[21] found in their study of 73 ECGs that atrial fibrillation and junctional bradycardia were associated with poor outcomes.

Circum-Rescue Collapse

Some years ago, physiologists postulated that the collapse that often occurred after victims were removed from hypothermic situations to warm environments was caused by an after drop in core temperature. However, research has shown this belief to be incorrect; the main problem appears to be sudden circulatory changes. This condition is now referred to as *circum-rescue collapse;* it most commonly occurs after rescue from immersion in water.[18]

In the water, an increased hydrostatic pressure around the victim's legs and trunk results in an increase in venous return and hence an increase in cardiac output. This increase in central volume is sensed as hypervolemia by the body, and thus, a diuresis and salt loss (natriuresis) occurs. Peripheral vasoconstriction occurs because of the relative cold temperate of the water, even in temperate climates, which results in a further increase in venous return and exacerbation of this response. In this way, the victim's intravascular volume becomes depleted.[19]

One suggested mechanism that leads to circulatory collapse is the stress on the myocardium from increased venous and arterial pressures that result in increased catecholamine release. Coupled with hypoxia, the increase in circulating catecholamines may provoke cardiac dysrhythmias. A second part to the theory is that vertical removal from the water causes both a sudden release in the hydrostatic pressure around the abdomen and legs and a consequent positional venous pooling in the lower limbs and reduced venous return to the heart. The resultant acute decrease in coronary perfusion may provoke ventricular fibrillation or acute myocardial ischemia, causing death.[17-19]

FROSTNIP AND FROSTBITE[35,37]

Frostnip, a superficial form of frostbite usually found on the face, nose, and ears, is manifested by numbness and pallor of the exposed skin. Management consists of warming the area with a warm hand or wrapping or covering the area for protection.

Frostbite results from the cooling of body tissue to the point of ice crystal formation[30] and most often involves the distal extremities. Destruction of the skin produces a more severe injury than frostnip. Although frostbite is commonly associated with below-freezing temperatures, it can be produced at above-freezing temperatures by wind, altitude, humidity, and prolonged exposure and can be exacerbated by impaired vascular integrity and decreased cardiac output.[34,51]

The injury caused by frostbite has been divided into four phases: the prefreeze phase, the freeze-thaw phase, the vascular stasis phase, and the late ischemic phase. This pathophysiology results in both intracellular and extracellular formation, cell dehydration and shrinkage, abnormal intracellular electrolyte imbalances, thermal shock, and denaturation of the lipid-protein complexes.[35]

Blood cells "sludge" in the vessels, and eventually circulation to the tissue ceases.[35] Frostbite is classified as first, second, or third degree. First-degree injury, superficial freezing without blistering or peeling, is characterized by hyperemia and edema. The tissue becomes mottled, cyanotic, and painful after rewarming. Second-degree frostbite produces blistering or peeling of the skin and is characterized by hyperemia and vesicle or bleb formation. When rewarmed, the skin is deep red, hot, and dry to touch. Third-degree frostbite is characterized by death of the dermis and even deeper tissue such as muscle and bone.[30]

Cauchy et al[6] recently proposed a new classification for grading the severity of frostbite injuries that is based on:

- Extent of initial lesion at day 0 after rapid rewarming.
- Bone scanning at day 2.
- Blisters at day 2.
- Prognosis at day 2.

This classification system describes the management and potential outcome of the frostbite injury based on the preceding descriptions. The authors suggest that the use of this system will[6]:

1. Provide earlier prediction of the final outcome of the frostbite.
2. Identify at day 2 the approximate level of amputation.
3. Precisely classify the frozen lesions and describe the management of the injury even without any specific knowledge of the topic on the part of the treating healthcare provider.

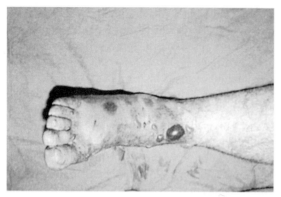

FIGURE 27-3 **Frostbite.** (From Sanders MJ: *Mosby's paramedic textbook,* ed 3, St Louis, 2007, Mosby/JEMS.)

Frostbite management has three stages.[4,6,35] The first stage is the most crucial and includes protection of the affected area from trauma or partial thawing. The second stage, rapid rewarming in a whirlpool bath, must occur in a controlled setting with constant observation. The third stage involves provisions for long-term care and follow-up.[4,6,35]

Prehospital care focuses on protecting the affected area from trauma and partial thawing (Figure 27-3). Superficial skin injury can be treated by removing any wet clothing and placing warm dry clothing on the injured area. The affected area should be kept frozen if any possibility of refreezing exists. The area must never be massaged. The patient should not be allowed to walk if the legs are involved unless it is a matter of survival.

Patients should be given ibuprofen and fluids and pain management provided with morphine or another appropriate narcotic.[4,6,35] The affected part needs to be carefully immobilized and protected from additional injury. Patients should be transported to a center familiar with the care of frostbite.

EPIDEMIOLOGY

Any individual becomes hypothermic given the proper circumstances, but specific groups are particularly vulnerable: infants, older individuals, alcoholic subjects, trauma victims, outdoor people, and those with CNS dysfunction.[1,3,14,27,28,32-36] The transport team must always consider hypothermia in assessment of patients in these high-risk groups.

INFANTS

Infants and neonates are particularly vulnerable to hypothermia. Mortality rates for neonatal cold injury range from 26% to 45%.[1,3,9] Hypothermia must be considered a threat in all out-of-hospital deliveries. The high mortality rate of infants is attributed to several causes:

1. The infant has less tissue insulation than the adult.
2. The large head in proportion to body size allows for greater heat loss.
3. Shivering occurs only at extreme degrees of hypothermia and may go undetected.
4. Limited energy stores are quickly exhausted.
5. Poor motor development may prevent infants from curling into a fetal position for protection.

In addition, the signs and symptoms of hypothermia in the infant are different from the adult and include lethargy, decreased appetite, facial and limb edema, and erythemic rather than blanching skin.

OLDER PATIENTS

Accidental hypothermia is common and often fatal in older subjects. Urban hypothermia is commonly seen in older subjects who do not have enough money for heat or warm clothing. People 75 years and older are estimated to have a five times greater chance of death from hypothermia than those younger than 75 years.[35] The reasons for the increased susceptibility of the elderly are many.

1. Older patients normally have a lower basal metabolic rate and body temperature.
2. Older patients have a decreased ability to adapt to temperature changes via vasoconstriction and shivering.
3. Older patients have a diminished perception of heat and cold.
4. Older patients are predisposed to other diseases such as diabetes or pneumonia that make them more susceptible to hypothermia.
5. Older patients are more susceptible to chronic dehydration.
6. Older patients have decreased metabolism of their essential medications as their renal and hepatic functions are decreased.

All confused and lethargic older patients should be assessed for hypothermia in addition to other problems, such as cerebrovascular accident or hypoglycemia.

ALCOHOL AND OTHER TOXIC STATES

Alcohol ingestion has been found to cause serious problems with thermoregulation. Many people consume alcohol with the mistaken belief that it will warm them. Many homeless people who become hypothermic are also intoxicated. Alcohol causes vasodilation, which contributes to additional heat loss. Alcohol ingestion also causes the patient to feel warm, perhaps by altering perception. Hypoglycemia is caused by alcohol ingestion and decreases the patient's ability to shiver and conserve heat. The effects of alcohol on thermoregulation are moderated by the temperature, the amount of alcohol ingested, the patient's nutritional status, body composition, and the patient's ability to tolerate the amount of alcohol ingested.[9,10]

Alcohol intoxication must be recognized as a dangerous cofactor for the patient with hypothermia. Intoxication is not uncommon in trauma patients.[9,10]

Other medications also cause hypothermia by impairing centrally mediated vasoconstriction. Barbiturates induce hypothermia in greater than therapeutic doses, whereas phenothiazines induce hypothermia even at therapeutic doses. Other drugs that can contribute to hypothermia include general anesthetics and tricyclic antidepressants. The toxic effects of any drug may not be significant while the person is hypothermic but become evident when liver, kidney, and metabolic function increase with rewarming. Interestingly, a combination of alcohol, barbiturates, and hypothermia prolongs brain survival even further than hypothermia alone.[54]

TRAUMA PATIENTS

Trauma victims are especially susceptible to hypothermia. Long delays in response time, extrications, stabilization at the scene, and transportation to the hospital contribute to the development of hypothermia. In addition, cold oxygen and intravenous (IV) fluids, removal of clothing, and continuous evaluations by numerous medical personnel add to the problem. The ability of trauma patients to thermoregulate may be disrupted by hypovolemia or head injuries. Burn patients are at high risk because skin integrity has been interrupted. All trauma victims should have temperature closely monitored.[2,22,28,32]

RECREATIONAL ACTIVITIES

Boaters, campers, sailors, hikers, anglers, mountaineers, and other outdoor people are at risk for hypothermia. Generally, such people are healthy but become victims of the environment, physical exhaustion, or their own carelessness. Outdoor hypothermia is categorized in two groups: immersion and no immersion. Examples of nonimmersion hypothermia include exposure to wind, rain, snow, and freezing temperatures. Immersion hypothermia occurs more rapidly than nonimmersion hypothermia; heat loss is 35% higher if the patient swims or treads water rather than stays still.[17,19] A person with immersion hypothermia may drown sooner because the level of consciousness decreases at 30°C.

CENTRAL NERVOUS SYSTEM DYSFUNCTION

Not only does CNS dysfunction increase susceptibility to hypothermia, but hypothermia also mimics the symptoms of CNS dysfunction. Cerebrovascular accidents are the most common CNS dysfunction to cause hypothermia. The transport team must determine if the patient with suspected cerebrovascular accident is hypothermic. Schizophrenia and senile dementia are occasionally accompanied by hypothermia. Whether hypothermia in these states is a consequence of hypothalamic dysfunction[23,27] or of psychosocial factors, such as homelessness and inattention to potential environmental danger, is unclear.

REWARMING TECHNIQUES[11,12,30,31,38,65]

Expert consensus is that the patient should be rewarmed as quickly as possible because the myocardium is refractory to therapy below 30°C. The three techniques for rewarming are: passive external, active external, and active internal. Only passive external, active external, and limited forms of active internal rewarming can be initiated in the air medical setting. Consequently, rapid transportation to a facility that can provide more extensive rewarming techniques is imperative. Transport personnel must be aware of the existence of these facilities in their service areas.

PASSIVE EXTERNAL REWARMING

Passive external rewarming is simple, inexpensive, and easily instituted. It is used only in mild hypothermia and when the patient can generate heat with shivering and vasoconstriction. The patient is placed in a warm environment, covered with blankets, and allowed to rewarm naturally. Passive external rewarming is available in any transport vehicle with the use of a blanket and a heater. Patients with long-term alcoholism have a lower mortality rate when passive external rewarming is used. Passive external rewarming increases core body temperature by 1°C per hour.[9]

ACTIVE EXTERNAL REWARMING

Active external rewarming involves placement of heat on the external surface of the body. Heated baths, thermal blankets, and packs to the groin, neck, and axilla and forced air devices such as the Bair Hugger are examples of active rewarming. Devices are also available that circulate warm water around the patient's body.

Afterdrop is a dangerous phenomenon that can occur in the initial stages of passive and active external rewarming. *Afterdrop* is defined as a decline of 1°C to 2°C in the core body temperature when cool blood from the extremities moves to the core.[58-62] Any action that moves blood rapidly from the extremities to the heart, including moving the patient or injudiciously applying heat to the periphery, can cause afterdrop and precipitate ventricular fibrillation. Savard et al[49] suggested another possible explanation for the afterdrop phenomenon: the myocardial irritability of afterdrop is caused by a blood chemical shift and not necessarily from a blood temperature shift.

ACTIVE INTERNAL REWARMING

Active internal rewarming delivers heat directly to the body core, thereby avoiding the dangers of afterdrop. The heart, lungs, and brain are warmed first and in turn rewarm of the rest of the body. Heated oxygen, IV fluids, hemodialysis and peritoneal dialysis, gastric lavage, mediastinal lavage (after thoracotomy), and cardiopulmonary bypass are all examples of active internal rewarming. The least invasive method of active internal rewarming is used when the patient has severe hypothermia but a stable cardiovascular condition. On the other hand, the most rapid active internal rewarming methods, such as cardiopulmonary bypass, are recommended if the patient has severe hypothermia and an unstable condition with cardiovascular collapse unresponsive to drugs and defibrillation. The *continuous arteriovenous rewarming* (CAVR) method, developed at the University of Washington, uses a modified bypass technique for rapid blood rewarming with a level one fluid warmer normally used for trauma resuscitation. The treatment is preferred for patients with profound hypothermia. A spontaneous pulse is necessary because the patient's intrinsic blood pressure drives flow through the countercurrent module. (In true cardiothoracic bypass, an external pump is built into the machine.) The catheters are placed into a femoral artery and venous cordis, and the blood is warmed as it flows through the countercurrent module. The CAVR method has rewarmed patients with profound hypothermia five times more rapidly (39 minutes versus 199 minutes) than standard methods and was shown to decrease mortality rate.

MANAGEMENT DURING TRANSPORT

Management of hypothermia has been controversial since Napoleon's chief surgeon, Baron Larrey, noted that hypothermic soldiers closest to the fire were the ones who died.[9] Hypothermia experiments in human subjects can be safely performed only to 35°C, and those in animals are not equivalent because the physiologic response of animals to hypothermia is different from that of humans. Consequently, current medical management of the patient with hypothermia is based mainly on anecdotal reports in the literature.

All patients with hypothermia should be transported, regardless of cardiopulmonary status. Using the old adage "A patient is not dead until warm and dead,"[15,54,55] *warm* is defined as 32°C. Severe hypothermia takes priority over any other problem except obstructed airway or major trauma with rapid exsanguination.

Danzl[9] recommends that preparation for the transport of a patient who is hypothermic include:

- Gentle removal of all wet clothing and application of dry clothing or insulation system.
- Keeping the patient supine and avoiding massaging of extremities.
- Stabilization of all injuries, including application of splints and covering of any open wounds.
- Initiation of intravenous fluids and administration of a fluid challenge.
- Active rewarming during transport, which should include heated oxygen and truncal heat. Any heating pack used should be properly insulated to avoid causing burns to the patient.
- Wrapping the patient in layers with access available to the airway, breathing, and monitoring equipment.

Management of the patient with mild hypothermia is relatively uncomplicated; covering the patient with blankets and allowing the patient to warm naturally prevents further heat loss. Management of the patient with severe hypothermia is more complicated and tests the expertise and knowledge of transport personnel.

GENTLE HANDLING

The patient must be handled gently during transport, and stimulation should be minimized. Any movement, particularly vertical lifting, has been shown to precipitate ventricular fibrillation. Rubbing or massaging the patient is contraindicated. Medical personnel should always cut clothing rather than pull it off. A patient with mild hypothermia must be kept quiet and not be allowed to assist with rescue. Vehicle vibration may also add to stimulation, and the patient should be placed in the vehicle so this can be avoided.

PREVENTION OF FURTHER HEAT LOSS

Prevention of further heat loss is paramount in the management of the patient with hypothermia. Limited exposure during assessment prevents heat loss during examination. The patient's wet clothing should be removed immediately to prevent conductive heat loss. The patient should be removed or protected from any wind source, including helicopter turbulence, which can produce wind up to 100 mph. Insulated and wind proofed blankets should be placed under and over the patient, with the face left exposed and the patient's head protected with a wool hat. An electric blanket is contraindicated because this form of active external rewarming can precipitate afterdrop. The cold railings of the stretcher conduct heat and should not be allowed to touch the patient during transport. Warm oral fluids should be considered for the conscious patient only after assessment for an active gag reflex. Aspiration can be a problem, especially if the size of the transport vehicle does not permit the patient to sit upright or at least at a 45-degree angle. Beverages containing alcohol are contraindicated.

ACTIVE INTERNAL REWARMING

The respiratory tract is a major area of heat exchange and evaporative loss. Administration of warm humidified oxygen effectively rewarms the heart, lungs, and brain by way of the bronchial circulation. In addition, the cilia become more active during rewarming and humidification and can assist in decreasing and mobilizing secretions. Warm humidified oxygen is easy to administer, safe, effective, noninvasive, and readily available in the air medical setting. Mask or bag-valve apparatus at 42°C to 46°C should administer 100% warm humidified oxygen. The rate of rewarming varies from 0.5°C/h to 2.0°C/h[9] to 3.5°C in 20 minutes.[25] A high flow rate is essential for this method to be effective. Core temperature increases an additional 0.3°C/h by increasing ventilatory rate by 10 L/min.[35] McCauley et al,[35] Danzl,[9] and Slovis and Bachvarov[51] have described various commercial products available.

Rehydration of the patient with hypothermia with warm IV fluids increases blood flow to the heart and decreases blood viscosity, vasoconstriction, potential of afterdrop, and the likelihood of cardiac arrhythmias.[9] Patients with hypothermia appear to have a better chance of survival when a bolus of warm IV normal saline solution is given before the patient is moved or externally rewarmed.[9] The transport team should establish an IV line in the largest vein available. If needed, a small amount of heat may be applied to the area to facilitate venous access. The fluid of choice is 5% dextrose in normal saline solution (D5NS) because lactated Ringer's solution is not fully metabolized by the liver in severe hypothermia.[9] D5NS can be made by adding 2 amps of D50 to 900 mL of normal saline solution. An adult patient may be infused with at least 200 mL/h, and the pediatric patient with at least 4 mL/kg/h, with adjustment if the patient needs additional fluid resuscitation. Pulmonary edema, jugular vein distention, and other problems associated with fluid overload are monitored. IV fluids are administered at a temperature of 40°C. Fluids can be warmed en route by wrapping them in a shirt, jacket, towel, or an electric blanket or other commercial warming devices. Some transport vehicles now come with environmental drawers that keep fluids warm during transport.

Monitoring Vital Signs

The patient's rectal temperature, heart rate, and respirations should be monitored carefully and on a regular basis. A special thermometer capable of registering to 20°C is necessary for the patient with hypothermia. An esophageal or tympanic thermometer is preferable, but they are impractical in the transport setting. Danzl[9] noted that rectal temperature lags behind actual core temperature and is influenced by leg temperature and placement of the rectal probe. Volunteers were placed in freezing cold water for 15 minutes, and all the classic signs of hypothermia were noted. However, Danzl discovered the body was able to compensate and core body temperature remained unchanged for at least 15 to 20 minutes; thus, he noted that rectal temperature lags behind actual core temperature and is influenced by leg temperature and placement of the rectal probe.[1,30,31]

Inaccurate assessment of the patient's respirations can lead to improper management and can precipitate life-threatening arrhythmias. The patient must be observed carefully for at least 1 full minute for the presence of respirations to be determined. A spontaneous respiratory rate of 4 to 6 bpm is adequate in hypothermia. An effective cardiac rhythm may be assumed if the patient is breathing spontaneously. Cardiac monitoring may be difficult because of muscle tremors. In fact, baseline oscillations on the ECG may be the only sign that the patient is shivering. Blood pressure may not be obtainable or may be inaccurate because of vasoconstriction. An ultrasound stethoscope may be of use in assessing the presence of a pulse or heartbeat.

Airway

The airway is opened without the use of adjuncts when possible, and intubation is performed only if airway reflexes are absent. Blind nasal intubation may be necessary if trismus is present.[7] The risk of cardiac arrhythmia may be decreased during intubation with preoxygenation and careful technique. Hyperventilation must be avoided because respiratory alkalosis can precipitate ventricular fibrillation. Fewer than 10 bpm successfully oxygenates the patient with hypothermia without causing respiratory alkalosis.[9]

Cardiac Resuscitation

Cardiac resuscitation in the patient with hypothermia is a controversial topic. The main concern is that chest compressions could be initiated on a patient with a slow but viable rhythm. External cardiac massage on a hypothermic bradycardic heart can precipitate ventricular fibrillation. Established ventricular fibrillation or asystole on the heart monitor is the only indication for prehospital CPR of the patient with severe hypothermia.[15] Maximal amplification should be used on the cardiac monitor to detect QRS complexes.

Some investigators believe that chest compressions should be withheld in any patient with a core temperature of less than 28°C.[14] Others believe that chest compressions should be reduced to half the recommended rate because metabolic demands are decreased in the hypothermic brain.[3,8] Strong evidence supporting these deviations from advanced cardiac life support (ACLS) guidelines for CPR is lacking. Although hypothermia does protect the brain from anoxic damage, this "safe period" has not been established, and brain damage occurs after cardiac arrest unless CPR is started.[54,55] Therefore, cardiac compressions should be started according to ACLS guidelines once ventricular fibrillation or asystole is established. If spontaneous respirations are present at any rate, a viable rhythm may be assumed, and CPR may be deferred. Danzl and Pozos[10] proposed that CPR be initiated in all cases except the following: (1) a do-not-resuscitate order is confirmed; (2) obviously lethal injuries are noted; (3) chest-wall compression is impossible; (4) rescuers are jeopardized during evacuation; or (5) signs of life are present. Again, a careful assessment of respirations and pulse for at least 1 full minute is imperative to avoid unnecessary and dangerous CPR.

Defibrillation is usually not effective until core temperature is greater than 28°C.

Pharmacologic Therapy

Little clinical evidence to confirm or rule out the effectiveness or complications of pharmacologic therapy has been noted.[9] Medications should be used with extreme caution. Decreased circulation pools medications in the extremities; a toxic reaction can occur when the patient is rewarmed and medication flows to the core. In light of this possibility, several authors have suggested withholding all medications from the patient with hypothermia.[9] Overzealous correction can precipitate ventricular fibrillation.

Pharmacologic manipulation of pulse, blood pressure, and respiratory rate should be avoided.[9] Medications should not be given orally or intramuscularly because of decreased absorption rates. Other medications should be deferred until the core temperature is 30°C.

Special Considerations

Transport personnel in the management of cold-related emergencies should consider the following principles:

1. Treat major trauma as the first priority and hypothermia as the second.

2. Remove all wet clothing and get the patient in dry blankets as quickly as possible.
3. Notify the receiving facility while en route to the scene, clinic, or hospital to give the receiving facility time to activate appropriate resources.
4. Insert a urinary catheter and gastric tube for long transports.
5. Avoid vasopressors. Consider them only if rewarming shock is unresponsive to fluids.
6. Continue CPR until the patient is rewarmed to 32°C.

DOCUMENTATION

The history of the incident should be documented, including the time and type of exposure, whether the patient was in cardiopulmonary arrest on arrival of the first responder, the management initiated before the arrival of transport personnel, and the heart rhythm, drug therapy, and rewarming techniques. Medical history is important if it is readily available.

Written assessment of the patient with hypothermia consists of a primary and secondary assessment, including all pertinent findings. The vital signs should be monitored and charted on a regular basis, preferably every 10 to 15 minutes, and should include rectal temperature and heart rhythm with strip readout. The patient and the rewarming techniques should be assessed continuously during transport.

SUMMARY

Dry warm blankets or transport blankets should be available in all transport vehicles. In responding to transport a patient with known hypothermia, the team should consider what methods may be needed to warm the patient and keep the patient warm during the transport process.

Expertise of transport personnel is tested when presented with a patient with severe hypothermia. Management requires gentle handling, accurate assessment of cardiopulmonary status, passive external rewarming to prevent further heat loss, and active internal rewarming with heated humidified oxygen and IV fluids.

COLD-RELATED EMERGENCIES CASE STUDY

A 7-year-old male unrestrained passenger was rejected from a vehicle and landed in a river. Paramedics were at the scene when the patient was extricated 1 hour later, and primary assessment revealed no breathing and no carotid or femoral pulse. Spinal protection was initiated, and the patient was gently moved to the ambulance, where CPR and ACLS procedures were initiated immediately. The patient was orally intubated with careful technique, and ventilations were assisted with a bag-valve mask. Two IV lines were started: one in the right jugular vein and one in the right antecubital space. Epinephrine was administered intravenously. Insulated warm packs were placed in the groin and armpits to initiate active external rewarming. A gastric tube was placed, and a small amount of pale yellow liquid was evacuated. Personnel at the scene ordered air medical transport of the patient immediately.

On the arrival of the transport team, reassessment revealed a young male patient (30 kg) lying supine on a backboard in the back of the ambulance; CPR was in progress, the skin was pale and cold to touch, and no capillary refill was noted. The patient was orally intubated, and breath sounds were clear. Good compliance was seen with ventilation. Cardiac monitor displayed pulseless electrical activity rhythm with a rate of 60 to 70 bpm with no associated femoral or carotid pulses. Rectal temperature was 24°C.

Physical examination revealed the following findings.

> *Neurologic: Pupils were fixed and dilated at 8 cm. There was no spontaneous movement of extremities, the child was areflexic, and Glasgow coma scale (GCS) was 3.*
>
> *Head: The head and neck were atraumatic, the nose and ears were clear, and the cervical spine had no palpable deformities. A small amount of pink frothy sputum from the endotracheal tube was seen, and the IV line to the right jugular vein was patent and secure.*
>
> *Chest: Breath sounds were equal, with scattered rales. The chest wall was intact with no visible trauma.*

> *Abdomen: The abdomen was distended and tense. Nasogastric tube placement was confirmed and secured.*
>
> *Extremities: The long bones were grossly intact, and IV access to right antecubital was patent and secure.*

The patient was gently loaded into the helicopter during continuing CPR and assisted ventilations. The pilot radioed to alert the emergency department of the patient's condition and requested the hypothermia team to remain on standby. In flight, the patient was managed in the following manner:

1. *Continuous reassessment of condition.*
2. *Continued CPR and assisted ventilations.*
3. *Warm humidified oxygen administered via bag-valve mask.*
4. *Warm IV fluid provided at a keep-vein-open rate.*
5. *Blankets added to prevent further heat loss.*
6. *Gastric tube to suction.*
7. *Cervical spine protection.*
8. *One additional dose of intravenous epinephrine.*

During the flight, the patient's condition remained clinically unchanged. Agonal respirations were noted toward the end of the flight. Rectal temperature rose to 28°C.

On arrival at the emergency department, the patient had a blood pressure of 98/60 mm Hg, with agonal respirations. Rectal temperature was 30°C. An increase in pink frothy sputum from the endotracheal tube was noted, and 3 cm of positive end expiratory pressure (PEEP) was added to the ventilator. A dopamine drip was started via pump at 16.6 μg/kg/min to maintain a systolic blood pressure between 90 and 100 mm Hg. All fluids were placed on IV warmers. The heart monitor displayed sinus tachycardia with palpable femoral and brachial pulses. Peritoneal lavage was started with warmed normal saline solution as a check for abdominal bleeding and to initiate active internal rewarming.

Initially, arterial blood gas (ABG) values (adjusted for rectal temperature) were pH 7.13, PCO_2 32, PO_2 50, actual HCO_3 11, base deficit 20, O_2 calculated 91, O_2 actual 89, K 2.9. Sodium 10 mEq was given along with potassium chloride 10 mEq IV. Peritoneal lavage was negative for blood. Chest radiography revealed right pneu-

mothorax, which was treated with a chest tube. Computed tomographic results of the head and neck were negative. The patient was transported to the critical care unit in fairly stable condition.

In the critical care unit, the patient was maintained on the ventilator with warm humidified oxygen. The dopamine drip was continued to maintain a stable blood pressure between 90 and 100 mm Hg systolic. The patient was placed between hypothermia blankets. The pupils remained fixed and dilated at 8 cm; no corneal reflex was present. There was slight spontaneous flailing of all extremities. ABGs were stabilized throughout the evening with small doses of sodium bicarbonate. The patient's blood pressure was stabilized with 18 μg/ kg/min dopamine. Rectal temperature increased slowly, finally stabilizing at 37°C. Four hours after admission to the intensive care unit, the patient had sudden deoxygenation, with the heart monitor displaying bradycardia. The patient's rhythm quickly deteriorated to ventricular fibrillation, and a cardiac arrest situation was called. Unfortunately, efforts failed, and the patient was pronounced dead after 1 hour of aggressive resuscitation.

REFERENCES

1. Antretter H, Muller LC, Cottogni M, et al: Successful resuscitation in severe hypothermia following near drowning, *Dtsch Med Wochenschr* 119(23):837-840, 1994.
2. Arthurs Z, Cuadrado D, Beekley A, et al: The impact of hypothermia on trauma care at the 31st combat support hospital, *Am J Surg* 191:610-614, 2006.
3. Bolte RG, Black PG, Bowers RS, et al: The use of extracorpeal rewarming in a child submerged for 66 minutes, *JAMA* 15(3):377-379, 1988.
4. Butler FK, Zafren K: Tactical management of wilderness casualties in special operations, *Wilder Environ Med* 9:64, 1998.
5. Caroline NL: *Emergency care in the streets*, ed 2, Boston, 1983, Little, Brown.
6. Cauchy E, Chetaille E, Marchand V, et al: Retrospective study of 70 cases of severe frostbite lesions: a proposed new classification scheme, *Wilder Environ Med* 12:248, 2001.
7. Crawshaw LI, Wallace H, Dasgupta S: Thermoregulation. In Auerbach P, editor: *Wilderness medicine*, ed 5, St Louis, 2007, Mosby.
8. Collins KJ: *Hypothermia: the facts*, New York, 1983, Oxford University Press.
9. Danzl D: Accidental hypothermia. In Auerbach P, editor: *Wilderness medicine*, ed 5, St Louis, 2007, Mosby.
10. Danzl DF, Pozos RS: Multicenter hypothermia survey, *Ann Emerg Med* 16(9):1042, 1987.
11. Davies DM, Miller EJ, Miller IA: Accidental hypothermia treated by extracorporeal blood-warming, *Lancet* 1036:May 13, 1967.
12. Dobson JAR, Burgess JJ: Resuscitation of severe hypothermia by extracorporeal rewarming in a child, *J Trauma* 40(3):483-485, 1996.
13. Ehrmantraut WR, Ticktin HE, Fazekras JF: Cerebral hemodynamics and metabolism in accidental hypothermia, *Arch Intern Med* 99:57, 1957.
14. Frakes M, Duquette L: Body temperature preservation in patients transported by air medical helicopter, *Air Med J* 27(1):37-39, 2008.
15. Giesbrecht GG: Prehospital treatment of hypothermia, *Wilder Environ Med* 12:24-31, 2001.
16. Giesbrecht G, Steinman A: Immersion in cold water. In Auerbach P, editor: *Wilderness medicine*, ed 5, St Louis, 2007, Mosby Elsevier.
17. Golden FS, Tipton MJ, Scott RC. Immersion, near-drowning and drowning, *Br J Anaesth* 79:214-225, 1997.
18. Golden FS, Hervey GR, Tipton MJ Jr: Circum-rescue collapse: collapse, sometimes fatal, associated with rescue of immersion victims, *Nav Med Serv* 77(3):139-149, 1999.
19. Golden F, Tipton M: *Essentials of sea survival*, Champaign, IL, 2002, Human.
20. Gordon AS: Cerebral blood flow and temperature during deep hypothermia for cardiovascular surgery, *J Cardiovasc Surg* 3:299, 1962.
21. Graham CA, McNaughton GW, Wyatt J: The electrocardiogram in hypothermia, *Wilder Environ Med* 12:232-235, 2001.
22. Gregory J, Flanbaum I, Townsend M: Incidence and timing of hypothermia in trauma patients, *J Trauma* 31:795, 1991.
23. Gregory RT, Patton JF: Treatment after exposure to cold, *Lancet* 1:377, 1972.
24. Hattfield ML, Lang AM, Han ZQ, et al: The effect of helicopter transport on adult patient's body temperature, *Air Med J* 18(3):103-106, 1999.
25. Hauty M, Esrig B, Long W: Prognostic factors in severe accidental hypothermia: experience from the Mt. Hood tragedy, *J Trauma* 27:1107, 1987.
26. International Commission of Alpine Rescue, Subcommission of Medicine: *Field and base treatment of cold injuries*, Presented at the Fifth International

Symposium on Mountain Medicine, Innsbruck, Austria, November 13, 1976.

27. Jolly T, Ghezzi K: Accidental hypothermia, *Emerg Med Clin North Am* 10(2):311, 1992.

28. Jurkovich G, Gaser W, Luterman A: Hypothermia in trauma victims: an ominous sign, *J Trauma* 27:1019, 1987.

29. Knowlton FP, Starling EH: The influence of variations in temperatures and blood pressure on the performance of the isolated mammalian heart, *J Physiol* 44:206, 1912.

30. Lloyd EL: Accidental hypothermia treated by central rewarming through the airway, *Br J Anaesth* 45:41, 1973.

31. Lloyd EL, Frankland JC: Accidental hypothermia: central rewarming in the field (correspondence), *Br Med J* 4:717, 1974.

32. Luna G, Maier R, Pavlin E: Incidence and effect of hypothermia in seriously injured patients, *J Trauma* 27:1014, 1987.

33. Lunardi N: Case review: ED management of hypothermia in an elderly woman, *Austral Emerg Nurs J* 8:165-171, 2006.

34. McAniff JJ: *The incidence of hypothermia in scuba-diving fatalities*, First International Hypothermia Conference, Kingston, Jamaica, January 23-27, 1980.

35. McCauley RL, Killyon GW, Smith DJ, et al: Frostbite. In Auerbach P, editor: *Wilderness medicine*, ed 5, St Louis, 2007, Mosby Eslevier.

36. Miller JW, Danzl DF, Thomas DM: Urban accidental hypothermia: 135 cases, *Ann Emerg Med* 9:456, 1980.

37. Mills WJ, Whaley R: Frostbite: experience with rapid rewarming and ultrasonic therapy, reprinted in *Lessons from History Wilderness and Environmental Medicine* 9:226, 1998.

38. Morrison JB, Conn ML, Hayward JS: Thermal increment provided by inhalation rewarming from hypothermia, *J Appl Physiol* 46:1061, 1979.

39. Okada M: The cardiac rhythm in accidental hypothermia, *J Electrocardiol* 17:123, 1984.

40. Okada M, Nishimura F, Yoshiro H: The J-wave in accidental hypothermia, *J Electrocardiol* 16:23, 1983.

41. O'Keefe KM: Accidental hypothermia: a review of 62 cases, *JACEP* 6:491, 1977.

42. Orr KD, Fainer DC: *Cold injuries in Korea during winter of 1950–1951*, Fort Knox, KY, 1951, US Army Medical Research Laboratory.

43. Proehl J: Environmental emergencies. In Kitt S, et al, editors: *Emergency nursing*, Philadelphia, 1995, Saunders.

44. Purdue GF, Hunt JL: Cold injury: a collective review, *J Burn Care Rehabil* 7(4):331, 1986.

45. Rango N: Exposure-related hypothermia mortality in the United States, 1970-1979, *Am J Public Health* 74:1159, 1984.

46. Rango N: Old and cold: hypothermia in the elderly, *Geriatrics* 35(11):93, 1980.

47. Rankin AC, Rae AP: Cardiac arrhythmias during rewarming of patients with accidental hypothermia, *Br Med J* 289:874, 1984.

48. Reuler JB: Hypothermia: pathophysiology, clinical settings and management, *Ann Intern Med* 89:519, 1978.

49. Savard GK, et al: Peripheral blood flow during rewarming from mild hypothermia in humans, *J Appl Physiol* 58:4, 1985.

50. Scime A, Grenier G, Huh MS, et al: Rb and p107 regulate preadipocyte differentiation into white versus brown fat through repression of PGC-1, *J Cell Metabolism* 1(5):283-295, 2005.

51. Slovis CM, Bachvarov HL: Heated inhalation treatment of hypothermia, *Am J Emerg Med* 2:533, 1984.

52. Smith DS: Accidental hypothermia: giving "dead" victims the benefit of the doubt, *Postgrad Med* 81(3):38, 1987.

53. Smith DS: *The cold water connection*, First International Hypothermia Conference, Kingston, Jamaica, January 23-27, 1980.

54. Steinman AM: The hypothermic code: CPR controversy revisited, *JEMS* 8(10):32, 1983.

55. Steinmann S, Shackford S, Davis J: Implications of admission hypothermia in trauma patients, *J Trauma* 30:200, 1990.

56. Tek D, Mackey S: Non-freezing cold injury in a marine infantry battalion, *J Wilderness Med* 4:353, 1993.

57. Tolman KG, Cohen A: Accidental hypothermia, *Can Med Assoc J* 103:1357, 1970.

58. Toner MM, McArdle WD: Human thermoregulartory response to acute cold stress with special reference to water immersion. In Fregly MJ, Blatteis CM, editors: *Handbook of physiology*, New York, 1996, Oxford University Press.

59. United States Coast Guard Station, Hypothermia, UCN 0075, New York, April 5, 1982.

60. Vaughn PB: Local cold injury-menace to military operations: a review, *Milit Med* 145:305, 1980.

61. Weast RC, editor: *Handbook of chemistry and physics*, ed 55, Cleveland, 1974, CRC Press.

62. Wilkerson JA, Bangs CC, Hayward JS: *Hypothermia, frostbite and other cold injuries*, Seattle, 1986, Mountaineers.

63. Wilson FN, Finch R: The effect of drinking iced water upon the form of the T deflection of the electrocardiogram, *Heart* 10:275, 1923.

64. White JD: Hypothermia: the Bellevue experience, *Ann Emerg Med* 11:417, 1982.

65. York-Clark D, Stocking J, Johnson J, editors: *Flight and ground transport nursing core curriculum*, ed 2, Denver, 2006, Air and Surface Transport Nurses Association.

HEAT-RELATED EMERGENCIES

Reneé Semonin Holleran

COMPETENCIES

1. Identify risk factors that contribute to heat-related illnesses.
2. Identify the different types of heat-related illnesses, including heat exhaustion and heatstroke.
3. Initiate the appropriate management of a heat-related illness in the transport environment.

Deaths attributed to heat-related illnesses have been reported for centuries. The Bible refers to persons who had heatstroke after working in hot fields 2000 years ago. In 24 BC, a Roman army was annihilated in the heat of the Arabian desert. The warriors of the Crusades were ultimately beaten in the Holy Land by heat and fever.[20] Incarceration in the infamous "Black Hole of Calcutta" resulted in high numbers of heat-related deaths.[9] During the summers of 1980, 1983, 1988, and 1995, severe heat waves in the United States resulted in multiple deaths from heatstroke.[4,6] Recent data related to heat illness have been obtained from pilgrims in Mecca, Saudi Arabia, in 1984 and 1985,[20,33] and military experience has provided extensive data on heat illness and the effect of heat on human physiology.[22] In Europe in the summer of 2003, 52,000 deaths were reported from heatstroke.[7]

Heatstroke is a true medical emergency that requires rapid diagnosis and treatment. The longer the body remains hyperthermic, the greater the damage and consequent increase in morbidity and mortality. The transport team, with quick recognition and immediate treatment of the heat illness, can do much to combat permanent organ damage and the sequelae of hyperthermia.[9,10]

INCIDENCE AND CAUSATIVE FACTORS

The very young and the elderly are at greatest risk of affliction with heat-related illness. Moderate forms of heat-related illness can cause discomfort but are of relatively short duration, with rare sequelae. Heat exhaustion and heatstroke are the two serious pathologic states of heat illness.

Even in relatively mild weather, heat illness can affect persons with predisposing risk factors; it can also affect persons who are unconditioned or not acclimatized and then pushed rapidly beyond their tolerance or physical capability, as can happen in military "boot camp" and with novice joggers. Even well-conditioned athletes are subject to heat illness if they are not properly acclimatized. Heat illness is second only to head injuries as a cause of death of US athletes.[4,5,8,9,20,21,23,25,30]

The mortality and morbidity statistics for heat illness do not reflect the true impact of this illness on the civilian population. Civilian statistics can be inferred from military experience. Records show that heat exhaustion affects 280 of 100,000 military recruits who undergo basic training in South Carolina.[21,26]

Many times, death from heatstroke goes unrecorded during heat waves. The patient often has an underlying cardiovascular, pulmonary, renal, or neurologic disease. During heat waves, deaths from myocardial infarction, pneumonia, kidney failure, and stroke climb sharply; these conditions are then recorded as the cause of death. The estimate of heat illness is postulated to be a dramatic underrepresentation of the true magnitude of this problem.[7,34]

Infants have a relatively small surface area for dissipation of heat. Parents often prevent heat loss by wrapping infants in blankets and clothing that are too heavy for a hot environment. The thermoregulatory ability of children lags behind other body systems in maturity and functional ability. Therefore, children are more predisposed to heat illness, and recognition and diagnosis of heat pathology are often made more difficult.[3,9,31]

Heat illness can develop in elderly persons under conditions that do not generally affect younger persons. As a person's age increases, physiologic ability to regulate temperature decreases. Older persons often do not notice temperature changes less than 2.3°C, probably because of sensory afferent deterioration.[17] The elderly population generally has a higher rate of cardiovascular and pulmonary disease, diabetes, and neurologic pathology, and they often take multiple medications. All of these conditions contribute to the increased likelihood of heat illness in persons in this age group.

Obese individuals also have a higher risk of heat illness. Heat loss is inversely proportional to body size and body weight. Adipose tissue has less ability to lose heat compared with nonadipose tissue because of decreased vascularity. Fat serves as an insulator, which is not conducive to heat loss.

Dehydration occurs because of a decrease in body water. As heat illness progresses, the circulatory blood volume decreases. When heat illness is superimposed on preexisting dehydration, the body has a severely limited volume reserve. The more severe the dehydration, the faster the physiologic compensation is exhausted. Fluid intake is crucial for the prevention of heat illness.

An increased endogenous heat load limits the body's ability to maintain normothermia in a hot environment. A classic endogenous heat source is fever. Fever is generally caused by pyrogens released from bacteria or viruses or by breakdown of cells caused by the infectious organism.

Two different mechanisms are involved in fever and heat illness. With fever, the thermal set point is elevated because of the induction of prostaglandin synthesis in the thermoregulatory center. Certain medications such as salicylates work well to inhibit the reactions that lead to elevation of the thermal set point and thus relieve hyperthermia caused by fever. With heat illness, the thermal set point remains normal. Hyperthermia occurs because of the body's inability to dissipate heat; normal defense mechanisms designed to protect the set point are overwhelmed. The medications used for fever medication do not work well in this setting and should not be used.[9-11,18]

Hyperactive states demand more energy. The increasing energy demand is met by an increase in metabolic activity. Endogenous heat increases as a byproduct of the increased metabolic rate. Strenuous physical exercise and seizures are examples of hyperactive states. Drugs can also lead to a hyperactive state and increase endogenous heat production.

Muscular exertion increases endogenous heat because of increased metabolic demand. Skeletal muscle is one of the major sources of heat production in the body. Muscular exertion often occurs outdoors under conditions in which the ambient temperature exceeds body temperature and high humidity is present. Hyperthermia can occur in this setting. "Weekend warriors," novice hard laborers, military inductees in physical training, football players who practice in the heat, and persons who use hot tubs unwisely can all predispose their bodies to heat illness.

Use of many prescription drugs and alcohol can also predispose a person to heat illness. Anticholinergic drugs reduce sweat gland secretions because of the blocking action of anticholinergics on transmission of sympathetic postganglionic nerve impulses to sweat glands. This cessation of sweating removes the body's chief agent of heat dissipation. Use of tricyclic antidepressants, phenothiazines, butyrophenones, thiothixenes, diuretics, and beta-blockers predispose the patient to heat illness.[9,18,21,30]

Other drugs associated with hyperthermia are glutethimide, those that induce hypersensitivity or idiosyncratic reactions (antibiotics, anticonvulsants, and hypertensives), and those that induce direct pyrogenic stimulation (bleomycin).[6,9,18,20,22]

Psychiatric patients often take anticholinergic drugs. Lithium and haloperidol have been reported to cause fatal hyperthermia. Haloperidol may reduce awareness or recognition of thirst.[16] Thioridazine (Mellaril) overdose is documented to cause hyperthermia.[8,13,16] The interaction of monoamine oxidase inhibitors with amphetamines, tricyclic antidepressants, or phenothiazines is a well-documented cause of hyperthermia. Psychiatric patients may lack the awareness or desire to care for themselves properly in hot environments.

Alcohol use is known to predispose most persons to heat illness.[18,30] The exact mechanisms of this phenomenon are complex. Alcohol is a vasodilator and may enhance external heat absorption. Use of alcohol interferes with the judgment and mental acuity necessary to care for oneself. Use of cocaine and lysergic acid diethylamide (LSD) has also been documented to cause fatal hyperthermia.[8,14]

One of the major organs that must be functional if heat is to be dissipated is the skin. Any pathologic process that disrupts skin integrity interrupts normal physiologic functions, or both conditions sharply limit heat dissipation. Sunburn and heat rash are relatively minor conditions that can have a drastic impact on physiologic compensation for heat stress. Major burns cause partial to total loss of skin function. Lack of ability to regulate body temperature is a complication of burn injury. Obviously, the burn victim may be a candidate for heat illness.[22]

Heat loss from the body occurs primarily through the evaporation of sweat. However, sweat trapped near the body in undergarments and below heavy clothing cannot evaporate because of lack of air circulation. Although adequate hydration ensures that you sweat enough, the mechanism is thwarted by saturated clothing. Differential humidity also plays a factor. In low humidity conditions, sweat evaporates readily. In people without adequate acclimatization, sweat production actually declines if the skin is wet, further blunting these cooling mechanisms.[32]

Patients with cystic fibrosis have a striking elevation of sweat electrolytes; the sodium and chloride content of their sweat is two to five times greater than that of healthy control subjects, and this occurs in 98% to 99% of affected children. These children are subject to massive sodium depletion in hot weather. Today, because of improved early diagnostic measures and treatment, many more patients with cystic fibrosis are living into early adulthood.

Lack of acclimatization predisposes a person to heat illness. On entering a warmer climate, exercise and general activity levels must be gradually increased. Persons vacationing in warm climates often overexert. Even well-conditioned athletes can be affected by heat-related illness if their training programs do not allow sufficient acclimatization before vigorous physical activity in hot humid weather.

Persons can become acclimated to a hot climate in 10 days with daily exposure to moderate work and heat.[8,14] With a less zealous routine, acclimatization occurs in several weeks. The recognition of the principle of acclimatization has led to a reduction of the incidence rate of heat illness for those who are exposed to hot or high-risk environments. Acclimatization can occur at any age; however, its effectiveness can be limited by any of the aforementioned predisposing factors. Recent experience in the Middle East has shown that full acclimatization can take several months and requires deliberate planning and varied work/rest/heat exposure schedules that initially avoid any activity during normal (daytime) work hours. Two different combat brigades using the traditional and the extended acclimatization strategies had 10% heat casualties and 0%, respectively.[32]

The most important physiologic adaptations during the acclimatization period include retention of salt and water, expansion of extracellular fluid volumes, and slight hemodilution.[8,15] Through these processes, sweating mechanisms improve. This improvement is characterized by early onset of sweating, an increase in the volume of sweat, and a lowering of electrolyte concentration in the sweat.[10,18,31-33]

The increase in the volume of sweat accompanied by a lowering of the threshold for the onset of sweating results in better heat dissipation. An increase in aldosterone production lowers the sodium content of sweat. Combined with a 7% increase in total body water, the increase in aldosterone lowers sodium content of sweat from 100 mEq/L to 70 mEq/L.[1] The chloride concentration in sweat falls from 40 or 45 mEq/L to as low as 15 or 20 mEq/L, and sweat volume rises from 1 to 3 L/h.[9,14]

After acclimatization, cardiovascular and metabolic proficiency is improved. Vasodilation occurs earlier and in greater magnitude. The heart rate is lower with a higher stroke volume, thus increasing cardiac output. Biochemical efficiency at the cellular level improves to the point that heat production for a given amount of work is less than in a person who is not acclimatized. Storage and utilization of glycogen are improved, which delays the onset of anaerobic metabolism with resultant lactic acidosis.

PATHOPHYSIOLOGIC FACTORS

NORMAL THERMOGENESIS

Human core temperature is closely regulated by a number of mechanisms to maintain a body core temperature of between 36°C and 38°C. Processes that alter temperature homeostasis result in pathologic changes at the cellular level. Rising body temperature, if unregulated, can exceed the critical thermal maximum and cause irreversible organ damage; death quickly ensues. The human thermal maximum is well documented to be 43°C.

Body core temperature is a species-specific genetically determined set point that is regulated by the hypothalamus. Temperature regulation is quite precise, with response to temperature changes as small as 0.2°C (1.6°F).[32] A "thermostat" in the pre-optic anterior portion of the hypothalamus receives information from various body thermoregulators. Peripheral and core temperature sensors in the skin, viscera, and nervous system tissues produce both thermal and endocrine signals. These signals are transmitted to the hypothalamus via neuronal and circulatory pathways. The thermostat then responds through a variety of negative feedback mechanisms to activate processes by which heat is lost or gained. These responses are mediated by means of the sympathetic nervous system.

Body heat production occurs because of two separate processes: endogenous metabolic processes and exogenous environmental exposure. Close regulation of body temperature is critical because the human body is dependent on relatively low temperature biochemical reactions at the microcellular level to sustain life.

Every body process produces exothermic heat. Normal basal cellular metabolism generates 50 to 60 kcal/h and causes a rise of 1°C/h if not dissipated by compensatory mechanisms.[10] Digestion of food is the source of body heat. Major heat-producing organs are the liver and skeletal muscle. Increasing bodywork raises body temperature. Maximal sustained exercise produces 600 to 900 kcal/h, which raises body core temperature 5°C/h without functional compensatory mechanisms.[25]

Exogenous (external) heat comes from the environment. Exposure to direct sunlight raises body core temperature 150 kcal/h. The amount of humidity present in the air directly affects the body's ability to disperse heat. Humidity limits cooling via evaporation, which is caused by a lack of an evaporation gradient from skin surface to air.

METHODS OF HEAT LOSS

Thermoregulation by the hypothalamus maintains normothermia by balancing heat production and heat loss. When thermoregulation breaks down because of excess heat generation (endogenous), inability to dissipate heat (pathophysiologic), overwhelming environmental conditions (high ambient temperature with high humidity), or a combination of these factors, hyperthermia results. Under normal conditions, 90% of the heat produced by the body is lost to the environment via the skin surface by conduction, radiation, convection, and evaporation.

Environmental temperature obviously has a direct effect on the patient. The higher the temperature, the more external heat is present. When the environmental temperature is equal to or greater than the body's temperature, passive heat loss through the means of conduction and radiation is decreased. *Radiant heat loss* occurs when the ambient temperature is lower than the body's temperature; conversely, the body readily absorbs radiant heat from the environment.

When air or water moves across the body surface, heat is lost via *convection*. An increase in the amount of air moving over the skin (forced convection) increases the amount of heat loss. The drier the air, the better the skin surface-to-air gradient, and the more heat that is lost.

The primary mechanism for heat dissipation is the *evaporation* of sweat. Through vaporization from the body surface, loss of 1 mL of sweat reduces body heat load by 1.7 kcal.[8,14,15,18,23,26,28] Under conditions of high ambient temperature and high ambient humidity, the skin is unable to provide effective cooling as the evaporation gradient is lost. At 75% humidity, evaporation decreases; at 90% to 95% humidity, evaporation ceases.[8]

The average person can produce up to 1.5 L of sweat per hour. Through conditioning and acclimatization, sweat production increases. The well-trained athlete can produce up to 3 L/h.[8,21,26]

Insensible heat loss also occurs; heat is lost with passage of urine and feces, and the respiratory tract can dissipate heat via convection and evaporation.

PHYSIOLOGIC COMPENSATION

Physiologic compensation begins in the hypothalamus. The exact chemical nature of thermoregulation is not yet fully understood. As endocrine and thermal sensors arrive from the heated periphery and core, the hypothalamic thermostat reduces bioamine concentrations. Final common pathway effectors probably include prostaglandins, central nervous system amines, and a host of other hypothesized candidates.[10,30]

On reception of effector "messages" from the hypothalamus and peripheral thermoreceptors, the cardiovascular system responds with peripheral vasodilation. Vasodilation maximizes the cooling surface and greatly decreases peripheral vascular resistance. In this manner, the cardiovasculature conducts heat to the surface of the body, where it can be released to the environment. When skin vessels dilate, blood flow shunted through the area can exceed 4 L/min.[9,18] With this increased flow, 97% of cooling occurs at the skin surface.[23]

HEAT PATHOPHYSIOLOGY

The initial response to heatstroke begins on a cellular level. Subcellular disruption directly causes cell destruction. Hypothermia also initiates apoptosis or programmed cellular destruction. The cells that produce the greatest number of apoptotic cells from hypothermia are the thymus, spleen, lymph nodes, and mucosa of the small intestine.[10]

On exposure to heat, the body initiates compensation by decreasing peripheral vascular resistance, thus shunting blood to the periphery. This action causes an increase in stroke volume and cardiac output, which increases demand on the heart. The healthy cardiovascular system can sustain this hyperdynamic state for a limited time; however, it eventually taxes the myocardium.

The purpose of this response is to cool the body. Heat is lost from the skin surface via evaporation of sweat. In severe heat stress, the body loses as much as 1.5 L/h, and even 3 L/h in extreme cases.[9,30] Over time, the circulating blood volume is reduced.

The cardiac output continues to drop as a result of the ensuing hypovolemia. Homeostasis becomes compromised. An altered hemodynamic state may develop that mimics high-output failure, such as that seen in sepsis. This results in hyperdynamic failure. In persons with heatstroke, structural damage to the heart is common, although not extensive. Rarely, acute transmural myocardial infarction or widespread myocardial damage may occur.[9,30]

Cardiac dysrhythmia and myocardial damage may occur because of subendocardial hemorrhage, rupture of muscle fibers, necrosis, and infarction. This pathology is second to increased cardiac workload and thereby increases myocardial oxygen demand. Not enough oxygen is available because of disruption of oxidative phosphorylation and a resulting shock state. Hypotension is usually a sign of severe or premorbid heat illness.[9,30]

The respiratory system initially responds with an increase in respiratory rate and depth to meet increased oxygen demand. This hyperventilation results in an initial heat loss from an increased volume of air moved over and through the respiratory tract. This evaporative loss decreases with increased respiratory fatigue. A high ambient humidity also limits this evaporative loss. An initial respiratory alkalosis develops as a result of the hyperventilation, with concurrent hypocarbia and the traditional muscle tetany. This tetany is the pathophysiologic basis for the ill-defined syndrome of heat tetany.

Ataxia, dysmetria, and dysarthria may be seen early in the onset of heatstroke because the Purkinje's cells of the cerebellum are particularly sensitive to the toxic effects of high temperature. Because these changes are seen in other neurologic events, such as stroke, heatstroke may not be recognized initially. Cerebral edema combined with associated diffuse petechial hemorrhages is often found in fatal cases.

When the hyperthermic insult is associated with status epilepticus and profound hypotension, the energy requirements of the brain increase. This in turn contributes to the spiraling core temperature, increasing up to four times the metabolic rate of the brain. The cerebral vessels dilate maximally, and thus, the blood flow is dependent on mean arterial pressure. The added effects of dehydration (hypovolemic source) produce a pathophysiologic state conducive to brain death and damage.

Kidney function is altered from the loss of sodium and water in sweat. The kidneys retain sodium, and thus, they retain water and excrete potassium. Renal dysfunction occurs because of hypovolemia and hypoperfusion. Urinary output drops, and acute renal tubular necrosis may ensue. If sodium losses are of sufficient severity, signs of hyponatremia may appear. A risk hypokalemia may develop because of the excretion of potassium in the urine.

The liver, which is particularly sensitive to temperature damage, is affected in nearly every case.[10,13] Liver function decreases by 20%. This decrease in function theoretically should aid in heat reduction because the liver is one of the major heat-producing organs. Prothrombin times become prolonged.[2,28] Reduced hepatic perfusion caused by shunting of blood to the periphery leads to hypoglycemia in 20% of patients with exertional heatstroke.[4,19] Interestingly, the pancreas is the only organ not damaged by the toxic effects of heat stress.[9]

During heat stress, the gastrointestinal tract undergoes direct thermotoxicity and relative hypoperfusion because of the shunt of blood to the periphery. Ischemic intestinal ulceration can also occur, which may lead to frank gastrointestinal bleeding.[9]

Muscle damage is evidenced by rhabdomyolysis. Muscle degeneration and necrosis occur as a direct result of extremely elevated temperature. Elevated creatine phosphokinase (CPK) values are a diagnostic hallmark of heatstroke because of this rhabdomyolytic process. The release of destructive lysosomal enzymes occurs as a result of extensive skeletal muscle damage. The release of lysosomal enzymes into the circulation may cause widespread capillary injury and lead to disseminated intravascular coagulation, acute respiratory distress syndrome, and acute renal tubular necrosis.[19] Muscle enzymes are greatly elevated.

ASSESSMENT PARAMETERS

The most common forms of heat illness, from least to most severe, are heat cramps, heat exhaustion, and heatstroke.

HEAT CRAMPS

Heat cramps of heavily exercised muscle occur during and after exercise in a hot environment and are an extreme inconvenience to the patient. These cramps usually occur in trained athletes and in physically fit, acclimatized persons. These persons sweat profusely and characteristically replace sweat losses with water and inadequate amounts of salt.

Hyponatremia ensues, which hinders muscle relaxation mechanisms. Usually, the muscles show the fasciculations of fatigue. A slight or moderate rise in CPK enzymes in serum is often observed. This rhabdomyolysis has not been shown to constitute an important clinical problem.[4,18,30] No permanent effects have been shown from heat cramps.

Heat cramps involve exquisitely painful sustained muscular contractions, most commonly involving the muscles of the lower extremity; however, any muscle group in the body can be affected. The patient usually reports heavy exercise in a hot environment, with onset of cramping after rest.

HEAT EXHAUSTION

Heat exhaustion is an ill-defined syndrome that can affect anyone. The brain cannot tolerate core temperatures greater than 40.5°C (104. 9°F).[18] The typical victim of heat exhaustion is usually not acclimatized to the environment and has worked in the heat for several days. Both infants and elderly bedridden patients are at higher risk of heat exhaustion because of their impaired ability to dissipate heat and communicate thirst.

Heat exhaustion, if allowed to proceed, results in heatstroke. An essential distinction between the two entities is that cerebral function is unimpaired in persons with heat exhaustion, aside from minor irritability and poor judgment. Body temperatures are lower, and the symptoms are less severe in persons with heat exhaustion.

This syndrome results from loss of water, loss of salt, or both. Pure forms of single loss of either water or sodium are rare. Water-depletion heat exhaustion, which results from inadequate fluid replacement, is more serious and develops in a few hours. Salt-depletion heat exhaustion develops over the course of several days.

Heat exhaustion is largely a manifestation of the strain placed on the cardiovascular system as it attempts to maintain normothermia. With sodium and water loss, the patient becomes dehydrated, tachycardic, and syncopal, with orthostatic hypotension. The patient's temperature is usually less than 38°C to 39°C (100.4°F to 102.2°F) and is often normal. The patient retains the ability to sweat, which gives rise to cool clammy skin. Headache and euphoria commonly occur because of dehydration and hypoperfusion. Mental status remains intact, although minor aberrations may be manifested. Flulike symptoms of nausea, vomiting, and diarrhea with muscle cramps may be present. Subjective symptoms include intense thirst, vague malaise, myalgia, and dizziness.

Laboratory values show classic signs of dehydration (elevated hematocrit, blood urea nitrogen [BUN], serum protein, and concentrated urine levels) with hyponatremia and hypokalemia. Liver function enzymes may be elevated. However, these signs may not occur until 24 to 48 hours after the heat injury.[8,18,30]

HEATSTROKE

Heatstroke is a life-threatening medical emergency in which the body's physiologic heat-dissipating mechanisms fail and body temperature rises rapidly and uncontrollably. The central core temperature exceeds 42°C. At 42°C and above, cellular oxygen demands surpass the oxygen supply, and oxidative phosphorylation is disrupted, which causes cell and organ damage throughout the body. The duration of the hyperthermic episode and the temperature reached may be the single most important factors in patient survival and prognosis.

The resultant damage of such severe hyperthermia has many causes. Central nervous system disruption with altered mental status is a key diagnostic criterion in heatstroke. Early in the course of heatstroke, some persons appear confused and show irrational behavior, or even frank psychosis; others become comatose or have seizures. The patient may have hot flushed skin, with or without sweating, vomiting, and diarrhea. Hyperventilation at rates up to 60 is universally seen. Respiratory alkalosis is often present with tetany and hypokalemia. Pulmonary edema is not uncommon.

The cardiovascular system responds by reaching maximal stroke volume. Because of the shunt through the dilated periphery, tachycardia is the only way to increase cardiac output. Heatstroke results in high output failure, with cardiac output of 20 L or more. Central venous pressure readings are elevated despite hypotension caused by decreased ventricular contractility over 40°C. The hyperdynamic state persists even after cooling. The electrocardiographic (ECG) results generally shows nonspecific ST-T changes with various atrial and ventricular arrhythmias.[10,29,31]

Blood studies should include arterial blood gas, complete blood cell count, platelets, prothrombin time/partial thromboplastin time (PT/PTT), electrolytes, BUN, creatinine, glucose, liver function tests (LVT), CPK, and LDH, and a urinalysis. White blood counts of 30,000 to 50,000 are not uncommon. The platelet count and PT/PTT are monitored for onset of hypocoagulability. Hypofibrinogenemia and fibrinolysis may occur and progress to frank disseminated intravascular coagulation (DIC).

The muscle enzymes in heatstroke are elevated in the tens of thousands—a diagnostic hallmark of heatstroke. Muscle breakdown occurs from direct thermal injury, clonic muscle activity, or tissue ischemia. In exertional heatstroke, CPK levels up to 1,500,000 IU/L have been reported. CPK levels greater than 20,000 IU/L are ominous and indicative of later DIC, acute kidney failure, and potentially dangerous hyperkalemia.[9,10,12,17]

Reduced renal blood flow from shock and dehydration leads to ischemic kidneys. Concentration of the urine may lead to accumulation of uric acid and myoglobin, which have the capacity to crystallize in renal tubules. Crystallization may lead to obstructive uropathy and the development of acute tubular necrosis. BUN levels are frequently elevated. Low serum osmolarity, moderate proteinuria, and machine oil appearance of the urine occurs in patients with exertional heatstroke.[9-11,18,26]

The liver is frequently damaged, and frank jaundice is noted. The development of early jaundice, less than 24 hours after onset, has a worse prognosis than delayed jaundice. The engorged vessels of the gastrointestinal tract may become ulcerated and hemorrhage massively.

Patterns of Heatstroke Presentation

Heatstroke is manifested in three distinct patterns: classic, exertional, and drug-induced. The three essential elements in the diagnosis of heatstroke are exposure to heat stress, internal or external; central nervous system dysfunction; and increased body temperature greater than 40°C.

Classic heatstroke, which tends to occur in the elderly, the ill, and infants, develops over a period of several days. It often occurs during heat waves and affects persons who do not have access to a cooler environment and fluids. Often, the patient is discovered in bed and is unresponsive. In these cases, the patient has hot, red, or flushed skin; has usually ceased sweating; and is significantly dehydrated.

Initial symptoms of classic heatstroke are similar to those of heat exhaustion: dizziness, headache, and malaise, with progression to frank confusion and coma. Fever, tachycardia, and hypotension are additional presenting signs. These patients also hyperventilate, which gives rise to respiratory alkalosis.

Exertional heatstroke usually occurs in young, fit, but unacclimatized persons who are often male athletes. Many such patients perform in hot and humid weather conditions that prevent adequate dissipation of generated heat. Of these patients, 50% still sweat profusely from the rapid onset; severe dehydration has not yet had time to occur.

Exertional heatstroke has a prodrome of chills, nausea, throbbing pressure in the head, and piloerection on the chest and upper arms. Concentration wanes, a subjective sense of physical deterioration is noticed, and the person feels increasingly hot, with decreased sweat production. Paresthesia is noted in the hands and feet.

Onset of irrational behavior then occurs. The face turns ashen gray, and the skin may feel relatively cool if sweat is still being produced. This effect is followed by seizures and collapse. Patients who have exertional heatstroke often have severe respiratory acidosis from lactate caused by muscle exertion and volume depletion. They also have significant rhabdomyolysis.[7,12,20]

Drugs that predispose a person to *drug-induced heatstroke* have been previously identified. Anticholinergic drugs such as phenothiazines, tricyclic antidepressants, antihistamines, antiparkinsonian agents, antispasmodics, and glutethimide inhibit sweating and thus interfere with heat dissipation. The side effects of some anticholinergic drugs include hyperkinesis and agitation, which result in an increase in body temperature. Drugs with cardiovascular actions (beta-blockers, diuretics, and antihypertensives) can inhibit or depress cardiovascular performance during increased demand that results from heat stress. Diuretics, especially if abused, can lead to dehydration. Amphetamines, neuroleptics, and possibly tricyclic antidepressants induce heatstroke because they increase the endogenous heat load.[7,22,23] Hyperthermia that results from interaction of monoamine oxidase inhibitors with tricyclic antidepressants and amphetamines has been noted.

Patients with drug-induced heatstroke have classic signs of heatstroke; the main difficulty is identification of the causative agent. Management should never be delayed by attempts to elucidate a comprehensive drug history.

INTERVENTION AND TREATMENT

PRIORITIES

The most critical goal and life-saving measure in heat illness is cooling the patient to rapidly decrease body temperature. Immediate treatment often leads to prompt recovery. The more rapid the cooling, the lower the risk of mortality. Morbidity and mortality are directly related to the duration and intensity (temperature maximum) of hyperthermia.

While the patient is cooled as rapidly as possible, maintenance of the ABCs of emergency care must not be forgotten. Because the patient may not have the ability to protect the airway, the transport team must effectively ventilate the lungs, oxygenate the blood, and maintain an adequate circulatory volume with an intact pump while carrying out continuous astute assessment through the duration of required therapy.

EQUIPMENT

No special equipment is needed to effectively treat patients with heat illness. Standard equipment for the provision of advanced life-support measures must be available.

Methods for cooling a patient range from use of simple ice packs to elaborate cooling tables. At this time, no method has proved to be superior to any other method. Recognition of the illness and prompt initiation of treatment are the most important tools in the management of heat illness.

INTERVENTIONS: MILD TO INVASIVE

Cooling can be accomplished in the prehospital setting first by removing the patient from the hot environment and especially away from hot surfaces, such as concrete and pavement, even if no shaded area is nearby. The transport team should remove the patient's clothing and wet down the patient.

Covering the patient with cool fluid and increasing the movement of air over the patient enhance heat loss by increasing the evaporative gradient. The transport team should open the windows of the ambulance or make use of the air circulation of helicopter rotors during transport to further increase air movement over the patient. In one study of three cases of heatstroke, the patients were sprayed with lukewarm water while they were exposed to the downwash of a helicopter's rotors.[14,21,24]

Heat cramps constitute a mild form of heat illness. Treatment consists of removal from the source of heat, rest, and fluid and electrolyte replacement. Oral replacement should be started by having the patient drink a balanced electrolyte solution. If oral intake is contraindicated, 1000 mL of normal saline solution is administered intravenously over a 1-hour to 3-hour period. Mild forms of heat exhaustion are treated in a similar manner. If the patient's body temperature is elevated, the transport team should cool the skin with fans and cool compresses.[12,19,23-26]

More severe cases of heat exhaustion necessitate parental rehydration. Laboratory values (renal electrolytes, BUN, and hematocrit) are best used to guide replacement. Fluid is titrated to cardiovascular status. Normal saline solution, half-normal saline solution, and dextrose-half-normal saline solution have all been used; no evidence exists of a clear superiority of any one of these fluids.[11,27] In 12 hours, patients generally feel well, have normal vital signs, and can be discharged without sequelae.

Heat exhaustion must be regarded on a continuum from the mild case, treated with simple cooling measures, to the severe case, which progresses to full-blown heatstroke. The most important treatment for heat illness is recognition of the hyperthermic insult and rapid initiation of cooling.

Controversy surrounds the question of which method is ideal for cooling the patient with heat-stroke. Several methods are considered to be of therapeutic benefit. Packing the patient in ice and immersing the body in cold water are historic methods of cooling.[22] However, ice water baths may actually cause vasoconstriction, decreased cutaneous blood flow, and capillary sludging, which promotes DIC. Furthermore, ice water may cause a shivering response, which is a heat-producing mechanism. Cold water enemas have been suggested and may help decrease core body temperature; however, they are usually not necessary.[17,32]

Other therapies involve the use of room-temperature water evaporated from the victim's skin surface by circulating air from a fan. The field treatment measure of ice packs placed in areas of maximum heat transfer (neck, axillae, and inguinal area) may also be continued with caution. The patient's skin must be closely monitored for injury from the ice.

Ice water immersion continues to be debated as to its value in rapidly cooling patients. Criticisms of this method include concern about vasoconstriction, shivering, patient discomfort, transport team discomfort, and difficulty in performing advanced cardiac life procedures such as defibrillation in the water. Moran and Gaffin[22] note that the technique may be useful because it is relatively easy to set up and perform. In the wilderness environment, cold water in a stream may be particularly useful. However, this procedure should be used with caution in the elderly.[22]

Cooling measures are ceased when body core temperature reaches 39°C (102°F). The core temperature then continues to fall to the normal range. If normal thermoregulatory mechanisms have been damaged by the thermic insult, a hypothermic overshot could result from further active cooling measures.[13]

Refractory hyperthermia necessitates more aggressive invasive methods. Ice-water gastric lavage has been reported to be effective both in a controlled canine model[26] and in actual victim treatment.[9,22] Gastric lavage has the advantages of rapid cooling and effective use of readily available equipment. Iced peritoneal lavage, hemodialysis, and cardiopulmonary bypass have been used as end attempts in severely refractory cases.[19,28-31] These increasingly invasive operative methods obviously require a great commitment of resources and have higher degrees of risk and complication rates.

TRANSPORT CARE

Heatstroke presents a complex patient management picture. If, when the transport team arrives, cooling measures have not been implemented or need augmentation, institution of the previously discussed interventions must be of the highest priority. As in any life-threatening case, a secured airway, institution of oxygenation, ventilation, and stabilization of cardiovascular status are mandated.

Endotracheal intubation is indicated for any patient who has a depressed sensorium because of the risk of emesis, aspiration, and seizure activity. Patients with heatstroke are often hypotensive because of dehydration and the physiologic compensation of extreme vasodilation. In most cases, the hypotension responds to cooling. Large amounts of fluids and inotropic agents are needed only when cooling results in no response.

In patients with normotensive conditions or in whom hypotension is readily resolved with cooling, normal saline solution is most often recommended; however, fluid choice should be made in consultation with medical expertise.[29] Vasoactive medications may need to be initiated for vascular support when fluid resuscitation is not effective. Because of complications of impaired cardiac function, pulmonary edema, congestive heart failure, adult respiratory distress syndrome, and acute kidney failure, fluid replacement is best guided with placement of a pulmonary catheter. Field guidelines for fluid replacement recommend infusion of normal saline solution until a systolic blood pressure of 90 mm Hg is obtained.[10] Solutions that contain glucose should generally be avoided to maximize absorption.[17]

In the light of the axiom that "the best defense is a good offense," monitoring the patient for multiple organ failure and prompt intervention on clinical manifestation of such failure are of utmost importance. Placement of a gastric tube accomplishes gastric decompression and monitors for the onset of gastrointestinal (GI) bleeding. Protect the GI tract: administer gastric protectants such as sucralfate in a slurry (1 g/10 mL water q 8 h) and consider antibiotics to prevent sepsis from bacterial translocation and GI mucosal damage.[17]

An indwelling urinary catheter should be inserted to monitor hourly urinary output and rhabdomyolysis. Because of the possibility of kidney impairment, the transport team must closely monitor and support kidney function. If urine output becomes more than 1 mL/kg after the patient is well hydrated, consider mannitol, dopamine, and furosemide intravenous (IV) bolus followed by 1 mg/kg/h infusion. After urine flow is initiated, fluid therapy should be continued at two to three times maintenance levels and titrated off.[17]

Liver failure is a frequent complication of heatstroke. When liver failure is combined with kidney failure, the choice of drugs used in treatment becomes difficult. DIC occurs in severe cases; most patients who die of heatstroke have evidence of DIC.[10] Standard treatment measures are instituted.[12] For prevention of DIC, administer heparin at 200 to 250 units/kg every 8 hours subcutaneously (SC).[17]

Electrolyte and acid-base imbalances may be manifested. Patients with low serum glucose levels are treated with glucose administration. Hyperkalemia and hypokalemia are common. Hypokalemia with respiratory alkalosis is transient and needs no treatment; hypokalemia with acidosis necessitates replacement therapy.[8,28] Hyperkalemia reflects cellular damage and acidosis.[20] Administer potassium chloride for hypokalemia correction at a rate of no more than 0.5 mEq/kg/h. Sodium bicarbonate may have to be given for severe metabolic acidosis (pH < 7.2). Sodium bicarbonate (0.3 × body weight [kg] × base deficit IV) should be given at 50% calculated dose, with subsequent blood gas determinations.[17]

Monitor ECG for arrhythmias. Seizures are treated with benzodiazepines. Use of prophylactic treatment has been considered because seizures may increase heat production, metabolic acidosis, and hypoxia. The neurologic status should be reevaluated constantly. If it deteriorates, consider mannitol (1 g/kg IV) and repeat corticosteroids every hour.[17]

MALIGNANT HYPERTHERMIA

Malignant hyperthermia is chemically induced either by anesthetic agents or by a depolarizing muscle relaxant (e.g., succinylcholine).[3,11,16,28] This disease is a genetic myopathy transmitted by an autosomal dominant gene. Malignant hyperthermia occurs in anesthetized patients at a ratio of approximately 1:15,000 in children and 1:50,000 in adults.[11] It is most common in male patients between ages 15 and 30 years. Malignant hyperthermia has been reported in all races but with less frequency in blacks; a muscle-mass gender influence increases the incidence rate in men. It is uncommon in patients over the age of 50 years and under the age of 2 years.[11] The triggering agents are anesthetics: potent inhalant agents (halothane, enflurane, isoflurane) and skeletal muscle relaxants (succinylcholine chloride and amide local agents).[8]

The primary disorder is a defect in the sarcoplasmic reticulum in skeletal muscle metabolism. The sarcoplasmic reticulum is a reservoir for calcium storage in the muscle cell. Under normal conditions, the sarcoplasmic reticulum releases calcium ions into the myoplasm, which causes skeletal muscle contractions. Contraction is sustained as long as a high concentration of calcium ions exists in the myoplasm. Relaxation occurs when a constantly functional calcium pump in the wall of the sarcoplasmic reticulum pumps calcium ions back into the reticulum.[3,8,11,16,28]

In malignant hyperthermia, either the sarcoplasmic reticulum is unable to reaccumulate calcium or an accelerated release of calcium occurs. The increase in intracellular calcium results in sustained muscle contractions, and a hypermetabolic state ensues. Increased oxygen consumption leads to decreased tissue oxygen saturation, which causes metabolic and respiratory acidosis. Increased heat production leads to hyperthermia.

The loss of muscle cell membrane integrity occurs, which complicates the existing problem. The cell ions and molecules follow their concentration gradients. Calcium continues to move into the myoplasm, sustaining and worsening the muscle contractions. Hyperkalemia, myoglobinemia, and elevated CPK levels occur in the serum.

Malignant hyperthermia is characterized by hyperthermia, sustained tetanic muscle rigidity and contractions, hypermetabolism, and muscle cell destruction. Signs and symptoms are dependent on the use or nonuse of succinylcholine chloride.

With the administration of succinylcholine chloride at induction, rigidity of the masseter muscle may make intubation impossible. Additional doses only worsen the rigidity. Muscle fasciculations normally observed with use of the drug may not occur. Unmovable joints with hard unindentible bellies may be noted.

Tachycardia is the most consistent first sign of malignant hyperthermia with the use of potent inhalation agents. Tachypnea, which results from hyperventilation caused by increasing acidosis, is the second sign. If the patient is not completely paralyzed, ventilatory efforts may be seen. Instability of systolic blood pressure is another consistent sign. Cardiac dysrhythmia and ensuing profound hypotension may occur. Cyanotic mottling of the skin, dark blood in the surgical field, and fever are late signs and indicate that the patient is already in crisis.

Immediate reversal of anesthesia and termination of surgery are mandated. Dantrolene sodium (Dantrium) is administered to maximize the survival of the patient. Dantrium, a skeletal muscle relaxant that acts by preventing the release of calcium ions from the sarcoplasmic reticulum, is the drug of choice. Dosage is 2.5 to 3.0 mg/kg to be administered as rapidly as possible. If no evidence of effectiveness (decreasing temperature) is seen, another dose of 1.0 mg/kg dantrolene should be given and repeated every 5 minutes until there is a response.[16]

Procainamide is the drug of choice for ventricular arrhythmia because it does not affect myoplasmic calcium. Lidocaine and cardiac glycosides are contraindicated because they increase myoplasmic calcium. Hyperthermia is treated with previously described cooling methods. The standard therapy for hyperkalemia is indicated. Late complications can include pulmonary edema, DIC, kidney failure, and recurrence of malignant hyperthermia that was initially responsive to treatment measures.

OTHER CAUSES OF HYPERTHERMIA

Although these syndromes are not commonly encountered in the transport environment, transport teams today are called to transport complicated critically ill and injured patients who may be need cooling measures as a part of their care.[1] Medications such as haloperidol or promethazine can cause akinesia, muscle rigidity, and hyperthermia. Serotonin syndrome may also be a cause of hyperthermia as the result of enhanced release of presynaptic serotonin caused by amphetamine or cocaine use; decreased serotonin uptake caused by medications such as selective serotonin uptake inhibitors; or by direct stimulation of the postsynaptic receptors caused by buspirone and sumatriptan.[8]

Anticholinergic and sympathomimetic poisonings can also cause hyperthermia. Drugs that can cause anticholinergic poisoning include antihistamines, belladonna alkaloids, and tricyclic antidepressants. Sympathomimetic poisoning can be caused by cocaine, amphetamines, and methamphetamines.[8]

SUMMARY

Heat illness presents as a continuum from mild to severe. Heat exhaustion, if untreated, may proceed to frank heatstroke, which is a life-threatening medical emergency. Causes of heat illness encompass endogenous, environmental, and drug-related pathologies. Malignant hyperthermia rarely occurs but has deadly consequences.

Prompt recognition of the problem and rapid cooling limit the severe sequelae associated with heat toxicity. Various cooling methods are used to limit the duration of exposure to hyperthermia. Research shows the length of exposure and maximum temperature reached are two critical criteria in the survival and recovery of patients with heatstroke.

Complications of heatstroke affect every organ system and can lead to multiple organ system failure. Liver and kidney failure are common. Neurologic complications are usually rare with prompt cooling to achieve euthermia. Cerebellar effects are the residual pathologies most often seen.

The onset of DIC, coma lasting more than 8 hours, cardiac dysfunction, hypotension, and high lactate and CPK levels are ominous signs and are usually predictive of mortality. Prevention of heat illness with adequate hydration; recognition of environmental, exertional, and physiologic risk factors; and proper acclimatization are important educational tools for the transport and potential of patients.

HEAT-RELATED EMERGENCIES CASE STUDY

The helicopter transport team was dispatched immediately to a rural hospital a distance of 60 miles from the base hospital. The dispatch information stated that a female patient in her middle 60s had collapsed and was unresponsive. The basic life-support unit reported seizure activity with no change in level of consciousness after tonic-clonic motor activity. The past week had been hot, with temperatures hovering between 90°F and 110°F and humidity registering 80% to 85%.

On arrival at the hospital, the patient's husband reported that they had arrived early that morning at an outlying lake for a fishing trip. He stated that their boat trailer became stuck on the ramp; as a result, he and the patient had to walk about 11 miles to get assistance to launch the boat. The patient tired and sat in the truck while the boat was launched.

After 2 hours of fishing, the patient had headache and nausea, which lasted for an hour. Her husband then noted "really strange behavior—she was talking funny and didn't remember she was in the boat." By the time he reached the shore, the patient was unresponsive. She subsequently had a seizure when the ground ambulance arrived. Because of the location of the boat dock, the weight of the patient, and the ground response time, the patient had been unresponsive for an hour before arrival at the rural hospital.

PHYSICAL FINDINGS

Obese female, weight 100 kg, age 64 years, supine on emergency department (ED) cart with red flushed skin surfaces. No response noted to any stimuli.

Vital signs: blood pressure (BP) 106/62 mm Hg; pulse 152 bpm, regular in rate and rhythm, sinus tachycardia; respiratory rate (RR) 40 bpm; temperature 40.8°C (105.5°F) rectally.

HEENT: PERRLA, no nuchal rigidity, mucous membranes dry, tongue leathery in appearance, upper airway patent.

Thorax: Symmetric expansion on inspiration, breath sounds clear and equal bilaterally, heart sounds normal S1 and S2, no murmur or rub noted, no trauma noted.

Abdomen: Obese, soft, no apparent guarding or tenderness, bowel sounds present but decreased, no organomegaly.

Extremities: No obvious trauma, no edema.

Neurologic: Glasgow Coma Score 4 (1–2–1), flaccid tone, no focal deficits noted, Babinski's sign negative bilaterally.

Skin: Hot, dry, red in color, no rashes or other abnormalities noted.

Current interventions: Oxygen 8 L via plain face mask; in-dwelling urinary catheter inserted; patient covered with damp bath blanket.

The patient's husband stated she had no medical allergies; she occasionally took Lasix for "fluid buildup"; her only medical history was mild heart failure.

LABORATORY AND RADIOGRAPHIC DATA

CBC: WBC 22,100; RBC 4.2; Hgb/Hct 14.6/42; differential normal.

ABG: pH 7.54; PCo_2 26; Po_2 97; HCO_2 26; O_2 sat 94: B.E. + 2; Na 142; K 3.2; Cl 100; CO_2 17; BUN 32; glucose 62; creatinine 1.2; CPK 25,000; LDH 730; amylase 142.

Urinalysis: Color dark greenish-brown; specific gravity 1.042; pH 7; ketones 3+; protein 2+.

PT/PTT and platelets: Within normal limits.

Chest radiograph: Within normal limits with heart size upper side of normal.

ECG (12-lead): Sinus tachycardia without ectopy; nonspecific ST-T changes.

TRANSPORT TEAM INTERVENTIONS

Before takeoff, the patient was endotracheally intubated because of neurologic depression and to prevent aspiration. Concurrent with cooling measures, a gastric tube was placed for stomach decompression, and ECG monitoring was instituted.

Immediate cooling measures consisted of stripping the patient and covering her with a wet sheet.

Ice packs placed in the axilla, neck, and inguinal areas were promptly replaced when they became warm.

Two large-bore lines were started for IV access because fluid replacement was begun, and the patient was closely monitored.

An indwelling urinary catheter was placed by the referral facility. Urinary output (UO) over the last hour was 20 mL. Because of decreased UO and abnormal urine character as a result of muscle rhabdomyolysis, renal diuresis was indicated; mannitol (1 mg/kg) was given to maintain adequate urine flow.

Further initial treatment was based on a review of the laboratory values. Respiratory alkalosis with hypokalemia was present; hypokalemia should clear with cooling. If signs of hypercarbia became evident, the patient would need ventilatory intervention. Hypoglycemia was corrected with the administration of dextrose (D50). CPK values over 20,000 alerted the transport to the probability of the development of DIC and multiple organ failure.

TRANSPORT ASSESSMENT

Continuous assessment of this patient for further signs of multiple organ failure was mandatory. Reassessment of the efficacy of cooling measures, airway patency, and neurologic status was especially important in the care of this patient. If seizure activity reoccurred, prompt termination with lorazepam would be indicated.

While in flight, the patient was kept moist with water and evaporation that was enhanced by directing air vents onto the body and flying with the windows open (permitted by the rotorcraft's design). The wet sheet was removed once the patient was loaded because it was warm and prevented evaporation. Ice packs were replaced as needed. When the patient's temperature reached 39°C (102°F), cooling measures were stopped.

Airway patency was ensured by frequent suctioning of the endotracheal tube and continuous assessment of respiratory status. If respiratory fatigue had become evident, ventilatory assistance would have been necessary. Oxygenation was assessed with pulse oximetry. Observation for increased pulmonary secretions, indicating pulmonary edema, was done in flight.

Electrocardiographic monitoring was necessary; advanced cardiac life support (ACLS) protocol was followed in the event of arrhythmia occurrence. Gastric output was observed for the presence of blood because GI bleeding is a frequent complication. Urine character and output were monitored to assess renal function.

Close attention and continuous ongoing assessment of the patient's condition for presenting signs of possible complications allowed the transport nurse to promptly initiate corrective and supportive care measures.

REFERENCES

1. Baker PS, et al: Hyperthermia, hypertension, hypertonia, and coma in massive thioridazine overdose, *Am J Emerg Med* 4:346, 1988.
2. Bledsoe BE, Benner RW: *Critical care paramedic*, Upper Saddle River, NJ, 2006, Pearson Prentice Hall.
3. Calvey N: Adverse drug reactions, *Anaesth Intens Care Med* 9(7):319-323, 2008.
4. Centers for Disease Control and Prevention: Heat-related illnesses and deaths—United States, 1994-1995, *MMWR* 44(25):465, 1995.
5. Chesney ML: Pediatric extertional heatstroke, *Air Med J* 22(6):6-8, 2003.
6. Drake DK, Nettina SM: Recognition and management of heat-related illness, *Nurse Pract* 19(8):43, 1994.
7. Earth Policy Institute: *Setting the record straight: more than 52,000 Europeans died from heat in summer 2003*, available at http://www.earth-policy.org, accessed June 2008.
8. Epstein Y, Hadad E, Shapiro Y: Pathological factors underlying hyperthermia, *J Thermal Biol* 29:487-494, 2004.
9. Gaffin SL, Hubbard R: Experimental approaches to therapy and prophylaxis for heat stress and heatstroke, *Wilder Environ Med* 4:312, 1996.
10. Gaffin SL, Moran DS: Pathophysiology of heat-related illnesses. In Auerbach P, editor: *Wilderness medicine: management of wilderness and environmental emergencies*, ed 5, St Louis, 2007, Mosby Elsevier.

11. Greany D, Brown MM: Malignant hyperthermia: a concern for critical care patients, *Focus Crit Care* 15:49, 1988.

12. Harker J, Gibson P: Heat stroke: a review of rapid cooling techniques, *Intens Crit Care Nurs* 11(4):198, 1995.

13. Hart LH, Dennis SL: Two hypothermias prevalent in the intensive care unit: fever and heatstroke, *Focus Crit Care* 15(49):235, 1988.

14. Hoffman JL: Heat-related illness in children. *Clin Pediatr Emerg Med* 2:203-210, 2001.

15. Holleran RS: *Prehospital nursing: a collaborative approach*, St Louis, 1994, Mosby.

16. Hopkins PM: Malignant hyperthermia, *Anaeth Intens Care Med* 9(6):244-246, 2008.

17. Hubbard RW, Armstrong LE: Hyperthermia; new thoughts on an old problem, *Phys Sportsmed* 17(6): 1989.

18. Huether SE, Defriez CB: Pain, temperature regulation, sleep and sensory function. In McCance KL, Huether SE, editors: *Pathophysiology*, ed 5, St Louis, 2007, Elsevier Mosby.

19. Karrimi FA, et al: Adult respiratory distress syndrome and disseminated intravascular coagulation complicating heat stroke, *Chest* 9(4):571, 1986.

20. Lee-Chiong TL, Stitt JT: Heatstroke and other heat-related illnesses: the maladies of summer, *Postgrad Med* 98(1):26, 1995.

21. Lim MK: Occupational heat stress, *Ann Acad Med (Singapore)* 23(5):719, 1994.

22. Moran DS, Gaffin SL: Clinical management of heat-related illnesses. In Auerbach P: *Wilderness medicine: management of wilderness and environmental emergencies*, ed 5, St Louis, 2007, Mosby Elsevier.

23. O'Brien DJ: Heat illness, *J Aeromed Healthcare* 2:6, 1985.

24. Pouton TJ, Walker RA: Helicopter cooling of heat stroke victims, *Aviation Space Environ Med* 58:358, 1987.

25. Proehl J: Environmental emergencies. In Kitt S, et al, editors: *Emergency nursing*, Philadelphia, 1995, Saunders.

26. Sidman RD, Gallagher EJ: Exertional heat stroke in a young woman: gender differences in response to thermal stress, *Acad Emerg Med* 2(4):315, 1995.

27. Syverud SA, et al: Iced gastric lavage for treatment of heat stroke: efficacy in a canine model, *Ann Emerg Med* 14:424, 1985.

28. Tek D, Olshaker JS: Heat illness, *Emerg Med Clin North Am* 10(2):299, 1992.

29. Tomarken JL, Britt BA: Malignant hyperthermia, *Ann Emerg Med* 16:1253, 1987.

30. Vicario S: Heat illness. In Marx J, editor: *Rosen's emergency medicine concepts and clinical practice*, ed 6, Philadelphia, 2006, Mosby Elsevier.

31. Wagner C, Boyd K: Pediatric heatstroke, *Air Med J* 27(3):118-122, 2008.

32. Walter BGB, Callahan CW, Hing M: The first enemy you meet; acclimatization and the mastery of desert heat, *Infantry Magazine*, Nov-Dec: 2004.

33. Yan YE, Zhao YQ, Wang H, et al: Pathophysiological factors underlying heatstroke, *Med Hypothesis* 67: 609-617, 2006.

34. Yaqua BA, et al: Heat stroke and the Mekkah pilgrimage: clinical characteristics and course of 30 patients, *Q J Med* 59:523, 1986.

DIVING EMERGENCIES

Reneé Semonin Holleran

COMPETENCIES

1. Perform a comprehensive assessment of the patient, including subjective and objective data on the diving emergency.
2. Anticipate and plan for the effects of transport on the patient with decompression illness.
3. Contact the Divers Alert Network website (http://www.diversalertnetwork.org) for advice on the care of the patient with a diving emergency.

Scuba (from "self-contained underwater breathing apparatus") diving is an increasingly popular pastime. The United States is now estimated to have more than nine million certified divers, with many more worldwide.[11] Diving activities are no longer restricted to coastal resorts but can be found in almost any body of water large enough to hold a diver and equipment. Diving is also a part of many occupations, including industry, military, scientific research, and search and rescue. Occasionally, an accident may even occur at a city aquarium, especially if envenomization is involved.[4,7]

Diving can lead to illnesses and injuries, some of them unique to the environment. Injuries and fatalities from diving may be reported at the Divers Alert Network (http://www.diversalertnetwork.org).

Generally, about 1000 injuries are reported each year; fatalities vary from year to year.[7]

Manifestations of diving injuries may not be noticed by the diver for 24 to 48 hours after a dive and may, in fact, be seriously potentiated by air travel. Thus, patients with diving-related problems may be seen many hours later and many thousands of miles from the original dive site.

Transport personnel encounter many types of scuba-related diving injuries, such as marine envenomation, near drowning, decompression illness, arterial gas embolism (AGE), middle-ear squeeze, and other forms of barotrauma. Of these diving injuries, decompression illness and AGE are medical emergencies that necessitate immediate recompression treatment. Air medical transport of the patient to a hyperbaric chamber is often necessary to avoid the significant morbidity and mortality that result from delays in treatment of these disorders. Transport personnel must therefore be able to diagnose and manage these diving emergencies in a timely manner.

This chapter provides a brief discussion of diving principles and the pathophysiology, clinical manifestations, and management of diving emergencies likely to be encountered by transport crews.

DIVING PRINCIPLES

A brief discussion of a few physical properties inherent to scuba diving is necessary for a thorough understanding of the pathophysiology underlying decompression illness and air embolism.

At sea level, a 1-square-inch column of air extending upward from the earth's surface to the edge of the atmosphere weighs 14.7 lb. Thus, the pressure exerted by this column of air at sea level is 14.7 lb/in^2 (psi) or 760 mm Hg, which is defined as 1 atmosphere of pressure (atm). As altitude increases, the column of air becomes shorter and the air pressure decreases. For example, at an altitude of 18,000 ft, the atmospheric pressure is half that at sea level: 380 mm Hg, or 0.5 atm. On the other hand, water is much denser than air, and a similar 1-square-inch column in seawater only has to be 33 ft (10 m) to exert the same amount of pressure as a 1-square-inch column of air. Because the density of water is uniform throughout, the proportional relationship of pressure and depth remains constant: pressure increases 1 atm for every 33-ft (10-m) column of seawater (Figure 29-1). For the scuba diver, the combined weights of the air and water columns must be taken into consideration. At a given depth underwater, the total pressure is the sum of the barometric pressure exerted by the column of air above plus the hydrostatic pressure exerted by the column of water. This total is the concept of absolute pressure or atmospheres absolute (ATA). Therefore, a scuba diver at a depth of 33 ft experiences an ambient pressure of 2 atm absolute pressure, or 2 ATA. Similarly, a scuba diver at 66 ft experiences an ambient pressure of 3 ATA.

As the diver descends from the water's surface, the effects of increasing ambient pressure on the scuba diver involve an understanding of the behavior of gases under conditions of varying pressure and volume. The following brief discussion concerns the primary gas laws of diving.[1,10,13,17,18]

BOYLE'S LAW

The first gas law is *Boyle's law,* which states that at a constant temperature and mass, the volume of a gas is inversely proportional to the total pressure. Simply stated, volume decreases as pressure increases; conversely, volume increases as pressure decreases. Figure 29-1 depicts the increase of gas volume as the pressure and depth decrease.

HENRY'S LAW

The second gas principle is *Henry's law,* which states that solubility is proportional to the partial pressure of a gas. As the pressure increases or decreases, the gas goes into or comes out of solution accordingly. This effect is the "soda bottle" phenomenon. When you release the pressure from the bottle by removing the cap, the dissolved gas comes out of solution (Figure 29-2).

DALTON'S LAW

The last gas principle is *Dalton's law of partial pressures,* which states that the total pressure of a mixture of gases equals the sum of partial pressures exerted by the constituent gases. The partial pressure is the pressure exerted by a single gas in a mixture as if it were the only gas in the mixture. Air comprises approximately 78% nitrogen, 21% oxygen, and 1% other gases. As illustrated in Figure 29-3, with an increase in the total pressure of the mixture, the pressure of each constituent gas is increased proportionately. At a depth of 99 ft (30 m), a scuba diver is under an ambient pressure of 4 ATA and is breathing compressed air with partial pressures of nitrogen and oxygen four times their value at the surface.

PATHOPHYSIOLOGIC FACTORS

Nitrogen is a relatively inert gas that is driven into solution according to Henry's law as the diver descends. The saturation of tissues with nitrogen depends on intrinsic properties, including tissue perfusion and solubility coefficients of the various

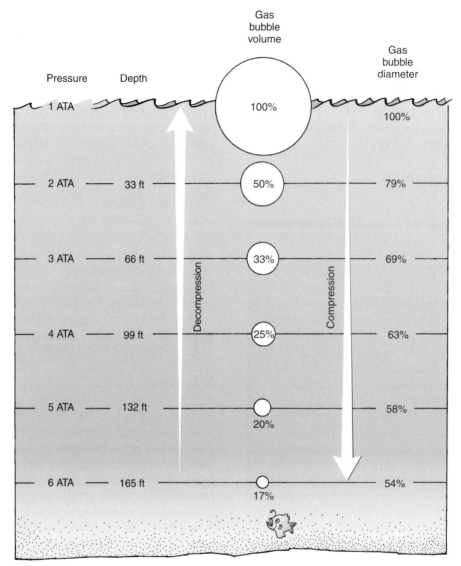

FIGURE 29-1   **Boyle's law.** (From Auerbach PS: *Wilderness medicine: management of wilderness and environmental emergencies,* ed 4, St Louis, 2001, Mosby.)

tissues.[11] The quantity of dissolved nitrogen in the tissues increases with the duration and depth of the dive.[8] If ascent of the scuba diver is too fast or the tissues are oversaturated with gas, the nitrogen is separated from solution rather than safely transported to the lungs for elimination. Tissue desaturation of nitrogen results in the formation of inert gas bubbles in venous blood and tissues on reduction in ambient pressure.[11]

DECOMPRESSION ILLNESS

The lesion that results from *decompression illness* has been a subject of debate for many years, although tissue ischemia is generally accepted to be the final common pathway.[8,11,19] Hallenbeck, Bove, and Elliott[9] demonstrated venous congestion with gas bubbles in the epidural venous plexus system of the spinal cord, most frequently in the lumbosacral region. The location of the intravascular lesion was consistent with the

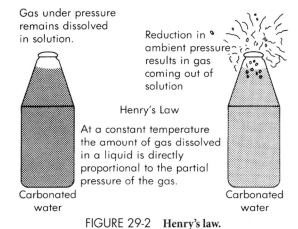

Gas under pressure remains dissolved in solution.

Reduction in ambient pressure results in gas coming out of solution

Henry's Law

At a constant temperature the amount of gas dissolved in a liquid is directly proportional to the partial pressure of the gas.

Carbonated water   Carbonated water

FIGURE 29-2 **Henry's law.**

corresponding neurologic symptoms.[9] The formation of bubbles in tissues and venous blood has multiple mechanical and physiologic consequences. Mechanical effects of bubble formation include intravascular or intralymphatic obstruction, cellular distention and rupture, and stretching of ligaments and tendons. These effects result in ischemia or infarction, edema formation, cell death, and pain. The physiologic consequences include activation of the intrinsic clotting pathway, kinins, and the complement system, which all result in platelet aggregation, increased vascular permeability, and microvascular sludging. The end results of all of these events are decreased tissue perfusion and ischemia.[11]

ARTERIAL GAS EMBOLIZATION

By far the most serious manifestation of pressure-related injuries or barotrauma is *arterial gas embolization* (AGE). The most classic presentation is a sudden onset of unconsciousness within minutes of reaching the surface after a dive. AGE is a leading cause of death among scuba divers.[2,5,11-18]

Divers need to exhale continuously and ascend slowly, or several consequences may occur. These consequences include the following:

- Air pushes through the lung tissues and enters the skin in the neck.
- Air pushes through the lung tissues and into the spaces between the lungs and causes a pneumothorax.
- Air is forced from the lungs into blood vessels and carried to vital organs.

In accordance with Boyle's law, gases in the lungs of a scuba diver expand as ambient pressure decreases during ascent. The greatest changes in pressure and volume occur at shallower depths. Pulmonary overpressurization syndrome and alveolar rupture can occur during an ascent from a depth as shallow as 4 ft if compressed air is held in the lungs.[1] Breath holding during an ascent, as with a panicked diver, or air trapping in a diseased lung results in lung overexpansion and rupture of alveoli. Air

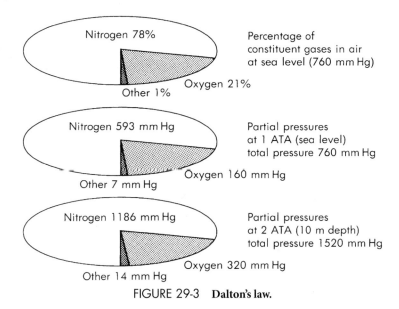

Nitrogen 78%

Percentage of constituent gases in air at sea level (760 mm Hg)

Oxygen 21%
Other 1%

Nitrogen 593 mm Hg

Partial pressures at 1 ATA (sea level) total pressure 760 mm Hg

Oxygen 160 mm Hg
Other 7 mm Hg

Nitrogen 1186 mm Hg

Partial pressures at 2 ATA (10 m depth) total pressure 1520 mm Hg

Oxygen 320 mm Hg
Other 14 mm Hg

FIGURE 29-3 **Dalton's law.**

bubbles from the ruptured alveoli are free to enter the pulmonary venous return to the left side of the heart for subsequent dissemination through the systemic circulation. Air bubbles can track in the lung parenchyma and tissue planes. The result may be interstitial and mediastinal emphysema or pneumothorax.[1]

Gas bubbles may enter the coronary arteries and produce myocardial ischemia or infarction. However, bubbles most often enter the carotid circulation, producing multiple areas of circulatory occlusion in the brain with resulting ischemia and infarction.

Because multiple cerebrovascular watersheds may be affected, a confusing clinical picture with multiple neurologic deficits may result. The patient may have seizures or become unconscious, which can confuse rescuers as to the seriousness of the patient's problem.[20]

CLINICAL MANIFESTATIONS

Diagnosis of a diving injury is usually made on the basis of the patient's history and clinical presentation.[15] Unfortunately, many of the signs and symptoms of decompression sickness (DCS) and AGE are nonspecific and may mimic other disease processes such as low back pain, arthritis, tendinitis, bronchospasm, stroke, and myocardial infarction. Because of the high morbidity and mortality that can result when treatment of DCS and AGE is delayed, diving accidents and injuries must be treated aggressively. The most common management error of these diving emergencies is failure to treat borderline cases.[16]

DECOMPRESSION SICKNESS

The signs and symptoms of DCS depend on the size and location of the ischemic insult. The most common presentation of decompression sickness may be headache, fatigue, limb or joint pain, skin rash and pruritus, and localized swelling. The patient may also have pain, numbness, tingling, and parathesias. Decompression sickness used to be divided into types I and II, but a better method is to look at the body systems that have been affected. Decompression sickness should be considered serious, and treatment quickly sought.[11] The joints commonly affected are the shoulders, elbows, hips, knees, and ankles. Box 29-1 shows a classification scheme based on the systems or tissues involved.[11]

BOX 29-1   Classification of Decompression Sickness

Type I
Local effects only: Limb bends (joint or limb pain), skin bends (skin rash or itch), lymphatic obstruction effects.

Type II
Cerebral manifestations: Fatigue, malaise, visual disturbances, headache, impaired coordination, motor and sensory disturbances ranging from minor neurologic impairment to major deficits (e.g., paraplegia, quadriplegia, hemiplegia, altered states of consciousness from drowsiness to coma, convulsions, and death).

Type III
Spinal manifestations: Any degree of any motor and sensory modality impairment, but commonly weakness and numbness of lower limbs and bladder and sphincter impairment.

Type IV
Pulmonary chokes: Pulmonary dyspnea, pain, cough, altered gas exchange.

Type V
Staggers: Mild to severe impairment of balance and coordination, often debilitating.

Type VI
Dysbaric osteonecrosis: Lytic bone lesions that result from long-term exposure to diving.

From Otton J: Medical problems of recreational diving, *Aust Fam Phys* 18(6):674, 1989.

Musculoskeletal decompression sickness, better known as "the bends," is the most common type of decompression sickness. Pain in the shoulders and elbows is a frequent symptom. The patient may have a burning or tearing pain in the affected joint. Rarely, the joint may be red and swollen.[11]

The diver may also have skin bends or *cutaneous decompression sickness.* The skin may display a variety of cutaneous manifestations including scarlatiniform or mottled rashes. The patient may also have itching or the sensation of ants crawling on the skin.[11]

Other symptoms of decompression sickness may involve any, or combinations, of the following symptoms: sensory and visual disturbances; dyspnea and nonproductive cough; paresthesia; paresis; fatigue and weakness; headache and nausea; chest, abdominal, or back pain; bowel and bladder dysfunction; shock; and loss of consciousness. Profound fatigue greater than the amount of exertion related to the dive is another symptom.[11]

Pulmonary Decompression Illness

Otherwise known as the "chokes" or type IV DCS, *pulmonary decompression illness* is the result of large volumes of emboli occluding end arteries in the pulmonary circulation. If the lesion is large enough, pulmonary artery pressure increases, which results in symptoms of dyspnea, chest pain, and nonproductive cough.[12] Pulmonary DCS is a rare but life-threatening manifestation of DCS that progresses rapidly to shock unless immediate hyperbaric treatment is administered.[7,11]

Arterial Gas Embolism

Manifestations of AGE usually begin during or in minutes of ascent. As described previously, AGE is a result of pulmonary overpressurization; therefore, symptoms occur at or shortly after the time of the insult. The manifestations of AGE are consistent with strokelike phenomena, and almost any sign of cerebral damage may be observed, from mild dizziness and motor and sensory deficits to severe impairment, coma, and death.[16] In a series of 42 cases analyzed by Kizer,[10] the most common symptom was asymmetric multiplegia or paralysis that involved the lower extremities. Other signs of AGE include altered mental status and personality changes, syncope, vertigo, dizziness, cardiac dysrhythmia or cardiac arrest, chest pain, apnea, cough, hemoptysis, and epistaxis.[3,4,10,17] Transport personnel should always suspect AGE whenever a scuba diver presents with an altered level of consciousness, respiratory distress, or signs of cerebral decompression illness.

Pulmonary decompression illness and arterial gas embolism should also be considered after explosive decompression of an aircraft. In addition, arterial gas embolism can occur in a patient who has escaped or been extricated from a submerged vehicle.

MANAGEMENT

The transport team must perform a primary and secondary assessment. Critical interventions should be performed.

A neurologic examination should be performed as a soon as possible after a diving incident. The initial neurologic examination guides the course of treatment and provides a baseline for comparison of whether treatment has been effective. The Divers Alert Network recommends documenting the time of this assessment. Assessment should include:

1. Orientation to person, place, time, and situation.
2. Eyes assessment: Are pupils equal, round, and reactive to light? Are extraocular eye movements intact?
3. Is there facial symmetry, and is movement intact? Have the patient grit the teeth, smile, and puff out the cheeks.
4. Is hearing intact?
5. Is the swallow reflex intact? Have the patient swallow and observe the Adam's apple.
6. Ask the patient to stick out the tongue. Is it midline?
7. Muscle strength: Have the patient shrug the shoulders against resistance and perform range of motion of upper and lower extremities, both passive and against resistance.
8. Sensory perception or cerebella function: Observe the gait both forward and backward, then the heel toe gait. Perform Romberg's test. Have the patient touch the index finger to the nose and then to your finger, moving your finger into different positions. Lastly, while the patient is lying down, have the patient slide the heel of each foot down the opposite shin.

Repeat the assessment every 30 to 60 minutes. Additional information can be found at http://www.diversalertnetwork.org/medical/neuroexam.asp.

Air embolism and decompression illness are medical emergencies and are managed similarly.[11] Recompression in a hyperbaric chamber is the only effective treatment for these diving emergencies. The Divers Alert Network (DAN) is located at Duke University in Durham, NC. Contact information for DAN, 24 hours a day, is on their website (http://www.diversalertnetwork.org). DAN can be reached internationally; these numbers and additional information are also available on the DAN website. DAN provides assistance in diagnosis and treatment and location of the nearest treatment facility. DAN may assist with ground and air transport arrangements. Another good resource is The Undersea and Hyperbaric Medical Society, which publishes a directory listing of all approved chambers in the United States and resources for international referral; the society can be contacted at 301-942-2980 or at http://www.uhms.org/.[7]

The following sequence is used for immediate treatment of a patient with a diving emergency:

1. Establish basic life support measures.
2. Place the patient in a supine position. The patient should remain in a supine position from the field and during transport.[11]
3. Administer 100% oxygen at high flow rates (10 to 15 L/min) through a nonrebreather mask to create a gradient for increased elimination of excess nitrogen.
4. Administer an isotonic fluid to correct underlying fluid deficits and maintain urinary output of 1 to 2 mL/kg/h.[11]
5. Protect the patient against hypothermia or hyperthermia.
6. Monitor pulmonary, cardiovascular, and neurologic status. Treat developing complications (e.g., pneumothorax, shock, seizures).
7. Avoid rough or excessive handling.
8. Give sedation and analgesics as needed.
9. Recent research has suggested that administration of lidocaine may improve recompression. However, the appropriate experts should be consulted.[11]

10. Transport the patient to the nearest hyperbaric treatment facility. Some patients with injuries may need resuscitation before transport to the chamber.
11. Provide the hyperbaric medical personnel with a detailed history of the dive (e.g., depth and duration), timing and onset of symptoms or complications, and treatment rendered. This information aids the hyperbaric medical personnel in determining proper management, such as time and pressure profiles. If a dive computer is available, the transport team should bring this along with the patient. The computer provides valuable information about the dive profile that may be useful in the patient's care.
12. Always consider the possibility of DCS or AGE in the patient's diving partners as well.

AIR MEDICAL TRANSPORT

Air medical transport of the patient to a hyperbaric chamber is often necessary to avoid significant morbidity and mortality resulting from delays in treatment. However, transportation via air ambulance or even ground ambulance over elevated terrain may exacerbate the patient's condition.[2] Patients should be transported in aircraft with cabins pressurized to 1 ATA, such as the Lear jet, Hercules C-130, Cessna Citation, or many commercial aircraft, but this may require flight at a lower altitude, at considerable fuel expense. If the aircraft cannot be pressurized to 1 ATA (e.g., a helicopter), it should be flown at the lowest and safest altitude possible, preferably below 1000 ft above sea level.[11] In some locations, a portable recompression chamber can be used to transport the patient from the field to the hyperbaric treatment center in a nonpressurized aircraft. The portable unit (with the patient inside) is mated to the larger static hyperbaric chamber while the patient is maintained under pressure.[6,16]

SUMMARY

The number of scuba-related injuries grows with the increasing number of scuba divers. Of these injuries, DCS and AGE are true medical emergencies that require immediate treatment in the nearest hyperbaric chamber. Delays in the treatment of these diving injuries may result in significant morbidity and mortality. Air medical transport teams may be called on to rapidly assess, manage, and transport patients with these life-threatening injuries. Knowledge of diving principles, pathophysiology, and manifestations of AGE and DCS aids the air medical transport team in developing proper management strategies.

DIVING EMERGENCIES CASE STUDY

An air ambulance was dispatched to the scene where a 19-year-old woman was reported to be unconscious. On arrival, the patient was found in a left lateral Trendelenburg's position. Bystanders reported that the patient was an inexperienced diver with a history of asthma. She had been scuba diving in a 12-ft swimming pool.

The patient was lethargic and incoherent. Her airway was patent with an intact gag reflex. Her color was pale with no cyanosis. She was dyspneic, with a respiratory rate of 40 bpm, heart rate of 120 beats/min, and blood pressure of 150/90 mm Hg. She also had symptoms of a left cerebral infarction, including impaired speech, right-sided paresthesia, and decreased motor strength in the right arm. Breath sounds were diminished over the right apex, with occasional expiratory wheezes.

Immediate management included 100% oxygen via mask, intravenous (IV) lactated Ringer's solution at 125 mL/h, and continuous cardiac, neurologic, and pulmonary monitoring. The patient was placed in a supine position. Cerebral AGE was the most likely diagnosis, but the transport team observed the patient for a possible closed-head injury as well. The patient was 10 minutes from the nearest recompression chamber, and the decision was made to immediately transport her via helicopter at a low altitude. Initial diagnosis by the transport team was based solely on history and clinical findings.

On the patient's arrival at the emergency department, assessment results remained unchanged. The patient had a blood pressure of 140/86 mm Hg, heart rate of 116 beats/min, and respiratory rate of 42 bpm, with an intact airway. Neurologic examination findings were unchanged. Cervical spine and computed tomographic (CT) scan of the head and neck showed negative results. The emergency physician confirmed a cerebral AGE. Endotracheal intubation was deferred because the airway was adequate, and the patient was taken immediately to the hyperbaric chamber.

Initial recompression therapy was performed to a depth of 6 ATA. The patient became increasingly coherent, with return of feeling to her right side. Vital signs remained stable during recompression therapy, and a patent airway was maintained. The patient needed two additional recompression treatments to a depth of 3 ATA and made a full recovery.

Recreational divers are found in every part of the country. In particular, knowledge of AGE embolism and decompression illness, the two most dangerous diving emergencies, is essential. Before embarking on any flight that involves a diving emergency, transport personnel must know the location of the nearest recompression chamber, along with transportation alternatives. This information can be obtained 24 hours a day on the Divers Alert Network (DAN).

REFERENCES

1. Arthur DC, Margulies RA: A short course in diving medicine, *Ann Emerg Med* 16:689, 1987.
2. Boettger ML: Scuba diving emergencies: pulmonary overpressure accidents and decompression sickness, *Ann Emerg Med* 12:563, 1983.
3. Davis JC: Decompression sickness in sport scuba diving, *Phys Sportsmed* 16(2):108, 1988.
4. DeGorordo A, Vallejo-Manzur F, Chanin K, et al: Diving emergencies, *Resuscitation* 59:171-180, 2003.
5. Dick AP, Massey EW: Neurologic presentation of decompression sickness and air embolism in sport divers, *Neurology* 35:667, 1985.
6. Divers Alert Network: *Provisional flying after diving guidelines*, available at http://www.diversalertnetwork.org/news/Article.aspx?newsid=787, accessed August 2008.

7. Divers Alert Network: *Divers helping divers*, available at http://www.diversalertnetwork.org/, accessed August 2008.

8. Francis TJ, Dutka AJ, Flynn ET: Experimental determination of latency, severity, and outcome in CNS decompression sickness, *Undersea Biomed Res* 15(6):419, 1989.

9. Hallenbeck JM, Bove AA, Elliott DH: Mechanisms underlying spinal cord damage in decompression sickness, *Neurology* 25:308, 1975.

10. Kizer KW: Disorders of the deep, *Emerg Med* 6:18, 1984.

11. Kizer KW, Van Hoesen KB: Diving medicine. In Auerbach P, editor: *Wilderness medicine*, ed 5, St Louis, 2007, Mosby Elsevier.

12. Leveritt SO, Bitter HL, McIver L: *Studies in decompression sickness: circulatory and respiratory changes associated with decompression sickness in anesthetized dogs, TDR 63-67*, Brooks AFB, 1963, TX USAF School of Aerospace Medicine.

13. Moon RE: Treatment of diving emergencies, *Crit Care Clin* 15(2):429-456, 2003.

14. Mebane GY, Dick AP: *Underwater diving accident manual*, ed 2, Durham, NC, 1982, National Divers Alert Network.

15. Repogle WH, et al: Scuba diving injuries, *Am Fam Pract* 37:135, 1988.

16. Spencer MP: Decompression limits for compressed air determined by ultrasonically detected blood bubbles, *J Appl Physiol* 40:229, 1976.

17. Strauss RH: Diving medicine, *Am Rev Respir Dis* 119:1001, 1979.

18. Strauss MB, Borer RC: Diving medicine: contemporary topics and their controversies, *Am J Emerg Med* 19:232-238, 2001.

19. Ward CA, McCullough D, Fraser WD: Relation between complement activation and susceptibility to decompression sickness, *J Appl Physiol* 62:1160, 1987.

20. Warren JP Jr, et al: Neuroimaging of scuba diving injuries to the CNS, *AJR Am J Roentgenol* 151:1003, 1988.

TOXICOLOGIC EMERGENCIES

Reneé Semonin Holleran

COMPETENCIES

1. Identify the common sources of poisoning.
2. Describe the care of the poisoned patient during transport.
3. Name three antidotes for specific poisons.

Each year, more than 2 million human poison exposures are reported to the American Association of Poison Control Centers (AAPCC). The AAPCC compiles the Toxic Exposure Surveillance System (TESS), the largest database of information about toxic exposures in the United States. More than 90% of these exposures occur in the victim's home. Others occur in locations such as the workplace, healthcare facilities, schools, and public areas.[5] More than half of the poisonings are found in children less than 6 years of age. Most poisonings continue to be unintentional. Intentional poisonings are generally related to suicide, misuse, and abuse. The age group with the most fatalities related to poisoning was the 20-year-old to 59-year-old age group.[5]

The human environment contains natural and manufactured toxins from plants, animals, chemicals, drugs, and chemotherapeutic agents. A new phenomenon that has been increasing over the past few decades is the nonmedical use of prescriptive medications, which has led to an increase in poisonings from medications that include sedatives, tranquilizers, opioids, and stimulants.[15]

Although multiple substances and various sources of toxins and poisons exist, only a limited number of antidotes are available. Table 30-1 lists most of the available antidotes that may be useful in the management of the poisoned patient.

The most important concept in the care of the patient who has been poisoned is supportive care. In addition to maintenance of the patient's airway, breathing, and circulation, the exposure to the toxin must be quickly stopped to prevent further harm to the patient. Some toxins can cause injury to caregivers, so appropriate decontamination must be accomplished before transport. Safety must be the number one concern when transporting a potentially poisoned patient.[1,21]

TABLE 30-1	Antidotes for Selected Poisonings
Toxin	**Antidote**
Opiates	Naloxone
Carbon monoxide	Oxygen
Cyanide	Amyl nitrate
	Sodium nitrate
	Sodium thiosulfate
Anticholinesterase	Atropine
Organophosphates	
Carbamates	
Methemoglobinemic agents	Methylene blue
Nitrates	
Chlorates	
Nitrobenzene	
Ethylene glycol	Ethanol
Acetaminophen	*N*-acetylcysteine
Heavy metals	BAL
	Disodium edetate
	Penicillamine
Iron	Deferoxamine
Anticholinergics	Physostigmine
Diphenhydramine	
Benzotropine	
Anticoagulants	
Coumadin	
Heparin	Vitamin K
Cardiac medications	Protamine
Beta-adrenergic blockers	
Calcium-channel blockers	Glucagon
Digoxin	Calcium
Tricyclic antidepressants	Digoxin Fab antibodies
	Sodium bicarbonate

From Wright RO, et al: Poison antidotes: guidelines for rational use in the emergency department, *Emerg Med Rep* 16(21):201, 1995.

Maloney and Pakiela[14] recently published a study that reviewed the air medical transport of patients with acute toxicologic emergencies. The three most common emergencies were carbon monoxide, acetaminophen, and antidepressant poisonings. The primary intervention provided by the transport team was endotracheal intubation.[14]

The purpose of this chapter is to discuss the general management of the poisoned patient, identify the pathophysiology of selected drugs, and describe the care of the poisoned patient during transport.

INTENTIONAL AND UNINTENTIONAL POISONING

Ingestion of or exposure to a toxic substance may be either intentional or unintentional. Determination of why the patient has become poisoned is important because it could make a difference in the care of the patient. A patient who intentionally took a lethal amount of a drug should be considered a potential safety risk by the transport team.[1]

Sources of unintentional exposure include therapeutic error (too much medication taken), bites and stings, environmental exposures, and food poisoning. Intentional poison exposures usually result from suicide attempts, abuse, and intentional misuse of medications.

The word *poisoning* denotes a toxic exposure that can be intentional, unintentional, or unknown to the patient. A patient or family member may have misread a label, taken too much of a drug, or accidentally become poisoned. A child may climb up and get into a medicine cabinet, ingest a bottle of aspirin, and be unintentionally poisoned. Criminals do not often use poisonous substances as a method of injuring or killing.[20]

An intentional overmedication or ingestion of a toxic substance is considered an *overdose*.[2,20,21,25] Poisoning generally occurs in the pediatric population. Patients who have overdosed or intentionally poisoned themselves are usually 12 years or older, although some cases suggest that children 5 years and older should be evaluated for intentional ingestion.[7,8]

The distinction between accidental and intentional toxic exposure is important. If the patient is suicidal, the transport team should take additional precautions to ensure a safe environment for the crew and the patient during transport.

GENERAL MANAGEMENT OF THE POISONED PATIENT

The initial management of any poisoned patient includes establishment of a patent airway, ventilation, and maintenance of adequate circulation.

The transport team should always ensure that whatever has poisoned the patient may not potentially cause harm to the team. Further evaluation consists of a detailed history about the event that led to the poisoning, a thorough physical examination, administration of antidotes as indicated, and transport to an appropriate healthcare facility for definitive care. The patient's family should be a part of the initial care because they may be able to offer important information about the incident. The emotional support of the patient, particularly a patient who has attempted suicide, should be included in the planning of care.

INITIAL MANAGEMENT

Shannon and colleagues[21] state that the initial approach to the management of a poisoned patient includes: stabilization; laboratory assessment; decontamination of the gastrointestinal tract, skin, or eyes; administration of an antidote if indicated; elimination enhancement of the toxin; and observation and disposition.

As with any other critically ill or injured patient, the ABCDEs (airway, breathing, circulation, disability, and exposure) take initial precedence. One exception in the case of the poisoned patient is the need to remove the victim from a toxic environment or toxic source before the ABCDEs can be assessed. If the patient has been sprayed with a toxic substance or the creature that caused envenomation is still in the immediate vicinity, the environment must be controlled and made safe before patient management so that the healthcare providers are not injured or poisoned.

Many toxins and poisons alter mental status and therefore may compromise the airway. Protection of the airway is particularly important if the toxin is to be removed via gastric lavage. During resuscitation, contamination of the rescuer with the toxic substance should always be avoided. Endotracheal or nasotracheal intubation is the preferred method of protecting the airway and preventing the possibility of aspiration.

Alterations in the patient's circulatory status may be profound and life threatening. Intravenous access and appropriate fluid resuscitation should be initiated. Blood pressure may need to be supported with vasoactive agents.

Depending on the type of poison or toxic exposure, decontamination may be needed before the patient can be transported. Generally, decontamination of the patient can be accomplished with soap and water. However, some toxins require specific decontaminates. The transport team must know and follow appropriate procedures to protect both themselves and the patient.[12,19,20]

ASSESSMENT
History
The history of the toxic exposure provides a vital method of identification of the type of substance responsible for the patient's symptoms. Poisoning or an overdose should be suspected in the following types of patients: a psychiatric patient, a trauma victim, a comatose patient with an unknown cause of coma, a young person with a life-threatening arrhythmia of undetermined origin, a patient rescued from a fire, a child with unexplained lethargy, and any person with suspicious or unusual behavior.[10,25] The history should include the type of substance or suspected substance that was taken, the exposure route, the time of the exposure, and the size or dosage of the exposure.

The patient may be exposed to a toxin through a number of routes. These include:

- Ingestion
- Dermal or skin contact
- Inhalation
- Ocular exposure
- Bite or sting
- Parenteral
- Aspiration

If a thorough history cannot be obtained, the environment in which the patient was found should be explored for clues to the cause of the poisoning. The transport team should look for bottles, containers, drug paraphernalia, animals, or items that may provide additional information about a suspected or unknown toxic substance. These items should be transported with the patient. Identification of witnesses to the event can add more information concerning what may have caused the poisoning or toxic exposure.[10,20]

Medical history, such as allergic reactions, previous surgeries, and past hospitalizations, should be noted. When possible, assessment of whether the patient has attempted suicide in the past is important.

In the care of the pediatric or elderly patient, the possibility of abuse or neglect must be kept in mind. A referral may be necessary to outside agencies, perhaps even the police, so that the patient's environment may be evaluated to see whether it is appropriate and safe.[16,20]

Symptoms of Poisoning and Toxic Exposures

Certain symptoms without a clear cause may suggest poisoning or overdose. Severe poisoning symptoms include coma, cardiac arrhythmia, metabolic acidosis, seizures, and gastrointestinal (GI) disturbances.[1-4,10,20] Many disease states may mimic overdose and should be considered in the differential diagnoses. Head injuries, encephalitis, meningitis, metabolic disturbances, and psychiatric diseases are easily mistaken for poisoning.

Physical Examination

The physical examination of a poisoned patient should include assessment of general appearance and pulmonary, cardiovascular, abdominal, and neurologic systems. The information obtained from physical examination not only helps determine the source of the toxic substance but also provides baseline data to follow the effects of the toxic substance and the particular interventions that have been initiated.

Baseline assessment data are particularly important in the determination of any changes in the patient's condition during transport. During transport, the toxic effects of the substance should be considered, as should the success or failure of initial treatments on the patient's condition.[13]

The physical appearance of the patient may give a clue to the type of poison or overdose the patient has taken. The presence of needle tracks, burns, bruises, lacerations, cutaneous bullae, erythema, petechiae, cyanosis, flushed skin, or bite marks may provide information to help diagnose the poison or toxic exposure.[4,8-10,20] Breath odors may suggest possible

TABLE 30-2	Odors Associated With Poisonings
Odor	**Possible Poison**
Sweet	Placidyl
	Acetone
	Chloroform
Bitter almond	Cyanide
Pear	Chloral hydrate
Garlic	Arsenic
Wintergreen	Methylsalicylate

poisoning or help rule it out for another cause. For example, the smell of oil of wintergreen can indicate salicylate poisoning. Table 30-2 lists odors associated with certain poisonings.[8,20]

Respiratory rate and pattern are also important assessment parameters. Auscultation of breath sounds is included in this assessment. Many toxins can cause respiratory arrest and impair the airway, with the potential for aspiration.

Assessment of the level of consciousness of the poisoned patient is secondary only to the patient's respiratory (and cardiovascular) assessments and may reveal a spectrum of altered sensorium. Hyperactivity, psychosis, somnolence, or coma may be manifested. Generalized seizures have been reported in many different cases of poisoning or overdose. Level of consciousness, pupillary response, motor and sensory function, and vital signs should also be included in the assessment.

An assessment of the patient's level of consciousness should go beyond orientation to person, place, and time. The patient's interaction with the environment can yield useful information about the patient's level of consciousness. Many drugs and toxic substances cause visual, auditory, or other sensory hallucinations and alter the patient's personality.

Pupil size, shape, and reaction are parts of the neurologic assessment. Constricted or dilated pupils may indicate drug or treatment effects. Motor and sensory functions are usually assessed together and may vary from normal activity to no movement at all. Seizure activity is not an uncommon complication from toxins and should be appropriately documented and treated.

The presence or possibility of an altered mental status occurring during transport necessitates the use of appropriate safety measures. Restraints and, in some cases, chemical restraint may be warranted to ensure safe transport.[1,13]

Cardiac monitoring should be performed and blood pressure and pulse quality frequently checked during transport. Hypotension, premature ventricular contractions, prolonged QT intervals, and a widened QRS complex are examples of some of the cardiac arrhythmia that may occur because of cardiac toxicity related to some poisonings.

Certain toxic substances cause GI disturbances such as nausea, vomiting, and severe abdominal pain. Iron, lithium, mercury, phosphorus, arsenic, mushrooms, organophosphates, and fluoride are examples of toxic substances that can cause GI disturbances. Phosphorus poisoning can cause luminescent vomit and flatus.[20] A gastric tube should be inserted before transport to prevent aspiration, especially if the patient has been given activated charcoal.

Laboratory Studies

Many substances responsible for adverse reactions, intoxications, and poisoning are difficult to identify. Serum levels are not reflective of tissue concentration or receptor interactions; therefore, levels of specific toxins may be incongruous with clinical manifestations.[20]

Laboratory evaluations such as complete blood count, electrolytes, whole blood glucose, liver function tests, and coagulation studies are frequently helpful. Many toxins are associated with leukocytosis or electrolyte alterations. An example is the hypokalemia associated with theophylline toxicity. Arterial blood gases are beneficial in determination of acidosis or alkalosis. Acidosis can be appreciated in tricyclic poisoning or late methanol or ethylene glycol poisoning, whereas alkalosis occurs in early salicylate intoxication.[8,20]

The treatment of poisoning with some drugs such as acetaminophen and aspirin necessitates determination of baseline serum levels and a repeat of these levels 3 to 6 hours after ingestion. Levels of some drugs may have to be monitored for several days after ingestion to ensure that they have been eliminated. Any blood, gastric contents, and urine that have been obtained for toxic analysis should accompany the patient for transport.

REMOVAL, ELIMINATION, OR DISRUPTION OF THE TOXIN

Ingestion, parenteral injection, ocular contamination, dermal exposure, inhalation, and envenomation are the major routes of intoxication.[19,20] The method of exposure must be established so that a method of removal or interruption can be chosen. Methods for reversal of the clinical effects of poisons include the use of antidotes, antivenin, supportive therapy, forced diuresis, charcoal, cathartics, whole bowel irrigation, hemoperfusion, and dialysis.[8,20] The most common method of removal is gastric lavage followed by administration of charcoal.

Ion-trapping diuresis is accomplished with alkalinization and acidification of the poisoned patient's urine. For alkalinization of urine, sodium bicarbonate is added to intravenous (IV) solution, and fluids are administered to yield a urine pH of 7.5. The patient must be monitored closely for complications from fluid and electrolyte imbalances.[20]

If the toxin has been inhaled, the individual should be removed from the source of the exposure. Administration of oxygen may be of use, particularly for the patient who has sustained carbon monoxide (CO) poisoning.

Contact poisons or toxins may enter the body through the skin, eyes, or mucous membranes. Removing the patient from the toxic environment, taking off the patient's clothes, and cleansing the affected area are the most important steps in the initial removal of the poison or toxic substance. Use of the correct irrigation fluid or fluids is important to prevent further injury to the patient. Attention also must be given to the proper disposal of the contaminated fluid and materials to prevent poisoning of the healthcare providers and the surrounding environment.

Antivenin administration, hemoperfusion, and dialysis should all be performed under the direction of a trained toxicologist or other healthcare professional acquainted with each procedure. Administration of antivenin in the prehospital environment is not recommended because of the potential of severe complications that may not be effectively managed.[6,17,18]

SUPPORTIVE AND EMOTIONAL CARE OF THE POISONED PATIENT

As noted previously, specific antidotes are limited compared with the numbers of the poisons and toxic substances disseminated in the environment. Frequently, supportive care directed at prevention of complications from the poison or toxic substance is the most that can be done for the patient.[20] Part of this supportive care may be the transport of the patient to a specific center with additional methods of care for the patient. Supportive care is based on the previous discussion of initial management, physical examination, and removal, elimination, or interruption of the toxic sequence.

The emotional care of the poisoned patient can be difficult. If the poisoning is intentional, the motive must be quickly discovered so that proper psychiatric and social care can be rendered. All procedures should be explained to the patient and a nonjudgmental attitude imparted when care is provided. If possible, the patient's family should be given some time with the patient before transport.

Protection of the patient from complications and respect for the patient as a human are important components of the care of the poisoned patient. E.J. Daniels[7] noted how insensitive nursing care can affect the poisoned patient:

> "The curtains hadn't been completely closed, and anyone and everyone walking by peered in, adding to my humiliation. I tried staring at everything but Brenda and the gaggy network of tubes in an attempt to keep my mind off the nauseating trauma. Alright. I have to put some medications down you. Try not to gag on it, because you really need it, keep this down. I'd never heard of any medicine that was pitch black! I felt like she had been flushing me out for hours. She hooked up a huge syringe to the end of the tube down inside of me. The thought of the tar going down my throat into my stomach was more repulsive than the gurgling sensation of lavage."[7]

SAFETY ISSUES IN THE TRANSPORT OF THE POISONED PATIENT

Safety is one of the most important issues to be addressed in the care of a poisoned patient during transport. Many intoxicants can cause hallucinations or violent behavior. Physical or chemical restraint to ensure safe transport should be a consideration when preparing the patient for transport.

Both physical and chemical (i.e., medications) restraints provide a means of safe control of the patient for transport. Decreasing excessive stimulation during transport with ear protectors may also reduce the possibility of dangerous or threatening patient behavior during transport. If neuromuscular blocking agents are used, adequate analgesia and sedation must be provided during transport.[1]

SUMMARY

The care of the poisoned patient who needs transport begins with management of the patient's airway and ventilation and maintenance of the cardiovascular system. Physical examination, including the patient's general appearance; assessment of the neurologic, respiratory, cardiovascular, and gastrointestinal systems; removal, elimination, or interruption of the toxic sequence; and supportive and emotional care are other important components of care of the poisoned patient.

Preparation for the transport of the poisoned patient includes decontamination; sampling of the toxic substance; transfer of laboratory work such as blood, urine, or vomitus; and informing the family of the transport destination.

Box 30-1 summarizes the care for the poisoned patient. The care of the poisoned patient must be approached in an organized manner to provide supportive care and prevent complications.

PHARMACOLOGIC PROPERTIES OF DRUGS

Therapeutic dose responses are affected by multiple variables including the rate of absorption, distribution, binding or localization in tissues, inactivation, and excretion. The *rate of absorption* is defined as the time needed for the chemotherapeutic agent to cross the enterovascular barriers and circulate in the cardiovascular system. Agents dissolved in solution are absorbed more rapidly than those in solid forms. Timed-release enteric-coated products are engineered to greatly decrease the absorption rate.

BOX 30-1	**Care of the Poisoned Patient by the Transport Team**

1. Provide basic and advanced life support after ensuring that the environment is safe for the transport team.
2. Remove the patient from the toxic environment.
3. When indicated, decontaminate the patient by removing clothing and washing off toxin.
4. Administer appropriate antidote when indicated.
5. Assess respiratory, neurologic, and cardiovascular status frequently.
6. Document or obtain baseline data.
7. Ensure the patient and transport team's safety in transport with the use of chemical or physical restraints. With use of chemical restraints, do not forget about analgesia and sedation.
8. Explain to the patient and family what is happening.
9. Transfer appropriate records and specimens.
10. Inform the patient's family of the patient's destination.

Medications given in higher concentration are absorbed more rapidly.

Gastric pH may deactivate or precipitate a drug. Areas of increased vascularity, such as the vagina or rectum, tend to absorb agents more rapidly. Topical exposure or inhalation of poisons reaches toxic levels quickly because of the large surface areas exposed to the intoxicants.

Most drugs are administered orally. Sites of absorption include the oral mucous membranes, stomach, duodenum, and small intestine. Sublingual administration usually promotes quick dissolution and rapid absorption. Absorption in the stomach is a passive process mediated by dissolution and diffusion. The nonionized form of a dissolved medication passes the mucosal barriers and enters the vascular compartment. Most drugs are either weak bases or weak acids. Gastric pH affects both dissolution and diffusion. Weak acids, such as salicylates and barbiturates, are predominantly nonionized in a strongly acidic environment; therefore, they are readily absorbed. Weak bases are in an ionized form in the stomach and are poorly absorbed. The intestinal pH. is less acidic than the stomach pH (pH, 5.3). Weak bases are readily absorbed, but weak acids cross the mucosal barrier less readily. In addition, the gastric mucosa is a lipoid membrane, which absorbs lipid-soluble substances, such as alcohol, rapidly. Factors that change gastric emptying time also alter the rate of absorption of a drug. IV injection is the most immediate and consistent blood concentration for any drug. After injection, a redistribution phase may significantly decrease the blood level of the drug. Absorption of medication given subcutaneously or intramuscularly depends on the site of injection, the solubility of the drug, and the vascularity of the injection area.

Once the drug is absorbed into the cardiovascular compartment, redistribution occurs throughout the body. Agents enter or pass through the various body-fluid compartments (plasma, interstitial, transcellular, vitreous, and cellular fluids). Medications are restricted in distribution by their ability to pass through cellular membranes.

Drugs may accumulate in storage depots because of protein binding, fat accumulation, and active transport. Medications are stored in equilibrium and released as plasma concentrations are reduced. Storage depots permit maintenance of plasma levels for long periods, prolonging pharmacologic effects. Anatomic components that act as storage depots include plasma proteins, connective tissues, tissue constituents (such as proteins, phospholipids, or nucleoproteins), adipose tissue, and transcellular fluids.

The mechanism responsible for drug transport across cell membranes may be an active or passive process. Passive transfer is diffusion driven by concentration gradients. Active transport is mediated by a carrier and requires expenditure of energy. The ultimate fate of a drug is metabolism and excretion. Biotransformation involves chemical reactions, classified as either nonsynthetic or synthetic. The nonsynthetic class involves oxidation, reduction, and hydrolysis. The parent drug is changed to a more active, a less active, or an inactive metabolite. Hepatocytic enzymes mediate most nonsynthetic reactions. Exceptions include nonenzymatic hydrolysis in the plasma, plasma cholinesterase and pseudocholinesterase, and synaptic metabolism of neurotransmitter analogs.

Synthetic reactions or conjugation occur in the liver or kidney. The process couples the parent drug or its metabolites to endogenous substrates (usually carbohydrates, amino acids, or inorganic sulfates). Conjugated drugs form inactive, highly ionized, water-soluble substances that are excreted in the urine. Conjugation is an active process that requires adenine triphosphate expenditure.

Active parent drugs and metabolites are excreted in the urine as a primary route of disposal. Drugs are also eliminated through excretion of feces. Metabolites are dissolved in bile, secreted into the alimentary tract, and passed through the GI tract. In addition, the unabsorbed parent drug is removed with fecal passage.

This discussion has focused on the incidence of poisoning; general considerations in the care of the poisoned patient; general management of the poisoned patient; signs and symptoms of toxicity; physical examination of the poisoned patient; useful laboratory studies; removal, elimination, or disruption of the poison; supportive and emotional care of the poisoned patient; transport nursing care of the poisoned patient; and the pharmacologic properties of drugs. The next part of this chapter focuses on the toxicity and treatment of toxicity of specific drugs. Information about each of these drugs is presented for quick reference.[20]

TOXICITY AND TREATMENT OF POISONING BY SPECIFIC DRUGS

ACETYLSALICYLIC ACID

Aspirin is one of the oldest nonprescription pharmaceutical agents. Its therapeutic popularity is mainly a result of its antipyretic and analgesic effects. In recent years, the effects of aspirin on platelets have been recognized as a preventive intervention for people who have had heart attacks and strokes. Single low doses (e.g., 80 mg) of aspirin taken daily are now prescribed.[20]

Aspirin can be taken orally, topically, or rectally. The most common route of toxicity is via ingestion. Many over-the-counter medications contain aspirin, and multiple sources of poisoning may be involved.

Salicylate toxicity initially manifests in an increased respiratory rate and hyperventilation.

Blood gas analysis usually reflects respiratory alkalosis. Clinical manifestations of mild intoxication include headache, vertigo, tinnitus, mental confusion, sweating, thirst, hyperventilation, nausea, vomiting, and drowsiness. Severe intoxication produces similar symptoms combined with base and electrolyte imbalances. Patients are agitated, restless, and uncommunicative and may have seizures or become comatose. Noncardiac pulmonary edema is observed in severe poisoning, whereas bleeding diatheses are less common.[20]

Treatment of salicylate poisoning involves gastric emptying, administration of oral-activated charcoal, and alkaline diuresis. Charcoal administration without gastric emptying has been found to be effective in the management of salicylate toxicity.[20]

Alkaline diuresis is performed to increase the pH of the patient's urine to improve free salicylate excretion. Supportive care and maintenance of vital functions are mainstays of treatment in this type of poisoning.[20]

The patient with severe poisoning may need hemodialysis. Hemodialysis not only enhances the removal of the toxic levels of the salicylate, but it can also correct the fluid, electrolyte, and acid-base imbalances that occur with salicylate toxicity.[20]

ACETAMINOPHEN

Acetaminophen, similar to aspirin, has antipyretic and analgesic properties. It is not chemically related to the salicylates. Acetaminophen has become a useful alternative to aspirin because it does not cause the GI and bleeding complications that can occur with aspirin use. Like aspirin, acetaminophen is contained in many over-the-counter drugs and may be administered orally or rectally. The main site of absorption is the small intestine, and the drug is uniformly distributed throughout most body fluids.[8,20]

Acetaminophen is a drug with a toxicity that is increased by the liver, rather than detoxified. The metabolite produced in the liver with metabolism of acetaminophen attaches to the hepatic cell membrane and injures the lipids bilayer if not neutralized by the antioxidant hepatic glutathione. When hepatic glutathione stores are depleted because of an overdose of acetaminophen, the metabolites are not neutralized and cause injury and death of the hepatic cells.[20]

The classic clinical course of toxic acetaminophen poisoning occurs in four stages. The initial stage of toxicity occurs 30 minutes to 24 hours after ingestion and produces anorexia, nausea, vomiting, malaise, pallor, and diaphoresis.

The second stage begins 24 to 72 hours after ingestion. Right upper quadrant pain and tenderness may result from liver enlargement. The levels of liver enzymes, serum bilirubin, and prothrombin time begin to increase 36 hours after ingestion. Oliguria may result from acute tubular necrosis.

The third stage begins 72 to 96 hours after ingestion and is the time of peak liver-function abnormalities. Anorexia, nausea, vomiting, and malaise return, and jaundice become apparent. Fatalities from acetaminophen poisoning usually occur during this stage and result from fulminant hepatic necrosis.

The fourth stage, or resolution period, occurs 4 days to 2 weeks after poisoning. Patients are asymptomatic, and liver function parameters return to baseline values.[8,20]

Ingestions of more than 7.5 g or 150 mg/kg are considered potentially toxic. The serum level of acetaminophen should be measured 4 hours after ingestion in any person who has ingested a potentially toxic dose of acetaminophen. If the acetaminophen level is still toxic at 4 hours after ingestion or the level cannot be assayed before 10 hours have passed since ingestion and the history suggests a toxic ingestion, N-acetylcysteine (NAC) should be administered. NAC is administered orally at an initial dose of 140 mg/kg. A maintenance dose of 70 mg/kg every 4 hours for 17 doses is then given.[20] NAC may be administered intravenously in the critically ill patient. Consultation with a toxicologist or local poison control should be done to provide the safest and most effective care for these patients.

ANTIDEPRESSANTS (TRICYCLICS)

Tricyclic antidepressants (TCAs) are widely prescribed in the United States. Their primary use is in the treatment of endogenous depression in adults; however, recent study has increased their use for school phobia, pain control, obsessive-compulsive behavior, and sleep disorders in children.[8,20] Overdose statistics show that cyclic antidepressants are one of the most deadly types of poisoning, with a high degree of morbidity and mortality in significant overdoses. Many tricyclic antidepressants are available throughout the United States.[8,13]

Tricyclic antidepressants are well absorbed in the GI tract. The parent compound and active metabolites are quickly bound to plasma proteins. TCAs exert their effects by inhibiting the amine pump mechanism responsible for the reuptake of norepinephrine and serotonin in adrenergic and serotonergic neurons. Cyclic antidepressants also block cholinergic receptors in the parasympathetic nervous system and exert antihistaminic properties.[8,13,20]

The clinical manifestations of TCA poisoning include mydriasis, tachycardia, dry mucous membranes, urine retention, and decreased peristalsis. Central nervous system (CNS) signs include confusion, agitation, hallucinations, seizures, and coma. Twitching, jerking, and myoclonic movements have also been reported. Generalized tonic clonic seizures are reported in 1% to 20% of TCA poisoning cases. Respiratory depression is common. The enhanced adrenergic stimulation of the myocardium and direct toxic effects of these agents result in many cardiovascular effects. Sinus tachycardia and mild hypertension occur early in poisoning. TCAs exert a quinidine-like cardiac action that depresses conduction velocity. QRS-interval widening, right bundle-branch block, and first-degree heart block are common findings. Acidosis occurs because of cardiac and respiratory depression.[8,13,20]

In TCA poisoning, support of vital functions is essential. Hypotension is initially managed with an IV infusion of saline solution. Pressor agents are used if hypotension is refractory to fluid challenges. α-Adrenergic agents are preferred. Physostigmine is not an antidote to cyclic antidepressant poisoning; however, some evidence shows that it may be of use in a small group of patients with cardiac stability for control of agitated delirium.[20]

BENZODIAZEPINES

Benzodiazepines became available in the United States in 1963 for control of anxiety. These drugs are now used to decrease anxiety and as sedative-hypnotics, muscle relaxants, and anticonvulsants. Generally, a toxic level of benzodiazepines must be quite high; however, benzodiazepines are often taken in combination with other poisons, such as alcohol, which can cause death.[20]

The syndrome of benzodiazepine toxicity is nonspecific. The clinical picture is usually mild compared with those of other sedative-hypnotic poisonings. Most oral poisonings result in drowsiness and coma.

Transport team members must keep in mind that other medications and alcohol can place the patient at risk of toxicity with administration of medications such as midazolam or lorazepam to manage a patient during transport.

The treatment of benzodiazepine poisoning begins with management of the patient's ABCDEs. Flumazenil can be administered to reverse the sedative, ataxic, anxiolytic, and muscle-relaxant effects of toxic benzodiazepine ingestion. However, this drug must be administered with caution because many patients with overdoses take combinations of drugs, some of which may cause seizures at toxic levels, such as TCAs. Flumazenil reverses the anticonvulsant effects of benzodiazepines, which leaves patients with polyoverdoses at risk for lack of seizure management.[24,25]

DIGITALIS

The term *cardiac glycoside* is used to describe a large group of drugs prescribed to treat heart failure. These drugs have been used throughout history, with early mention of the compound found in ancient writings in the year 1500 BC. *Digitalis* has become the most familiar of the group. It is derived from the dried leaf of the foxglove plant *Digitalis purpurea*.[20]

Several factors contribute to digitalis poisoning, including patient age, severe heart disease, electrolyte imbalances, and drug therapy such as the use of diuretics.[20]

Clinical manifestations of digitalis toxicity are classified as cardiac and noncardiac. Cardiac manifestations are the result of depression through the sinoatrial and atrioventricular nodes and alteration of impulse formation. Noncardiac signs and symptoms include fatigue, vascular weakness, anorexia, nausea, vomiting, diarrhea, confusion, restlessness, insomnia, drowsiness, hallucinations, frank psychosis, blurred vision, photophobia, and yellowhalo visual effects.[20]

Treatment of digitalis toxicity includes support of vital functions and possible correction of the underlying cause (e.g., correction of an electrolyte imbalance). Advances in immunotherapy have yielded digoxin-specific antibody fragments (Fab) that neutralize digoxin toxicity. Fab fragments are indicated if conventional supportive care to life-threatening dysrhythmias and hyperkalemia fails. Fab fragments bind to digoxin, and the Fab-digoxin complex is excreted in the urine.[20]

OTHER DRUGS
Cocaine

Cocaine continues to be a drug of abuse in the United States. The cocaine problem varies with geographic location; however, few places in the United States have escaped difficulties related to illegal drug use.[20]

Cocaine is a naturally occurring alkaloid, the only source of which is the leaves of the evergreen shrub *Erythroxylon coca*. The leaves contain 0.5% to 2.5% cocaine. The plant is native to Peru, Bolivia, and Colombia but is now a major cultivated cash crop in many Central and South American countries. The crystallized cocaine is extracted from the coca leaf in the hydrochloride salt form. Cocaine hydrochloride is usually transported in a 90% to 95% pure form until it reaches its intended destination, where the drug is diluted and adulterated for street sale. Street cocaine generally varies in potency from 2% to 30% purity. Common adulterants are mannitol, lactose, and local anesthetics such as lidocaine, procaine, and tetracaine. Many times, street samples contain no cocaine at all but are combinations of caffeine, amphetamines, codeine, phencyclidine (PCP), and other local anesthetics.

Several routes are used for cocaine abuse. The easiest and most popular method of misuse is nasal inhalation or "snorting." The blood concentration after snorting increases rapidly for approximately 20 minutes, peaks at 1 hour, and then slowly subsides for several hours. Cocaine may also be injected intravenously. Because blood levels peak after 3 to 5 minutes, this method can be very toxic and lethal. In addition, cocaine can be combined in a mixture that may contain a flammable solvent that is ignited. Smoking cocaine may lead not only to toxicity but also to severe burn injuries.[20]

Crack is the "cooked and dried" version of freebase cocaine. When cocaine is mixed with baking soda and water and then heated in an ordinary pot, the impurities used to cut the drug are removed. The resulting mixture dries into a hard substance that is broken into small chunks or "rocks," which are white or yellowish-white in color. The user then smokes the rocks.[20]

Another popular method of cocaine use is for the male to apply the drug topically to his penis before sexual intercourse. Because cocaine is a local anesthetic, the desired effect of this practice is prolonged erection. Cocaine is absorbed in the female's vagina, and intoxication can occur.[4]

The drug is metabolized by the liver and excreted by the kidney.[20] Cocaine stimulates both the peripheral and central adrenergic nervous systems. Cocaine produces euphoria and a mild-to-moderate CNS stimulation manifested by decreased fatigue, excitement, and a general feeling of well-being. The user tends to be talkative, physically active, and sociable and may experience slight tachycardia, mydriasis, slight diaphoresis, and tremor.

Death from cocaine results from cardiovascular and respiratory collapse. Metabolic acidosis, hyperthermia, status epilepticus, or ventricular arrhythmias are seen in the severely poisoned patient. Fatalities may occur from any method of abuse. Unexplained sudden death may occur after IV injection, but most fatal cases follow a progressive downhill course over 30 to 60 minutes. Death can also occur as a result of the effects of agents used to mitigate cocaine effects (especially heroin) or from the untoward effects of adulterants or substituted drugs.[20]

The main objectives in treatment of acute cocaine poisoning are to support the respiratory system, control hypertension, suppress malignant cardiac arrhythmias, correct metabolic acidosis, reduce hyperthermia, and minimize seizure activity.[13,20]

Hallucinogens

Two types of drug poisoning that cause hallucinations are *phencyclidine* (PCP) and *lysergic acid diethylamide* (LSD). PCP was initially developed as a general anesthetic in 1958. Because of the postanesthetic reactions that occurred with its use, it has not been used legally since 1965. PCP now is manufactured in "kitchen" laboratories.

The drug may be smoked, snorted, or ingested and is distributed to all tissue compartments, metabolized by the liver, and excreted through the kidneys. Its effects can last up to 48 hours.[24] PCP can produce bizarre and dangerous behavior. In larger doses, it can cause psychosis, hostility, and coma. A common neurologic sign of PCP intoxication is nystagmus.[24]

Treatment consists of supportive care. Air medical transport of patients who have taken PCP or any hallucinogen demands close observation. Patients may become hostile, belligerent, and destructive. Sedative or neuromuscular blocking agents with airway control may be necessary to safely transport these patients.

Lysergic acid diethylamide is the most potent hallucinogen known. Psychiatrists initially used the drug in the 1950s as an aid in clinical psychotherapy. Abuse became popular during the 1960s, with illicit use reaching epidemic proportions in 1965.[20]

Lysergic acid diethylamide can be taken both orally and nasally. The dose needed to produce hallucinations is between 0.5 and 1.0 µg/kg, and the intensity of its effect is dose dependent.[13] Absorption of the drug is rapid, and LSD is distributed to all tissues, including the brain. Initial effects occur in 30 to 40 minutes, and peak effects occur in 1 to 2 hours. LSD is metabolized in the liver, and small amounts are excreted unchanged in urine.[20]

Psychologic effects follow ingestion of LSD in 30 to 90 minutes. These effects are generally pleasurable, and the person is usually able to function and is aware of the drug-induced illusions. Occasionally, a person may have an intense panic reaction ("bad trip") that includes frightening hallucinations and loss of the knowledge that the symptoms are caused by a transient drug effect. Such a person may become confused, aggressive, suicidal, or violent. Particularly frightening and uncontrollable experiences are linked to the contamination of LSD with other drugs, such as amphetamines.[20]

As with the patient who has taken PCP, extreme caution should be taken during the transport of these patients. Use of ear protectors, sedation, and prophylactic restraints may be necessary before transport.

Designer drugs continue to appear on the street, for example, ecstasy or 3,4-methylenedioxymethamphetamine (MDMA) a substitute amphetamine. Each of these medications causes different signs and symptoms and generally requires supportive care. However, safety must remain the number one concern when transporting these patients for additional care.[20]

ALCOHOL

Alcohol (ethanol) is the most widely used and abused drug in America. It is often involved in poison emergencies because it is frequently used with other drugs.

Ethanol alcohol is rapidly absorbed from the stomach, small intestine, and colon. Food reduces the rate of absorption by 2 to 6 hours. Once ethanol is ingested, equilibration is rapid, and distribution uniformly occurs throughout all bodily tissues and fluids. Passage across the placenta has been documented.[8,20]

Ethanol metabolism occurs mainly in the liver. Ethanol is oxidized by alcohol, which is a CNS depressant. Acute intoxication produces psychomotor retardation, reflex slowing, lethargy, sleep, and ultimately, coma and death. Initially, respirations are stimulated as a result of the production of carbon dioxide. However, with increasing concentrations of alcohol, respirations are dangerously depressed. Ethanol enhances cutaneous blood flow, which causes heat loss through vasodilation. Excessive amounts depress the central thermoregulatory mechanism, adding to the hypothermia effects. Ethanol stimulates gastric secretions, which causes an irritation of the gastric mucosa. In addition, ethanol causes diuresis mediated through inhibition of antidiuretic hormone, which decreases renal tubular reabsorption of water.[8,20,24]

Patients respond differently to alcohol poisoning. Table 30-3 correlates signs and symptoms of alcohol intoxication with blood alcohol levels.[15] The lethal dose of alcohol in children is considered 3 g/kg and in adults is 5 to 8 g/kg.

Care of the alcohol-poisoned patient consists of supportive care. Such patients may become combative, and precautions should be taken for appropriate restraint before transport.

TABLE 30-3	**Assessment of the Severity of Alcohol Intoxication by Blood Alcohol Level**
Blood Alcohol Level	**Signs and Symptoms**
Mild (0.05%-0.15%; 0.5-1.5 mg/mL)	Decreased inhibitions
	Slight visual impairments
	Slight muscular incoordination
	Slowing of reaction time
Moderate (0.15%-0.3%; 1.5-3 mg/mL)	Definite visual impairment
	Sensory loss
	Muscular incoordination
	Slowing of reaction time
	Slurred speech
Severe (0.3%-0.5%; 3-5 mg/mL)	Marked muscular incoordination
	Blurred or double vision
	Approaching stupor
	Sometimes hypoglycemia with hypothermia
	Conjugate deviation of the eyes
	Extensor rigidity of the extremities
	Unilateral or bilateral Babinski's sign
	Convulsions and trismus
	Fatalities begin to occur
Coma (>0.5%; >5 mg/mL)	Unconsciousness
	Depressed respirations
	Decreased reflexes and complete loss of sensation
	Deaths are frequent

From Dreisbach RH, Robertson WO: *Handbook of poisoning: prevention, diagnosis and treatment,* Norwalk, CT, 1987, Appleton & Lange.

Ethylene Glycol

Ethylene glycol is an odorless water-soluble solvent most commonly used in permanent-type antifreezes and coolants. Ingestion usually occurs in the inquisitive toddler or the subject desperate to commit suicide. Ethylene glycol is rapidly absorbed and reaches peak blood levels in 1 to 4 hours after ingestion. Large doses result in an inebriated patient without the odor of alcohol. Ethylene glycol approximates ethanol in CNS toxicity; however, its metabolites produce profound systemic effects.[20,23]

Ethylene glycol is hepatically metabolized. It eventually breaks down into four main byproducts that include formic and oxalic acid. Most investigators believe that these byproducts are responsible for the pathology seen in ethylene glycol toxicity.[20,23]

Signs and symptoms of ethylene glycol ingestion include nausea, vomiting, ataxia, stupor, coma, convulsions, nystagmus, depressed deep-tendon reflexes, myoclonic jerks, hypothermia, and low-grade fever. A profound anion-gap metabolic acidosis is a hallmark of this poisoning, but it only occurs after metabolism has begun. Severe hypocalcemia from chelation of calcium may produce tetany and cardiac compromise. Other complications of ethylene glycol poisoning include kidney failure and pulmonary edema.[20,23]

Serum and blood levels guide treatment for ethylene glycol ingestion. If history suggests a significant ingestion, an IV ethanol drip should be initiated before the ethylene glycol level is determined. Ethanol blocks the conversion of ethylene glycol to its toxic form. Dialysis is used to remove the ethylene glycol because metabolism is retarded and renal excretion of the parent compound is poor.

Fomepizole (Antizol)[23] is also an antidote for ethanol toxicity. It prevents the formation of toxic metabolites. The advantages of fomepizole use include:

- Intermittent administration.
- Decreased mental status changes compared with the use of alcohol.
- Reduced likelihood of the patient needing admission to a critical care unit.

Carbon Monoxide

Carbon monoxide (CO) is a colorless, odorless, tasteless gas yielded by the incomplete combustion of carbonaceous material. Sources include car exhaust, space heaters, defective fireplace flues, flame-type water heaters, improperly vented gas ranges and furnaces, coal and oil furnaces, poorly ventilated charcoal and gas grills, and fires of all types.[10,20]

Carbon monoxide poisoning should be suspected in any patients with unexplained symptoms who may have been exposed to machinery running in an enclosed poorly ventilated space; to a furnace that is new or run for the first time when the weather changes; or to smoke in an enclosed space. It may also be suspected with unexplained symptoms in multiple people in the same living space. Animals are more sensitive than humans to CO poisoning and may have been ill long before their human owners.

Carbon monoxide combines with the hemoglobin molecule in the red blood cell. The affinity of hemoglobin for CO is approximately 200 times that for oxygen. Not only does CO compete with oxygen for hemoglobin, but also the presence of carboxyhemoglobin greatly impedes the dissociation of oxygen from hemoglobin. This leads to a decreased partial pressure of oxygen in the blood and diminished gradient for oxygen diffusion from the red blood cell to the tissues, which results in tissue anoxia. Arterial hypoxia results from any of the following conditions: pulmonary venous admixture from an uneven ventilation/perfusion relationship; marked inhibition of the circulatory system; direct effect of CO on the pulmonary tissue, which results in increased capillary permeability and decreased production of surfactant; and a change in the oxyhemoglobin dissociation curve with a shift to the left.[10,20]

The concentration of CO in the blood has been found to relate poorly to the clinical features observed in the person who has been exposed. Figure 30-1 describes the symptomatology of CO poisoning related to CO saturation in the blood.[10,20]

The treatment of acute CO exposure is oxygen delivery. Carboxyhemoglobin dissociates and converts to oxyhemoglobin if high concentrations of oxygen are provided. Hyperbaric therapy has also been found to be extremely successful for patients with levels of 40% at the exposure site and emergency unit levels of 25%.[10,20,22]

The treatment of the patient in transport with CO poisoning includes management of the patient's airway so that high-flow O_2 can be delivered. A neurologic assessment is helpful before treatment and

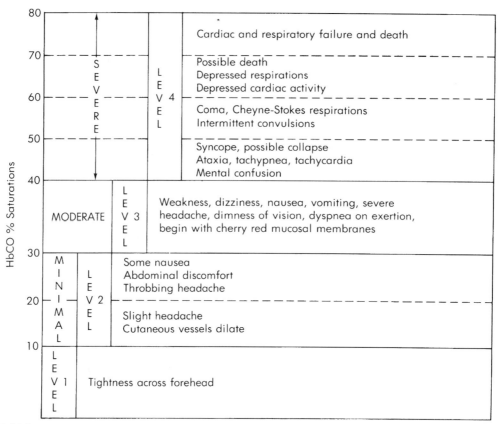

FIGURE 30-1   **Signs and symptoms of various blood levels of carboxyhemoglobin (HbCO).** (Modified from Elo T: *Carbon monoxide: quick reference to clinical toxicology,* Philadelphia, 1980, Lippincott.)

once treatment has been begun with high-flow oxygen. In addition, the patient must be observed and treated for such hypoxic side effects as seizures.

SNAKEBITES

Responding to the needs of a victim of *snakebite* may not be one of the most common flights encountered by the transport nurse; however, knowledge of how to care for such patients can decrease complications and save lives. Many thousands of snakebites are reported in the United States each year. Venomous snakes inflict about 7000 of those bites. This number of bites is a "guess." Unfortunately, people still die of envenomation.[3,6,11,17,18,22]

Venom is a special category of poison that must be injected by one organism into another to produce a harmful effect.[17] It is secreted by special epithelial cells in certain organisms and is stored in the lumina or exocrine glands. It comprises multiple substances, some of them toxic. The toxins may affect particular body systems such as the neurologic, hematologic, and cardiovascular systems.[3,6,11,17,18,22]

The effects of venom are dependent on the pharmacologic complexity of the venom and the action that the venom exerts on the tissues. The location of the venom injection also affects the spread of the venom. Bites to the leg may be more serious than to the face because muscle movement spreads the venom throughout the body. However, any bite in the area of a vessel could potentially spread the venom more quickly.[3,6,11,17]

The most prevalent venomous snakes in the United States are the pit vipers, which include the true rattlesnakes, the copperheads, and the water moccasins. These snakes are found throughout the country with the exception of Maine, Alaska, and Hawaii.[3,6,11,17]

The coral snake is another venomous snake found in the United States. The eastern coral snake is found in North and South Carolina, Florida, Louisiana, Mississippi, Alabama, Georgia, and Texas.

In addition to the venomous snakes native to the United States, poisonous snakes have been collected from all over the world. A bite from any one of these snakes may be fraught with complications or may even be instantly fatal.

The following subsections describe the venomous snakes, the initial treatment of snakebites, transport nursing care of patients with snake bites, and the role of the transport team in the care of these victims.

RECOGNITION OF VENOMOUS BITES

Figure 30-2 compares venomous and nonvenomous snakes. The most prevalent type of venomous snake in the United States is the pit viper. Only trained people should handle live snakes; even a dead snake can envenomate a careless person.[16-18]

Pit vipers belong to the *Crotalidae* family (as shown in Figure 30-2) and have a pit midway between the eye and nostril on each side of the head. This pit is a heat-sensing organ that helps the snake locate its prey. This particular characteristic, unlike others in Figure 30-2, is a 100% consistent characteristic in the identification of pit vipers.[16-18]

Envenomation by a pit viper usually results in symptoms of localized pain, swelling, and edema in the bitten area. Other symptoms include diaphoresis and chills, paresthesia, nausea, hypotension, faintness, weakness, muscle fasciculations, local ecchymosis, and coagulopathies.[16-18]

The second largest family of snakes in the world is the *Elapidae,* which contains some deadly species. These include cobras, mambas, and the eastern coral snakes. One of the distinguishing characteristics of these snakes is their color.

Envenomation by a coral snake may result in a neurotoxic course. Systemic manifestations include drowsiness, euphoria, weakness, nausea, vomiting, fasciculations, dysphagia, salivation, extraocular muscle paresis, hypotension, and cardiopulmonary failure.[16-18]

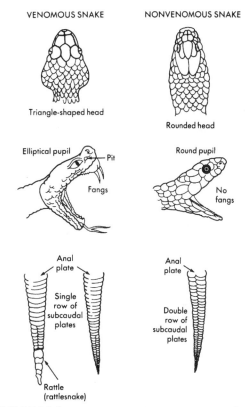

FIGURE 30-2 **Venomous and nonvenomous snakes.** (From Otten M: Venomous animal injuries. In Marx JA, et al, editors: *Rosen's emergency medicine: concepts and clinical practice,* ed 6, St Louis, 2006, Mosby.)

INITIAL MANAGEMENT OF SNAKEBITES

Envenomation does not always occur with a snake bite. Estimates are that 20% to 30% of crotalid bites and 50% of elapid bites do not result in penetration; such bites are called dry bites.[6] The literature contains lengthy and controversial (and many emotional) discussions over the appropriate management of snakebite.[3,6,18] In the following discussion of the general management of patients with snakebite, it is important to emphasize that experts should be consulted when questions arise about the care of patients with snakebite. Many of the authors cited in this chapter are available for consultation, as is the local poison control center. Identification of the snake is important so that appropriate treatment can be initiated. Many patients have received unnecessary treatment for nonvenomous bites.[3,6,11,16,18]

If the snake has not been secured, the patient should be moved to a safe environment. The patient must be kept calm and the affected part immobilized. These two interventions decrease the circulation of venom throughout the patient's system. Specific prehospital care of the patient with snakebite is based on the type of envenomation that has occurred. For elapid envenomation, the wound should be cleansed, a compressive bandage applied, the extremity immobilized, and the patient transported. The care of viper envenomation should include cleansing of the wound, immobilization of the affected part, no use of compression techniques, and transport of the patient.[7,26]

The airway, ventilatory, and circulatory status of the patient should be constantly evaluated. Two large-bore IV lines should be started, preferably in an area away from the bite. The patient must be observed closely for progression of symptoms from a localized reaction at the wound site to a systemic reaction.

When possible, blood samples for baseline laboratory work should be drawn before transport. These tests may include a complete blood count, coagulation studies, electrolytes, blood urea nitrogen, creatinine, and urinalysis. Included in the coagulation studies should be fibrin split products and fibrinogen levels.[17,18]

If the patient shows signs of severe envenomation, such as edema that has progressed 30 cm in 1 hour of the bite, shock, kidney failure, pulmonary edema, bleeding, or paralysis, administration of antivenin should be started.[17,18] The size of the patient needs to be considered in relation to the amount of venom that the person may be able to tolerate. A child or small adult may be more severely affected.

Snake antivenin is prepared from the serum of horses hyperimmunized against a specific venom or venoms. Unlike other drugs, the dosage of antivenin should be based on clinical findings rather than on the age and weight of the patient. Skin testing for hypersensitivity with epinephrine at the patient's bedside is recommended before antivenin is administered.[17,18] Administration of steroids and other medications to decrease the risk of anaphylaxis is used by some healthcare providers. Again, it cannot be overemphasized that experts are available via a number of communication routes and should be consulted.[3,6,16]

When antivenin is given, the package instructions should be followed and resuscitation equipment kept in close range. Patients should be monitored continuously for anaphylactic reactions.

Serum sickness may develop after antivenin administration. The incidence rate of serum sickness varies from 10% to 80% of all patients given antivenin therapy.[17] The symptoms of serum sickness have occurred up to 3 weeks after antivenin administration. They include fever, rash, nausea, vomiting, and neurologic symptoms. Treatment of serum sickness includes antihistamines and steroids.[17]

TRANSPORT CARE OF PATIENTS WITH SNAKEBITE

The transport team may become involved in the care of the patient with snakebite by directly responding to the scene of the injury or by transporting the patient to more definitive care. Experts in the care of snakebites note that rapid transport of these patients to a hospital or to a person who can manage the injury is imperative in saving lives and preventing complications. Box 30-2 summarizes care to be provided for the patient bitten by a snake.[17]

SUMMARY

The transport of the poisoned patient generally involves support of the patient's airway, breathing, and circulation. Few antidotes are available for the poisoned patient, and generally the transport team may have limited resources to determine the cause of the poisoning.

The transport team should always ensure safety before transport begins so they do not become victims of the poison as well. A patient who has deliberately taken poison must be appropriately retrained before transport.

The transport care of the poisoned patient can be interesting (i.e., discovering the poison responsible) and challenging (i.e., ensuring the best care).

BOX 30-2	Transport Care of the Patient Bitten by a Snake

1. Provide a safe environment for the transport team and patient.
2. Provide basic and advanced life support.
3. Obtain as much information as possible about the type of snake that has envenomated the patient.
4. Immobilize the affected part.
5. Keep the patient calm.
6. Notify the appropriate receiving facility. Consult an expert when patient management questions arise.
7. Establish a large-bore IV line.
8. Watch for local and systemic effects from the snakebite.
9. Administer analgesia for pain.
10. Bring the dead snake in a secure container for identification, if possible.

TOXICOLOGY
CASE STUDY 1

HALLUCINOGENIC TOXICITY

A 16-year-old boy ingested a plant known as monkshood after being told by his friends that he would have a "good trip." The plant that he ingested was a potent alkaloid. He immediately began hallucinating and then went into status epilepticus. The transport team was dispatched to assist in patient care and to transport the patient.

On the arrival of the transport team, the patient's seizures had subsided after administration of 5 mg diazepam. However, the patient was screaming and had to be physically restrained. An IV line was started, and the patient was intubated with the use of rapid-sequence induction. Ten milligrams vecuronium and 2 mg lorazepam were given for safety and sedation.

Blood pressure was 80 mm Hg systolic via palpation, pulse was 130 beats/min and irregular (the monitor showed atrial fibrillation), and respirations were being assisted because of the vecuronium. A fluid bolus of 200 mL of normal saline solution was infused. The patient's blood pressure increased to 100/50 mm Hg. The patient was prepared for transport. Restraints were applied, and a headset was placed on the patient to decrease outside stimulation.

During transport, the patient sustained cardiac arrest, going into coarse ventricular fibrillation.

He underwent successful electroconversion with 360 W/s. Atrial fibrillation continued after resuscitation. A lidocaine bolus was administered and a lidocaine drip initiated per advanced cardiac life support protocol.

The patient had no additional problems during transport and was admitted to the medical intensive care unit of the receiving facility. The toxicologist continued supportive care, including correction of the metabolic acidosis and maintenance of sedation. The patient regained consciousness 48 hours later and was discharged home within 5 days of the incident.

TOXICOLOGY
CASE STUDY 2

VICTIM OF A SNAKE BITE

The transport team was asked to transport via helicopter a 4-year-old boy who had sustained a snake bite. The child stated he had been playing in a field when a "brown snake with sharp teeth bit him." An adult did not witness this incident.

The child was alert and oriented. His vital signs were stable. The referring physician reported that the child had two puncture wounds at the side of his right foot. Localized swelling was also noted.

The care of this patient included assessment of whether the bite was venomous. Because copperheads are native to the area and fang marks were visible, the transport nurse had to assume that the child had been bitten by a pit viper. The wound had been cleansed and immobilized. The transport nurse placed an IV line and started a cardiac monitor. A tetanus shot was administered because the child had never been immunized.

During flight, the transport nurse monitored the child for signs and symptoms of localized and systemic poisoning, including increasing edema in the bitten extremity, nausea and vomiting, hypotension, and excessive bleeding.

An important role for the transport team in the care of snakebite envenomation is the timely delivery and initiation of antivenin in areas where it is not readily available. However, this child, as in about 50% of snakebites, only sustained a dry bite. He was admitted for observation and discharged later without complications.

REFERENCES

1. Air and Surface Transport Nurses Association: *Transport nurse safety in the transport environment*, Denver, 2006, ASTNA.
2. American Health Consultants: Special report on overdose patient in the ED, *ED Nursing* 3:77, 2000.
3. Auerbach P, editor: *Wilderness medicine*, ed 5, St Louis, 2007, Mosby Elsevier.
4. Brewer JD, Meves A, Bostwick M, et al: Cocaine abuse: dermatologic manifestations and therapeutic approaches, *J Am Acad Dermatol* 59:483-487, 2008.
5. Bronstein AC, Spyker DA, Cantilena LR, et al: 2006 Annual report of the American Association of Poison Control Centers' national poison data system (NPDS), *Clin Toxicol* 45(8):81-917, 2007.
6. Callahan M: Challenging paradigms is risky business: reflections on CC Snyder's: a definitive study of snakebite, *Wilder Environ Med* 12:273, 2001.
7. Daniels EJ: *Any other song*, Bowie, MD, 1980, Brady.
8. Emergency Nurses Association: *Emergency nursing pediatric course*, ed 3, Des Plaines, IL, 2004, ENA.
9. Foulke GE: Identifying toxicity risk early after antidepressant overdose, *Am J Emerg Med* 13(2):123, 1995.
10. Goldstein M: Carbon monoxide poisoning, *J Emerg Nur*. In press. Available at www.sciencedirect, accessed August 2008.
11. Jurkovich G, et al: Complications of Crotalidae antivenin therapy, *J Trauma* 28:1032, 1988.
12. Kitt S, et al: *Emergency nursing: a physiologic and clinical perspective*, Philadelphia, 1995, Saunders.
13. Lemke TL, Wang R: Emergency department observation for toxocologic exposures. *Emerg Med Clin North Am* 19(1):155-167, 2001.
14. Maloney GE, Pakiela JA: Characteristics of patients transported by an aeromedical service for acute toxicologic emergencies: a five year experience, *Air Med J* 27(1):48-50, 2008.
15. McCabe SE, Cranford JA, West BT: Trends in prescription drug abuse and dependence, co-occurrence with other substance use disorders and treatment utilization: results from two national surveys, *Addictive Behaviors* 33:1297-1305, 2008.
16. McNally J, Boesen K, Boyer L: Toxicologic information resources for reptile envenomations, *Vet Clin* 11:389-401, 2008.
17. Norris RL, Ling LJ, Wang R: Snake venom poisoning in the United States: assessment and management, *Emerg Med Rep* 16(10):87, 1995.
18. Norris RL, Bush SP: Bites by venomous reptiles in the Americas. In Auerbach P, editor: *Wilderness medicine*, ed 5, Philadelphia, 2007, Mosby Elsevier.
19. Peterson ME: Toxic exotics, *Vet Clin* 11:375-387, 2008.
20. Proehl J, editor: *Emergency nursing procedures*, ed 4, Philadelphia, 2009, Saunders Elsevier.
21. Shannon MW, Borron SW, Burns MJ: *Haddad and Winchester' clinical management of poisoning and drug overdose*, ed 4, Philadelphia, 2007, Saunders Elsevier.
22. Snyder CC, Pickins JE, Knowles RP, et al: A definitive study of snakebite, *Wilder Environ Med* 12:276, 2001.
23. Stolpe M, et al: Preliminary observations on the effects of hyperbaric oxygen therapy on western diamondback rattlesnake (Crotalus atrox) venom poisoning in the rabbit model, *Ann Emerg Med* 18:871, 1989.
24. Weinman S: A new antidote in review: Fomepizole (Antizol), *J Emerg Nurs* 24:333, 1998.
25. Wright RO, et al: Poison antidotes: guidelines for rational use in the emergency department, *Emerg Med Rep* 16(21):201, 1995.
26. York-Clark D, Stocking J, Johnson J: *Flight and ground transport nursing core curriculum*, Denver, 2006, Air and Surface Transport Nurses Association.

Selected Patient Populations

CHAPTER

31

THE PREGNANT PATIENT

Teri Campbell

COMPETENCIES

1. Perform a focused assessment of the pregnant patient, which includes subjective and objective data related to the patient's pregnancy.
2. Identify normal physiologic changes that occur during pregnancy.
3. Perform a focused assessment of the fetus before and during transport.
4. Initiate appropriate interventions for the patient in preterm labor.
5. Discuss common indications for transport of the high-risk obstetric case.

Complications that arise during pregnancy and place the pregnant patient at risk have many causes. Some complications may be related to the pregnancy itself, others may be related to preexisting medical conditions that may be aggravated by the pregnancy, and yet others may be related directly to the fetus.

Transport team personnel who provide care for the obstetric patient at risk must be prepared to assess obstetric factors so that stabilizing care can be provided in preparation for transport. For recognition of the pathologies associated with pregnancy, the transport clinician must have an understanding of normal physiologic changes that occur during pregnancy. The well being of the fetus and the mother must be considered. Identification of risk factors, early detection of possible complications, and interventions by the team during the transport can ensure a more favorable outcome for both the mother and the fetus. The transport team must be prepared to perform an obstetric assessment, determine strategies for transport, perform fetal monitoring, and initiate appropriate interventions. Complications are numerous and are usually multifocal. They can include, among other things, amniotic fluid embolism, delivery complications, diabetes in pregnancy, hemorrhagic complications, multiple gestation, pregnancy-induced hypertension (PIH) and related disorders, preterm labor (PTL) and related issues, and trauma in pregnancy.[21] The information gained with the general obstetric assessment (Box 31-1) aids the transport team in setting priorities for care during the transport.[2,4,7,8,13] The old cliché in transport and

---

BOX 31-1	**General Obstetric Assessment**

1. Age of patient: Age (for teenagers and for women over age 35 years) predisposes the obstetric patient to many complications.
2. Gravida/para: Gravid: The number of times pregnant, regardless of outcome. Parity is broken down into four sections. The first assessment is the number of term deliveries (after 36 weeks gestation), and the next section is the number of deliveries before 36 weeks gestation but less than 20 weeks. The next section is the number of abortions and miscarriages. The final section is the number of now living children. This more specific assessment of parity provides a tremendous amount of obstetric history. For example, a woman has been pregnant six times. She has two term deliveries, one preterm delivery, two abortions, and one baby who died of sudden infant death syndrome (SIDS). Her G/P is: G6 P 2122.
3. Estimated date of confinement (EDC): The EDC can be estimated from the first day of the last menstrual period (LMP) by using Nägele's rule: Count back 3 months from the LMP and then add 7 days. The due date is accurate within 2 weeks. Palm operating programs have free versions for calculating LMP/EDC and gestational age.
4. Ultrasound scan: Has the patient had an ultrasound scan? How many? In the event of an uncertain or unknown LMP or irregular menses, an ultrasound scan performed between 12 and 30 weeks is reliable for dating the pregnancy within 2 weeks. An ultrasound scan can confirm the EDC estimated by the LMP. Early ultrasound scans performed before 12 weeks are accurate for dating within 1 week. An ultrasound scan is invaluable with any question about placental location, amount of amniotic fluid present, fetal presentation, expected fetal growth, or anomalies.
5. In addition to inquiry into medical history and allergies, obstetric history is of particular significance. The following information may be of some predictive value for the outcome of the current pregnancy:
   a. Did the patient deliver vaginally or by cesarean section? Has she had a vaginal birth after a cesarean section? Observe for the location and extent of any abdominal scars.
   b. Did she or the baby experience any delivery complications?
   c. Did she experience any complications associated with any past pregnancies?
   d. Has she had any preterm deliveries? At what gestation did she deliver, and what was the outcome?
   e. Has she had either spontaneous or elective abortions? Was a dilation and curettage required?
   f. How many living children does she have? What were the birth weights and genders of each child?
   g. Has less than 1 year elapsed between the last delivery and commencement of the current pregnancy?
   h. What was the length of her last labor?
6. Pertaining to the current pregnancy:
   a. Is the patient having contractions? If so, when did the contractions begin? Has there been a change in the intensity or frequency of contractions? Is there accompanying backache, pelvic, or rectal pressure? How strong do the contractions palpate and how do they compare with patient reporting? What are the frequency, duration, and regularity of the contractions?
   b. Is any vaginal bleeding or bloody show present? Is there active bleeding? Attempt to help the patient quantify the bleeding by the number of towels, pads, or amount of clothing soaked before arrival and observe for evidence of dried blood on the perineum, legs, and soles of the feet. Was the bleeding painless or associated with contractions or abdominal pain? Was the blood bright red or dark? Was mucus combined with the blood (bloody show)? When did the bleeding begin? Was there any previous activity that may have precipitated the bleeding?

BOX 31-1 **General Obstetric Assessment—cont'd**

   c. Does the patient report leaking fluid vaginally? Does the patient believe her "bag of waters" has ruptured? Was there a gush or an intermittent trickle? A small leakage of clear fluid may be confused with urinary incontinence. Leakage of amniotic fluid is uncontrollable. What time did it happen? What color was the fluid: meconium-stained, dark (presence of blood in the fluid), or clear? Was an odor present? Is the Chux pad under the patient wet or pooling with fluid?

   d. Does the patient smoke? If so, how much? Is there any evidence of alcohol or substance abuse? Attempt to ascertain from the patient the frequency and time of last usage.

   e. Has the patient had an adequate weight gain? Does she appear malnourished or obese?

   f. Has the patient had consistent prenatal care, no prenatal care, or limited prenatal care (three or fewer visits)? Obtain prenatal record if available because it provides a tremendous amount of obstetric information including history, ultrasound scan reports, laboratory reports, vital signs, etc.

   g. Has there been any change in fetal activity in the past several days?

   h. Is the patient currently taking any medications? If so, what is she taking and when was the last dosage?

   i. Is the patient having any current medical problems or problems with this pregnancy?

   j. Have any diagnostic tests been done?

7. Assess initial vital signs, including temperature: The blood pressure (BP), pulse, and respirations should be assessed every 15 minutes or as indicated. The obstetric patient should be positioned in the left lateral recumbent position before the BP is taken. When the patient is in the supine position, the gravid uterus may cause obstruction of the inferior vena cava, diminishing venous return to the heart, which may lead to supine hypotension. Consequently, uteroplacental blood flow is decreased, placing the fetus at risk for compromise.

8. Fetal heart tones (FHT): If the patient is currently being monitored with electronic fetal monitoring (EFM), evaluate the fetal heart rate (FHR) baseline and variability, observing for accelerations and decelerations. FHR should be assessed with Doppler scan if EFM is unavailable. FHR auscultations should be assessed every 15 minutes or less if any irregularities are noted. For strip interpretation, refer to the discussion in this chapter on fetal monitoring.

9. Fundal height (FH): FH should be measured in centimeters from the symphysis to the fundus. The fundal height roughly correlates to the gestation of the pregnancy in weeks. In the presence of hydramnios, multiple gestations, a large-for-gestation fetus, or a fetus with intrauterine growth restriction, the fundal height may not correlate with the gestation, signaling the possibility of complications. If no tape measure is available or the patient is unable to provide information, such as in the case of a trauma, assess the fundus in relation to the umbilicus. If the fundus is above the umbilicus, it is estimated the pregnancy is 20 to 24 weeks gestation.

10. Lightly palpate the fundus for strength, frequency, and duration of contractions: The fingertips can indent the fundus freely with mild contractions and slightly with moderate contractions; firm tension is noted with strong contractions. Between contractions, palpate the abdomen for localized or generalized tenderness and observe the patient's coping response to the contractions. Gestures, posture, and facial expressions in response to contractions and verbal description should be noted. If the patient is in labor, observe for indications of advancing labor such as apprehension, restlessness, increasing difficulty coping with the contractions, screaming, nausea and vomiting, bearing-down effort, increase in bloody show, or a bulging perineum.

11. Roughly determine the fetal position with abdominal palpation: With the fingertips and palms, lightly palpate the fundus for the head or buttocks, moving down the sides to identify the fetal spine and small parts, and palpate the lower uterine segment for the presenting part. If the fetal position remains unclear, the fetus may be in a transverse lie. The FHT is heard most clearly over the fetal spine.

12. Assess cervical status as indicated by the presence of contractions: If the amniotic membranes are intact, cervical status just before departure should be documented. If the membranes are ruptured, a sterile vaginal examination (SVE) should never be attempted unless delivery is deemed imminent. In the presence of hemorrhage, an SVE should never be attempted unless a placenta previa has been ruled out with ultrasound scan. During transport, an SVE is not indicated unless signs of advancing labor are noted.

13. Observe for the presence of other risk factors that predispose the obstetric patient to complications.

emergency medical service (EMS) was that all energies should be concentrated on the mother because "if you don't save the mother, you can't save the baby." Although this adage is true in global terms, the transport team must be aware of maternal and fetal therapies that can improve survivability and decrease morbidity of the fetus as well as the mother.

DETERMINATION OF TEAM COMPOSITION FOR TRANSPORT OF THE PREGNANT PATIENT

Determination of the members of the transport team who transport the pregnant patient continues to generate controversy. Many pregnant patients are transported by teams composed of personnel who transport a variety of patients.[11] However, at times, the patient's or fetus's condition may warrant personnel with high-risk obstetric or neonatal experience. Dedicated maternal transport teams may be considered ideal from a patient care stand point but are often cost prohibitive or unavailable for many transport programs. The challenge becomes the adequate training of nonspecialty teams in competent assessment and care of the high-risk obstetric case. This controversy is not dissimilar to the training of transport teams in care for specialty patients who need intraaortic balloon pumps, left ventricular assist devices (LVADs), and other specialized equipment. Some suggested guidelines include[3,16]:

- A patient who is not in labor but needs transport for complications of pregnancy, such as preeclampsia or third-trimester bleeding, can probably be transported by a team with maternal and neonatal experience or a general transport team that has had high-risk obstetric (HROB) training from obstetric specialists.
- A patient not in labor but with severe preeclampsia ideally should be transported by a maternal transport team.
- A patient in labor may need both a maternal and a neonatal transport team. If this is not feasible or practical, the transport team may consider delaying the maternal transport and waiting until the baby is delivered. At this

time, the neonate can be safely transported in a controlled environment. Individual program-directed guidelines are imperative in assisting with transport timing decisions.

If the transport team does not routinely transport high-risk obstetrical cases, the Commission on Accreditation of Medical Transport Systems[9] recommends that the team members receive training in neonatal resuscitation. The transport vehicle should allow access to both the mother and the child in the case of a delivery during transport. Each transport program should have a policy and procedure in place that addresses when transport of a pregnant patient is and is not appropriate and what team members should provide care during transport. In addition, facilities are recommended to offer high-risk obstetric education, through the receiving facility or outside educators. Education directly leads to increased competency and confidence.

If transport services do include specialty teams as a part of their service, they must be sure that these individuals receive annual training and are equipped and dressed for transport. This training should include[9]:

- Use of restraint systems in the transport vehicle.
- Safety and survival skills.
- Emergency egress training.
- Postaccident/incident training.

Contraindications for initiation of maternal transport should be considered before leaving a referring facility. These contraindications include[1,8]:

- Inability to stabilize the mother's condition, for example, inability to control bleeding.
- Acute fetal distress.
- Imminent delivery, especially in a vehicle that does not allow access to both the mother and child.
- Lack of maternal and neonatal experience by the transport team or no experienced personnel available to accompany the team.
- Hazardous weather conditions that may prolong the transport time.

GENERAL STRATEGIES FOR TRANSPORT

The primary survey and obstetric physical assessment should be completed in a very short time because of concerns with the crew and the patient being out of belts for adjustment of the external fetal monitor. The primary survey is completed as it is in every other patient. The obstetric assessment is completed in the secondary survey. Pertinent information obtained from the patient may be gathered as the situation permits during the course of the transport. In a life-threatening situation for the mother, the fetus, or both, lifesaving measures must take precedence. During transport, or preferably before, the team should perform the following assessments and interventions[3,8,19]:

1. Place the patient in a left lateral or right lateral recumbent position or displace the uterus with a wedge if the patient cannot be turned. Displacing the uterus from the inferior vena cava provides optimal return to the heart for maintenance of adequate mean arterial pressure (MAP).
2. Note the patient's temperature if possible. The American College of Obstetricians and Gynecologists (ACOG) recommends assessment of vital signs every 15 minutes for any patient in labor or at high risk.
3. Note fetal heart tones (FHTs). Initiate continuous electronic fetal monitoring (EFM) if available and applicable. Concerns for continuous fetal monitoring en route include vibration and movement that cause an intermittent fetal heart rate (FHR) tracing, the EFM monitoring of maternal heart rate and not the fetal heart rate, and the need for the crew members and patient to be out of belts for monitor adjustment. FHR assessment with Doppler scan should be performed at least every 15 minutes per ACOG guidelines. Document fetal movement as either present or absent. Documentation should also include current fetal movement patterns to previous fetal movement patterns. For example, is the fetus moving the same amount, more or less compared with usual movement patterns? Decreasing fetal movements may indicate progressive hypoxia and decreasing perfusion. In addition, the uterus must be palpated for contractions with assessment for frequency and duration and subjective assessment of strength.
4. Start an intravenous line with a large-bore 18-gauge or 16-gauge catheter and blood tubing. Use lactated Ringer's or a 0.9 normal saline (NS) solution with an infusion rate of up to 125 mL/h or titrate volume with consideration for renal, cardiac, and pulmonary status. A maintenance solution of D5LR may be used with patients who do not need intravenous fluid (IVF) boluses.
5. Provide supplemental oxygen with a nonrebreather mask as indicated by FHR pattern or maternal condition.
6. Monitor oxygen status with pulse oximetry, maintaining a level of 98% to 100%.
7. Have a qualified clinician assess uterine contractions and cervical status before departure. Although the assessment is subjective, a commonly used tool is palpation of the fundus during contractions. If at the peak of the contraction, the fundus palpates similar to the consistency of a nose, the contraction is considered mild. If the contraction palpates as firm as the chin, it is considered a moderately strong contraction; and if it palpates as firm as a forehead, it is considered a strong contraction. Keep in mind that this assessment is subjective and patient perceptions should also be taken into consideration. Sterile vaginal examinations (SVEs) may be inappropriate for patients with ruptured bag of membranes or for concerns with infection. Sterile speculum examinations are more appropriate for this patient population.
8. Note and quantify any bleeding. Blood loss should be assessed as objectively as possible. Use pad counts, weighing of blue chux pads, or actual description on the pad (i.e., a 1×4-inch stain). Clots can be measured in a graduated cylinder or suction canister. Assess whether blood loss is associated with any pain or contractions.
9. Observe for leaking of fluid vaginally. Note the color and odor of the fluid and presence or absence of contractions.

Emotional and psychologic support provided to the obstetric patient at risk and her family is as vital an aspect as the emergency care provided.

The team should encourage the patient to express and verbalize her anxiety, fear for the fetus, and concern regarding complications. The transport team should assess the patient's knowledge of the situation, encourage questions, and use the opportunity for patient education. The vocabulary used should be based on the education and employment background of the patient. Because most patients have never been transported via air or ground ambulance, the team should explain all medications, procedures, and equipment to allay apprehension about the unfamiliar circumstances. The team should also reassure family members about the current condition of the patient and answer any questions they may have regarding the diagnosis, treatment, or destination. This is true of *all* patients.

INFERIOR VENA CAVA SYNDROME

The inferior vena cava (IVC) was once described by a cardiovascular surgeon as having the consistency of a wet paper towel roll. Use this description to imagine the weight of the fetus, amniotic fluid, placenta, and uterus compressing the inferior vena cava. Keep in mind that the IVC is responsible for transporting venous blood from the lower part of the body back to the right atrium where it can travel through its normal cardiac flow and then be returned to the central circulation as oxygenated blood. When a gravid (pregnant) patient lies supine, she quite effectively compresses the IVC. Venous blood return is dramatically decreased, which causes a logical decrease in cardiac output. If blood is not brought to the heart, the heart does not have volume to pump out. This condition is called the *inferior vena cava syndrome* (IVCS). IVCS greatly mimics hypovolemic shock. Patients present with hypotension (decreased cardiac output [CO]), reflexive tachycardia (as a result of decreased CO), skin parameter changes (cool diaphoretic skin), and potential mental status changes (decreased cerebral blood flow leads to nausea, vomiting, and decreased level of consciousness [LOC]). Decreased blood flow to the uterus occurs secondarily. The limited amount of blood is shunted to the mother's vital organs, sacrificing the fetus. Unfortunately for the fetus, the uterus is *not* considered a vital organ. If fetal monitoring is in place, signs of fetal distress are seen as a result of hypoplacental perfusion. Luckily, for awake and alert patients, IVCS is rarely a problem because they cannot tolerate lying supine if the weight of the gravid uterus is enough to compress the IVC. The patients experience nausea and naturally flip themselves to their sides. This action increases the patency of the IVC, and the patients feel better as venous blood is returned. The greatest potential problem occurs when the pregnant patient is obtunded or unconscious, for example, a trauma patient. Appropriately, EMS puts these patients on a LBB and cervical collar. A towel roll under the backboard in the area of the patient's hip relieves the compression of the IVC. At this time, the patient's condition should dramatically improve as blood is now able to return to the heart. If the patient is indeed in hypovolemic shock, then an objective assessment can now be made (e.g., left or right side). For years, we have all learned that the pregnant patient has to be on her *left* side to increase venous and placental blood flow. The IVC lies slightly to the right midline under the uterus. In theory, if the patient is turned to the left, the IVC is the most patent. We now know that the IVC is also patent if the patient is tilted or turned to the right. In addition, if the patient cannot be turned, the uterus can be manually displaced by gently pushing or pulling it to the left and off the IVC. IVCS is the most common mistake healthcare professionals make in the care of the pregnancy patient. We are not accustomed to "tilting" our patients, and this condition is often forgotten. Prevention is key because these patients already have compromised conditions. This is a great example of how an intervention cannot only improve the maternal condition but can also save the life of the fetus.

FETAL MONITORING BEFORE AND DURING TRANSPORT

Fetal monitoring may be accomplished with intermittent Doppler scan auscultation, which is used most frequently for short transports, and with EFM, used for longer transports (approximately 30 minutes or more). An external ultrasound scan device records FHTs, and a tocodynamometer detects subjective uterine activity.[11,12,16,17] The mode of FHR assessment, be it continuous or intermittent via

Doppler scan, is often program and institution dependant. One has not been clearly identified over the other as superior during transport. The ACOG does not make a statement on which method of fetal monitoring is recommended. However, they do state that FHR assessment should be done a minimum of every 15 minutes during transport.

Continuous assessment of fetal well being is best accomplished with *electronic fetal monitoring*. FHTs are recorded simultaneously with uterine activity. The EFM works by sending ultrasound waves into the uterus; the monitor detects the fastest moving objects, which are typically the valves on the fetal heart. This information or sound is returned to the monitor where it is converted to a number on the graph paper. The monitors have a program designed to detect heart rates between approximately 50 and 190 bpm. A limitation of the EFM is that if the FHR nears the lower limits of the monitor capacities the EFM may erroneously detect the motion of one heart beat as two separate beats. This error is called "doubling" the FHR; the monitor paper graphs the FHR at twice the actual heart rate. Conversely when the FHR nears the upper limits, the monitor may only recognize every other motion as a heartbeat and "halving" of the FHR occurs. So, how does one accurately assess the FHR with an EFM? The key is the audible signal on the monitor. The audible signal of the monitor remains accurate and can be compared against the printed FHR tracing to confirm accuracy. In addition, the maternal pulse should be compared with the FHR tracing to confirm that the maternal signal is not being traced. This error has occurred in circumstances in which the fetus is dead in utero and the EFM then monitors the maternal aorta fluctuations and misinterprets them as a fetal heart rate. Subtle changes in the FHT are often the earliest indication of hypoxia caused by uteroplacental insufficiency or umbilical cord compression. Recognition of normal FHR tracing permits abnormalities to be realized quickly. Appropriate intervention should be aimed at correcting or alleviating the source of insult; at a minimum, actions should improve placental/uterine perfusion.

Historically, conflicting interpretations have been seen. Most of this conflict has revolved around nomenclature, classification, and significance of EFM patterns. As a result of these inconsistent interpretations, the National Institute of Child Health and Human Development (NICHD) developed a defined terminology and classification system. This system was later adopted by the ACOG and Association of Women's Health, Obstetric and Neonatal Nurses (AWHONN). This chapter reflects all of the NICHD nomenclature.

BASELINE ASSESSMENT

The first parameter to be assessed is the *FHR baseline*. The baseline is the average of the FHR and typically is between 110 and 160 bpm. The baseline is assessed over a minimum 10-minute period. In addition, it is assessed between contractions and periodic or episodic changes. Periodic changes are accelerations or decelerations that occur to the fetal heart rate as a result of contractions. Episodic changes are accelerations/decelerations that occur in the FHR as a result of fetal movement. The FHR baseline is the approximate mean FHR rounded to increments of 5 bpm over a 10-minute period. In any 10-minute section, a minimum of a 2-minute period of no contractions or periodic or episodic changes is needed to determine the FHR baseline. Evaluation of the FHR baseline is a critical step in FHR interpretations. It allows interpretation of trends that occur in the baseline and can reflect subtle changes in the fetal environment.

FETAL HEART RATE ABNORMALITIES
Variability

Fluctuations in the FHR reflect interplay between the sympathetic and parasympathetic branches of the autonomic nervous system. A constant pull from the sympathetic nervous system increases the heart rate and from the parasympathetic nervous system decreases the heart rate. These normal variations between each fetal heartbeat give the FHR tracing its "squiggly" appearance. *Variability* is the single most important factor in prediction of fetal well being, based on EFM monitor interpretation. Fetal movement remains the number one nonmonitor indicator of fetal well being. Similar to assessment of the baseline, variability can only be assessed between contractions and episodic and periodic changes (Figure 31-1).

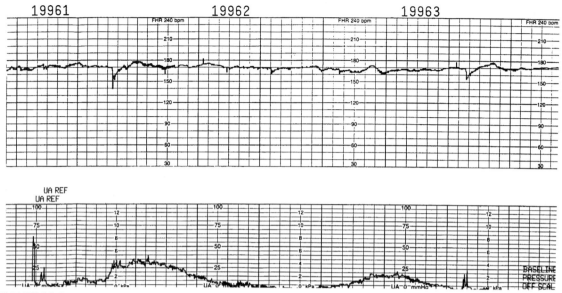

FIGURE 31-1   **Reduced variability and tachycardia.** Note the almost absent beat-to-beat variability and reduced long-term variability as recorded by fetal scalp electrode; also note the tachycardic baseline.

Moderate variability is indicative of an adequately oxygenated, normal PH, mature and intact autonomic nervous system. *Moderate variability* is defined as fluctuations in the FHR that range between 6 and 25 bpm. The presence of moderate variability is reassuring because it indicates that the fetus is tolerating blood flow changes within the uterus.

Minimal variability is defined as fluctuations in the FHR that are equal to or less than 5 bpm. This variability is often associated with fetal hypoxia and acidosis. However, benign or expected minimal variability can occur in certain clinical situations; for example, the fetal variability can decrease if the mother has received any narcotics. Narcotics are a central nervous system (CNS) depressant; anything that decreases the maternal CNS can decrease fetal CNS as it passes through the placenta. As the maternal drug is metabolized and excreted, the effects on the fetus should also be seen to diminish. *Persistent minimal variability* is not associated with maternal drug use, and other causes of decreasing variability must be assessed. Another common reason for minimal variability is immaturity in gestational age, which is associated with CNS immaturity. Fetuses

that are less than 32 weeks gestation show less variability because the autonomic nervous system (ANS) may not yet be fully developed. Fetal arrhythmias and cardiac or CNS anomalies may also be responsible for minimal or absent variability. These causes show variability changes from the time monitoring is initiated. The most common reason for benign minimal variability is fetal sleep patterns. The fetus has frequent sleep periods that range from 20 to 40 minutes. A key assessment pearl is that although fetal sleep patterns are common, they are transient in nature and rarely last longer than 40 minutes. In addition, moderate variability should be documented before and after the sleep pattern. As blood flow decreases across the placenta or umbilical cord, less oxygen is available for the fetus. If the hypoxic events are corrected, the fetus usually tolerates them well. However, if the cause of decreased perfusion is not corrected, an eventual decrease in variability is noted. Careful evaluation of the FHR tracing reflects trending of decreasing variability (minimal or absent), which is a warning sign that the fetus is losing compensatory mechanisms and fetal hypoxia and acidosis are increasing. Interestingly, the incidence rate of actual fetal acidemia in the presence of minimal or absent variability and decelerations is only 23%.[16] However, the presence of these signs still remains an indicator for intervention. This intervention includes measures to increase placental and uterine perfusion, such as maternal position change, intravenous (IV) fluid bolus to increase maternal volume/perfusion, and application of supplemental O_2.

Increased or *marked variability* of more than 25 beats of fluctuation may be one of the earliest signs of hypoxia. Although it may also be an indication of increased fetal activity, constant assessment and reevaluation is necessary. If continuous EFM is used during transport, the clinician should keep in mind that a greater degree of variability may be recorded than is actually present because of vibrations from the vehicle. Special notice of long-term variability and other reassuring signs must be made, including the presence of fetal movement. Variability should be assessed with NICHD terminology such as moderate, minimal, absent, or marked (see Table 31-1).

Periodic Changes/Episodic Changes

Periodic changes are changes that occur in the FHR tracing related to uterine contractions. *Episodic changes* are changes in the FHR tracing that are not related to uterine contractions and are often related to fetal movement. The FHR may accelerate, decelerate, or not respond.

TABLE 31-1	**NICHD Terminology**	
NICHD	**Fluctuation**	**Indications**
Moderate	6-25 bpm	Well-oxygenated, nonacidotic, intact/mature CNS
Minimal	≤5 bpm	Hypoxia, acidosis, sleep patterns, maternal drug use, cardiac or CNS insult, prematurity
Absent	Undetectable from baseline	Hypoxia, acidosis, sleep pattern, maternal drug use, cardiac or CNS insult
Marked	>25 bpm	Fetal movement or early hypoxia

Acceleration.   Accelerations above the baseline are usually associated with fetal movement but may occur during contractions (Figure 31-2). Because the hypoxic fetus with metabolic acidosis is unable to accelerate its heart rate, accelerations are viewed as a sign of fetal well being. The true definition of *acceleration* is a transient increase above the baseline greater than 15 bpm for 15 seconds or longer and typically lasting less than 2 minutes in duration. This definition is applied for fetuses that are greater than 32 weeks in gestation. The definition of acceleration for a fetus younger than 32 weeks is a transient increase over baseline of greater than 10 bpm for at least 15 seconds and typically less than 2 minutes. *Uniform accelerations* are accelerations that occur with each contraction and are uniform in shape and size. This acceleration pattern may be associated with breech presentation or early and mild cord compression. In very early labor, the contractions are not strong and the fundus or top of the uterus gently compresses the breech during contractions, which causes a sympathetic response and accelerations are noted. Later, as the contractions increase in strength and the head of the fetus is pushed down into the pelvis, uniform decelerations are seen, discussed in the section on early decelerations.

Although the presence of accelerations and moderate variability are excellent monitor signs of fetal well being, fetal movement remains the best nonmonitor indicator of fetal well being. Only well-oxygenated fetuses with normal pH levels have consistent fetal movement patterns. Certainly all fetuses have different movement patterns that are unique to themselves. During transport, the clinician should assess the current movement pattern compared with the usual movement pattern. For example, a fetus that is known to have movements of at least 15 times an hour that is now reported to have only moved once in the past 2 hours shows a significant deviation from normal patterns and further assessment and documentation are necessary. The transport team should take note of fetal movements, whether the mother has noticed a decrease, increase, or no change in fetal movement. Decreased fetal movement is indicative of hypoxia. Although a decrease in fetal movement may be anticipated, such as in the event of maternal trauma and blood loss, the transport team is expected to inform the maternal fetal medicine physicians of this change in fetal status.

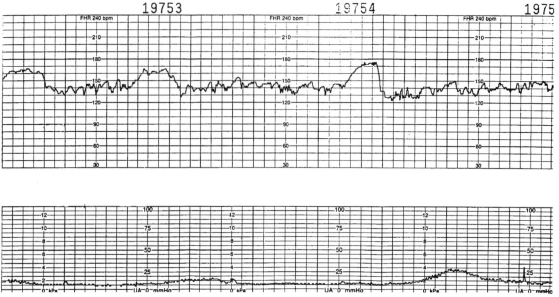

FIGURE 31-2   **Accelerations.** With use of an ultrasound scan transducer, accelerations of approximately 20 beats above the baseline may be noted. Long-term variability is present, and the FHR baseline range is approximately 135 to 145 bpm.

Variable Deceleration.   *Variable decelerations* can occur at any time during a contraction (Figure 31-3). The shape may also vary and is frequently V-shaped or W-shaped. The decelerations are known as variable because of the varied shape and timing.

Cord compression is typically responsible for these decelerations. However, they may also occur from head compression as a result of vagal stimulation in the second stage of labor (pushing). Physiologically, as the cord is compressed, blood flow through the

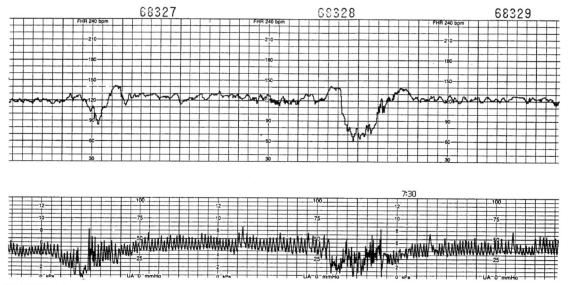

FIGURE 31-3   **Variable decelerations.** Note the variable decelerations in the presence of average variability. The accelerations before and after the deceleration (also called shoulders) are a reflection of adequate variability.

umbilical cord is decreased. Baroreceptors cause a short increase in the FHR to compensate. The blood flow is further impeded, and a sharp decrease occurs in the FHR. As the umbilical cord compression is relieved, the FHR responds with a quick increase above the baseline in an attempt to increase oxygenation status. After a short period of time, typically less than 5 to 10 seconds, the FHR returns to baseline with moderate variability. Initially, variables may have a characteristic appearance; frequently, a short acceleration is observed, followed by a rapid deceleration for some seconds and then a rapid rise and a short acceleration before a return to the FHR baseline. The short period of increased FHR before and after the deceleration is known as *shoulders*. Shoulders are associated with moderate variability and indicate that the fetus still has the ability to compensate with varying amounts of placental blood and available oxygen. Shoulders are considered a reassuring characteristic associated with variable decelerations. If the fetus continues to have variable decelerations that are progressively more consistent or deeper in nadir, often this compensatory response is lost and only the sharp deceleration is seen without shoulders noted. The abrupt onset and sharp decline with usual rapid return to baseline makes these decelerations easily identifiable. Cord compression may occur in a variety of circumstances. After the membranes rupture, less fluid is available to cushion the cord. Variables usually occur in response to uterine contractions but also may occur in response to fetal movement in the absence of contractions when membranes are ruptured. If a nuchal cord, short cord, or cord entanglement is present, variables usually result.

In the past, these decelerations have commonly been described as mild, moderate, or severe, depending on the drop in FHR. However, to remain consistent with NICHD nomenclature, a more conclusive method is to describe the deceleration. This description should include the depth (nadir), duration, shape, and return variability status. A better indicator of the fetal response is reflected in the FHR baseline, variability, and changes in the variable decelerations. Signs that the fetus is losing its ability to tolerate the stress of repeated cord compression or that the cord compression is becoming more severe include a deeper deceleration that lasts longer, a slow return to baseline, loss of shoulders, and decreased variability. *Overshoots* are another type of acceleration seen with variable decelerations. These differ from shoulders in the sense that these accelerations are seen only *after* the variable deceleration as the compromised fetus attempts to improve oxygenation status. These offshoots are typically well above baseline. Offshoots are associated with minimal to absent variability and are considered nonreassuring. In interpreting the tracing, careful observations of any changes in FHT reveal more than what has just occurred during the last contraction.

Late Decelerations. *Late deceleration* begins at or after the apex (peak) of the contraction. They gradually decelerate in a uniformed "U" shape and return to the FHR baseline well after the contraction is over (Figure 31-4). By definition, late decelerations must be recurrent, which means they occur in greater than 50% of all uterine contractions (National Institute of Child Health and Human Development [NICHD]).[3] Physiologically, during a normal contraction, a minimal amount of oxygen always crosses the placenta. A healthy fetus can tolerate this decrease in oxygen via its oxygen reserves. A compromised fetus that has experienced prolonged or chronic hypoxia does not have oxygen reserves available and therefore cannot tolerate the decrease oxygen availability found during contractions. Not until the contraction is over and the maternal-fetal exchange can resume does the FHR return to baseline. Late decelerations always mean *uteroplacental insufficiency:* either the placenta, the fetus, or the uterus presents with conditions that interfere with normal exchange of oxygen between the mother and fetus. Use the analogy of a child being dunked in a pool. The child tolerates the dunking early on, but if it continues, the child becomes fatigued, loses O_2 reserve, and ends up gasping every time he surfaces. When a contraction is stronger, the insufficiency is greater and the deceleration is proportional. However, "size does not matter." With severe hypoxia, the myocardial depression may be such that the heart is unable to decelerate in response to the stress of the contraction, and very subtle late decelerations are seen accompanied by a flat FHR baseline. Simply stated, the fetus becomes so hypoxic and acidotic that it

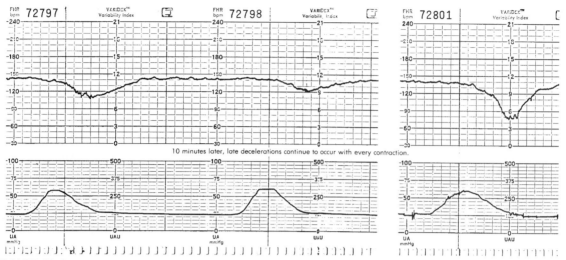

FIGURE 31-4   **Late decelerations.** Note the onset of deceleration at the apex of the contraction. Also note the minimal variability, slow recovery, and the proportional deceleration observed.

cannot render a response to the impeded blood flow. The fetus is too sick to "wave the white flag." A FHR tracing that is tachycardic with minimal or absent variability and subtle late decelerations is considered an ominous FHR tracing and interventions must be made to improve fetal oxygenation. These interventions include measures to increase placental perfusion, such as maternal position change, supplemental O_2 via a nonrebreather mask, IVF boluses, and possible delivery, if improvement is not noted.

Uteroplacental insufficiency may result from numerous maternal and fetal conditions, such as pregnancy-induced hypertension (PIH), diabetes mellitus (DM), cardiovascular or kidney disease, chorioamnionitis, smoking, a fetus that is past maturity, and fetal hydrops. Uteroplacental insufficiency may also result from decreased placental perfusion in placental abruption or previa, uterine hypertonus as a result of oxytocin stimulation, and hypotension. As with variable decelerations, evaluation of late decelerations with respect to FHR baseline, variability, and changes noted over time is necessary in evaluation of the well being of the fetus. Even an otherwise healthy well-oxygenated fetus can experience late decelerations in the presence of acute hypotension and hypoxia. An example of this is a mother that is obtunded and was laid flat on her

back on a back board. This position alone can cause IVCS and rapid decrease in maternal venous blood return, which then causes maternal hypotension that leads to profound fetal hypotension and results in late decelerations. Once the maternal position is tilted to the right lateral position (RLP) or left lateral position (LLP), the blood flow improves and the late decelerations resolve.

Early Decelerations. *Early decelerations* are innocuous decelerations that begin close to the beginning of the contraction and end close to the end of the contraction. These decelerations appear to mirror the contractions. As the head is compressed, the vagus nerve is stimulated and causes a parasympathetic response that leads to a deceleration. The deceleration ends as the contraction ends because the vagus nerve (head) is no longer compressed. Early decelerations are usually associated with moderate variability and are considered benign in nature. These decelerations frequently occur in active labor when the cervix has dilated 4 to 7 cm, or they may be seen in early labor with breech presentation because, in this position, the head is compressed into the pelvic cavity with contractions. A transport consideration is that a sterile vaginal examination (SVE) or sterile speculum exam (SPE) should be preformed before transport to rule out

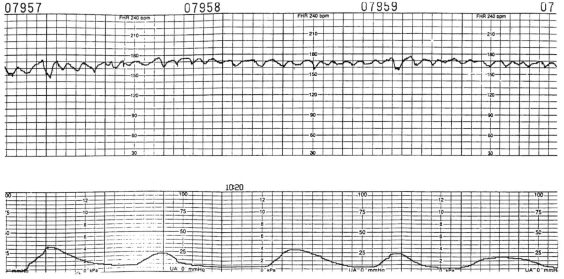

FIGURE 31-5 **Sinusoidal pattern.** Note the jagged, nonuniform pattern observed after intravenous administration of butorphanol (Stadol), 1 mg, which resolved spontaneously after 20 minutes.

advanced cervical dilation. In FHR interpretation, late decelerations should not be confused with early decelerations. Accurate placement of the tocotransducer over the fundus ensures that contractions are recorded correctly. Also, consider other reassuring attributes such as moderate variability and the presence of accelerations or fetal movement to help discern early from late decelerations.

Sinusoidal. *Sinusoidal* is a rare FHR pattern in which a uniform sine wave pattern occurs. This FHR remains within normal baselines but has an obvious unusual appearance. It is often described as an undulating pattern that is saw-toothed in appearance. Possible causes of this pattern are fetal hypovolemia or anemia; it may occur in cases of erythroblastosis fetalis, accidental tap of the umbilical cord during amniocentesis, fetomaternal transfusion, placental abruption, or another type of accident. Variability is absent or minimal, and accelerations are not seen. When this pattern is recognized, rapid delivery is usually recommended unless the underlying pathology can be corrected. For example, in the case of severe fetal anemia, a blood transfusion can be administered to the fetus via a percutaneous umbilical cord sampling (PUBS) procedure. Once the anemia is

resolved, the sinusoidal pattern is resolved. However, a more commonly observed FHR pattern is a pseudosinusoidal or undulating pattern that is not pathologic (Figure 31-5). This pattern is linked to maternal drug administration, both prescribed and illicit.

Bradycardia. An FHR of less than 110 bpm for a period of 10 minutes or longer is defined as *bradycardia*. Bradycardia can occur as result of numerous acute or chronic conditions and can be hypoxic or nonhypoxic in nature. Many term fetuses and those past maturity may have a stable baseline between 100 and 120 bpm, reflecting a more mature fetal neurologic system that is more parasymphathetically controlled. In the absence of hypoxia, adequate variability and accelerations are also noted.

Bradycardia is a response of increased parasympathetic tone and is reflected by a decrease in fetal cardiac output in the presence of hypoxia. The fetus can tolerate sustained bradycardia for only a short length of time before becoming acidotic. Bradycardia can be acute as a result of severe cord compression. It can occur minutes before delivery when the cord is drawn into the pelvis in the second stage or with a cord prolapse. Bradycardia can also occur with hypertonic or tetanic contractions as seen with placenta abruptio and any event that causes maternal hypotension. In the presence of chronic hypoxia, bradycardia is usually a late occurrence. Evaluation of variability determines how the fetus tolerates the stress.

Tachycardia.   A FHR of more than 160 bpm for a period of 10 minutes or longer is considered *tachycardia*. Tachycardia is a response of increased sympathetic tone and is reflected by a compensatory mechanism to increase cardiac output in the presence of transient hypoxia. A decrease in variability is generally associated with tachycardia. This decreased variability and increased rate is reflective of the fetus returning to a more primitive or sympathetic response. Fetal tachycardia may be maternal or fetal in origin. Factors that contribute to tachycardia include smoking, maternal fever, use of beta-sympathomimetic agents, fetal anemia, fetal hypovolemia, fetal tachydysrhythmias, chorioamnionitis, and maternal hyperthyroidism.

Fetal distress is a loose term that implies that the fetus is in danger of hypoxia and metabolic acidosis. Late and variable decelerations are sources of stress to the fetus, whereas variability is an indicator of how the fetus tolerates the stress.

Assessment of FHR tracings should follow a systematic approach with these sequential steps:

Assessment of baseline.
Assessment of variability with NICHD standards.
Assessment of periodic/episodic changes, including accelerations or decelerations.
Assessment for the presence of tachycardia or bradycardia.

At any time that the transport team considers that the FHR tracing is not reassuring, medical control or receiving maternal fetal medicine physicians must be contacted for further orders. Interventions should be made to improve placental perfusion, including maternal position change, supplemental O_2 via a nonrebreather mask, and IVF boluses. If the transport team is unsure of the FHR interpretation, the FHR strip can be faxed to the receiving facility for interpretation. If the FHR is not reassuring en route, medical control should be contacted (if possible) and diversion should be considered for signs of ominous fetal distress.

Nonreassuring signs of fetal well being include a significant increase or decrease in the FHR baseline during a period of several hours, a wandering baseline, a spontaneous decrease in variability or a decrease in variability as labor progresses, bradycardia or tachycardia with reduced variability, subtle late decelerations, or any combination of these signs.

Abnormal FHR tracings are observed in situations of congenital anomalies. Frequently, variability is reduced or absent, and tachycardia or bradycardia may be noted. Table 31-2 summarizes comparative signs of acute and chronic distress. Whatever the mechanism of insult to the fetus, the plan of action for possible fetal distress is intrauterine resuscitation.

The key formula (LOCK) is as follows:

L: Place the patient in the left lateral or right lateral recumbent position.
O: Provide supplemental oxygen, via 100% nonrebreather mask.
C: Correct or improve contributing factors.
K: Keep reassessing the FHR and intervene when indicated.

CONTRIBUTING FACTORS TO FETAL DISTRESS

Interventions that must be performed by the transport team when signs and symptoms of fetal distress are present are as follows:

1. Hypotension: Initiate a 500-mL intravenous fluid bolus, depending on the condition of the patient. If the patient has no comorbidities that promote pulmonary edema, the maternal patient can receive 2 L of crystalloids to improve maternal and placental perfusion. Correct for supine hypotension with a change to the left lateral or right lateral position, uterine displacement, or a towel roll under the backboard.
2. Hypertonic or tetanic contractions: Consider the use of terbutaline, 0.25 mg, administered subcutaneously or via intravenous push. Check to ensure that the patient's heart rate is less than 120 bpm before administering the medication.

TABLE 31-2	**Comparison of Signs of Chronic and Acute Distress**
Chronic Distress (Occurs Over Time)	**Acute Distress (Occurs Suddenly)**
Mechanism of insult	
Uteroplacental insufficiency	Umbilical cord compression or uteroplacental insufficiency
Signs of IUGR, decreased fetal movements	Initially, no indication of fetal compromise
Contributing factors	
PIH (preeclampsia)	Cord prolapse
Cardiac or kidney disease	Placental abruption
Severe anemia	Hypotension (vena cava compression, epidural anesthesia, hemorrhage)
DM (class B-R)	Hypertonic contractions
Postdate pregnancy	Placenta previa with hemorrhage
Rh isoimmunization	
Chorioamnionitis	
Smoking	
Fetal response (progression differs depending on circumstances)	
Tachycardia	Variable decelerations
Increased variability	Prolonged decelerations
Decreased variability	Tachycardia
Late decelerations	Increased variability
Bradycardia	Decreased variability
	Late decelerations
	Bradycardia

IUGR, Intrauterine growth restriction.

The terbutaline can be repeated every 10 minutes for three doses; however, program protocol should always guide therapy.

3. Rule out cord prolapse. A sterile vaginal examination is used to confirm the presence of a cord. Lift the presenting part of the cord to relieve the cord compression and reposition the patient, following recommendations provided in this chapter.
4. Assess for placental abruption or other complications that may affect the FHR.
5. Change the position of the mother. If the left lateral position does not relieve the cord compression as indicated by continued variable decelerations, reposition the mother to the right side, to the hands and knees, or last, to the knee-chest position. A transport consideration is the inability to restrain the maternal patient in the knee-to-chest position in some vehicles, especially small helicopters.
6. Assess for signs of maternal hemorrhage. Changes in FHR, including tachycardia and loss of variability, are often the first signs of maternal blood loss. The maternal patient has 40% to 50% more blood volume at term and therefore can mask signs of hypovolemia. In addition, the maternal patient shunts blood to her vital organs, and the uterus is *not* considered a vital organ.

If the patient is located in an outlying area where the transport time is expected to be lengthy, evaluation of the FHT for reassuring signs of fetal well being aids in the decision to transport the mother or to deliver the fetus at the referring facility to increase the chance of fetal survival. With this in mind, the accepting maternal fetal medicine physicians make the ultimate decision of whether or when to transport. At times, the primary reasons for transport are maternal and fetal conditions that cause a nonreassuring FHR tracing. In these circumstances, a nonreassuring FHR strip does not preclude or exclude maternal transport. Appropriate indications for maternal/fetal transport are if the referring facility is unable to offer specialized or high-risk obstetric services or a neonatal intensive care unit (NICU). Likewise, if the transport is expected to be short and the time needed by the referring facility to prepare for a cesarean section is longer than the estimated transport time, maternal transport is recommended. The intent of the transport is to attain the most expedient delivery of the mother and fetus in a facility most capable of dealing with the mother and fetus at risk. Studies show improved neonatal outcomes if the fetus is delivered at a perinatal network with a level III nursery.

The transport team may consider use of Doppler scan auscultations or EFM for transports. Advantages and disadvantages are found with both methods. Doppler scan auscultation is performed a minimum of every 15 minutes. This method does not allow for assessment of variability but can assess for FHR and responses to contractions if auscultation is performed during and after contractions. Continuous EFM allows for assessment of variability; however, vibration of the aircraft may artificially add artifact. Remember that this can be a problem in any transport vehicle. Because of position constraints in the aircraft, the EFM may slip and monitor maternal heart rate, which causes the transport team and patient to frequently be out of belts so the monitor can be adjusted. The FHR strip should clearly identify when maternal heart rate is monitored so it is not later assessed to be fetal distress. Trained and competent individuals must accomplish this monitoring. The age-old controversy with continuous fetal monitoring during transport is what to do with the information found. For example, if the fetal condition acutely deteriorates into fetal distress, is there adequate time to divert to another facility? Does diversion to another facility outside of the level III hospital offer services other than the referring facility? Both forms of monitoring are accepted by the ACOG as appropriate and safe. Regardless of the method chosen, if the FHR reflects acute or chronic signs of deterioration or distress, appropriate interventions must be made to alleviate the cause and to increase uterine/placental perfusion. These interventions and their responses need to be documented.

NORMAL PHYSIOLOGIC CHANGES IN PREGNANCY

For true appreciation and recognition of the pathologies that may be associated with pregnancy, a review of normal physiologic changes is necessary. This review of systems is brief and highlights key areas.[5,6,10,14,19]

Airway: The failure rate with oral intubation is four times higher in the pregnant patient than in the nonpregnant patient. The trachea of the term pregnant patient tends to be anterior, and the epiglottis is reported to be friable.

Hematalogic: By term, the maternal blood volume has increased by 40% to 50%. The greater increase is in plasma then in red blood cells (RBCs), platelets, etc. As a result, a normal dilutional anemia is often associated with pregnancy. In cases of maternal blood loss, maternal hypotension is often not noted until the patient has lost approximately 30% of the blood volume because of the extra volume created during the pregnancy. Platelets and fibrinogen slightly increase during pregnancy and cause the pregnant patient to be in a hypercoagulable state, which allows faster and more efficient clotting to prevent hemorrhage after delivery.

Respiratory: Tidal volume increases by about 40%, and respiratory rate slightly increases; thus, pregnant women have compensated respiratory alkalosis. Alveolar ventilation increases by 65%.

Cardiac: CO increases by about 50% (related to the increased blood volume). Heart rate (HR) slightly increases by about 10 beats by term. Blood pressure is normotensive (for the patient) in the first trimester, decreased in the second trimester, and returned to normotensive in the third trimester. This change is greatly related to a pregnancy hormone called relaxin. A key assessment point is that the blood pressure should never be elevated over 140/90 mm Hg during pregnancy. If it is, a pathology is always indicated.

Gastrointestinal: Slowing of peristalsis and resulting constipation occur. The stomach empties slowly, and the pregnant patient is at a high risk of aspiration with altered levels of consciousness. This effect is also related to the hormone relaxin. Because of this effect, a pregnant woman is always considered to have a full stomach no matter when her last meal was. Increased salvation is common and frequent suctioning may be needed in the case of oral intubation. An increased incidence of cholelithiasis is found during pregnancy.

Renal: Increased renal filtration of glucose and sodium occurs during pregnancy. BUN and CR levels are both lower during pregnancy. Elevated levels of either renal function laboratory tests indicate pathology. Protein is a large molecule and should not be passed renally in the absence of pathology.

Uterus: The uterus becomes the largest intraabdominal organ. Uterine and placental perfusion increases to 600 to 800 mL of blood per minute at term. A very high risk of maternal hemorrhage is found in the presence of uterine or placental injury.

Musculoskeletal: The abdominal viscera become stretched and distended because of the growing uterus. These distorted viscera may cause abdominal pain to be referred. The effects of the hormone relaxin also cause the symphysis pubis cartilage to slightly separate, thereby increasing pelvic instability. The gravid uterus causes the patient's center of gravity to be altered, and an increase in falls may be noted. The thoracic cavity also expands during pregnancy to allow greater lung expansion because the lungs have less distance to elongate as a result of the gravid uterus.

Liver: The liver is the only organ to not increase efficiency during pregnancy. Hepatic function values remain the same as nonpregnant values. However, if elevations of serum glutamate oxaloacetate transaminase (SGOT)/serum glutamate pyruvate transaminase (SGPT), or aspartate aminotransferase (AST)/alanine aminotransferase (ALT), are noted, significant pathology is implied.

COMPLICATIONS OF PREGNANCY AND DELIVERY

In the following discussions regarding complications of pregnancy and delivery, general obstetric assessment and implementation of general guidelines for transport are assumed to have already been performed, including assessment of fetal well being.

AMNIOTIC FLUID EMBOLISM/ ANAPHYLACTIC SYNDROME OF PREGNANCY

Amniotic fluid embolism is now known as *anaphylactic syndrome of pregnancy*. Previous thought was that amniotic fluid gained access to the maternal circulation during labor or delivery or immediately after delivery, resulting in obstruction of the pulmonary vasculature. In addition, particulate matter in the amniotic fluid, such as meconium, lanugo hairs, fetal squamous cells, bile, fat, and mucin, was also thought to embolize. The belief now is that the process is more likely to be an anaphylactic reaction to the amniotic fluid and the fetal cells they contain. Treatment is primarily supportive and usually necessitates immediate intubation, mechanical ventilation, pressor administration, and treatment of coagulopathy. In the United States, amniotic fluid embolism causes 10% of maternal deaths. The complication is very rare and is frequently fatal, with a maternal mortality rate nearing 90%. Amniotic fluid embolism is often initially misdiagnosed as result of the vague clinical picture of surviving patients and missed autopsy findings in fatal cases. Unfortunately, the rapid progression of this syndrome is associated with a high maternal mortality that is often not diagnosed until postmortem.

Etiology and Pathophysiologic Factors

The route by which amniotic fluid enters the circulatory system of the mother is not clear. The most frequently suggested sites of entry are lacerations in the endocervical veins during cervical dilation and lacerations in the lower uterine segment, the placental site, and uterine veins at sites of uterine trauma. Under the pressure of uterine contractions, amniotic fluid gains access to the circulatory system of the mother and travels quickly to the pulmonary vasculature, where embolization and anaphylactic reaction quickly ensue.

Factors that have been associated with amniotic fluid embolism include uterine rupture, cesarean section, and the use of uterine stimulants to induce labor, which produces hypertonic contractions. Other factors that place the obstetric patient at risk are a large fetus, placenta previa, placental abruption, intrauterine fetal death, meconium in the amniotic fluid, multiparity, precipitous delivery, knee-chest position, and maternal age of more than 30 years.

Disseminated intravascular coagulation (DIC) is a complication that can be expected, although the pathway is unclear. Uterine atony and postpartum hemorrhage are also frequent complications. Acute cor pulmonale, right heart failure, and pulmonary edema follow.

Assessment

Of the predisposing factors that the patient may have, sudden acute dyspnea is the most characteristic symptom, followed by profound cyanosis and sudden shock. Other symptoms may include chest pain, restlessness, anxiety, coughing, vomiting, pulmonary edema with pink frothy sputum, seizures that are frequently confused with eclamptic seizures, and coma. If the patient has delivered, the transport team should watch for symptoms of postpartum hemorrhage caused by uterine atony.

Because of the extremely rare occurrence of amniotic fluid embolism and the rapidity of onset of symptoms with deterioration, the transport team may be unsure of the clinical picture. If dyspnea appears in a patient who is in a tumultuous labor with ruptured membranes, amniotic fluid embolism is recommended to be suspected. Tachycardia, hypotension, and tachypnea indicate the severity of the embolic process. Urine output may be decreased (less than 30 mL/h), which indicates inadequate renal perfusion. Blood is shunted away from the uterus to the vital organs, and FHR changes indicative of placental insufficiency are observed. Severe fetal distress may be present. DIC can be suspected if petechiae, hematuria, bruising, or bleeding from intravenous sites is observed. Coagulation study results confirm DIC. Chest radiograph may show infiltrates.

Strategies for Transport

In the event that an obstetric patient with amniotic fluid embolism/anaphylactic syndrome of pregnancy is transported, supportive care should be provided. Although the clinical picture may not be clear, treatment focuses on the alleviation of presenting symptoms. The transport team should provide supplemental oxygen with a 100% nonrebreather mask if the patient is not already intubated. Positive end-expiratory pressure may be necessary because of a high association with acute respiratory distress syndrome (ARDS). The transport team can provide circulatory support with additional intravenous fluids and likely will need numerous lines or a multilumen central line. The transport team may initiate blood replacement in an attempt to correct hypovolemia, blood loss, and coagulopathy. This syndrome most commonly occurs postpartum, but if the patient is still gravid, the FHTs should be monitored for signs of severe distress.

If the fetus has been delivered, oxytocin, 20 to 40 units, may immediately be added to 1000 mL intravenous solution for uterine atony. Frequent fundal massage should be performed by supporting the lower uterine segment with one hand while massaging the fundus with the other. Morphine or fentanyl can be administered intravenously for apprehension, dyspnea, and pain. An antiemetic should be considered if the mother is nauseated or has vomited. The transport team should expedite the transport and, if the transport will be extended because of distance, weather, or other issues, consider delivering the baby.[1,21]

DELIVERY COMPLICATIONS

Delivery complications can be predicted in some situations and may be quite unforeseen in others. A neonatal nurse, or at a minimum, a transport nurse trained in a neonatal resuscitation program (NRP), should always be included on transports when delivery is a possibility.

The information about assessment and suggested transport care that follows makes specific reference to the complication only. General obstetric assessment and general transport principles are assumed to be considered before transport.

Breech Presentation

Breech presentation is the noncephalic (head) part of the fetal body presenting into the bony pelvis. The body often can be felt through the cervix on vaginal examination. With a breech presentation, the buttocks may descend first, with the legs flexed on the fetal abdomen and the feet alongside the buttocks (*complete breech*); the legs may also be extended upward (*frank breech),* or one or both feet or knees may be present (*footling* or *incomplete breech).* At or near term, the incidence rate of breech is 3% to 4%. Because of the effects of gravity, most fetuses are cephalic or vertex. However, before 34 weeks gestation, the incidence is considerably higher.

Etiology and Pathophysiologic Factors.

Breech presentation is more likely to occur in situations with uterine abnormalities, such as a septum that extends part or all of the way from the fundus to the cervix (septate uterus) or a Y-shaped uterus (bicornuate uterus). The belief is that as the pregnancy progresses, the uterine cavity provides the most room for the fetus's bulkier and more movable parts, with the extremities in the fundus of the uterus and the cephalic presenting. Before 34 weeks gestation, the head of the fetus is disproportionately larger than the body, favoring the breech presentation. For the same reason, the hydrocephalic fetus has a high incidence of breech presentation.[11,12]

Other factors that appear to predispose to the breech presentation are grand multiparity, a previous breech delivery, multiple gestation, hydramnios, oligohydramnios, placenta previa, uterine tumors, and congenital anomalies.

Complications associated with breech presentation are inherent because of the position of the fetus. With the buttocks and lower extremities presenting, cord prolapse, cord entanglement around the extremities, and cord compression are more likely to occur. When delivery is managed too forcefully, birth trauma may result. Trauma to the fetal cervical spine and brachial plexus and fractures of the humerus, clavicle, skull, and neck may occur. A common concern with breech presentation is that the body of the neonate can be delivered but the head is too large to fit through the pelvis. This condition is called cephalopelvic disproportion (CPD).

The fetus in breech presentation is at higher risk for birth asphyxia (hypoxia, hypercapnia, and metabolic acidosis) compared with the fetus that has a vertex presentation. Head entrapment is a complication that occurs when the buttocks and lower extremities of the premature fetus pass through a cervix that is not completely dilated and is inadequate for the head to be delivered without trauma, asphyxiation, or both for the infant.

Assessment. Although the possibility of breech presentation may be determined either through vaginal examination or ultrasound scan, this does not have any bearing on the transport of the obstetric patient unless the patient is in active labor or the membranes are ruptured. In the event that vaginal delivery is inevitable, the transport team must be prepared to assist in a potentially difficult delivery. Vaginal delivery is imminent when the fetal buttocks are bulging the perineum and one or both legs are visible.

Strategies for Delivery. Essentially, the fetus in a breech presentation should not be touched until the umbilicus has spontaneously delivered. However, the risk of hypothermia is great for these babies, and a dry warm towel should be wrapped around the torso to prevent heat loss and allow for greater control when handling a slippery baby. The team should disengage the legs if one or both have not delivered spontaneously. This maneuver can be accomplished by hooking a finger on the leg by the groin and gently reducing the leg so it is extended outside the mother's body. Caution must be taken to avoid palpating the exposed umbilical cord. At one time, it was taught to palpate the cord to assess the FHR. However, this palpation could cause venospasm and the umbilical cord could clot off. Recommendations now are that the umbilical cord should be covered with a moist gauze dressing. At this point, the arms can usually be delivered by hooking the index finger over each of the baby's shoulders in turn (Figure 31-6). After the shoulders have been delivered, the baby's trunk is rotated so that the back is anterior (facing up), and gentle steady downward traction is applied until the hairline is visible. The body can now rest on the palm of one hand and forearm with the index and middle fingers supporting the baby's mouth and chin to maintain flexion of the head. With the other hand supporting the back and shoulders, the body can then gently be brought upward while another member of the transport team applies gentle suprapubic pressure to facilitate the delivery of the head with a minimal amount of neck traction (Figure 31-7).

Application of suprapubic pressure can be controversial because it can lead to uterine rupture if the pressure is extreme. If gentle suprapubic pressure is not

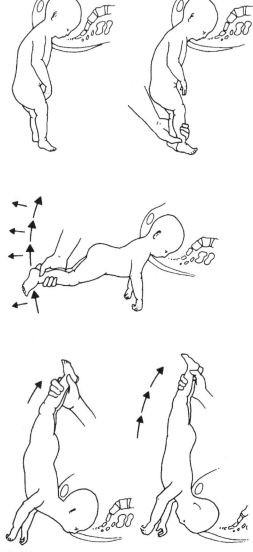

FIGURE 31-6   **Breech extraction.** Upward traction to effect delivery of the posterior shoulder, followed by freeing the posterior arm. (From Hickman M: *Midwifery,* ed 2, Oxford, 1985, Blackwell Scientific Publications.)

sufficient to deliver the baby, then the procedure must be stopped. Care must be taken to achieve slow and controlled delivery of the head, allowing the chin, face, and brow to sweep over the perineum. As soon as the baby's mouth has been delivered, the airway should be cleared with a bulb syringe; then, the rest of the head can be gently and slowly delivered. These deliveries can

be traumatic for the neonate. Preparation for resuscitation should be initiated before delivery.

Because breech delivery is a rare occurrence for the transport team, the tendency may be to act in haste when this situation arises. The team should guard against haste because it increases the risk for birth trauma.[11,12]

HEMORRHAGIC DELIVERY COMPLICATIONS

Once excessive bleeding occurs, quick intervention is necessary to minimize further blood loss. Postpartum hemorrhage, uterine inversion, placenta previa, placenta abruptio, PIH, and uterine rupture are delivery complications that predispose the patient to postpartum hemorrhage and risk of hypovolemic shock. Care should be directed at correcting the cause of the hemorrhage and then managing the hypovolemic shock and associated complications such as DIC.

Postpartum Hemorrhage

Blood loss in excess of 500 mL after delivery is defined as *postpartum hemorrhage* (PPH). The blood loss frequently occurs in the first few hours after delivery but can occur more than 24 hours later. PPH occurs in approximately 5% of all deliveries.

Etiology and Pathophysiologic Factors.

Postpartum hemorrhage is a blood loss of greater than 500 mL or more for a vaginal delivery and 1000 mL for a cesarean delivery. Estimates of blood loss must be accurate. Some studies have shown that estimated blood loss was approximately half the amount actually lost. Techniques used to improve objective blood loss measurement are pad counts, weighing of chux pads, or collection of blood clots in a graduated cylinder or suction canister. Uterine atony is the major cause of postpartum hemorrhage. Normally, bleeding from the placental site is controlled when the interlacing muscle fibers of the uterus contract and retract in conjunction with platelet aggregation and clot formation in the vessels of the decidua. This occurs immediately after delivery of the placenta as the uterus involutes to spontaneously clamp off uterine blood vessels that once perfused the placenta. Factors that predispose to uterine atony and prevent compression of the

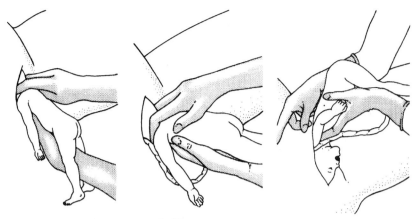

FIGURE 31-7 **Delivery of head with use of Mauriceau's maneuver.** Note that as the fetal head is being delivered, flexion of the head is maintained with suprapubic pressure provided by an assistant and simultaneously with pressure on the maxilla by the operator as traction is applied. (From Hickman M: *Midwifery,* ed 2, Oxford, 1985, Blackwell Scientific Publications.)

vessels at the implantation site predispose to postpartum hemorrhage. Uterine atony can occur after a prolonged or tumultuous labor or after general anesthetic is used. The uterus that is overdistended as a result of multiple gestation, uterine tumors, hydramnios, or a large fetus is more likely to be hypotonic after delivery. Multiparity, chorioamnionitis, previous PPH, placenta previa, and use of labor stimulants place the obstetric patient at increased risk for uterine atony and PPH.

As the uterus fills with clots, it is increasingly unable to contract and retract normally, compounding the problem of hemorrhage. In addition, when the placenta and membranes are retained, the same circumstances are created. An abnormally adherent placenta (placenta accreta) or incomplete separation may be the cause.

Another common cause of PPH is lacerations that result from delivery. Undetected lacerations of the cervix, vagina, perineum, or lower uterine segment are all sources for hemorrhage. Hemorrhage as a result of lacerations is usually limited and is rarely severe. However, constant seepage over a few hours can amount to an appreciable loss. Application of forceps may be the reason for the hemorrhage. When a patient has had a previous cesarean section followed by a vaginal delivery, dehiscence of an old uterine scar with hemorrhage may result. Lacerations should be suspected when hemorrhaging occurs in the presence of a firmly contracted uterus. Coagulopathy associated with DIC, placental abruption, and PIH are other causes of PPH. Idiopathic thrombocytopenia or von Willebrand's disease as preexisting coagulopathies predispose to PPH.

Hemorrhage may also result from a combination of sources. Hemorrhage from uterine atony may be coupled with hemorrhage from a cervical laceration.

Assessment. The transport team should determine the source of the hemorrhage. Abdominal palpation may reveal a boggy, enlarged, and soft uterus. Persistent vaginal bleeding from slight to profuse is noted with uterine atony. The team should also examine the patient for the presence of lacerations in the perineal area. Assessment for cervical, vaginal, and lower uterine segment while en route may be difficult or impossible.

Strategies for Transport. A team member should palpate and vigorously massage the fundus. One hand should cup the fundus; the other provides support to the lower uterine segment just above the symphysis pubis. Often, clots are expressed, and frequent massage alone may be all the stimulation that is needed for the uterus to adequately contract and retract. Fundal massage should be performed at least every 5 to 15 minutes, and the location of fundus in relation to the level of the umbilicus, the degree of firmness, and the vaginal flow should be noted. For example, if the fundus is at the level of the umbilicus, it is documented as U/U. If the fundus is 2 cm (finger breaths) above the umbilicus, it is noted as 2/U. A full bladder is often the reason that the uterus remains boggy and cannot involute. The puffy full bladder lies directly beneath the uterus and interferes with its ability to contract. Simply having the patient void or inserting a Foley catheter for the transport tremendously decreases uterine bleeding. When the uterus is firm, it palpates like a small grapefruit and vaginal bleeding is greatly decreased. If on repeated assessment, the uterus becomes boggy again, the uterus palpates as soft and mushy and increased vaginal bleeding with clots is usually noted. Treatment is to again perform uterine massage. The awake and alert patient can be taught this treatment and can perform it herself. Also of note is that fundal massage can be painful for patients and pain relief medications should be offered and titrated to relieve pain.

Rapid infusion of 20 to 40 units of oxytocin in 1000 mL lactated Ringer's solution, or methylergonovine 0.2 mg administered intramuscularly or intravenously, is recommended. Methylergonovine should be used cautiously in patients with PIH because of the pressor effects that may result in further elevated blood pressure.

The integrity of the cervix, vagina, perineum, and lower uterine segment should be documented at the referring facility. Inspection of the placenta after delivery reveals missing fragments, membranes, or both that may be retained. The team should assess blood loss and inspect the perineum; little external bleeding is observed in the presence of a pelvic hematoma. Blood from lacerations tends to be brighter red. Uterine bleeding from either a relaxed or boggy uterus or from retained parts also is bright to dark red and has numerous large clots. Maternal patients are in a hypercoagulable state. Do not pack the vagina if lacerations are seen. Instead, apply a peripad and have the patient squeeze her legs together. The pad can also be applied to the external genitalia to manage bleeding. If at any time the patient loses the ability to clot or if petechia or bleeding from IV sites becomes apparent, the presence of DIC must be investigated (Figure 31-8).

UTERINE INVERSION

Complete inversion of the uterus is extremely rare and occurs when the entire uterus turns inside out, extending out through the cervix and into the vagina where it

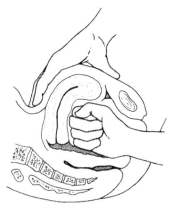

FIGURE 31-8   This technique is very invasive; hence, the transport nurse may avoid use of this procedure. As a last line of action it is usually effective in controlling PPH as a result of uterine atony. Note the placement of the fist in the anterior fornix. (From Hickman M: *Midwifery*, ed 2, Oxford, 1985, Blackwell Scientific Publications.)

is visible. The uterus can partially invert with the fundus turned inside out. *Partial inversion* is not as obvious and may initially be more difficult to determine.

Etiology and Pathophysiologic Factors

Inversion may occur spontaneously after a contraction or with increased abdominal pressure caused by coughing or sneezing, and it often occurs as the result of overly aggressive management of the third stage of delivery (delivery of the placenta). Predisposing factors include excessive cord traction, fundal pressure, excessive cord traction with a placenta accreta, fundal implantation of the placenta, and uterine atony. The lesson to be learned here is do *not* pull on the umbilical cord to deliver the placenta after the baby is delivered. Within 5 to 20 minutes, the placenta spontaneously separates with a gush and lengthening of the cord. At this time, it can gently be guided out through the vagina.

Assessment

Vaginal bleeding, which may be profuse after delivery and accompanied by sudden and severe lower abdominal pain, may rarely be caused by uterine inversion. Abdominal palpation may reveal a defect in the fundus, or it may not be palpable at all, being nonglobular in shape. Signs of hypovolemic shock may develop quickly.

Strategies for Transport

If uterine inversion is recognized immediately before the uterus has had a chance to contract down and the cervix to constrict, manual replacement may be possible. Without attempting to remove the placenta, pressure should be applied with the fingertips and palm of the hand to push the fundus upward and through the cervical canal (Figure 31-9). This procedure can be extremely painful for the patient.

While the attempt at manual replacement is being made, analgesics should be administered and the procedure and the necessity for it should be explained to the patient.[11,12]

Removing the placenta before attempting to replace the uterus may increase the hemorrhaging. The placenta will deliver unless some degree of placenta accrete exists, and oxytocin should be administered immediately. The best preventive measure is allowing spontaneous delivery of the placenta. If the uterus cannot be safely replaced, it should be covered with sterile moist gauze and immediate transport should ensue because surgical procedures are needed. Diversion of transport should be considered if the patient's condition is hemodynamically unstable and diversion is available and appropriate.

UTERINE RUPTURE

A spontaneous or traumatic disruption of the uterine wall, known as *uterine rupture,* can occur. If the laceration is extensive and comes in direct contact with the peritoneal cavity, it is a complete rupture. The rupture most frequently occurs in a weak area of the myometrium, usually at the site of a previous incision. Examples of previous incisions include a previous caesarian section scar, a scar from a myomectomy, or a scar from the result of rapid deceleration forces.

Etiology and Pathophysiologic Factors

Before further discussion of uterine rupture, differentiation between rupture and dehiscence of a scar is necessary. *Rupture* refers to the separation of an old incision and possibly an extension into previously uninvolved myometrium, with rupture of membranes. Fetal parts may extend through the rupture into the peritoneal cavity. Hemorrhage is usually present from the edges of the separation and may be massive. A *dehiscence* does not involve the fetal membranes and may not even involve the entire previous scar. Bleeding may be minimal or bloodless. Dehiscence occurs gradually, whereas rupture occurs as a sudden event. A dehiscence may become a rupture with labor or trauma.

Factors that predispose to uterine rupture include previous surgery involving the myometrium, previous cesarean section with a higher incidence of a "classic" vertical scar being involved, use of labor stimulants, trauma, previous rupture, overdistention of the uterus as a result of multiple gestation or hydramnios, and grand multiparity. Uterine rupture usually occurs during labor but can occur before the onset of labor. Uterine rupture can be seen with an unscarred uterus resulting from blunt trauma. This trauma is most likely a rapid deceleration injury in which pressures inside the uterus are too high as a result of sudden impact and rupture occurs. Uterine rupture may also occur as a result of internal trauma, such as perforation with an instrument (e.g., a difficult forceps delivery); from external pressure, such as from an external version of the breech fetus; or from overly vigorous fundal pressure during delivery attempts.

In situations in which the patient has had a previous cesarean section, the probability of rupture is much greater when the scar traverses the body of the uterus vertically (classical incision) than when the scar involves the lower uterine section transversely. Dehiscence occurs more frequently without subsequent complications when the scar is low and transverse.

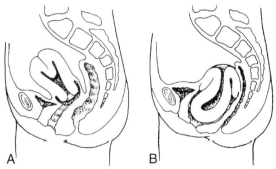

FIGURE 31-9   **Uterine inversion. A,** First degree; **B,** second degree. Note the abdominal depression where the fundus would normally be and vaginal palpation of the fundus at the cervical opening. Continued pressure with the fingertips encourages reversion of the fundus. Note the stages of inversion in the inset. (From Hickman M: *Midwifery,* ed 2, Oxford, 1985, Blackwell Scientific Publications.)

The degree of hemorrhage and extent of possible complications depend on the location and extent of the rupture. If the rupture does not involve the large arteries, the hemorrhage is less severe. If the rupture is complete, the mortality rate for the fetus is high. Potential complications are postpartum infection, injury to the bladder, potential for hysterectomy for uncontrolled bleeding, hypovolemic shock, kidney failure, DIC, and death.

Assessment

Signs and symptoms of uterine rupture include severe sudden continual abdominal pain and signs of hypovolemic shock. Contractions may cease or may increase in intensity and frequency. Shoulder or chest pain may result from the collection of blood under the diaphragm (Kehr's sign). Generalized tenderness with rebound pain or vaginal bleeding is likely when the rupture occurs in the lower uterine segment. However, many of these patients are obtunded from blood loss and are unable to report pain. Most bleeding is intraabdominal, and the abdomen may be distended. Frequent assessment of fundal height may be an indication that the uterus is filling with blood. Use a marker to mark the top of the fundus with ink, and frequently reassess the fundal height. Palpation of the uterus also reveals a firm or hardening uterus, which is reflective of accumulating blood. Remember the maternal patient carries 40% to 50% more blood at term and is able to compensate for a longer period of time before maternal vital sign changes are noted. The maternal patient can be in class III shock before any blood pressure change is noted. Another text book description of uterine rupture is that the clinician should be able to palpate fetal parts as the uterine wall integrity is lost. Although this may or may not be true, this is a *secondary* assessment, and because of tremendous blood volume losses, it is unlikely the clinician has moved beyond the primary survey.

Strategies for Transport

Rapid recognition of the signs and symptoms of uterine rupture often mean the difference between life and death for the obstetric patient. Surgical intervention is necessary, and care is supportive. Oxytocin, 20 to 40 units in a 1000-mL solution administered intravenously, may incite uterine contraction with vessel constriction and reduce the bleeding after delivery of the fetus. Serial abdominal measurements can be made to further assess intraabdominal bleeding. Acute fetal distress with increasingly severe variable decelerations, late decelerations, minimal to absent variability, or absent FHT is observed.

A history of previous cesarean sections and observation of abdominal scar is of primary importance. Although the scar noted may be low and transverse, documentation is needed to determine the location of the scar on the uterus. For the patient in labor who has had a previous cesarean section, the first sign of placental abruption may actually be rupture. Tocolytics may be considered for patients with a previous classical incision that is at risk for contracting or is currently contracting. Appropriate medical staff must be contacted for direction and management.

PRECIPITATE DELIVERY

Precipitate delivery occurs when the labor is abnormally rapid with strong contractions and rapid cervical dilation and descent of the presenting part. Delivery usually occurs in 2 to 3 hours from the start of contractions. The transport team's goal is to prevent an expulsive delivery and minimize trauma to both the mother and the fetus. Possible complications include uterine rupture, amniotic fluid embolism, PPH, and lacerations. Other concerns for precipitous delivery involve the neonate. This rapid and forceful delivery can lead to an increased need for resuscitation at birth and a higher incidence of birth trauma. These neonates are literally "shot out" and often need some respiratory assistance with bag-mask-valve (BVM) devices until they can acclimate to life outside the uterus. Transport professionals may not be able to control the labor, but they should have some control over the delivery. An uncontrolled delivery can cause cerebral hemorrhage in the neonate because of rapid changes in pressure. The baby's head should be guided with application of a small amount of pressure.

RETAINED PLACENTA

Normally, the placenta separates spontaneously in 5 to 20 minutes after delivery of the fetus. Signs of separation include lengthening of the exposed cord and a gush of blood; the uterus appears to "ball up." Slow gentle downward traction is usually all that is needed to assist the delivery of the placenta. When no signs of separation occur and hemorrhage is not evident, transport can be accomplished with the placenta retained. Encouraging the mother to breastfeed promotes separation of the placenta and involution of the uterus. When the placenta is partially retained, postpartum hemorrhage results. Frequent fundal massage must be initiated until surgical services can be obtained.

SHOULDER DYSTOCIA

After delivery of the head, the anterior shoulder pushes against the symphysis, creating a situation commonly referred to as *shoulder dystocia*. In most circumstances, the head is the largest diameter of the fetus. Occasionally, the shoulders have a larger diameter. The obvious concern is that the head will fit through the pelvic bones and the shoulders will be unable to. The condition becomes apparent when the head is pulled down against the perineum and the shoulders do not follow with gentle traction. This is called turtling. The head extends out during a contraction but then retracts after the contraction is over because the shoulders prevent further progression. The incidence of shoulder dystocia increases significantly with birth weight.

Etiology and Pathophysiologic Factors

Several predisposing factors have been linked to shoulder dystocia. However, shoulder dystocia can occur quite unexpectedly without obvious associated factors. The complication occurs more frequently with the presence of a large fetus or with a macrosomic fetus such as those found with gestational diabetes. Other risk factors include patients with a contracted pelvis, maternal obesity, or a prolonged second stage of labor, including deliveries that require instruments for delivery.

Possible complications of shoulder dystocia include brachial plexus damage and fractured fetal clavicle. Fetal hypoxia can occur when the cord is drawn into the pelvis and compressed.

Assessment

In any situation of imminent delivery, unless the fetus is expected to weigh 2500 g or less, shoulder dystocia is a possibility. However, any fetus greater than 4000 g is at a considerably higher risk. After the head has been delivered and inspection for a nuchal cord has been performed, the delivery of the anterior shoulder should be attempted. If the anterior shoulder is unable to be delivered, consider the possibility of shoulder dystocia. Careful considerations for preparation for a difficult delivery, anticipated neonatal resuscitation, and possible diversion should be initiated.

Unnecessary haste and overly aggressive force should be avoided because of the increased possibility of birth trauma to the fetus. Excessive lateral flexion of the neck and overly vigorous traction of the head and neck increase the risk of damage to the brachial plexus.

Strategies for Delivery

Once the team member is aware of the situation, the head may be observed to retract against the perineum. Fundal pressure aggravates the shoulder impaction and should be avoided. If an episiotomy has not been made, a generous mediolateral episiotomy is recommended. The McRoberts maneuver, a simple maneuver that increases the diameter of the pelvis by stretching the pelvic joints, should be tried next. With the patient's legs flexed at the knees, the maternal nurse should help the patient draw her knees up and toward the chest (dorsal knee-chest position) and continue, with gentle downward traction of the head. Once the anterior shoulder clears the symphysis, the posterior shoulder usually delivers without resistance. The key to success in this position is to have the mother's knees as far back to her shoulders as possible. Next, gentle application of suprapubic pressure can be applied by another member of the air medical crew (the shoulder may be palpated suprapubicly). Gentle downward traction of the head should be applied concurrent with gentle suprapubic pressure. Suprapubic pressure should never be excessive because it can lead to uterine rupture and bladder trauma. The team should not persist if the shoulder does not slip under the symphysis.

Delivery of the posterior shoulder can also be attempted with rotation of the posterior shoulder downward and into the left posterior quadrant. With release of the posterior arm and shoulder, the anterior shoulder follows. As a last resort, the infant's clavicle may be deliberately broken; however, when this is done, the chance of damage to the brachial plexus is increased. Vaginal delivery increases the risk for perinatal mortality and morbidity by 3%.[3,11]

UMBILICAL CORD PROLAPSE

Overt *cord prolapse* occurs when the cord slips down into the vagina or appears externally after the amniotic membranes have ruptured. When the cord slips down into or near the pelvis, adjacent to the presenting part, it is not palpable on vaginal examination (occult prolapse). The cord may also have slipped down to a position in which it is palpable through the cervix but in intact membranes (forelying prolapse). Varying degrees of prolapse may occur. The weight of the presenting fetal part causes compression of the umbilical cord. The amount of fetal distress is directly related to the degree or compression.

Etiology

Circumstances that cause maladaptation of the presenting part to the lower uterine segment or prevent descent of the presenting part into the pelvis predispose the obstetric patient to cord prolapse. These factors include breech presentation, transverse lie, premature rupture of membranes (PROM), a contracted pelvis, unengaged large fetus multiparity, hydramnios, multiple gestations, a long cord, and preterm labor. Complications include severe fetal distress and fetal death.

Assessment

Cord prolapse occurs suddenly and requires quick identification of the problem and quick action. Identification of the obstetric patient who is vulnerable to cord prolapse is of primary importance. Clinical signs of prolapse include sudden fetal bradycardia and severe recurrent variable decelerations that do not respond to a change in maternal position, administration of oxygen, or hydration. Compression of the cord between the presenting part and the pelvic tissues causes the FHT patterns that are observed.

Strategies for Transport

Actions necessary in the event of cord prolapse include elevating the presenting part off the cord with a hand in the vagina that must remain there during the entire transport to prevent further cord compression. The mother should be positioned in a Trendelenburg's or knee-chest position to further reduce pressure on the cord. The cord may spontaneously retract, depending on the degree of prolapse, but should never be manually replaced because severe compression may occur. Intervention to elevate the presenting part off the cord must be maintained during the transport and through delivery. The cord should be gently wrapped in moist gauze and then wrapped in plastic to prevent it from drying out.

The transport team should provide supplemental oxygen via nonrebreather mask. A tocolytic agent, such as terbutaline 0.25 mg administered subcutaneously or via intravenous push, should be given to slow the contractions and reduce the pressure on the cord during contractions. When the cord compression is relieved, the fetus is able to recover from the hypoxic event in utero as long as the compression does not recur.

If cord prolapse occurs when the patient is en route, the receiving facility should be alerted to prepare for an emergency cesarean section. On occasion, the FHR pattern is normal or shows minimal abnormalities. This results from no cord compression from the presenting fetal parts. The only symptom evident is the prolapsed cord; however, the interventions are the same.

DIABETES IN PREGNANCY

Basically, *diabetes mellitus* (DM) is a disease in which the body is unable to produce or sufficiently use insulin to metabolize glucose. The disease is complicated by faulty metabolism of fats and proteins for energy. The course and outcome of a pregnancy complicated by diabetes depend on the severity of the disease process.

Etiology and Pathophysiologic Factors

This discussion of diabetes in pregnancy is limited primarily to how diabetes, whether gestational or a preexisting condition, is affected by the pregnancy and how the pregnancy affects the patient with diabetes. Pregnancy is considered a diabetogenic state in which the patient has an increased need for glucose and protein and fat are metabolized to aid in the demand for higher glucose requirements. During pregnancy, the metabolism of the mother adapts to provide fuel for the growing fetus and for her own increased metabolic needs. Early in pregnancy, during the period of rapid growth of the embryo, the mother's blood glucose level decreases. The obstetric patient who has diabetes may have hypoglycemia.

At approximately 24 weeks of gestation, the diabetogenic effects of pregnancy begin. Increased hormonal activity exerts an antiinsulin effect that results in a decreased responsiveness to insulin and a rise in the level of blood glucose. Increased production of insulin by the pancreas counteracts the antiinsulin effects of the hormones, and normal blood glucose levels are maintained. If, as a result of an acquired or inherited defect in beta cell function, maternal insulin secretion fails to keep pace with the demand, a further increase in blood glucose levels occurs. At this point in the pregnancy, gestational diabetes is frequently recognized and diagnosed. For the woman who is already diabetic, an increase in insulin requirement occurs and remains increased until after delivery.

The obstetric patient with a pregnancy complicated by DM is at an increased risk compared with the remainder of the pregnant population for development of PIH and related disorders, hydramnios, infections such as vaginitis, urinary tract infections, and pyelonephritis. Delivery via cesarean section and preterm delivery also occur with increased frequency because of macrosomia or fetal distress. As commonly found with patients with diabetes, vascular changes can affect perfusion. The placentas of women with diabetes tend to have decreased perfusion and more calcification. This in turn leads to decreased fetal perfusion and higher risks of intrauterine growth restriction (IUGR) and fetal distress.

The fetus of a mother with diabetes is at increased risk as well. Complications associated with the fetus include congenital anomalies, IUGR, macrosomia, delivery trauma, fetal distress, hypoglycemia, hypocalcemia, hyperbilirubinemia, respiratory distress, and intrauterine death. *Macrosomia* refers to a fetus that is large for gestational age with increased fat deposition and an enlarged spleen and liver. Macrosomia is seen more commonly when the mother has gestational DM or DM without vasculopathy. Congenital anomalies are seen more frequently when pregnant women with diabetes are in poor control of their diabetes.[4,11,12]

Assessment

Assessment of the patient with diabetes includes screening for the presence of risk factors linked to DM. All pregnant women with diabetes need to be assessed so the disease can be classified. Assessment by the flight nurse should include the following:

1. *Obstetric history:* Assess for the possibility that a previous pregnancy was complicated by undiagnosed diabetes. Has the patient had gestational DM with a previous pregnancy, or does she have a family history of DM? Has she delivered an infant that weighed more than 4000 g? Has she had unexplained perinatal losses, stillbirths, or traumatic deliveries? Has more than one pregnancy been complicated by PIH? PIH as a multipara? Does she have a history of hydramnios or preterm delivery? Is she older than 35 years?

2. *Current pregnancy:* Does the patient have signs and symptoms of DM? Is glycosuria present? Are results of a glucose challenge test abnormal? Is the patient obese? Has the patient had recurrent urinary tract infections or vaginitis? Does the patient have chronic hypertension? What are the results of ultrasound scans or other diagnostic tests? Is the diabetes controlled with diet or insulin? What is the patient's current insulin regimen? Note: If the patient has not received prenatal care with this pregnancy, most of this information is not known.

3. *History of preexisting condition:* What class is the DM, as determined by the age of onset, duration of the disease, and evidence of vasculopathy? Does the patient have cardiovascular or kidney disease? Has there been good control of the diabetes during the pregnancy? What is the patient's current insulin regimen?

Strategies for Transport

In addition to following the general guidelines for transport care, careful assessment is needed for the obstetric patient with gestational DM or diabetes because of changing metabolic demands. The transport team should obtain a diabetic history from the patient and assess for complications associated with DM in pregnancy. The time of her last meal and last insulin injection are also important to record.

If the patient is in labor, simultaneous continuous insulin and glucose infusions stabilize maternal levels and may reduce neonatal hyperglycemia. The insulin may be adjusted after delivery on the basis of blood sugar levels, and the insulin demand decreases after delivery. The patient is given nothing by mouth. Blood glucose levels are evaluated every 1 to 2 hours and maintained at a level of 80 to 120 mg/dL (or to whatever range is desired by maternal fetal medicine physicians or endocrine physicians), with insulin as indicated by the patient's blood sugar.

The transport team should obtain a blood glucose reading just before transport. Because labor increases metabolic needs, the team should be aware of the signs and symptoms of hypoglycemia and hyperglycemia and should never administer terbutaline to a patient with insulin-dependent diabetes because of the transient hyperglycemic response seen with terbutaline. Caution is also advised with the administration of magnesium sulfate because many patients with DM have decreased renal function. Magnesium sulfate is cleared through the kidneys. In addition, many diabetic patients have the comorbidity of PIH.

HEMORRHAGIC COMPLICATIONS
Placental Abruption

Placental abruption can be defined as the premature detachment of a normally implanted placenta from the uterine wall. The separation may occur over a small area with little evidence or can separate totally with devastating results. The incidence of abruption varies widely, depending on the source. Of considerable significance is the incidence of recurrence with subsequent pregnancies.[3]

Etiology.   The primary cause of placental abruption is largely unknown. Hypertension, whether chronic or PIH, and previous abruption are two factors that are known to greatly increase the risk of placental abruption. Other factors that place the obstetric patient at risk include abdominal trauma, an unusually short umbilical cord, amniocentesis, multiparity, age over 35 years, uterine anomalies or tumors, and sudden uterine decompression (such as when a twin is delivered and the other twin remains in utero, or when a hypertensive crisis is acutely resolved). Other risk factors include cigarette smoking, and substance abuse, especially abuse of cocaine.[18]

Pathophysiologic Factors.   Hemorrhage occurs from the arterioles that supply the decidua (lining of uterus), causing a retroplacental hematoma. Placental separation takes place at that site and may continue with the hemorrhage. As the hemorrhage continues, more vessels are disrupted, which leads to increased hemorrhage and further separation. Placental separation can be an avalanche that continues to total separation or suddenly stops for reasons unknown. Sometimes a clot blocks the hemorrhage. The decidua is rich in thromboplastin, and clotting occurs rapidly. When vaginal bleeding is observed, the blood is usually dark because of the rapid clotting and the distance it takes to reach the vagina and be seen externally. If separation occurs at the margin of the placenta (Figure 31-10) or if the amniotic membranes are dissected from the decidua as a result of the hemorrhage, vaginal bleeding is observed. No vaginal bleeding is observed if the hemorrhage is completely concealed behind the placenta. Use the mental imagery of a fried egg: the yellow yolk is the the abruption, and the white egg is the attached placenta. Bleeding is certainly associated with the abruption; it is just occult and cannot escape vaginally to be seen.

As the hemorrhage continues and a retroplacental clot forms, enough pressure may be exerted to force blood through the membranes, giving the amniotic fluid a port wine color, or into the myometrium, causing a condition called Couvelaire uterus. The uterine tone is increased, and irritability is noted. Contractions are frequently present. Blood is a known irritant and often leads to uterine irritability or contractions. The process is a vicious circle: as the bleeding increases, the incidence of contraction increases; as the incidence of contractions increases, so does the incidence of bleeding.

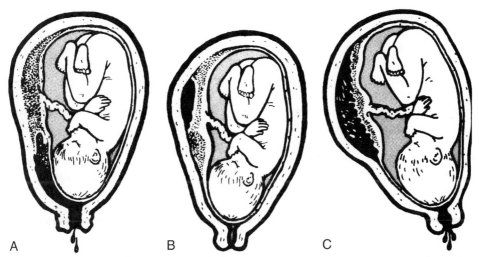

FIGURE 31-10 **Examples of placental abruption. A,** Placental separation occurs at the margin of the placenta; **B,** and **C,** separation originates from a central area behind the placenta. (Illustrated by Vincenza Genovese, Phoenix, AZ. From Gilbert ES, Harmon JS: *High-risk pregnancy and delivery,* St Louis, 1986, Mosby.)

A common complication of placental abruption is DIC. Other complications include postpartum hemorrhage, anemia, postpartum infection, hypovolemic shock, kidney failure, and fetal distress or death. As placental perfusion is altered, the risk for fetal hypoxia and acidosis is increased. The factors that predispose to placental abruption may occur preterm, predisposing to preterm delivery.

Placenta Previa

Placenta previa occurs when the placenta becomes implanted in the lower uterine segment and as a result covers or partially covers the internal cervical os. A marginal or low-lying previa extends to or close to the internal os but does not cover any part of it. Placenta previa occurs approximately once in every 200 to 400 deliveries. The incidence of placenta previa is higher preterm. As the pregnancy progresses, the fundus hypertrophies and the lower uterine segment elongates, which allows the placenta to migrate away from the internal os toward the fundus. In reality, the placenta does not move; it is merely carried up towards the fundus as the uterus grows.

Etiology. Although the exact cause is unknown, a higher incidence of placenta previa is seen with uterine scarring. A previous cesarean section, dilation and curettage, increased parity, multiparity with short intervals, and a previous occurrence of placenta previa can scar the uterus. Other factors that place the obstetric patient at risk for placenta previa include previous chorioamnionitis, multiple gestation (for which a larger surface area is covered by the placenta), fetal erythroblastosis, maternal age over age 35 years, substance abuse, previous myomectomy, and uterine tumors.

Pathophysiologic Factors. Normal placental implantation usually occurs in the fundus or body segment of the uterus. Defective perfusion of the decidua has been suggested to favor implantation of the placenta in the lower uterine segment. Because less vascularization exists in the lower uterine segment, the placenta compensates and tends to grow thinner and larger, thus covering a larger area and thereby increasing perfusion.

Before the onset of labor, the cervix begins to soften, efface, and dilate. These cervical changes disrupt the placental attachment, tearing the vessels, and hemorrhage results. Bright red vaginal bleeding is observed; it is initially painless and is not initially associated with contractions. The primary episode usually involves less than 250 mL of blood and tends to cease spontaneously as clot formation rapidly occurs. Recurrence is unpredictable. Generally, the greater the extent to which the internal os is covered, the sooner the initial episode occurs. In addition, subsequent bleeds that are larger than the one prior are not uncommon.

Potential complications of placenta previa include complications similar to those of placental abruption, such as DIC, hypovolemic shock, kidney damage (from hypoperfusion), anemia, postpartum infection, postpartum hemorrhage, and fetal distress or death. A common complication of placenta previa and the resulting bleeds is preterm labor. As with other areas in the body, blood is an irritant. And as with abruptions, bleeding leads to uterine irritability and contractions, and contractions lead to more bleeding. Because hemorrhage may occur at any time without warning or precipitating events, the risk is increased with premature delivery. Furthermore, placenta accreta is a rare complication of placenta previa. With placenta acreta, the placenta (chorionic villi) attaches to the myometrium. Normal placental attachment is to the endometrium.

Assessment of Placental Abruption and Placenta Previa

Generally, the clinical findings of placental abruption vary in degree with the extent, or percentage, of the placental separation and clot formation behind the placenta. Onset of symptoms may be gradual in mild cases to sudden and without warning in severe situations. In cases of vaginal bleeding after 20 weeks of gestation, placenta previa should be considered.

Uterine Assessment (Placental Abruption). Symptoms of placental abruption may range from slight abdominal tenderness and lower back discomfort with a mild abruption to severe unceasing abdominal pain in a large abruption. Sudden severe pain without vaginal bleeding may be indicative of retroplacental hemorrhage into the myometrium. The bleeding is occult because it is behind the placenta and it is trapped. However, most presentations of placenta abruptio include vaginal bleeding. Typically, the blood is dark and clotted because of the distance it must travel from the fundus to the cervix. A key assessment point is that the color of the vaginal bleeding is related to how old the blood is not the source of the bleeding (abruptio versus previa). The intensity, frequency, and duration of contractions may vary from contractions with a slight increase in uterine tone to hypertonic (Figure 31-11) or tetanic contractions. *Tetanic contractions*

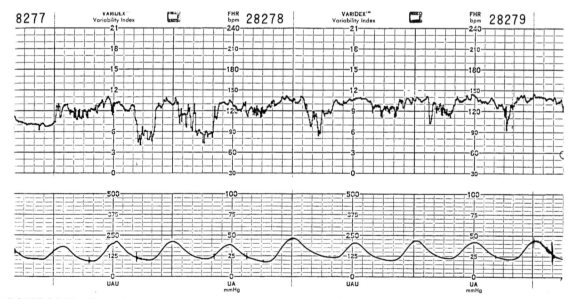

FIGURE 31-11   **Abruption pattern.** Note the increased uterine tone documented with the use of an internal uterine pressure catheter (IUPC). Hypertonic contractions are occurring approximately every minute with virtually no period of relaxation between contractions. Note the distressed fetal response. An emergency cesarean section was performed with Apgar scores of 2 and 7 at 1 and 5 minutes, respectively.

are very strong contractions that typically last longer than 90 seconds and have minimal resting tone in between. Assessment should include palpation of the uterus for the frequency, duration, strength, and sustained uterine tone associated with contractions. The uterus is often described as board like, primarily because of the tetanic contractions and the accumulation of blood within the uterus. A classic presentation of placenta abruptio is profound abdominal pain that appears disproportionate to the contractions palpated. Although not a rule, often the larger the abruption, the more severe the abdominal or uterine pain. With moderate to large abruption, labor tends to progress rapidly and the risks for precipitous delivery and fetal distress are greater. Preparation must be taken for immediate vaginal delivery, or in the case of extensive hemorrhage, cesarean delivery. Radio or call ahead to the receiving facility so appropriate preparation can be made. If determination of when a contraction begins or ends is difficult and the abdomen is rigid, the patient is in profound pain and, especially with the presence of vaginal bleeding, a placental separation should be suspected.

Uterine Assessment (Placenta Previa).
Contractions may or may not be present with placenta previa. The onset usually occurs during or after the hemorrhage because of increased uterine irritability. Blood is an irritant, and as a result, the uterus may become irritable or contract.

Assessment of Blood Loss (Placental Abruption).
When placental abruption occurs, vaginal bleeding may vary from absent or minimal to profuse. The amount of vaginal bleeding is not an indicator of the degree of separation or of total blood loss but of the location of the separation. Assessment of a concealed hemorrhage includes any change in fundal height as an indication of continued hemorrhage. The fundus can be marked to provide a quick visual indicator of increasing uterine size. However, rising fundal height is a late sign and often requires a substantial amount of blood to accumulate in the uterus. Early signs of maternal bleeding are reflected in the FHR with an increasing baseline and loss of variability noted. Maternal tachycardia is then noted. Approximately one third of the maternal blood volume is lost before significant changes are seen in the maternal blood pressure. The bleeding may continue until delivery of the placenta, or it may stop spontaneously. The bleeding from placenta abruptio is often unpredictable. An abruption may be classified as chronic and have a constant but minimal amount of spotting or bleeding. Other abruptions may have an initial separation and bleed but then do not progress. Still other abruptions have an initial separation and then unpredictably continue to separate to varying percentages. The larger the percentage of placental separation, the more unstable the abruption.

Assessment of Blood Loss (Placenta Previa).
Blood loss can be more accurately estimated with placenta previa, for which only external hemorrhage is observed. Placenta previa is characterized by repetitive and frequently more extensive bleeding episodes. Objective measurements of blood loss should always be used. Methods to use are pad counts, weighing of towel or chux pads, and collection of blood in graduated cylinders or suction canisters.

Ultrasound Scan.
An ultrasound scan can confirm the location of the placenta. If ultrasound scan is not available, a previa cannot be ruled out. A sterile vaginal examination may stimulate profuse bleeding by dislodging a clot and should never be done. With cervical changes that accompany active labor, occasionally an increase in bloody show is noted and may appear excessive, which may lead the transport professional to believe that a placenta previa is present. If unsure, do not attempt a vaginal examination. If the increased source of bleeding is indeed from an active bloody show, then signs of imminent delivery are also present. If available, ultrasound scan may also be used to rule out the presence of an abruption. However, not all abruptions are visible with ultrasound scan and the diagnosis may be made based on clinical presentation.

Assessment of Vital Signs.
Signs of maternal hypovolemic shock may not be present until a blood loss of approximately 30% has occurred.

However, before any change in vital signs, shunting away from the placenta to the vital organs occurs, and FHT indicative of placental insufficiency is seen. FHR changes often include increasing or tachycardic baseline and loss of variability.

Assessment of Fetal Heart Tone.   Fetal distress as a result of placental separation or placenta previa occurs primarily from placental insufficiency (hypertonic uterus, maternal hemorrhage, or decreased placental perfusion) or fetal hemorrhage as a consequence of placental separation. The team must observe for the early signs of fetal hypoperfusion, as just mentioned, and late decelerations and bradycardia.

Assessment of Urinary Output.   Urinary output of 60 to 100 mL/h suggests adequate renal perfusion and, indirectly, adequate circulating blood volume. Urinary output of less than 30 mL/h suggests decreased circulatory volume. Insertion of a urinary catheter is recommended for any circumstances in which maternal hypoperfusion or hypovolemia is suspected.

Assessment of Coagulopathy.   The transport team should observe for petechiae, hematuria, bruising, or bleeding from intravenous sites.

Assessment for Impending Shock.   Because of the normal physiologic changes of pregnancy, early symptoms of hypovolemia may be masked. Careful assessment of serial vital signs aids in differentiating expected blood pressure, pulse, and respirations from symptoms of impending shock. Symptoms include tachypnea, decreased blood pressure, increased pulse rate (rapid and thready), oliguria, cyanosis, pallor, and clamminess.[3,19,21] Current research suggests that trending MAPs may be more helpful in assessment of signs of shock then pure blood pressure measurement.

Strategies for Transport (Abruption and Previa)

The transport team should use the following strategies for transport of patients with abruption or previa:

1. Implement general guidelines for transport care after the primary survey and obstetric assessment are completed. Assess for contractions, the extent of hemorrhage, and estimated blood loss. Determine fundal height or mark the fundus, with frequent reassessment. Recognition of concealed bleeding is confirmed by noting an increase in the fundal height and with earlier signs of blood loss such as changes in the FHR, vital signs, and LOC.

2. Administer tocolytics as recommended. Refer to the discussion in this chapter regarding preterm labor for specifics about labor suppressants. Program-specific guidelines for tocolysis should be followed. Any deviation should be discussed with medical control or accepting maternal fetal medicine physicians. Maternal bleeding is a contraindication for use of beta mimetics because they cause maternal and fetal tachycardia and blur the assessment of maternal hemorrhage.

3. Assess vital signs every 15 minutes or more frequently as needed. Note any subtle changes that may indicate hypovolemia. Check capillary refill as needed to assess for peripheral perfusion. Initiate EFM, if available, to monitor FHT for changes indicative of impending fetal distress. Provide supplemental oxygen, IV fluids, and maternal position change.

4. Observe for signs of DIC. Administration of fluid and blood or blood products may be necessary for the patient with active hemorrhage or shock.

5. Expedite transport if the patient's condition deteriorates. Consider diversion for active hemorrhage or fetal distress. Notify the medical director and receiving hospital to prepare for a possible emergency cesarean section delivery.

DISSEMINATED INTRAVASCULAR COAGULATION

Disseminated intravascular coagulation (DIC) is a serious and deleterious complication of pregnancy. When accelerated coagulation and activation of the fibrinolytic system occur simultaneously in pregnancy, DIC occurs as a secondary event activated by hemorrhagic complications, such as placental abruption and placenta previa, or by delivery complications, such as ruptured uterus, uterine inversion, and postpartum hemorrhage. Also indicated are traumatic labor and delivery, amniotic fluid embolism, abortions, and sepsis. DIC is also a complication of trauma in pregnancy, retained dead fetus syndrome (more than 3 weeks since intrauterine death), and hydatidiform mole.

Treatment is primarily supportive and often includes initially removing or treating the circumstance that caused the DIC, such as delivering the dead fetus. Secondarily, blood products, such as packed red blood cells, fresh frozen plasma (FFP), and cryoprecipitate, may be given to correct the coagulopathy. After the delivery of the fetus and after the patient's primary complication has been eliminated or improved, further intervention may not be needed unless the hemorrhage has been severe.[3,19,21]

MULTIPLE GESTATION

A pregnancy with more than one fetus is a *multiple gestation*. Twins occur in 1 in 80 to 90 births, and triplets occur in 1 in 8000 births. The use of fertility medications and in vitro fertilization has increased the occurrence of multiple gestations.

Etiology

Embryologically, twins may result from multiple ovulations, in which two distinct ova are fertilized (dizygotic, or fraternal), or from one separate ovum that subsequently divides into two (monozygotic, or identical). Either or both processes can also result in triplets, quadruplets, and so on. The incidence of dizygotic twins is influenced by heredity, maternal age, race, and treatment for infertility, whereas the frequency of monozygotic twins is relatively constant.

In vitro fertilization and fertility medications also contribute to the incidence of multiple fetuses.

Previous delivery of twins, maternal family history of fraternal twins, advanced maternal age, infertility treatment, and multiparity all increase the chance of multiple gestations.

Pathophysiologic Factors

Pathophysiology is related to the complications associated with multiple gestations. The large area of the uterine surface covered by the placenta is suspected in several complications. Portions are more likely to implant in the lower uterine segment where less vascularity is found, increasing the chances of IUGR, or at or near the cervical os, increasing the chances of placenta previa. The superabundance of chorionic villi appears to predispose the obstetric patient to PIH, especially in a first pregnancy.

Other complications may be caused by uterine overdistention and hemodynamic and endocrinologic changes associated with multiple gestations. The mother is placed at risk for anemia, glucose intolerance, hydramnios, dysfunctional labor associated with uterine overdistention, and dystocia. In addition, multiple gestations predispose to PROM, preterm labor and delivery, placental abruption, cesarean section, uterine atony and resulting postpartum hemorrhage, and malpresentations. The fetuses are at risk for congenital anomalies, cord prolapse or entanglement, vasa previa, twin-twin transfusion, discordant fetal growth, and intrauterine death.

The greatest threat to multiple gestations is premature labor and delivery. One theory for this is overdistention of the uterus caused by multiple fetuses. The average gestational age for onset of labor is about 36 weeks for pregnancies that have spontaneous multiple gestations. Multiple gestation pregnancies as a result of infertility often deliver before 36 weeks gestation.[11] In addition, the incidence of PIH is significantly higher in pregnancies with multiple gestations.

Assessment

Multiple gestations are usually suspected when a discrepancy develops between the gestational age determined by the obstetric patient's last monthly period and the uterine size determined by regular fundal measurements. When the expected size of approximately 1 cm per week of gestation is exceeded, investigation may be warranted. If twinning is suspected, an ultrasound scan confirms or disproves the presence of more than one fetus. Although ACOG states that early ultrasound scans are not necessary for low-risk pregnancies, they are often considered expected by obstetric patients. As a result of frequent and early ultrasound scans, multiple gestations are diagnosed commonly in the first trimester.

Strategies for Transport

The transport team must be aware that any multiple gestation is a pregnancy at risk and must assess for additional risk factors associated with a multiple gestation.

The primary survey is completed as it is for any patient with assessment of airway, breathing, circulation, disability, and exposure. The secondary assessment is the complete head-to-toe assessment with the addition of the general obstetric assessment. Assessment for the patient with multiple gestation includes a thorough assessment of preterm labor with palpation of the uterus for contractions and cervical examination if the patient is contracting. Other assessment priorities involve specific assessment of comorbidities such as PIH or DM. Fetal monitoring of multiple gestations during transport can be accomplished with continuous or intermittent FHR assessment via Doppler scan, dependent on availability and transport protocols. Of special note: Multiple gestations should be identified as "A," "B," "C," etc, and not as "1," "2," and "3." In addition, location should also be described in relationship to the quadrants of the uterus. Numbering indicates birth order, which is not determined until the actual delivery. For example, a triplet pregnancy may have a fetus in the left lower quadrant (LLQ), the right upper quadrant (RUQ), and the right lower quadrant (RLQ). The babies are labeled as A: RLQ; B: RUQ; and C: LLQ. This distinction avoids confusion for monitoring purposes as the fetuses do not get mixed up. Caution must be taken to monitor each fetus separately. Because of close fetal lie, a single fetus may be inadvertently monitored in more than one location. For example, triplet A may be monitored in the RUQ and may also be picked up in the LLQ. Clinicians think they are monitoring two separate fetuses, but they are actually monitoring one fetus, twice. Ultrasound scan may help to guide monitoring of separate fetuses. When the babies are actually delivered, the first fetus delivered is "1," the second is "2," etc.

The drug of choice in the treatment of preterm labor is magnesium sulfate ($MgSO_4$) because it has been observed that an increased incidence of pulmonary edema is associated with use of beta-sympathomimetic agents in women with multiple gestations.

PREGNANCY-INDUCED HYPERTENSION AND RELATED DISORDERS

Pregnancy-induced hypertension refers to a group of hypertensive disorders that have their onset during pregnancy and resolve after pregnancy. Gestational hypertension develops after 20 weeks gestation without evidence of hypertension. PIH is characterized by hypertension, proteinuria, and edema. It may develop before 20 weeks gestation in cases of trophoblastic disease. Eclampsia refers to the development of clonic and tonic seizures in a patient with preeclampsia. Persistent hypertension not associated with pregnancy that develops before 20 weeks of gestation is considered to be chronic and is called essential or primary hypertension. Chronic hypertension as a preexisting condition may be complicated during pregnancy by superimposed preeclampsia. HELLP syndrome (hemolysis, elevated liver enzymes, and low platelets) is considered a complication of severe preeclampsia. The incidence of PIH complicates 5% to 10% of pregnancies.[11]

ETIOLOGY

The absolute cause of PIH is unknown. Current theories point to nutritional deficiencies, immunologic deficiencies, genetic predisposition, response to chorionic villi exposure, chronic intravascular coagulation, and other factors. Certain factors are known to predispose the obstetric patient to development of PIH. Primarily, PIH is a disease of the primigravida, the teenaged primigravida, or the primigravida over 35 years of age. The patient with DM, preexisting cardiovascular or kidney disease, hydramnios, family history of PIH, or no prenatal care is also at risk. Other predisposing factors include pregnancy that is exposed to a superabundance of chorionic villi, such as with multiple gestation, hydatidiform mole, or fetal hydrops, or poor nutritional status, large fetus, or Rh incompatibility.

PATHOPHYSIOLOGIC FACTORS

In patients with PIH, the disease process actually begins many weeks before the onset of any symptoms and is theorized to begin when the pregnancy is in the early weeks of gestation. A chain reaction of events is initiated as, for unknown reasons, an increased sensitivity to angiotensin II develops. As a result, vasospasm occurs, particularly arteriolar vasospasm, which initiates vasoconstriction and leads to increased peripheral resistance and eventually to hypertension. Blood perfusion to all body organs is decreased, and the function of the placenta, kidneys, liver, and brain is significantly impaired. Without forgetting the essential problem of vasospasm, the following pathophysiology is characteristic of PIH.

Uteroplacental Changes

Compromised uterine and placental blood flow can lead to degeneration of the placenta and necrosis. With chronic decreased blood perfusion, IUGR can result. During labor, fetal distress of varying degrees can be seen, caused by uteroplacental insufficiency. As a consequence of decreased uterine blood flow, uterine activity is increased and uterine irritability and preterm labor is frequently seen. An old fashioned phrase used to describe preeclampsia is *toxemia*. The belief was that the fetus was "toxic" to the mother, and the only treatment at the time was delivery.

Renal Changes

Decreased renal blood flow decreases glomerular filtration rate and in turn decreases urinary output. Cellular changes are observed in the glomerular capillary endothelial cells. The cells swell, producing narrowing of the capillary lumens, and lesions develop, causing the proteinuria (primarily albumin) seen in preeclampsia. Plasma uric acid is typically elevated as a result of the decreased uric acid clearance by the kidneys. In addition, creatinine clearance and blood urea nitrogen aid in the evaluation of kidney function. With decreased kidney function, sodium and water are retained. In conjunction with a decreased circulating albumin and a decrease in colloid osmotic pressure, fluid is shifted from the intravascular space to the extracellular space, which gives rise to edema that may range from slight to severe. In addition, increased sensitivity to angiotensin occurs as angiotensin I converts to angiotensin II; this conversion stimulates renin release, which causes aldosterone to be secreted. As this occurs, more salts and water are retained. This entire process is an attempt for the kidneys to improve their own renal perfusion and does initially pull more fluid into the intravascular space; however, because of osmotic changes in the blood vessels, much of the fluid leaks into the extravascular space.

Hematologic Changes

Because of fluid shifts caused by osmotic changes, hemoconcentration is seen with a rise in hematocrit levels. An increase in the hematocrit level noted after an initial assessment may signal a deteriorating condition. The normal hypervolemia of pregnancy is decreased or nearly absent when preeclampsia is present. The pregnant patient still has a tremendous amount of volume in her body; it just is no longer in the intravascular compartment where it belongs. Also observed is intravascular platelet and fibrin deposition, which occurs in response to vessel wall damage as the disease progresses. In addition, hemolysis and coagulopathy in patients with severe PIH is more frequently associated with HELLP syndrome and the development of DIC as severe complications of preeclampsia.

Hepatic Changes

Reduction in blood flow to the liver impairs liver function. Swelling of the capsule (the fibrous sheath that completely covers the liver) and subcapsular hemorrhage may occur. Necrosis and damage to liver tissue are seen with elevated liver enzyme levels. In rare cases, subcapsular hemorrhage can be so extensive that the liver capsule can rupture with massive hemorrhage into the peritoneal cavity. Epigastric pain (right upper and mid upper quadrant pain) is associated with hepatic swelling. This epigastric pain is caused by hepatic swelling but is often misdiagnosed as heartburn, an accepted symptom associated with pregnancy. Many patients with preeclampsia have epigastric pain, but few have liver rupture. Subcapsular hemorrhage is a rare occurrence but is associated with a higher morbidity and mortality.

Cerebral Changes

Although cerebral perfusion is not initially impaired, osmotic changes and vasospasm give rise to cerebral edema, hemorrhage, and central nervous system irritability, evidenced by hyperreflexia, headaches, visual disturbances, clonus, nausea and vomiting, decreasing LOC, and clonic and tonic seizures.

Retinal Changes

Retinal arteriolar spasms, ischemia, and edema as a result of decreased perfusion are the sources of the visual disturbances seen in preeclampsia. Blurring, scotoma (blind or twinkling spots in the vision), and diplopia (double vision) may occur. Retinal detachment is a rare occurrence. Questions related to blurred vision or visual changes are key in assessment of patients with preeclampsia because they rarely offer this information. Most lay pregnant patients believe the visual changes "are just part of being pregnant"; they do not comprehend the pathology associated.

Pulmonary Changes

Changes in pulmonary capillary permeability can occur, predisposing to pulmonary edema in severe cases of PIH. A key assessment pearl is frequent assessment of lung sounds at a minimum of once an hour, especially true if the patient is currently on magnesium sulfate, which may also increase the risk of pulmonary edema.

COMPLICATIONS

Complications of PIH, some of which have already been discussed, include eclampsia, placental abruption, pulmonary edema, DIC, HELLP syndrome, hemolytic anemia, thrombocytopenia, preterm delivery and prematurity, and IUGR. Seldom-observed and grave complications include retinal detachment, kidney failure, cerebral hemorrhage, liver rupture, heart failure, intrauterine death, and rarely, maternal death.

As a general rule, the predisposition for the development of complications increases as the disease state deteriorates. Although prompt treatment should stabilize the condition, complications and progression to eclampsia can occur.[3,11]

Eclampsia

Eclampsia can occur before labor, during labor, or early in the postpartum period. It is defined as seizures that occur in patients with severe PIH. Headache, visual disturbances, epigastric pain, apprehension, anxiety, and hyperreflexia with clonus in a patient with severe PIH are signs of impending eclampsia. Symptoms of CNS irritability are present, and the more severe the symptoms, the more likely the patient is to have progression into eclampsia. However, 20% of all patients with eclampsia had seizures before CNS symptoms.

Seizures are characterized by clonic and tonic activity and may begin around the mouth in the form of facial twitching. The seizure may be so forceful that the patient may fall from the bed. Respirations cease during the seizure but may spontaneously resume as the seizure activity quiets. Commonly, respirations must be supported initially during the seizure and into the postictal period via BVM. Often, elective intubation is performed to further protect the patient's airway. Coma frequently ensues, and the patient remembers little of the events immediately before and after the seizure. The length of the coma varies, with the patient gradually becoming responsive. Frequently, labor spontaneously begins and progresses rapidly. As with many other severe medical states in pregnancy, the maternal host is essentially saying, "I am sick…get this kid out of me." Although the mechanism remains unclear, delivery of the fetus improves the maternal medical/obstetric status. With severe PIH, the risk for the mother continuing with the pregnancy and the risk of a premature delivery for the fetus are heavily weighed. Decisions regarding timing of delivery are based on these factors and responses from medications such as magnesium sulfate and steroid administration to mature fetal lungs. Pulmonary edema may develop. Massive cerebral hemorrhage and death can occur as a result of eclampsia, but the incidence is rare (Table 31-3). Primary treatment of the eclamptic seizure is with benzodiazepines. Drugs such as lorazepam are titrated until the seizure is eliminated. Magnesium sulfate is used to prevent the next seizure by raising the seizure threshold and is not an anticonvulsant. Stop the seizure first, and then prevent the next one with magnesium sulfate after the patient's condition has been stabilized and the magnesium sulfate can be safely administered via bolus and maintenance dosing.

TABLE 31-3   **General Guidelines for Determining the Severity of the Disease Process***

	Mild	Severe	Impending Eclampsia
Blood pressure (mm Hg)	≥140/90; Diastolic increases ≥15	Diastolic, >100	Diastolic, >100
Proteinuria (dipstick)	2+/3+	3+/4+	3+/4+
Urinary output (mL/h)	>30	<20-30	<20-30
Edema	+1/+2	+3/+4	+3/+4
Pulmonary edema	Not present	May be present	Present
Headache	Not present	May be present	Present
Visual disturbances	Not present	May be present	Present
Epigastric pain	Not present	May be present	Present
Hyperreflexia and clonus	Not present	May be present	Present

*Some crossover of clinical findings can occur, and not all findings are absolute for each category.
Data from Magee LA: Management of hypertension in pregnancy, *Br Med J* 318:1332-1336, 1999.

HELLP Syndrome

The HELLP syndrome was first identified and described as a serious complication of preeclampsia by Weinstein in 1982. *H* stands for hemolysis, which is confirmed with the evidence of red cell fragments and irregularly shaped red cells on peripheral blood smears. The belief is that as red cells pass through the constricted vessels that have sustained wall damage with platelet and fibrin deposition, red cell integrity is altered and many cells are lysed. As a result, hyperbilirubinemia is frequently seen. Hemorrhagic necrosis is a serious complication of HELLP. Hepatic infarction may occur as a result of gross ischemia and obstruction of blood flow from the fibrin deposits. *EL* stands for elevated liver enzyme levels. Elevated serum glutamicoxaloacetic transaminase and serum glutamic-pyruvic transaminase values are observed. *LP* stands for low platelet count. Consumptive thrombocytopenia (a platelet count lower than 100,000/mm^3) unaccompanied by any other coagulation factor abnormalities is characteristic of the HELLP syndrome. Management of HELLP syndrome is primarily supportive and includes control of hypertension, bed rest, frequent fetal evaluation, and careful assessment of hepatic, glucose, and coagulation studies. DIC is a significant risk of HELLP.

ASSESSMENT

The "big three" in assessment of PIH include hypertension, edema, and proteinuria. Easy assessment pearls start at the top and work their way down. Assessment should include the presence of a headache (HA), blurred vision (visual changes), epigastric pain, uterine contractions, or irritability; FHR assessment for uterine perfusion; assessment of deep tendon reflexes (DTRs) on upper and lower extremities; and assessment of clonus (muscle fasciculations seen on the shin when the foot is sharply dorsiflexed) and generalized body edema (most commonly found in dependant areas such as the left side or sacral if the patient is lying that way). Traditional assessment also includes measurement of the blood pressure (with trending of MAP), measurement and dip of urine output, and review of laboratory tests such as compete blood cell count (CBC), platelets, liver assessment (serum glutamate oxaloacetate [SGOT]/serum glutamate pyruvate transaminase [SGPT]), glucose, and coagulation studies.

Hypertension

Hypertension is a rise in systolic pressure of 30 mm Hg or a rise in diastolic pressure of 15 mm Hg on the basis of previously known pressures or a blood pressure of 140/90 mm Hg or higher. Current beliefs put more emphasis on the blood pressure of 140/90 mm Hg because this is the point at which destructive endothelial changes are seen. The diastolic pressure is a more reliable predictor of the disease process. The blood pressure should be taken with the patient in the left lateral recumbent position. Hypertension associated with PIH is labile and may change in the time it takes to retake the blood pressure. Careful assessment of trending MAPs may be a more reliable indicator of worsening pathology then blood pressure measurement alone.

Edema

A sudden excessive weight gain of more than 2 lb in a week or 6 lb in a month is primarily attributable to fluid retention. Nondependent edema of the eyelids, face, and hands is characteristic of PIH. Pitting edema of the lower extremities is common. Assessment of edema is subjective, especially as clinicians do not know what patients looked like before pregnancy. For more objective assessment of overall body edema, ask a family member or the patient herself if she looks "puffy." For evaluation of edema, see Table 31-4.

Proteinuria

Proteinuria usually develops after hypertension and edema. Proteins are large molecules, and proteinuria reflects significant renal deterioration.

The transport nurse should observe the patient for evidence of the following: (1) central nervous system irritability (headache, hyperreflexia evaluated with deep tendon reflexes and ankle clonus [see Table 31-4], nausea, vomiting, apprehension, and anxiety); (2) impaired renal function (oliguria and proteinuria); and (3) hepatic involvement (epigastric pain [unmistakable from uterine contractions], malaise, nausea, vomiting, and in extremely rare conditions, jaundice).

STRATEGIES FOR TRANSPORT

Minimization of the effects of vasospasm and hypertension and prevention of seizures and other complications are critical. Maintenance or improvement of uteroplacental blood flow minimizes the risk of insult to the fetus.

The primary survey, including assessment of airway, breathing, circulation, disability, and exposure, is done initially. The obstetric assessment is completed in the secondary survey after

TABLE 31-4 **Assessment of Edema and Hyperreflexia**	
Evaluation of Edema	**Score**
Minimal edema of lower extremities	+1
Marked edema of lower extremities	+2
Edema of lower extremities, face, and hands	+3
Generalized massive edema, including abdomen and sacrum	+4
Evaluation of Hyperreflexia	**Grade**
None elicited	0
Sluggish or dull	+1
Active, normal	+2
Brisk	+3
Brisk with transient clonus	+4
Brisk with sustained clonus	+5

Assessment of edema should include description and scoring with regard to location, onset, and duration, any sudden increase in swelling noticed, and any pitting edema.
Assessment of hyperreflexia is usually accomplished with eliciting patellar deep-tendon reflexes. Clonus can be assessed at the same time with swift dorsiflexion of the foot. Clonus indicates neuromuscular irritability, and each beat should be counted.
Data from Seidel HM, et al: *Mosby's physical examination handbook,* St Louis, 1999, Mosby.

all of the life threats identified in the primary survey. The transport team should follow general guidelines for transport care and assess for PIH and risk factors and complications associated with PIH. A history of the onset of any symptoms provides insight in the consideration of the full clinical picture.

The fetus is at increased risk for uteroplacental insufficiency. The maternal transport professional should observe the FHR tracings. Evaluation should include observation of variability, the presence or absence of acceleration or deceleration, and baseline trending. Assessment of fetal movement and trends of fetal movement reflect fetal status.

The maternal transport professional should place a urinary catheter to monitor urinary output and proteinuria when symptoms indicate severe preeclampsia. As a result of renal deterioration, strict assessment of urine output must be made hourly. When assessing for proteinuria, avoid contamination with vaginal discharge (blood, amniotic fluid, and bacteria) to avoid inaccurate results.

Sensory stimulation is almost impossible to eliminate during transport. However, keeping lights dimmed, voices low, and sirens turned off and turning the cardiac monitor audible signal to low or off may help to decrease noxious stimuli. The transport team must be prepared to intervene in the event of an eclamptic seizure, albeit unpredictable. Magnesium sulfate, benzodiazepines, and airway supplies should be readily available.[15,21]

A coagulopathy is suspected if petechiae, hematuria, bruising, or bleeding from the intravenous sites is noted. Because these are late signs, symptoms of shock may rapidly ensue. If available, a review of laboratory values, including a CBC with platelets, prothrombin time (PT), partial thromboplastin time (PTT) and fibrinogen, reflects progression to DIC earlier than clinical signs.

The transport nurse should evaluate pulmonary status for signs of pulmonary edema. Lung sounds and pulse oximetry (SpO_2) should be evaluated hourly. If acute pulmonary edema with respiratory distress occurs, morphine can be administered intravenously. Furosemide (20 to 40 mg administered intravenously over 2 to 3 minutes) can be given.

Outside of acute pulmonary edema, furosemide is not commonly used in obstetrics. Furosemide crosses the placenta and can cause decreased perfusion to the placenta. The medical plan to minimize the disease includes a thorough knowledge of the action, dosage, administration, and adverse reactions of the medications that may be used in the management of PIH.

Magnesium Sulfate

Magnesium sulfate acts at the neuromuscular junction to slow transmission of impulses. By displacing calcium, it interferes with the release of acetylcholine, blocking nerve transmission to the muscle. This action, in addition to raising the seizure threshold, is thought to prevent seizures. Fifty grams of $MgSO_4$ can be added to 500 mL lactated Ringer's solution (or 40 g added to 1000 mL) with a bolus of 4 to 6 g given slowly over 15 to 30 minutes, followed by 2 to 4 g/h infusion is highly recommended via infusion pump as the side effects of magnesium toxicity can be lethal. Therapeutic serum magnesium levels range from approximately 4 to 8 mEq/L (1.5 to 2.5 mEq/L is normal). When therapeutic levels are achieved, deep tendon reflexes are depressed but not absent. Loss of deep tendon reflexes may indicate a toxic level. Loss of lower DTRs (patella) without loss of upper (bicep) reflexes is not uncommon; it is not necessarily a sign of toxicity but does reflect higher serum magnesium levels. Changes in LOC, respiratory depression with potential for arrest, and cardiac arrest are seen with highly toxic levels (greater than 10 to 15 mEq/L). While a patient is receiving intravenous $MgSO_4$, hourly assessment of deep tendon reflexes is essential. Respirations should also be closely monitored and the infusion stopped if they reach less than 12 per minute with poor respiratory effort associated with decreasing LOC. Other respiratory concerns include the risk of pulmonary edema. Pulse oximetry should be used during transport.

The antidote for magnesium toxicity is calcium gluconate. Calcium stimulates the release of acetylcholine, stimulating nerve transmission to the muscle. Figuratively, calcium and magnesium are on a teeter totter. As serum magnesium levels increase, the serum calcium levels are driven down. Conversely, if calcium levels are increased, the magnesium levels decrease as do the associated pathologic side effects of magnesium toxicity. The recommended dosage of calcium gluconate is 1 g of a 10% solution administered intravenously over at least 3 minutes. If one ampule is not enough to reverse the side effects of hypoventilation, another ampule may be given and titrated to effect. The goal is spontaneous respiration, a return of DTRs, and a responsive LOC. If calcium is administered too rapidly, bradycardia and arrhythmias may occur.

Magnesium sulfate is not an antihypertensive agent. However, a transient drop in blood pressure after initiation of treatment is frequently seen and can be attributed to smooth muscle relaxation. Adverse reactions include flushing, sweating, nausea and vomiting, and drowsiness. A decrease in FHR variability may be observed because magnesium is a known CNS depressant. Magnesium sulfate is primarily excreted in the urine, and toxicity may develop rather rapidly in the patient with significantly impaired kidney function. The urinary output should exceed 30 mL/h while the patient is receiving the infusion. If urinary output drops below 30 mL/h, consultation with appropriate medical control or the receiving physician should be made because they may want to decrease the maintenance infusion. Magnesium should be used cautiously in patients with renal or cardiac disease.

Labetalol

Labetalol is a selective beta-blocking agent that decreases systemic vascular resistance without changing cardiac output. The standard dosage is 20 mg administered via intravenous push over 2 minutes; the dose may be repeated every 10 minutes until the maximum dosage of 300 mg has been given.[12] Large subsequent doses of labetalol should be avoided because profound drops in blood pressure can acutely occur. As with non-pregnant patients, labetalol can be an "unforgiving" drug in the sense that if the blood pressure drops to a hypotensive state it is slow to return to normotensive pressures. The effects of a rapid decrease in maternal blood pressure can be profound on the uterus and placenta. Both are not considered vital organs and are the first to feel the effects of hypoperfusion. The MAP should be evaluated and used to trend the decrease in maternal blood pressure. The MAP should not be dropped more than 20% to avoid causing placental hypoperfusion and increasing the risks of placental abruptio.

Hydralazine

Hydralazine acts by relaxing arterioles and decreasing vasospasm. As a result, it reduces blood pressure and stimulates cardiac output. Blood perfusion to the brain, kidneys, liver, and uterus is thus improved. Hydralazine is recommended with diastolic pressure 110 mm Hg or greater for prevention of cerebrovascular accident. Transport protocol should be followed regarding titration of hydralazine. During administration, the blood pressure should be taken every couple of minutes because the onset of action is 5 to 10 minutes. If the diastolic pressure falls below 90 mm Hg, uterine blood flow may be further reduced, placing the fetus at risk. Profound decreases in maternal blood pressure not only decrease placenta perfusion but also increase the risk of placenta abruptio. The MAP should not be decreased more than 20%. Adverse reactions include reflex tachycardia, headache, palpitations, dizziness, nausea, and vomiting. Hydralazine is contraindicated in cases of lupus erythematosus and tachycardia.

Benzodiazepines

Benzodiazepines are classified as antianxiety/sedative medications but are known to prevent or arrest seizure activity, although the exact mode of action is not known. They also produce mild sedation and muscular relaxation. Benzodiazepines should be administered parentally, but in an extreme emergency when intravenous access is not possible, they may be given rectally. They are the first line drug for active eclampsia. Adverse reactions include transient bradycardia, hypotension, and hypoventilation. If respirations are profoundly decreased, the antidote is flumazenil. If flumazenil is indicated, cautious and judicious administration allows for the return of spontaneous respirations without the return of seizures.

PRETERM LABOR AND RELATED ISSUES

Regular and rhythmic contractions that produce progressive cervical changes after week 20 of gestation and before week 37 are considered to be *preterm labor*. Although contractions are included in this definition, note that many patients with preterm labor do not feel or perceive these contractions. Preterm delivery occurs in 6% to 12% of all deliveries. Preterm labor does not always result in preterm delivery; however, the rate of preterm delivery has not decreased in recent years and statistics have actually shown a modest increase in the incidence of PTL. With improved prenatal care, reduction of risk factors, patient education, and earlier diagnosis and treatment of preterm labor, it is hoped that the next decade may realize a decrease in the rate of preterm delivery.

ETIOLOGY

Although many factors predispose the obstetric patient to preterm labor, a few single identifiable causes exist. Infection has been recognized as a primary cause of preterm labor. Although the pathways frequently differ, sources of infection may include urinary tract infection, pyelonephritis, vaginitis (particularly bacterial), chorioamnionitis, and viral infection. Another identifiable cause is PROM (spontaneous rupture before the onset of contractions and before week 37). Other factors include previous preterm delivery (the single most frequent contributing factor), uterine anomalies, poor nutritional status, poor perineal hygiene, poor weight gain, no prenatal care, less than 1 year between the last delivery and commencement of the current pregnancy, substance abuse, PIH, cigarette smoking, diabetes, chronic cardiovascular or kidney disease, previous induced or spontaneous abortion, abdominal trauma, a long commute to work, a high stress level at work or home, physical stress, overdistention of the uterus as a result of multiple gestation, hydramnios, uterine tumors, age (teenaged or more than 40 years), placenta previa or placental abruption, cervical incompetence, women exposed to diethylstilbestrol in utero, a retained intrauterine device, a history of pelvic inflammatory disease, and fetal anomalies, distress, or death.[11,17]

Single or multiple factors may initiate preterm labor. When multiple factors are present, the obstetric patient is at greater risk. Many cases have no identifiable causes. Numerous factors are theorized to lead to the progression of preterm labor and delivery.

PATHOPHYSIOLOGIC FACTORS

In any situation in which uterine blood flow is reduced or impaired, an increase in uterine irritability can be noted and may result in the onset of labor. Viral infections with symptoms of fever, nausea, vomiting, or diarrhea may predispose to preterm labor primarily because of dehydration, which reduces uterine blood flow. Other similar conditions in which uteroplacental perfusion is compromised include PIH, diabetes, cardiovascular or kidney disease, overdistention of the uterus, heavy smoking, placental abruption, or placenta previa.

Hormonal influence contributes to increased uterine activity and the onset of labor. Prostaglandin release is associated with PROM, bacterial infections, abdominal trauma, and overdistention of the uterus. In at least half the patients who have PROM, labor begins in 48 hours. Meconium-stained amniotic fluid (indicating possible fetal distress) contains high levels of oxytocin, which can initiate labor. The fetus is also believed to play a role in the activation of preterm labor, but little is known of this contribution.

When a patient has cervical incompetence, the cervix is unable to support and maintain the growing pregnancy to term and often dilates without perceptible contractions. Cervical incompetence is characterized by premature, painless, bloodless cervical dilation in which the membranes can bulge and rupture. Obstetric history of numerous second trimester losses or "painless" preterm labors and deliveries is suspect. Another concerning presentation is the patient with vaginal fullness or pressure, which is often caused by the presenting fetal part causing lower uterine segment pressure. The lower the fetus, the more pressure on the cervix and the more likely preterm delivery will occur. Even vague symptoms need to be evaluated. Advanced cervical dilation and rupture of the amniotic fluid lead to certain delivery. Congenital defects and traumatic injury to the cervix may result in cervical incompetence. Probable causes of cervical injury include trauma during a previous childbirth, cervical dilation after elective or spontaneous abortion, or gynecologic procedures. Another physiologic abnormality in which cervical anomalies and cervical incompetence are known to occur is maternal exposure to diethylstilbestrol (DES). For cases of known or suspected cervical incompetence, a cervical cerclage may be placed at 12 to 14 weeks gestation. This cervical cerclage is a purse-string suture that is applied through the cervix and then tied off. Its intent is to maintain cervical integrity so the cervix is not prematurely opened. Any patient with a cervical cerclage that has preterm labor is at risk of cervical dilation and tearing of the cervix. Maternal fetal medicine physicians or the receiving physician should be consulted, and decisions regarding aggressive tocolysis or removal of the cerclage and delivery by the referring facility are made before transport.

The complications associated with preterm labor and delivery predominantly affect the fetus. However, the side effects of tocolytic medications to maintain the pregnancy primarily affect the mother. Birth trauma and the complications associated with the transition to extrauterine life for the premature infant are primary. These complications include immature lungs, risks of infection, thermoregulating issues, intracerebral bleeding, etc. Neonatal sepsis can result from numerous unknown and known sources such as PROM. The intact bag of water prevents bacteria and flora from the vagina from ascending into the uterine cavity. The severity of the complications seen depend in a great measure on the gestational age of the neonate.

Maternal complications include adverse reactions to labor-suppressing agents, complications associated with cesarean section (increased incidence with preterm labor), endometritis, septicemia, and septic shock related to prolonged PROM and chorioamnionitis. In addition, other maternal risks include comorbidities or obstetric complications associated with the current pregnancy.

Tocolytics are used to stop contractions. Research has not shown that tocolysis has been successful in maintaining pregnancy. As a result, current belief patterns are use of tocolytics not to greatly extend the pregnancy but rather to allow the administration of glucocorticoid steroid for the benefit of the fetus (see Box 31-2).

ASSESSMENT

Preterm labor should be suspected if the patient has a history of contractions 10 minutes apart or less for a period of 1 hour or longer. Another definition is more than six contractions in a 1-hour period. The transport team should assess for factors associated with preterm labor, remembering that the incidence of preterm labor increases with the number of predisposing factors. Contractions should always be palpated on the fundus or at the top of the uterus. Despite where the patient "feels" the contractions, they all initiate in the fundus and diminish as they reach the cervix. Contractions are most easily palpated in this area also. Although obstetric patients are reliable historians, they do not always perceive contractions. The smaller the uterus is related to gestational age, the less typical the contractions feel. Often, preterm labor patients deny they are having contractions. However, on the monitor or with palpation, contractions are evident. Further investigation reveals that the patient feels little in her uterus or abdomen but has a lower backache that comes and goes. Other common reports of preterm contractions are colicky abdominal pain similar to that with diarrhea, suprapubic cramping, pressure that comes and goes, or a feeling "like the baby is balling up." These vague symptoms are one reason that preterm labor is often not discovered until advanced cervical dilation has occurred. The patient is unaware of contractions until she is far progressed into labor, which also highlights the need to *palpate* the uterus for contractions, even when the patient denies contractions, particularly during transport. Dependent on how often the contractions occur, the uterus should be palpated every 5 minutes for a patient still contracting to every 15 to 30 minutes for patients who are acontracile. Reports of the palpation should be noted in the patient record. This palpation time allows for palpation of fetal movement, which also should be documented.

Cervical Dilation/Effacement Patterns

Cervical dilation patterns vary from primiparas to multiparas. Primiparas tend to have *effacement* or thinning of the cervix before dilation occurs. The multipara patient often has dilation before significant effacement

---

BOX 31-2	**Common OB Medications**

This brief review of common medications used in the treatment of the high-risk obstetric patient is intended to identify only key information.

Pitocin (oxytocin): Used after delivery of placenta to promote uterine involution/prevent postpartum hemorrhage; 20 to 40 units/1000 mL wide open (or) 10 to 20 units IM.

Magnesium sulfate ($MgSO_4$): TX PIH: $\downarrow$ seizure threshold to prevent eclampsia. Transient $\downarrow$ in BP. TX PTL: $\downarrow$ CA influx into cells, decreasing smooth muscle ability to contract.
- $MgSO_4$ level: Therapeutic: 4.8 to 8.4; Toxic: ~10; assess patient.
- Draw level 2 h after bolus and then q 6 h.
- Loading dose: 2 to 4 g/100 mL over 20 min. Patient will have systemic burning, SOB, N/V, feeling miserable. *Warn the patient.* Apply cold packs to decrease side effects.
- Maintenance dose: 20 to 40 g/1000 mL. Usually 1 to 3 g/h.
- Assessment: ABCs, lung sounds, bicep/patellar reflexes, UO, (PIH) HA, blurred vision, epigastric pain.
- Toxic: Loss of reflexes, $\downarrow$ RR, $\downarrow$ LOC, $\downarrow$ UO, $\downarrow$ BP.
- Antidote: Calcium gluconate 10%, 1 to 2 amps.

Terbutaline/brethine: Beta mimetic, relaxes smooth muscles by decreasing gap junction.
- Side effects: Maternal/fetal: tachycardia, hypotension, hyperglycemia, pulmonary edema.
- Contraindications: Maternal cardiac disease, brittle diabetic.
- Dose: 0.25 mg SQ/IV q 4 h or per protocol. 2.5 mg PO, q 4 h. Hold for HR > 120.
- Laboratory tests: Check glucose, EKG for chest pain. Confirm maternal/fetal HR difference.

Indomethacin: Prostaglandin synthesis inhibitor. Prevents cytokine production thought to start labor.
- Side effects: Maternal/fetal: $\downarrow$ renal blood flow, $\downarrow$ UO, $\downarrow$ liver enzymes, $\downarrow$ AFI.
- Contraindications: After 32 weeks, delays closure of PDA.

Nifedipine: Ca++ channel blocker. Limits influx of Ca++ into cells, decreasing ability to contract. Decreases strength/effectiveness versus frequency of uterine contractions.
- Side effects: Hypotension, tachycardia, palpitations.
- Dose: Load 30 mg, then 20 mg q 4-8 h.
- Vital signs: Hold for HR >120 and BP < 100/60.

Approved Antihypertensives in Pregnancy
- Hydralazine: Initial dose, 5 to 10 mg IV push; Labetalol: Initial dose, 20 mg slow IV; Methyldopa: Aldomet.
- Diuretics: HCTZ.
- Lasix: Rarely and cautiously used (crosses placenta barrier).

Contraindicated in Pregnancy:
- ACE inhibitors (fetal deformity, IUFD).
- Nitroprusside (Nipride), metabolizes into cyanide for the fetus.

Glucocorticoid steroids: betamethasone: Matures fetal lungs, decreases neonatal IVH, $\downarrow$ RDS.
- Side effects: Maternal, $\uparrow$ WBC, caution with PROM.
- Dose: 12 mg q 12 to 24 h times 2 doses. Benefits last 1 week.

---

occurs. For example, the preterm labor patient who is a primipara and is 2 cm dilated, 100% effaced, +1 station is a higher concern than the multipara who is 2 cm dilated, 10% effaced, and −2 station. Because of predictable dilation and effacement patterns, the primipara shows more signs of active labor. Of note is that cervical status is always reported in this way: dilation/efface-ment/fetal station (e.g., 3/90/−1). The last parameter is measurement of the presenting fetal part in relation to the ischial spines, which are protruding bones on the lower pelvis. These spines can be palpated through the vaginal basement, and the presenting part is compared with the location of these protrusions. If the presenting fetal part, usually the head, is at the level of the spines, the baby is reported as a 0 station. One fingerbreadth (or 1 cm) above the spines is −1, etc. If the presenting part is 1 fingerbreadth below the spines, the position is reported as +1 station, etc. For perspective, the head begins to crown at +3 station and is delivered at +4. The transport team is not expected to be proficient in these examinations. However, they are expected to understand the implications of the examinations.

Vaginal mucus may be the first sign of cervical dilation. The mucus plug that fills the cervical canal can be dislodged by cervical changes. The cervix is considered completely dilated when it is approximately 10 cm. An important transport consideration is that with premature gestations the fetus is small and may fit though a cervix that is not completely dilated. For example, a 500-g, 23-week fetus may fit through a cervix that is only 6 to 7 cm dilated.

Spontaneous Rupture of Membranes

With any history of possible spontaneous rupture, a sterile speculum examination (SSE) is used to verify the presence of amniotic fluid leaking from the cervix and collecting in the posterior fornix of the vagina (the area underneath the cervix posteriorly). If an SSE has already been performed, the transport team should note documented results. Many transport professionals may not feel competent to perform a speculum examination. Assessment can be completed by the referring facility or fluid assessment can be obtained from fluid leaking on the external vagina. Three factors, positive pooling, positive nitrazine, and positive ferning, definitely confirm *spontaneous rupture of the membranes* (SROM). Ultrasound scan is also a useful tool when assessing amniotic fluid volumes. Pooling of fluid is seen in the vaginal vault. If none is seen, the team may encourage the patient to cough; the increased pressure usually results in the release of amniotic fluid. A sample from a site as close to the posterior fornix as possible turns nitrazine paper dark blue (alkaline) in the presence of amniotic fluid. Vaginal secretions are acidic in nature and do not affect the paper. The transport team should aware that blood, cervical mucus, and povidone-iodine are alkaline in nature and can give a false-positive reading. Finally, a small amount of the fluid can be spread on a slide and allowed to dry completely. A frond crystallization

pattern of dried amniotic fluid (with a high concentration of sodium chloride) is seen with microscopic examination; it is similar to a Boston fern in appearance. Because a microscope may not be available in small outlying areas and there may not be time to perform this procedure, the transport team must depend on the presence of pooling and positive results of a test for nitrazine. If rupture is confirmed or suspected, a sterile vaginal examination (SVE) should be avoided, unless delivery appears imminent, to prevent introducing microbes from the vagina into the cervical canal, which can place the patient at an increased risk for infection. If a gross rupture has occurred, if the patient has a history of a large volume loss, or if continual leaking is observed, a sterile speculum examination is not necessary if it does not alter the plan for nursing care. The transport team should keep in mind that with a decreased amount of amniotic fluid, the umbilical cord is at risk for compression and variable decelerations may be seen, with or without contractions.

If a rupture has not occurred, an SVE confirms whether any cervical changes have taken place. The cervix does not have to dilate before changes can be noted. Normally, the cervix is firm, long, and closed. Any softening or effacing, which may occur before dilation, indicates cervical changes. If this is not the initial episode of preterm labor, the transport team should assess for the history of onset, current medications, other treatment such as home monitoring or bed rest, and patient compliance. Frequently, the present episode can be linked to increased activity, failure to take medication altogether, or inconsistency in following the medication regimen.

The transport team should observe the patient for any indications of the presence of infection. Symptoms of urinary tract infection, pyelonephritis, or both include dysuria, frequency of urination, fever, and flank tenderness, pain, or both. Evidence of poor perineal hygiene may be a factor not only in the development of a urinary tract infection but in vaginal infections and chorioamnionitis as well.

The transport team may assess the patient for possible chorioamnionitis; symptoms include fever, tachycardia, fetal tachycardia, uterine tenderness not associated with contractions, purulent vaginal discharge, and an elevated white blood cell count. If results of laboratory tests from the referring facility are available, the laboratory tests indicated are a complete blood count with differential and cervical cultures for β-hemolytic streptococcus and *Neisseria gonorrhoeae*. However, most are initially asymptomatic. Commonly, the infected uterus is tender to palpation; this often an early clinical sign. The most common route for infection is the ascending route from the vagina to the cervix. For this reason, sterile vaginal examinations are avoided in the presence of PROM. Evidence indicates that the presence of bacteria in the vagina may locally dissolve the membrane; the bacteria then gain access to the fluid and cause a chorioamnionitis that dissolves the membrane, and SROM results. With no evidence of prior infection, the incidence of infection after SROM greatly increases if the membranes have been ruptured longer than 24 hours.

STRATEGIES FOR TRANSPORT

Primary goals for transport include minimization or prevention of complications, treatment of current pathologies, and improvement in or maintenance of uterine perfusion.

The primary survey and secondary survey, including the general obstetric assessment, should be done first. The transport team should then follow these general guidelines for transport care:

1. Assess fetal well being. This assessment includes review of the FHR tracing for baseline, variability, and presence or absence of accelerations or decelerations. This also includes the assessment of the presence or absence of fetal movement and comparison with usual movement patterns.

2. Determine the contraction pattern. Determine the phase of labor and assess whether transport can safely be attempted or whether delivery should be accomplished at the referring facility. In the event of an imminent delivery, call for the neonate team (unless *you* are the neonate team also), notify the medical director, and help the referring facility prepare for delivery.

3. Determine the status of the amniotic membranes. With questionable history of fluid leakage and contractions that have slowed or stopped altogether, absolute determination of rupture is not needed before transport if it does not alter the plan for nursing care.

4. Determine cervical status. Determine the number of SSEs done at the referring facility, especially if an SSE was done in the presence of ruptured membranes. Assess the amount of cervical change accomplished since admission to the referring facility. Remember that once labor is established, the multiparous woman frequently has progression at a faster rate than a primipara and may need rapid transport. Sterile speculum examinations may be more appropriate for patients with PROM to prevent ascending infections.

5. Maintain the patient in the left lateral or right lateral position. Not only do these positions improve uterine perfusion, thus decreasing uterine irritability, but they also decrease pressure on the cervix from the presenting part and may protect against further cervical changes. Having the patient stand, sit, or bend can place pressure against the cervix and should be avoided during transport. Load the patient so she is facing you in your vehicle.

6. Assess for infection. Observe for symptoms of urinary tract infection, pyelonephritis, vaginitis, chorioamnionitis, or signs of viral infection. These signs may include uterine tenderness, vaginal discharge, an elevated white count, uterine contractions, fetal tachycardia, maternal fever, and maternal tachycardia.

7. Assess for cervical incompetence. An incompetent cervix can be suspected if the patient has vague symptoms accompanied by disproportionate cervical changes. Obstetric history in these cases is of particular importance. Placing these patients in the left lateral position with hips slightly elevated may further reduce any pressure on the cervix.

8. Administer or continue tocolytic agents as prescribed. Following transport protocols, tocolytics may be titrated to effect if they are within accepted parameters and are tolerated by the mother and fetus. Suppression of labor is always attempted to "buy time" for the transport. Current goals of "buying time" are 48 hours. The belief is that tocolytics do a poor job at maintaining the pregnancy and that the primary goal

is to delay delivery until steroids can be given to aid in the maturation of the fetal lungs. Optimal neonatal outcome can be anticipated when the delivery occurs in a hospital that is prepared for the intensive care of premature infants. If hydration and positioning to the left lateral have not slowed or arrested labor, tocolytic agents can be administered. The medications used most frequently in suppressing labor are magnesium sulfate and terbutaline.

TRAUMA IN PREGNANCY

Minor accidental injuries are common during pregnancy. The gravid uterus, loosened joints, altered center of gravity, shortness of breath, dizziness, increased fatigue, and edema all contribute to minor accidents, including falls.

Serious accidental injuries during pregnancy place not only the obstetric patient but also the fetus at risk. Serious injuries during pregnancy are fortunately less common. The most common etiologies of serious obstetric trauma are motor vehicle crashes, falls, stabbings, burns, and domestic violence. The fetus is well protected in the confines of the uterus because it is surrounded by amniotic fluid, which serves as an excellent shock absorber. Physical trauma to a fetus is extremely rare, except as a result of direct penetrating wounds or extensive blunt trauma. The fetus is at greatest risk for fetal distress and intrauterine death as a result of hypoperfusion from maternal trauma and death. The obstetric patient is more vulnerable to hemorrhage because of the increased vascularity surrounding the gravid uterus. Early signs and symptoms of hypovolemia may be masked by the normal physiologic changes of pregnancy. As a result, blood is shunted away from nonvital organs, including the uterus, which threatens the well being of the fetus. In dealing with a trauma patient who is pregnant, the best interest of the fetus is served by prompt assessment and interventions on behalf of the mother. Although the fetus does not survive if the mother does not survive, measures can be taken to improve fetal viability. Some of these measures include preventing inferior vena cava syndrome by tilting the patient to

the left or right and increasing uterine/placental perfusion by increasing IVFs, correcting blood or volume losses, and applying 100% O_2. Pregnant patients are sensitive to volume, and particularly in the occurrence of trauma, active volume replacement must be initiated early.[19]

The pregnant trauma patient needs to be appropriately immobilized for transport. Placing a small roll under the right side of the backboard and tipping the backboard 30 degrees displaces the uterus to the left or right side. Stretcher straps should be placed low and tight over the pelvis. The pregnant trauma patient is at high risk of aspiration because of the hormones of pregnancy. Early intubation should be considered. No contraindications for rapid sequence intubation (RSI) exist during pregnancy; however, be aware that the baby is also paralyzed until neuromuscular blocking (NMB) agents wear off. This is not a concern if the fetus remains in the uterus because it is oxygenated via the placenta and umbilical cord. The concern for paralytics in the neonate is in the event of an immediate cesarean delivery.

PERIMORTEM CESAREAN SECTION

Controversy exists over whether a perimortem caesarean section is of any value in the transport environment. Some anecdotal reports are found of these types of deliveries, but with limited survival of either the infant or the mother. Indications for this procedure may include the following[19,20]:

- Gestational age of the fetus (24 to 26 weeks at the youngest gestation, extending to term).
- Limited amount of time since maternal arrest. Some investigators suggest within 5 minutes of maternal arrest as ideal timing to improve fetal outcomes, but anecdotal reviews have reported fetal survival up to 20 to 30 minutes after maternal arrest. However, fetal/neonatal neurologic outcomes diminish with longer arrest to delivery time.

Experienced personnel should perform the procedure, and they must be prepared to perform neonatal resuscitation. An important transport note is to call ahead. The receiving perinatal hospital needs to be alerted to the possibility of a perimortem section so they are prepared to perform it or prepared to receive a likely compromised neonate. Another transport pearl is to perform perfect CPR. In the best case scenario, CPR provides only 25% of circulating blood volume. CPR of poor quality provides less than this. Current American Heart Association (AHA) guidelines advocate "Push hard, Push fast." To aid with adequate chest compressions, the backboard should be elevated approximately 30% from behind the area of the head and chest with manual displacement of the uterus. The ACLS OB course recommends keeping the patient supine to increase cardiac compression and having another clinician manually displace the uterus to minimize IVCS, which may be ideal over the lateral displacement of the mother and uterus (alone) because it allows for better compression of the heart. This positioning prevents IVCS and still allows adequate compressions of the heart against the spine. In the event of maternal ventricle fibrillation or ventricular tachycardia, no contraindications exist for defibrillation or cardioversion. Current ACLS algorithms should be followed during the arrest of adult pregnant patients. However, the ACLS OB course recommends that amiodarone be held until the baby is delivered because the fetus has delayed metabolism of amiodarone and resulting hypotension. Many retrospective studies suggest that early emergency cesarean delivery improves both maternal and fetal outcome.

SUMMARY

The transport of the patient who is pregnant requires experience and skills so that both the mother and fetus may benefit. If the mother does not receive appropriate care, the baby suffers; but at times, the patient or the fetus's condition may warrant personnel with specific abilities not generally obtained by a general transport service.

Each transport service must ensure that they are competent and capable of providing care for both the mother and fetus. This can be accomplished with education obtained from specialists in high-risk obstetrics, information from NRP, and clinical time.

PREGNANT PATIENT TRANSPORT CASE STUDY

A 22-year-old G 6 P 0 4 1 4 is at 28 4/7 weeks gestation. She presents to the emergency department (ED) with symptoms of a backache and "pressure on her bottom." The patient is rapidly transferred to the labor and delivery department (L&D) where she is placed on a monitor. FHR baseline is 155 bpm with minimal variability. No accelerations or decelerations are noted at this time. Cervical examination reveals the cervix is 4/80% /+1. Contractions are noted via tocotransducer to be every 4 to 5 minutes, lasting 40 to 60 seconds. The patient does not feel contractions but states her back hurts every 4 to 5 minutes. Per palpation, the contractions are assessed to be moderately strong. What information does her gravidity and parity reveal? What are your transport priorities? Are you concerned that the FHR variability is minimal? What other assessment can be made to assess fetal well being? What does the cervical examination reveal? What medications, if any, would you consider initiating?

Her gravidity reveals that she has had numerous pregnancies in a short period of time (she is only 22 years old) and that all of her deliveries have been preterm. The best indicator of preterm delivery is a strong history of previous preterm deliveries. Your transport priorities should be to start with a primary and secondary survey that includes an obstetric assessment. After this is done, and contraindications are ruled out, aggressive tocolysis and administration of steroids should be considered. That a fetus of such early gestation would have minimal to moderate variability, as a result of CNS immaturity, is not unusual. However, continued assessment of the FHR pattern, including observation for acceleration or deceleration, should be noted. In addition, assessment of fetal movement is the number one, nonmonitor method of assessing fetal well being. The cervical examination reveals that she had advanced dilation and that successful tocolysis with extended duration of the pregnancy is unlikely. The pressure she is feeling in her "bottom" is most likely related to the low fetal position (+1 station) and pressures felt into the lower uterine segment and the vaginal vault. The goal of tocolysis is primarily to extend the pregnancy another 48 hours so tocolytics can be given to benefit the fetus. The most common tocolytic chosen is magnesium sulfate. Most likely a bolus of 2 to 4 g will be given over 20 to 30 minutes and then followed by a maintenance dose of 2 to 4 g/h. The magnesium can be titrated until tocolysis is achieved, as long as it is within medication parameters and the mother does not have loss of DTRs or hypoventilation.

REFERENCES

1. Air and Surface Transport Nurses Association: *Transport nurse advanced trauma course*, Denver, 2006, ASTNA.

2. American Academy of Pediatrics: *Air and ground transport of neonatal and pediatric patients*, Elk Gove, IL, 2007, AAP.

3. American Academy of Pediatrics and American College of Obstetrics and Gynecologists: *Guidelines for perinatal care*, ed 6, Elk Grove, IL, 2007, AAP/ACOG.

4. Barrett NA, Yentis SM: Outreach in obstetric critical care, *Best Pract Res Clin Obstet Gynaecol* 22(5):885-898, 2008.

5. Benorub GI: *Obstetric and gynecologic emergencies*, Philadelphia, 1993, Lippincott.

6. Bickley LS: *Bate's guide to physical examination and history taking*, ed 9, Philadelphia, 2007, Lippincott Williams and Wilkins.

7. Campbell J: *International trauma life support for prehospital care providers*, ed 6, Upper Saddle River, NJ, 2008, Pearson Prentice Hall.

8. Clark SL, Cotton DB: *Handbook of critical care obstetrics*, Boston, 1994, Blackwell.

9. Commission on Accreditation of Medical Transport Systems: *Standards*, ed 7, Andersonville, SC, 2006, CAMTS.

10. Cunningham GF, et al: *Williams obstetrics*, ed 19, East Norwalk, CT, 1993, Appleton-Century-Crofts.

11. Gilbert E: *The manual of high risk pregnancy and delivery*, ed 4, St Louis, 2007, Mosby Elsevier.

12. Hill CC, Pickinpaugh J: Trauma and surgical emergencies in the obstetric patient, *Surg Clin North Am* 88:421-440, 2008.

13. Jones AE, Summers RL, Deschamp C: A national survey of the air medical transport of the high-risk obstetric patients, *Air Med J* 20(2):17-20, 2001.

14. Kopecky J: Obstetric transport and airway management, *Hosp Aviat* 13-18, 1989.

15. Magee LA: Management of hypertension in pregnancy, *Br Med J* 318:1332, 1999.

16. Menihan CA, Kopel E: *Electronic fetal monitoring: concepts and applications*, Philadelphia, 2008, Wolters Kluwer/Lippincott Williams and Wilkins.

17. Simpson KR, Creehan PA: *Perinatal nursing*, Philadelphia, 2007, Wolters Kluwer Lippincott Williams and Wilkins.

18. Smith J: The dangers of prenatal cocaine use, *Matern Child Nurs J* 13:174, 1988.

19. Smith LG: The pregnant trauma patient. In McQuillan, Makic MF, Whalen E, editors: *Trauma nursing: from resuscitation through rehabilitation*, ed 4, Philadelphia, 2009, Saunders Elsevier.

20. Strong T, Lowe R: Perimortem cesarean section, *Am J Emerg Med* 5:489, 1989.

21. York-Clark D, Stocking J, Johnson J: *Flight and ground transport nursing core curriculum*, ed 2, Denver, 2006, Air and Surface Transport Nurses Association.

CARE AND TRANSPORT OF THE NEONATE

Christine Tijerina

COMPETENCIES

1. Perform an initial assessment of the neonatal patient.
2. Perform the necessary interventions to maintain the neonate's airway, breathing, and circulation after delivery.
3. Recognize the normal transitional stages to extrauterine life and identify a neonate's inability to transition appropriately.
4. Prepare the neonate for transport with use of appropriately sized equipment.
5. Maintain the same or higher level of care during transport.

The *neonatal patient* is defined as any newborn infant less than 28 chronologic days of age or 28 days beyond the due date in the case of preterm infants. A *term pregnancy* is typically 38 to 42 weeks. *Premature infants* are commonly defined as infants born before 37 weeks gestation, and *postterm infants* are born later than 42 weeks gestation.

Neonates have unique anatomy, physiology, and pathophysiology that require advanced knowledge and understanding of these differences for appropriate care. The depth of knowledge of neonatal specialty needed by transport personnel is directly related to the mission profile of the team. Medical transport providers who care for neonates in any out-of-hospital environment must have training

in the stabilization and care of the types of infants they may transport. Attention to both appropriate team composition and the availability of specialized equipment and medications is necessary to ensure safe transport of these patients.

Medical transport providers may care for neonates in a prehospital setting or an interfacility transport setting. For neonatal patients born or presenting in a nonmedical environment, such as a home or car, the immediate stabilization needs of the infant (thermoregulation, resuscitation, stabilization, and expedient transport to the nearest appropriate medical facility) are stressed. Interfacility transport of neonates requires an emphasis on maintaining the equivalent level of care or a higher level of care during stabilization and transport to the receiving hospital. Competency in neonatal care protocols and procedures, and recognized expertise in the field, is an essential component of neonatal transport care.

The American Academy of Pediatrics offers some specific criteria for the composition and training of the neonatal transport team. In addition, this organization also provides guidelines for the minimum equipment that should be used for safe stabilization and transport of the neonate. Box 32-1 includes a summary of Neonatal Transport Guidelines.

FETAL CIRCULATION AND TRANSITION

The scope of this chapter allows only a brief overview of fetal circulation and transition to extrauterine life. In utero, the placenta and fetus are nourished by an umbilical vein that carries highly oxygenated blood to the right atrium via the ductus venosus and the inferior vena cava. The right and left ventricles both pump at systemic pressures into the aorta (Figure 32-1).[15] A large percentage of this blood is directed across the foramen ovale to the left atrium, left ventricle, and ascending aorta to perfuse the coronary arteries and the brain with the most highly oxygenated blood in fetal circulation. Some of the blood from the umbilical vein along with blood returning from the superior vena cava flows through the tricuspid valve to the right ventricle

and out through the pulmonary valve. Most of the blood flow from the right ventricle shunts from the pulmonary artery through the ductus arteriosus and into the descending aorta as a result of the high pressure of the pulmonary vasculature system. The shunted blood mixes with the remainder of the blood coming from the left side of the heart.

The transition to extrauterine life begins the moment the neonate takes its first breath. The expansion of the lungs and exposure to oxygen at birth causes the pulmonary vascular resistance to fall and allows a rapid increase in pulmonary blood flow and a consequent decrease in flow across the ductus arteriosus. Simultaneously, as the umbilical cord is clamped, the low-resistance placental circuit is removed and an increase in systemic resistance occurs. This increase in afterload, and the increased return to the left atrium from the pulmonary circuit, helps to close the flap-like foramen ovale.

Careful ongoing assessment and early intervention are critical during this time period because subtle changes can indicate undiagnosed congenital cardiac diseases. Neonatal hypoxia, hypoglycemia, hypothermia, sepsis, stress, and acidosis can all interfere with the normal progression of this transition period.[9,23,24] Common findings at this time may include intermittent grunting, mild retracting, and tachypnea and poor feeding.[31] The infant must be observed and monitored closely until all these symptoms have been addressed or resolved.

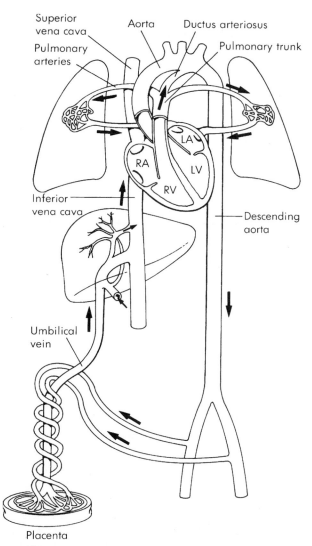

FIGURE 32-1   Normal fetal circulation and major fetal flow patterns. (From Heymann MA: Biophysical evaluation of fetal status: fetal cardiovascular physiology. In Creasy RK, Resnik R, editors: *Maternal fetal medicine*, Philadelphia, 1984, Saunders.)

INITIAL PRIORITIES: DELIVERY ROOM MANAGEMENT

ASSESSMENT OF THE INFANT

The initial assessment should be brief and focus on identification and treatment of life-threatening issues related to airway, breathing, or circulation. One essential component of the initial assessment is the Apgar score. The Apgar score, developed in 1953

by Dr Virginia Apgar (Table 32-1),[1] is a basic rapid evaluation of the infant's immediate adaptation to extrauterine life. Evaluation of color, respiratory effort, heart rate, body tone, and responsiveness to stimuli provides an immediate guidance of how the transition to extrauterine life is progressing. Apgar scores are measured at 1 and 5 minutes after birth. Early studies correlated low 5-minute Apgar scores with poor neurologic outcome[8]; however, later

Score	Sign		
	0	**1**	**2**
Appearance, color	Blue, pale	Centrally pink	Completely pink
Pulse, heart rate	None	Less than 100 beats/min	Greater than 100 beats/min
Grimace, reflex	No response	Grimace	Cough, gag, cry
Activity/attitude	Flaccid/limp muscle tone	Some flexion	Well-flexed/active motion
Respiratory, effort	None, irritability	Weak/irregular	Good, crying

TABLE 32-1   **The Apgar Score**

studies have shown that the Apgar score is not an accurate indicator of neonatal asphyxia as defined by metabolic acidosis.[22,32] If, however, the neonate's condition continues to be depressed after 5 minutes of age, continuation of Apgar assignment for up to 20 minutes after delivery while necessary care interventions are provided can be useful.[20]

CLEARING THE AIRWAY

The airway should be cleared with either bulb syringe, DeLee, or a 10F to 14F suction catheter with use of a mechanical suction immediately on delivery of the neonates head and before the infant's first breath. The oropharynx should normally be cleared before suctioning of the nares because stimulation may cause the infant to gasp and aspirate secretions present in the oropharynx. Stimulation of the vagus nerve from suctioning too vigorously and too deeply may result in severe bradycardia; therefore, suctioning after the initial clearing of the airway should be done on an as-needed basis. The Neonatal Resuscitation Program (NRP) recommends that no greater than 100 mm Hg of negative pressure should be used to avoid injury to the neonate.[20]

Aspiration of meconium-stained fluid into distal airways may significantly contribute to morbidity and mortality. Infants presenting with depressed condition with inadequate respiration, poor tone, or a heart rate (HR) less than 100 beats/min should have the trachea intubated and suctioned with an endotracheal tube and a meconium aspirator before positive-pressure ventilation. If the baby looks good (i.e., breathing well, HR > 100 beats/min, good muscle tone) and is covered in meconium, suctioning of only the mouth and nose may be prudent. The NRP states "Some previous recommendations have

suggested that endotracheal suctioning should be determined by whether the meconium has 'thick' versus 'thin' consistency. While it might be reasonable to speculate that thick meconium might be more hazardous than thin, there are currently no clinical studies that warrant basing suctioning techniques on meconium consistency."[20] The incidence of meconium aspiration syndrome can be greatly reduced with effective clearing of the airway of affected infants.[6,34]

Initiation of Breathing

Most neonates initiate spontaneous breathing without intervention. Neonates that do not initiate breathing on their own may require only minimally invasive interventions such as opening the airway and positioning to stimulate breathing. Neonates that are breathing spontaneously but remain centrally cyanotic may need initial oxygen support delivered with blow-by oxygen, face mask, or nasal prongs. If the neonate does not begin spontaneous effective respiration or the heart rate remains below 100 beats/min after opening and clearing the airway, stimulating the infant and providing supplemental oxygen with assistive manual ventilations should be initiated at a rate of 40 to 60 breaths/min with the minimal amount of oxygen to support oxygenation. Adequate ventilation should be evaluated with auscultation of breath sounds and observation of chest excursion and heart rate. The infant should respond to adequate ventilation with an improvement in color, heart rate, and tone.

Neonates are at high risk for pulmonary air leaks, thus ventilating pressures should always be monitored with a manometer. Although pressures up to 30 to 40 cm H_2O may be initially necessary to open the lungs, the lowest pressures possible to maintain adequate chest rise and oxygenation should be used. Once the infant has established spontaneous respiration and a heart rate of 100 beats/min and is centrally pink, the team should reevaluate the amount of support needed.

If no response in heart rate and color is seen after 30 seconds of assistive manual bag and mask ventilation, then cardiopulmonary resuscitation (CPR) should be initiated while preparations for endotracheal tube (ETT) intubation are made. Because the placement of the endotracheal tube leaves little room for error, careful and immediate evaluation for right or left mainstem or esophageal intubation should be done and adequacy of ventilation should be assessed. In addition to the presence of improved color, increasing heart rate indicating successful intubation, confirmation of ETT placement with the use of a color metric CO_2 detector is recommended to confirm ETT placement.[20] Table 32-2 contains a guideline of endotracheal tube size and insertion depth.

CHEST COMPRESSIONS

Chest compressions should be initiated if the heart rate remains below 60 beats/min or does not increase after 30 seconds of assisted manual ventilation. Two methods are recommended for chest compressions on the neonate: the thumb technique and the two-finger technique. Resuscitation for neonates should be performed at a rate of 120 "events" per minute. Ninety compressions plus 30 breaths should occur. The status of the infant should be reassessed after 30 seconds of resuscitation. If the child's heart rate is above 60 beats/min, compressions can be stopped. If chest compressions are not effective, epinephrine should be administered.[20]

The thumb technique involves the caregiver encompassing the infant's chest with both thumbs used to depress the infant's sternum. The baby should be placed on a firm surface for delivery of effective compressions. The two-finger technique uses the tips of the caregiver's middle finger and either the index finger or the ring finger of one hand to compress the sternum. The other hand can be used to support the infant's back. With both the thumb and the two-finger technique, the infant's chest should be depressed to a depth of approximately one third of the anterior-posterior diameter of the chest. The chest should be allowed to recoil completely by releasing pressure so that the heart can refill.[20]

DRUG SUPPORT

Drugs are rarely needed in the delivery room resuscitation of the newborn if adequate ventilation has been established. If the heart rate continues below 60 beats/min despite adequate ventilation and compressions for a minimum of 30 seconds or if no heart rate is found, the transport team should instill 0.3 to 1 mL/kg of 1:10,000 solution of epinephrine down the endotracheal tube per protocol (Table 32-3). To ensure that the epinephrine reaches the lungs, it may be diluted in or flushed with 1 to 2 mL of normal saline solution for smaller volumes based on weight. Intravenous (IV) access should be attained as soon as possible, and the medication delivered intravenously rather than through the endotracheal tube. Current NRP guidelines for resuscitation in the delivery room recommend emergent low line placement into the umbilical vein as the most accessible parenteral route (Box 32-2).[20] If the heart rate remains below 60 beats/min, subsequent doses of epinephrine may be given every 3 to 5 minutes through the endotracheal tube or established IV line.

TABLE 32-2	**Endotracheal Tube Size Selection**		
Weight (kg)	**Endotracheal Tube (size)**	**Depth of Insertion (cm from upper lip)**	**Suction Catheter (size)**
1	2.5	7	5F
2	3.0	8	6F
3	3.5	9	8F
4	4.0	10	8F-10F

TABLE 32-3	Neonatal Emergency Drug Dosages		
Drug	**Indication**	**Dose**	**Route**
Naloxone (neonatal Narcan)	Narcotic depression	0.1 mg/kg	IV/UVC/IM/ETT
Epinephrine (1:10,000)	Bradycardia, cardiac arrest	0.01 mg/kg - 0.03 mg/kg	ETT/UVC/IV
Sodium bicarbonate, 4.2% (0.5 mEq/mL)	Metabolic acidosis	1-2 mEq/kg given slowly to reduce risk of intraventricular hemorrhage	UVC/IV (always clear line before and after administration)
5% Albumin	Hypotension volume restoration	10 mL/kg over 5-10 min	UVC/IV
Lactated Ringer's	Hypotension volume restoration	10 mL/kg over 5-10 min	UVC/IV
Dextrose 10%	Hypoglycemia	2-4 mL/kg (list over 5 to 10 min)	UVC/IV

IM, Intramuscular; *UVC*, umbilical venous catheter.

BOX 32-2   Umbilical Vein Catheterization

The neonatal transport nurses should place the umbilical vein catheter with aseptic technique. The umbilical stump and surrounding skin should first be cleansed with an approved protocol that describes preparation of the area. For example, use alcohol first, then povidone-iodine (Betadine), and let the povidone-iodine dry for at least a minute; povidone-iodine can be wiped off when the procedure is completed. Drapes are then applied to create a sterile field. A 5F catheter is usually adequate and can normally be placed in all sizes of infants; it is prepared by either attaching the catheter directly to a three-way stopcock or trimming the flared end of the catheter and inserting a blunt needle adapter. The blunt needle adapter is then connected to the three-way stopcock and flushed with solution.

Umbilical tape is tied snugly around the base of the cord to provide control of bleeding during the procedure. The umbilical stump can be cut approximately 1 cm above the skin line. The neonatal transport nurse can then identify the two thick-walled constricted arteries (4-o'clock and 8-o'clock positions) and the thinner-walled larger vein (12-o'clock position). A pair of curved iris forceps may be helpful in identifying and opening the lumen of the vein.

The neonatal transport nurse then inserts the catheter tip in the lumen and gently advances it. Stabilizing the cord by gently holding the cord at the base or applying traction with a clamp on the Wharton's jelly may be helpful. The umbilical vein normally runs in a cephalad direction. Directing the catheter in that line may assist in ease of entry. The venous catheter should be inserted only as far as necessary to obtain blood return, which is normally 2 to 3 cm. Further catheter advancement may result in a placement in the liver and consequent hepatic damage from medication injections.

The umbilical catheter can then be secured with a "goalpost" tape bridge. A purse-string suture around the Wharton's jelly tied to the catheter controls bleeding and assists in securing the catheter.

Complications of this procedure include infection, hemorrhage, air emboli, and thrombus formation; therefore, the procedure should only be undertaken after appropriate training under supervision and then performed with extreme care.

Hypovolemia should be suspected with a history of bleeding or if the infant has poor response to resuscitation, pallor, or weak poorly palpable pulses that persist despite adequate ventilation. If hypovolemia is suspected, volume expanders should be given. As soon as possible, a blood sample should be evaluated for partial pressure of oxygen (PaO_2), partial pressure of carbon dioxide ($PaCO_2$), and pH. If an arterial sample is not available, a venous sample is still valuable, particularly for $PaCO_2$ and pH.[33]

Maintenance of Body Temperature

As soon as possible after delivery, the infant should be dried, wet linens removed, and an external heat source provided, such as radiant warmers or double-walled isolette. If an external heat source is not immediately available, particular attention must be paid to ambient temperature, and the neonate should be swaddled in warm blankets with the head covered with a stocking cap if possible. The only circumstance in which thermoregulation efforts may be delayed is in the presence of meconium-stained amniotic fluid. These neonates should not be stimulated until the airway has been cleared with direct suctioning of the trachea to avoid the possibility of aspiration of any meconium that may be in the trachea.

Glucose Requirements

Neonates are susceptible to hypoglycemia because of immature glucose control mechanisms and decreased glucose substrate stores. The definition of hypoglycemia in the newborn may be variable depending on the reference. In actual practice, most clinicians consider a serum glucose of less than 40 mg/dL to represent hypoglycemia.[23,25] The infant who needs resuscitation or has conditions that necessitate transport to a higher level of care is generally at higher risk for hypoglycemia (Box 32-3). Infants identified as high risk should have screening

| BOX 32-3 | Risk Factors for Hypoglycemia |

Small for gestational age (SGA)
Hypothermia or cold stress
Respiratory distress
Congenital heart disease
Large for gestational age (LGA)
Infant of a diabetic mother
Rh incompatibility
Beckwith-Wiedemann syndrome
Nesidioblastosis
Islet cell adenomas
Sepsis
Asphyxia

glucose levels as soon as possible after delivery and every 30 minutes to 1 hour until normal serum levels have been achieved. Further discussion of glucose monitoring and stabilization is included in this chapter.

EVALUATION

If the neonate has not responded to the initial priorities of delivery room management, the transport team must reevaluate the clinical assessment and management of the infant. Common reasons for an inadequate response to resuscitation include the following:

1. Mechanical problems
   a. Inadequate oxygen supply
   b. Inadequate ventilation
2. Endotracheal tube malposition
   a. Tube in esophagus
   b. Tube in right or left mainstem bronchus
   c. Obstructed tube
3. Unrecognized clinical problem
   a. Congenital cardiac disease
   b. Electrolyte imbalances
   c. Congenital airway abnormality
   d. Pneumothorax
   e. Diaphragmatic hernia

NONINITIATION OR DISCONTINUATION OF RESUSCITATION

The International Guidelines for Neonatal Resuscitation for 2000 presents recommendations for the noninitiation or discontinuation of resuscitation, which include[27,37]:

- Birth weight less than 500 g.
- Confirmed trisomy 13 or 18.
- Congenital hydrocephalus.
- Gestational age less than 24 weeks.
- No response to ongoing adequate resuscitative efforts.
- Severe fetal growth retardation.

Each transport team should have policies and procedures that outline the management of these issues.

DETAILED ASSESSMENT AND ONGOING STABILIZATION

The goal of assessment and stabilization before transport is to ensure safe and optimal transport conditions for a neonate who has achieved or is being managed to support adequate vital signs, perfusion, optimal blood gases, and normal glucose and electrolyte levels. This goal is not always attainable, but every attempt should be made to maximize patient status and achieve stability before transport.

Assessment of the newborn should include history, clinical examination, and laboratory data. Obstetric information obtained should include the estimated day of confinement (EDC) based on the mother's dates and clinical data, maternal age, gravity, parity, abortions, fetal demise, neonatal deaths, number of living children, length of rupture of membranes, and complications of the pregnancy, labor, or delivery. Maternal medications (both during pregnancy and during perinatal period), Group B *streptococcus* (GBS) status and associated treatment, any maternal infections, and any maternal illicit drug use should also be obtained. Neonatal history should include Apgar scores, resuscitation efforts, initial physical examination, and subsequent course. Laboratory data and radiographic studies should also be reviewed.

GESTATIONAL AGE EXAMINATION

Basic knowledge of gestational age is helpful when considering the anatomy and physiologic immaturities of preterm infants. The transport team's role in determination of the gestational age is obtaining a thorough maternal and delivery history. Most often the gestational age is determined before the transport team's arrival with one of a variety of assessment tools. One example of an assessment tool is included in Figure 32-2.

PHYSICAL EXAMINATION

A considerable amount of baseline information can be obtained strictly through observation of the infant before disturbing the infant. This observation should include:

1. Heart: Rate, rhythm, heart sounds, murmurs, extra sounds.
2. Chest: Symmetry and adequacy of air entry, rales, rhonchi, wheezes.
3. Abdomen: Bowel sounds, organomegaly, masses.
4. Femoral pulses: Quality.
5. Signs and symptoms of distress: Color, respiratory effort, posture, and tone.
6. Obvious morphology.

Once the baseline examination has been established, the rest of the examination should proceed with an organized systematic approach. For example, the transport team might examine the infant beginning from the head and working downward. The essential components of a detailed examination are outlined as follows:

1. Head: Symmetry, shape, caput succedaneum, cephalhematoma.
2. Fontanelles/sutures: Fontanel number, fullness, depression, and size; suture mobility.
3. Symmetry of face: Development, shape, movement.
4. Ears: Shape, position of face, presence of skin tags.
5. Eyes: Shape, position, size, pupils, hemorrhages.
6. Mouth: Cleft palate, teeth, abnormalities, presence of micrognathia (in the event of the need for airway management).
7. Neck: Webbing, length.
8. Nose: Symmetry, septum, patency.
9. Clavicles: Masses, intactness.
10. Chest: Size, symmetry, shape.
11. Umbilical cord: Number of vessels.
12. Genitals: Development, testes, urethral and vaginal openings.
13. Anus: Patency, meconium.
14. Spine: Masses, symmetry, dimples.
15. Extremities: Symmetry, development, movement, pulses.
16. Hips: Range of motion.
17. Reflexes: Root, suck, Moro's, grasp.
18. Tone: Flaccid, normal, jitteriness, flexion.

In the transport setting, the potential value of each part of the examination must be weighed against any stress it may cause to an already compromised infant and current physiologic stability.

A.	VARIABLES					
SOMATIC	Nipple formation	Nipple barely visible; no areola 0	Well-defined nipple; areola <0.75 cm 5	Areola stippled not raised >0.75 cm 10	Areola raised >0.75 cm 15	
	Skin texture	Thin, gelatinous 0	Thin and smooth 5	Smooth, medium thickness, superficial peeling 10	Slight thickening, superficial cracking & peeling of hands & feet 15	Thick and parchment like 20
	Ear form	Pinna flat & shapeless 0	Incurving of part of edge 8	Partial incurving of whole of upper pinna 16	Well-defined incurving of pinna 24	
K= 204 days	Breast size	No breast tissue 6	Diameter <0.5 cm 5	Diameter 0.5 - 1 cm 10	Diameter >1 cm 15	
	Plantar creases	No creases 0	Faint red marks over anterior ½ 5	Definite red marks over anterior ½, indentations over anterior ⅓ 10	Indentations over anterior ½ 15	Deep indentations over more than anterior ½ 20
B. SOMATIC AND NEUROLOGIC	Scarf sign	0	6	12	18	
K= 200 days	Head lag 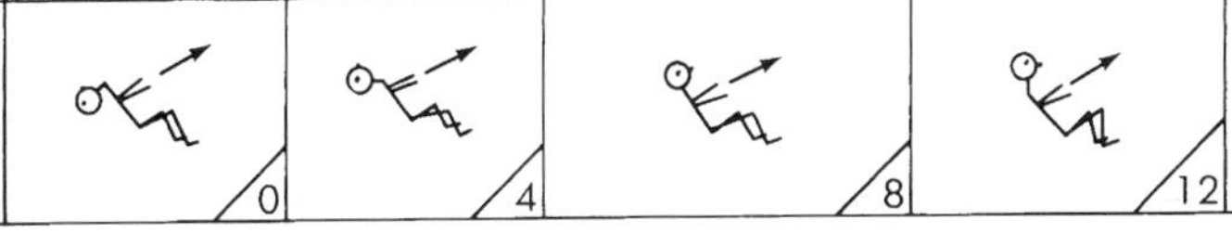	0	4	8	12	

Variables and assigned scores in the modified Dubowitz method for assessment of gestational age. A. Gestational age in days = 204 + total somatic score (for neurologically depressed infants). *B.* Gestational = 200 + total combined somatic and neurologic score (for healthy infants).

FIGURE 32-2 **Cappurro's method for assessment of gestational age.** (From Cappurro H, et al: A simplified method for diagnosis of gestational age in the newborn infant, *J Pediatr* 93:121, 1978.)

Respiratory Management: General Considerations

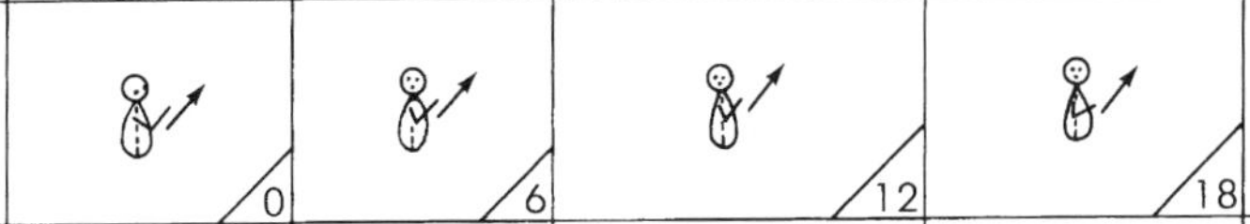

The primary component of respiratory management is ensuring correct opening, positioning, and clearing of the airway. Because most ill neonates who need transport have some degree of respiratory compromise, the transport team must perform careful and continuous assessment of respiratory status. The presence of retractions, grunting, and nasal flaring may indicate a condition of decreased lung compliance. Both central and peripheral color should be evaluated for the presence of cyanosis. Adequacy of central oxygenation should be checked with evaluation of mucous membranes. The absence of central cyanosis typically indicates adequate pulmonary blood flow and gas exchange. Peripheral cyanosis, however, may reflect problems with either oxygenation or perfusion. If the infant is centrally oxygenated (pink) but peripherally cyanotic (purple), then the child should be evaluated to determine the cause of the poor perfusion. As a basic principle, sufficient oxygen should be supplied to ensure central oxygenation. Acrocyanosis is a self-limiting condition in which the neonate's hands and feet and circumoral area may remain cyanotic for 24 to 48 hours after birth. Acrocyanosis may be a normal finding for the first 24 to 48 hours or it could suggest poor cardiac output, vasoconstriction, or cold stress; careful assessment, both physical and diagnostic, of fluid balance and environmental stressors may help identify causes of cyanosis.

Oxygen is a drug with risks and side effects associated with its use. Current technology, including use of pulse oximetry and end tidal carbon dioxide monitoring devices, greatly enhances the ability to titrate oxygen delivery based on patient response and need. Oxygen can be supplied with a number of methods: blow-by administration, head hoods or tents, nasal cannula, continuous positive airway pressure (CPAP), or endotracheal tube insertion. Blow-by or free-flow oxygen near the baby's face can be used on a short-term basis but has two main drawbacks: first, accurate measurement of the exact percentage of oxygen that the baby is receiving is impossible; and second, the flow of cold oxygen into the nenoate's face may result in increased inappropriate heat-generating responses and vagal stimulation. Hood oxygen allows for accurate measurement and stabilization of oxygen supply to the newborn but restricts accessibility to the newborn's head without disturbing the oxygen concentration and is not practical for transport. Continuous positive airway pressure can be delivered via alternate modes that include nasal prongs, nasopharyngeal tube, and endotracheal tube. An endotracheal tube obviously provides the most effective delivery of CPAP, but it requires the invasive procedure of intubation. Positive-pressure ventilation requires the placement of an endotracheal tube, with its inherent potential complications, but it can be done safely in the hands of a skilled practitioner.

In selection of the mode of oxygen delivery, the transport team must weigh both the benefits to be gained and the risks incurred with the selected approach. Once respiratory support has begun, continuous observation and reevaluation must be accomplished to maintain the correct level of support. Adjustments must be made to accommodate changes in the infant's pulmonary compliance.

Diminishing compliance without an appropriate adjustment in oxygen support may result in hypoxia with hypercarbia. Improvement in compliance could result in hyperoxia, hypocarbia, and potentially air leaks with a resultant decrease in cardiac output. Any infant treated with positive pressure is at an automatic increased risk for air leaks, including pneumothorax, pneumomediastinum, and pulmonary interstitial emphysema. Uncommonly, pneumoperitoneum and pneumopericardium could also occur. Any sudden deterioration in an infant receiving positive-pressure ventilation should prompt immediate evaluation for a displaced endotracheal tube or pulmonary air leaks. Evaluation should include assessment of breath sounds, shifting of the point of maximal intensity (PMI), transillumination of the chest, and chest radiograph.[28] Mechanical problems with the oxygen delivery system should also be immediately ruled out. Excess air must always be removed from the stomach with a nasogastric or orogastric tube because a distended stomach could interfere with adequate ventilation.

BLOOD PRESSURE AND PERFUSION

Hypotension and *poor perfusion* are also common problems in the neonate. Assessment of circulatory status should begin with an evaluation of the obstetric history, which may suggest a cause for either hypovolemia or myocardial dysfunction. Historical facts suggestive of hypovolemia as a basis for poor perfusion may include compression of the cord or a history of blood loss during the pregnancy, labor, or delivery. Infants with a history of asphyxia may have both hypovolemia and myocardial dysfunction. Assessment should include arterial pressures, central venous pressures, extremity versus core temperatures, capillary refill greater than 3 seconds in the presence of a normal temperature, and evaluation of pulse volume. The presence of progressive metabolic acidosis in a well-ventilated and oxygenated infant and evidence of cardiomegaly on radiographic films may be indicative of an asphyxial cardiomyopathy.

Treatment is aimed at the return to adequate perfusion of the tissues to prevent continued metabolic acidosis. If the transport team suspects hypovolemia, treatment may include infusion of 10 mL/kg of an isotonic crystalloid solution such as normal saline solution.[20] Fluids should be infused slowly because a rapid increase in systemic blood pressure carries the risk of sudden rise in pressure in vascular beds, which could potentially cause capillary rupture and hemorrhage and possible intracranial bleeding. If myocardial dysfunction is suspected, the transport team may consider administration of inotropic agents per protocol. Whichever treatment is instituted, careful monitoring of arterial pressures is essential both to monitor results and to prevent complications. Neonates have limited ability to control their own cardiac output.

THERMOREGULATION

The neonate is at high risk for *hypothermia* because of large surface area compared with body mass and poor thermal insulation. Premature or hypoxic neonates are at increased risk for cold stress because of decreased stores of brown fat available for generation of heat production.[29] Hypothermia in the neonate is usually an iatrogenic condition, almost always preventable; if untreated, it can be contribute to neonatal death. A neonate can have a normal central temperature with axillary or skin temperature measurements and still be cold stressed with a cool skin temperature. Side effects of cold stress and hypothermia include increased oxygen consumption, hypoxemia, acidosis, and pulmonary vasoconstriction. In addition, the infant increases glucose consumption, which may result in hypoglycemia and increases the probability of mortality and morbidity.

The neonate maintains body temperature through basal metabolism, muscular activity, and chemical thermogenesis. The infant's primary mechanism of heat production in response to cold stress is chemical thermogenesis with metabolizing brown fat stores. This process requires increased oxygen consumption and increased glucose utilization.[17] Compared with the adult, the neonate has a limited ability to produce heat by shivering, an increased oxygen consumption, and a limited ability to dissipate heat through sweating.

An understanding is essential of the mechanisms of heat production and loss and interventions for maintaining a neutral thermal environment during stabilization and transport. The neutral thermal environment is the range of environmental temperatures at which the neonate maintains a normal body temperature with minimal metabolic activity and oxygen consumption.[4,7,30,45]

The optimal temperature ranges for the newborn are:

Skin: 36.0°C to 36.5°C.
Axillary: 36.5°C to 37.0°C.
Rectal: 36.5°C to 37.0°C.

Temperature must be frequently monitored during transport via skin temperature probes in transport isolettes and with intermittent axillary measurements if an isolette is not available. Lacking this capability, the temperature should be assessed at 15-minute intervals as a minimum standard. Rectal temperatures are not recommended as a preferred method of thermoregulation monitoring during transport because of the high risk of perforation of the rectum.

Heat losses occur through convection, conduction, evaporation, and radiation, as follows:

Radiation: Heat transfer between the body and surrounding objects (e.g., isolette walls).
Convection: Heat transfer dependent on air flow over the body (e.g., a cold delivery room, emergency department, aircraft, or ground transport vehicle).
Evaporation: Heat transfer to water in the state change from liquid to gas (e.g., a wet infant).
Conduction: Heat transfer between the body and objects in contact (e.g., a scale).

During transport, the team must anticipate the effects of environmental conditions. The neonate can lose significant amounts of heat through radiation to cold isolette walls. Convection and evaporation are the most probable mechanisms of heat loss in neonatal transport. The management of the infant's thermal environment requires a careful balancing of heat losses and heat sources. Double-walled neonatal transport isolettes with active warming capabilities should be standard equipment for any neonatal interfacility transport. Interventions for reducing heat loss include keeping the infant dry; swaddling in warm blankets, foil, or plastic; using heat shields and stocking caps; and preventing drafts. Heat sources may be most effective when used in combination. Available sources, including radiant heat, warmed air, and application of commercial products such as chemical mattresses and plastic wrap, are beneficial in preparing the neonate for transport. Caution to carefully follow manufacturer's use guidelines should be taken with any commercial heat-generating products to prevent overheating or burns. Clear plastic wrap or commercial products can be applied directly to the infant with avoidance of the head and airway to prevent suffocation to minimize further heat loss. When transporting a neonate in severe cold conditions, thermal covers may be used over double-walled transport isolettes to further maintain a neutral thermal environment for the neonate. In addition, back-up systems to provide for the thermoregulation needs of neonates (such as chemical mattresses, Mylar blankets, and hot packs) should be available in the event of equipment failure during transport or transport vehicle breakdown, particularly in cold weather operations. The neonate must also not become hyperthermic. *Hyperthermia* has been associated with perinatal respiratory depression.[26,27] Ambient temperatures in aircraft during the hot summer months can increase to over 100°F. Careful monitoring of the neonate's temperature is essential to ensure the neonate is not overheating. Reducing or turning off the heat source on isolettes may be necessary to maintain a neutral thermal environment.

FLUIDS, CALORIES, AND ELECTROLYTES

Maintenance of fluid, electrolyte, and glucose balances in the newborn requires careful precise calculations to meet the neonates requirements followed by close observation and evaluation. The main sources of neonatal fluid loss are insensible water loss and urinary output (UO). In the sick neonate, UO should be measured as accurately as possible with urine bags, diaper weights, or catheterization. With appropriate fluid intake, UO should be 1 to 2 mL/kg/h with specific gravities of approximately 1.008 to 1.012. During the first week of life, the infant should be anticipated to lose 5% to 15%

of birth weight.[2] Subsequent changes in the baby's fluid intake are based on evaluation of these criteria. Insensible water loss increases significantly in the extremely premature or extremely low birth weight infant. Radiant warmers, elevated environmental temperature, and respiratory distress increase insensible water loss. The use of heat shields and warm humidified air delivered through the ventilator can significantly minimize these losses.

The neonatal patient typically needs approximately 60 to 80 mL/kg/d on the first day of life. This requirement increases by approximately 10 mL/kg/d on the first subsequent day of life. Premature infants, particularly those weighing less than 1500 g, should be given special consideration to potential increased fluid needs. Insensible water losses, immature skin surfaces, and prolonged exposure to radiant warmers can increase fluid requirements by as much as 50%.[2]

The need for electrolyte evaluation before transport must be determined based on the age of the newborn, the length of the transport, and the presence of risk factors for electrolyte imbalance. The addition of electrolytes to IV fluids is usually not necessary in the first 12 to 24 hours, although calcium is sometimes added depending on laboratory results. Serum electrolyte levels should be checked before any additional electrolytes are added. The transport team should precisely calculate the infant's fluid requirement, including any abnormal losses, because either too much or too little fluid can be detrimental to the progress of the infant. High fluid intake including flushes and medications in these infants may contribute to an increased incidence of patent ductus arteriosus.[2]

The healthy term infant normally reaches the nadir of serum glucose level at approximately 2 hours after birth. Glucose screening is therefore recommended to be conducted in all healthy term infants at 1 to 2 hours of age. Oral reestablishment of serum glucose is the preferred method; however, most critically ill stressed neonates cannot tolerate oral intake. IV fluids of 10% dextrose in water can be used to maintain glucose needs for infants who cannot tolerate oral intake. The infant weighing less than 1000 g should receive 5% dextrose in water because of intolerance of higher glucose loads, which could result in hyperglycemia.

Hypoglycemia may be treated in several ways depending on the severity of the deficiency. A bolus of 200 to 400 mg/kg (2 to 4 mL/kg) of 10% dextrose in water may be slowly given to return the serum glucose to the normal range. Glucose management can typically be maintained with maintenance IV fluids. If the hypoglycemia is not profound, the transport team may elect to respond by increasing the maintenance fluids to increase glucose delivery without the use of a bolus. A decision to increase fluid rate or dextrose concentration must be made on the basis of the fluid tolerance of the individual baby and medical control direction or protocol.

A peripheral vein may be used to administer solutions that contain glucose concentrations up to 12.5% dextrose. At concentrations of 12.5% dextrose and higher, a central venous line should be considered. Treatment of extremely resistant hypoglycemia may include the use of corticosteroids, glucagon, epinephrine, and diazoxide. Administration of these drugs, however, is beyond the scope of this chapter.

Hyperglycemia, blood glucose levels greater than 125 mg/dL, is most commonly seen in the infant weighing less than 1000 g or in infants whose hypoglycemia has been overcorrected. Management of hyperglycemia in infants of less than 1000 g can usually be handled with the use of 5% dextrose as a maintenance fluid. Hyperglycemia in the infant who is being treated for hypoglycemia can be avoided by administering the appropriate amount of glucose. In general, hyperglycemia is managed by individual program protocol or medical direction.

Glucose monitoring should be conducted frequently during transport to ensure that glucose homeostasis is maintained. A point of care glucose check should be assessed within 15 to 30 minutes after changing IV fluids containing dextrose or increasing or decreasing infusion rates. All abnormal results should be monitored and reported per protocol or medical direction.

PATHOLOGIC CONDITIONS OF THE NEONATE

One of the major roles of the transport team is to assist in identifying potential differential diagnoses and developing a management plan for the neonate who needs transport. The assessment of the neonate serves to identify the basis for formulating the differential diagnosis. The maternal and birth history should include the development and timing of symptomatology and the progress of the condition. Integration of historical data with the physical examination and evaluation of laboratory and radiographic data is essential to further support the diagnosis and treatment options.

RESPIRATORY DISORDERS
Diaphragmatic Hernia

Diaphragmatic hernia occurs early within the first few weeks of gestation when the pleuroperitoneal cavity fails to close. Abdominal contents migrate into the thoracic cavity, compressing developing lungs and causing pulmonary hypoplasia. Early detection of this defect is essential to the initiation of appropriate therapy and surgical intervention. Typical classic presentation of neonates with diaphragmatic hernia includes early onset of respiratory distress with deterioration between the 1-minute and 5-minute Apgar scores in the delivery room. Clinical signs include dyspnea, unequal breath sounds, a shift in the PMI, and potentially scaphoid abdomen. Although scaphoid abdomen is listed as a classic sign, it is frequently not evident in the delivery room.

Because any distention of the bowel further compromises respiratory function, the transport team should insert a large-bore (10F) orogastric tube and initiate low intermittent suction. Positive-pressure ventilation with a face mask should be avoided. When ventilation is necessary, immediate endotracheal intubation should be performed. These infants are at high risk of severe hypercarbia and pneumothoraces; therefore, ventilatory management is aimed at maximizing ventilation while minimizing barotrauma, if possible. Persistent pulmonary hypertension and shock frequently complicate the management of these infants. In the transport setting, an additional member should be added to the team to potentially decrease the stabilization time. Diaphragmatic hernia used to be considered a surgical emergency. Recent studies have supported delaying surgery to allow for a period of physiologic stabilization.[21] The efforts of preoperative stabilization are aimed at optimizing oxygenation, maintaining an adequate systemic blood pressure, and reducing the associated pulmonary hypertension.

Meconium Aspiration Pneumonia

Although aspiration of meconium is the most severe form of aspiration pneumonia, the neonate may also aspirate amniotic fluid or blood at the time of delivery. Typically, *meconium aspiration* occurs in term or postterm infants and may occur while the infant is in utero. The presence of meconium in the amniotic fluid should alert the medical team to the possibility of acute or chronic in utero asphyxia. Common symptoms of neonates with meconium or other substance aspiration include the appearance of a hyperinflated chest and tachypnea. Radiographic findings may reveal bilateral patchy densities. The presence of meconium in the bronchial tree causes obstruction to airflow and pneumonitis. Common complications in meconium aspiration syndrome include pulmonary air leaks and persistent pulmonary hypertension. The goals of respiratory management of the neonate with aspiration pneumonia are maintaining oxygenation, avoiding acidosis, and minimizing high airway pressures. Antibiotic therapy is frequently started in these infants until sepsis has been ruled out as the cause of in utero meconium release.

Surfactant Deficiency

The most common cause of respiratory distress in the preterm infant is *respiratory distress syndrome* (RDS), formerly known as hyaline membrane disease (HMD). This condition is primarily caused by a deficiency of surfactant; however, RDS can also occur in the presence of extreme stress such as severe hypoxia. The primary function of lung surfactant is to lower surface tension at the air-water interface of the alveoli, thereby preventing atelectasis and improving compliance. Surfactant decreases surface tension in the alveolus during expiration, which allows the alveolus to maintain a functional residual capacity. The absence of surfactant results in poor lung compliance and atelectasis. Infants with *surfactant deficiency* have progressive respiratory distress symptoms such as increased work of breathing, accessory muscle use, retractions, nasal flaring and

grunting, and increased oxygen support as a result of poor lung compliance. Increased respiratory effort necessary to maintain respiration results in lethargy. Characteristic radiographic findings include reticular granular pattern in the lungs and hypoexpansion. The severity of the illness varies from minimal respiratory support with hood oxygen to maximal support with the ventilator.

Exogenous surfactant was approved for use by the Food and Drug Administration (FDA) in 1990. Ten years of extensive clinical studies showed that exogenous surfactant treatment substantially reduces mortality and the incidence of air leak, although it does not appear to reduce other complications such as bronchopulmonary dysplasia and intraventricular hemorrhage. Both natural surfactant extracts and synthetic preparations are available. Each team should have working protocols and procedures for administration of surfactant. Administration of exogenous surfactant may result in rapid changes in lung compliance, subsequent overventilation, and air leaks unless close monitoring and adjusting of ventilator settings occur.

Pulmonary interstitial emphysema is common in those infants who need high levels of ventilatory support. Added complications of the disease include development of chronic lung disease as a result of ventilatory support and persistent patent ductus arteriosus. These complications may be decreased with use of the lowest possible ventilatory settings and avoiding excessive fluid administration during transport.[3,12,14]

Pneumonia

Pneumonia is often associated with a history of prolonged rupture of membranes of at least 12 hours before delivery. However, respiratory infection can occur in the fetus even in the presence of intact membranes. Symptoms of amnionitis and fetal infection, including maternal fever or elevated white count, purulent or foul-smelling fluid, fetal tachycardia, loss of beat-to-beat variability, or premature labor, are also suggestive. Signs of infection in infants may be present immediately at birth or may be delayed for 1 to 2 days. In addition to respiratory symptoms of tachypnea, apnea, grunting, nasal flaring, and retracting, systemic symptoms may also be present. Systemic symptoms may include hypotonia, hypotension, poor perfusion, lethargy, and seizures. An elevated or extremely low white blood cell count may or may not be present. Radiographic examination may resemble either RDS with a uniform granularity or aspiration with patchy lung fields. Management includes maintenance of adequate oxygenation and ventilation, antibiotic therapy, and cardiovascular support.

Pulmonary Air Leaks

Air leaks including pulmonary interstitial emphysema (PIE), pneumothorax, and pneumomediastinum are most commonly related to excessive positive-pressure ventilation used during resuscitation or the use of positive airway pressure treatments.[28] The infant with an air leak may appear nearly asymptomatic, with only muffled heart tones or absent/diminished breath sounds, or the infant's condition may deteriorate rapidly, necessitating immediate intervention. Assessment includes evaluation of breath sounds, shift in the location of point of maximum impulse (PMI), positive transillumination of the chest, and radiographic confirmation.

Neonates with minimal symptoms may need only a one-time needle thoracentesis and hood oxygen, or no treatment other than close monitoring may be adequate. Infants with severe distress with clinical indication of a tension pneumothorax need immediate resuscitation and emergent needle decompression or thoracentesis without delay for radiographic diagnosis. In the transport setting, transport medical personnel must consider the impacts of flight physiology by anticipating increasing symptoms from an untapped pneumothorax if the transport requires moving the child at high altitudes. A chest tube should be considered before any air transport of a neonate with a significant air leak or with a tension pneumothorax. Before departing the referring hospital, the flight nurse must also evaluate the effectiveness of the use of either a one-way valve or suction on the chest tube.

Persistent Pulmonary Hypertension in the Newborn

Persistent pulmonary hypertension in the newborn (PPHN) is a syndrome characterized by persistent elevated pulmonary vascular resistance that results in right-to-left shunt at the ductus arteriosus or the foramen ovale and leads to hypoxemia in the presence of a structurally normal heart.[10] This disease process is most commonly seen in near-term infants with severe asphyxia, meconium aspiration syndrome, congenital diaphragmatic hernia sepsis, or other respiratory distress that results in hypoxia. The clinical differentiation between cyanotic heart disease and PPHN can be difficult to make in the transport setting. Demonstration of right-to-left shunting at the ductus with preductal and postductal simultaneous arterial blood gas levels is helpful in the diagnosis of this problem. Treatment is aimed at maintenance of adequate oxygenation until the pulmonary vasculature resistance begins to drop, which normally occurs in the first several days. Infants who are more severely affected may need extremely high inspiratory pressures and rates to maintain adequate oxygenation. Maintenance of the systemic blood pressure (BP) higher than pulmonary pressure through adequate circulating volume and cardiac output discourages right-to-left shunting. Ongoing studies of the pulmonary vasodilatory effects of inhaled nitric oxide have been promising; the method is now used by most transport teams.[20,26,27] Nitric oxide is a potent vasodilator that acts specifically on the pulmonary bed. This allows for pulmonary bed relaxation without the systemic vasodilation effects of other medications. Nitric oxide has an extremely short half life and works quickly. Use of nitric oxide with high frequency oscillatory ventilation (HFOV) is extremely beneficial for patients with underinflation or lung disease. Patients transported with nitric oxide should be treated with minimal stimulation and be given sedatives and paralytics to minimize oxygen consumption and maximize treatment effects.

These risks need to be weighed against the complications of hypoxemia in determination of what percentage of oxygen to supply. The team should err on the side of caution and administer the minimum amount of oxygen to maintain oxygen saturations between 88% and 92%, especially in premature infants. Individual team protocols should direct the use of oxygen in the neonatal population. The infant of 34 weeks or less gestational age has a decreased incidence of persistent pulmonary hypertension.

However, concern for irreversible side effects is increased if these newborns are maintained in a hyperoxic state. Thus, adequate oxygenation in these infants without long periods of hyperoxia should be ensured.

Neonatal Heart Disease

The diagnosis and management of the infant with *congenital heart disease* can be a major challenge in the transport setting. Frequently, the referring staff and transport team do not have the benefit of echocardiography and must rely on history, clinical examination, laboratory, and radiographic results. A detailed history of the onset of symptoms from the referring staff is critical to planning and implementing appropriate care during transport (Table 32-4). An obstetric history that would indicate an infant at risk for pulmonary disease is important in determining whether the condition is pulmonary or cardiac in nature. Maternal history of diabetes, lupus, or exposure to viral illness is an important indicator that the infant may be at greater risk for congenital heart disease. High-risk factors for pulmonary disease include prematurity, postmaturity, meconium-stained fluid, prolonged rupture of membranes, maternal diabetes, neonatal asphyxia, or cesarean section.

Typically, tachypnea with low $PaCO_2$ may be indicative of nonpulmonary causes of respiratory distress such as cardiac anomalies or metabolic or neurologic disorders. Clinical signs suggestive of respiratory disease include retractions, grunting, poor air exchange, and unequal air entry. Tachypnea accompanied by increased PCO_2 may indicate pulmonary conditions such as respiratory distress syndrome, infectious processes, or transient tachypnea of the newborn.[18] Immediate onset of respiratory symptoms at birth is likely to indicate the presence of pulmonary disease because few babies are born in active heart failure.

The initial symptoms of serious congenital heart disease in the newborn are cyanosis, cyanosis with heart failure, heart failure without cyanosis, cardiogenic shock, and arrhythmias within the first week of life. Clinical examination includes a complete examination of the cardiorespiratory system and a search for evidence of other anomalies. Findings suggestive

TABLE 32-4   Top Five Diagnoses at Different Ages

Age on admission: 0-6 days (N = 537)

Diagnosis	
D-Transposition of great arteries	19%
Hypoplastic left ventricle	14%
Tetralogy of Fallot	8%
Coarctation of aorta	7%
Ventricular septal defect	3%
Others	49%
Total	100%

Age on admission: 7-13 days (N = 195)

Diagnosis	
Coarction of aorta	16%
Ventricular septal defect	14%
Hypoplastic left ventricle	8%
D-Transposition of great arteries	7%
Tetralogy of Fallot	7%
Others	48%
Total	100%

Age on admission: 14-28 days (N = 177)

Diagnosis	
Ventricular septal defect	16%
Tetralogy of Fallot	7%
Coarctation of aorta	12%
D-Transposition of great arteries	7%
Patent ductus arteriosus	5%
Others	53%
Total	100%

From Fyler D, Lang P: Neonatal heart disease. In Avery GB, editor: *Neonatology*, Philadelphia, 1987, Lippincott.

of cardiac disease include cardiac murmur, hepatomegaly, decreased or unequal pulses, hyperactive precordium, arrhythmias, and poor perfusion. Tachypnea without other signs of respiratory distress such as grunting and retracting may also be an indication of early heart failure. The early signs of congestive heart failure are tachypnea and tachycardia, which make distinguishing pulmonary inefficiencies from cardiac disease difficult in the cyanotic tachypneic newborn. Laboratory data that may be helpful include a comparison of oxygenation in room air and 100% oxygen. The infant who is hypoxic in room air but has a partial pressure of oxygen (PaO_2), greater than 150 in 100% oxygen is more likely to have pulmonary disease than cyanotic heart disease with a fixed right-to-left shunt. Preductal and postductal oxygen saturation monitoring can be used as a supportive diagnostic tool. Preductal oxygen saturation monitoring uses placement of an oxygen saturation monitor probe on the right hand for 3 to 5 minutes; the oxygen saturation is recorded, and then the probe is moved to either foot for the postductal oxygen saturation reading. If a greater than 10% saturation difference is found between the two sites (either higher or lower), the findings should be reported to the medical control officer. Preductal oxygen saturations higher than lower extremity saturations may indicate right-to-left shunting across the ductus arteriosus. Preductal oxygen saturations lower than lower extremity saturations may indicate transposition of great vessels.[18] Once the determination has been made that cyanosis in the newborn is caused by a fixed right-to-left shunt, the transport team should attempt to differentiate between shunting caused by persistent pulmonary hypertension and anatomic heart disease.

Defects with cyanosis and decreased pulmonary blood flow, such as severe pulmonary stenosis, tetralogy of Fallot with severe pulmonary stenosis or atresia, and tricuspid atresia with significant pulmonary stenosis, require maintenance of the ductus arteriosus for mixing of oxygenated and deoxygenated blood or for improvement of intercirculatory mixing as in transposition of the great vessels. Cyanotic or acyanotic systemic obstructive lesions, aortic stenosis, hypoplastic left heart syndrome, critical coarctation of the aorta, and interrupted aortic arch require prostaglandin E1 administration to maintain a right-to-left shunt through the ductus arteriosus, which supports systemic circulation.[19]

Administration of oxygen is necessary to improve oxygenation and decrease pulmonary vascular resistance.[19] If oxygen administration is ineffective in maintaining oxygen saturations greater than 75% in infants with suspected congenital heart disease, efforts to improve pulmonary blood flow before transport may require initiation of prostaglandin E1.[11] Prostaglandins are normally used when the patient's condition is deteriorating, as indicated by the presence of metabolic acidosis, or when deterioration is anticipated before completion of the transport. The most common side effect with the use of prostaglandin E1[16] that complicates transport is apnea or hypoventilation. The length of the transport and the difficulty of endotracheal tube placement during transport must be considered in the decision of whether to place an endotracheal tube before transport when prostaglandins are begun. Other side effects with the use of prostaglandin E1 include fever, vasodilation with flushing, and diarrhea. Uncommonly, the vasodilation may result in systemic hypotension that necessitates intervention.

Nonductal-Dependent Lesions

The four predominant cyanotic *nonductal-dependent cardiac lesions* are: tetralogy of Fallot without significant pulmonary stenosis or pulmonary atresia, truncus arteriosus, total anomalous pulmonary venous return, and Ebstein's anomaly without significant pulmonary stenosis or functional pulmonary atresia. These defects are not primarily reliant on a patent ductus arteriosus for survival; they typically have some form of structural atrial, ventricular, or arterial/venous structural defect that allows mixing of oxygenated and deoxygenated blood.

The presence of clinical and laboratory evidence of heart failure dictates the interventions used to stabilize the patient's condition during transport. Clinical symptoms may include audible murmur, hepatomegaly, decreased pulses, capillary refill greater than 3 seconds, mottled color, peripheral cyanosis, tachycardia, and cool extremities. Diagnostic indications should include identification of cardiomegaly on radiographic findings and metabolic acidosis in laboratory studies. The primary intervention available for the failing myocardium is inotropic drug support. Basic general approach for congenital cardiac disease is oxygenation and respiratory and hemodynamic support to maintain tissue perfusion. Management of the infant with congenital heart disease during transport involves treatment of the symptomatic failing heart.[19]

GASTROINTESTINAL DISORDERS

The transport team deals primarily with gastrointestinal disorders related to obstruction, either functional or anatomic; infection; or externalized abdominal contents. Obstructions of the gastrointestinal (GI) tract can occur anywhere from the esophagus through the anus. The management of all of these disorders primarily centers on decompression of the bowel, fluid management, antibiotic therapy, and respiratory support.

Esophageal Atresia

Findings related to identification of *esophageal atresia* include inability to pass an oral gastric tube to the stomach, excessive oral secretions, and feeding intolerance. An obstetric history of polyhydramnios should increase suspicion of upper GI obstruction. Of patients with esophageal atresia, 92% have an associated tracheoesophageal fistula; approximately 8% of infants with esophageal atresia have no tracheoesophageal fistula. Esophageal atresia with a fistula to the tracheal tree from both the upper and the lower pouch occurs approximately 1% of the time. An H-type fistula that connects an intact esophagus and tracheal tree occurs approximately 4% of the time. These conditions may be more difficult to diagnose, with more subtle initial symptoms of choking or coughing during feedings. They also require more detailed radiographic studies with a contrast-medium dye. Diagnosis can be confirmed with radiographs taken while a radiopaque catheter is curled in the upper esophageal pouch. Careful evaluation of the rest of the GI tract, the cardiovascular system, and the genitourinary system should be completed because of frequent associated anomalies.[13] Approximately 85% of fistulas occur between the lower esophageal pouch and the trachea. These fistulas allow air to pass from the respiratory tree into the stomach and gastric acids to reflux into the bronchial tree. These infants are at high risk for aspiration either from the oropharynx refluxing from the upper esophageal pouch or aspiration of gastric contents from the lower tracheoesophageal fistula. Positive-pressure ventilation distends the stomach via the fistula and may interfere with ventilation or result in gastric perforation if adequate esophageal/gastric decompression is not maintained. The presence of air in the stomach or intestines confirms the presence of a lower esophageal fistula. A transport team that suspects that an infant has esophageal atresia should immediately elevate the head of the bed and place a double-lumen suction tube in the upper esophageal pouch. This tube should be placed to suction. Management of these infants during transport should feature the following:

1. Intermittent suction of the upper esophageal pouch.
2. Elevation of the head of the bed to prevent gastric reflux.
3. Intravenous fluid therapy for fluids and glucose.

Intestinal Obstructions

Common initial symptoms for *intestinal obstruction* include bilious vomiting, abdominal distention, feeding intolerance, large quantities of gastric contents at delivery, absence of an anal opening, and lack of stooling in the first 24 hours. Obstetric history with a high obstruction may reveal polyhydramnios. Although the presence of bilious vomiting may be related to other causes, intestinal obstruction should be presumed until ruled out. Abdominal distention may be present depending on the level of the obstruction. Presence of tenderness, metabolic acidosis, or decreasing platelets may indicate a bowel necrosis or peritonitis and should be treated as an urgent problem.

Diagnosis can usually be made through radiographic evaluation. Radiographic studies should be carefully evaluated for perforation of the bowel. Urgent cases include malrotations with volvulus and those with associated peritonitis, perforation, or suspected bowel necrosis.

Management includes decompression of the bowel with intermittent large-bore gastric suction, IV fluids, antibiotic therapy as indicated, and respiratory support. These infants may have large fluid requirements because of large interstitial fluid losses. Severe abdominal distention may compromise respiratory status. Evaluation of these neonates should include assessment of oxygen needs and ventilatory capacity with appropriate measures taken to correct deficits. In severe cases of peritonitis, sepsis and shock may also be present and should be treated appropriately.

Necrotizing Enterocolitis

Although the cause of *necrotizing enterocolitis* (NEC) remains controversial, ischemia of the bowel predisposes the infant to this disease process. NEC is an acquired disease characterized by areas of the bowel that have become necrotic. Infants at particular risk include those with asphyxia, especially small, ill, preterm infants.[5] Early recognition of risk factors and symptoms allows for early treatment, which minimizes the incidence of necrosis of the bowel. Early symptoms include feeding intolerance with increased gastric aspirates, bile-stained gastric aspirates, abdominal distention, and Hematest-positive stools. Progression of the disease results in increasing abdominal distention to the point of tautness, grossly bloody stools, abdominal wall erythema, and abdominal tenderness. Radiographic findings include intestinal distention, thickening of the bowel wall, and the classic sign of air in the bowel wall (pneumatosis intestinalis); the absence of these radiographic findings, however, does not rule out the diagnosis of necrotizing enterocolitis. These infants are at risk for peritonitis, bowel perforation, and disseminated intravascular coagulation.

The infant at risk for NEC as a result of severe birth asphyxia or with early symptoms of NEC should be maintained on nil per os (NPO), gastric decompression, IV fluids, and antibiotics to allow the bowel to recover. The presence of thrombocytopenia may indicate underlying disseminated intravascular coagulation and may necessitate treatment with platelet infusions.

Omphalocele/Gastroschisis

Although omphalocele and gastroschisis are two separate entities, their treatment during transport is essentially the same. An *omphalocele* is an arrest of development of the abdominal wall, with the abdominal contents remaining externalized. The defect is covered by a membrane in utero, although the sac may be broken during delivery. The size of the defect may vary from a small hernia to inclusion of a large percentage of the abdominal contents. *Gastroschisis*, on the other hand, is a defect in the abdominal wall that has otherwise completed its development. The defect allows for protrusion of abdominal contents. Because the defect is normally

very close to the umbilicus, it is frequently mistaken for an omphalocele. This defect, however, is not covered by a membrane. The defect occurs early in gestation, so the intestines may appear edematous with adhesions because they have been floating in the amniotic fluid for some time.

Both groups of infants are at risk for infection, large fluid losses, impaired bowel perfusion, and hypothermia. Treatment includes immediate wrapping of the defect with moist saline gauze and plastic wrap or, alternatively, placement of the neonate in a bowel bag to prevent fluid losses. The infant must be maintained on NPO status, and gastric suction should be applied to maintain decompression of the bowel. If the abdominal opening is extremely small, the patient may be at a high risk for bowel ischemia as a result of the constriction of blood flow. Caring for the child on his or her side may help to reduce tension on the bowel and improve circulation. Careful monitoring and maintenance of temperature in normal range are essential in the management of these children. This increased need for thermogenesis also places them at risk for hypoglycemia and requires closer observation of blood glucose. They may also need increased fluid intake, particularly in the case of the gastroschisis or omphalocele with ruptured membranes.

NEONATAL INFECTIONS

The most common neonatal infections that necessitate treatment on transport include pneumonia, both viral and bacterial; sepsis; and infrequently, meningitis. Pneumonia has been addressed in the subsections on respiratory illnesses. The infant with sepsis may have mild and subtle onset of symptoms or a fulminating course that results in rapid progression to shock. Symptoms include temperature instability, either hypothermia or hyperthermia; apnea and bradycardia ("As & Bs"); lethargy; poor feeding; tachypnea; hypoglycemia; and cyanosis. An infant with any of these symptoms must be evaluated for potential sepsis. If the infant has meningitis, seizures must be added to the list of common presenting signs.

Evaluation of these infants includes a complete blood cell count with differential. A low absolute neutrophil count and an elevated ratio of immature to total neutrophils, although not diagnostic, increase the level of suspicion for bacterial sepsis. Samples for blood cultures should be obtained with strict aseptic technique. Although the definitive diagnosis of septicemia requires positive blood culture results, infants with highly suspicious signs should be started on an appropriate antibiotic regimen. In addition to antibiotic therapy, supportive therapy should be provided as needed. Infants with overwhelming sepsis may be in shock and need support of blood volume and myocardial function. In the case of meningitis with seizures, examination of the cerebrospinal fluid is indicated but usually can be delayed until after the transport. However, antibiotic therapy and treatment for the seizures should be begun as soon as possible on transport.

NEUROLOGIC DISORDERS
The primary neurologic disorders that necessitate therapy during transport include cranial enlargement, neural tube defects, and seizures.

Cranial Enlargement
Cranial enlargement may either be benign or caused by a number of pathologic conditions that include hydrocephalus, intracranial hemorrhage, intracranial cysts and tumors, or other encephalopathy. Differentiation of etiology requires careful evaluation of history, skull films, computed tomographic (CT) scan, and transillumination. If the history indicates a difficult delivery and intracranial bleeding is suspected, the infant should be evaluated for anemia. From a transport perspective, management of these disorders is primarily supportive, with response to secondary dysfunctions in the respiratory or cardiovascular systems. Careful monitoring for seizures or subtle changes in patient status is essential to identify status change indicating an emergent condition.

Neural Tube Defects/Encephaloceles
Failure of development of the neural tube early in gestation may result in a number of defects including anencephaly, meningomyelocele, meningocele, and encephalocele. These defects may include nervous tissue. The primary concern during transport is prevention of infection in the case of the open lesion. A moist sterile dressing should be applied and the infant positioned off the defect for transport.

Seizures
Seizures occur frequently in ill newborns, either as a primary or secondary disorder. Because of the immature nervous system of the newborn, infants rarely exhibit the generalized tonic-clonic seizures seen in adults and older children. Seizures in the newborn can be divided into four categories[22]:

1. *Subtle:* This type of seizure is frequently overlooked by caretakers. It may consist of repetitive mouth or tongue movement, bicycling movements, eye deviation, repetitive blinking, staring, or apnea.
2. *Clonic* (multifocal or focal): Clonic seizures are characterized by repetitive jerky movements of the limbs, which may move from limb-to-limb in a disorganized fashion.
3. *Tonic* (generalized or focal): Tonic seizures may resemble posturing seen in older infants and children and be accompanied by disturbed respiratory patterns and may include tonic extension of limbs or tonic flexion of upper limbs and extension of lower limbs.
4. *Myoclonic:* Myoclonic seizures are characterized by multiple jerking motions of the upper (common) or lower (rare) extremities.

Seizure activity is frequently confused with jitteriness in the newborn. *Jitteriness* may be distinguished from seizures in the following ways:

1. Jitteriness is sensitive to stimulus, whereas seizures are not.
2. Jitteriness is characterized by tremors rather than the slow and fast phases of seizure activity.
3. Jitteriness can normally be stopped with flexing of the limb, as opposed to seizures, which do not respond to this maneuver.

In treatment of neonatal seizures, identification of the cause is important (Box 32-4). Careful examination of the obstetric and neonatal history may reveal risk factors for seizure disorders. Physical examination should be performed, along with laboratory studies including glucose, calcium, phosphorus, magnesium, sodium, and potassium. The glucose level should be checked immediately with the bedside test strip. If hypoglycemia is present, it

---

| BOX 32-4 | **Causes of Neonatal Seizures** |

Birth trauma or intracranial hemorrhage
Hypoxic or ischemic encephalopathy
Hypoglycemia
Hypocalcemia
Hypomagnesemia
Hypophosphatemia
Hyponatremia or hypernatremia
Pyridoxine deficiency
Amino acid disturbances
Neonatal injection of caine derivatives
Bacterial meningitis
Central nervous system abnormalities
Drug withdrawal

---

should be corrected immediately with an infusion of glucose. If a correctable metabolic cause is not identified, seizures should be treated according to established protocols or after consultation with the appropriate physician. A number of medications including phenobarbital, phenytoin (Dilantin) or fosphenytoin (Cerebryx), and benzodiazepines such as lorazepam (Ativan) may be used. Serious side effects from these drugs may include respiratory or cardiovascular depression.[20]

EQUIPMENT

The transport of the neonate requires a skilled team and proper equipment. Box 32-5 contains a list of neonatal equipment designed for critical care interfacility neonatal transport. The equipment selected for a scene-response team could be much abbreviated.[1] In addition to the equipment listed, the transport team should use safety and best industry practice for securing neonates with a five-point safety harness. Term infants without thermoregulation issues can be safely transported in an approved five-point car seat that is secured onto the stretcher in the rear

---

| BOX 32-5 | **Neonatal Equipment Inventory** |

Respiratory Equipment
Laryngoscope handle with blades, sizes Miller 0 and
   Miller 1
Spare laryngoscope bulbs and batteries
Endotracheal tube stylet
Anesthesia resuscitation bag, 0.5 L
Anesthesia resuscitation bag, 1.0 L
Oxygen tubing
Pressure manometer
Infant self-inflating bag
Pediatric self-inflating bag
Masks for resuscitation bags, 1 each, premature, term,
   and infant
Endotracheal tube, sizes 2.5, 3.0, 3.5, and 4.0
Benzoin
Tape
Suction catheter and glove sets, sizes 5/6F, 8F, 10F, and
   12F
Bulb syringe
Extra-small, small, and large CPAP nasal prongs, 1
   each CPAP hats with ties
Gastric tubes, 10F, 12F
Feeding tubes, 5F and 8F
Thoracentesis

Large-bore catheters
Heimlich valve
Scalpel no. 11
Suture, 3-0 and 4-0 silk
Vaseline gauze
Stopcock
T-connector
Chest tubes, 8F and greater
Christmas tree adapters

Intravenous Therapy Equipment
Intravenous fluids
IV pump tubing
Blood tubing
Umbilical artery catheters, sizes 3.5 and 5.0
IV extension tubing
T connectors
Steri drape
Three-tail connector
Syringes, sizes from 1 mL through 60 mL
Peripheral IV catheters: 24 gauge, 22 gauge, and 20
   gauge
Heparin locks
Three-way stopcock and stopcock plugs

Continued

BOX 32-5	Neonatal Equipment Inventory—cont'd

Intraosseous needles
Medication additive labels
Arm boards, sizes premature and infant
Assorted tape
Umbilical tape
Umbilical artery catheterization/thoracotomy set, including two sterile drapes, iris forceps, needle holders, scissors, curved forceps, tongue tissue forceps, sterile 2 × 2s, umbilical tape, scalpel, and blade
Blood pressure cuffs, neonate and infant (size 1-5)

Thermoregulation and monitoring equipment

Stocking hat
Plastic wrap
Portawarmer/chemical mattress
Silver swaddler/bubble wrap/plastic wrap
Thermometers
Limb leads
Chest electrodes
Heart monitor lead wires
Capillary tubes
Chemstrips
Lancets
Arterial transducer tubing

Miscellaneous

Blood culture bottles
Scissors and hemostat
Flashlight
2 × 2s
Limb restraints
Safety pins
Rubber bands
Pacifier
Cotton balls
Sterile glove packs
Neonatal stethoscope
Trash bag

Sterile plastic bags for gastroschisis, omphalocele, and dressings for spinal dysraphism
Glass filter needles
Camera with instant film
Parent information books, permits, transport documents, and maps

Medications

Epinephrine, 1:10,000
$NaHco_3$, 4.2%
Narcan
Dopamine
Dobutamine
Phenobarbital
Phenytoin
Midazolam
Fentanyl
Ketamine
Morphine
Vecuronium
Xylocaine, 1%
Heparin, 1000/mL
0.9% Normal saline dilutent
Sterile water dilutent
Flush solution
Antibiotics
Antivirals
Albumin
D50W
Atropine
Amioderone
Calcium gluconate
Calcium chloride
Exogenous surfactant
Methylprednisolone sodium succinate
Furosemide
Amrinone
Isoproterenol
Digoxin
Prostaglandin E1

facing position. If a team engages in multiple simultaneous transports, a full set of functioning equipment and appropriate caregiver skill mix is necessary for each neonate that is transported. Providing the most therapeutic environment for the transport of critically ill neonates is essential. Maintenance of a thermal-neutral, minimal-stimulation environment is best to reduce complications of the transport environment. Mini muffs or other suitable hearing protection should be used for all neonates that are exposed to loud or vibratory environments, such as during rotor-wing transports.

SUMMARY

Medical transport providers caring for neonates in any out-of-hospital environment must have training in the stabilization and care of the types of infants they may transport Attention to both appropriate team composition and the availability of specialized equipment and medications is necessary to ensure safe transport of these patients. Competency in neonatal care protocols and procedures, and recognized expertise in the field, is an essential component of neonatal transport care.

NEONATAL CASE STUDY 1

Baby B was a 38-week, 3200-g, appropriate-for-gestational-age female born to a 24-year-old gravida 2, para 1 (now 2), living child 1 (now 2), A+ married woman. Medical history was unremarkable. Normal prenatal course was seen during this pregnancy. At 38 weeks by date, an elective repeat cesarean section was performed. Membranes were ruptured at delivery with clear fluid. Apgar scores were 7 at 1 minute and 9 at 5 minutes, with suctioning, O_2 blow-by, and stimulation in the delivery room. Baby's early course was reported to be unremarkable in level I. She was breastfeeding in room air. Transport was called at 18 hours of age for sudden deterioration with respiratory rate of 78 breaths/min and pale, cyanotic, poorly perfused infant with diminished pulses. Lower extremity pulses appeared to be weaker than upper extremity pulses. Arterial blood gas in 40% oxygen by hood was PaO_2 of 52, $PaCO_2$ of 38, pH 7.28, with a base deficit of 11. Complete blood cell count with differential was in normal limits. Provisional diagnosis was coarctation of the aorta with a closing ductus.

Predeparture differential diagnosis in the referring facility by the transport nurse included the following:

1. *Rule out sepsis.*
2. *Respiratory distress/rule out pneumonia versus PPHN versus aspiration.*
3. *Rule out congenital heart disease.*

Transport considerations included the distance of the trip, which was 1600 miles round trip, with an approximate trip time of 8 hours. Prostaglandin E1 would be taken in the event the child had a ductal-dependent congenital heart defect. The transport team anticipated the need for full support; a neonatal nurse practitioner and a respiratory therapist were dispatched.

On arrival at the referring hospital, the infant was observed to be pale pink in a 78% hood in a crib. Further history from the nursing staff included an early nursery course remarkable for intermittent mild tachypnea with respiratory rates in the range of 60 breaths/min and slight duskiness with agitation. The chest radiographic findings at 18 hours of age revealed increased perihilar streaking, fluid in the right fissure, and a normal cardiothoracic ratio. The radiographic film was otherwise unremarkable. Both history and radiographic findings were consistent with mild retained fetal lung fluid and borderline oxygenation.

The infant was placed on a radiant warmer with automatic temperature control. Transcutaneous PO_2 and PCO_2 monitors were placed. Physical examination was remarkable for a lethargic term infant who was pale pink in 78% oxygen by hood. Pulses were decreased in all extremities but equal with upper extremity blood pressures of 58 mm Hg via palpation and lower blood pressure extremities of 50 mm Hg via palpation. Capillary refill was 4 seconds with slight mottling. Heart tones were normal with no murmur or extra sounds noted. Respiratory rate was 82 breaths/min; breath sounds were equal and clear with shallow air exchange. Peripheral IV fluid was infusing with D10W at 80 mL/kg/d. Blood glucose level was 60. O_2 was increased to 85%, secondary to transcutaneous PuO_2 of 50 with an increase to PaO_2 of 54 and $PaCO_2$ of 36. After consultation with the attending physician at the receiving hospital, 10 mL/kg of 5% albumin was begun via slow push through the peripheral IV line. An umbilical artery catheter was placed, and blood culture obtained. Continuous blood pressure monitoring was begun via umbilical catheter. Blood pressure after volume was 64/42 mm Hg; capillary refill was 3+ seconds. Simultaneous preductal and post-ductal pulse oximeters were placed with results of 93% preductal and 85% postductal, indicating a shunting of blood at the ductal level.

Oxygen was increased to 100% by hood with no increase in transcutaneous PO_2. Blood pressure remained at 60/36 mm Hg. A second 10 mL/kg of 5% albumin was administered with increase in blood pressure to 72/45 mm Hg and decrease in capillary refill time to 3 seconds.

An endotracheal tube was inserted, and hand ventilation was used to test for response to hyperventilation with decrease of $PaCO_2$ to 26. Transcutaneous monitoring TCM began to increase, rising to transcutaneous $PtcO_2$ of 78, with a transcutaneous $PtcCO_2$ of 26. The patient was placed on peak inspiratory pressure (PIP) support of 24 over positive end expiratory pressure (PEEP) support of 4, a rate of 60, and a 100% attempting to match hand ventilation. Arterial blood gas results revealed a PaO_2 of 80, $PaCO_2$ of 25, pH 7.43, and a base deficit of 6. Transport diagnoses included:

Health care maintenance for a 38-week appropriate-for-gestational-age female. Plan: Fluids of D10W were continued at 80 mL/kg, and blood glucose levels were checked every 1 to 2 hours and remained stable throughout.

Respiratory distress; rule out PPHN. Plan: Blood pressure was monitored continuously throughout transport with a plan to support blood pressure with dopamine and volume as needed to prevent right-to-left shunting. Rule out sepsis. Plan: Antibiotics begun before transport.

Departure: The neonatal nurse practitioner and the referring physician spoke with the family, updating the patient's condition, current treatment, potential complications, and risks of transport. Transport consent was signed. The parents were also provided with information regarding intensive care nurseries and the specific information on the receiving nursery, including phone numbers, the attending physician, and policies regarding phone information and visiting. A Polaroid photograph of the baby was left with the parents. After the baby was put in the transport isolette, she was taken to the parents' room where the parents were encouraged to see her and touch her before departure. The parents were offered the option of having one parent accompany the baby to the receiving hospital, but this was declined. Oral gastric tube was placed before transport to empty the stomach of any air or contents. Care during transport included cardiorespiratory monitor, continuous skin temperature monitoring, continuous blood pressure monitoring, and vital signs with axillary temperature every half hour throughout the trip. The baby was in stable condition and tolerated the transport well.

Neonatal Case Study 2

Baby H was a 28-week, 1430-g appropriate-for-gestational-age male born to a gravida 5, para 3, who had no prenatal care. Previous history includes maternal IV drug abuse with denied use during pregnancy. The mother smoked a half pack of cigarettes per day. Prenatal laboratory data were unavailable.

The mother came to the emergency department in labor, where she was completely dilated with bulging membranes. Terbutaline was given 1 hour before delivery but did not stop labor. Phenobarbital was also given before delivery. The membranes were ruptured 30 minutes before delivery, and an attempt was made at a vaginal delivery, but the baby's presentation had changed to a transverse lie. A cesarean section was performed with the mother receiving epidural anesthesia.

Infant cried spontaneously and appeared to be about 28 weeks of gestational age by examination. Apgar scores were 6 at 1 minute and 8 at 5 minutes. A 2.5 ETT was inserted. Initial ventilator settings were 20/4, rate 50, 100% fractional concentration of oxygen in inspired gas (FiO_2); arterial blood gases were pH 7.18, $PaCO_2$ 59, and PaO_2 43. Umbilical artery and umbilical vein catheters were placed. Initial chest radiographic films revealed ETT down the left mainstem and air leak *around ETT; reintubation was performed with 3.0 ETT. Second chest radiographic film revealed bilateral reticular granular pattern with ETT down the right mainstem; ETT was pulled back. The umbilical venous catheter was in the liver and was discontinued. Blood samples for culture and complete blood cell count were sent to the laboratory with these findings: complete blood cell count: white blood cell count 10.1 with 26% neutrophils, 61% leukocytes, 12M 1B, hematocrit 51, hemoglobin 17.1%, platelets 278,000. Initial blood glucose level was 80. Antibiotics were given at 3:30 AM.*

Attending physician called for transport because of inability to care for a premature infant on a ventilator. Transport team arrived 1 hour and 19 minutes after transport initiated. Predeparture differential diagnosis by transport nurse included:

1. *Premature appropriate-for-gestational-age male infant.*
2. *Respiratory distress, probable RDS versus group B streptococcal pneumonia.*
3. *Rule out sepsis.*
4. *Rule out maternal drug use.*

Transport considerations included ventilatory management and thermoregulation because of the infant's extreme prematurity.

On arrival at the referring hospital, the patient was on a radiant warmer with temperature 37°C axillary, heart rate 163 beats/min, respiratory rate (RR) with ventilator, blood pressure 46/18 mm Hg. Ventilator settings were 24/4, rate 60, 60% FiO$_2$ with arterial blood gases of pH 7.37, PaCO$_2$ 34, and PaO$_2$ 288. Pulse oximeter reading was 99. The team received report, and radiographic films were viewed.

Because the umbilical venous catheter was discontinued, the neonatal nurse practitioner began a peripheral IV line for maintenance fluids. After discussion with the attending physician, it was decided to give exogenous surfactant. In-house time was lengthened because the patient's condition needed to be monitored in-house for at least a half hour after surfactant was given. Patient's ventilator settings were weaned with physical parameters (i.e., chest excursion, auscultation, and monitoring of transcutaneous readings and pulse

oximetry). A second arterial blood gas sample was sent for determination of values 20 minutes after the surfactant. The values were as follows: pH 7.40, PaCO$_2$ 29, PaO$_2$ 142 on 22/4, rate 50, and 40% FiO$_2$. Transport diagnosis included:

1. *Health care maintenance for a 28-week appropriate-for-gestational-age male. Plan: Fluids of D10W in the IV line and normal saline solution in the umbilical artery catheter continued at 80 mL/kg/d. Blood glucose levels were checked every 1 to 2 hours and remained stable throughout.*
2. *Respiratory distress, presumed HMD. Plan: Continue to wean ventilator as indicated by previous physical and monitor observations.*
3. *Rule out sepsis. Plan: Antibiotics were begun during transport.*
4. *Rule out maternal drug use. Plan: A urine toxicology screen would be sent when patient voided.*

Care during transport included all measures mentioned in Case 1. The patient's condition was stable, but he became agitated and began breathing against the ventilator. Fentanyl was given for sedation, and the patient did not "fight the vent." On arrival at the hospital, report was given to the attending physician and bedside nurse. Care was transferred to the staff.

REFERENCES

1. American Academy of Pediatrics: *Guidelines for air and ground transport of neonatal and pediatric patients*, ed 3, Elk Grove Village, IL, 2006, AAP.
2. Babson SG, Behrman RE, Lessel R: Live-born birth weights for gestational age of white middle class infants, *Pediatrics* 45:937, 1970.
3. Bell EF, Oh W: Fluid and electrolyte management. In Avery GB, Fletcher MA, MacDonald M, editors: *Neonatology*, ed 4, Philadelphia, 1994, Lippincott.
4. Berg TJ, et al: Bronchopulmonary dysplasia and lung rupture in hyaline membrane disease: influence of continuous distending pressure, *Pediatrics* 55:51, 1975.
5. Buetow KC, Klein SW: Effect of maintenance of normal skin temperature on survival of infants of low birthweight, *Pediatrics* 34:163, 1964.

6. Cappurro H, et al: A simplified method for diagnosis of gestational age in the newborn infant, *J Pediatr* 93:120, 1978.

7. Carson BS, et al: Combined obstetric and pediatric approach to prevent meconium aspiration syndrome, *Am J Obstet Gynecol* 126:712, 1976.

8. Day RL, et al: Body temperature and survival of premature infants, *Pediatrics* 34:171, 1964.

9. Dubowitz LMS, Dubowitz V, Goldberg C: Clinical assessment of gestational age in the newborn infant, *J Pediatr* 77:1, 1970.

10. Flanagan MF, Fyler DC: Cardiac disease. In Avery G, Fletcher MA, MacDonald M, editors: *Neonatology*, ed 4, Philadelphia, 1994, Lippincott.

11. Fox WW, Duara S: Persistent pulmonary hypertension in the neonate: diagnosis and management, *J Pediatr* 98:505, 1983.

12. Freed MD, et al: Prostaglandin E1 in infants with ductus arteriosus-dependent congenital heart disease, *Circulation* 64:899, 1981.

13. Greenough A, Dixon AK, Roberton NRC: Pulmonary interstitial emphysema, *Arch Dis Child* 59:1046, 1984.

14. Guzzetta PC, et al: Surgery of the neonate. In Avery GB, editor: *Neonatology*, ed 3, Philadelphia, 1987, Lippincott.

15. Hart SM, et al: Pulmonary interstitial emphysema in very low birthweight infants, *Arch Dis Child* 58:612, 1983.

16. Hill A, Volpe JJ: Neurologic disorders. In Avery G, Fletcher MA, MacDonald M, editors: *Neonatology*, ed 4, Philadelphia, 1994, Lippincott.

17. Hill JR, Rahimtulla KA: Heat balance and the metabolic rate of newborn babies in relation to environmental temperature, and the effect of age and weight on basal metabolic rate, *J Physiol* 180:239, 1965.

18. Karlsen K: *The S.T.A.B.L.E. Program: post-resuscitation/pre-transport stabilization care of sick infants: guidelines for neonatal healthcare providers*, ed 5, Park City, UT, 2006, Learner Manual.

19. Karlsen K: *The S.T.A.B.L.E. cardiac module: recognition and stabilization of neonates with severe CHD*, Park City, UT, 2003.

20. Kattwinkel J, editor: *Textbook of neonatal resuscitation*, ed 4, Elk Grove Village, IL, 2000, American Academy of Pediatrics.

21. Kinsella JP, Abman SH: Recent development in the pathophysiology and treatment of persistent pulmonary hypertension of the newborn, *J Pediatr* 126:853, 1995.

22. Langer J, et al: Timing of surgery for congenital diaphragmatic hernia: is emergency operation necessary? *J Pediatr Surg* 23:731, 1988.

23. Lubchenco LO, Hansman C, Boyd E: Intrauterine growth in length and head circumference as estimated from live births at gestational ages from 26 to 42 weeks, *Pediatrics* 37:403, 1966.

24. Martin M, Paes BA: Birth asphyxia: does the Apgar score have diagnostic value? *Obstet Gynecol* 72:120, 1989.

25. Nelson N: Physiology of transition. In Avery G, Fletcher MA, MacDonald M, editors: *Neonatology*, ed 4, Philadelphia, 1994, Lippincott.

26. Niermeyer S: Evidence-based guidelines for neonatal resuscitation, *NeoReviews* 2:38, 2001.

27. Niermeyer S, Waldemar C, Boyle D, et al: What is on the horizon for neonatal resuscitation? *NeoReviews* 2:51, 2001.

28. Phibbs RH: Delivery room management. In Avery G, Fletcher MA, MacDonald M, editors: *Neonatology*, ed 4, Philadelphia, 1994, Lippincott.

29. Philips JB, editor: Neonatal pulmonary hypertension, *Clin Perinatol* 11:515, 1984.

30. Pildes R, et al: The incidence of neonatal hypoglycemia-a completed survey, *J Pediatr* 70:76, 1967.

31. Primhak RA: Factors associated with pulmonary air leak in premature infants receiving mechanical ventilation, *J Pediatr* 102:764, 1983.

32. Scopes JW, Ahmed I: Range of critical temperatures in sick and premature newborn babies, *Arch Dis Child* 41:417, 1966.

33. Shaul DB, Horth SB: Temperature regulation in preterm infants: role of the skin-environment interface, *NeoReviews* 2:282, 2001.

34. Streeter NS: *High-risk neonatal care*, Rockville, MD, 1986, Aspen.

THE PEDIATRIC PATIENT

Reneé Semonin Holleran

COMPETENCIES

1. Identify the differences between the pediatric and adult patient.
2. Perform a primary and secondary assessment of the pediatric patient in preparation for transport.
3. Provide an overview of some selected pediatric illnesses and injuries.
4. Identify the equipment necessary to perform a competent pediatric transport.

The care and transport of the ill or injured pediatric patient requires an ability to quickly assess and treat acute changes in a child's condition. Consideration of the critical anatomic and physiologic differences in this population is paramount for safe and effective intervention. An understanding of normal growth and development in children is an invaluable tool for the pediatric practitioner.

A DEVELOPMENTAL APPROACH TO PEDIATRIC ASSESSMENT

The assessment of an ill or injured child is for all intents and purposes not dissimilar to the evaluation of an adult. The challenge in caring for children is the impact of growth and development on a variety of clinical factors. A child's age can present challenges in ability to communicate verbally, response to invasive procedures, and ability to be separated from a family member, and it may be a risk factor for traumatic injury. For proper treatment of children with illness and injuries and, more importantly, for teaching parents and children to avoid injury, growth and developmental factors must be used as a foundation for clinical care. Table 33-1 summarizes age-specific development and injury patterns.

Although not addressed in Table 33-1, children, regardless of age, are at risk for emergent complications that arise from infectious disease and metabolic or endocrine disorders. These conditions are discussed briefly later in this chapter. Box 33-1 contains examples of developmental approaches to the pediatric patient.[5,6]

TABLE 33-1	Age-Specific Development and Injury Patterns	
Age	**Development**	**At-Risk Injuries**
Infant, 0 to 4 months	Feeding, holding, bonding and dependence on caregivers.	Aspiration, SIDS, bathing injuries (burns, near drowning), environmental exposures (heat and cold), abuse/neglect/homicide/sexual assault, MVCs without proper restraint.
Infant, 4 to 8 months	Introduction of solid foods, teething, rolling side to side, sitting up, crawling.	Falls, electrocution from cords/outlets, foreign body aspiration, toxic ingestions, MVCs without proper restraint, burns, near drowning, abuse/neglect/homicide/sexual assault, lacerations, fractures, head and spine injuries.
Infant, 8 to 12 months	Crawling, walking, increased motor coordination (opening doors, latches, etc).	Falls, aspiration, foreign body ingestion, toxic ingestion, pedestrian versus vehicle injuries, near drowning, electrocution, MVCs without proper restraint, burns, suffocation, abuse/neglect/homicide, lacerations, fractures, head and spine injuries.
Child, 15 months to 3 years	Walking well and running, increased climbing skills, increased use of riding toys, use of utensils and cup, advanced motor skills (latches, doorways, match/lighter use). Emotionally, have increased desire for autonomy but have stranger anxiety. Beginning to speak simple sentences.	Falls, strike by vehicle as pedestrian or bike rider, burns, suffocation, near drowning, toxic ingestions, foreign body aspiration, electrocution, MVCs without proper restraint, abuse/neglect/homicide, lacerations, fractures, head and spine injuries.
Child, 4 to 9 years	Bike riding, swimming skills, entry into school systems; use of tools, firearms, and weapons. Increased exposures to nonfamily members, involvement in team sports. Use of seat belts. Emotionally continue to increase autonomy with heightened body awareness and sensitivity to invasive examinations/procedures. Rapidly increasing verbal skills.	Toxic ingestions, foreign body aspiration, electrocution, MVCs without proper restraint, abuse/neglect/homicide/sexual assault, lacerations, fractures, head and spine injuries.
Child, 10 to 12 years	Rapid physical growth, learning complex social skills, beginning of alcohol/tobacco/drug experimentation, increased sexual experimentation, and involvement in largely physical team sports. Use of motorized vehicles. Emotionally, have heightened awareness in gender differences, intense need for privacy, sense of responsibility, and need to be involved in decision making. May experience clinical depression.	Falls, strikes by vehicle as pedestrian or vehicle rider, burns, near drowning, toxic ingestions, drug/alcohol overdose, foreign body aspiration, electrocution, MVCs without proper restraint, abuse/neglect/homicide/sexual assault, suicide, complications of pregnancy or contraception, lacerations, fractures, head and spine injuries.

TABLE 33-1	**Age-Specific Development and Injury Patterns—cont'd**	
Age	**Development**	**At-Risk Injuries**
Child, 12 to 16 years	Increased incidence of risk-taking behaviors, increased autonomy in decisions of daily living, begin car driving, begin part-time jobs, increased sexual behavior, increased drug/alcohol/tobacco use. Emotionally, have increased body image disturbances, increased need for independence/decision making. May suffer from clinical depression.	MVCs, falls, occupational injuries, strikes by vehicle as pedestrian or bike rider, burns, near drowning, toxic ingestions, drug/alcohol overdose, foreign body aspiration, electrocution, abuse/neglect/homicide/suicide/sexual assault, complications of pregnancy or contraception, lacerations, fractures, head and spine injuries.

SIDS, Sudden infant death syndrome; *MVC*, motor vehicle collisions.

PEDIATRIC RESUSCITATION

The resuscitation of the pediatric patient involves knowledge and skills that each transport team member needs to have. Some transport programs use specialty teams to care for the child during transport. However, many pediatric transports are still provided by teams who do not specialize in pediatrics but have received additional education and training for working with this group of patients. Specialized pediatric critical care transport teams can bring expertise in the assessment and stabilization of critically ill pediatric patients and when available they should be considered for the transport of complex pediatric cases.

Pediatric resuscitation begins with the use of an algorithm that outlines pediatric advanced life support. The following is a more detailed description of the components of that algorithm and a discussion of the transport of the ill or injured pediatric patient.

PEDIATRIC AIRWAY MANAGEMENT/RESPIRATORY DISTRESS

The most important clinical skill for any clinician involved in pediatric care is the ability to assess respiratory distress and intervene appropriately. Most life-threatening complications in pediatric care are related to inadequate oxygenation and ventilation.

PEDIATRIC AIRWAY ANATOMY

Pediatric airway anatomy differs from adult anatomy in the following ways (see Figure 11-14 in Airway Management Chapter):

- Airway diameter in children is smaller when compared with adults.
- The tongue (especially in infants) is proportionately larger.
- The larynx is anteriorly located in infants and children.
- The epiglottis is long and narrow and angled away from the trachea.
- The vocal cords are attached lower anteriorly.
- In children younger than 10 years, the narrowest portion of the trachea is at the cricoid process.

The clinical implications of these differences are as follows[3]:

- Small amount of edema or obstruction can markedly decrease air exchange.
- Posterior displacement of the tongue may cause airway obstruction.
- Control of the tongue with the laryngoscope may be difficult.
- The angle between the base of the tongue and the glottic opening is more acute, which makes straight blades more efficacious in visualization of the glottis.
- Control of the epiglottis with the laryngoscope blade may be more difficult.

BOX 33-1 Developmental Stages and Approach Strategies for Pediatric Patients

Infants
Major Fears
Separation and strangers.

Approach Strategies
Provide consistent caretakers.
Reduce parent anxiety because it is transmitted to the infant.
Minimize separation from parents.

Toddlers
Major Fears
Separation and loss of control.

Characteristics of Thinking
Primitive.
Unable to recognize views of others.
Little concept of body integrity.

Approach Strategies
Keep explanations simple.
Choose words carefully.
Let toddler play with equipment (stethoscope).
Minimize separation from parents.

Preschoolers
Major Fears
Bodily injury and mutilation.
Loss of control.
The unknown and the dark.
Being left alone.

Characteristics of Thinking
Highly literal interpretation of words.
Unable to abstract.
Primitive ideas about the body (e.g., fear that all blood will "leak out" if a bandage is removed).

Approach Strategies
Keep explanations simple and concise.
Choose words carefully.
Emphasize that a procedure helps the child be healthier.
Be honest.

School-Age Children
Major Fears
Loss of control.
Bodily injury and mutilation.

Failure to live up to expectations of others.
Death.

Characteristics of Thinking
Vague or false ideas about physical illness and body structure and function.
Able to listen attentively without always comprehending.
Reluctant to ask questions about something they think they are expected to know.
Increased awareness of significant illness, possible hazards of treatments, lifelong consequences of injury, and the meaning of death.

Approach Strategies
Ask children to explain what they understand.
Provide as many choices as possible to increase the child's sense of control.
Reassure the child that he or she has done nothing wrong and that necessary procedures are not punishment.
Anticipate and answer questions about long-term consequences (e.g., what the scar will look like, how long activities may be curtailed).

Adolescents
Major Fears
Loss of control.
Altered body image.
Separation from peer group.

Characteristics of Thinking
Able to think abstractly.
Tendency toward hyperresponsiveness to pain (reactions not always in proportion to event).
Little understanding of the structure and workings of the body.

Approach Strategies
When appropriate, allow adolescents to be a part of decision making about their care.
Give information sensitively.
Express how important their compliance and cooperation are to their treatment.
Be honest about consequences.
Use or teach coping mechanisms such as relaxation, deep breathing, and self-comforting talk.

From Sanders MJ: *Mosby's paramedic textbook*, ed 2, St Louis, 2000, Mosby.

BOX 33-2	**Airway Adjuncts for Respiratory Distress in the Pediatric Patient**

Nasal cannula: Children rarely tolerate flows > 4 L/min. Not humidified.
Simple oxygen mask: Can deliver 35% to 60% O_2 at 6 to 10 L/min.
Nonrebreathing mask with reservoir: Can deliver 95% to 100% O_2 at 10 to 12 L/min.
Face tent or shield: Can deliver 40% O_2 at 15 L/min. Allows access to face without interruption of oxygen flow.
Oxygen hood: Plastic shell that encompasses the child's head. Can deliver 80% to 90% O_2 at 10 to 15 L/min. Usually not large enough for children over 1 year old.
Oropharyngeal airway: A plastic flange that displaces the tongue from the posterior pharynx and provides an oral channel for ventilation and suction. The oral airway should be placed with a tongue depressor and direct visualization in the unconscious child in whom other airway maneuvers (jaw thrust and chin lift) have been unsuccessful at opening the airway. The proper size is determined with external measurement. With the flange at the level of the mouth, the tip should reach the angle of the jaw. Airways range from 4 to 10 cm in length.
Nasopharyngeal airway: A plastic or rubber tube that provides a conduit for air or oxygen from the nares to the posterior pharynx. It also allows for suctioning from the posterior pharynx. These airways are better tolerated in responsive patients. Proper size is again determined externally. The airway is approximated to equal the length from the tip of the nose to the tragus of the ear. A properly sized nasopharyngeal airway should not cause blanching of the external nares. These airways should be lubricated before placement.

- A blind endotracheal tube placement may become caught at the anterior commissure of the vocal cords.
- Properly sized endotracheal tubes have a minimal air leak with ventilation.
- Airway adjuncts for respiratory distress are listed in Box 33-2.

INITIAL MANAGEMENT OF RESPIRATORY DISTRESS/ARREST IN THE PEDIATRIC PATIENT

- Open the airway. This can be accomplished with a jaw thrust or chin lift maneuver.
- Support breathing. This can be accomplished with any of the preceding adjuncts dependent on clinical severity of the respiratory distress.

ADVANCED MANAGEMENT OF RESPIRATORY DISTRESS IN THE PEDIATRIC PATIENT

Some patients may present with or progress to respiratory distress and need more aggressive support. These patients can be supported with bag-valve-mask (BVM) ventilation (Box 33-3) with or without endotracheal intubation. A pediatric resuscitation bag is shown in Figure 33-1.

Endotracheal Intubation

Endotracheal intubation is the most effective and reliable method of airway control for a variety of reasons,[1-5] including:

- The airway can be isolated, which ensures adequate ventilation and oxygen delivery.
- The potential for aspiration is decreased.
- Ventilations with chest compressions can be provided more efficiently.
- Inspiratory times and pressures can be controlled.
- Positive end expiratory pressure (PEEP) can be delivered.
- Endotracheal medications can be administered when access cannot be achieved.
- Pulmonary toilet can be accomplished.

Indications for endotracheal intubation include[1-5,8,13-17]:

- Functional or anatomic airway obstruction.
- Loss of airway protective reflexes.
- Excessive work of breathing, which may lead to fatigue or respiratory insufficiency.
- Need for high inspiratory pressures or PEEP.
- Need for mechanical ventilatory support.

BOX 33-3   Bag-Valve-Mask Ventilation

- Bag-valve-mask ventilation is a two-handed technique or preferably a two-person technique. With one hand or person securing the mask to the child's face, the other provides bag ventilation.
- The technique is best performed with proper positioning. The child should be managed with a head tilt/chin lift maneuver while care is taken not to depress the submental area. Depression of the submental area may cause airway obstruction. Patients with suspected cervical spine injury should be managed with the cervical spine in a neutral position. Infants are often best managed in a neutral sniffing position, whereas toddlers benefit from a roll or towel placed under the head and neck to provide optimal airway patency. A variety of head and neck positions may be attempted to find the optimal position for effective ventilation.
- All bag-valve-mask ventilation should be provided with 100% oxygen, which is best achieved with the use of self-inflating bag-valve devices with an attached reservoir. Anesthesia bags may also be used but require greater training and experience to use successfully.
- An oropharyngeal or nasopharyngeal airway (depending on the patient's level of consciousness) is helpful in providing more effective oxygenation/ventilation.
- Gastric distention is common during bag-valve-mask ventilation. This distention may worsen respiratory embarrassment and lead to emesis. Relief of this distention with a gastric tube is extremely important in the pediatric population.
- In the unconscious or extremely sedated patient, application of cricoid pressure (Sellick's maneuver) may limit gastric distention and passive regurgitation.
- A resuscitation bag should not have a pop-off valve or one that is easily occluded for proper ventilation of patients with poor lung compliance or airway resistance.
- A manometer that attaches to the self-inflating bag can be helpful in assessment of pressure ventilation during resuscitation.

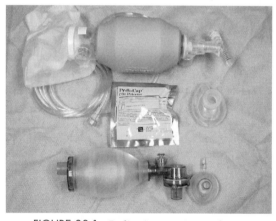

FIGURE 33-1   **Pediatric resuscitation bags.**

- Potential for any of the preceding if patient transport is anticipated.
- As a route for resuscitative medications when access cannot be achieved.

Endotracheal intubation is a skill that requires as much clinical judgment as it does manual skill.

Pediatric practitioners must always assess for and anticipate respiratory distress. The ability to determine which patients will need aggressive ventilatory support is an indispensable talent. The cricoid process is the narrowest portion of the trachea in children less than 8 to 10 years of ages. Thus, uncuffed endotracheal tubes are the most appropriate choice in this group (Figure 33-2). However, in certain circumstances, such as a near drowning, where lung compliance may be poor, a cuffed tube may be indicated. If a cuffed tube is used by the transport team, they must pay attention to the endotracheal tube size, the position of the tube, and the cuff inflation pressure. The cuff inflation pressure should be kept less than 20 cm of water.[3] A variety of ways are used for selection of proper endotracheal tube size, including[3]:

- Matching the outside diameter of the endotracheal tube to the child's little finger.
- Matching the outside diameter of the endotracheal tube to the child's nares.

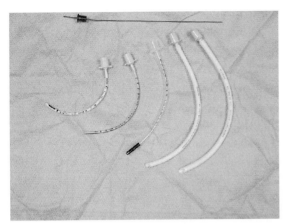

FIGURE 33-2   **Pediatric uncuffed endotracheal tubes.**

- Oxygen delivery system
- Bag-valve resuscitation bag without pop-off valve
- Resuscitation masks of various pediatric sizes
- Oral and nasopharyngeal airways of various pediatric sizes
- Suction devices, including pediatric-sized catheters
- Pulse oximeter with pediatric probes
- Cardiac monitor
- If sedation and paralytics are used, rescue medications (i.e., naloxone) should also be available
- Pediatric endotracheal tubes (Figure 33-2) and pediatric laryngoscope blades
- Pediatric stylettes
- End-tidal CO_2 detectors (disposable or in line)
- Securing tape or device

- Use of length-based resuscitation tapes (Broselow tapes) reliable to approximately 35 kg.
- For children older than 2 years, the formulas:

$$\text{endotracheal tube size} = \frac{(16 + \text{age in years})}{4}$$

or

uncuffed endotracheal tube size (mm ID)

$$= \left(\frac{\text{age in years}}{4}\right) + 4$$

or

cuffed endotracheal tube size (mm ID)

$$= \left(\frac{\text{age in years}}{4}\right) + 3$$

Multiplying the internal diameter of the endotracheal tube (ET) by 3 can approximate the proper depth of endotracheal tube placement (i.e., a 3.5-mm ET × 3 is inserted 10.5 cm).

Preparation for endotracheal intubation is the most overlooked but often the most important part of the procedure. Proper preparation for problems that may arise can often prevent life-threatening complications during this procedure. The necessary equipment is listed in Box 33-4.

Immediately after intubation, proper tube placement can be verified clinically with a variety of means:

- Observation of symmetric chest movement.
- Auscultation of bilateral breath sounds high in the axillae.
- Absence of breath sounds over the stomach.
- Positive end-tidal CO_2 readings via colormetric detectors or capnography.
- Chest radiograph results, when clinically possible, should verify proper tube placement.

Esophageal obturator airways and oxygen-powered breathing devices are both discouraged in the pediatric population because of variability in patient sizes.[1-4]

Loading and unloading an intubated child into an aircraft or ground vehicle can place a child at risk of extubation. If change is seen in the child's condition, the mnemonic DOPE may be of help in identification of a problem. The components include[3,5]:

D: Displacement of the tube from the trachea.
O: Obstruction of the tube.
P: Pneumothorax.
E: Equipment failure.

Needle Cricothyroidotomy

A rare occurrence in the pediatric population is the necessity for control of the airway via surgical means.[3,5] A surgical airway can be placed through the cricothyroid membrane on children over the age of 11 years (see Chapter 11), but *needle cricothyroidotomy* is recommended for children younger than this (Figure 33-3).

Indications for needle cricothyroidotomy include:

- Complete airway obstruction.
- Severe orofacial injuries.

- Laryngeal transection.
- Inability to secure the airway with less invasive means.

The procedure for needle cricothyroidotomy is shown in Box 33-5.

Complications of needle cricothyroidotomy include:

- Inadequate ventilation that leads to hypoxia and death.
- Aspiration (blood).

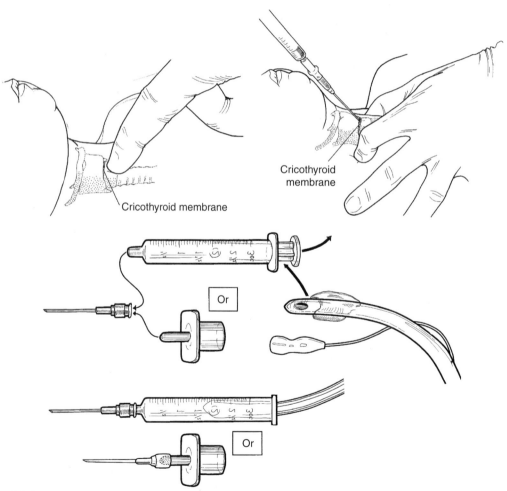

FIGURE 33-3   **Needle cricothyrotomy.** (From Dieckmann R, et al: *Pediatric emergency and critical care procedures,* St Louis, 1997, Mosby.)

BOX 33-5	**Needle Cricothyroidotomy**

1. Place the patient in a supine position.
2. Assemble a no. 14-gauge, 8.5-cm, over-the-needle catheter to a 10-mL syringe.
3. Surgically prepare the neck with antiseptic swabs.
4. Palpate the cricothyroid membrane between the thyroid and cricoid cartilage.
5. Stabilize the trachea with the thumb and forefinger to prevent lateral movement.
6. Puncture the skin in the midline over the cricothyroid membrane with the no. 14-gauge needle attached to the syringe. A small incision with a no. 11 blade may facilitate passage of the needle.
7. Direct the needle at a 45-degree angle caudally.
8. Carefully insert the needle into the lower half of the cricothyroid membrane, aspirating as the needle is advanced.
9. Aspiration of air signifies entry into the tracheal lumen.
10. Remove the syringe and stylette while gently advancing the catheter downward into position, taking care not to perforate the posterior trachea.
11. Oxygen can then be delivered in a variety of ways. Commercial jet insufflators are available for this purpose. Oxygen can also be supplied by attaching the adapter from a no. 3.0 endotracheal tube to the catheter and ventilating with a resuscitation bag. Finally, oxygen tubing can be cut with a hole toward the end of the tubing, which is then attached to the catheter hub. Once attached to an oxygen source of 50 psi or greater, oxygen can be delivered by occluding the hole with your thumb. Regardless of the oxygen delivery source, inspiration should be provided for 1 second while passive exhalation is provided for 4 seconds.

- Esophageal laceration.
- Hematoma.
- Posterior tracheal wall perforation.
- Subcutaneous or mediastinal emphysema.
- Thyroid perforation.

Needle cricothyroidotomy does not protect the patient's airway from passive aspiration. Also, because of its limited lumen size, it is more effective in oxygenation than in ventilation. Needle cricothyroidotomy is a temporary measure until endotracheal tube placement or removal of the obstruction can be achieved.

SELECTED DIAGNOSES WITH RESPIRATORY DISTRESS IN THE PEDIATRIC POPULATION

ASTHMA

Asthma is the most common chronic illness in the pediatric population. The incidence rate of asthma continues to climb worldwide. A variety of environmental and immunologic factors appear to contribute to this increase.

Clinical Presentation

Expiratory wheezing is a hallmark finding in the patient with an acute asthmatic attack. In a severe asthma exacerbation, air exchange may be so limited that wheezing is not appreciated (e.g., silent chest). The patient also has sensitive but nonspecific signs of respiratory distress, including retractions, nasal flaring, cyanosis, accessory muscle use, and eventually altered mental status. Peak expiratory flow also is diminished and should be measured to gauge both acuity and patient's response to therapy. Patient history may reveal past exacerbations that necessitated the use of home medications. The number and frequency of home treatments are important indicators of acuity. In addition, hospital admission, especially intensive care, is another important piece of history that should be collected in determination of the potential severity of the respiratory difficulty.

Treatment

The primary goals of asthma treatment are reversal of hypoxemia and control of contributing inflammatory responses. First-line therapy continues to be supplemental oxygen and the use of beta-adrenergic and anticholinergic aerosols.[18] The most common are Albuterol and ipratropium bromide delivered via a nebulizer.

The frequency of administration of these medications is a much-debated subject. As with any clinical intervention, patient response should be closely monitored. A key component of asthma therapy is the control of inflammation, which is now believed to contribute to chronic airway changes. Acute inflammation is controlled with steroid therapy.

CROUP

Croup is the common term for a viral infection that affects the larynx but may extend into the trachea and bronchi.

Clinical Presentation

Patients generally present with a history of fever and coryza (cold symptoms). As the illness progresses, inspiratory stridor may be present as may a characteristic "barking" cough. If the inflammation extends to the bronchi, rhonchi and wheezing may also be present. Care must be taken to rule out epiglottitis and retropharyngeal abscess because the presentations can be similar.[8]

Treatment

Treatment for croup is primarily supportive and centers on treatment of dehydration and the respiratory distress. In rare severe cases, upper airway edema or obstruction may necessitate endotracheal intubation for ventilation and airway protection. Medications include racemic epinephrine aerosols, intramuscular (IM) or oral (PO) dexamethasone, and prednisolone.

EPIGLOTTITIS

Epiglottitis is a rare but life-threatening bacterial infection of the epiglottis and surrounding structures. Epiglottitis has become increasingly rare with the advent of immunization for *Haemophilus influenzae*, which is the causative agent in 90% of epiglottitis cases.[8]

Clinical Presentation

Epiglottitis is second only to croup as a cause for infectious stridor. The course of epiglottitis is differentiated from other presentations because of its abrupt nature. Symptoms often occur rapidly and cause parents to seek medical attention in 24 hours of the initial symptoms. Patients present with fever, stridor, labored respirations, and often drooling, because of supraglottic edema. The appearance of these children is also helpful in diagnosing of epiglottitis. They are often anxious and present in a classic tripod position, sitting forward with their arms supporting them with their jaws thrust forward. This position is assumed by the patient to increase air entry. Clinicians must recognize this presentation because of the life-threatening nature of airway involvement.

Treatment

The focus of treatment with epiglottitis is rapid recognition and treatment of airway obstruction. Patients in extremis must have the airway controlled before any other intervention, including laboratory work and intravenous access. Before dealing with these patients, creation of a well-defined epiglottitis algorithm is crucial. A lateral neck radiograph may be helpful in delineating epiglottitis from the much more common causes of stridor and respiratory distress. If endotracheal intubation is indicated, the support from anesthesiologist or ear, nose, and throat (ENT) staffs is invaluable. Use of the operating room with inhalation induction and rapid access to tracheostomy equipment is the optimal method of airway control. In situations without this support, endotracheal intubation should only be undertaken by staff capable of securing the airway, surgically if necessary. Airway control before transport is best for the patient with epiglottitis. Current antibiotic recommendations include cefuroxime, cefotaxime, and ceftriaxone.[18]

All patients with epiglottitis need intensive care admission.

FOREIGN BODY ASPIRATION

Aspiration of foreign bodies into the respiratory system can create difficult diagnostic challenges. Aspiration into the upper airway may be immediately life threatening with obvious clinical symptoms, whereas aspiration into the lower respiratory tract may have varying degrees of severity. Sixty-five percent of lethal aspirations occur before the age of 2 years, and special consideration for education should be given to parents of these children. Foods most frequently associated with aspiration are hot dogs, candy, nuts, and grapes.

Upper Airway Aspiration

Clinical Presentation. Patients with *upper airway* foreign body aspiration generally present in severe respiratory distress. The history includes rapid onset of stridor, tachypnea, and in some cases, total airway obstruction.

Treatment. Complete airway obstruction should be managed initially with basic life support (BLS) measures, such as the Heimlich maneuver in older children and chest thrusts in infants. If the child's condition is apneic, attempts at ventilation should also be provided. Failure of BLS measures should be followed by laryngoscopic visualization and attempts at removal. Unresolved total upper airway obstruction is an indication for needle or surgical cricothyroidotomy, depending on the child's age.

Lower Airway Aspiration

The majority of *lower airway* foreign body aspirations occur in children under 3 years of age. The difficulty in treatment of these aspirations is the wide range of presentations and the difficulty in imaging nonradioopaque objects. A high index of suspicion must be maintained for at-risk age groups (6 months to 3 years) with respiratory distress.

Clinical Presentation. As stated previously, presentations can range from essentially asymptomatic to severe respiratory distress. A careful history is often helpful in diagnosis. Common presentations include new-onset coughing and wheezing. Less than half of these events are diagnosed on the day of aspiration. If sought, a history of a recent choking or aspiration episode is usually found in 75% of cases.

Treatment. If an object is found with radiographic or if a strong likelihood of aspiration is found by history, bronchoscopy with removal of the aspirated object is the standard of care for these patients.

BRONCHIOLITIS

Bronchiolitis is a lower respiratory tract infection (primarily viral) that is one of the more common causes of new-onset wheezing in children. *Respiratory syncytial virus* (RSV) is the causative agent in most cases, but *Haemophilus parainfluenzae* and *Mycoplasma pneumoniae* have also been isolated.

Clinical Presentation

Wheezing is the most common presenting symptom, often with an accompanying 2-day to 5-day course of coryza and cough. These patients are often tachypnic, with respiratory rates reaching 80 to 100 breaths/min in some cases. Nonspecific signs of respiratory distress such as nasal flaring and intercostal retractions are also present. Most cases occur in the winter months, with the majority of infections in children from ages 2 to 8 months. Apnea in children younger than 3 months is also characteristic of RSV infections.[8]

Treatment

Once other causes for wheezing have been ruled out (asthma, foreign body aspiration, pneumonia), care is generally supportive. Supplemental oxygen, antipyretics, and adequate hydration are all helpful for patients in mild distress. Children may benefit from nebulized albuterol aerosols and oral albuterol solution. Oral albuterol solutions are not indicated for patients who do not respond to aerosol therapy. Corticosteroids are not indicated for the treatment of bronchiolitis. Patients in severe distress who are unresponsive to therapy may need intubation and mechanical ventilation.[8]

PNEUMONIA

Pneumonia, an inflammation of the pulmonary parenchyma, can be caused by a variety of bacterial, fungal, and viral agents. Discussion of all of the causative agents is beyond the scope of this module, so this process is discussed in general terms.

Clinical Presentation

Bacterial pneumonia generally has a rapid onset with accompanying high fevers, chills, and cough. The patient with bacterial pneumonia may also have grunting respirations, decreased breath sounds, and tachypnea, which are all nonspecific signs. *Viral pneumonia*, in contrast, has a more gradual onset over 2 to 4 days with cough coryza and low-grade fevers. Patients with viral pneumonia may also have rales, grunting respirations, tachypnea, and decreased breath sounds. In truth, bacterial and viral pneumonia are difficult to distinguish based on clinical examination results alone. Leukocytosis over 15,000/mm is a more predominant finding in bacterial pneumonia and weighs against a viral diagnosis.[9,10] A chest radiograph can be helpful in diagnosis. Bacterial pneumonia often shows a lobar consolidation, whereas viral pneumonia causes hyperaeration or diffuse interstitial infiltrate without consolidation.

Treatment

Treatment involves supportive measures with appropriate antibiotic therapy for bacterial infections. Dehydration and hypoxia are common complications of pneumonia, so adequate intake, whether oral or intravenous, and supplemental oxygen may be essential. Antipyretics lower fevers and increase patient comfort. Drugs most commonly used in children for antipyretics include acetaminophen and ibuprofen.[18]

Sensitivity to these drugs should be determined before administration. Currently, little data exist on the lower age limits for ibuprofen therapy, so caution should be used in younger children (<6 months). The practice of alternating these medications in patients is also being investigated. Supplemental oxygen for children in distress is indicated. As with other respiratory illnesses, some children may need intubation and mechanical ventilation, depending on the severity of pulmonary dysfunction. *Streptococcus pneumoniae* and *H. influenzae* remain the major bacterial causes for pediatric pneumonia. Medication therapy is dependent on the causative microorganism.

Children who need hospital admission for pneumonia include[5]:

- Children <1 year old.
- Patients with respiratory compromise.
- Patients with pleural effusion.
- Patients with pneumatocele.
- Patients with failure to respond to antibiotic therapy.
- Patients with dehydration.

CONGENITAL HEART DISEASE AND METABOLIC ACIDOSIS

Two other causes of acute respiratory distress in children that may be encountered by the transport team are congenital heart disease and metabolic acidosis.

Congenital Heart Disease

Because of varying rates of closure of the ductus arteriosus, clinical presentations of respiratory distress from *congenital heart disease* can be seen anywhere from a few days to 6 weeks after birth. The list of both cyanotic and acyanotic lesions that can cause respiratory distress in newborns is too lengthy for discussion in this chapter. Cardiac processes should be kept on the list of differential diagnoses for children in this age group.[5]

Metabolic Acidosis

Tachypnea from *metabolic acidosis* is a common clinical finding in pediatric patients. Respiratory buffering of acidosis may be the most obvious clinical finding in these situations. Tachypnea without an obvious cardiac or respiratory source should be further investigated to rule out metabolic acidosis.[5]

Causes of metabolic acidosis in children include:

- Diarrheal dehydration (most common cause).
- Diabetic ketoacidosis.
- Renal failure (acute or chronic).
- Inborn errors of metabolism.
- Poisons (salicylate, ethanol, methanol, ethylene glycol).
- Lactic acidosis (hypoxia, sepsis, shock).
- Hyperalimentation.
- Enteric fistulas.
- Ureterosigmoidostomy.
- Drugs (e.g., mafenide [Sulfamylon], ammonium chloride, amphotericin, acetazolamide).
- Dilution (rapid volume expansion).

Identification and management of the cause of the acidosis must occur quickly. Supplemental oxygen including intubation and mechanical ventilation may be necessary during the acute treatment phase of these disorders.

PEDIATRIC TRAUMA

Outside of the immediate perinatal period, trauma and accidents continue to be the leading cause of death in all pediatric age groups. Although this section focuses on specific injuries and treatment, education aimed at the prevention of these avoidable injuries should always be the focus for emergency care providers and transport team members.

PHYSIOLOGIC AND PSYCHOLOGIC CONSIDERATIONS

Pediatric patients have several unique physiologic, psychologic, and anatomic characteristics that must be considered when dealing with the acutely injured child.

Size and Body Surface Area

Because of children's smaller size and surface area, energy from traumatic injuries imparts more force per unit of body area. The relative lack of body fat, the decreased elasticity of connective tissue, and the close proximity of internal organs to surface tissue all increase the potential for multiple injuries in this population. Increased body surface area also lends itself to increased thermal loss. Hypothermia becomes a major clinical concern.[1-7]

Skeletal Structure

Incomplete calcification of the child's skeleton predisposes children to underlying soft tissue and organ injury without obvious overlying bony deformity. Multiple growth centers in the pediatric skeleton may also have clinical implications in care. Skeletal fractures in children, especially in the thorax, should heighten clinical suspicion of a high-energy injury with resultant trauma to underlying structures.[1-5]

Psychologic

Children of different ages present with different emotional and developmental needs. Familiarity with these issues allows the clinician to tailor the clinical approach and anticipate the patient's needs. Injuries and stress may cause regression in psychologic behavior, which in turn can complicate clinical management.

Long-Term Effects of Traumatic Injury

The effect of traumatic injuries on the growth and development of pediatric patients should never be underestimated. Evidence suggests that more than 50% of children with multisystem injuries have cognitive and personality changes up to a year after injury. Social, affective, and learning disabilities have all been linked to serious injuries in children. Damage to growth plates, amputations, or physical scars can have a lasting impact on not only physical function but emotional well being as well. Pediatric injuries also create considerable strain on the family. Difficulties with finances, parental relationships, and sibling relationships are common issues with childhood injuries.[1-5,11]

Support from family services, social work, and psychologists or psychiatrists is invaluable in these situations.

THE PRIMARY SURVEY

The ABCDE algorithm (airway, breathing, circulation, disability, and exposure) for the initial survey of trauma in adults is also applied to pediatric patients. Again, consideration of unique physiologic and anatomic differences is critical for proper assessment and care. Just as with the adult patient, the child's cervical spine needs to be appropriately immobilized.

Airway and Cervical Spine Protection

The establishment and maintenance of an open airway is critical to prevent complications in the pediatric population. Effective oxygenation and ventilation cannot take place until this is achieved.

An open airway is the number one priority in care. In children, a disproportion in size is found between the child's head and mid face. Placing the child in a "sniffing" position, with the mid face placed superiorly and anteriorly, is the optimal alignment for airway protection. With traumatic injuries, care must be taken to maintain a neutral position of the cervical spine during opening of the airway. (Immobilization of the cervical spine is addressed in the Disability section of the primary assessment.) Padding of the backboard under a child's shoulders and posterior thorax also aids in neutral alignment of the cervical spine (Figure 33-4).

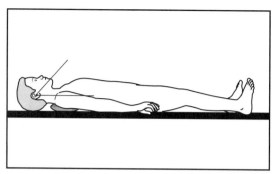

FIGURE 33-4   **Proper positioning of a child on a backboard.** (From Emergency Nurses Association: *Emergency nursing pediatric course: provider manual,* ed 2, Des Plaines, IL, 1998, ENA.)

The airway in the unresponsive child should be opened with the cervical spine protected. If the child is profoundly unconscious, an oral airway aids in keeping the tongue out of the hypopharynx. An oral airway should be placed with direct visualization with a tongue blade to prevent oral trauma and subsequent bleeding.

Once the airway is opened and suctioned for debris or secretions, supplemental oxygen should be provided. Patients with inadequate respiratory rates, impaired ventilation, or an inability to protect the airway from secretions or emesis should have the airway protected with endotracheal intubation. Before mechanical control of the airway, patients should be oxygenated via face mask or assisted bag-valve-mask ventilations.

Nonelective nasal intubations should not be performed on children less than 12 years of age because the acute angle to the glottis makes this an extremely difficult procedure for maintaining neutral cervical spine position. Needle or surgical cricothyroidotomy (dependent on age) may be necessary for airway protection for patients who cannot be successfully intubated.[5,12]

Many clinicians use rapid sequence induction (RSI) protocols as a part of airway management. Generally speaking, these protocols outline the use of intravenous medications to optimize patient condition for endotracheal intubation. Accurate weights are necessary to provide proper dosages during this procedure. Controversy exists over which specific medications are best for traumatically injured children. Many protocols use atropine sulfate as the initial medication to block vagal responses to laryngoscopic instrumentation. Hypoxia is a major cause of bradycardia in the pediatric patient, so bradycardia during any airway procedure should be treated promptly with assisted ventilation with supplemental oxygen. Atropine is then followed by a short-acting sedative and a short-acting neuromuscular blocking agent. Many medications fulfill these requirements and can be safely used in children. The medications used in RSI and management of the pediatric airway are discussed in more detail in Chapter 11.

Rescue airways such as the Combitube have limitations that may preclude their use in children. However, supraglottic airway devices such as laryngeal mask airways (LMAs) are available in all sizes from neonatal to young adult. Familiarity with the contraindications for use of these devices is necessary before use with pediatric patients. Information about these devices is contained in Chapter 11.

Breathing

After control of the airway and cervical spine has been achieved, attention is then turned to oxygenation and ventilation of the patient. All trauma patients need supplemental oxygen. Assessment of effectiveness of breathing and ventilation can be determined with a variety of factors.

Subtle findings of respiratory distress are often missed in pediatric patients. Respiratory rate is the initial factor assessed. Children have varying normal rates of respiration depending on age. An infant breathes 40 to 60 times per minute, whereas older children have normal respiratory rates of 20 breaths per minute. Tachypnea is an early but nonspecific sign of respiratory distress. Bradypnea is a late sign of distress and often heralds impending cardiorespiratory arrest. In assessment of children, the respiratory rate, when viewed with other physical findings, often provides a much more accurate assessment of ventilation.

Work of breathing increases in children with respiratory distress. Increased work of breathing can present with any of the following clinical findings[5]:

- Nasal flaring.
- Retractions (intercostal, subcostal, substernal, clavicular, and suprasternal).

- Head bobbing.
- Grunting respirations.
- Tripod positioning.
- Paradoxic respirations (seesawing respirations with increased dependence on the diaphragm).
- Pallor.
- Increased drooling or inability to control secretions.
- Decreased gag reflex.
- Altered respiratory rate (tachypnea, bradypnea, or apnea).
- Snoring.
- Stridor.
- Adventitious breath sounds (wheezing, rales, or rhonchi).
- Decreased or absent breath sounds.
- Cyanosis (late sign of distress).

Any of these findings necessitate support with supplemental oxygen and may necessitate, depending on the severity of distress, assisted ventilation with a bag-valve-mask or endotracheal intubation.

Selected Traumatic Injuries That Contribute to Respiratory Distress. Injuries to the thorax are a common cause of respiratory distress after traumatic injuries. Physiologic differences in children change the patterns of injury. A child's ribs are more cartilaginous, so rib fractures are uncommon, whereas injuries to underlying structures (i.e., pulmonary/cardiac contusions) occur more frequently. The pediatric mediastinum is more mobile and easily shifted, which can contribute to ventilatory and cardiovascular compromise. The thinness of the chest wall makes respiratory assessment more difficult because breath sounds may be referred from one area of the chest to another, diagnosis of atelectasis and pneumothoraces difficult.[5]

Tension Pneumothorax. *Tension pneumothorax* occurs when air enters the pleural space on inspiration but cannot escape on expiration. Rapidly rising intrathoracic pressures can lead to rapid ventilatory and cardiovascular collapse. This complication is life threatening. A tension pneumothorax is characterized by decreased or absent breath sounds on the affected hemothorax, dyspnea, hypotension, neck vein distention, cyanosis, and as a late sign, tracheal deviation. Subcutaneous emphysema may be appreciated with tactile examination of the chest. Intubation and mechanical ventilation may put trauma patients at risk for this complication because intrathoracic pressure increases with positive-pressure ventilation. Tension pneumothoraces are diagnosed with clinical not radiographic examination.

Treatment for Tension Pneumothorax. Initial treatment is with needle decompression with a large-bore intravenous (IV) catheter placed into the intrapleural space at the second intercostal space at the midclavicular line of the affected hemothorax. Tube thoracostomy with a chest tube appropriate for size and age at the fifth intercostal space at the anterior midaxillary line of the affected hemothorax is definitive treatment. Chest tubes should have a one-way flutter valve attached or be placed to water seal drainage to prevent reaccumulations of air. Tension pneumothoraces should always be treated before transport.

Simple Pneumothorax. A *simple pneumothorax* occurs when air enters the pleural space and causes a loss of negative pressure between the visceral and parietal pleura. This loss of pressure leads to partial or total lung collapse. A simple pneumothorax is characterized by decreased breath sounds over the affected hemothorax, dyspnea, hyperresonance of the affected hemothorax, and chest pain with radiation to the shoulders. Respiratory distress is also seen. Subcutaneous emphysema may be appreciated with tactile examination of the chest.

Treatment for Simple Pneumothorax. Treatment consists of placement of a chest tube appropriate for size and age to the fifth intercostal space, at the anterior midaxillary line of the affected side. An alternative site for chest tube placement is the second intercostal space at the midclavicular line of the affected hemothorax. Chest tubes should be attached to one-way flutter valves or water seal drainage to prevent reaccumulation of air. An anterior approach is inappropriate if both air and fluid are suspected in the pleural space. Suspected pneumothoraces that do not cause severe respiratory or cardiovascular compromise should be confirmed radiographically because other conditions (e.g., traumatic diaphragmatic hernia) may have similar clinical findings. All pneumothoraces greater than 20% or any pneumothorax present in patients who need positive pressure ventilation should be treated with tube thoracostomy before transport.

Open Pneumothorax. *Open pneumothorax* occurs when an open wound allows free movement of air into and out of the pleural space. Collapse of the lung and impaired ventilation result. An open pneumothorax is characterized by the presence of a penetrating chest wound, dyspnea, chest pain, and hyperresonance and decreased breath sounds over the affected hemothorax. An audible "sucking" sound may be heard during inspiration and expiration.

Treatment for Open Pneumothorax. Treatment of this complication requires treatment of both the lung collapse and the penetrating wound. A sterile occlusive dressing, taped on three sides, should be immediately placed over the wound. The dressing is taped on three sides to allow for venting of the pleural space by lifting the dressing should reaccumulation of intrapleural air occur. If untreated, reaccumulation of pleural air can lead to tension pneumothorax. After the wound is treated, a chest tube should then be inserted as discussed previously to treat lung collapse and prevent tension pneumothorax during transport. This chest tube should be placed remotely from the penetrating wound to decrease the risk of intrathoracic infection.

Hemothorax. *Hemothorax* occurs when blood accumulates in the pleural space. In adults, accumulation of more than 1500 mL of blood in the pleural space is considered a *massive hemothorax*. In pediatrics, the amount of blood loss is dependent on weight. A greater than 10% loss is a major complication. A hemothorax is characterized by dyspnea, chest pain, decreased or absent breath sounds over the affected side, and dullness to percussion of the affected hemothorax. Signs of shock (related to the blood loss) may also be present.

Treatment for Hemothorax. Treatment for this complication also requires a two-pronged clinical approach. The affected hemothorax must be decompressed and drained with a chest tube appropriate for age and size placed in the fifth intercostal space of the anterior midaxillary line. The chest tube then needs to be placed to water seal drainage with suction. Controversy surrounds how much blood should be drained from the pleural space before the thoracostomy tube is clamped. Advanced trauma life support (ATLS) guidelines state the tube should be clamped after 1000 mL of blood is removed in adult patients. Pediatric patients have a circulating volume of 80 mL/kg. The 1000 mL in adults represents one fifth of the circulating volume (in an average-sized patient), so a similar 20% loss in children (depending on size) may require thoracostomy tube clamping. Remember that tube clamping is a temporizing measure until open thoracotomy can be performed. Fluid resuscitation for blood loss with crystalloid and possibly transfusion therapy also needs to be initiated in these patients. Fluid resuscitation is discussed in depth in the Shock and Shock Management section of this module.

Flail Chest. *Flail chest* occurs when rib fractures of more than two ribs at more than two sites cause a segment of the chest to lose continuity with the rest of the thoracic cage. Flail chest injuries are uncommon in children because of the lack of rib calcification, but they can occur with adolescents. A flail chest is characterized by paradoxic chest wall movement of the affected segment during inspiration and expiration, chest pain, dyspnea, hypoxia, and cyanosis.

Treatment for Flail Chest. Treatment of flail chest injuries centers around support of ventilation, provision of humidified oxygen, and careful fluid administration to prevent overhydration. The underlying pulmonary contusion is the primary concern of this injury. Without the presence of systemic hypotension, great care should be taken to prevent overhydration. These injuries can be difficult to manage because the affected lung is sensitive to both overresuscitation and underresuscitation. Some patients need intubation for ventilatory support. IV or epidural analgesia to control the severe pain of this injury is also beneficial in support of the patient's ventilatory status.

Pulmonary Contusion. *Pulmonary contusion* occurs when lung parenchyma is traumatically injured causing leakage of blood and fluid into the interstitial spaces. Pulmonary contusions are characterized by dyspnea, tachypnea, bloody sputum, and possibly obvious chest wall injuries. Clinical appreciation of pulmonary contusions on examination can be difficult, and a high index of suspicion should be maintained for patients with thoracic injuries or those involved in rapid deceleration injuries. Radiologic changes may not be present until 24 hours after injury.

Treatment for Pulmonary Contusion. The treatment of this injury involves fluid resuscitation as noted previously and support of the patient's ventilatory status. Use of steroids and diuretics for these injuries remains controversial.

Diaphragmatic Rupture. *Diaphragmatic rupture* occurs when a traumatic injury causes a defect in the diaphragm, allowing for herniation of abdominal contents into the thoracic cavity. Some injuries may only cause small diaphragmatic tears that take time (even years) to develop into diaphragmatic herniations. Most of these injuries occur in the left hemothorax because the liver serves as protection for the right hemidiaphragm. Herniation of abdominal contents causes compression of the ipsilateral lung and possible shift of mediastinal structures. Intestinal or gastric obstruction or ischemia may also occur.

Diaphragmatic ruptures are characterized by dyspnea, dysphagia, chest pain, sharp shoulder pain, auscultation of bowel sounds over the lower thorax, and decreased breath sounds over the affected hemothorax. Radiographic studies may show shift of thoracic structures, the presence of the gastric silhouette above the diaphragm, and if present, the radiopaque gastric tube curled in the lower left chest.

Treatment for Diaphragmatic Rupture. The definitive treatment for diaphragmatic rupture is surgical repair. Clinical support of ventilation and gastric decompression is necessary before surgical intervention or transport. If the child is to be transported via air, adequate gastric decompression must be provided during transport.

Tracheobronchial Injuries. *Tracheobronchial injuries* occur when blunt or penetrating trauma causes a tear in the trachea or bronchus, allowing air to enter the pleural space or mediastinum. These injuries are characterized by palpable subcutaneous emphysema (in the neck, face, and thorax), dyspnea, hemoptysis, and absent breath sounds to the affected hemothorax. Hamman's sign, which is a crunching sound auscultated to the anterior chest that is synchronized to the patient's heartbeat, may also be appreciated. A pneumothorax that reaccumulates after chest tube insertion and placement to water seal drainage and suction should heighten a clinician's suspicion for tracheobronchial injuries.

Treatment for Tracheobronchial Injuries. Intubation with placement of the tube distal to the injury site should be accomplished. This procedure can be extremely difficult in the transport setting because the level of injury may be difficult to appreciate and fiberoptic support is rarely available. Patients may need more than one chest tube placed on the affected hemothorax, and they may need them placed both anteriorly and laterally as described previously. All of these patients must be closely monitored for development of tension pneumothorax during transport. Surgical intervention for repair of these injuries is necessary.

Sternal Fractures and Rib Fractures. Both *sternal fractures* and *rib fractures* are fortunately rare in children but may be present in adolescents. Injuries to these areas with or without fracture should always raise concern for damage to underlying structures (i.e., cardiac and pulmonary contusions, aortic injuries). These injuries are characterized by pain to the injured area, splinting of respirations, dyspnea, ecchymosis, and possibly crepitus.

Treatment for Sternal Fractures and Rib Fractures. Treatment for these fractures centers on ventilatory support and appropriate analgesia. Clinical examination for damage to underlying structures should always take place.

Circulation

The third step in trauma assessment is determination of the circulatory status of the patient. In traumatic injuries, this assessment centers primarily on the estimation and treatment of fluid and blood loss that accompanies traumatic injuries. Again, physiologic differences in pediatric patients make this assessment more difficult than in adults. Knowledge of the normal parameters of heart rate, blood pressure, and respiratory rates in various age groups is essential for accurate diagnosis. Physical examination combined with a history of the injury mechanism is extremely helpful in identification of patients who need circulatory support.

Physical Examination.   Clinical signs and symptoms of fluid and blood loss in pediatric patients after traumatic injuries include the following:

- Altered level of consciousness. In preverbal children, this may be manifested as an inability to recognize parents or caregivers.
- Decreased response to stimuli or the environment. This is often identified by decreased pain response to procedures such as IV starts or reduction of fractures.
- Restlessness or anxiety.
- Confusion or irritability.
- Dry mucous membranes or absence of tears.
- Tachypnea.
- Tachycardia. In the early stages of shock, tachycardia with a widened pulse pressure may be the only clinical finding in patients with fluid or blood loss.
- Changes in skin color. This includes patients who appear ashen, pale, mottled, or cyanotic.
- Capillary refill greater than 3 seconds. This can be an extremely sensitive measure of circulatory status in children. Care must be taken in examination of the hypothermic patient because hypothermia may increase capillary refill time without fluid or blood loss.
- Changes in the quality of pulse pressures. Peripheral pulses in severe shock are weak and thready.
- Cool diaphoretic skin.
- Difficulty in obtaining a blood pressure. With vasoconstriction from catecholamines release and decreased cardiac output, blood pressure readings may be difficult to obtain

in pediatric patients. Children can remain normotensive in moderate to severe shock because of sustained catecholamine response. Blood pressure can be the vital sign least reflective of circulatory status in children. Other clinical indicators as listed previously are often much more sensitive. Hypotension and bradycardia after traumatic injuries in children are ominous clinical findings and need to be treated aggressively.
- Decreased or absent breath sounds.
- Decreased urine output. Placement of a urinary catheter early in the care of traumatically injured children is essential for assessment of circulatory status and effectiveness of resuscitation. End organ perfusion (i.e., kidneys) decreases with fluid or blood loss and is reflected with oliguria or anuria. Maintenance of 1 to 2 mL/kg/h of urine output is the goal of circulatory support in the pediatric patient.

Circulatory compromise in children can often be subtle and must be found with a careful physical examination. Waiting for major changes in vital signs or laboratory studies increases patient morbidity and often makes resuscitation more difficult.

Monitoring of the patient is required during assessment and resuscitation of traumatically injured children. Cardiac monitoring and pulse oximetry monitoring can aid in initial assessment and monitoring of ongoing patient status.

A normal pulse oximetry reading does not preclude a patient's need for supplemental oxygen and may not accurately reflect tissue oxygenation.

Laboratory studies that may be helpful in assessment of the circulatory status of trauma patients include:

- A complete blood cell count, especially hematocrit levels.
- Serum or finger or heel stick glucose measurement.
- Electrolytes.
- Arterial and venous blood gases. Decreasing pH indicates acidosis developing from oxygen debt and anaerobic metabolism. Elevated $PaCO_2$ indicates respiratory acidosis and

impaired ventilation, and a decreased PaO_2 is indicative of hypoxia. Decreased HCO_3^- indicates buffering of acidosis. The blood gas measurement can be a helpful tool in the initial assessment of ventilation and fluid status in the injured child.

- Lactate level.
- Urinalysis for measurement of specific gravity.

Diagnostic studies that may be helpful in assessment of circulatory status of trauma patients include:

- Chest radiography for evaluation for hemothorax, aortic injury, or pulmonary contusion.
- Head and cervical spine computed tomographic (CT) scan for evaluation of intracranial bleeding and spinal cord injury.
- Abdominal and pelvic CT scan.
- Pelvis radiography for evaluation for pelvic fractures.
- Long-bone radiography, especially of the femurs, which can account for significant blood loss.

After determination of circulatory status, care is focused on prevention of further fluid loss (i.e., controlling bleeding) and replacement of fluid or blood loss. Fluid resuscitation is discussed at length in the Shock and Shock Management portion of this chapter.

Selected Traumatic Injuries That Can Lead to Fluid or Blood Loss or Circulatory Compromise.
Any injury that causes bleeding or fluid loss has the potential to cause compromise if not treated. The following injuries are of greatest concern for major blood or fluid loss in the pediatric trauma patient.

Head Injuries and Scalp Lacerations.
Epidural bleeding (bleeding between the skull and dural meninges) and *subdural bleeding* (bleeding between the dura and the brain) can cause lethal amounts of blood loss in pediatric patients. Pediatric patients have an estimated circulating volume of 80 mL/kg. Combined with the fact that infants have a proportionately larger amount of blood volume in the head, this can lead to hypovolemia with relatively small amounts of intracranial hemorrhage. Infants with fontanelles and open cranial sutures may have increased bleeding and intracranial pressure. The vascularity of the head and scalp can also lead to hypovolemia from scalp lacerations, and aggressive fluid resuscitation may be necessary. The support of circulatory status takes precedence over management of increased intracranial pressure with fluid restrictions. (Head injuries are discussed in depth in the Disability section of trauma care.)

Facial and Mandibular Injuries.
As with the scalp, the bony structures of the skull are very vascular and can bleed profusely when injured. Patients with Le Fort fractures or open mandibular fractures may need aggressive resuscitation. Clinical findings are often obvious, with frank external bleeding noted. After airway control is achieved, some patients may need oral and retropharyngeal packing to control bleeding. Marked facial swelling and ecchymosis may also be present with these injuries.

Treatment of Facial and Mandibular Injuries.
Treatment is focused on basic support and involves maintenance of a clear and secure airway and bleeding control. Patients often need fluid resuscitation but may also need transfusion therapy, depending on the response to crystalloid support.

Massive Hemothorax.
This injury is discussed in depth in the preceding section.

Cardiac Injury.
Injuries to the heart can be caused by either blunt or penetrating traumatic forces and cause a variety of pathologic conditions.

Cardiac Tamponade.   *Cardiac tamponade* occurs when blunt or penetrating injury causes bleeding from the heart (cardiac rupture), the pericardial vessels, or the great vessels to accumulate in the pericardial sac. Very small amounts of blood in a child can interfere with cardiac activity. Fortunately, removal of these same small amounts can drastically improve cardiac function. Clinically, cardiac tamponade is diagnosed by the presence of muffled heart tones, hypotension, and distended neck veins (Beck's triad). Remember that other clinical conditions, such as hypovolemia, or environmental concerns, such as noise, can make this diagnosis difficult.

Cardiac tamponade should be considered in all patients with blunt or penetrating thoracic injuries. Pulseless electrical activity in the absence of tension pneumothorax and hypovolemia is highly suggestive of cardiac tamponade. Kussmaul's sign (a rise in venous pressure with inspiration) and pulsus paradoxus (a decrease of >10 mm Hg of systolic blood pressure with inspiration) are extremely difficult to assess in the transport setting but can be indicative of cardiac tamponade.

Treatment of Cardiac Tamponade. Treatment of this injury is rapid pericardiocentesis to decompress the pericardium. Before initiation of pericardiocentesis, one should ensure that the patient has not responded to fluid resuscitation to raise venous pressure. A subxiphoid approach with a spinal needle or an over-the-needle catheter attached to a 30-mL syringe with a three-way stopcock is the preferred method of aspiration. The needle is directed to the pericardium at a 45-degree angle during aspiration. Cardiac monitoring to assess for ventricular arrhythmias or irritability is required. Because the pericardium is self healing, aspiration of a small amount of blood may be all that is necessary as a temporizing measure to definitive surgical care. Controversy surrounds leaving a needle or catheter in place during transport because risks of inadvertent cardiac damage may outweigh the benefits.

Myocardial Contusion. *Myocardial contusion* occurs when blunt force is delivered to the myocardium, causing injury. With relatively smaller amounts of subcutaneous fat and cartilaginous ribs, children are at great risk for this injury. Patients with this injury often have chest pain. Definitive diagnosis can only be made with direct inspection of the myocardium. Because this is rarely done, clinicians must assess for complications of myocardial contusion, which include hypotension, conduction abnormalities, or wall motion abnormalities on echocardiography. Common arrhythmias include premature ventricular contractions, unexplained sinus tachycardia, atrial fibrillation, and bundle branch blocks (primarily on the right). Electrocardiographic examination results may show ST segment abnormalities and may indicate myocardial infarction.

Treatment of Myocardial Contusion. Treatment of myocardial contusion is supportive. Patients need at least 24 hours of cardiac monitoring. The risk for sudden arrhythmia decreases greatly after 24 hours. Significant arrhythmias should be treated with advanced cardiac life support (ACLS) and pediatric advanced life support (PALS) protocols, and cardiology consultation may be indicated.

Traumatic Aortic Disruption. *Traumatic aortic disruption* occurs when the aorta is damaged from rapid deceleration, most commonly seen in motor vehicle crashes and falls from great heights. Traumatic aortic disruption is often rapidly fatal, but survival is increased with rapid detection and surgical intervention. Most survivors of this injury have partial lacerations at the level of the ligamentum arteriosum and survive because of contained hematoma at the site. Unexplained persistent hypotension is usually not related to this injury, and other bleeding sources should be sought.

A transected aorta that bleeds freely into the left chest can cause profound hypotension but is quickly fatal (in minutes) without operative intervention. Clinical signs and symptoms of this injury are often absent, and a high index of suspicion must be maintained for patients with mechanisms of injury that involve rapid deceleration. Chest radiographic findings that may be indicative of major vessel injury are listed in Box 33-6.[2]

BOX 33-6 | **Chest Radiographic Findings That May Indicate Major Vessel Injury**

A widened mediastinum
Obliteration of the aortic knob
Deviation of the trachea to the right
Obliteration of the space between the pulmonary artery and the aorta
Depression of the left main stem bronchus
Deviation of the esophagus or the gastric tube to the right
Widened paratracheal stripe
Widened paraspinal interfaces
Presence of a pleural or apical cap
Left hemothorax
Fractures of the first or second rib or scapula

False-positive and negative radiographic findings are possible, so any patient with the possibility of aortic injury should be further evaluated with radiography. Angiography continues to be the gold standard for diagnosis, but CT scan of the chest and transesophageal echocardiography may also show aortic injury.

Treatment of Traumatic Aortic Disruption. Treatment of this injury is operative repair either with resection and grafting or primary repair. Hemothoraces should be treated as described previously, and fluid resuscitation should be provided based on patient need.

Abdominal Injuries.   Blunt trauma is the cause of most abdominal injuries in children. Anatomic differences in children predispose them to injuries. These differences include a less-developed abdomen that results in less protection from injury, a more protuberant abdomen that places vital organs closer to impacting forces, and a small thorax with compliant ribs that decreases protection to the liver and spleen.

Abdominal examination can be extremely difficult in the pediatric population because fear of examination or pain from distracting injuries interferes with assessment. Preverbal children are unable to describe or relate pain. Abdominal findings can be subtle and are often missed on initial examination. A high index of suspicion should always be maintained with patients with multisystem injury.

Spleen and Liver Injuries.   These solid organs are the most commonly injured in pediatric abdominal trauma. Disruption of the vascular supply to these organs can result in massive hemorrhage. Clinical signs may be subtle but may include point and rebound tenderness, radiation of pain to the left shoulder in splenic injuries, ecchymosis or abrasion to the upper quadrants, lower rib fractures, and abdominal distention. Signs of shock may be present with significant injury.

Treatment of Spleen and Liver Injuries.   Treatment of these injuries requires fluid resuscitation (discussed in the Shock and Shock Management portion of this module) and surgical evaluation. Splenectomy is undesirable in children because of the increased rates of sepsis in children after splenectomy. Prompt transport to an institution with pediatric surgical capabilities is imperative with these patients.

Stomach Injuries.   Stomach injuries rarely occur as a result of trauma but can occur with lap belt, air bag, and handlebar injuries. A greater concern in the pediatric trauma patient is gastric dilation from crying or assisted ventilation. Gastric distension can lead to circulatory and respiratory embarrassment if untreated. All pediatric patients with multisystem injury or those who need assisted ventilation should have their stomachs decompressed with a gastric tube to prevent these complications. Gastric tubes can be used if the patient does not have known or suspected facial or head injuries.

Pancreatic and Duodenal Injuries.   Pancreatic and duodenal injuries occur in children as a result of rapid deceleration, often in conjunction with lap belt use or falls onto handlebars. These injuries are extremely difficult to diagnose clinically and need to be ruled out radiographically in patients at risk. Clinical examinations can be variable, but these injuries should be suspected with the previously noted mechanisms or obvious trauma to the abdomen. Treatment of these injuries is supportive and requires surgical evaluation.

Genitourinary Injuries.   Although injuries to the genitourinary system are rarely fatal, they may be accompanied by hemorrhage and shock. The kidneys in pediatric patients are less protected by fat and are more mobile than in adults, increasing the risk for injury. Fortunately, because of its anatomic position in children, the bladder is less likely to be injured by pelvic fractures. The genitourinary system in children can be injured by vehicle restraints in deceleration injuries or by falls with direct blunt trauma.

As with many abdominal injuries, a high index of suspicion must be maintained for patients with mechanisms of injury likely to cause trauma to the genitourinary system. Clinical findings may be subtle, and hematuria is an insensitive predictor of injury. Treatment of these injuries is supportive and may require surgical evaluation. However, most pediatric abdominal trauma is handled without surgery.

Pelvic Fractures. Pelvic fractures are rare in young children but can be common traumatic injuries in late adolescence. Mechanisms of injuries include motor vehicle crashes and falls with direct blunt trauma. Lethal retroperitoneal hemorrhage can accompany these fractures and requires prompt immobilization and aggressive fluid resuscitation.

Clinical findings include obvious visual asymmetry, instability and pain to palpation, pain with adduction of the legs, and ecchymosis. As noted, these findings may also present with profound hypotension and shock.

Treatment of Pelvic Injuries. Controversy surrounds the most appropriate method of stabilizing these fractures for transport. Each transport program should have pediatric protocols to guide pelvic support during transport. Military antishock trousers (MAST) may be still be used, but many programs no longer have access to them.

Stabilization with sheet strapping and external fixators is another splinting option dependent on fracture patterns and orthopedic surgeon availability. Pelvic fractures without hemodynamic instability may only need close observation during transport.

More aggressive immobilization, as discussed previously, should be reserved for patients with clinical signs of fluid loss. Fluid resuscitation with both crystalloids and blood products may be necessary.

Femur Fractures. Fractures of the femur, much like fractures of the pelvis, can cause significant amounts of blood loss in children. Femur fractures are rarely isolated injuries and are often part of a constellation of multisystem damage. Clinical findings include shortening of the affected leg, obvious deformity of the femur, pain to palpation at the site, and ecchymosis. Wounds in the areas of suspected or obvious fracture should heighten concerns for open fracture at the site.

Treatment of Femur Fractures. After assessment of neurovascular function and administration of appropriate analgesics, fractured femurs should be aligned and immobilized. Traction splints, air splints, or a variety of commercial splints can be used for immobilization. If air splints are used for transport, monitoring for pressure gains and losses during altitude changes is important. After alignment and immobilization, a neurovascular assessment should be repeated. Fluid resuscitation with crystalloids and blood products may be necessary. Antibiotic coverage should be considered with the presence of open wounds.

Disability

The fourth step in the primary assessment of injured children is the evaluation of injuries that cause patient disability.

Head injuries and spinal cord injuries are the primary sources of disability in the pediatric trauma patient. Head injuries continue to be the leading cause of death in traumatically injured children. Anatomic differences in children that predispose them to head injuries include head size that is disproportionate to body surface area, open fontanelles and cranial sutures that allow for increased intracranial swelling, and poorly developed neck and upper extremity musculature that offer less protection to the head and neck.

A rapid neurologic assessment provides immediate information on patient condition and provides a baseline for further evaluations. A neurologic examination is especially important if paralytics or sedatives are used in patient care. Factors that are evaluated in a rapid neurologic assessment include level of consciousness, pupillary response, and gross motor function.

Level of Consciousness. Determining level of consciousness in older verbal children is the same as the assessment in adults. Use of the AVPU mnemonic (A, awake and alert; V, only responsive to verbal stimuli; P, only responsive to painful stimuli; and U, completely unresponsive) is a quick and reliable method of primary neurologic assessment.

Evaluation of the preverbal child becomes more challenging. Factors that can be assessed for preverbal children include level of alertness, response to painful stimuli, interaction with caregivers and family members, ability to be consoled, the presence of abnormal eye movements (i.e., disconjugate gaze), and motor responses to tactile stimuli.

A modified Glasgow coma score for infants may be helpful in this assessment. Presence of a high-pitched cry and bulging tense fontanelles are also indicative of head injuries in infants. Continued emesis after traumatic injury is also suggestive of head trauma.

Pupillary Response. The pupils should be assessed for size, equality, and light response. Unequal pupils and sluggish or no reaction to light may be indicative of intracranial hypertension. Direct trauma to the eye may also cause pupillary dysfunction, so ocular findings should be correlated with the rest of the neurologic evaluation.

Motor Responses. Children with intracranial hypertension may have decreased or abnormal responses to pain. Decorticate and decerebrate posturing may be present. Flaccidity with severe head injury and paralysis from spinal cord injuries may be found on initial examination. Inspection and palpation of the head, neck, and spine should be performed to assess for lacerations, hematoma, cerebral spinal fluid (CSF) or bloody drainage from the ears or nose, depressed skull fractures, or step off in the spinal column.

All inspection and palpation should be performed with protection of the cervical spine and logrolling with spinal precautions. Although evaluation of the spine and back are not technically part of the primary survey, these assessments are best performed with the patient placed on a backboard, which is necessary for transport protection of the cervical spine. Specific head injuries are discussed in a previous section of this curriculum, so this section focuses on treatment specific to pediatric patients with head injuries.

Airway Control and Ventilation. Children with Glasgow coma scores of 8 or less, with ongoing seizure activity, or with deteriorating neurologic status should be intubated so that adequate oxygenation is assured. Care must be taken to prevent the development of low CO_2 levels (hypocarbia) or high CO_2 levels (hypercapnia) because both can be detrimental to resuscitation. The use of capnography during transport can be helpful in these patients.

Circulation. An overlooked facet of treatment in the head-injured patient is blood pressure support. Hypoxia and hypotension are the leading causes of neurologic deterioration in the head-injured patient. As noted previously, hypotension can be caused directly from head injury. Blood loss in the head or from other injuries that impede circulation should be treated appropriately. Preservation of stable mean arterial pressures is important to provide adequate cerebral perfusion and oxygenation.

Diuresis and Seizure Control. Diuresis and the control of posttraumatic seizures are extremely controversial topics in the care of pediatric head injury. Little consensus on the application of these measures without CT scan results can be found in the literature. If diuresis and seizure control are deemed necessary, the medications listed in Box 33-7 have been safely used in children. These agents should be used with neurosurgeon consultation.

Positioning. Elevation of the backboard to 30 degrees unless precluded by other injuries may aid in decreasing intracranial pressure.

Environmental Issues. Control of noise, especially in the transport setting, is important in controlling acute elevations in intracranial pressures. Unless precluded by patient injury, earplugs or muffs can decrease noise stress on patients. Adequate sedation and pain management can decrease intracranial pressure.

BOX 33-7	**Drugs Used for Diuresis and Seizure Control**

Diuresis
Mannitol 20% solution IV bolus
Furosemide

Seizure Control
Lorazepam may be given rectally
Diazepam may be given rectally
Midazolem may be given rectally
Phenytoin or fosphenytoin
Phenobarbital

Caution should be used in the patient with hypotension because these agents can aggravate hypovolemia. Electrolyte imbalances may also result and should be monitored.

Reevaluation. Constant monitoring and reevaluation of the patient with neurologic impairment is necessary in transport to assess for deterioration of patient status and effectiveness of medical interventions.

Spinal Cord Injuries. Spinal cord injuries are rare in children, but prevalence increases in adolescents. These devastating and often preventable injuries are rarely seen as an isolated injury but often are combined with complex injury patterns. Careful patient assessment becomes critical in identification of injuries because patients may not be able to assist with the examination.

Specific to children, spinal cord injury without radiographic abnormality (SCIWORA) is not uncommon. Any child with neurologic dysfunction on examination needs neurosurgical evaluation.

As with many injuries, anatomic differences in children may predispose them to specific spinal injuries. These differences include a large head with weak neck muscles that result in less protection of the cervical spine and horizontal facets combined with ligamentous laxity that allow more movement of the spine.

Clinical findings of any level of motor or sensory impairment should heighten concern for spinal injury. Spinal care specific to pediatric patients is discussed next.

Spinal Protection. The most important intervention in the transport of children with known or suspected spinal cord injury is proper spinal protection. Before application of cervical collars and a backboard, jewelry and necklaces should be removed to prevent interference with radiologic examinations and possible pressure injuries. Care should also be taken to remove sharp debris such as glass from the patient to prevent further injury.

A firm cervical collar should then be placed while a second person maintains manual stabilization of the cervical spine. An improperly sized collar can interfere with respiration or cause inappropriate extension of the cervical spine. A properly fitted cervical collar has the child's chin resting in the chin piece; the collar is below the child's ears and rests on the clavicles. Infants may be too small for a properly fitted cervical collar. In these circumstances, a towel roll may be used to immobilize the cervical spine. A towel roll must prevent flexion and extension and align the cervical spine in a neutral position. If a towel roll cannot achieve these goals, manual control may need to be continued.

Once a cervical collar has been applied, the child is then logrolled onto a backboard (see Figure 33-4). One person should provide manual control of the collared cervical spine, with another person at the child's shoulders and hips and another at the child's hips and legs. Opposite the patient, one person should be in place to position the backboard. The person controlling the cervical spine may then lead the command to turn the patient as a unit onto his or her side. As stated previously, this is an opportune time for a caregiver not involved in logrolling the patient to inspect and palpate the patient's back and spine, assessing for injuries or pain.

Children younger than age 8 years have disproportionately large heads, so padding beneath the shoulders on the board is necessary to keep the cervical spine in a neutral position. The backboard can be positioned at a 30-degree to 45-degree angle and the child then rolled onto it.

Once the patient is centered on the board, lateral stabilization of the cervical spine with blanket rolls or blocks and securing of the head with straps or tape should be performed. The final step in spinal immobilization is securing the body to the board with straps (securing the chest, hips, and knees). Straps should be secure enough to allow turning the board from side to side without movement of the patient's body. This turning may be necessary in the nonintubated patient who has periods of emesis during transport.

Suction should be readily available for any patient secured to a backboard. A neurologic examination should precede and follow all spinal immobilization procedures.

Removal of a Child from a Child Safety Seat with Maintenance of Spinal Immobilization. Children with an unstable airway or respiratory or circulatory compromise should be removed from the safety seat to a backboard to allow for appropriate intervention.[5] The procedure for accomplishing this is as follows:

- Initiate manual protection of the cervical spine.
- Remove or cut the shoulder harness, and move the safety bar out of the way.
- Position the child safety seat at the foot of the backboard. Tip the child safety seat back, and lay it down on the backboard.
- One person then slides his or her hands along each side of the patient's head until they are behind the patient's shoulders. The head and neck are now supported laterally by that person's arms. A second person should then take control of the patient's body.
- On the instruction of the person holding the head, slide the child out of the safety seat to the backboard and immobilize as described previously.
- Instruct parents or caregivers to replace the seat involved in the crash. Some auto insurance companies reimburse this cost.

Exposure and Environment

The fifth and final portion of the primary examination of traumatically injured children is exposure (to identify obvious injuries) and assessment of environmental issues on patient condition.

Hypothermia. The most pressing environmental concern for pediatric patients is the effects of hypothermia. *Hypothermia* may be caused both by environmental exposure and by therapeutic interventions such as rapid fluid infusion.

Hypothermic insults can be rapid, as with submersion injuries, or gradual, as a result of exposure to ambient temperature. The clinical signs of hypothermia are subtle, especially in the unresponsive patient, and a high index of suspicion in patients at risk is essential. The effects of hypothermia in children can be devastating, particularly during resuscitation. Diagnosis and treatment of hypothermia from both injury and therapy requires vigilance by clinicians.

The increased body surface area of children combined with their decreased energy stores puts them at greater risk for hypothermia. Hypothermia can be described as *mild* (35°C to 32°C), *moderate* (32°C to 30°C), or *severe* (temperature <30°C). Clinical signs of hypothermia are listed in Box 33-8.

Management of Hypothermia. Management of hypothermia is dependent on the level of hypothermia encountered. Attention to the ABCDEs of the primary survey remains important. Intubation, CPR, and intravenous access may be necessary for patients in cardiorespiratory arrest. Chest compressions may cause organized cardiac rhythms to convert to ventricular fibrillation. The existence of an organized rhythm may represent sufficient circulation in patients with decreased metabolism, and CPR may not be indicated. In the absence of an organized cardiac rhythm, CPR should be initiated and continued throughout the rewarming process. The exact role and benefit of CPR in the hypothermic arrest remains controversial.

The initial and often most overlooked factor in rewarming is the removal of the patient from cold stresses. Patients should be removed from the cold environment, have wet clothing removed, and be covered with warm blankets. Warmed supplemental oxygen should be provided via mask if spontaneous

---

BOX 33-8	**Clinical Signs of Hypothermia**

Decreased core temperature (<35°C). Temperatures should be measured rectally or with temperature-sensing indwelling catheters to provide the most accurate clinical information. Some clinicians believe any level of hypothermia in the pediatric trauma patient is detrimental and requires treatment.

Changes in mental status.

Cool, mottled skin.

Shivering in mild to moderate hypothermia. Children have limited energy stores for effective shivering, and the absence of shivering in patients with decreased core temperatures is concerning.

Variable vital signs (dependent on level of hypothermia). Cardiorespiratory arrest is not uncommon in severe hypothermia.

Coagulopathies with moderate to severe hypothermia.

respirations are present or via bag-valve-mask if respiratory support is indicated. Contributing factors to hypothermia such as hypoglycemia, shock, and occult injuries should be considered and treated if present. Mild and moderate hypothermia is treated with passive external rewarming, whereas severe hypothermia requires active core rewarming (Box 33-9).

Cardiac irritability and asystole are not uncommon in severe hypothermia. Cardiac drugs and defibrillation are usually not effective in core temperatures below 28°C. Rewarming to temperatures above 28°C is therefore recommended before initiation of these interventions. Dopamine is the only inotrope that retains some degree of action in the patient with hypothermia. Attempts at rewarming should not delay transport to a critical care setting.

Heatstroke.   Another environmental emergency in children that merits discussion is heatstroke. *Heatstroke* is a life-threatening complication of environmental thermal stress. Mortality has been reported in ranges from 17% to 70%, depending on the patient's age and the degree of heat stress. Children left in cars for extended periods, athletes, children with cystic fibrosis, and children intoxicated with drugs or alcohol are at increased risk related to impairment of heat dissipation.

BOX 33-9	**Rewarming Measures for Hypothermia**

Passive External Rewarming Measures

Placement in a warm room environment
Warmed humidified oxygen
Warm blankets and clothing
Warmed intravenous fluid

Active Core Rewarming Measures*

Warmed peritoneal lavage
Warmed thoracic and pleural lavage
Hemodialysis and extracorporeal membrane
    oxygenation
Cardiopulmonary bypass

*Active core rewarming is best performed in a critical care setting.

Clinical Presentation of Heatstroke.   The symptoms of heatstroke include:

- Core temperature > 41 °C.
- Hot dry skin.
- Circulatory collapse.
- Severe central nervous system (CNS) dysfunction or seizures.
- Rhabdomyolysis or acute renal failure.

Treatment of Heatstroke.   Treatment for heatstroke is as follows:

- Remove the patient from heat stress, remove clothing, and immerse the patient in cool or iced water. All patients should be transported in air-conditioned vehicles. Monitor and protect the airway during immersion therapy.
- Moisten the skin with water and direct fans onto the patient's skin to increase convection and evaporative heat losses.
- Support circulation with room temperature crystalloid infusion initially. Inotropic support with dopamine or dobutamine may also be necessary.
- Although rare, electrolyte and glucose imbalances should be evaluated and treated.
- Myoglobinuria not cleared with fluid resuscitation may necessitate diuresis with mannitol or furosemide.

Patients with heatstroke should be rapidly transported to a critical care setting. Cooling procedures should continue during transport.

Near Drowning.   Near drowning is an environmental emergency that, although not exclusive to the pediatric population, is responsible for a large number of pediatric deaths and morbidity. Drowning is often the second or third leading cause of death in warm and water-oriented portions of the country. Males are much more frequently injured than females, and older infants and toddlers represent a disproportionate number of cases. Although swimming pools and natural bodies of water are often recognized as dangerous, other more innocuous situations such as bathtubs, buckets, and rain barrels are overlooked.

Teaching to parents and at-risk age groups as described previously in this module is imperative because of the frequently poor outcome of these injuries.

After submersion, patients may or may not aspirate fluid. Regardless of aspiration, hypoxemia is the major contributing factor to death and disability in these children. Although many body systems can be affected, the primary sites of insult are the central nervous and pulmonary systems. If fluid is aspirated, pulmonary gas exchange is impaired and quite often, increased capillary permeability leads to pulmonary edema. The aspirated fluid and resultant pulmonary edema leads to decreased pulmonary compliance, increased airway resistance, elevated pulmonary artery pressures, and decreased pulmonary flow. These factors cause a rapid decrease in the partial pressure of arterial oxygen related to the perfusion of nonventilated alveoli. Metabolic acidosis then follows the marked tissue hypoxia.

Hypoxemia is rapidly followed by unconsciousness and anoxia. Irreversible damage to the CNS occurs in 4 to 6 minutes. The role of the diving reflex in CNS preservation in these injuries is controversial. Although this reflex is much stronger in pediatric patients, many authors now believe that the diving reflex may only be helpful in those patients who become rapidly hypothermic as a result of cold-water submersion. Cardiovascular complications such as dysrhythmias and myocardial depression occur as a result of myocardial ischemia, acidosis, hypothermia, and intravascular volume changes.

Management of the Near-Drowning patient.
Pediatric survivors of near drowning almost universally have two things in common: limited submersion times and excellent initial resuscitative care.

On removal from the water, the airway should be secured and supplemental oxygen (100%) applied. Oxygen can be delivered via mask, BVM, or endotracheal intubation, depending on the patient's respiratory effort. Even patients who are awake and seemingly uninjured should receive supplemental oxygen to minimize the risk of hypoxemia and its related complications. If the patient is intubated, PEEP should be provided in an attempt to ameliorate atelectasis.

After oxygen and ventilatory support, reversal of metabolic acidosis should be addressed. This condition may improve with adequate ventilation but may also necessitate fluid resuscitation, inotropic support, and sodium bicarbonate therapy. Arterial blood gases are invaluable in guiding therapy and assessing the effectiveness of interventions.

Almost all children involved in submersion injuries, regardless of the time of year, have hypothermia. Rewarming as outlined previously should be provided for these patients.

After stabilization of the blood pressure, fluid restriction (one-half maintenance) and diuresis with furosemide (0.5 to 1.0 mg/kg/IV) for pulmonary edema may be indicated. Antibiotics are not indicated unless bacterial infection is documented.

Steroids in the initial resuscitation of these patients are also not indicated. Rarely, ongoing hemoglobinuria necessitates forced diuresis in these patients. Hyperglycemia and hypercapnia should be avoided because they contribute to CNS complications.

Predicting the eventual prognosis for these patients is extremely difficult in the acute setting. Many factors, including submersion time, water temperature, speed of resuscitation, and age of the child, seem to play a role in recovery. Emotional support of families during this period is a vital component of patient care.

SECONDARY SURVEY
After completion of the primary survey, a complete head-to-toe evaluation should be completed to assess for non–life-threatening injuries. This evaluation requires inspection, palpation, and where appropriate, auscultation and percussion of all body regions. Ideally, this survey should take place during transport rather than at the scene of injury.

Assessment for lacerations, fractures, abrasions, ecchymosis, ocular and dental injuries, and areas of swelling or edema are included in the secondary survey. Any part of the body not fully assessed during the primary survey should now be evaluated for injury. A full set of vital signs should also be completed.

If time permits, dressing of wounds and immobilization of fractures can now take place. Frequent reassessment of the patient's primary survey and effectiveness of medical interventions should be ongoing during transport. Neurovascular assessments before and after immobilization of fractures are necessary.

A patient weight either by caregiver history or by use of a length-based resuscitation tape should be ascertained. Cardiac monitors and pulse oximeters (if not already in place) should be applied. A radio report to receiving facilities should also be completed at this time.

NONACCIDENTAL TRAUMA OR NEGLECT

The ability to detect maltreatment and neglect is, unfortunately, a necessary skill for any person involved in the care of children. Careful consideration of patient findings and caregiver history is crucial in identification of children in need of intervention.

Abuse can be physical, emotional, or sexual. Acts that deprive children of their basic needs (e.g., food, clothing) are more appropriately termed *neglect*. All states have statutes that require the reporting of suspected maltreatment or neglect. Familiarization with local statutes and community support options is important.

Physicians, nurses, police officers, social workers, prehospital personnel, and other adults who interact with children should all be aware of historical and physical findings that are indicators for abuse or neglect. These findings are listed in Box 33-10. Keep in mind that some of these injuries can occur in the absence of abuse. A careful history of mechanisms and supervision is critical in children with these clinical findings.

BOX 33-10	**Indicators of Child Abuse or Neglect**

Historical Indicators of Maltreatment

Caregiver history incongruent with the mechanism of injury and actual injuries
Caregiver history incongruent with child's developmental abilities
Delay in seeking medical treatment
Patterned or unusual marks on the child's body
Injuries of various age or injuries of multiple types
A caregiver who denies knowledge of how an injury occurred
A caregiver whose response to the child's injury is not appropriate
A caregiver who expresses overconcern or underconcern for the seriousness of the child's injury
A recent change in caregivers
No preexisting medical condition that describes the child's injury
Inconsistencies or changes in the history provided
Emphasis of unimportant details or unrelated minor problems by the caregiver
Previous treatment for suspicious or unexplained injuries
Caregivers who seek medical attention for the child's injuries in other area hospitals
Bypassing a closer emergency department to seek care at a department further away
Tension or hostility between caregivers or tension or hostility directed at the child or staff
An uncooperative caregiver
Injuries that could have been prevented with closer supervision

Clinical Signs and Symptoms of Maltreatment

Behavioral
Inappropriate reactions to procedures
Frightened of caregiver

BOX 33-10	**Indicators of Child Abuse or Neglect—cont'd**

Goes easily to strangers; uncharacteristic for child's age

Extreme apprehension with other children's crying

Bruises

Potentially inflicted bruises include:

- Bruises to the face, neck, chest, abdomen, back, flank, thighs, or genitalia
- Bruises in various stages of healing
- Bruises suggestive of being struck by an object
- Pinch marks; pairs of crescent-shaped bruises
- Fingerprint or thumb patterns
- Bruises suggestive of being kicked
- Bruises to the mouth, gums, or buccal mucosa

Multiple or symmetric bruises or marks

Burns

Characteristics of intentionally inflicted burns include:

- Immersion burn; circumferential and often symmetric "stocking" pattern burns to the feet, "glovelike" pattern burns to hands, doughnut pattern burn to buttocks
- Burns with sharply demarcated edges without splash burns
- Ligature or rope burns to wrists, ankles, torso, or neck
- Cigarette or cigar burns, especially on typically concealed areas
- Contact burns; dry uniform print may be in configuration of an object used to cause the burn (e.g., grill)
- Symmetric burns
- Splash patterns in unusual sites (e.g., genitalia) or splash patterns with separated areas
- Burn to the dorsum of the hand

Delays in seeking treatment

Bites and other marks

Characteristics of potentially inflicted marks include:

- Down-turned lesions at the corners of the mouth, caused by being gagged
- Human bites; crescent-shaped bruises with circular lesions; individual tooth marks may be present; a distance greater than 3 cm between the third tooth or canine on each side indicates a bite caused by an adult or child older than 8 years of age

Head injuries suggestive of abuse:

- Skull fractures; multiple complex or bilateral skull fractures in an infant
- Cerebral edema with retinal hemorrhage (common in shaken baby syndrome)
- Subdural hematoma or subarachnoid hemorrhage
- Traction alopecia and scalp swelling from hair pulling

Skeletal fractures suggestive of abuse:

- Multiple fractures in different stages of healing or untreated healing fractures
- Unusual fractures; ribs, scapula, sternum, vertebrae, distal clavicle
- Metaphyseal injuries that have the appearance of tufts, chips, or "bucket handles" causing arcs of bone
- Spiral fractures of long bones
- Transverse fractures
- Repeated fractures at the same site
- Multiple, bilateral, or symmetric fractures

Modified from Emergency Nurses Association: *Emergency nursing pediatric course: provider manual*, ed 3, Des Plaines, IL, 2004, ENA.

SEXUAL ABUSE

Children who suffer *sexual abuse* may present vague somatic symptoms or behavioral changes. Sexual abuse should always be considered in patients with equivocal clinical findings. Other children may present for care after revealing abuse to a caregiver.[5]

Sign and symptoms of sexual abuse include the following:

- Clinical signs may be absent.
- Trauma to the genitals or rectum.
- Abnormal discharge from the vagina or penis.
- Bleeding from the rectum or abnormal bleeding from the vagina.
- Foreign bodies to the vagina, urethra, or rectum.
- Vaginal or rectal pain, itching, or discomfort.
- Sexually transmitted diseases beyond the period of the newborn.
- Pregnancy in young adolescents.
- Psychologic issues, which could include low self esteem, feelings of detachment, helplessness and self blame, fear of criticism or rejection, or intrusive images.

Care in the transport setting should include treatment of medical issues with psychologic support of the patient.

SHOCK AND SHOCK MANAGEMENT

The clinical presentation of *shock* in the pediatric patient can be extremely subtle. Clinicians therefore must be proficient in both history taking and physical examination to allow for prompt and effective intervention. Although many etiologies of shock exist, the underlying pathology is inadequate tissue oxygenation. The goal of all shock management is the support of both oxygen delivery and cardiac output.

ETIOLOGIES OF SHOCK

The several etiologies of shock include:

- Hypovolemic: Caused by a decrease in circulating blood or fluid volumes. Common causes include hemorrhage, vomiting, diarrhea, diabetic ketoacidosis, and burns.

- Cardiogenic: Caused by an inability of the myocardial tissue to provide an adequate cardiac output. Common causes include congenital heart disease, cardiomyopathy, drug intoxication, or cardiac arrhythmia.
- Distributive: Caused by vasodilation and peripheral pooling of blood. Common causes include sepsis, neurologic injuries, brain stem injury, anesthetic agents, anaphylaxis, and drug intoxication.
- Obstructive: Caused by obstruction in or compression of the great vessels, the aorta, or the heart. Common causes include pericardial tamponade, tension pneumothorax, mediastinal masses, or congenital anomalies.

ASSESSMENT AND DIAGNOSIS

Because of the subtle presentation in the early stages of shock, a careful history is extremely important in patients with suspected shock.[5,12] Important historical data include:

- Obvious bleeding or history of blood loss.
- Vomiting and diarrhea.
- Decreased fluid intake.
- Obvious sites of fluid loss, such as burn injuries.
- Congenital heart disease.
- Potential source or risk factors for infection.

Clinical signs and symptoms of shock include[5,12]:

- Altered level of consciousness. This can present in a variety of ways. Any alteration in level of consciousness should be attributed to decreased cerebral perfusion unless proved otherwise. Possible presentations of altered levels of consciousness include an inability to recognize caregivers, decreased levels of responsiveness to the environment, restlessness, anxiety, confusion, and irritability.
- Tachypnea.
- Tachycardia.
- Hypotension. This is an extremely late sign of shock in the pediatric patient because of the aggressive response to catecholamine release.

In early shock, the patient may be normotensive or have only a widened pulse pressure. Hypotension and bradycardia should always be recognized as ominous signs and aggressively treated.

- Changes in skin color. Similar to level of consciousness, skin changes have variable presentations. Children in shock may present with pale, mottled, ashen, or cyanotic skin. Environmental temperature can also cause skin color changes, so these findings should be taken into context with the remainder of the physical examination.
- Changes in pulse quality. Pulses may become weak, thready, or absent.
- Cool diaphoretic skin.
- Difficulty in obtaining a blood pressure.
- Decreased or absent bowel sounds.
- Decreased or absent urinary output.

Many of the preceding clinical signs and symptoms are not specific to shock and need to be considered in relation to history and patient presentation. Measures of end-organ perfusion such as level of consciousness, urinary output, heart rate, and pulse quality may be the most helpful assessment factors in patients with suspected shock.

Diagnostic aids for children in shock include:

- Cardiac monitor.
- Pulse oximeter. Poor perfusion may impede accurate oximetry readings. A normal oximetry reading does not preclude a patient's need for supplemental oxygen because oximetry is not a true measure of tissue oxygenation.
- Chest radiography to rule out cardiomegaly, pulmonary infection, or the presence of pneumothorax or hemothorax.
- Laboratory studies to assess complete blood count, glucose, and electrolyte levels. A lactate level should always be obtained.
- Urinary catheter for accurate measurement of urinary output.
- Arterial or capillary blood gases are helpful in assessment of acidosis caused by oxygen debt and anaerobic metabolism. They also assist with determining the ventilatory status of the patient. Serial blood gases can be used to gauge the effectiveness of clinical intervention.
- Cultures of blood, body fluids, sputum, cerebrospinal fluid, wounds, and indwelling devices for determination of sources of potential infection.
- Urinalysis for assessment for the presence of blood, ketones, bacteria, and glucose and for specific gravity measurements.

TREATMENT OF SHOCK

Regardless of the etiologic basis for shock, the basic tenets of care remain the same: provision of supplemental oxygen, support of ventilation, and support of an adequate cardiac output. The manner in which these goals are achieved is dependent on patient illness or injury. Methods of oxygenation and ventilation and treatment for specific injuries (i.e., tension pneumothorax) have been discussed previously in this module. The direct cause of shock should be treated while patient support is provided. This section deals with fluid resuscitation and support of cardiac output.

Hypovolemic Shock

The goal in supporting cardiac output in *hypovolemic shock* is the replacement of lost circulating volume. A child only has 80 mL/kg of circulating volume, so small amounts of fluid or blood loss can cause serious physiologic effects. Before fluid resuscitation can begin, venous access must be obtained. Sites for venous access in children include[4,9,10]:

- Percutaneous peripheral attempts (limited to two attempts).
- Intraosseous needle placement.
- Saphenous vein cutdown.
- Percutaneous placement in the femoral vein.
- Percutaneous placement in the subclavian vein.
- Percutaneous placement in the external jugular vein. This site should not be used if a cervical collar is applied.
- Percutaneous placement in the internal jugular vein.

Fluid Resuscitation in Hypovolemic Shock.

After venous access is obtained, resuscitation should quickly follow. Resuscitation begins with a 20-mL/kg bolus of warmed Ringer's lactate or normal saline solution. Because only approximately one third of crystalloid infusions remains in the intravascular space, this bolus may need to be repeated two or three times.

When beginning the third fluid bolus, consideration to giving 10 mL/kg of type-specific or O-negative packed red blood cells should be entertained. Children who need aggressive fluid resuscitation as described should receive consultation with a pediatric surgeon or intensivist, depending on the etiology of the hypovolemia. Transfer to an appropriate center should not be delayed. Fluid resuscitation can be continued during transport.

Children should be closely monitored for improvement in hemodynamic status during fluid resuscitation. Signs of hemodynamic improvement include[5]:

- Improved capillary refill.
- Slowing of the heart rate to the age-appropriate rate with improvement in other physiologic signs.
- Increased pulse pressure.
- Return of normal skin color.
- Increased warmth of extremities.
- Clearing of sensorium.
- Increased systolic blood pressure (>80 mm Hg).
- Urinary output of 1 to 2 mL/kg/h. Urinary output varies with age. Urinary output for newborns to 1 year of age is 2 mL/kg/h, for toddlers is 1.5 mL/kg/h, and for older children is 1 mL/kg/h.

After fluid resuscitation, maintenance fluids must be provided on a kilogram–body weight basis.

The formula for calculation of intravenous maintenance fluid is:

- First 10 kg of body weight: 100 mL/kg/24 h
- Second 10 kg of body weight: 50 mL/kg/24 h
- Any weight greater than 20 kg: 20 mL/kg/24 h

With use of this formula, a 40-kg child needs 1900 mL over 24 hours (1000 mL for the first 10 kg, 500 mL for the second 10 kg, and 400 mL for the remaining 20 kg) or an hourly IV rate of 80 mL/h.

Prevention of hypothermia as a result of fluid resuscitation is imperative. The use of warmed fluids, warmed room environments, and judicious patient exposure should all be included in the care of these patients.

Cardiogenic Shock

Support of patients with *cardiogenic shock* is focused on the improvement of cardiac output. In comparison with hypovolemic shock, these patients more often need intravenous inotropic medications for output support. The need for inotropic support does not preclude the need for fluid resuscitation.

The role of fluid resuscitation may be difficult to ascertain in patients with cardiac dysfunction. An initial 20-mL/kg bolus of Ringer's lactate or 0.9 normal saline solution (NS) is generally safe in most patients. Colloids may be more efficient volume expanders in patients with cardiac dysfunction, but the risk of sensitivity reactions and complications of colloid administration should be considered. Obviously, if the cardiac output is compromised by cardiac arrhythmia, prompt correction of the arrhythmia following ACLS/PALS protocols is indicated.

Patients at risk (congenital heart disease, viral cardiomyopathy, drug ingestions) should all have consideration given for inotropic support early in the course of care. Correction of electrolyte imbalances and acid-base imbalances may also be necessary in these patients. Laboratory studies are needed to aid in diagnosis and treatment.

Inotropic agents that may be indicated for the treatment of cardiogenic shock include epinephrine hydrochloride, dopamine hydrochloride, and dobutamine hydrochloride. Other medications that may be indicated in the treatment of patients with cardiogenic shock include amiodarone, lidocaine hydrochloride, sodium bicarbonate, and glucose. Blood gases should be used as guide. Hypoglycemia should be monitored with evaluation of whole blood glucose.

Invasive monitoring, which allows for central venous pressure monitoring, arterial pressure measurement, and cardiac pressure monitoring, can be extremely helpful in both diagnosis and treatment of these patients. Measures of patient improvement are identical to those discussed with hypovolemic shock. Maintenance fluids may be decreased depending on underlying cardiac function.

Distributive Shock

Management of patients with *distributive shock* requires an astute and skilled pediatric clinician. Distributive shock often combines the need for fluid resuscitation with the need for inotropic support. The balancing of these interventions can vary dramatically from patient to patient. Sepsis is by far the most common cause of distributive shock, but CNS dysfunction in the poisoned or traumatically injured patient should also be considered.

As in hypovolemia, aggressive fluid replacement is always necessary in patients with distributive shock. The underlying cause of the shock should be addressed while fluid and inotropic support are provided. If sepsis is suspected, antibiotic therapy should be anticipated and discussed with both the referring and the receiving physician. The range of possible infectious sources in pediatric patients is beyond the scope of this module, but concern for caregiver exposure in transport bears discussion.

As in cardiogenic shock, invasive pressure monitoring can be extremely helpful in determination of the appropriateness and effectiveness of fluid or inotropic agents. Sepsis should be managed with specific protocols based on current evidence.

The use of antipyretics (acetaminophen or ibuprofen) in sepsis and methylprednisolone in acute spinal injuries may also be indicated. In addition to the laboratory values discussed previously, evaluation of leukocytosis and white blood cell count differentials are also indicated in the patient with suspected sepsis.

Obstructive Shock

The initial goal in management of *obstructive shock* is the determination of the etiology of the obstruction. Some etiologies are amenable to emergent intervention (i.e., tension pneumothorax or pericardial tamponade), whereas others are much more complicated (i.e., coarctation of the aorta in a newborn). As with most shock therapies, patients with obstructive shock usually are helped with judicious fluid resuscitation and some may need inotropic support.

The roles of fluid resuscitation and inotropic support vary depending on the etiology of the obstruction and the ability of the clinician to treat the obstruction. The most important factor is prompt diagnosis of the obstruction and emergent intervention. In the trauma patient, careful physical examination coupled with a patient and injury history can assist in diagnosis.

The prompt diagnosis of shock and appropriate clinical intervention are valuable skills in any clinician involved in the care of children.

PREPARATION FOR TRANSPORT

The preparation for transport of the pediatric patient should include use of the appropriate restraint system for transport. Each state has regulations that describe the type of device that should be used, based on the weight of the child. Restraint can be particularly challenging depending on what illness or injuries the child has. However, the transport team must ensure that the child is appropriately restrained (Figure 33-5) whether transported via ground or air.

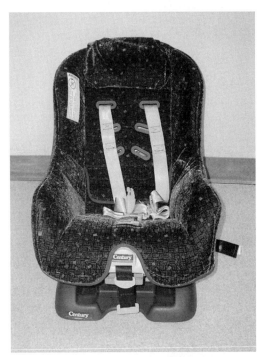

FIGURE 33-5 **Infant and toddler car seat.**

The family should always be included. There is probably no greater cause of fear and anxiety in a parent than the illness or injury of a child. Even though as transport personnel we must focus on the needs of the child, the family cannot be ignored. Each program determines whether a family member can accompany the child during transport. Policies and procedures should be in place related to providing information for the family and how they may accompany the child, if they are allowed. A further discussion of the role of the family in transport is contained in Chapter 38.

SUMMARY

The care of ill and injured children is a challenging facet of transport care. Decisions based on an understanding of growth and development and physiologic differences in this population are essential for reducing pediatric morbidity and mortality.

CASE STUDY

An 8-year-old bicycle rider without a helmet was struck on a residential road by a passenger car traveling at approximately 35 miles per hour. Local emergency medical services (EMS) arrived 8 minutes after the incident, and helicopter transport was requested. The transport team arrived on the scene 15 minutes after the crash to find an 8-year-old girl supine on the roadway and receiving assisted ventilation by EMS. Decerebrate posturing was also noted on initial examination. The patient had, by EMS report, suffered two episodes of emesis, and suctioning of the airway was difficult because of trismus.

The patient's airway was partially obstructed with emesis, and modified jaw lift maneuvers did little to improve airway patency. The patient was spontaneously breathing at 6 to 8 breaths per minute but was supported by EMS at a rate of 16 to 18 breaths per minute with a bag-valve-mask and 100% oxygen. Cervical immobilization was provided manually by EMS. A strong radial pulse was palpated at a rate of 140 beats per minute. The child's skin was moist and cool with a capillary refill of 5 seconds.

With use of a length-based tape, the child's weight was estimated at 24 kg, and preparation for rapid sequence induction and endotracheal intubation was begun. An IV of 1000 mL 0.9 normal saline solution had been initiated by first responders with an 18-gauge needle in the patient's right antecubital area and was infusing. Fluid boluses of 20 mg/kg had been administered.

An intravenous dose of weight-based atropine was given, followed by lidocaine 36 mg. Etomidate 8 mg was given IVP, and cricoid pressure was applied. After etomidate administration, succinylcholine 48 mg was also given intravenously, and flaccid paralysis was quickly achieved. After effective neuromuscular block, suction of the oropharynx was performed, and the patient was orally intubated with a 6.0 endotracheal tube, secured at the lip line at 18 cm. After intubation, breath sounds were auscultated bilaterally, and chest expansion was equal. No breath sounds were auscultated over the epigastrium, and end-tidal carbon dioxide was detected with a disposable CO_2 detector.

While a cervical collar and lateral immobilization were placed and the patient was secured to a padded backboard, a repeat primary survey revealed an airway protected by an endotracheal tube, a respiratory rate of 16 via bag-valve-mask ventilation with 100% oxygen, and a pulse rate of 150. The skin remained moist and cool with a 5-second to 7-second capillary refill. A saline bolus of 500 mL was begun. The patient remained decerebrate with midrange reactive pupils. At this point, the child was loaded into the aircraft and evacuated from the scene.

En route to the hospital, a second intravenous line was initiated with 1000 mL 0.9 normal saline solution and an 18-gauge needle in the patient's right forearm. A secondary survey of the patient revealed a large hematoma to the left temporoparietal area with bloody drainage from the left ear. No Battle's sign or raccoon eyes were appreciated. No nasal discharge was noted. The face and teeth were stable to palpation. The neck was supple, and the trachea was midline. The clavicles and shoulders were without obvious injury. The chest continued to expand symmetrically, and no crepitus or instability *was appreciated. The patient's abdomen was flat with abrasions to the left upper quadrant. The pelvis was stable to palpation, and femoral pulses were weak but palpable. No obvious injury to the lower extremities was seen, but decerebrate posturing continued. Examination of the upper extremities revealed a deformity of the left forearm, but all peripheral pulses were palpable.*

After completion of the third fluid bolus, vital signs were blood pressure 114/60 mm Hg, pulse 110 beats/min, and respiratory rate 16 breaths/min via bagvalve-mask ventilation. The end-tidal CO_2 detector continued to detect exhaled carbon dioxide.

Five minutes from arrival at the pediatric trauma center, the patient had a generalized tonic-clonic seizure that was quickly resolved with administration of 2.4 mg of intravenous lorazepam. A repeat neurologic examination revealed continued decerebrate posturing and a dilated 8-mm left pupil and a right pupil of 2 mm.

Neither pupil was reactive to light. After report to the receiving facility, the patient was hot offloaded from the aircraft and admitted directly to the emergency department for evaluation.

An emergent CT scan revealed a large left epidural hemorrhage that required emergent operative evacuation. An abdominal CT scan after evacuation of the epidural revealed a small splenic laceration that did not require operative intervention. A radial/ulnar fracture of the left arm required closed reduction and was casted.

The patient was extubated on postoperative day 2 and was transferred from the intensive care unit on postoperative day 4. Ten days after injury, the patient was discharged home neurologically intact. Her prognosis for a full recovery was excellent.

REFERENCES

1. American Academy of Pediatrics: *Air and ground transport of neonatal and pediatric patients*, ed 3, Elk Grove Village, IL, 2007, AAP.
2. American College of Surgeons, Committee on Trauma: *Advanced trauma life support for doctors: student manual*, ed 8, Chicago, 2008, American College of Surgeons.
3. American Heart Association: Part 12: pediatric advanced life support, *Circulation* 112:IV-167–IV-187, 2005.
4. de Caen AR, Reis A, Bhutta A: Vascular access and drug therapy in pediatric resuscitation, *Pediatr Clin North Am* 55: 909-927, 2008.
5. Emergency Nurses Association: *Emergency nursing pediatric course: provider manual*, ed 3, Des Plaines, IL, 2004, ENA.
6. Engel JK: *Pediatric assessment*, ed 5, St Louis, 2006, Mosby Elsevier.
7. Fleisher GR, Ludwig S: *Pediatric emergency medicine*, ed 4, Philadelphia, 2000, Lippincott, Williams & Wilkins.
8. Froh DK: Alterations of pulmonary function in children. In McCance KL, Huether SE, editors: *Pathophysiology: the basis for disease in adults and children*, ed 5, St Louis, 2006, Elsevier Mosby.
9. Horowitz R, Rozenfeld RA: Pediatric critical care interfacility transport, *Clin Pediatr Emerg Med* 8: 190-202, 2007.
10. Kleinman ME, Srinivasan V: Postresuscitation care, *Pediatr Clin North Am* 55:943-967, 2008.
11. Kortbeek JB, Ali J, Brenneman F, et al: Advanced trauma life support: ed 8, the evidence for change, *J Trauma Injury Infect Crit Care* 64(6):1638-1650, 2008.
12. Moloney PA: Pediatric trauma. In McQuillan KA, Makic MB, Whalen E, editors: *Trauma nursing from resuscitation through rehabilitation*, Philadelphia, 2009, Saunders Elsevier.
13. McCowan CL, Swanson ER, Thomas F, et al: Outcomes of pediatric trauma patients transported from rural and urban scenes, *Air Med J* 27(2):78-83, 2008.
14. Nolan JP, Neumar RW, Adrie C, et al: ILOR consensus statement, *Resuscitation* 79:350-379, 2008.
15. Orenstein JB: Prehospital pediatric airway management, *Clin Pediatr Emerg Med* 7:31-37, 2006.
16. Sanders M: *Mosby's paramedic textbook*, ed 3, St Louis, 2007, Elsevier Mosby.
17. Soar J, Deakin CD, Nolan JP, et al: European resuscitation council guidelines for resuscitation 2005: section 7: cardiac arrest in special circumstances, *Resuscitation* 67S1:S135-S170, 2005.
18. Turkoski BB, Lance BR, Bonfiglio MF: *Drug information handbook for advanced practice*, ed 9, Hudson, OH, 2008, Lexi-Comp, Inc.

ADDITIONAL REFERENCES

Jaimovich DG, Vidyasagar D: *Handbook of pediatric and neonatal transport*, ed 2, St Louis, 2002, Mosby.
Slota M, editor: *AACN core curriculum for pediatric critical care*, ed 2, available at www.aacn.org bookstore, accessed February 2009.
Verger J, Lebel RM: *AACN procedure manual for pediatric acute and critical care*, Philadelphia, 2007, Saunders.

MILITARY PATIENT TRANSPORT

Christopher T. Paige, Timothy L. Hudson

Special thanks to Teresa Duquette-Frame, Kathleen Flarity, Debra Krupa, and George Brand of their expertise and guidance.

COMPETENCIES

1. Describe military patient transport systems used during humanitarian and combat action.
2. Describe military patient movement through levels of care provided within the military medical system.
3. Identify different levels of military medical capability provided by each service (Air Force, Army, and Navy).
4. Identify military patient transport platforms (air and ground).
5. Identify the military medical training needed for transport personnel.
6. Recognize special military patient transport situations (search and rescue, peacetime).

This chapter describes the United States military patient transport system during combat operations. Not unlike the US medical system, the deployed military healthcare system is an integrated system that accomplishes triage and emergency treatment and then transports the patient to the appropriate level of care or returns the member to duty. In essence, the military builds a state-of-the-art trauma system in some of the most austere and dangerous locations for humanitarian or wartime

contingences.[3] At the point of injury (POI), first aid is initiated. The patient is then rapidly transported through multiple medical support levels to include emergency medical response (Figure 34-1), advanced trauma surgery (Figure 34-2), and patient transport (Figures 34-3 and 34-4) towards hospital admission.

Within the Department of Defense, the Air Force, Army, and Navy each have their own independent service surgeons general and doctrines. In the past, by design, the different medical services generally

The opinions or assertions contained herein are the private views of the authors and are not to be considered as official or as reflecting the views of the Department of the Army, Department of the Air Force, Department of the Navy or the Department of Defense. Cleared for release by H. Pearson PAIRS case # AETC-2008-0140.

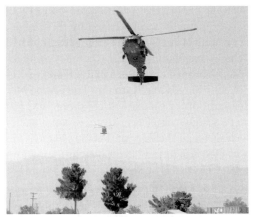

FIGURE 34-1   Two Army UH-60 Black Hawks arriving on scene to emergently evacuate injured soldiers.

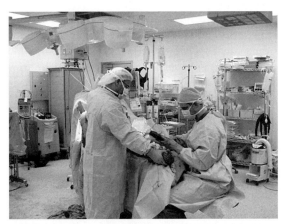

FIGURE 34-2   Military patient in advanced trauma surgery in forward location.

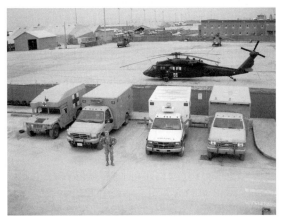

FIGURE 34-3   Some military ground and air intratheater transport capabilities.

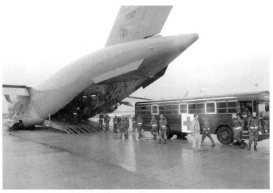

FIGURE 34-4   Loading patients for intertheater patient transportation on Air Force C-17.

"took care of their own," with each service caring for its members (i.e., Army soldiers seeing Army providers) and the Marines being cared for by the Navy. This system made sense because each of the military services is charged with a unique mission. The Navy and Marines primarily are tasked with the oceans and coastal areas, the Army with land security, and the Air Force with aerospace. However, today's military operations are vastly more complicated, with the Navy, Marines, Army, and Air Force frequently sharing missions in and around the battle space in what are called Joint Operations. In addition, coalition partners and host nation military resources are frequently embedded together in operations. Joint Operations present a challenge to the military patient transport system. The interdependent Air Force, Army, and Navy medical transport capabilities must be interoperable and interchangeable.[11]

LEVELS OF CARE

To best understand US military patient transport, one must first understand the different levels of patient care. After being introduced to the military medical levels of care, one can more easily understand the different transportation platforms, capacities, and resources found in the combat arena.

The *military levels* refer to the capability of care and are in sequential order of a patient's movement through the military medical system. Figure 34-5 shows how traditional combat injuries move from a forward line of troops (front), level I, to definitive care (rear), level IV. This can be somewhat confusing at first

Forward line of troops

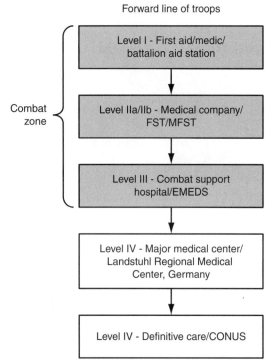

FIGURE 34-5   **Patient movement through levels in traditional battle lines; front, or forward line of troops.**

as it is directly opposite to the civilian system of trauma levels. In the military system, the lower the level, the less capability to provide the patient with a full compliment of medical and surgical services. The purpose of creating graduating levels is for service members to be evaluated, treated, and released to duty at the lowest level possible. If medical care needed by the service member cannot be administered at a certain level of care, then they are transported to a higher level. Of note, in the urban environment, like Afghanistan and Iraq, where there is no "front," transportation of a patient directly from level I to level III care for definitive care is not uncommon (Figure 34-6).[8] In recent conflicts surgical intervention has been moved closer to combat, which has blurred the lines between levels I and II. The levels presented here are adopted from the Army model but are similar among each service.

POINT OF INJURY CARE

Point of injury care begins with patient assessment and triage, conducted immediately to identify whether life-saving measures must be taken. These measures encompass actions such as maintenance of airway, hemorrhage control, and prevention of shock. POI care is accomplished by the individual first on scene, which can be a nonmedical provider.

The *nonmedical provider* (combat soldier or marine) is trained to perform first-aid procedures to begin early life-saving treatment. The primary focus is stabilization of the patient condition and transport to a higher level of care. This is not the only care available to the warrior. The *corpsman* or *medic* is a trained emergency medical technician with the combat team that is on scene to provide trauma care. In addition to emergency care, many are trained in public health, disease prevention, and evaluation of diseases and injuries that are not related to battle.

LEVEL I

For support of the many medical needs of a security force, small medical teams are placed far forward near combat operations *(level I)*.[8] They are commonly referred to as *Battalion Aid Stations* (BASs). The team includes a physician, physician assistant, and medics. Traditionally, surgical intervention is minimal at the BAS. Recently, in an effort to bring more surgical capability closer to the POI, trauma teams that were built into the level II facility were brought forward and attached to the BAS. The Marines (staffed by Navy medical providers) moved a Forward Resuscitative Surgical System (FRSS) attached to the BAS, as did the Army with their Forward Surgical Team (FST) during the Iraq War in 2003.[7] This shift forward of surgical capability has blurred level I and level II care by increasing surgical capability closer to the POI.

LEVEL II

Level II care has more capabilities than the BAS. These facilities, like level I, are 100% mobile (Figure 34-7). They do, however, have limited inpatient bed capacity with increased access to primary care, laboratory, emergency dental, combat stress/mental health, optometry, and basic radiography and can be augmented with surgical assets. Each service has similar but slightly modified capability at level II. The patient is triaged to determine transport priority based on current medical assets and the patient's condition. At times, patients can be treated and returned to duty. Usually this decision is made immediately or before 72 hours.[8] If needed, emergent care, including resuscitation, is provided and more complete medical and surgical measures are taken. Because the level

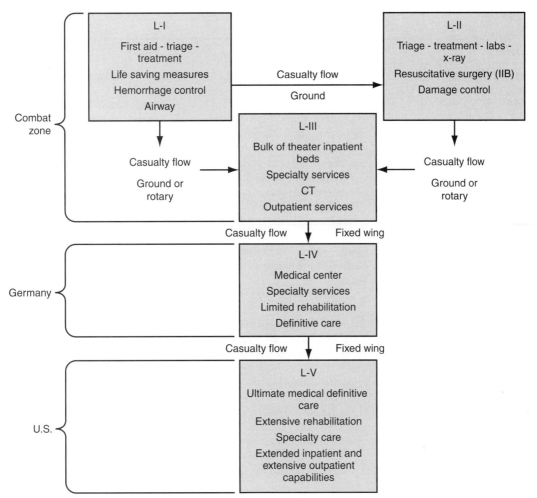

FIGURE 34-6   **Patient movement in urban environments such as Afghanistan and Iraq.**

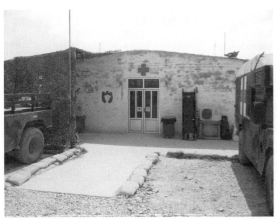

FIGURE 34-7   **Emergency entrance to level II facility.**

II facility is close to combat operations, the relative safety of the tactical situation at times dictates what extent of medical care can be administered. Recent data suggest minimal intervention at level II (2 hours or less) provides a better outcome.[5]

The Navy can place an Amphibious Ready Group (ARG) offshore during a humanitarian crisis or war. This ARG can include up to six ships with assault helicopters on their decks. These helicopters are used for assault but can double as both amphibious assault and patient transport platforms. One ship in the ARG is called a Casualty Receiving and Treatment Ship. It has up to 48 beds, six operating rooms (ORs), and 17 intensive care beds. See Box 34-1 for more information on level II capabilities among the services.

BOX 34-1	**Level II Capabilities**

US Army

Treatment Platoon

- Basic/emergency treatment is continued.
- Packed Red Blood Cells (type O, Rh positive and negative), limited radiography, laboratory, and dental.
- 20 to 40 cots with 72-hour holding.
- No surgical capability.

Forward Surgical Team (FST)

- Continuous operations for up to 72 hours.
- Life-saving resuscitative surgery, including general, orthopedic, and limited neurosurgical procedures.
- Twenty-person team with one orthopedic and three general surgeons, two nurse anesthetists, critical care nurses, and technicians.
- Operational within 1 hour of arrival at the supported company.
- May be transported by ground, fixed-wing, or helicopter; some are airborne deployable.
- Two operating tables for a maximum of 10 cases per day and for a total of 30 operations within 72 hours.
- Postoperative intensive care for up to 8 patients for up to 6 hours.

US Air Force

Mobile Field Surgical Team (MFST)

- Five-person team (general surgeon, orthopedist, anesthetist, emergency medicine physician, and OR nurse/technician).
- Ten life-saving/limb-saving procedures in 24 to 48 hours from five backpacks.
- Designed to augment an aid station or flight line clinic.

Small Portable Expeditionary Air Medical Rapid Response (SPEARR) Team

- Ten-person team: five-person MFST, three-person critical care transport/two-person preventive medicine team (flight surgeon, public health officer).
- Stand alone capable: 7 days.
- Ten life-saving/limb-saving procedures in 24 to 48 hours.
- Designed to provide surgical support, basic primary care, postoperative critical care, and preventive medicine for early phase of deployment.
- Highly mobile unit, with all equipment fitting in a one pallet-sized trailer.

Expeditionary Medical Support (EMEDS) Basic

- Medical and surgical support for an airbase, sick call, resuscitative surgery, dental care, limited laboratory and radiography capability.
- Twenty-five staff includes SPEARR.
- Four holding beds/one OR table.
- Ten life-saving/limb-saving procedures in 24 to 48 hours.
- Can augment: 10 beds/56-person staff (EMEDS + 10).

US Navy

Forward Resuscitative Surgical System (FRSS)

- Rapid assembly, highly mobile.
- Resuscitative surgery for 18 patients within 48 hours without resupply.
- One OR, two surgeons (general/orthopedic).
- No holding capability.
- No intrinsic evacuation capability.
- Typically augmented with an en route care team to allow for evacuation capability.
- Also requires host unit for logistics and security.

Surgical Company

- Provides surgical care for a Marine Expeditionary Force. Basis of allocation is one per infantry regiment.
- Three ORs, 60-bed capability.
- Patient holding time up to 72 hours.
- Stabilizing surgical procedures.

Casualty Receiving and Treatment Ships (CRTS)

- Provides medical care for an Amphibious Ready Group.
- Helicopter assets with casualty receiving capability.
- Laboratory, radiography.
- Fleet Surgical Team: three to four physicians, one surgeon, one certified registered nurse anesthetist, and support staff.
- Augment: two orthopedic, two general surgeons, and oral maxillofacial surgeon with dental unit.
- Excellent casualty flow capability because of large helicopter flight deck.
- Forty-seven to 48 beds, four to six ORs, 17 intensive care beds.

After stabilization, the patient is packaged for transport to the next level of care (level III), a Combat Support Hospital (CSH; pronounced "cash"; Army) or a Fleet Hospital (Navy).

LEVEL III

Level III medical assets are the highest level of medical care available within the combat zone and contain the majority of hospital beds within the theater.[8] These level III facilities are similar in capability to a US civilian trauma center. Most are modular (Figure 34-8), with the exception of the Fleet Hospital. Modular build allows medical planners to tailor medical personnel and size of facility to actual or predicted requirements. The Fleet Hospital comes with up to 500 beds and is comparable with the Army level III hospital. It is equipped to provide resuscitation, initial wound surgery, and postoperative treatment. Patients at a level III hospital are stabilized for continued transport through the system or returned to duty. Level III capability is similar between the services and has proven to be interoperable, interchangeable, and interdependent with deployment rotations.[8] The Army CSH level III facilities can have up to 248 beds, which are usually divided into 48 intensive care unit (ICU) beds and 200 intermediate care beds (medical/surgical). Patients who need minimal care are handled by a 120-bed Minimal Care Medical Detachment. The

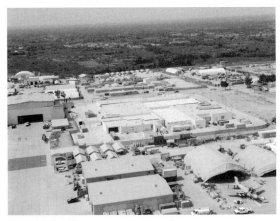

FIGURE 34-8 **Level III facility. Note proximity to airport for intertheater movement back to level IV or V facility.**

surgical capability can provide up to six OR tables with a maximum of 96 operating hours per day. Surgical services include general, orthopedic, urologic, dental, and oral maxillofacial. Units include a robust blood bank, laboratory, radiology (to include computed tomographic [CT] scan and magnetic resonance imagery [MRI]), nutrition, and physical therapy and a specialty clinic section. This clinic provides patient services including sick call for staff and attached units. It also provides preventative medical surveillance capability to monitor disease and nonbattle injury. This clinic also provides outpatient psychiatry and inpatient neuropsychiatric consultation services.

In the corps CSH, the hospital Company A (84 beds) and hospital Company B (164 beds), with support in headquarters sections and transportation element, are completely functional hospital companies. Company A provides hospitalization for up to 84 patients and consists of two wards that provide critical care nursing for up to 24 patients and three wards that provide intermediate care nursing for up to 60 patients. Company B provides hospitalization for up to 164 patients, consisting of two wards that provide critical care nursing for up to 24 patients and seven wards that provide intermediate care nursing for up to 140 patients.

An Air Force level III, traditionally the Expeditionary Medical Support Hospital (EMEDS) +25, is a 25-bed facility. It includes 84 personnel and two OR tables that can accomplish 20 operations within 48 hours. The Air Force EMEDS +25 capability can be increased by the addition of specialty teams such as vascular/cardiothoracic; neurosurgery; obstetrics/gynecology (OB/GYN); ear, nose, and throat; and ophthalmology.

LEVEL IV

Traditionally, *level IV* medical care was provided by field hospitals within theater but outside combat operations. Iraq and Afghanistan operations have patients transported directly from level III assets to a fixed facility, Landstuhl Regional Medical Center in Germany (Figure 34-9). Humanitarian operations (a natural disaster, such as tsunami, hurricane, earthquake) frequently use the naval ship Mercy or Comfort as a level IV platform (Figure 34-10).

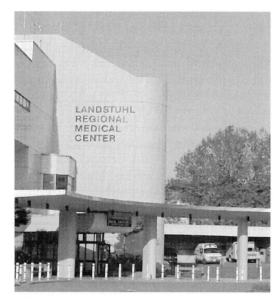

FIGURE 34-9   **Landstuhl Regional Medical Center, a level IV facility.**

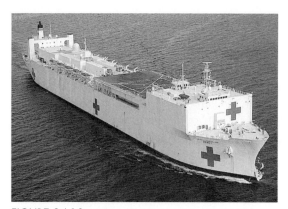

FIGURE 34-10   **Level IV hospital ship, T-AH Mercy, used when medical care is needed near shore.**

The level IV facility is designed for treatment and evaluation of patients with the goal of return to duty. If patients are unable to return to combat duty, they are transported to their home unit or to one of the level V hospitals in the United States.

LEVEL V
Level V hospitals, located in the United States, provide complete medical care and maintain all general and specialty capabilities. These include

Department of Defense hospitals such as Bethesda National Naval Medical Center and Walter Reed Army Medical Center. The focus in these facilities is on medical, surgical, rehabilitative, and convalescent care.

MILITARY PATIENT TRANSPORTATION

Within the military medical system, during combat operations, patient transportation involves moving patients intratheater and intertheater.[12] This movement takes the full effort of the military medical system. For example, it is not unusual for a wounded Marine to be treated initially by another Marine, followed by a Navy corpsman, an Army surgeon, and an Air Force flight nurse, all during transport through levels I to V. Common means of military patient transport are summarized in Table 34-1 and discussed in the following sections.

INTRATHEATER: LEVEL I TO LEVEL III
Point of Injury Care Providers
En route care is a continuation of care during transport.[12] En route care builds with critical care capability as the patient moves through the system. Rapid care and transport helps return individuals to their units or moves them out of theater to a facility that can provide more definitive care.[9] To provide rapid care, medical and surgical assets have been moved closer to combat operations. Each soldier is trained in first aid, "self aid and buddy care," or combat casualty care. Ideally, help comes from an embedded medical specialist: the team "doc," a Navy corpsman or Army combat medic with specific training for resuscitation, triage, and packaging for transport. They are trained in combat arms as well as emergency medical treatment. These professionals are trained in spinal stabilization and extrication, advanced airway support (e.g., intubation and cricothyrotomy), and emergency surgical procedures, such as chest decompression, use of tourniquet, and emergency laceration repair to stop bleeding.

Notable differences between the Army and Navy are found in regards to how they support en route casualty evacuation. For the most part, the US Army uses a dedicated medical evacuation platform (air or ground

TABLE 34-1	**Common Means of Military Patient Transport**		
	Title	**Level**	**Litter Spaces/Seats Available**
	Fireman's Carry	Intratheater CASEVAC or MEDEVAC	One example of carries from POI
	North Atlantic Treaty Organization (NATO) Litter	Intratheater and Intertheater POI through level V MEDEVAC and Aeromedical Evacuation	All transport platforms are designed to NATO litter specifications
	M997 4 litter HMMWV	Intratheater POI to level III CASEVAC or MEDEVAC	4 Litter (max) 8 Ambulatory (max) Combination of litter/ ambulatory 2/4
	Black Hawk UH-60A	Intratheater POI to Level III CASEVAC or MEDEVAC	6 Litter (max) 7 Ambulatory (max) Combination of litter/ ambulatory 3/4 (max)

(Continued)

TABLE 34-1	Common Means of Military Patient Transport—cont'd		
	Title	**Level**	**Litter Spaces/Seats Available**
	Sea Knight CH-46	Intratheater POI to Level III CASEVAC or MEDEVAC	15 Litter (max) 25 Ambulatory (max) Combination of litter/ ambulatory 6/15 (max)
	Ambus	Intratheater MEDEVAC	20 Litter (max) 44 Ambulatory (max)
	Hercules C-130	Intratheater Level III to IV Aeromedical Evacuation	74 Litter (max) 92 Ambulatory (max) Combination of litter/ ambulatory 50/27
	Globemaster C-17	Intertheater Level III to V Aeromedical Evacuation	36 Litter (max) 102 Ambulatory (max) Combination of litter/ ambulatory 36/54

TABLE 34-1	**Common Means of Military Patient Transport—cont'd**		
	Title	**Level**	**Litter Spaces/Seats Available**
	KC-135	Intertheater Level III to V Aeromedical Evacuation	15 Litter (max) 50 Ambulatory (max) Combination of litter/ ambulatory 15/24
	Osprey CV-22	Air Force Special Operations	9 Litter 24 Ambulatory
	MRAP Ambulance or RG33 Heavy Armored Ground Ambulance (HAGA)	Intratheater From POI to Level I to III	4 Litter 8 Ambulatory
	Mercy T-AH	Intertheater Intratheater Level III	1000 Hospital beds (max) Combination of services 21 Operating rooms/20 recovery 80 Intensive care beds 900 Medical/surgical

ambulance) that is staffed with trained flight medics or nurses (medical evacuation or MEDEVAC).[6] The Navy often uses transport vehicles designed for multiple use (air or ground). This use of vehicle of opportunity (not necessarily fitted for a medical specific mission) is called casualty evacuation (or CASEVAC).

Casualty Evacuation

Once POI care is provided and the decision to transport has been made, a number of options are exercised. Usually, the most rapid option is referred to as casualty evacuation or *CASEVAC*. These patients are moved from the POI to medical treatment with a military vehicle of opportunity. With minimal defense systems, when the scene is unsafe, a medical transport platform is not typically brought into active combat zones.[1] CASEVAC transport to a level I to III facility may or may not be coordinated or announced. CASEVAC is frequently used in military operations in urban terrain because of the limited number of landing zones for rotor-wing medical evacuation platforms. At times, application of first aid/buddy aid and rapid transport to the nearest treatment facility in a vehicle of opportunity is faster and safer. Basically, the military on-scene are prepared to 'load-and-go' to the nearest medical facility.

Ground Transportation

The US Army has the largest intratheater medical ground evacuation capability for collecting, regulating, and caring for US military personnel. Numerous medical *ground transport* platforms exist. These platforms are largely dedicated field ambulance vehicles that are operated by two basic emergency medical technicians with typical basic life support (BLS) medical supplies and equipment similar to that found in a civilian ambulance.

Traditionally, casualties are first taken to a BAS or medical platoon. From the POI, the casualty can be taken to one of these areas directly on a military stretcher called a North Atlantic Treaty Organization (NATO) litter (see Table 34-1) or more frequently by tactical vehicles such as the armored High Mobility Multipurpose Wheeled Vehicle (HMMWV; pronounced HUMVEE), Stryker, or Mine Resistant Ambush Protected (MRAP) vehicle (RG33 Heavy Armored Ground Ambulance [HAGA]).

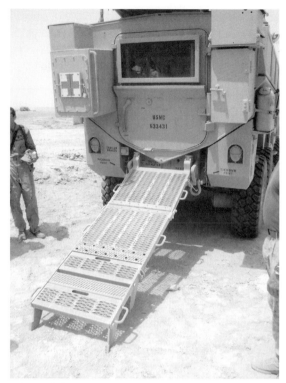

FIGURE 34-11   **Ramp used to load patient into a HAGA.**

If available, a HAGA (Figures 34-11 and 34-12) is used in a high-risk environment. Soft-skinned ambulances such as the M996 or M997 (see Table 34-1) are not used forward of a BAS because of limited protection against small-arms fire.

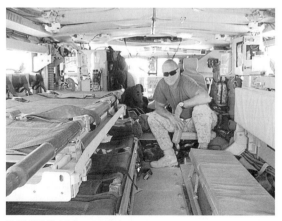

FIGURE 34-12   **Litter mounted on *top* and *bottom left* in a HAGA (patient litter system).**

Based on the combat situation, a casualty could be transferred from a BAS to a level II or level III facility with an M996 or M997. However, this transfer is occurring less because of the urban environment of current conflicts. The risk from improvised explosive devices (IEDs) and ambush attacks has made it necessary to use armored transport vehicles for casualty transport to a protected forward operating base.

The wheeled ambulance is designed for field use; it can operate on paved and secondary roads, trails, and cross-country terrain and can operate in all weather conditions. Electrical power access is provided to operate the onboard medical equipment. Before evacuation of casualties, the medical personnel must configure the evacuation platform to accommodate the types and number of patients. After configuring the platform, they prioritize, load, and appropriately secure the casualties to ensure safe transport and patient access during evacuation. Casualties are normally loaded head first in the field ambulance. However, if the casualty requires access to a specific injured side, the patient can be loaded feet-first. A M996 ambulance can accommodate two litter patients and one ambulatory. The M997 and the M113 tracked ambulance can accommodate four litter patients and one ambulatory or a total of eight ambulatory.[10]

Medical Evacuation

Medical evacuation or *MEDEVAC* involves the rapid movement of a patient with a medically staffed and equipped vehicle. A classic example of this is the UH-60 Black Hawk, the MEDEVAC workhorse of the Army (Figure 34-13).

The transport can be from a battlefield (on scene) to a medical treatment facility or movement between medical treatment facilities. A nurse does not generally accompany a MEDEVAC to the POI or level I location. Care is provided by flight medics between levels of care unless the patient being transported is in critical condition. In a critical care transport, a critical care nurse and a flight medic accompany the patient. Critical care patients from a level I or II FST or FRSS frequently have abdomens left open and can be chemically paralyzed, sedated, and ventilated. The transport route is frequently unsafe, and control of the combat area of operations (air and surface) is a challenge.[4] Enemy attacks during transport are pos-

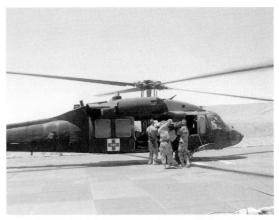

FIGURE 34-13   **UH-60 Black Hawk helicopter.**

sible. This risk requires the provider to wear combat gear (weapon, ammunition, Kevlar helmet, body armor) and fly or drive with rapid evasive moves, which makes care an exponential challenge.[6] In 2007, the US Army conducted more than 12,000 helicopter patient transports in Afghanistan and Iraq in support of combat operations. Most of these transports (more than two thirds) were casualties who needed surgery. These transports included level II to III transports and transports between level III facilities.[6]

Airmedical Evacuation

Airmedical evacuation (AE) is an Air Force–specific mission that uses fixed-wing resources to rapidly evacuate the sick and wounded under the care of qualified AE crew members both intratheater and intertheater. AE uses an integrated multiplatform capability. The crews are universally qualified on multiple aircraft and can provide care on any of the following: C-130 or C-17, for intratheater, and C-17 or KC-135, for intertheater (see Table 34-1).

Airmedical evacuation crews, flight nurses, and airmedical evacuation technicians (AETs) provide en route medical support necessary to reduce the loss of life, limb, and eyesight (Figure 34-14). The specific number of crew members depends on the length of the flight, patient acuity, and number of patients. Typically, an urgent or priority intratheater mission is shorter in flight time and will be called to care for only a few patients. This therefore requires one flight nurse and two AETs. A standard crew for other missions

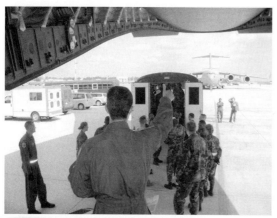

FIGURE 34-14   **MCD directing a patient on load (on ramp of C-17).**

that may be carrying larger patient loads for longer flight times is two flight nurses and three AETs. The AE environment is dynamic, and each crew member is required to maintain professional expertise, accountability, knowledge, and skill to manage patients in flight. The team leader, one of the flight nurses known as the medical crew director (MCD), is responsible for operational medical mission management.

For transport of critical patients, the AE crew may be augmented by specialty teams. One example is the Critical Care Air Transport Team (CCATT). This team consists of one physician, one critical care nurse, and a cardiopulmonary technician. An augmentation to the AE team, the CCATT works with and receives mission operational direction from the MCD.

Augmenting specialy teams to the AE system has resulted in rapid critical patient transport. Moving an injured patient from a level 1 to a level V facility in the continental United States (CONUS) was a process that sometimes took more than a month during the Vietnam War. Today it is not unusual to take only 36 hours. The speed of the process, combined with improvements in body armor and surgical care, has made a life-saving difference in survival rate among wounded soldiers. Some of the success is from the location of AE crews close to level I to III facilities, CCATT development, and the effective and efficient use of airframes.[2]

Other specialty teams that may augment AE include the US Army Flight Burn Team from Brooke Army Medical Center in San Antonio, the Lung Team from Landstuhl Regional Medical Center in Germany, and the Neonatal Unit teams located throughout the military medical system.

HOW PATIENT TRANSPORT IS INITIATED

INTRATHEATER

A call to "911" is not used in a combat zone, but the ability to get MEDEVAC capabilities on scene is just a call away. All combat movements are monitored on a communication channel by an operations center. If casualties are sustained or reinforcements are needed, the operations center is notified and reinforcements are dispatched. If a helicopter evacuation is necessary, the operations center establishes a location and the medical requirements are relayed through a MEDEVAC request. This method is most common from point of injury to level II or III care but can include interfacility transfers as well between equally rated facilities (level III to III). This may be done because a fixed-wing transport is needed and the other facility is located near an airfield. For the longer transports, the Air Force is notified for fixed-wing assets.

Air Force patient movement (Figure 34-15) begins when a patient movement request (PMR) is made from the attending physician to the validating flight surgeon. The flight surgeon is located in the Patient Movement Requirements Center (PMRC), with a flight nurse, administrative technician, and medical service officer. The PMRC assists the referring physician creating the PMR and patient preparation for flight. The PMRC then contacts the Air Operations Center (AOC), specifically the Aeromedical Evacuation Control Team (AECT). The AECT is staffed by aeromedical evacuation technicians and nurses who work with the C-130, KC-135, and C-17 pilot and crew representatives. The process can have an aircraft and AE crew on the way in 1 hour.

INTERTHEATER

Intertheater aeromedical evacuation is accomplished the same way as intratheater AE. The facility contacts the PMRC. A patient movement request is submitted. The AECT finds an aircraft. The patient is then moved out of the combat theater and to a level IV or V facility for definitive care.

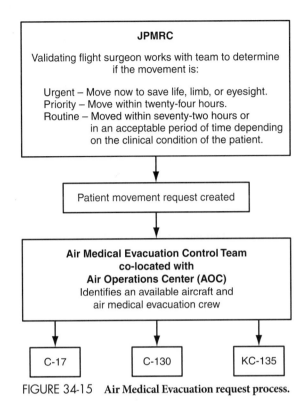

JPMRC

Validating flight surgeon works with team to determine
if the movement is:

Urgent – Move now to save life, limb, or eyesight.
Priority – Move within twenty-four hours.
Routine – Moved within seventy-two hours or
in an acceptable period of time depending
on the clinical condition of the patient.

Patient movement request created

**Air Medical Evacuation Control Team
co-located with
Air Operations Center (AOC)**
Identifies an available aircraft and
air medical evacuation crew

C-17   C-130   KC-135

FIGURE 34-15   **Air Medical Evacuation request process.**

TRAINING

POINT OF INJURY CARE PROVIDERS

Moving medical treatment closer to each service member is best accomplished by requiring each service to train for trauma. Training starts with basic first aid. The focus is on teaching each member of the service (Soldier, Sailor, Marine and Airman) how to care for themselves or their buddy if they are injured. The Air Force calls it Self Aid/Buddy Care, the Army Self Aid/Buddy Aid, the Navy First Aid, and the Marines Basic Life Saving First Aid. The Combat Life Savers Course is given to combat Marines. The military is trained in a course called Tactical Combat Casualty Care. Although the training varies slightly, each course focuses on stopping bleeding, cardiopulmonary resuscitation, procedures (e.g., needle decompression), and communicating for help and transport. For the medical specialist in each service, further trauma training is provided.

The Army sends combat medics through a course called Health Care Specialist for nearly 5 months. A medic assigned to a MEDEVAC unit is trained at the US Army's flight medic course where the focus is enhancement of basic trauma life support skills from the POI to initial treatment locations.[6] The Navy sends corpsman to a basic corpsman course and then augments that training with specific war medical skills with assignment to a Marine unit.[13] In addition to the trauma training, special training is provided for chemical, biologic, and radiation exposure.

Maintenance of currency is accomplished through civilian continuing education programs, online training, and different symposiums and conventions. In addition, the Air Force, Army, and Navy have contracted with city trauma centers around the United States to exercise trauma skills before transfer to combat zones.

GROUND TRANSPORT

Currently, no ground transport formal courses are sponsored by any of the services. Most medics and nurses are trained on the job.

ROTOR-WING TRANSPORT

Initially, limited training was provided for the hospital-based critical care nurse in transporting patients in rotor-wing aircraft. In 2004, the US Army initiated the Joint Enroute Care Course (JECC) to give a more formal orientation to transport nursing. This training is accomplished by the Army Medical Department Center and School Program of Instruction at Fort Rucker, Ala. The JECC provides trauma transport training to Joint Service, Coalition Forces, Department of Defense (DoD), and other Federal Government organizations. It teaches patient transport specifics for rotary wing. The 10-day course includes didactic and practical applications of flight transport trauma management concepts, effective communication, crew resource management, and roles of the transport provider.[6] In addition to flight patient care, flight physiology, water survival, combat survival, emergency egress, and communications are covered.

FIXED-WING TRANSPORT

The fixed-wing military transport training is an Air Force responsibility. Developed in the 1940s, this 21-day course covers patient considerations, the stresses of flight, altitude physiology, a systems review of altitude-related illnesses, and the effects of altitude on other diagnoses. Included is a review of the AE system, communication of patient needs, and the roles of supporting agencies. In addition, there is a focus on the equipment used in the AE system and the logistics of patient movement items (monitors, suction machines, etc) and how they are maintained in such a large system. The course is combined with a 2-week survival course that covers combat survival, evasion, and water survival. Finally, local training at home station is accomplished to complete AE qualification. The airframes focused on during training include the C-130, C-17, and KC-135. This course is open to all services and frequently has Army, Navy, Department of Homeland Security, and allied nation health providers in attendance.

SPECIAL OPERATIONS

Each of the services has Special Operations capabilities: Army Special Forces; Navy Sea, Air, Land (SEALs); and Air Force Para Rescue Jumpers (PJs). Each is trained in nonconventional assisted recovery. These teams may be tasked to recover a prisoner of war or someone who has been shot down behind enemy lines. The Army calls this Personnel Recovery, the Navy terms it Tactical Recovery of Aircraft and Personnel (TRAP), and the Air Force refers to it as Combat Search and Rescue (CSAR).[11] Each rescue team has a member that is trained to the paramedic level. These specialists work on platforms that combine combat tactics with medical capabilities. Common search and rescue vehicles are the HH-60G Pave Hawk (Army), the CV-22 Osprey (Air Force), and the MH-46 Sea Knight (Navy; see Table 34-1).

DEPARTMENT OF HOMELAND SECURITY

US Coast Guard

Similar to combat search and rescue, the US Coast guard has the capability to move patients from an austere environment (out at sea) to a hospital. With search and rescue being an almost daily operation,

these professionals are trained to the paramedic level. The common transport vehicles are the HH-65 Dolphin and the HH-60 Jay Hawk.

US Immigrations and Customs Enforcement

The Department of Homeland Security (DHS) has found itself in need of transporting illegal aliens and arrested foreigners that are sometimes ill. The DHS sends nurses to the Air Force Flight Nurse Course in San Antonio for training. They commonly use fixed-wing aircraft and employ nurses with transport backgrounds as Immigrations and Customs Enforcement employees.

PEACETIME OPERATIONS

Military Operations Other Than War

In times of natural disaster or humanitarian relief, either in the United States or abroad, the US military medical system can be mobilized. Requests from individual state governments or other nations for medical assistance are frequent to the US military. Support may include search, recovery, care, and transport from special operations assets or any of the available medical platforms mobilized in war.

Local Agreements

When not at war, the military frequently uses civilian services for patient transport. Many communities have memorandum of agreements sharing resources. These agreements allow the military (a Federal agency) to respond to emergencies outside the "gate" of a military reservation or to transport patients from the Military Treatment Facility (MTF) to a local hospital with a higher level of care. In addition, these agreements set lines of communication and levels of support that can be provided if a local community is overwhelmed in a mass casualty situation. These agreements increase the capabilities for the local community in a disaster response. In addition, they allow the military transport system to bring patients needing further treatment "downtown." Frequently, unit deployments account for varied reliability in this relationship. A civilian ambulance company that responds to emergencies on military reservations is not unusual, even if it has an organic well-trained, robust medical transport capability.

SUMMARY

Whether in times of war or humanitarian crisis, the military medical system is planned, deployed, and constructed from the ground up to support military action. The medical system must be able to support this action anytime, anywhere in the world. Within the military medical system, the Air Force, Army, and Navy work to combine different military medical transport platforms that move patients rapidly from point of injury to definitive care. Soldiers, Marines, Airmen, and Sailors know if they are ever injured, even in the most remote location, they will be rapidly triaged, treated, and transported to the highest level of medical care necessary. The interdependence of the Air Force, Army, and Navy patient transport system is supported by highly skilled and trained transport medical personnel. By providing joint interoperable and interchangeable platforms, military patient transport saves lives.

REFERENCES

1. Butler FK Jr: Tactical medicine training for SEAL mission commanders, *Military Med* 166(7):625-631, 2001.
2. Butler FK Jr, Holcomb JB, Giebner SD, et al: Tactical combat casualty care 2007: evolving concepts and battlefield experience, *Military Med* 172(11 suppl):1-19, 2007.
3. Eastridge BJ, Jenkins D, Flaherty S, et al: Trauma system development in a theater of war: experiences from Operation Iraqi Freedom and Operation Enduring Freedom, *Military Med* 61(6):1366-1373, 2006.
4. Gawande A: Casualties of war: military care for the wounded from Iraq and Afghanistan, *N Engl J Med* 351(24):2471-2475, 2004.
5. Holcomb JB, Stansbury LG, Champion HR, et al: Understanding combat casualty care statistics, *J Trauma* 60(2):397-401, 2006.
6. Hudson TL, Morton RT: Critical Care Transport in a Combat Environment: Building tactical trauma transport teams pre-deployment and intra-theater. (unpublished).
7. Peck M: Golden hour surgical units prove worth, *Military Med Technol* 7(5), 2003.
8. Szul AC, Davis LB: Levels of medical care. In Walter Reed Army Medical Center, editor: *Emergency war surgery: third United States revision*, Washington, DC, 2004, Department of the Army.
9. US Department of the Army: *TRADOC pamphlet 525-66, military operations force operating capabilities*, Washington, DC, March 2008, available at www.tradoc.army.mil/tpubs/pams/p525-66.pdf, accessed May 2008.
10. US Department of the Army: *Field manual 8-10-6: medical evacuation in a theater of operations; tactics, techniques, and procedures*, Washington, DC, 1992, US Department of the Army.
11. US Department of Defense: *Joint publication 3-50, personnel recovery*, Washington, DC, January 2007, available at: http://www.fas.org/irp/doddir/dod/jp3_50.pdf, accessed May 2008.
12. US Department of Defense: *Joint publication 4-02, doctrine for Health Service Support in Joint Operations*, Washington, DC, July 2001, available at www.dtic.mil/doctrine/jel/new_pubs/jp4_02.pdf, accessed May 2008.
13. US Department of the Navy: *Bureau of Naval Personnel Web Connection*, Millington, TN available at http://buperscd.technology.navy.mil/bup_updt/508/nec/8000_8999.htm, accessed June 2008.

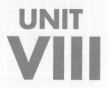

UNIT VIII

Patient Care Issues

CHAPTER

35 EVIDENCE-BASED PRACTICE, RESEARCH, AND QUALITY MANAGEMENT

Cheryl Erler, Reneé Semonin Holleran

EVIDENCE-BASED PRACTICE

Worldwide attention has been focused on the need for healthcare providers to be accountable for delivery of safe quality care based on scientific information and knowledge of "best practices." Evidence-based medicine (EBM) is a term that originated in the 1980s at McMaster Medical School, Hamilton, Ontario. Canada, Australia, and Great Britain are credited with the early EBM movement to promote healthcare best practice decisions. *Evidence-based medicine*, as defined by Sackett and colleagues,[12] is the conscientious, explicit, and judicious use of current best practice information for making decisions about the care of patients. *Evidence-based practice* (EBP) includes integration of individual clinical expertise with the best available clinical evidence from systematic research.[5] EBP is a problem-solving approach to the delivery of healthcare that combines the best evidence from well-designed studies with a clinician's expertise and a patient's preferences and values.[1,2] A number of EBP models for nursing care are found in the literature,

two of which are the Advancing Research and Clinical Practice Through Close Collaboration (ARCC) model, developed by Melnyk and Fineout-Overholt, and the Iowa model, developed by Titler and colleagues.[9]

The EBM process involves categorization of clinical practices according to the strength of the evidence. The general categories include systematic reviews, clinical evidence, and clinical practice guidelines. Levels of evidence (Box 35-1) are also referred to as the hierarchy of evidence. Systematic reviews and metaanalyses of randomized clinical trials (RCTs) are considered the strongest level of evidence (level I), and opinions and reports of expert committees are considered the weakest (level VII).[9]

Evidence-based practice guidelines provide direction for dealing with many common clinical situations. A number of electronic resources provide access to systematic reviews and evidence-based practice guidelines. The following sources disseminate high-quality reviews of healthcare interventions: the Cochrane Database of Systematic Reviews (CDSR);

BOX 35-1	**Levels of Evidence**

Level I	Systematic reviews
	Metaanalyses of randomized controlled trials (RCTs)
	Evidence-based clinical practice guidelines based on systematic reviews of RCTs
Level II	Well-designed RCTs (one or more)
	Single nonrandomized trials
Level III	Noncontrolled trials without randomization
	Systematic reviews of correlational/observational studies
Level IV	Well-designed case-control and cohort studies
	Single correlational/observational studies
Level V	Systematic reviews of descriptive and qualitative studies
Level VI	Single descriptive or qualitative studies
Level VII	Opinions of authorities or reports of expert committees

From Melnyk BM, Fineout-Overholt E: *Evidence-based practice in nursing and healthcare: a guide to best practice*, Philadelphia, 2005, Lippincott, Williams & Wilkins.

the Johanna Briggs Institute for EBP and Midwifery; and the Database of Abstracts of Reviews of Effects, or DARE. A number of professional health care organizations publish clinical practice guidelines; these can be accessed through the National Quality Measures Clearinghouse and the Agency for Healthcare Research and Quality (AHRQ).[1,5-7] Although systematic reviews are considered the highest level of evidence, some have design flaws. The practitioner needs to ask the following questions when evaluating any study:

- Is the study of high scientific merit, and does it have an appropriate research design?
- Are results consistent from study to study?
- Are all clinical outcomes, including benefits and potential harm, addressed?

- Does my patient population of interest correspond to patients described in the studies?[5]

For identification of best practice information, the clinician needs to formulate an appropriate clinical question that narrows the scope of the literature search. PICO, a model developed by faculty at McMaster University, Ontario, is a strategy used for framing the clinical question. PICO is an acronym in which *P* stands for patient or population of interest, including diagnosis, age, and gender; *I* is for intervention, such as a medication or treatment; *C* is for comparison (not every question has a comparison component); and *O* is for outcome, which may include a primary and secondary outcome (Box 35-2).[2] A sample clinical question might

BOX 35-2	**PICO (Patient/Population, Intervention, Comparison, Outcome) Model for Evaluation of a Study's Clinical Utility**

Components of the Clinical Question	Patient	Intervention	Comparison (optional)	Outcome
	Description of the patient or population of interest	Intervention or therapy of interest (e.g., medication, treatment) or prognostic factor	Alternative medication, treatment, etc, for comparison	The clinical outcome, including a timeframe if appropriate
Example	In patients with anxiety	Does music therapy	Or support groups	Reduced hospital visits

be, "Do patients with traumatic brain injury who are intubated during prehospital transport have fewer metabolic acid-base disturbances than patients who are not intubated?" This question involves a comparison group, but not all questions do. In a search of the literature, limiting electronic searches to articles with the terms "evidenced-based" or "systematic reviews" can help narrow your search.[13]

RESEARCH

Research is systematic inquiry that uses disciplined methods to answer questions or solve problems with an ultimate goal of developing, refining, and expanding a body of knowledge.[10] The goal of healthcare research is validation of existing knowledge or discovery of new knowledge that provides the evidence or direction necessary to guide quality clinical practice. Nurses are responsible for using knowledge gained through research to define and refine critical care transport practices. The field of critical care transport is a relatively new area of research compared with other medicine and nursing specialties. It offers a wide spectrum of potential research questions based on method of transport and patient populations transported. Clinical practice can serve as a rich source of research ideas that include clinical observations, validation of treatment guidelines, testing of new procedures, replication of previous studies, and identification of gaps in existing medical or nursing literature. Additional areas for research in critical care transport include, but are not limited to, staff education, program administration, patient safety, economic concerns, development of a safety culture, healthcare delivery systems, and quality evaluation.

The research process is consistent across all disciplines. However, research studies are often accorded greater credibility when the research team is multidisciplinary. Approaches to research may be qualitative or quantitative. *Quantitative research* includes systematic collection of numeric information; *qualitative research* involves systematic collection of subjective data. The selection of one or the other or both methodologies typically depends on the question of interest. Research may also be grossly classified as basic or applied. *Basic research* is conducted to expand a body of knowledge; *applied research* is

performed to find answers or solutions to existing problems. Applied research tends to be of greater immediate utility for defining best practices.[10]

Before initiation of the research process, a fundamental understanding of common terms is essential. Box 35-3 contains definitions of several useful research terms. The initial step in the research process is identification of the question of interest. The question should be clear and specific. For example, what is the incidence rate of hypothermia in patients transported via air? Another research question might focus on identification of the relationship between an independent variable (the intervention variable) and one or more dependent variables (the outcomes measured). Such a question might read, what is the relationship between hypovolemia and hypothermia? An example of a qualitative study questions is, how do family members of patients transported via air perceive the level of care provided? Once a specific question has been selected, a literature review can be conducted to identify existing studies and determine their levels of evidence. Pertinent studies then need to be critiqued for research strength and may be evaluated with established critique guidelines that focus on each step of the research process. Some questions to consider include:

1. How many subjects are in the study, and how was sample size determined?
2. Was the research design appropriate to answer the research question?
3. What are the results of the study? Are the results valid? Can they be generalized to my setting?
4. Will the results of the study impact clinical care or project design?

The research design forms the general structure of the study; multiple designs may be used. A common mistake made by novice researchers is failure to fit the research question to the appropriate study design. An example is use of a quantitative design (seeking to make statistical predictions) when a qualitative design (an in-depth exploration of subjective information) would better answer the research question. Box 35-4 lists several common research designs. Experimental study design elements include manipulation, randomization, and control.

BOX 35-3	**Definition of Terms**

Cluster sampling: A process in which the sample is selected by randomly choosing smaller and smaller subgroups from the main population.

Convenience sampling: A process in which a sample is drawn from conveniently available subjects.

Internal validity: The degree to which the changes or differences in the dependent variable (the outcome) can be attributed to the independent variable (intervention or group differences). This is related to the degree to which extraneous variables are controlled.

Judgmental sampling: Another name for purposive sample.

Population: All subjects of interest to the researcher for the study.

Purposive sampling: A process in which subjects are selected by investigators to meet a specific purpose.

Quota sampling: A process in which the subjects are selected by convenience until the specified number of subjects for a specific subgroup is reached. At this point, subjects are no longer selected for that subgroup, but recruitment continues for subgroups that have not yet reached their quota of subjects.

Sample: The small portion of the population selected for participation in the study.

Sampling: The process used for selecting a sample from the population.

Simple random sampling: A process in which a sample is selected randomly from the population, with each subject having a known and calculable probability of being chosen.

Snowball sampling: A process in which the first subjects are drawn by convenience; these subjects then recruit people they know to participate, and they recruit people they know, etc.

Stratified random sampling: A process in which a population is divided into subgroups and a predetermined portion of the sample is randomly drawn from each subgroup.

Systematic random sample: A process in which a sample is drawn by systematically selecting every nth subject from a list of all subjects in the population. The starting point in the population must be selected randomly.

Threats to Validity

Assignment of subjects: Changes in the dependent variable are a result of preexisting differences in the subjects before implementation of the intervention.

Biophysiologic measures: Measures of biologic function obtained through use of technology, such as electrocardiographic or hemodynamic monitoring.

Blocking: Assignment of subjects to control and experimental groups based on extraneous variables. Blocking helps to ensure that one group does not get the preponderance of subjects with a specific value on a variable of interest.

Concurrent validity: Criterion-related validity where the measures are obtained at the same time.

Construct validity: A form of validity where the researcher is not as concerned with the values obtained by the instrument but with the abstract match between the true value and the obtained value.

Content validity: Concern with whether the questions asked, or observations made, actually address all of the variables of interest.

Criterion-related validity: The results from the tool of interest are compared with those of another criterion that relates to the variable to be measured.

Determination of stability: Only appropriate when the value for the variable of interest is expected to remain the same over the time period examined.

External validity: The degree to which the results can be applied to others outside the sample used for the study.

Face validity: The instrument looks like it is measuring what it should be measuring.

Hawthorne effect: Subjects respond in a different manner just because they are involved in a study.

History: Natural changes in the outcome variable are the result of another event inside or outside the experimental setting but are attributed to the intervention instead.

Instrumentation: Changes in the dependent variable are the result of the measurement plan rather than the intervention.

Internal consistency: The degree to which items on a questionnaire or psychological scale are consistent with each other.

Interrater reliability: The degree to which two or more evaluators agree on the measurement obtained.

(Continued)

BOX 35-3   **Definition of Terms—cont'd**

Loss of subjects: Changes in the dependent variable are a result of differential loss of subjects from the intervention or control groups.

Maturation: Changes in the dependent variable are a result of normal changes over time.

Observation: The activity of interest is observed, described, and possibly recorded via audiotape or videotape.

Predictive validity: Criterion-related validity where measurement with one instrument is used to predict the value from another instrument at a future point in time.

Psychological scale: Usually a number of self-report items combined in a questionnaire designed to evaluate the subject on a particular psychological trait, such as self esteem.

Reliability: The degree of consistency with which an instrument measures the variable it is designed to measure.

Self report: The variables of interest are measured by asking the subject to report on the perception of the value for the variable.

Stability: Determination of the degree of change in a measure across time.

Validity: How well the tool measures what it is supposed to measure.

BOX 35-4   **Classifications of Research Designs**

1. True experimental
2. Quasiexperimental
   Cohort
   Group sequential
   Cross sectional
3. Nonexperimental
   Case-control
   Historical
   Surveys, questionnaires
   Case series
   Case reports

According to Thompson and Panacek,[14] *manipulation* is the ability of the researcher to interact with study subjects to effectively direct the independent variable. Manipulation is evidenced in interventional studies in which one group receives an intervention while a control group does not. *Randomization* assures that all subjects have an equal chance of assignment to either the control or the experimental group. *Control* refers to the researcher's ability to limit the influence of confounding or extraneous variables. Studies with a true experimental design contain all three of these elements. However, most clinical studies are not true experiments and are therefore classified as quasiexperimental studies, because one or more of these three key elements is missing.

Once a research project involving human subjects has been designed, an *institutional review board* (IRB) must review and approve the study. The function of an IRB is to ensure that subject rights are protected. Some IRBs also evaluate the validity and methodology of the research proposal. Whenever human subjects are involved in research, informed consent or a consent waiver must be obtained from the IRB. One of the roles of an IRB is to ensure that researchers have honored the tenets of informed consent, which include verifying that the patient shown decision-making ability, that the patient was not coerced, and that the study has been thoroughly explained. Subjects must be free to refuse participation without jeopardizing access to treatment. All subjects need to be assured of anonymity and their right to withdraw from the study at any time. Research in the prehospital environment can make obtaining timely informed consent difficult. Exceptions have been made for life-threatening situations. In 1996, a Waiver of Informed Consent Guidelines for emergency research was established under federal rule (21CFR 50.24).[15] The federal guidelines, referred to as the Final Rule, outline qualifying criteria for subjects (Box 35-5).[4] Researchers must ensure that the criteria for these exceptions have been included in the research proposal.

After a research design has been selected, the sample identified, and data collected, the data need to be analyzed and the results interpreted. The specific research design dictates the techniques used to for data analysis. *Descriptive statistics* summarize quantitative data

Emergency Exception to Informed Consent

- Subject is in life-threatening situation.
- Subject is unable to consent because of condition.
- No time to contact legally authorized representative for subject.
- Available treatments are untested or deemed unsatisfactory.
- Possibility must exist that subject will benefit from treatment.
- Prior community consultation and public disclosure of study protocol.

From *Title 21 Part 50 Section 24: exception from informed consent requirements for emergency research*, available at http://www.cfsan.fda.gov/~lrd/cfr50.html. accessed 9/3/08.

and allow the researcher to describe what occurred in the sample. *Inferential statistics tests* are used to determine differences between two or more samples. Qualitative data require nonstatistical analysis procedures. A major problem for clinical researchers is interpreting research findings; numbers can be used to say many things. Also, in interpretation of results, some findings of statistical significance may have little or no clinical significance. Any conclusions drawn from the data must actually be supported by the data.[8,14]

The final component of clinical research is presentation of the data. Professional associations and journals afford many opportunities to share results and link study conclusions to the work of other researchers. Research in the transport environment can present some unique challenges, including: coordination of study protocols with other departments, institutions, and agencies; inability to control the study environment; the simultaneous need for urgent care delivery; and complications associated with obtaining and assuring informed consent.[5]

The final component of clinical research is dissemination of the data. Professional associations and journals afford a great opportunity to present findings and link studies and conclusions. Dissemination of findings contributes to the weight of evidence necessary for practice.

Research in the transport environment can present some unique challenges, including coordination of study protocols with other departments and

institutions, an uncontrolled environment, the need for urgent acute care delivery, and the complications of obtaining and assuring informed consent. Communication and collaboration are key to assembling a research team and identifying issues to facilitate a smooth research process.

QUALITY MANAGEMENT

Patient transport has become a crucial part of modern healthcare. As the healthcare system faces dwindling financial resources, ongoing financial justification and proof of improved patient outcomes is necessary to justify the high cost of transport services. For many transport programs, *quality management* (QM) is often viewed as a time-consuming activity with little measurable impact on actual patient outcomes. This section provides an overview of the QM process for transport programs and suggests several practical methods for evaluation of patient transport and improvement of systems of care.

DEFINITION OF TERMS: QUALITY ASSURANCE VERSUS CONTINUOUS QUALITY IMPROVEMENT

A veritable alphabet soup of quality terms has glutted healthcare. For the sake of clarity, it is important to define the terminology. *Quality assurance* (QA) implies a traditional approach to outcome evaluation. It includes such activities as monitoring specific indicators and comparing results with predetermined thresholds or standards. Unfortunately, healthcare providers sometimes perceive traditional QA in a negative light because it is associated with the perception that individuals are doing a poor job or are not complying with certain standards. As an alternative to traditional QA, *continuous quality improvement* (CQI), *total quality management* (TQM), and many derivations of these concepts have been used in the healthcare arena over the past few decades. These terms are often used interchangeably, but they embrace essentially the same concepts. The CQI approach is radically different from traditional QA, but not all individuals who use the terms appreciate the differences.

Quality assurance, CQI or TQM should always occur within a no-blame culture. Transport team members may reluctant to acknowledge breeches in protocols, incidents, or events if they sense that someone will be punished. However, accountability should never be underplayed. Mistakes may occur, but intentional high risk behaviors should not be tolerated.

Continuous quality improvement and QA practices differ radically in approaches to motivation, leadership, methodology, and organization. Traditionally, healthcare providers have been motivated to perform QA activities primarily to meet externally mandated regulatory requirements (e.g., The Joint Commission). Conversely, the focus of CQI activities is to please customers. We are in an era of choice in healthcare, and patients are informed consumers with discriminating tastes in healthcare services. Although few choices may be available in emergency transport situations, patients and their families have certain expectations of healthcare providers, regardless of the setting.

General components of a quality management program include[11]:

- Program mission statement.
- Program vision statement.
- Program value statement.
- Goals and objectives.
- Delineated critical success factors.
- Definition of the scope of practice of the transport program.
- Decision on an approach to QM.
- Chosen methodology.
- Established reporting procedures.
- Development of recommendations for action.
- Establishment of evaluation intervals.

The role of a leader in a CQI program differs dramatically from that of a leader in a QA program. In a QA program, quality initiatives are typically the responsibility of a middle manager, or QA coordinator. The entire responsibility for ensuring quality is relegated to this individual. In a CQI program, accountability for quality rests with the organization's leaders, who must be committed to the CQI initiative in both word and deed.

Perhaps the greatest difference between the CQI and QA approaches is the methodology used. The QA approach has typically focused on retrospective audits, quality indicator monitoring, and less-than-rigorous studies. With this approach, decisions can be made based on weak data and personal opinions. CQI methodology relies on statistics and facts, not feelings and assumptions. In addition, CQI methodology stresses a standardized problem-solving approach designed to yield predictable evidence-based results.

Finally, the organizational culture in a program committed to CQI is fundamentally different; all processes and plans are centered around the customer (patients and families). Quality customer service is a core value in CQI organizations. Employees are empowered to meet the needs of the customer by implementing changes and making decisions without being unduly encumbered by bureaucratic rules and regulations.

QUALITY MANAGEMENT MODEL FOR AIR MEDICAL TRANSPORT

The Commission on Accreditation of Air Medical Transport Systems (CAMTS) provides a framework for the development of a quality management program for a medical transport program. A summary of these components are contained in Box 35-6.[3]

Despite some inherent limitations, traditional QA activities have merit in the medical transport environment. Transport programs might be inclined to discard QA methods completely to adopt an exclusive CQI approach, but a combination of the two methods may be the most effective way to evaluate and improve care. Both QA and CQI methodologies

---

BOX 35-6	**Components of QA Program from the Commission on Accreditation of Air Medical Transport Systems**

- QM flow chart
- QM program linked to risk management
- Written QM plan
- Regularly scheduled QM meetings
- Monitoring and evaluation process driven by:
  - Aspects of care
  - Indicators and thresholds or other criteria
- Evidence of action plans
- Evidence of the reporting of QA activities
- Evidence of outcome studies
- Evidence of annual goal establishment

can be integrated into a program's overall QM strategy. QA activities can serve as a stimulus for multidisciplinary CQI teams because the transport process encompasses multiple phases and persons. The remainder of this chapter uses the term quality management, or QM, to imply a blending of the best aspects of traditional QA and CQI.

Assignment of Accountability: The Staff-Based Approach to Quality Management

Medical transport services managers are ultimately accountable for their program's quality activities. However, involvement of all transport team members in the QM program, (from inception through monitoring, data collection, change, and evaluation) is the only way to achieve commitment at all levels. Managers can delegate many activities to committees or individuals, such as a QM coordinator, but top-down support and involvement are essential components of an effective QM program. Executive level involvement is demonstrated by financial support for individuals assigned QM responsibilities. These individuals must receive adequate training and be allowed paid time away from routine duties to complete QM activities and projects. Some medical transport services hire QM coordinators who are assigned the bulk of the QM workload. Whether the QM coordinator is a full-time staff member or an individual who works part time, one individual must be accountable for overseeing the process. Failure to assign accountability results in disorganization and lack of QM program direction.

The success or failure of a medical QM program is also related to the degree to which team members are involved in its development, implementation, and ongoing maintenance. If a QM program is conceived and implemented with little or no involvement on the part of those who deliver care, it is likely to be perceived negatively. If, on the other hand, all team members are given an opportunity to contribute to QM program development, personal investment on the part of the staff improves the chances of program success.

The Quality Management Committee

Development of a QM committee is one way to promote staff involvement in the QM process. The QM committee approach promotes "ownership" of the QM program on the part of the transport team. The participation of transport team members may be used as part of the program's clinical advancement system. Committee membership may be determined by application, appointment, or election. Whatever the approach, members must be committed to the goals of the committee. Bylaws that address QM committee structure, reporting mechanisms, voting privileges, attendance requirements, and so on can serve to heighten members' sense of commitment to the aims of the committee.

QUALITY MANAGEMENT PROGRAM ORGANIZATIONAL STRATEGIES

The most effective QM programs are well organized and multifaceted. Programs that rely too heavily on one monitoring method risk missed opportunities for improvement. However, management of multiple or simultaneous studies and indicators can be overwhelming. A written QM plan is an effective organizational tool. The plan provides the infrastructure for quality initiatives and facilitates a systematic and organized monitoring and evaluation process. The development of such a plan is straightforward; however, certain essential components must be included.

First, the content of the QM plan must be based on the transport program's scope of service, which describes the types of patients transported and how they are transported. For instance, a flight program that transports 80% of its patients from the scene of injury has a different scope of care than a neonatal transport program. A statement that clearly summarizes the essence of the services provided by the particular program and by its crew members could read: "LifeFlight provides rapid assessment, diagnosis, and treatment of critically ill or injured patients of all ages from the scene of injury and between care facilities." With this statement as a framework, QM personnel can begin to develop standards, identify high-risk high-volume aspects of care, and target appropriate strategies to monitor them.

Identification of Important Aspects

Important aspects of care to evaluate include areas that are high risk, problem prone, or high volume. Events with these characteristics have the greatest impact on patient outcome, costs, and program functioning. Care interventions such as physical assessment, documentation, medication administration, invasive procedures, and response to requests for service are examples of important aspects of medical transport care.

Indicator Development

Indicators are well-delineated objective measures of compliance with a particular standard. Potential indicators of physical assessment after endotracheal intubation are:

1. Bilateral breath sounds are documented on all patients after intubation.
2. Esophageal intubations are recognized and corrected.

Thresholds and Benchmarks

The final step in development of a written QM plan is establishment of the level at which lack of compliance with a given standard or quality indicator is considered unacceptable and necessitates intervention. This level, usually expressed as a percentage, is known as the *threshold*. Some experts prefer the use of the term *benchmark* when implying an externally determined performance level. National professional associations have sometimes published suggested thresholds, but little research has supported their validity. Whether this will change in the future remains to be seen. However, lack of current data does not preclude a transport program from identifying its own thresholds and benchmarks.

When no national data are available with which to validate a certain level of performance, how does one realistically assign thresholds? First, thresholds must be attainable and practical. Thresholds that are so high they cannot be met are unrealistic. Conversely, there are high-risk indicators for which failure to meet the standard 100% of the time could result in deleterious patient outcomes. For example, the threshold for the indicator "esophageal intubations are recognized and corrected" should be 100%.

Establishment of Priorities for Monitoring and Evaluation

A written QM plan outlines all general categories of care monitored in a given time period, how often these aspects of care are monitored, and the methods used. Actual implementation of these activities can be daunting. A prioritization tool is needed to determine which activities should be undertaken first. A *decision matrix* is a simple but valuable way to prioritize QM efforts. It is usually most effective when completed by a group, such as the QM committee, or a similar planning structure. The following example describes the use of a decision matrix.

The XYZ Transport Program QM committee meets the first week of January to establish quality initiatives for the coming year. During this meeting, group members brainstorm to identify both clinical and operational nursing, paramedic, respiratory therapy, administration, aviation, medical, mechanical, and communications issues. As a result of their brainstorming, the QM committee targets 10 important opportunities for improvement. Areas of concern include: interfacility bedside times, intubation success rates, medical control contact documentation, maternal transport team composition, chest pain management documentation, fetal monitor interpretation, refueling turnaround times, compliance with transport guidelines, referral hospital satisfaction, and pediatric fluid management. To decide which of these issues will be addressed first during the coming year, the QM committee consults a decision matrix and identifies their five highest priority issues to determine where they need to focus the greatest efforts.

Utilization Appropriateness

A comprehensive transport program QM plan monitors appropriate indicators and uses findings from monitoring activities as a stimulus for the inclusion of all who are involved in the transport process. Another component of a comprehensive QM program is the evaluation of transport appropriateness. Utilization evaluation is an essential piece of the greater quality picture, yet this important element is often overlooked by many transport services.

The criteria for a medically appropriate transport are controversial and remain to be validated. Several professional organizations have proposed utilization appropriateness criteria.[3] Each program must develop a mechanism to screen for transport appropriateness, both prospectively and retrospectively. In development of criteria, several general considerations should be kept in mind. First, does the patient's condition dictate the need to minimize scene or interhospital transport time? Second, what distances, local geography, or traffic conditions might justify various transportation alternatives? Third, what is the availability of appropriate vehicles and personnel? Fourth, what are the prevailing weather conditions that might interfere with air or ground transport? And finally, what are the costs of various transportation alternatives?[2] With these considerations as a framework, the transport program can develop criteria for appropriate use of medical transport resources.

LEGAL CONSIDERATIONS FOR QUALITY MANAGEMENT

One of the most underacknowledged considerations in the development of a QM program involves the legal issues that surround the quality evaluation process. Laws that protect QM activities and personnel involved in data collection from the threat of subpoena and liability vary significantly from state to state. In fact, in some states, the confidentially of QM documentation has been challenged. This section examines the importance of state discoverability, immunity, and admissibility laws to the QM process and the legal protection of individuals involved in QM activities.

For an understanding of the ramifications of state legislation on the QM process, a few legal terms must be defined. *Discovery* is a term used to describe the acquisition of information and evidence before a trial, via oral or written deposition or other means. Laws governing rules of procedure and evidence vary significantly by state. *Admissible evidence* is anything that is allowed as evidence by a court. Information not typically considered discoverable is not automatically precluded from admissibility if it comes to light by means other than the formal discovery process. For example, if a plaintiff's attorney stumbles on undiscoverable QM data stored in sloppy personnel files or carelessly placed in patient records, certain states allow this information to be admitted as evidence.

A *subpoena* is a directive from the court requiring a witness to appear before the court. A subpoena can also force a witness to produce any written evidence that may be pertinent to the case. The difference between subpoena and discoverability becomes problematic because they are two separate legal processes. State laws that prevent discoverability may not necessarily prevent subpoenas. These issues are further confused by the often unclear and ambiguous language used in these laws, which leaves interpretation up to individual courts.

State laws defining the protection of QM data and QM activities from discoverability, subpoena, and admissibility should have considerable impact on the planning, design, and implementation of a transport service's QM plan. These laws have implications regarding the protection of both the healthcare providers monitored and the data derived from QM activities. Without protective legislation, persons who initiate QM activities place themselves and their colleagues at risk. In addition, transport programs that implement QM plans with inadequate knowledge of peer-review statutes in their state place the transport service at risk. Each transport program should consult with an attorney to determine the rules within their service area.

Once a transport program has adequate knowledge of applicable discoverability and peer-review statutes, several additional precautions need to be taken to ensure protection under the law. Examples of activities include:

1. Written memoranda regarding adverse patient outcomes, medication errors, and reasons for transport delay (whether valid or otherwise) should not be circulated through the transport program for review.
2. Written documentation of such incidents should never be kept in employee personnel files, which may be discoverable and admissible in court.
3. Data derived from QM studies should be contained within the QM system. A helpful method is to title all QM data, reports, and summaries with "XYZ Transport Service's Quality Management Program: Confidential."
4. If the actual number of the state's peer-review protective statute and its wording are known, the transport program can affix this wording to all documents relating to QM.

5. Explicit discussion of sensitive patient care information should not occur in the open forum of the transport service's weekly or monthly chart review. This practice, though it has educational merit, places all crew members who hear about the incident at risk for subpoena.

6. Any memoranda or other written materials, such as incident reports, should not make references to the source of the data.

Laws that affect QM activities are diverse and often ambiguous. Statutes in many states have gone unchallenged. Because of complexities in law, program administrators must obtain legal assistance when tackling these issues.

SUMMARY

Research provides a way to identify, describe, and communicate evidence-based practice related to the care of patients during critical care transport. It provides a systematic approach to review and analysis of data to develop clinical practice guidelines. Critical care transport research can be particularly challenging because of the environment in which it is conducted and the challenges faced when studying critically ill and injured patients. However, without research, justification of patient transport and improvement of care to those we serve are difficult.

Documentation and evaluation of care in the transport environment remain among the greatest challenges a program must face. This section has proposed a framework for a quality evaluation process that is both practical and comprehensive. As healthcare moves into the 21st century, these tools are invaluable for documenting the value of medical transport services.

REFERENCES

1. Agency for Healthcare Research and Quality: Database of abstracts of reviews of effects (DARE), available at http://www.ahrq.gov, accessed September 2008. http://www.library.ucsf.edu/db/record.html?idrecord=29.
2. *The well built clinical question: the EBM process*, available at http://www.hsl.unc.edu/Services/Tutorials/EBM/Question.htm, accessed September 2008.
3. Commission on Accreditation of Air Medical Transport Systems (CAMTS): *Accreditation standards*, ed 6, Andersonville, 2006, CAMTS.
4. Erler CJ, Thompson CB: Ethics, human rights and clinical research, *Air Med J* 25:110-113, 143, 2008.
5. *Evidence based clinical practice tutorial: Edward G. Miner Library*, University of Rochester Medical Center, available at http://www.urmc.rochester.edu/HSLT/Miner/resources/evidence_based/EBHC_tutorial2.cfm, accessed September 2008.
6. *National Quality Measures Clearinghouse*, available at http://www.guideline.gov/browse/xrefnqmc.aspx, accessed September 2008. *Evidence based practice: levels of evidence and the systematic review*: Cushing/Whitney Medical Library, available at http://www.med.yale.edu/library/nursing/education/sysdata.html, accessed September 2008.
7. International Organization for Standardization: *Quality management principles*, available at http://www.iso.org/iso/qmp, accessed November 2008.
8. *Johanna Briggs Institute EB Medicine*, available at http://mrw.interscience.wiley.com/cochrane/cochrane_clsysrev_articles_fs.html, accessed September 2008.
9. Melnyk BM: Integrating levels of evidence into clinical decision making, *Pediatr Nurs* 30(4):323-325, 2004.
10. Polit DF, Beck CT: *Nursing research: generating and assessing evidence for nursing practice*, ed 8, Philadelphia, 2008, Wolters, Kluwer/Lippincott Williams & Wilkins.
11. Robinson KJ, Kamin R: Quality management for transport programs. In Blumen IJ, editor: *Principles and direction of air medical transport*, Salt Lake City, 2006, Air Medical Physicians Association.
12. Sackett DL, Rosenberg WM, Gray JA, et al: Evidence based medicine: what it is and what it is not, *BMJ* 312:71-72, 1996.
13. *The Cochrane Library for Healthcare Decision Making*, available at http://mrw.interscience.wiley.com/cochrane/cochrane_clsysrev_articles_fs.html, accessed September 2008.
14. Thompson CB, Panacek EA: Research study designs: experimental and quasi-experimental, *Air Med J* 25;242-246, 2006.
15. *Title 21 Part 50 Section 24: exception from informed consent requirements for emergency research*, available at http://www.cfsan.fda.gov/~lrd/cfr50.html, accessed September 2008.

LEGAL ISSUES

Reneé Semonin Holleran

COMPETENCIES

1. Identify the elements of malpractice.
2. Describe the impact of the Consolidated Omnibus Reconciliation Act, the Emergency Medical and Active Labor Act, and the Health Insurance Portability and Accountability Act on patient transport.
3. Identify the components of professional practice.

Knowledge of legal principles is necessary for members of the transport team. Registered nurses and other members of the transport team practice in a unique setting in which they must become familiar with a myriad of regulations, legal principles, and laws. Examples include the scope of practice of transport team members, Federal Aviation Administration (FAA) and Federal Communications Commission (FCC) regulations, and state and local regulations that direct ground transport vehicles. The education and training of the transport team must include information on the various laws and regulations pertinent to the practice. Specific laws such as the Consolidated Omnibus Reconciliation Act (COBRA) and the Emergency Medical and Active Labor Act (EMTALA) provide guidelines and regulations of which the transport team must be aware to provide safe and competent patient care.

AN OVERVIEW OF THE LAW

Law comprises all of the rules and regulations by which a society is governed. *Statutes* are laws made by governmental bodies; they vary from state to state. Statutes must comply with applicable federal law. The various acts applicable to nursing practice (e.g., the state nurse practice acts) are examples of statutory law. Statutes frequently require written rules and regulations for enforcement. Administrative agencies write *administrative law*, the rules and regulations that enforce the statute. The State Boards of Nursing are administrative agencies that promulgate administrative law.[8,13] *Case law*, or *judicial law*, varies from state to state. Legal issues brought before the courts are interpreted based on the facts of a particular case.

Criminal law permits legal action to be filed by the state for behavior that is offensive or harmful to society. Transport nurses may be charged with a criminal offense for a violation of either the State Nurse Practice Act or safe nursing practices (e.g., a charge of assault for treating a patient who explicity refused or withdrew consent, or a charge of criminal negligence when a serious medical error caused a patient's death). *Civil law,* in contrast to criminal law, permits an action to be filed by an individual for monetary compensation. *Tort law* is used most commonly in civil cases related to medical and nursing care. Compensation is requested for the person wrongfully injured by the actions of another.[6,8,20]

Negligence and malpractice are often incorrectly used as interchangeable terms. *Negligence* is a deviation from accepted standards of performance.[5,7,8,13-18] *Malpractice* is based on a professional standard of care and the professional statutes of the caregiver.[10,13,16,17] The same types of acts form the basis for negligence and malpractice.

Standards of care are another important concept of which transport teams must be aware. Standards of care are created in multiple ways, including by law, regulation, or case law. Numerous standards of care are applied to patient transport. Many come from professional associations such as the Air and Surface Transport Nurses Association (ASTNA). These standards are used to determine whether the care provided in the transport process is the generally accepted or expected care that should occur in similar circumstances. These standards are routinely used by legal experts and presented to juries in determination of whether malpractice has occurred.[1,20,21]

ELEMENTS OF MALPRACTICE

The elements of malpractice that must be present are shown in order of priority in Box 36-1. First, a *duty* must be present. The duty may be a contract, statute, or voluntary assumption of care of a patient by a transport nurse.[5,8,13,20] A duty is created by the development of a nurse-patient relationship and not merely employment status.[6]

Once a duty is established to exist, the second element is a *breach of duty.* Breach of duty may occur as a result of malfeasance (act of commission) or nonfeasance (act of omission).[8,13,20] Administration of the wrong medication is malfeasance, whereas failure to follow a procedure is nonfeasance.

BOX 36-1	**Elements of a Malpractice Case**

Presence of duty
Breach of duty
Foreseeability
Causation
Injury
Damages

The third element is *foreseeability;* that is, one could reasonably expect certain events to cause specific results.[3,8]

The fourth element in malpractice is *causation.* A reasonable cause-and-effect relationship must be shown between the breach of duty and injury.[3,5,13,20]

The two types of causation are: (1) in fact; and (2) proximate. *Proximate cause* occurs when the result is directly related to the act. *Cause in fact* occurs when the breach of duty owed causes the injury.

The fifth element is *injury.* The patient must be harmed physically, financially, or emotionally in a discernible way.[3,5,13,20]

The sixth element is *damages.* Damages are compensatory in nature and may be of different types. *General damages* are inherent to the injury itself. *Special damages* are losses and expenses incurred as a result of stress and emotional pain produced by the injury. *Punitive damages* are requested for an alleged malicious intent or willful or wanton misconduct.[8,22,23]

In certain circumstances, the doctrine of *res ipsa loquitor,* "let the thing speak for itself," is used. The elements that must be proved are causation, injury, and damages. Commonly, *res ipsa loquitor* is used in situations in which the patient was unconscious or in surgery at the time the injury occurred.[13,20]

STATUTE OF LIMITATIONS

Filing a lawsuit is under a *statute of time limitations.* Generally, if malpractice is alleged after a traumatic injury, the statute of limitations is 2 years; in cases of disease, it is at the time discovered.[5,8] The exception is in pediatric cases. The statute of limitations is extended until the minor is emancipated or reaches the age of majority (established by state law).[8]

TYPES OF LIABILITY
Intentional Torts or Criminal Acts

Assault or battery, or both, may be either *criminal* or *tort* (civil). *Assault* is placing an individual without consent in a situation in which he or she fears immediate bodily harm. *Battery* is the touching of a person without his or her consent. Battery can also occur with the touching of anything connected with a person (clothing, purse, jewelry) without consent.[3,4] Damages for battery may be punitive or nominal as well as compensatory.[8,20]

Other types of intentional torts are, briefly, false imprisonment, the unjustifiable detention of a person without his or her consent, and invasion of privacy, a key concept in issues related to confidentiality. The patient has the right to privacy of medical information. Photographs may not be taken and information may not be released without consent. Some situations are newsworthy, and the public's right to know can exceed the patient's right to privacy.[8] Obviously, knowledge of statutes and knowledge of relevant laws related to consent is vital. Defenses used against intentional torts are consent (discussed later in this chapter), self defense, defense of others, and necessity.[8,20]

Quasiintentional Torts

A *quasiintentional tort* protects an individual's interest in a person's reputation, privacy, and freedom from legal action that is unfounded.[1] It is a legal action that arises from damages inflicted on a person's reputation or privacy. Examples of such a tort include defamation of character, libel, and breach of confidentiality. Tort law does not actually protect a person; it just provides an avenue through the courts to seek compensation for damages done.

Vicarious Liability

Vicarious liability is defined as one party being responsible for the actions of another. The doctrine of *respondeat superior*, "let the master respond," has been used frequently when nurses are accused of malpractice. As a result of this doctrine, the employer has an obligation to ensure that employees perform duties in a competent safe manner. Two elements must be shown: (1) the injured party must prove that the employer had control over the employee; and (2) the negligent act occurred in the scope and course of the employment.[6] Vicarious liability can be found with either malfeasance or nonfeasance of the employee.

Recently courts have attached judgments directly against institutions for corporate negligence. Hospitals have found themselves accountable as an entity when the duty is owed directly to the patient and not through employees. Types of corporate duties attached directly to the institution are outlined in Box 36-2.[13-17]

Product Liability

An increase has been seen in *product liability* cases, which are mixtures of tort and contract law. The sale of a product places the manufacturer, processor, or nonmanufacturing seller at risk for a product liability case should injury to a person or person's property occur. Delivery of a service without the sale of the product is generally not substantial enough for a successful product liability suit. However, court decisions have been inconsistent in separating the sale of product from delivery of a service.[8] *Collective liability* may occur when several manufacturers have participated in a cooperative activity. *Alternative liability* occurs when two or more manufacturers commit separate acts.

ABANDONMENT

The principles related to abandonment are important to flight nurse practice. *Abandonment* occurs with unilateral termination of the nurse-patient

---

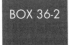 **BOX 36-2** | **Examples of Corporate Duties Owed Directly to Patient**

Duty of reasonable care in maintenance and use of equipment

Availability of equipment and services

Duty of reasonable care in selecting and retaining employees

Adoption and assurance of compliance with rules related to administrative responsibility for patient care

Selection and retention of medical staff

relationship without consent from the patient.[7] Abandonment can also occur if the care of the patient is transferred to someone less qualified.[7,9] Questions may arise regarding abandonment any time there is a demonstration of disregard for the patient's welfare, unreasonable practices, or both.[7] The various types of air medical transports should be reviewed by each program and evaluated to ensure that potential abandonment issues are addressed. George[8] suggested that the act of dispatching an ambulance was presumptive of voluntary assumption of a duty to a patient. This assumption should be considered in development of communication center protocols.

CONSENT ISSUES

Many medical tort claims are related to *consent issues*.[5] *Informed consent* requires more than a patient's signature on a consent form. The suggested treatment must be presented to the patient with a discussion of all material risks, consequences, and available alternatives.[1,5] If the patient refuses the first treatment option, other treatment options should be explained. Informed consent requires understanding on the part of the patient.

Consent can be written or oral. Nurses are frequently asked to obtain signatures on consent forms. Before the patient signs, the nurse should determine that the patient understands the purpose of the consent. *Expressed consent* occurs with written or oral acknowledgment. *Implied consent* occurs when a patient is compliant with a request (extending arm for phlebotomy, allowing placement of nasal prongs, and so on). Implied consent is frequently operational in emergency situations. Most consent statutes allow for treatment of life-threatening emergencies if the patient is unable to consent because it is the reasonable thing to do.[5] One should be cautious, however, not to exceed the limits of implied consent. If the patient is physically or mentally incapable of consenting, implied consent is operative in the case of a true emergency. In the absence of a true emergency, consent should be obtained before treatment from a person who is authorized to consent.[5]

Consent for treatment of minors is reserved for a parent or legal guardian. Implied consent is used for minors with life-threatening emergency conditions. The parents or legal guardian should be contacted as soon as possible for notification and consent. Most states have laws related to emancipated minors who can consent before the age of majority. In addition, minors may be allowed to consent for treatment of certain conditions such as sexually transmitted diseases, pregnancy, and substance abuse.[5]

Refusal to consent or *withdrawal of consent* is sometimes a murky question. A common issue is the refusal of a blood transfusion because of religious beliefs. If the treating physician believes that a blood transfusion is necessary and the patient refuses, an attempt can be made to obtain a court order. However, in the field, the competent patient's wishes must be respected. The court uses a balancing test to weigh one right against the other. The court leans to the right of the patient to make a knowing choice in refusing consent. The exception is in the case of minors. If the court is convinced a child needs lifesaving measures, compelling state's interest in the child usually overrides the parent's interest.

DOCUMENTATION

The purpose of documentation is to document care and treatments given, assist with continuity of care between health professionals, establish a record of patient care so that it can be reviewed for continuity and continuing education and research, provide data for reimbursement and cost analysis, and legally protect the caregiver.

The medical record of a patient belongs to the hospital or transport service, although the patient has a right to the information contained therein.[1-3,20] The *medical record* is the documentation of the patient's course of treatment. It serves as a means of communication between various providers of service. It protects the legal interests of the patient, the hospital, and the healthcare practitioner.[1-3,20] The patient's privacy must be protected in these situations. The Health Insurance Portability and Accountability Act (HIPAA) and transport are briefly discussed later in this chapter. The contents of the medical record should be factual and based on objective data.[20]

The medical record should be:

- Brief, concise, accurate, and thorough.
- Clearly written and legible.
- Without judgmental terms.
- Timely.

Abbreviations are strongly discouraged today. The Joint Commission offers guidelines on the use of abbreviations. Only approved abbreviations should be used. The entries should be readable, concise, and complete.[20] The patient description should be objective and include the patient's appearance, signs and symptoms, and interventions and responses. Documentation should occur in a timely fashion. If an untoward incident occurs, an event report should be completed and appropriate personnel notified. Today, several computer-based transport records are available; however, these programs must provide the components of patient documentation pertinent to the transport service using the program. The several advantages to computer-based documentation include the ability to read the documentation, time stamping of procedures and medication administration, recordkeeping of transport team interventions, and retrieval of data for research and continuous quality improvement. The transport record should "tell the story" of the transport process. Documentation of any deviations from protocols and orders obtained from medical control is also important.[20]

Only designated personnel should review charts, and such review must comply with relevant privacy legislation. Records are an important component of the continuous quality improvement process and a way to document transport team competencies.

HEALTH INSURANCE PORTABILITY AND ACCOUNTABILITY ACT

The *Health Insurance Portability and Accountability Act* (HIPAA) became effective in 1996. It is a federal law that is intended to protect patient health information and simplify the means by which healthcare providers electronically file and transmit healthcare claims.[1,21] These safeguards currently apply to all protected health information, including electronic, written, and photographic. The HIPAA law has three different rules with specific compliance guidelines. The *Transaction and Code Set Rule* (TCS) is primarily related to billing and requires that the transport team ensure that the appropriate information is documented to enhance this process. The *Privacy Rule* designates that private health

information (PHI) about the patient be safeguarded and restricted. Finally, the *Security Rule* outlines how PHI should be protected, including encryption of transmitted data and physical security of a facility where PHI is stored. HIPAA has presented a challenge to transport teams who must be careful and consistent in how information about the patient is provided and used. Implications to transport teams include [1,21]:

- Transport team members must undergo mandatory HIPAA training.
- Oral and written information about the patient must be protected. Information about the patient should be appropriately stored.
- Patients should receive a Notice of Privacy Practices (NPP). This notice is not given during the transport process but should be provided after the emergency has passed.
- Transport teams may share PHI about the patient with providers at a scene and at a referring hospital without a patient's consent, contact a base station and provide radio reports, provide follow-up on the patient for quality improvement purposes, and provide selected information with involved law enforcement.

Information may also be shared without the patient's consent when information is needed related to the monitoring and controlling of communicable disease, injury, or disability; to disclosure for compiling statistics, such as for births and deaths; to reporting of adverse events to the Food and Drug Administration (FDA) and disclosure to government oversight committees; to disclosure to evaluate work place injuries; and to organ donation programs and certain law enforcement personnel. Examples of information that may be shared with law enforcement personnel include child maltreatment, PHI sought through the court system, and disclosure of limited information in the process of identifying a suspect. Transport team members must become aware of the implications of HIPAA to the patients that they transport and their practice.[1,21]

Consolidated Omnibus Budget Reconciliation Act/ Emergency Medical and Active Labor Act

The *Consolidated Omnibus Budget Reconciliation Act* (COBRA) was passed in 1986. This contained the Emergency Medical Treatment and Active Labor Act of 1986.[1-3,6,8,9,13,14,16,18-20] In this law is the *Emergency Medical and Active Labor Act* (EMTALA), the anti-dumping statute. The essential components of the EMTALA include[19]:

1. All patients who present to an emergency department should receive a nondiscriminatory medical screening to determine whether a medical emergency is present.
2. A patient with a medical emergency must be stabilized within the capabilities of the transferring hospital and within reasonable probability that no material deterioration in the patient's clinical condition will occur.
3. If the patient must be transferred for further care, a receiving hospital must have accepted the patient and have the appropriate equipment and staff available to care for the patient.
4. The referring hospital must send all copies of medical records, diagnostic studies, and informed consent documents, and the patient must be transported with the appropriate vehicle and personnel.

If the patient's condition is unstable, the transfer certification must address[19]:

a. Patient's condition.
b. Benefits of transfer.
c. Risk of transfer.
d. Specific information about the receiving facility, including that patient report was called to the receiving facility.
e. Description of the mode of transportation.
f. Patient or designate must sign a consent and certify how the transfer was initiated (patient request, physician request, or other).
g. The form should be witnessed, and the patient or designate must sign that he or she understands the risks and benefits of transfer.

In 1990, the COBRA law underwent further revisions that broadened who is subject to the law. The law now includes all participating physicians and any other physician responsible for the examination, treatment, or the transfer of the participating hospital.[19] Further clarification of EMTALA was released by the Department of Health and Human Services, Centers for Medicare and Medicaid Services (CMS) in September of 2003. The document was titled "Clarifying Policies Related to the Responsibilities of Medicare-Participating Hospitals in Treating Individuals with Emergency Medical Condition (Final Regulation).[19] Violations of COBRA/EMTALA legislation include financial penalties and potential loss of government funding.

The transport team needs to be aware of potential violations (e.g., a transfer that may be based on financial reasons instead of patient need) and notify the appropriate authorities when a violation has occurred.[19]

Clarification of Hospital Helipads

In 2004, site review guidelines from EMTALA helped to clarify the use of hospital helipads by emergency medical services (EMS) personnel.[20] An ambulance may meet a helicopter team on hospital A's helipad for transfer to hospital B without triggering any EMTALA obligation unless the ambulance crew requests medical assistance from hospital A.[20] If medical assistance is requested, hospital A becomes responsible for EMTALA compliance.

If hospital A owns the ambulance that requests the assistance of the helicopter on hospital A's helipad, hospital A has an EMTALA obligation if the patient is transported from the scene of an emergency response, subject to the exceptions under the "ambulance rule."[20]

Diversion

In the past 15 years, emergency department and hospital patient *diversion* has become a major issue in the United States. Initially, it was seen in larger cities, but it has now become an issue across the entire country and even the world.[4,11] Causes of diversion include use of the emergency department by non-urgent cases; inadequate staffing; decrease in the number of emergency departments (EDs) available in given areas of the country; use of ancillary services, such as computed tomographic (CT) scans; and hospital bed shortages. No matter the cause, diversion does have an impact on transport programs.[4,11,12,19-21] According to EMTALA, hospitals with specialized services such as trauma and burn centers do not have a "right" to divert; however, they can use diversion to help manage patient flow. Hopefully, this assists with keeping patients safe and improving quality of care.[20]

Transport teams must be aware of diversion policies in the communities in which they serve and be a part of how these policies are developed. This awareness also includes the role of the transport program in the event of a disaster.

Mission diversion as explained by Williams[20] is not specifically involved with EMTALA regulations. However, similar to the resource issues identified in ED overcrowding and diversion, many times a transport program may have to direct limited resources to meet multiple responses. Transport programs should have written policies and procedures about how and when missions are diverted, what priorities are used to determine who or what missions may be diverted, who makes the decision to divert or redirect the patient, how are the transport teams notified, and what type of documentation is used.

Diversion is a challenging issue for the 21st century. No simple solutions exist, and the problems will take awhile to solve. Diversion impacts patient transport and patient care. Transport personnel and services must be aware of its consequences, participate in decision making related to diversion, and have policies and procedures to address it.

MEDICAL DIRECTION DURING INTERFACILITY PATIENT TRANSFERS

Who is responsible for the patient during transport is an important legal concept that must be understood by transport team members. Transfer of patients from one institution to another has become a fundamental part of patient care today. The chapter on patient preparation for transport identified some of the multiple reasons a patient may need transfer and

transport. The section in this chapter describes the federal regulations related to patient transfer and transport as pointed out by EMTALA. According to COBRA/EMTALA, unless otherwise specified, patient care during transport is the responsibility of the transferring physician and hospital. The transferring physician is responsible for[1-3,14,15,18,22,23]:

- Identifying the appropriate receiving facility.
- Writing transfer orders.
- Identifying the appropriate transport team, equipment, and treatment that are needed during the transport process.

The authority that governs patient care during transport varies from state to state and is based on the type of transport team that is with the patient. Medical responsibility for the patient should be arranged before the transport process is initiated. For example, our transport team is composed of a nurse and a physician. Because a physician is present, medical direction can come from that person. Other options for medical direction during transport include:

- Transferring physician assumes medical direction.
- Receiving physician assumes medical direction.
- Medical director of the transport service assumes medical direction.
- Responsibility may be shared and predefined with a transfer of medical direction en route because of long distances (e.g., on international transports).

Transport teams should have policies, procedures, and protocols in place to address medical direction during transport. The transport service and their medical director are responsible for providing safe competent care during the process.

SCOPE OF PRACTICE

Statutes, rules, or a combination of the two defines the *scope of practice*. Some of the statutes that govern members of the transport team include the scope of practice as stated in State Nurse Practice

BOX 36-3	**Elements of Nurse Practice Acts**

Definition of professional nursing
Requirements for licensure
Exemptions
Licensure across jurisdictions
Disciplinary action and due process requirements
Creation of Board of Nursing
Penalties for practicing without a license

Acts or Emergency Medical Services statutes. The Nurse Practice Acts establish licensure requirements for nurses. Most states require mandatory licensure before either the title or actions are permitted. Exceptions are generally related to students, new graduates, and transport through a state's jurisdiction.[7,8] Box 36-3 illustrates the common elements of nurse practice acts as an example of a scope of practice.[6]

Chapter 4 describes the roles of specific members of the transport team. Most of these members practice in an expanded role. Before practicing in an expanded role, transport team members should review the pertinent nurse, emergency medical services, medical, and pharmacy practice acts; attorney general's opinions; and recent judicial decisions that govern their practice.[7,8] The institution's policies and procedures should be investigated and followed to ensure that the scope of practice for the transport team is clearly defined. This is also done with the transport services medical director. The Commission on Accreditation of Medical Transport Systems (CAMTS) outlines in its standards the role of the medical director.[5]

In addition to scope of practice, the standards of care that govern the professional practice of the transport team members must be reviewed. *Internal standards* are set by the role of the team member, job descriptions, and policies and procedures. *External standards* are established by state boards of nursing, professional and specialty organizations, and federal guidelines.[7,8,20] In cases of purported deviation from the standard of care, the external standards may be submitted as evidence, expert witnesses used, or both. Professional publications may be submitted to assist the jury in understanding the expected standard of care.[5,7,8,20]

The Air and Surface Transport Nurses revised "Practice Standards for Flight Nursing" in 1995. A summary of these standards is presented in Box 36-4. The transport nurse practice standards are an example of external standards. The International Association of Flight Paramedics and the Association

BOX 36-4	**Standards of Professional Performance**

Standard I. Quality of Care

The flight nurse systematically and continuously evaluates the quality, appropriateness, and effectiveness of client care and nursing practice in the air medical transport environment.

Measurement criteria:

1. The flight nurse participates in quality management activities to evaluate care in the transport environment. Such activities may include but are not limited to:
   A. Delineation of scope of care.
   B. Development of standards of care.
   C. Identification of aspects of care important for quality monitoring.
   D. Identification of indicators used to monitor quality and effectiveness of care delivered by flight nurses.
   E. Data collection to monitor quality and effectiveness of client care.
   F. Data assessment to identify opportunities for improving flight nursing practice and client care.
   G. Formulation of recommendations to improve flight nursing practice and client outcomes.
   H. Action to improve care and service.

BOX 36-4	**Standards of Professional Performance—cont'd**

    I. Evaluation.

    J. Report of findings.

2. The flight nurse uses the results of the quality management activities to initiate appropriate changes in client care procedures and flight nursing practice.

3. The flight nurse uses the results of the quality management activities to initiate appropriate changes in air medical services.

4. The flight nurse uses the results of the quality management activities to initiate appropriate changes throughout the healthcare delivery system.

5. The flight nurse identifies safety concerns.

6. The flight nurse ensures that appropriate infection control measures are implemented according to: (1) Centers for Disease Control and Prevention (CDCP) guidelines; (2) Occupational Safety Health Administration (OSHA) standards; and (3) individual program and institution procedures.

7. The flight nurse advises appropriate personnel if actual or potential risk exists from exposure to infectious organisms.

8. The flight nurse participates in ongoing infection control educational activities.

Standard II. Performance Appraisal

The flight nurse evaluates his or her own nursing practice.

Measurement criteria:

1. The flight nurse engages in performance appraisal on a regular basis, identifying areas of strength and areas for professional/practice development.

2. The nurse seeks constructive feedback regarding his or her own practice.

3. The flight nurse takes steps to achieve goals identified during performance appraisal.

4. The flight nurse participates in peer review as appropriate.

Standard III. Education

The flight nurse acquires and maintains knowledge necessary for competent flight nursing practice.

Measurement criteria:

1. The flight nurse successfully completes an initial training or orientation program, which includes didactic and clinical topics pertinent to flight nursing practice and specialty areas of practice.

2. The flight nurse participates in ongoing educational activities pertinent to flight nursing practice and specialty areas.

3. The flight nurse seeks learning experiences to maintain a knowledge base and clinical skills necessary for flight nursing practice.

4. The flight nurse maintains documentation of educational activities.

Excellence criteria:

1. The flight nurse independently seeks advanced learning experiences to expand knowledge base and clinical skills to enhance flight nursing practice.

2. The flight nurse attains advanced educational degrees.

Standard IV. Collegiality

The flight nurse contributes to the knowledge base of peers, colleagues, and healthcare providers.

Measurement criteria:

1. The flight nurse shares knowledge and skills with colleagues and other healthcare providers.

2. The flight nurse provides peers with constructive feedback regarding their flight nurse practices.

3. The flight nurse contributes to an environment that is conducive to clinical education of other healthcare providers.

(Continued)

BOX 36-4 | Standards of Professional Performance—cont'd

Excellence criteria:

1. The flight nurse organizes educational presentations for other healthcare providers to promote optimal healthcare for the community.

Standard V. Ethics

The flight nurse's decisions and actions on behalf of clients are determined in an ethical manner.

Measurement criteria:

1. Flight nurse practice is guided by the American Nurses Association's Code of Ethics.
2. Flight nursing practice is guided by the Nurse Practice Act as defined by each state.
3. The flight nurse delivers care in a nonjudgmental and nondiscriminatory manner that is sensitive to client diversities.
4. The flight nurse provides information to assist the client or significant other in making an informed decision for transfer.
5. The flight nurse is a client advocate.
6. The flight nurse maintains client confidentiality at all times.
7. The flight nurse delivers care in a manner that preserves and protects client autonomy, dignity, and rights.
8. The flight nurse uses available resources to help formulate ethical decisions.
9. The flight nurse uses available mechanisms to identify and resolve ethical issues related to client care.

Standard VI. Collaboration

The flight nurse collaborates with the client, significant others, and other health care providers in providing client care.

Measurement criteria:

1. The flight nurse communicates with the client, significant others, and health care professionals regarding client care and nursing's role in the provision of care.
2. The flight nurse consults with health care providers for client care, as needed.
3. The flight nurse makes referrals, including provisions for continuity of care, as needed.

Standard VII. Research

The flight nurse enhances and supports practice through the use of research findings.

Measurement criteria:

1. The flight nurse incorporates into practice validated research outcomes.
2. The flight nurse disseminates validated research findings to others.
3. The flight nurse complies with ethical research principles.
4. The flight nurse uses the results of validated research to initiate changes in air medical services.

Excellence criteria:

1. The flight nurse initiates and actively participates in formal research through participation in one or more of the following areas: (1) research design; (2) grant application; (3) research analysis; (4) abstract presentation; and (5) research contribution to literature.

Standard VIII. Resource Utilization

The flight nurse considers factors related to safety, effectiveness, and cost in planning and delivering care.

Measurement criteria:

1. The flight nurse practices safety measures through applied knowledge of:
   A. General aviation safety procedures.
   B. FAA rules and regulations pertaining to safety.

BOX 36-4	**Standards of Professional Performance—cont'd**

C. Emergency aircraft equipment and procedures.

D. Ground operations.

E. Safe use of client care procedures and equipment used in the aircraft environment.

F. Scene hazards.

2. The flight nurse evaluates factors related to safety, effectiveness, and cost when two or more practice options would result in the same expected client outcomes.

3. The flight nurse assigns or delegates care based on the needs of the client and the knowledge and skill of the provider.

4. The flight nurse assists the client and significant others to identify and secure appropriate services.

From National Flight Nurses Association: *Standards of flight nursing practice,* St Louis, 1995, Mosby.

---

of Air Medical Physicians provide additional examples of external standards that guide the practice of patient transport.[5,7,8,20]

SUMMARY

Knowledge of the law and legal doctrine is a necessary component of the transport process. Transport team members must be familiar with both the internal and professional standards that describe their scope of practice and profession. Ignorance of the law harms not only the healthcare provider but also the patients that they serve.

REFERENCES

1. Air and Surface Transport Nurses Association: *Transport nurse advanced trauma course,* ed 4, Denver, 2006, ASTNA.

2. American Academy of Pediatrics: *Air and ground transport of neonatal and pediatric patients,* ed 3, Elk Grove Village, IL, 2007, AAP.

3. Bitterman RA: *Providing emergency care under federal law: EMTALA,* Dallas, 2000, American College of Emergency Physicians.

4. Burt CW, McCaig LF, Valverde R: Analysis of ambulance transports and diversions among US emergency departments, *Ann Emerg Med* 47(4): 317-326, 2006.

5. Cisar NS: Informed consent: an ethical dilemma, *Nurs Forum* 30(303):20, 1995.

6. Commission on Accreditation of Medical Transport Systems (CAMTS): *Standards,* ed 7, Andersonville, SC, 2006, CAMTS.

7. Cushing M: *Nursing jurisprudence,* East Norwalk, CT, 1988, Appleton & Lange.

8. George JE: *Law and emergency care,* St Louis, 1980, Mosby.

9. Guido GW: *Legal issues in nursing: source book for practice,* East Norwalk, CT, 1988, Appleton & Lange.

10. Hepp R: *Standards of flight nursing practice,* St Louis, 1995, Mosby.

11. Hoot NR, Aronsky D: Systemic review of emergency department crowding: causes, effects and solutions, *Ann Emerg Med* 52(2):126-136, 2008.

12. Khaleghi M, Loh A, Vroman D, et al: The effects of minimizing ambulance diversion hours on emergency departments, *J Emerg Med* 33(2):155-159, 2007.

13. Lazar RA: *EMS law: a guide for EMS professionals,* Rockville, MD, 1989, Aspen.

14. Mitchiner JC, Yeh CS: Emergency medical treatment and active labor act, *Nurs Clin North Am* 37(1): 19-34, 2002.

15. Shelton SL, Swor RA, Domeier RM, et al: *Medical direction of interfacility transports,* Lenexa, KS, 2000, NAEMSP.

16. Southard P: COBRA legislation: complying with ED provisions, *J Emerg Nurs* 15:23, 1989.

17. Southwick AF: *The law of hospital and health administration,* ed 2, Ann Arbor, MI, 1988, Health Administration Press.

18. Swor RA, Storer D, Domeier R, et al: *Medical direction of interfacility patient transfers,* Dallas, 1997, American College of Emergency Physicians.

19. Teshome G, Closson FT: Emergency medical treatment and labor act: the basics and other medicolegal concerns, *Pediatr Clin North Am* 53:139-155, 2006.
20. Williams A: Legal issues in air and ground medicine. In Blumen IJ, editor: *Principles and directions of air medical transport*, Salt Lake City, 2006, Air Medical Physicians Association.
21. York-Clark D, Stocking J, Johnson J, editors: *Flight and ground transport nursing core curriculum*, Denver, 2006, Air and Surface Transport Nurses Association.
22. Youngberg BJ: Medical-legal considerations involved in the transport of critically ill patients, *Crit Care Clin* 8(3):501, 1992.
23. Youngberg BJ: Legal issues related to transport. In McCloskey K, Orr RA, editors: *Pediatric transport medicine*, St Louis, 1995, Mosby.

ETHICAL ISSUES

Reneé Semonin Holleran

Many of us went through our professional training with limited exposure to ethical decision making. Then, we went through training that persuaded us that we could save everyone. So, when we have to make difficult transport decisions, we have to do it based on previous experience or with use of preestablished protocols whose development we may or may not have been allowed to participate in.

Today, transport team members are faced with many ethical dilemmas, including who to transport, when resuscitation is futile, and the use of technology. One of the most commonly faced dilemmas by all transport teams is when not to transport a patient. Research has documented that the outcomes of patients who sustain cardiac arrest before reaching the hospital are dismal, and patient transport is expensive.[2-9,11,17] Currently, transport programs make "no-transport" decisions on the basis of a number of factors.

Other ethical challenges may include being asked to transport patients in unsafe environments, for example, when the weather is less than optimal. Some transport teams are forced to make decisions about whether to transport a patient with equipment or problems that they have inadequate experience handling because of competition or fear of revenue loss.

This chapter offers an example of a framework that may be used to make ethical decisions. It also contains information about a common problem encountered in the transport environment: to transport or not to transport. The case study at the end of this chapter provides an outline that may be used to generate discussion about ethical problems that may be encountered by the transport team.

ETHICAL DECISION MAKING IN THE TRANSPORT ENVIRONMENT

Ethical decisions are generally made based on a set of specific values, which include[1,10]:

- *Patient autonomy:* Allowing patients to make decisions about their healthcare.
- *Beneficence* versus *malfeasance:* The benefit of the transport outweighs the potential harm the transport could cause.
- *Veracity:* Honesty, telling the truth, open patient care and healthcare provider relationships. Veracity should also extend to statement of purpose for the transport program.
- *Justice:* Fairness for the patient and, at times, the community that the transport program serves.

The American Nurses Association[1] has provided a Code of Ethics for Nurses for decades. The most recent version offers a framework on which a nurse may practice. Concepts expressed include:

- Nurses must practice with compassion and respect for the inherent dignity, worth, and uniqueness of every individual unrestricted by their diversity.
- A nurse's primary commitment is to the patient.
- Nurses must strive to protect the health, safety, and rights of the patient.
- Nurses are responsible and accountable for their nursing practice.
- Nurses owe the same duties to themselves as to their patients to preserve integrity and safety, maintain competence, and continue personal and professional growth.

Nursing is involved nationally and internationally in the shaping of social policy and in efforts to meet healthcare needs.

Examination of these values is important when making decisions about patient care in the transport environment. Unfortunately, multiple demands may influence the transport decision, including competition, lack of experience, and concern about employment.

The availability of equipment, advanced life support skills, and personnel has contributed to the development of a *technologic imperative.*[5,10] In other words, because we have it, we must use it. Patients, families, and communities have come to expect that everything is available for everyone.

Iserson and colleagues[10] have developed a model that can be used to make ethical decisions in the transport environment. This model includes:

- Problem perception: Is there a problem?
- List alternatives: Identify solutions and barriers.
- Choose an alternative.
- List the consequences of the actions chosen.
- Consider one's own personal beliefs when making the decision.
- Evaluate the decision.

Ethical decision making is a dynamic process. The transport team cannot ignore previous experience or the personal beliefs of the team members and those with whom the team is working. These things are never easy, but they cannot be overlooked.

TO TRANSPORT OR NOT TO TRANSPORT

As healthcare costs continue to increase, the cost of patient transport and appropriate use of services have become important issues that many transport programs must address. Deciding when to transport patients who have sustained cardiac arrest, whether as a result of trauma or a medical problem, continues to be one of the most difficult dilemmas faced by many transport programs. Research has shown that survival rates of patients who have out-of-hospital cardiac arrests range from 1.9% to 5%. Many survivors sustain severe neurologic injury, and the quality of their life is impaired.[9-18]

Data from a 10-year period of transport of patients who needed cardiopulmonary resuscitation during air medical transport indicated that only 1.9% of these patients survived. The injuries sustained by the patients ranged from those from motor vehicle crashes to gunshot wounds to the head. The only intervention provided by the flight team that was not provided by emergency medical services was the administration of blood. The average cost of each flight was $2671.[8]

In a study from the University of Louisville,[9] researchers found that six patients (2.4%) of patients with traumatic arrest survived. The air medical costs for these patients averaged $2600. The researchers concluded that patients with cardiac arrest who have obvious severe brain injury and those who have been in arrest for longer than 30 minutes should not be resuscitated.[9]

Whether to transport a patient who may be dead in the field remains a difficult decision and has profound ethical implications. Air medical transport illustrates one example of a technologic imperative, or the "unquestioning impulse to use any available technologic intervention."[5] The public also has come to expect both emergency medical services and transport programs to come to the rescue of all who need medical assistance, which attaches additional pressure to the decisions that must be made related to the transport of a patient who is in full arrest.

An ethical practice model suggested by Drought and Liaschenko[5] may serve as a framework for the decision of whether to transport or pronounce the patient dead and not transport. The practice model is based on the practice account of morality and is composed of the following: (1) the practice knowledge is obtained from dealing with concrete problems, not abstract or hypothetic situations (e.g., the knowledge that patients who sustain blunt cardiac arrest in the field have less than a 1% chance of survival has been obtained from actual cases); (2) the knowledge that is obtained from practice is shared with other practitioners, such as the fact that multiple studies have shown that the survival rate of patients who have an out-of-hospital arrest is less than 5%[2-4,8-18]; (3) this knowledge has implications for all types of transported patients; and (4) it is dynamic; that is, research is continuous to describe the problem.[5]

The transport team must always be critical when making an ethical decision related to the transport of patients who have sustained cardiac arrest. *Critical* means thoughtful and reflective of the means, goals, and implications of this practice.[5] The transport team must consider the feelings of those who have been caring for the patient; the wishes of the patient's family, if present; and whether everything has truly been done for the patient.

Education, critical examination of the facts, and evaluation of one's personal values related to death and dying should assist the transport team in developing guidelines for when not to transport and with difficult transport decisions. Case presentations, literature reviews, and the use of clinical guidelines are some methods that may be used to make moral practice decisions. Figure 37-1 presents a protocol that is used to pronounce patients dead in the field. As pointed out by Mattox,[13] "both society and trauma resuscitators [must] accept that the patient who has a fatal injury [should] die with dignity, not being subject to extensive and expensive resurrection techniques."

SUMMARY

Ethical decision making can be challenging in the transport environment. It must encompass care values, compassion, accountability, and commitment to the people served by the transport service. Transport teams should discuss troubling patient transports. Decision-making protocols should include all members of the transport team, the patients, and the communities that they serve.

As healthcare technology progresses and presents us with new challenges, we must never lose sight of the rights of our patients. In addition, we must never lose sight of our duties to ourselves to provide care in a safe supportive professional transport environment.

UNIVERSITY OF CINCINNATI HOSPITAL UNIVERSITY AIR CARE NURSING	
Policy	Page __1__ of ____

Policy: Pronouncing Patients Dead-Scene	
File: p-10-a	**Date Originated:** 11/86
Revised: 5/90	**Reviewed:** 4/92, 4/94, 4/95,
Previous Reviews/Revisions: 11/86 - 11/91	4/98, 4/00, 4/02
Precautions:	
Responsibility:	
Equipment:	

Purpose:
To provide guidelines for the pronouncing dead of patients by the University Air Care Flight Physician at the scene of an accident, injury, or illness.

Procedure:
A. Due to the presence of a physician on the University Air Care Team, a patient may be pronounced dead in the field in the following circumstances:
1. If in the judgment of the University Air Care Physician the patient is clinically dead with no chance of survival.
2. The requesting agency, rescue personnel, and family members *if and when present* are comfortable with the decision to terminate resuscitative efforts.
3. There are no medical-legal contraindications to pronouncing the patient dead in the field, such as in homicide or suicide cases.
B. The following are specific situations that if present would generally prohibit pronouncing a patient dead in the field:
1. Rescue personnel have been working diligently to save the victim's life and feel that the patient should be transported to a higher level of care.
2. Invasive surgical procedures such as chest tube insertion have been accomplished by the University Air Care Team.
3. Advanced skills for establishing an adequate airway such as endotracheal intubation and cricothyrotomy may be necessary to determine the likelihood of survival for a patient. These procedures do not preclude pronouncing a patient dead in the field but if accomplished should cause the University Air Care Team to carefully consider all the factors associated with pronouncing a patient dead in the field.
4. A patient **may not** at any time be pronounced dead in the aircraft or on the helipad.
5. In the event that a flight nurse is flying without a physician, they **cannot** pronounce a patient dead.
6. Whenever there is a question as to whether a patient should be pronounced dead in the field, contact should be made with the Emergency Medicine Faculty.

Reviewed by: _____

_____
Senior Administrator, Patient Care Services

FIGURE 37-1   **Example of protocol used in air medical program when a patient is pronounced dead.**

CASE STUDY

The transport team of a large tertiary care facility has been requested to perform intraaortic balloon pump (IABP) transports from a small community hospital. The team has already had several complicated referrals from the cardiologist at the referring community hospital, including care that had been initiated by the referring cardiologist that was actually harmful to patients. The cardiologist wishes to insert the IABP, and the team is concerned about the safety and consequences of his request. In addition, a machine would have to be purchased and the transport team trained in its use.

With the model suggested by Iserson and his colleagues,[10] the transport team discussed this issue.

Problem perception:

Is there a need for this service to implement an IABP transport program?

List alternatives:

Two services can currently provide IABP transport, but they are not under the direction of the cardiologist at the tertiary center.

The cardiologist at the referring hospital has guaranteed the receiving cardiologist at least 175 patients who may need open heart surgery if IABP transport is available.

A machine would have to be purchased.

The transport team would have to be trained.

The amount of transports that the service may do will increase.

List the ethical values that may be related to the problem:

Patient autonomy: The patient may not receive all the facts to make a decision or be afforded the opportunity to do so.

Beneficence versus malfeasance: The flight time to the referring facility is less than 20 minutes. Patient delay to transfer is greater than 60 minutes to the receiving facility when the IABP is put in.

Preparation for transport is greater with the machine in place.

The referring cardiologist could offer only one study that suggested that this procedure was beneficial in patients with stable conditions.

Choose one alternative:

An individual trained in the use of the equipment should be on each transport.

List consequences:

The 30-minute delay in transport waiting for additional team member.

Scan personal values:

Professional: This type of transport requires training and competencies not readily available at the receiving facility. Most programs that do the transport recommend that the service complete a minimum of 60 transports per year.

Compare consequences with values:

Patient injury is a potential risk because of lack of experience.

Make the decision:

A trained person must accompany each IABP transport. From the transport service or a perfusion sit/CVICU RN?

Evaluation: What is this evaluation based on? What was the decision the crew was comfortable with?

Only five transports have been completed. Transport team members feel comfortable with their decision.

REFERENCES

1. American Nurses Association: *Code of ethics for nurses with imperative statements*, Washington DC, 2005, ANA, available at http://nursingworld.org/ethics/code, accessed August 2008.
2. Blumen I, editor: *Principles and direction of air medical transport*, Salt Lake City, 2006, Air Medical Physician Association (AMPA).
3. Cummins RO, Hazinski MF: The most important changes in the ECC and CPR guidelines 2000, *Resuscitation* 23:431, 2000.
4. Dries D: Recent progress in ACLS, *Air Med J* 19:38, 2000.
5. Drought TS, Liaschenko J: Ethical practice in a technological age, *Crit Care Nurs Clin North Am* 7(2).297, 1995.
6. Eisenberg M: Charles Kite's essay on the recovery on the apparently dead: the first scientific study of sudden death, *Ann Emerg Med* 23:1049, 1994.
7. Eisenberg M, Pantridge J, Cobb L, et al: The revolution and evolution of cardiac care, *Arch Internal Med* 12:1, 1996.
8. Falcone RE, et al: Air medical transport for the trauma patient requiring cardiopulmonary resuscitation: a 10-year experience, *Air Med J* 14:197, 1995.
9. Fulton R, Voigt W, Hilakos A: Confusion surrounding the treatment of traumatic arrest, *J Coll Surg* 181:209, 1995.
10. Iserson K, Sanders A, Mathieu D: *Ethics in emergency medicine*, Tucson, AZ, 1995, Galen Press.
11. Jecker N: Ceasing futile resuscitation in the field: ethical considerations, *Arch Internal Med* 152(2):3035, 1992.
12. Marco C: Resuscitation research: future directions and ethical issues, *Acad Emerg Med* 8:839, 2001.
13. Mattox K: "Ideal" posttraumatic parameters, *J Trauma* 34(5):734, 1993.
14. Morrison L, Verbeek P, Vermeulen M, et al: Derivation and evaluation of a termination of resuscitation clinical prediction rule for advanced life support providers, *Resuscitation* 74:266-275, 2007.
15. Naess AC, Steen E, Steen P: Ethics in treatment decisions during out-of-hospital resuscitation, *Resuscitation* 33:245, 1997.
16. Ong M, Tan E, Ng F, et al: Comparison of termination guidelines for out-of-hospital cardiac arrest in Singapore EMS, *Resuscitation* 75: 244-251, 2007.
17. Pepe P, Swor R, Ornato J, et al: Resuscitation in the out-of-hospital setting: medical futility criteria for on-scene pronouncement of death, *Prehosp Emerg Care* 5:79-87, 2001.
18. Safar P: On the future of reanimatology, *Acad Emerg Med* 7:75, 2000.

THE FAMILY AND TRANSPORT

Reneé Semonin Holleran

COMPETENCIES

1. Perform a focused assessment of the needs of families before, during, and after transport.
2. Identify the advantages and disadvantages to allowing the family to accompany the patient during transport.
3. Describe methods to meet the needs of the family.

Patient care during transport is generally focused on meeting the physiologic needs of an acutely ill or injured patient. However, the patient is generally a part of a family, although the definition of the term may vary. A family may be described in legal, cultural, religious, or personal terms. The families of today are as diverse as the people who live in them.[5]

Although transport team members are accustomed to the transport environment and process, they should not forget that this experience is new and often frightening for the family members of a seriously ill or injured person. The transport team must consider care of the family to be an extension of patient care and not an additional task that needs to be accomplished. The support that healthcare professionals provide to the patient's family during the initial stages of the patient's crisis can be invaluable. Contact with a transport team or emergency department (ED) employees may be the family's

first interaction with healthcare personnel in this emergency. The family's perception of the response of these healthcare providers can be the impetus to either healthy or ineffective coping. Ideally, early interventions aimed at decreasing the family's stress should be performed to prevent the breakdown of the family structure.[9,10,15]

Death of the patient, unfortunately, is an inherent part of the transport process. Some patients die before transport, and the role the family may play in this dying process can make patient care particularly arduous for the transport team. Whether the family is allowed to be present during resuscitation attempts is an issue that has been gaining attention from both healthcare professionals and the public. Families now demand to be a part of the resuscitation so that they can at least say goodbye to their loved ones no matter where the resuscitation takes place.[16,19-25]

This chapter presents the advantages and disadvantages of allowing the family to accompany the patient during transport, the importance of family presence, and how to meet the needs of the family involved in transport.

FAMILY ISSUES RELATING TO TRANSPORT OF THE PATIENT

Family members of critically ill or injured patients are already under stress,[3] and the need to transport the patient on a fixed-wing aircraft, helicopter, or ground vehicle adds to that level of stress.[17] Decisions concerning care must be made quickly, and the patient's family members often feel uninformed and unsure, especially if they have limited medical knowledge. Because time is a factor, the family has no opportunity to elicit medical information and request second opinions.

Family members may feel uncomfortable relaying concerns about the transport to the healthcare providers and transport team. Some concerns are related to the medical treatment rendered or even the safety of transport (Figure 38-1). Other concerns may include[17,24]:

- Separation from their loved one for the duration or distance of the transport.
- Uncertainty about the events that necessitated transfer and transport of the patient.

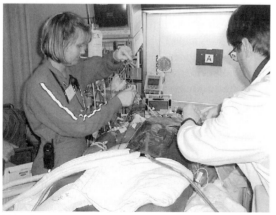

FIGURE 38-1   **Example of a critically ill patient on a left ventricular assist device who needs to be transferred to another facility for care.** (Courtesy Stanford Life Transport.)

- Lack of understanding of the medical diagnosis.
- The referring physicians, nurses, and transport team members are unfamiliar to the family and patient.

Because most patients who need critical care transport have injuries or illnesses that are sudden and unplanned, family members usually do not have time to prepare for the emergency. If they have never been exposed to this type of crisis, they may not have the coping skills needed to effectively manage the stress entailed.[10]

REFERRING FACILITY

The transport team should make every effort to speak with the patient's family before leaving the referring facility. This interaction may be as simple as an introduction, such as "Hi, my name is Jane Doe, and I am the transport nurse who will be with your family member during the transport." During this interaction, the team can assess the family. The team can then alert personnel at the receiving hospital's social or pastoral service department if it appears that the family may need their assistance. The transport team can also take this opportunity to determine the family's plans for traveling to the receiving hospital and get an estimate of their time en route. Family members should be notified of the transport vehicle's intended destination, and they should be told where to report once they arrive at the receiving facility. If necessary, directions to the receiving hospital can be given to the family. Many transport programs provide individual maps for this purpose. When possible, the family should be provided with a specific individual name or place they may ask for when arriving at the receiving facility. The transport team can offer to contact the family via cell phone at the conclusion of the transport. This practice is particularly useful with pediatric patients to help alleviate parental anxiety.

The transport team may pause before leaving the institution to allow family members to say goodbye to the patient. This is especially important if the patient's injuries are life threatening; in this case, the family may not have another opportunity to speak to the patient before he or she dies. In this author's experience, the opportunity to say goodbye to the patient is greatly appreciated by the family. In most cases, depending on the severity of the patient's injuries, the transport can be delayed for a few minutes without negative effects on the patient's outcome. These simple interactions between the family and the transport team are invaluable in helping to alleviate the family's stress.

Fultz and colleagues[13] conducted a study to identify the information needs of family members regarding air medical transport. The information needs rated as very important by family members included what was wrong with the patient, why the patient had to be flown to another facility, and where the patient could be found at the receiving hospital. Box 38-1 lists important needs that most family members perceived as being unmet.[13] The results of this research are important no matter how the patient is transported. Transport programs should use this information as a guide when providing care to the family to better care for the needs of the patient's family.

RECEIVING FACILITY

Information concerning the patient's family members should be communicated to the receiving hospital to facilitate continuity of care. The social services department of the receiving hospital can be alerted to cases in which their services may be especially needed. Personnel at receiving hospitals want to know whether the family plans to travel to their hospital. Because large distances must sometimes be covered by ground, an estimated time of arrival is useful. Knowledge of the family's plans can be helpful in case the patient's condition deteriorates and consent to perform particular procedures is needed.

The hospital may need to know the family's wishes for treatment if the patient's condition is life threatening. Organ procurement issues can be considered if the staff knows when and if the family intends to arrive. These issues are particularly important if the patient is a minor.

Family members frequently leave the referring facility as soon as the decision is made to transfer the patient, and they may arrive at the receiving hospital ahead of the patient. In this case, the referring nurse can notify the receiving hospital of the family's departure for their facility. If the receiving hospital is aware of the family's intended time of arrival, they can direct the family to the appropriate area in the hospital.

TRANSPORTING FAMILY MEMBERS

Family members frequently ask whether they can travel to the receiving facility with the patient. In this era, patients and families are more assertive in making their requests known to the medical community. Research continues to show that patients, families, and healthcare providers can benefit from family presence.[1,2,21,22]

The decision to transport a family member is based on multiple factors, some more important than others. The personal feelings of a team member should not interfere with a decision on what is best for the patient and family. The entire transport team should provide input, but safety should always be the overriding principle. In air medical transport, the pilot has the final word. Safety for the entire team is the primary factor on which to base this decision when concern exists about the possibility of family interference.

| BOX 38-1 | **Family Needs of Patients Transported via Helicopter** |

Family members of patients who need helicopter transport perceived that they lacked the following:
1. The opportunity to see the patient before he or she was put in the helicopter.
2. Information about who would take care of the patient in transport.
3. Information about the safety of air transport.
4. Directions to the receiving hospital.
5. Knowledge about how the patient fared during the transport.

From Fultz JH, et al: Air medical transport: what the family wants to know, *J Air Med Trans* 431, 1993.

BOX 38-2	**Examples of Inclusion/Exclusion Criteria for Determination of Whether Family Members Should Accompany a Patient During Air Medical Transport**

Inclusion of family members during air medical transport may be desirable in the following cases:
The referring facility is far from the receiving facility, and the family has no other means of transportation.
The patient is near death, and the family wishes to be with the patient during his or her last moments.
The patient is a child and would benefit from being accompanied by a parent.
The family and the patient both strongly want the family to accompany the patient.
  Exclusion of family members during air medical transport may be desirable in the following cases:
Inclusion of the family member will interfere with patient care.
The family member's weight exceeds permissible parameters.
The family member is overly anxious and poses a danger to the safety of the transport.
The landing zone is walled in on three sides, and the pilot must do a vertical takeoff.
A crew member has a concern about a family member.
Weather conditions are marginal.
The family member has a fear of flying.
The family member gets motion sickness.
The distance between the two facilities is short.
The patient's condition is unstable and requires extensive care.

Other factors the team may take into consideration when deciding whether to transport members of the patient's family are the patient's age, the seriousness of the patient's condition, other transportation available to the family, and the length of the transport time. Box 38-2 provides examples of inclusion and exclusion criteria for transport of family members.

Some transport vehicles, particularly air medical, are not capable of carrying an additional passenger because of performance factors or space limitations. Although the aircraft may have the capability of carrying extra passengers, some limitations, including engine power, effects of weather on equipment performance, and the amount of weight the aircraft can safely carry, determine whether an additional passenger can be brought aboard.

Parents often ask whether they can accompany their child on the transport. Determination of whether the presence of the family member will pose a problem during transport is important because of an inappropriate level of anxiety. All family members exhibit some anxiety, and thus, anxiety should not rule out the possibility of the person going on the transport. The determination must be made on the basis of whether inclusion of the family members will interrupt the transport team's duties if they

sit in the front or interfere with care to the patient if they sit in the back. It cannot be stressed enough that if transporting the family member in any way jeopardizes safety or care, the family member should not be transported.

The transport team may want to exclude the family from the transport when the weather is marginal. This factor can apply to either a ground or an air vehicle. Diversions or precautionary landings require extra concentration on the part of the pilot; thus, interference with flying can occur if the pilot has to explain what is happening or calm a worried passenger. Ground vehicle drivers need to be able to address their full concentration on roads that may be ice covered or if visibility is impaired by fog.

Once the determination to transport family members is made, they need a safety briefing by the pilot in an air medical vehicle or the driver in a ground vehicle. The family member should be directed to the transport vehicle for the briefing while the patient is being prepared for the transport; this gives the pilot or driver an appropriate amount of time to conduct the safety briefing. The extra passenger can be belted in the seat and be ready for departure. If this is done before the patient reaches the vehicle, the transport is not delayed.

Edgington[8] conducted a survey of all air medical programs in North America to investigate whether family or friends are taken on transports. The results showed that 60% of the programs carried extra passengers. The helicopter programs that carried family members did not advertise that they did so, and they transported them on less than 5% of their transports. Extra passengers were taken more frequently on transports of children. Fixed-wing aircraft programs transported family members on 35% to 95% of their transports. One fixed-wing aircraft program located in the Midwest claimed to carry family members on almost every transport. A program located in the West indicated that offering to transport family members was important because their transferring sites were so remote that the family refused to consent to the transfer unless they were allowed to accompany the patient.[8]

Forty percent of the programs surveyed did not transport family members. Box 38-3 summarizes the reasons that influenced the decision by these programs not to transport family members. Of the programs surveyed, the ones that carried extra passengers listed the benefits of transporting family members. Box 38-4 lists some of these benefits. Problems with the transfers were rare; only three problems were listed. On one transport, a child experienced respiratory arrest and the parent was asked to assist in ventilation. In the other two cases, the passengers experienced airsickness. One program in Oregon has a pretransport screening form to determine a prospective rider's suitability for transport. The form included questions about whether the potential passenger had had "recent alcohol or drug consumption, inner ear problems, pregnancy, back or joint trouble, and recent blood donation or dental work."[8]

Many times the transport team must make a split-second decision as to whether the family can be transported with the patient. Experience helps to make this decision process easier. No specific rules exist for including or excluding the family. Each situation must be assessed separately. In many instances, family members are not allowed to accompany the

---

BOX 38-3   Reasons for Deciding Against Transport of Family Members

Liability concerns
Lack of useful load on the aircraft
Exposure of the family to invasive medical procedures
Operator restrictions
Lack of insurance for passengers
Prohibition by the program's operations manual
Concerns about a lack of time to properly brief family members
Concerns about increased stress for the medical team as a result of having a family member on the aircraft

From Edgington BH: Transporting the family and other concerned parties aboard air medical aircraft, *J Air Med Trans* 11-13, 1992.

BOX 38-4   Benefits of Transporting a Family Member

The family member may provide emotional support for the patient.
The family member is available to sign releases for further treatment and to fill in gaps in the patient's medical history.
The family member may be able to act as a translator.
Organ procurement questions can be resolved more quickly.
The medical team may have the opportunity to explain the patient's prognosis and disposition to the family.

From Edgington BH: Transporting the family and other concerned parties aboard air medical aircraft, *J Air Med Trans* 11-13, 1992.

transport team. The possibility of transporting family members should not automatically be ruled out by the transport team because at times it is appropriate and would be beneficial if the team made an effort to include the family.

If family members accompany the transport team, the risk of increased emotional difficulty always exists for the transport team. However, the benefits to the patient and family when emotional support is provided far outweigh the emotional risks to the transport team. One must always look at each situation for what provides the best care for both patient and family.

FAMILY PRESENCE DURING RESUSCITATION

The presence of family members during attempts to resuscitate a patient is an emotionally charged topic that is gaining the attention of healthcare practitioners and the public. Whether families should be allowed to view resuscitation is a topic of controversy among the medical community. Providing emotional support for family members can be difficult. Before health care providers determine the stance they will take on this issue, they should familiarize themselves with the literature, discuss the issue with others who have participated in a resuscitation attempt with family members present, and ask themselves the following question, "If my child or family member needed to be resuscitated, would I want to be there?" Box 38-5 lists other questions that

practitioners should consider when dealing with this issue. A major point to keep in mind is that in most situations, the risks to the health care provider in emotionally supporting the family do not outweigh the benefits that are provided for the family.

The mission statement or philosophy of most institutions is probably amenable to having family members present during a resuscitation attempt. The practice standards of the Air and Surface Transport Nurses Association state that the transport nurse should possess the skills to effectively communicate with the patient's family.[25] This statement easily applies to all members of the transport team.

The Emergency Nurses Association (ENA) has issued a position statement in support of the option of family members being present during invasive procedures or resuscitation attempts.[9] The ENA believes that allowing family members to be present during resuscitation attempts facilitates the grieving process. The ENA also believes that families have a right to be together and that this allows the patient and family members to support each other.[6,9]

The vision of the American Association of Critical Care Nurses (AACN) is that they work toward a patient-driven healthcare system in which critical care nurses make their optimal contribution. The AACN interviewed many nurses who indicated that listening and learning from patients and families is the key to accomplishing this vision. The information obtained from patients and families could then be used to challenge conventional care and ultimately change individual practice. The AACN realizes that activities that alter both the system and

---

BOX 38-5	**Questions to Be Considered by Healthcare Providers in Evaluation of Whether Family Members Should Be Present During Resuscitation Attempts**

1. How do you feel about allowing family members to participate in a resuscitation attempt?
2. Have you ever facilitated family participation in a resuscitation attempt?
3. Have you ever experienced a situation in which family members participated in a resuscitation attempt?
4. What, if anything, makes you feel uncomfortable about participation of family members in a resuscitation attempt?
5. What, if anything, would make you feel more comfortable about participation of family members in a resuscitation attempt?

From Emergency Nurses Association: *Presenting the option for family presence*, Park Ridge, IL, 2005, The Association.

the individuals are necessary for this vision to come true. The AACN wants nurses to look at the hospital experience "through the patient's eyes," which, they realize, requires enormous effort.[14]

Although nurses have historically professed to be patient and family advocates, little research supports this statement. When Gorden[14] interviewed Dracup, she cited her previous study on family visitation issues, which found that nurses and families were not in concert with each other. Dracup and Beau[14] examined whether nurses' perceptions of family needs were similar to the actual needs of the families. The results of their survey showed that nurses did not always know what the family wanted. The recommendation was made that nurses continually ask family members what they want, instead of nurses assuming they know what the family wants. Dracup discussed two other issues with Gorden: first, families want to visit patients more frequently in the intensive care unit, yet 80% of hospitals continue to successfully restrict visiting hours; and second, regarding the issue of family members present during resuscitation attempts, presence in the room during a code or when the patient dies is far less upsetting for some persons than sitting alone and frightened in a waiting room or living with the haunting memory that a husband, wife, or child died alone.[14,18]

Nurses' persistence and vision have now influenced other organizations such as the American Heart Association and the American College of Surgeons. In new guidelines, the role of the family is expanded, and family presence is an important consideration to the delivery of care.[5]

When family members are encouraged to become involved in the situation, they feel supported and useful and have a sense of some control, which enhances the healthcare provider–family relationship. Family members who are frustrated and angry because they do not know what is happening to the patient are actually harder to manage and take more time than those who are kept informed. Healthcare providers must keep in mind that family members may not feel comfortable expressing their feelings, especially if they think these feelings are contradictory to the nurse's feelings. Asking family members what is best for them helps the transport team attain the goal of being a family advocate.[3-8]

Time and societal influences have changed views about healthcare and healthcare management. Most family members like to be involved in every aspect of the patient's life, except when it comes to hospitalization. Healthcare has marginalized the role of both the patient and family in the care.[24]

At one time, the issue of whether a father should be allowed in the delivery room during the birth of his baby was controversial; many healthcare professionals voiced their opposition and resisted this change in policy. Currently, fathers, siblings, and extended family members are often present in birthing rooms. Fathers are even allowed in the operating room when a cesarean section is performed. This routine practice is not questioned today, and families and healthcare providers have adjusted to this change in practice. An obstetric nurse denying a family member access to a mother giving birth is unheard of today. It may be just a matter of time before it is common practice for family members to be present during a resuscitation attempt; it is hoped for the family's benefit that this process of change will begin sooner rather than later.[24]

FAMILY PRESENCE PROGRAM

Foote Hospital in Michigan[6] is a pioneer in the family presence program. The Foote Hospital program was initiated because of two instances in which family members refused to leave the patient during a resuscitation attempt. After these two instances occurred, a survey was sent to the families of patients who had been resuscitated in the Foote Hospital ED. The survey asked whether they would have wanted to be present during the resuscitation attempt of their family member if they had been given the opportunity. Seventy-two percent of the respondents indicated that they would have liked to have been present. These results showed the staff at Foote Hospital the need for a formalized family presence program.[6] Foote Hospital approached the issue by developing a formalized program. Initially, a chaplain or social worker provides the family with information about the condition of the patient and determines whether the family would like to view the resuscitation attempt. During the time that the chaplain or social worker is with the family, the medical personnel perform any necessary invasive procedures. After the invasive procedures have been completed, the chaplain or social worker accompanies the family into the resuscitation room and stays with them to provide support and information. Because the medical staff has very little responsibility for providing support to the family, they can then keep their attention focused on the resuscitation. If further invasive procedures are needed, family members are asked to step out of the room.[6]

The nurses at Foote Hospital, who were informally surveyed before the program was initiated, had two main concerns: (1) that the family would interrupt patient care; and (2) that outward expressions of grief by family members would make it difficult for nurses to perform their job. They also had a fear that they would be observed doing or saying something that would upset the family.[4] Box 38-6 lists reasons that healthcare providers give for not wanting family members to be present during resuscitation attempts. Stress for the family is another concern cited by nurses.

The literature confirms that family members have a desire to be present during resuscitation attempts and that this process helps them in their grief work.[6] After Foote Hospital's program was established, a survey revealed that three of four staff members supported the program. They believed that the program benefited the family even if it was emotionally harder for the staff. Follow-up research with family members who were present during resuscitation attempts showed that the program was successful and that it helped in the grief process. Many family members commented that they were glad to see that everything possible was done for their loved one. One family member commented that he was glad to be able to say goodbye before the person died.[6]

IMPLICATIONS FOR PATIENT TRANSPORT

All healthcare providers have opinions on the issue of whether family members should be present during a resuscitation attempt. Most beliefs on this issue are at opposite ends of the spectrum; few people have middle-of-the-road opinions. Many of those who oppose family presence have admitted that they have never participated in a resuscitation attempt with a family member present. Their feelings are based on what they perceive might happen instead of on reality. Persons who have experience with resuscitation with family members present generally state that they believe it is good for the family and that they only occasionally have problems with the family.

Anecdotes from the Foote Hospital program recount families who have actually been involved in the decision to end a resuscitation attempt. The family was witness to the attempt and was able to say, "Yes, everything was done for my family member. Everyone worked very hard, and it is obvious that the attempts to save the life were futile."[6] This scenario cannot happen if family members are left alone in a waiting room and are not informed about what is happening. Difficulty in grasping the reality of the unknown hinders the grieving process.

Some healthcare providers are more comfortable with providing emotional care than are others. Some nurses allow family members to visit patients for extended periods of time, whereas others restrict visits to the exact amount of time mandated by the facility or even less. Some doctors take the time to talk to the patient's family members and keep them updated, whereas others avoid contact with the family.

BOX 38-6	**Reasons Given by Healthcare Providers for Excluding Family Members During Resuscitation Attempts**

The family may disrupt or interfere with patient care.

Outward expressions of grief by family members might make control of their own emotions difficult or impossible for staff members.

The experience may be too traumatic for the family.

From Emergency Nurses Association: *Resolution 93-02: family presence at the bedside during invasive procedures and/or resuscitation,* Park Ridge, IL, 1993, The Association.

If family presence programs are to be successful, everyone's needs must be addressed. Physicians and nurses who find emotional care difficult to provide have the most difficult time adjusting to this change. Helping them with the transition is essential.

Campbell and colleagues[4] found that nurses and physicians differ on how they handle death. Nurses tend to view death more as a natural part of life and associate it with positive terminology, such as rebirth, tranquility, and victory. Physicians, who tend to view death negatively, use words such as unsafe, alone, forgotten, and cold to describe the experience. Gender was not differentiated in this study. An argument could be made that gender instead of the profession of the respondents was the factor that led to different attitudes toward death because most nurses are women and most physicians are men. In addition, male nurses have been influenced in their education mainly by female professors, and female physicians have been influenced mainly by male professors. Historically, women take a different approach to interpersonal and emotional events than do men. In general, men are much more uncomfortable handling and discussing issues surrounding death than are women. When gender is taken into consideration, in general, nurses appear to be best equipped as patient and family advocates and at assisting physicians in determination of what is best for the family. Nurses should be the family's voice when communicating with physicians, and if necessary, they should create the atmosphere necessary to have family members present.

Transport team members and emergency personnel, because of the nature of their work, are exposed to situations in which family members may be in close proximity during the resuscitation process. Nurses have a wealth of information on this topic that comes from personal experience, and they should relate these experiences to other healthcare providers. Nurses should be on the forefront of supporting family presence; this support can play an important role in changing practice.

If family members are to be allowed in the resuscitation room, the code scenario of hospitals has to change. The code scenarios of transport teams are a good example for them to follow. When transport teams resuscitate a patient outside the helicopter or fixed-wing aircraft in the presence of prehospital care providers or referring hospital personnel, the code is conducted in a professional manner. Because transport team members are never on their "own turf," the care they provide is open for scrutiny by all bystanders. Less noise and chaos are generally present during a resuscitation attempt by a transport team than in a hospital simply because fewer people are present. Transport nurses can attest to the fact that a code can be successfully run with fewer people than are used in a hospital. Speaking in normal calm tones during a code seems to have a calming effect on those present; thus, simply decreasing the noise level during a resuscitation attempt lessens the degree of chaos.

One factor the transport team must consider when giving emotional care to the family outside the hospital is the lack of ancillary support services, such as social services or pastoral care. The transport team must adjust to this lack of support services and find other innovative ways to provide care to the family without jeopardizing patient care.

Birth and death are both private life processes that belong to the patients and their families. Healthcare providers do not have the right to interfere in either of these processes. People should be able to die with peace and dignity with their families at their sides.

Although not everyone is prepared to view resuscitation attempts, the literature supports the fact that many persons wish families to be present when attempts are made to resuscitate a family member. Presence at resuscitation attempts is helpful for grief work. Transport nurses and all transport team members should be patient advocates in the true sense of the word by asking the family what they want and by helping them to achieve their goals.[11,12]

BEREAVEMENT AFTER SUDDEN DEATH IN THE FIELD

When patients are pronounced dead in the field or are not transported from a referring facility, their families may not be able to benefit from support services available when patients are taken to the receiving facility. Family members often have many questions after the death of a loved one. If family members are at the scene, the transport team should make an attempt to interact with them. If at all possible, the family should be encouraged to view the patient's body at the scene.

The initial shock experienced by family members may prevent them from knowing what questions to ask. The team can talk to the family about the facts that led up to the incident and explain the possible injuries that caused the death. Family members often do not remember what was said to them as much as they remember the attitude of the person who was talking to them. Table 38-1 lists interventions that healthcare professionals may use in their initial responses to crises.

Common responses of family members to the death of a patient are anger and hostility. These feelings are the result of a lack of control, frustration, and helplessness over the events surrounding the illness and death. Expressed anger often disguises underlying fears and anxieties that need to be addressed. Angry persons often discourage healthcare professionals from helping them, thus leaving them feeling lonely and isolated. Rando[21] believes that if the family accepts the death, the grief experience is more quickly resolved, and the feelings of anger, hostility, and guilt are diminished.

Transport teams can help the family to understand that the advanced care that their team delivered was the best care possible. The public may not be aware that the transport team is capable of providing the same care that is delivered in an ED; they may be under the impression that the best care

TABLE 38-1	**Interventions for Initial Family Responses to Crisis**
Family Responses	**Interventions**
Anxiety, shock, fright	Give information that is brief, concise, explicit, and concrete.
	Repeat information and frequently reinforce; encourage families to record important facts in writing.
	Ascertain comprehension by asking family members to repeat the information they have been given.
	Encourage or allow ventilation of feelings, even if they are extreme.
	Maintain constant, nonanxious presence in the face of a highly anxious family.
	Inform the family of the potential range of behaviors and feelings that are the "norm" for crisis.
	Maximize control in the hospital environment as much as possible.
Denial	Identify the purpose that denial serves for family (e.g., does it buy them "psychologic time" for future coping and mobilization of resources?).
	Evaluate the appropriateness of the use of denial in terms of time; denial becomes inappropriate when it inhibits the family from taking necessary actions or when it impinges on the course of treatment.
	Do not actively support denial, but do not dash hopes for the future either (e.g., "It must be very difficult for you to believe your son is nonresponsive and in a trauma unit").
	If denial is prolonged and dysfunctional, more direct and specific factual representation may be essential.
Anger, hostility, distrust	Allow for ventilation of angry feelings, clarifying the thoughts, fears, and beliefs that are behind the anger; let them know it is "okay" to be angry.
	Do not personalize the family's expression of these strong emotions.
	Institute family control in the hospital environment when possible (e.g., arrange for a set time and set person to give information about the patient and answer questions).
	Remain available to families while they vent these emotions.

TABLE 38-1	**Interventions for Initial Family Responses to Crisis—cont'd**
Family Responses	**Interventions**
	Ask families how they can take the energy in their anger and put it to positive use for themselves, for the patient, and for the situation.
Remorse and guilt	Do not try to "rationalize away" guilt for families.
	Listen, support their expression of feeling and verbalizations (e.g., "I can understand how or why you might feel that way; however…").
	Follow the "however" with careful, reality-oriented statements or questions (e.g., "None of us can truly control another's behavior"; "Kids make their own choices despite what parents think and want"; "How successful were you when you tried to control this behavior with that before?" "So many things have happened for which there are no absolute answers").
Grief and depression	Acknowledge the family's grief and depression.
	Encourage family members to be precise about what it is they are grieving and depressed about; give grief and depression a context.
	Allow the family appropriate time for grief.
	Recognize that grieving is an essential step for future adaptation; do not try to rush the grief process.
	Remain sensitive to your own unfinished business and hence, comfort or discomfort with the family's grieving and depression.
Hope	Clarify with family members what their hopes are, individually and with one another.
	Clarify with families what their worst fears are in reference to the situation; are the hopes or fears congruent? Realistic? Unrealistic?
	Support realistic hope.
	Offer gentle factual information to reframe unrealistic hope (e.g., "With the information you have or the observations you have made, do you think that is still possible?").
	Assist families in reframing unrealistic hope in some other fashion (e.g., "What do you think others will have learned from the patient if he doesn't make it?" "How do you think she would like for you to remember her?").

From Kleeman KM: Families in crisis due to multiple trauma, *Crit Care Nurs North Am* 1(1):25, 1989.

possible is that which is given in the hospital. They may believe that the role of the transport team is to provide rapid transport and that the gold standard of care is provided in the hospital.

The transport team is responsible for giving care to the victim and emotional care to the family. If at all possible, the transport team should assist the prehospital care providers in talking with the family. Because of the nature of transport operations, the team cannot always stay at the scene and assist the family. If the team cannot stay, the team's assessment of the family may be an impetus for initiating a referral for follow-up. If the base station is associated with a hospital, the social services department

may be able to assist with the follow-up. The team may be involved with this follow-up at a later date by calling the family and repeating some of the medical information that the family either did not understand or were not capable of comprehending at the time of the patient's death.

SUMMARY

Emotional care of the family is an important part of patient transport. The transport team may need additional education and increased awareness of their potential impact in this area. Understanding the diversity of patients and their families aids in providing care. The development of policies and procedures that address the needs of families related to transport must be a part of every transport program. Family care is an integral part of transport practice, and that advocacy role is what makes a difference in what we do.

THE FAMILY AND TRANSPORT CASE STUDY

A 68-year-old man with a history of a leaking abdominal aneurysm was to be transferred to another facility for repair of the aneurysm. On arrival of the transport team, they found a gravely ill man in hypovolemic shock. He was alert but in severe distress. The transport team decided to intubate the patient to assist with oxygenation and began administration of packed red blood cells. The patient requested to speak with his daughter before intubation. A few minutes were provided, and the patient was able to ensure that his wife's needs would be met if he should die.

The daughter, who was a nurse at the referring facility, asked to accompany the patient in transport. The pilot approved this transport, and she was briefed and placed in the front seat of the BK 117. During transport, the patient's condition improved. He arrived at the referring facility with stable vital signs; however, when in transport to the operating room, his blood pressure markedly decreased and he became bradycardiac. His daughter accompanied the transport team to the operating room. She held her father's hand and spoke to him. The patient did well in surgery, and both he and his daughter returned to visit the team. Both felt that her presence made a difference in his survival.

REFERENCES

1. Bassler PC: The impact of education on nurses' beliefs regarding family presence in a resuscitation room, *J Nurses Staff Dev* 15:126, 1999.
2. Boie ET, Moore GP, Brommett C, et al: Do parents want to be present during invasive procedures performed on their children in the emergency department? A survey of 400 parents, *Ann Emerg Med* 34:70, 1999.
3. Caine RM: Families in crisis: making the critical difference, *Focus Crit Care* 6:184, 1989.
4. Campbell TW, Abernethy V, Waterhouse GJ: Do death attitudes of nurses and physicians differ?, *Omega* 14(1):43, 1983.
5. Cummins RO, Hazinski MF: The most important changes in the international ECC and CPR guidelines 2000, *Resuscitation* 46(1-3):431, 2000.
6. Doyle CJ, et al: Family participation during resuscitation: an option, *Ann Emerg Med* 16:673, 1987.
7. Drought TS, Liaschenko J: Ethical practice in a technological age, *Crit Care Nurs Clin North Am* 7(2):297, 1995.
8. Edgington BH: Transporting the family and other concerned parties aboard air medical aircraft, *J Air Med Trans* 11(2):11, 1992.
9. Emergency Nurses Association: *Position statement: family presence at the bedside during invasive procedures and cardiopulmonary resuscitation*, Park Ridge, IL, 2005, ENA.
10. Emergency Nurses Association: *Trauma nursing core course*, ed 6, Des Plaines, IL, 2007, ENA.
11. Falcone RE, et al: Air medical transport for the trauma patient requiring cardiopulmonary resuscitation: a 10-year experience, *Air Med J* 14:197, 1995.
12. Fulton R, Voigt W, Hilakos A: Confusion surrounding the treatment of traumatic cardiac arrest, *J Am Coll Surg* 181:209, 1995.
13. Fultz JH, et al: Air medical transport: what the family wants to know, *J Air Med Trans* 12(11-12):431, 1993.
14. Gorden S: Inside the patient-driven system, *Crit Care Nurse Suppl* 3-28: 1994.
15. Guzzetta C, Clark A, Wright J: Family presence in emergency medical services for children, *Clin Pediatr Emerg Med* 7:15-24, 2006.
16. Jecker N: Ceasing futile resuscitation in the field: ethical considerations, *Arch Int Med* 152(2):3035, 1992.
17. Kleeman KM: Families in crisis due to multiple trauma, *Crit Care Nurs Clin North Am* 1(1):25, 1989.
18. Macnab A, George S, Sun C: The cost of family oriented communication before air medical interfacility transport, *Air Med J* 20(4):20-22, 2001.
19. Mattox K: "Ideal" posttraumatic parameters, *J Trauma* 34(5):734, 1993.
20. Meyers TA, Eichhorn DJ, Guzzetta CE, et al: Family presence during invasive procedures and resuscitation, *Am J Nurse* 100:32, 2000.
21. Rando T: *Grief, dying and death: clinical interventions for care givers*, Champaign, IL, 1984, Research Press Co.

22. Sacchetti A, Carraccio C, Leva E, et al: Acceptance of family member presence during pediatric resuscitation in the emergency department: effect of personal experience, *Pediatr Emerg Care* 16:85, 2000.

23. Von Rueden KT, Hartsock R: Nursing practice through the cycle of trauma. In McQuillan KA, Von Rueden K, Hartsock R, et al, editors: *Trauma nursing: from resuscitation through rehabilitation*, ed 3, Philadelphia, 2002, Saunders.

24. Williams J: Family presence during resuscitation: to see or not to see, *Nurs Clin North Am* 37(1):211-220, 2002.

25. York-Clark D, Stocking J, Johnson J: *Transport and ground transport nursing core curriculum*, Denver, 2006, Air and Surface Transport Nurses Association.

MARKETING THE TRANSPORT PROGRAM

Kevin High

COMPETENCIES

1. Identify the components of a marketing plan for a transport program.
2. Describe marketing activities that may be used by a transport program.
3. Articulate the mission of a transport program.

This chapter presents an overview of the marketing process components and how marketing relates to the transport program.

Marketing is a planned, multistep, strategic process and not a single or isolated event; it is continuous and persistent and part of the job description of every individual in the organization.

The main components of a marketing plan are the mission statement of the program, market research, market planning, and public relations. Each component is one carefully interwoven building block in the overall marketing plan. The critical elements of the marketing process are quality of service, high performance of the transport system, and customer relations.

Marketing activities should be designed so that the end results are measurable. This design is important for the transport manager in evaluating current and past marketing activities and setting strategies for future market potentials. Marketing plans, just like continuous quality improvement programs, need to be continuously evaluated. Marketing is not the distribution of program paraphernalia, such as calendars, pens, and buttons. The expenditure of resources for such materials must be carefully planned, budgeted, and evaluated in terms of other marketing activities that are significantly more important. Marketing is not primarily a sales activity. Rather, it is the preparation and delivery of information and support to those on whom the program depends. Through marketing, the program attempts to influence the decision-making and buying practices of the users. The transport program has no control over these external agencies. However, through the informational value of the marketing program's public relations function, the manager can influence user selection.[1,3,6]

A *marketing plan* is a written document that describes the strategies necessary to successfully penetrate, capture, and retain market share of the patient referral area. Essentially, it is the foundation on which the transport program's other operating plans are built.

Unfortunately, transport programs have a history of initiating operations with a limited scope of market planning. The Commission on Accreditation of Medical Transport Systems (CAMTS) educational plan may serve as a starting point and a framework for a marketing plan. CAMTS recommends that each transport program have a professional and community education program or printed information with the target audience to be defined by the medical transport service. The information provided by the transport service should be trustworthy and may include[4]:

- Hours of operation.
- Capabilities of the medical transport personnel.
- Types of aircraft or ground interfacility vehicles used and operational protocols specific to type.
- Coverage area for the transport service.
- Preparation and stabilization of the patient.

Unfortunately, beyond the CAMTS regulatory recommendations, marketing may be viewed administratively as a luxury to be addressed later because it requires time, personnel, and financial support. Quick program start-ups as a response to competition have often left strategic planning processes on the back burner.

The budget line item for marketing, advertising and public relations, and program promotion is not unusually the lowest allocation in the overall transport program. In addition, the sponsor hospital's marketing resources and marketing departments, which are assigned responsibility for promoting the transport service along with an array of other hospital services and programs, often neutralize transport managers.

Thus, the involvement of the transport manager may be limited and often quite latent. At a minimum, the transport program leader must strive to influence the informational environment in which the marketing department makes decisions that can affect the program's success. The program leader must educate the marketing department on the program's mission, customer base, and focus, which are often very different from typical healthcare entities to which they are accustomed.

MISSION OF THE TRANSPORT PROGRAM

A program's *mission* is generally expressed as a broad statement that defines the roles and purpose of the organization and the environment in which it operates. The mission reflects the primary reasons for the organization's existence.

Mission and scope may refer to the nature of the program's product and activities in terms of its ability to serve its market area. The mission statement should address the basic questions "What business are we in?" and "What markets should we serve?"

The transport programs mission should have the following characteristics:

- Safe operation of the transport vehicle, along with the safety of the transport personnel and patient, are priority one.
- The focus of the transport program should align with the sponsoring hospital or institution or corporation (if applicable).
- The mission should define what types of individuals and organizations the program serves and how (modes of transport).

The mission statement gives clarity to the transport program with regard to what it does and whom it serves. Through the mission, the program can communicate its identity to its staff and the outside community. In essence, the mission statement is the foundation for the behavior of the organization. The mission statement should drive the goals of the transport program.

A primary mode for success in marketing is to segment the multiple macromarkets into homogeneous micromarket segments. This subclassification allows implementation by the management of an affordable focused plan of action.

IDENTIFICATION AND SEGMENTATION OF THE MARKET

Market segmentation is concerned with finding, identifying, and serving consumer and user groups in the organization's service area. A transport program's service area can be divided into groups of people with similar needs and characteristics to which the program can provide specific services. The focus should be on the system activator (i.e., someone who has the ability to make a transport request). This core principle is often forgotten. Marketing efforts are often focused on potential patients or end users of the service, which in most cases cannot or do not have the authority to request a transport.

Market segmentation reveals who the customers are and prioritizes the provision of information addressed to their specific needs. In the typical transport program, the two main segments are prehospital providers and hospital personnel (Table 39-1).

As Table 39-1 illustrates, transport programs have two groups of people they generally serve. Each of these groups has different needs and desires. Note that the table does not contain patients who receive direct care; more often than not, these individuals cannot and do not make a transport request. Expenditure of resources on this group has a low marketing yield with respect to boosting transport requests. Each of the noted groups should be the recipients of marketing efforts; however, efforts need to be tailored to each group.

CREATION OF AN EFFECTIVE MARKETING PLAN

The transport manager must first identify the potential activators of the service. The identification process is relatively simple. The steps are as follows:

- Create a list of every agency, organization, and healthcare facility within a 50–nautical mile radius of the transport vehicle's base of operations.
- Divide these into two groups: prehospital providers and hospital providers.
- Begin building the customer database (Box 39-1).
- Focus efforts within this area and target the individuals within the database.

Gathering data on individuals of influence within the area can be tedious. System activators must be identified and added to a customer database (see Box 39-1).

TABLE 39-1	**Two Groups of People Transport Programs Generally Serve**	
	Hospital Personnel	**Prehospital Personnel**
Disciplines	Physicians	911 Dispatchers
	Nurses	Firefighters
	Administration	EMTs, paramedics
	Case managers	Law enforcement officers
Focus	Interhospital transport	Scene transport
High value issues	Patient safety	Speed/response time
	Quality/level of care	Aircraft/vehicle capability
	Timely/appropriate feedback	Timely/appropriate feedback

EMTs, Emergency medical technicians.

BOX 39-1	Customer Database 101

Introduction

Whether you are using some type of sophisticated customer management software or just a piece of paper, there are a few things to keep in mind when building a customer database.

Decide on the Platform

The transport manager may use anything from a ring notebook to a software program; whatever platform is chosen, it should be easily accessible for everyone within the organization. However, this information should be kept and stored securely. A simple software spreadsheet template makes a great beginning database and can be stored on a network and accessed from the Internet.

Keep It Simple

An Internet-based system is the easiest and most accessible system but can be technically overwhelming at times. The goal should be first and foremost to gain and store information. Ideally, the transport program should want to harness the power of that information.

Gather the Right Data on the Right Customer

- Initially focus on each hospital, EMS agency, and 911 center within the contiguous counties (counties that

are adjacent to your transport aircraft or vehicle base county).
- Initial focus within hospitals should be on the Emergency Department (ED) Director, Medical Director, Intensive Care Unit (ICU) Director, and Charge Nurses.
- Focus on 911 centers should be aimed at Manager/Shift Supervisors.
- Focus on EMS agencies should revolve around the Director/Chief and division/shift leaders.
- Within each county are five to 10 must-see/must-know customers within the three institutions; find out who they are and how to contact them.
- Obtain basic information; name, address, email address, and fax and phone numbers for each individual.

Focus Constantly

Initial focus needs to be on leadership of these adjacent areas or areas within a 50–nautical mile area of the base. Concentrate only on agencies, facilities, and individuals that can use the transport service.

A marketing plan for a new base startup can be particularly challenging; moving into a new market space and dealing with new customers requires a comprehensive plan. A sample plan is shown in Table 39-2.

MARKET RESEARCH

Market research is a systematic analysis of the market to obtain objective data relevant to the goals or objectives of the transport program. Market research facilitates informed management decision making. Data from market research help identify and solve marketing problems, but these data are not a substitute for management decision making.[1-4]

As stated previously, market research is focused on people from agencies that have the ability or option to activate a patient transport. Having projected the largest potential group of activators, a survey instrument such as a questionnaire can be developed to obtain information from each specific market segment (physicians, law enforcement agencies,

and so on) about the perceived servicing needs of the transport program. From this information, marketing strategies can be formulated.

In addition to the questionnaire, the transport manager can use staff to interact with activators in a community. One activity can be small focus groups. Something as simple as brief discussions at local hospital medical staff meetings, or in groups as small as a 911 dispatcher meeting, may elicit important market information. Whether the interview method or survey instrument is used, questions should be constructed in such a manner that an objective analysis can be made on the data gathered.

COMPETITION

As of January 2008, the Association of Air Medical Services (AAMS; www.aams.org) put the number of rotor-wing aircraft within the United States at more than 800. Several states have more than 30 aircraft that operate from within their border. Competition

TABLE 39-2 **Example of Marketing Plan**		
30 Days Before Base Opening	**First 30 Days of Operation**	**First 90 Days of Operation**
• Assemble marketing team • Begin market space study • Begin formulation of database • Focus strictly on referral area, within 50 nautical miles from base • After identifying customers, meet with each of them as quickly as possible within this time period • Plan at least one open house for customers or in combination with media day • Write press release announcing first full day in service; send this to local media and within database	• Conduct at least one visit to one of the target agencies/facilities within this time period • Conduct one transport vehicle site visit to each county within market space; tie in local media and dignitaries if possible • Begin teaching basic safety/ utilization class for EMS personnel within target area • Begin teaching basic utilization/ patient packaging class for hospital personnel within the target area	• Revisit or complete initial visits to identified customers • Continue teaching basic safety/ utilization class for EMS personnel within target area • Continue teaching basic utilization/ patient packaging class for hospital personnel within target area • Begin quarterly regional educational events that are rotated throughout market space • Write "first 100 days" press release • Expand database beyond initial leadership within market space

between transport programs for market share is stronger than ever. Marketing efforts by transport programs must be sophisticated and focused.

In the case of competing programs, market research can objectively identify the perceived strengths and weakness of each of the transport services. A simple SCOT analysis (strengths, challenges, opportunities, and threats) performed internally can be helpful.

The transport manager must set forth policies and procedures for dealing with competing programs. These policies and procedures should include the following core concepts:

- Established "rules of engagement" or codes of professional conduct and interaction between the programs.
- Some type of regular and open dialogue with the leadership from the competitor program.
- Specific processes in place to address operational safety and mutual response incidents.

In a competitive environment, a transport program can easily lose its focus, which can lead to complacency and inattention to the details of everyday operation and clinical care. The transport manager must keep the team focused on the business at hand and not on what the competitor may or may not be doing. The competitor's actions are beyond your control.

INTERNAL ENVIRONMENTAL SUPPORT

Transport programs that have sponsoring hospitals or institutions are uniquely tasked with gaining and maintaining the support of their respective supporting organizations or entities. These individuals can be thought of as internal customers. At times, these customers can be more challenging than dealing with external customers. Oftentimes, these internal customers allocate some or all of the resources that support the transport service.

The internal customers and the internal environment need as much care, support, and organizational framework to function in as possible. Key leaders should be brought on board to help develop marketing strategies for the transport service. Other internal institutional resources, such as the marketing department or training and development, can be used in planning to develop marketing strategies for establishing collaborative relationships with neighboring and system hospitals. The sponsor institutions' resources or strengths in marketing or staff development may well be a supportive asset to the smaller community hospitals' development or participation in a healthcare network or system. These internal customers must be addressed, especially hospital leaders and administration and physicians. Quarterly events, such as an open house, an educational event, or dinner, can help the transport program build goodwill internally. These internal efforts must be sustained and persistent.

EXTERNAL MARKET STRATEGIES

Marketing strategies generally revolve around making personal contact with customers, sponsoring events, and performing or providing educational opportunities. A successful marketing or outreach contact can be defined as follows.

A successful marketing or outreach contact results in the beginning or the sustaining of a relationship with the customer. Specific steps need to be followed for a contact to be successful for both the program and the customer. Generally speaking, the six steps to an outreach or marketing contact are[6]:

1. Research and Intelligence Gathering: You must do your homework. Do the research beforehand on your target: their likes, dislikes, affinities, danger points, etc. Review any preinformation you have on the customer.
2. Message: Know the message you want to give to the customer. "LifeFlight gives superior care" or "Statran offers the best pediatric care."
3. Meeting preparation: Be prepared. Besides working on the message, you need to be prepared to provide answers, information, etc, to the customer. If you are chairing the meeting with a partner, have a plan on how to best communicate the message.
4. Meet: Do the meeting; make it short, or as long as the customer allows, and maximize the time. Before leaving, learn the best avenue for communicating with the customer.
5. Follow up: Follow up is as important as the meeting itself. A personal thank you note or sending of requested information is mandatory.
6. Report: Record any information, findings, and actions into your database. Notify colleagues of any actionable items.

Core outreach and marketing ground rules are outlined in Box 39-2.[7,9] Other external marketing strategies include sponsoring events for customers such as transport vehicle site visits, participating in health fairs, etc.

The transport manager should consider public relations a part of the overall marketing plan while keeping in mind that other marketing activities are much more likely to yield requests for transport. The public relations activities of the transport program involve those tasks that foster positive regard for the program. *Public relations* are the building of goodwill and the enhancement of relations with the community and users of the service, in effect, the "image-building" aspect of the overall marketing plan.[9]

Public relations policy should be consistent with and driven by the organization's mission and goals. The policy objectives should ensure two-way communication between the program and the internal and external communities. The image-building results of a good public relations program may be difficult to measure. This is the biggest obstacle for the transport manager to overcome in justifying the budget needs for the public relations aspect of the marketing plan.

The benefits of public relations are important not only to boosting transport requests but also to cooperation and two-way communication with the community. The two basic elements of the public relations program to be explored are community involvement and publicity.

Community Involvement

Obtaining successful community support uses the same techniques used in networking with hospitals. Enlisting local resources such as government representatives by making them part of the team essentially makes or breaks the service's welcome to their jurisdiction. The transport manager should be knowledgeable about local government activities and recognize opportunities for transport personnel to support these activities.

The range of community activities for involvement of the team is limited only by management's imagination. Possible areas include [2,5,9]:

1. Medical programs. The program can cosponsor CPR or wellness training with local emergency medical services (EMS), fire department, and hospital personnel. Opportunities to support primary healthcare activities, such as

BOX 39-2   Outreach and Marketing Contact Ground Rules

What to Do

Provide decision makers and system activators with information that enables them to have the ability to define, defend, and differentiate your program from competitors; by doing so, you give your customers information to reposition your competitor for you.

What Not to Do

Do not directly discredit competitors. Participating in discourse that discredits other programs reflects more on your program than it does on theirs.

Make Everything Local

Your contact has mainly local interests and a local sphere of influence. Use specific local incidents, transports, and patients to emphasize your points. Be informed on local issues and nuances that that may affect your program or your customer.

Know Local Statistics, Facts, and Demographics

How many flight requests does your program get from the target? How many scene transports versus interfacility? What is the patient/payer mix in that area? You must know your "numbers."

Talk to the Right Person

You have a finite amount of time and effort to do outreach and marketing. Use your time and efforts wisely. Focus your efforts on individuals who have

the authority to trigger transport requests (system activators). Fortify and leverage your relationships with system activators first.

Do Not Underestimate the Importance of Ancillary and Auxiliary Staff

The customer's staff can be a big influence on decisions and decision making. Treat all staff with respect and dignity.

Know the Customer

Know everything about the target, their position within their organization, their responsibilities, clinical and operational interests, allies and opponents and personal history. *Everyone* has a story; know your target's story.

Rules for the Outreach Contact

- Be on time.
- Be positive and identify yourself properly.
- Dress appropriately, wear a name tag, be a professional.
- Remember to be a resource; provide material, education, and food.
- Be polite, be patient, and be gracious.
- Always tell the truth.
- Do not directly discredit the competition.
- Make the competition's arguments and answer them.
- Know your message and stay on it.
- Follow up with a thank you note.

---

immunization clinics in remote areas, should also be considered, or injury prevention programs, such as Prom Promises, should be supported.

2. Educational assistance. An effective method for promoting goodwill is to provide scholarships, speakers, equipment, and other assistance to local high schools, colleges, and universities.

3. Recreation and sports. Sponsoring sporting events, such as golf outings or long-distance runs to raise money for charity, can enhance the organization's image in the communities it serves.

4. Fund-raising drives. Participation by the organization in fund-raising activities to support local charities is good public relations.

5. Leadership activities. Transport personnel can become active in the Chamber of Commerce,

professional associations, and political advisory groups.

6. A ride-along program. This program allows members of referring EMS agencies or hospitals the opportunity to observe a patient transport and tour the transport team's facilities.

Educational events fulfill several roles; they provide participants with information and continuing educational credits and provide a venue for transport personnel to showcase clinical expertise. Any event provides a venue to interact with customers, make an impression, and gather information. In addition, these events allow the transport service to provide safety training for the hospital personnel that use their services, including helipad safety, loading and unloading the aircraft, or ground transport vehicle.

Training and education events and seminars are often efficient marketing tools. Generally, they work because they offer the personal contact needed to present the program's expertise and services in a low-key, nonthreatening environment (Figure 39-1; Box 39-3). The training and education of prehospital personnel, if considered part of an overall marketing plan, should receive adequate funding and support to make this effort successful. These events are great venues to build relationships and pass along information in a more relaxed environment.

Training and education can be separate activities of the transport program yet complement marketing strategies. By identifying the needs of prehospital personnel through surveys or personal communication, the nurse manager may discover a market demand for specific programs to improve the level of prehospital care. Many of these programs should be conducted in conjunction with local training, physicians, or community hospitals. Specifically in the rural communities, hospitals may appreciate and need the additional support of the air medical team and its sponsor hospital resources to provide

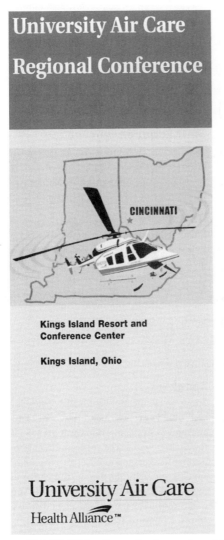
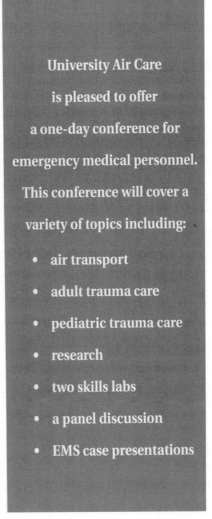

FIGURE 39-1 **Example of a seminar.** (Courtesy of University Air Care, Cincinnati, Ohio.)

BOX 39-3   Educational Event Management 101

Introduction

The following are some general guidelines and principles for events that involve a transport program's customer base, either for educational or public relations purposes. The following are guidelines only and may be tailored to each program or situation.

Program Format

A variety of formats for educational or public relations events is possible. This document outlines some basic formats and formulas that can assist you in event planning. Whatever type of format you choose should be used consistently for each and every event.

Every educational event should offer interdisciplinary continuing education units and should be 1 to 2 hours in length.

Cancellation Policy

Some type of cancellation policy with a specific deadline should be implemented. Lack of interest or participation is not really a reason to cancel. It is up to your program to promote the event to generate interest. A cancellation policy for inclement weather is advisable. Use of the hosting town or county school's weather closure policy as a guideline is a good idea.

Educational Topics

Topics should cover a wide variety of medical, pediatric, and trauma emergencies encountered by physicians, prehospital providers, and emergency personnel. Topics presented should be pertinent to the practice of the attendees.

Evaluations

A standard evaluation form should be used for course evaluation. Evaluations are given to the participants before the event and collected after the last presentation.

Evaluations must meet all continuing education requirements of the respective state and local licensing agencies. A standard certificate should be awarded to participants at the end of each session.

Teaching Aids

Teaching aids should consist of handouts, slides, and computer presentation programs. Use of extemporaneous speakers or speakers that are not familiar with presentations via PowerPoint should be avoided.

Event Personnel

An advance person or coordinator should direct the event. This person serves as the spokesperson for the program and directs all activities related to it. The coordinator should delegate staff to specific tasks within the format and make sure that they are completed. The coordinator serves as a point of contact within the agency for all things related to the event.

The coordinator also interacts with the point of contact from hosting agencies and is in charge of event production. The coordinator is responsible for executing the tasks outlined in the checklist or delegating staff to them.

Ancillary Staff

A minimum of one to two other staff should be at each event. They can be used for registration, venue set up, etc.

Staff Requirements

Staff members should arrive on time and be prepared to stay after the event is completed. Staff should be paid for both travel and actual time at the event along with mileage (or in accordance with policy).

Dress Code

Ideally, all transport staff should have a homogeneous look and be well dressed. Leadership must establish a dress code and enforce it.

Guidelines

- Duty uniform with name badge.
- Slacks with collared shirt.
- No blue jeans.
- No ball caps.
- No t-shirts.

Speakers

Speakers can be any healthcare professional that can provide pertinent and timely information to the audience. Physicians, nurses, and EMS providers are the main group to recruit from. Do not overlook nonmedical professionals. Law enforcement or specific specialty speakers are often informative and draw large crowds. Speakers from the sponsoring institution or agency or speakers that have ties to the sponsor (alumni, former employees, etc) are often good choices.

| BOX 39-3 | **Educational Event Management 101—cont'd** |

Provide specific instructions and guidelines for the speakers (see checklist) and give expectations as to presentation content, time limits, etc. Make sure they delivery their presentation at the appropriate cognitive level (i.e., do not let the speaker talk over the audience's head). The agency or institution providing continuing education credit for the event may require the speaker to have a list of objectives and provide a resume or curriculum vitae.

Be sure the speaker adjusts the material to the cognitive level of the audience. Provide the speaker with a map or directions and a phone number to call for emergencies. Emphasize preparation, find out audiovisual needs, and have a backup speaker or plan in place in case the speaker cancels.

Food and Drinks

Typically, one of the biggest challenges in producing an event is the food and drink equation. The program's goal in providing food and drink at an event should be as follows:

- Choose a menu format that can be provided easily and consistently.
- Choose a menu format that requires minimal effort on the part of the staff.
- Choose a menu format that is widely available throughout the referral area.
- Choose a menu format that appeals to the customer base.

Guidelines for Food and Drink

The coordinator or a designate should make arrangements for the delivery of food and drink before the day of the event.

The food item should also be cheap, popular, and readily available. Be sure the food item meets those criteria.

Venue and Room Set Up

Ideally, the venue should have a room for the class and a separate area for registration and food and drink set up.

Several tables are needed: one table for registration, two to three for food and drink, and another for handouts and marketing items.

Venue Requirements

The absolute requisites for any event venue are as follows:

- Climate-controlled room capable of seating 30+ people.
- One extension cord and power strip.
- Easily accessible restrooms.
- Two to four tables.

Postevent Actions

- Keep one staff member available to answer questions and interact with students.
- Police area for trash and bag all food items, drink cans, etc.
- Take down all signs and posters.
- Pack equipment.
- Secure and lock venue.
- Leave the venue in as good a shape as you found it.

Event Follow Up

- Send a thank you note to the host agency and point of contact.
- Summarize all evaluations and note any pertinent suggestions or feedback for future events.
- File and report the evaluations as per your CE accrediting agency's regulations.

---

continuing education opportunities for prehospital and hospital staff. Networking programs such as these have a subtle but positive public relations effect. They can have a dramatic impact on creating the desired team approach and collaboration with the air medical service through recognition of the valued role of each primary caregiver.

The Commission on Accreditation of Medical Transport Systems[4] recommends that each program have a community outreach program. As a part of this program, the transport service should support joint continuing education programs and operational programs that may include:

- Hazardous materials recognition and response.
- Disaster response and triage.
- Advanced trauma care.
- Interface of the transport team with other regional resources.
- Crash recovery (extricating personnel from specific types of aircraft and knowledge of the location of certain components in an airframe of specific aircraft make and model).

The team approach must also be emphasized on any scene response. Before the initiation of the request for service, the air medical program personnel and prehospital personnel should have decided who is in charge. Coordination on the scene directly reflects collaboration that has already taken place.

Many air medical services have follow-up and callback programs for user agencies. These programs should be constructed so that they focus on quality improvement (QA) activities for both organizations. A comprehensive QA program reviews the clinical, operational, and aviation components of each mission. The services should each independently evaluate performance against mutually developed standards and share their discoveries about the positive areas and areas for future improvement. The manager should develop the comprehensive collaborative quality improvement program with a progressive and positive tone. Focusing feedback on predetermined standards, rather than on emotionally charged assumptions, creates clarity for communication and avoids a negative policing attitude that might otherwise be conveyed.

Each transport program also needs a planned and structured safety program that is provided on a regular basis to agencies that use the air transport service. The components of this program should include[4]:

- Identifying, designating, and preparing an appropriate landing zone (LZ).
- Personal safety in and around the helicopter for all ground personnel.
- Procedures for daylight operations, conducted by the air medical team, specific to the aircraft.
- High and low reconnaissance.
- Two-way communication between helicopter and ground personnel to identify approach and departure obstacles and wind direction.
- Approach and departure path selection.
- Procedures for the pilot to ensure safety during ground operations in a landing zone with or without engines running.
- Procedures for the pilot to have ground control during engine start and departure from a landing site.

Many of the marketing strategies involve the external environment of the medical transport service. In brief, strategies look at opportunities for expansion of services and carefully critique areas in which services may be threatened. The air medical program depends on external sources over which it has little control. Without control, the focus turns to providing information, influence, and support to achieve the desired outcomes.

PUBLIC RELATION EVENTS AND ACTIONS

PUBLICITY

Through *publicity*, the program can develop good relations with media audiences by informing them about the organization, its services, and its contributions to the communities. To be effective, publicity must be newsworthy and have special interest for the media's audiences.

Publicity begins with the development of appropriate topics that enable the organization to translate corporate mission and goals into publicity goals. Such goals may include gaining the competitive edge over other services, influencing the decisions of service users, and improving relations in specific communities.

Through a strategic use of publicity, the organization can maintain a continuous flow of program information to the community. Publicity is a proven technique for achieving specific corporate objectives with a smaller financial investment than other marketing methods. "Free" publicity that is used in conjunction with paid advertising and other marketing methods is especially effective. Remember, however, that the success of a publicity program is reflective of its role in the overall marketing plan.

Working with the press and media has often been outside the responsibilities of the transport manager in hospital-based programs. However, inadequate or inappropriate press relations directly reflect the transport program. Thus, the transport manager must become involved with the press and media either directly or indirectly through the hospital's normal network. Proactively, the transport manager should form a positive relationship between the media and the program.

Methods of Publicity

The transport manager has several options for effectively communicating the objectives and performance of the program through the use of the media. Several methods for obtaining publicity are as follows.

Press Releases. The *press release* is the foundation of the publicity program. It is an inexpensive method for the dissemination of program news through the media. Releases contain a brief description of the subject, often accompanied by a diagram.

The media generally welcomes press releases, and releases can be an especially successful means of stimulating positive coverage and increasing the visibility of the program. One can significantly increase the chances of generating coverage of events that are of marginal news value by minimizing the effort needed by reporters. The release should be well written in a style appropriate for the media. The transport manager should meet the media contacts personally and, after sending releases, make follow-up courtesy calls. Releases should be sent as far in advance of the event as possible to facilitate scheduling. Photographs of the program in action may increase the likelihood of media coverage, especially in smaller newspapers.

Feature Articles. Generally longer than press releases, *feature articles* include materials such as a case history of the program (or product news item), an explanation of how the product is properly used, or a description of how the product helped solve a specific problem. Photographs are an asset to the article.

The chances of having an article accepted are dramatically increased by developing strong working relationships in the media. A major part of publicity work is in establishing and maintaining rapport with the media representatives.

Press Conferences. Through effective *press conferences*, program management has the opportunity to disseminate news about the program and its services. These events can be somewhat complex and intimidating and therefore require extensive planning and preparation for successful execution. Transport managers should look to their sponsor hospital or agencies resources for involvement in planning and executing a press conference.

Trade Shows. The opportunity to disseminate information about the program to a specific audience can be enhanced by participation at *trade shows*. The types of shows to consider including in the public relations budget should be reflective of the primary users of the program, such as hospital associations, physicians' conferences, EMS conferences, and public safety agency trade shows.

Public Speaking Engagements. Participation as a public speaker is important to both community involvement and publicity aspects of the public relations program. This public relations tool can keep the transport program's name visible in the community while enabling the program to publicize its objectives. Steps involved in the process of using speakers from the sponsor or participating hospital effectively include identifying speaker opportunities, accessing the primary program users, constructing presentations to ensure consistency in the message delivered, and developing the list of probable questions that will be asked.

Press Relations Day. Representatives of the media can be invited for a formal luncheon to encourage open dialogue and conversation. The agenda should include expectations of both the transport program and the media in terms of information that is needed for a successful news release and explanation of why some information cannot be made available (i.e., patient confidentiality). The transport manager can create the appropriate environment in which the media learn that the program will provide the information needed in the constraints of patient privacy. The media can provide feedback on how best to supply information, including the framework and content for news releases, and how to hold a press conference. Establishing a collaborative relationship between the press and the program aids in future coverage but should not carry the expectation that the program will be shown favoritism by the news media.

ADVERTISING

Oftentimes, public relations, publicity, and advertising are all thought of as the same thing; they are not. *Advertising* a transport program can yield transport requests, but only if it is focused on the right target group: system activators. A giant billboard along the side of a highway is seen by a multitude of people; yet how many of them have the authority to make a request for transport services? Properly targeted advertising in hospital periodicals, EMS journals, and such is a much more advantageous way to advertise the transport program. Advertising must be carefully integrated and should support the objectives of the marketing plan.

EVALUATION OF RESULTS IN A PUBLIC RELATIONS PROGRAM

The means by which to monitor and evaluate the public relations program are recording activities and measuring success. The record of activities should include the number of press releases mailed versus the number used and by whom; press conferences and speaking engagements, including numbers and lists of participants for future follow-up; and newsletters and brochures produced with documentation of follow-up activities, including solicitation of feedback regarding material content.

Measuring the success of the public relations program is somewhat difficult in that the results are generally seen in changes of attitudes of the program activators. A successful program may result in increased service utilization, but this is not a reliable indicator because it is dependent on an event that is triggered external to the targeted audience. Success may be measured through appropriate use, tracking the numbers of times one service is used versus that of a competitor, and monitoring ground transports that potentially were appropriate to be flown. Other program outputs can be measured on the basis of projections of the response expected through marketing the speaker's bureau versus actual numbers of programs delivered.

THE MARKETING PROCESS

The marketing plan begins with an analysis of the results of market research, public relations activities, strengths identified in the internal and external environment, identification of the market segments, program goals, and ultimately the program mission. Specific objectives are derived from this information that focus program management and staff on the development of a plan that will have specific measurable outcomes.

Marketing has to be consistent and persistent; it should be one of the disciplines of the transport program, just like clinical operations, safety, communications, and aviation.

Marketing process can fail for a multitude of reasons, but more often than not failure revolves around a lack of execution, or failure to execute on consistent transport system performance and marketing actions or initiatives. There is no secret ingredient to having a successful marketing process outside of commitment to documenting and following it. The marketing plan should be simple, clear, and open to accommodating new strategies. The effectiveness of the plan should be evaluated on a regularly scheduled basis.

Poor communication of the marketing plan internally also adds to the demise of successful marketing strategies. A collaborative goal-setting and strategic-planning process involving internal and external organizational players is critical to the success of the plan.

SUMMARY

Approaching marketing as a process with each of the components developed to support the transport program's mission and goals is important. Integrated into the marketing process are strategies specific to the activities of the transport program.[7,8] Patient transport involves a great deal of one-on-one contact with EMS agencies and hospitals. Perception of how the transport team works with the referring personnel is a primary component of marketing the transport program. A well-functioning professional transport system performing consistently day in and day out is the best marketing tool available.

Providing transport in a timely seamless way based on the mission of the transport program is the best way transport programs can serve their patients and those who use their services.

REFERENCES

1. American Academy of Pediatrics: *Air and ground transport of neonatal and pediatric patients*, ed 3, Elk Grove Village, IL, 2007, AAP.
2. Blumen I, editor: *Principles and directions of air medical transport*, Salt Lake City, 2006, Air Medical Physicians Association.
3. Association of Air Medical Services (AAMS): *News/views newsletter*, May 2004.
4. Commission on Accreditation of Medical Transport Systems: *Standards*, ed 6, Andersonville, SC, 2006, CAMTS.
5. Cowan-Danovaro M, Griffith R: CALSTAR celebrates 15 years of community service, *Air Med* 4(3):18, 1998.
6. High RK, Yeatman J: Developing an educational outreach program, *J Emerg Nurs* 23(3):256-258, 1997.
7. Jones J: EMS night out and LifeFlight, *The Vanderbilt Reporter Magazine* May 2003.
8. Rodenberg JH, Rodenberg H: Part 3: the business plan: cornerstone of success, *Air Med J* 17(4):174, 1998.
9. York Clark J, Stocking J, Johnson J: *Flight and ground transport nursing core curriculum*, Denver, 2006, Air and Surface Transport Nurses Association.

40 ACCREDITATION FOR AIR AND GROUND MEDICAL TRANSPORT

Eileen Frazer

Accreditation means to give authority or reputation; to trust; to accept as valid or credible. Most medical professionals are familiar with the term accreditation because of the organization that accredits hospitals, the Joint Commission. The history of accreditation for hospitals is an interesting one that laid the foundation for other accrediting agencies to follow.

HISTORY OF THE JOINT COMMISSION

In 1915, the American College of Surgeons (ACS), recognizing the need to standardize patient care in hospitals, allocated $500.00 to establish standards to promote quality patient care.[5] Hospitals in 1915 were not necessarily places patients went to be cured but places patients went to die. Medical knowledge was minuscule compared with today's world. Penicillin had not yet been discovered, and although aseptic technique was used in surgery, no effective medications were available to manage postoperative infections.[7]

By 1917, the ACS developed a one-page list of requirements they called Minimum Standards for Hospitals.

An on-site inspection was developed by the ACS in 1918 to determine whether hospitals with more than 100 beds could meet compliance with the Minimum Standards for Hospitals. More than 700

hospitals throughout the United States were evaluated in the first year, and only 89 (13%) met the requirements of the Minimum Standards. Although these results were dismal, the inspection raised the awareness of the medical community, who were ready to accept the need for standardization and a verification process to improve quality.

More than 3000 hospitals were voluntarily surveyed by 1951. With the growth and overwhelming success of voluntary accreditation for hospitals, the ACS organization became overwhelmed and invited other organizations to participate. The Joint Commission on Accreditation of Hospitals (JCAH) was chartered in 1951 with the ACS and the following participating organizations: the American College of Physicians, the American Medical Association, the Canadian Medical Association, and the American Hospital Association.

Later in the 1950s, the Canadian Medical Association withdrew to form its own national organization, and JCAH expanded to include healthcare outside the hospital environment, such as home health, mental health, and ambulatory healthcare. This expansion eventually resulted in a name change to the Joint Commission on Accreditation of Healthcare Organizations (JCAHO), known as *the Joint Commission* today.

THE "WHITE PAPER" CALLS FOR IMPROVED EMERGENCY MEDICAL SERVICES

The Joint Commission was well established before standards even existed for medical transport. In fact, problems in transport were not even identified until 1966 when the *White Paper* entitled "Accidental Death and Disability: The Neglected Disease of Modern Society"[2] was published by the National Academy of Science. At that time, helicopter transport for the civilian population was unheard of, and standardization did not exist for ground transport vehicles or for the medical attendants who accompanied patients. Untrained personnel in the back of a mortician's vehicle did 50% of ground transports. Fire, police, or volunteer groups did the other 50% of the transports.

The *White Paper* triggered legislation that specifically addressed emergency medical services (EMS) and even suggested the use of helicopters.[5]

The Maryland State Police Aviation Division developed the earliest known public service helicopter system in 1969. A few hospital-based helicopter programs were seen by the mid 1970s, but the growth of these types of services did not really peak until the mid 1980s. At this time, hospitals were regionalizing, with specific hospitals recognized as centers of excellence in one or more specialty areas. Trauma center designation often included a helicopter program or access to a helicopter program, which was an added impetus to the growth in the number of helicopter services.

Also, the Vietnam experience proved a sharp decrease in mortality rates because of the rapid response of helicopters in transporting the injured from the field to definitive care. From a civilian perspective, the Golden Hour theory by Dr R. Adams Cowley of the Shock Trauma Unit of Baltimore proposed that a critically injured patient had a precious 60 minutes to obtain definitive surgical treatment after an injury to survive.[8] The Golden Hour theory and the Vietnam experience[6] were frequently touted as reasons for a hospital, especially a trauma center, to start a helicopter service.

In 1980, a new organization, the Association of Hospital Based Emergency Air Medical Services (ASHBEAMS; the name was later changed to the Association of Air Medical Services [AAMS]) was formed. This organization started as a forum for administrators and personnel to get together and network with other hospital-based helicopter programs. No standards were available at this time, so those assigned to start up a hospital-based helicopter program usually had no air transport experience, no pattern to follow, and no awareness of the potential hazards and managers who understood the risks even less. The aviation component (aircraft, pilots, and maintenance) was contracted from an aviation vendor. Pilots were usually Vietnam survivors who were still operating under the oath they practiced in the military—complete the mission. Care providers were thrust into the unfamiliar aviation environment without standardized transport training and with the ingrained attitude that the patient, not safety, always comes first. Clearly all were well intentioned, but as more and more accidents began to occur, it was recognized that the profession needed standardization, not unlike the ACS recognized the need for standards in hospitals in the early 1900s.

In 1985, 16 air medical accidents with 12 fatalities occurred.[4] The Federal Aviation Administration (FAA) was concerned, and the press began to alert the public. At the time, ASHBEAMS had minimal guidelines addressing patient care issues, but when the press started to focus on the number of air medical accidents, ASHBEAMS began to meet with other national groups, such as the Helicopter Association International (HAI), the National Flight Nurses Association (NFNA), National Flight Paramedics Association (NFPA), and the National EMS Pilots Association (NEMSPA), to develop consensus standards on safety and operational practices.

In 1986, the ASHBEAMS Safety Committee started a peer review safety audit called Priority One, with use of the safety guidelines that had been developed through the consensus process of the organizations listed previously. Priority One was beta-tested at Duke University in Durham, NC, and at the Staff for Life Program in Columbia, Mo. As a result of these visits, the Safety Committee found that patient care standards specific to the transport environment were needed as were the safety guidelines to make the process complete. Therefore, a feasibility study was performed to determine the need and viability of an accreditation program specifically for air medial transport.

Part of the feasibility study involved dialogue with the Joint Commission and other accrediting bodies. Many organizational leaders felt that the Joint Commission should incorporate transport standards into its accreditation process and then layer in the air medical profession, which would negate the expense and effort needed to create another accrediting agency. However, the Joint Commission was not interested in responsibility for standards addressing the aviation environment, stating that it was completely out of their field of expertise. Also, in the late 1980s, helicopter services were starting to be outsourced or privately owned and no longer sponsored or based at hospitals. Typically, fixed-wing medical transport services were privately owned and operated by an aviation company with no connections to hospitals. Both types of services were completely outside the realm of the Joint Commission.

ACCREDITATION ORGANIZATION FOUNDED FOR AIR MEDICAL TRANSPORT

In 1989, with the feasibility study completed and presented, ASHBEAMS members voted to fund start-up costs for an air medical accreditation agency. Conceptually, this organization would be separate and independent of ASHBEAMS and would be made up of member organizations, so each member organization had equal representation on the Board of Directors.

The following seven organizations met on July 13, 1990, in Kansas City, Mo, to form the Commission on Accreditation of Air Medical Services (CAAMS): the American College of Emergency Physicians, the Association of Air Medical Services, the National Association of Air Medical Communication Specialists, the National Association of EMS Physicians, the National EMS Pilots Association, the National Flight Nurses Association (now called Air and Surface Transport Nurses Association [ASTNA]), and the National Flight Paramedics Association.

The Commission on Accreditation of Air Medical Services was formally incorporated in the state of Pennsylvania as a nonprofit organization. The mission of CAAMS was and is to improve the quality of patient care and safety of the transport environment. Along with the tools for the new organization's foundation, such as the articles of incorporation, policies, and bylaws, the most important task for the new board was to develop the accreditation standards.

All accrediting organizations have a similar process of site visits, usually every 3 years, to verify compliance with standards. But the standards are what define the site survey process. Medical transport services that apply for accreditation are awarded or are withheld from accreditation based on compliance with the accreditation standards. Therefore, the standards must be attainable, measurable, and consistent with current practice.

ACCREDITATION STANDARDS

To gain acceptance of the accreditation standards, CAAMS used guidelines and standards from many of the organizations mentioned previously (ASHBEAMS, HAI, NFNA, NEMSPA, and NFPA) to begin the process. In an attempt to create a document that would address both safety and patient care issues, the CAAMS board studied the National Transportation Safety Board's (NTSB) accident reports to determine whether a standardized practice, policy, or procedure could have prevented an accident. The CAAMS board also worked with officials from the FAA who were specifically assigned to be a liaison with the air medical profession.

In some cases, the accreditation standards exceeded FAA regulations, and in some cases, the regulation was copied into a standard to provide needed emphasis on a particular issue. For example, an FAA regulation is that personnel and passengers must be seat belted for all takeoffs and landings.[1] However, during site visits, medical personnel would often tell site surveyors that if they were busy with the patient on liftoff or landing, they did not bother with the seat belts. Indeed, in some of the survivable air medical accidents, several medical attendants received serious back and spinal injuries because they were not secured in their seat belts on liftoff.

Before the first edition of Accreditation Standards was published in 1991, numerous drafts were mailed to organizations and individuals affiliated with the air medical transport profession. CAAMS also held a public hearing at the air medical transport conference in September 1990 in Nashville, TN, to gather opinions and suggestions for the draft of standards that were distributed.

Accreditation Standards are revised every 3 years to keep abreast of current practice. The following broad topics included in the Accreditation Standards are each supported by specific criteria (Box 40-1).

SITE SURVEYORS

Several accrediting agencies in related healthcare fields were willing to share copies of their policies and qualifications for site surveyors when CAAMS was developing its new accrediting agency. One of those organizations, the Commission on Accreditation of Rehabilitation Facilities (CARF), was very generous and allowed the Executive Director of CAAMS to participate in its site surveyor training course. Subsequently, the course developed by the CAAMS Site Surveyor Selection Committee was based on the principles of CARF's program. Originally, in 1991, there were 35 applicants for the 12 site surveyor positions. Applicants were chosen based on the requirements and on their level of experience. Applicants were required to have a minimum of 4 years experience and a background in two of the four following categories: aviation, communications, medical, and management, with a heavy emphasis on management experience. The first site surveyor training class was held in 1991, with classes repeated every 2 to 3 years to keep up with attrition and site-visit demands.

PAST AND FUTURE CHALLENGES

In 1997, CAAMS changed its name to the Commission on Accreditation of Medical Transport Systems (CAMTS) to capture a wider range of potential applicants and to accommodate the need for standards and accreditation for critical care ground services. Many of these ground MICU services consisted of pediatric and neonatal specialty teams, and many were part of an already existing air service. The

---

BOX 40-1	**Accreditation Standards**

General Standards*
Medical Section
Medical Direction and Clinical Supervisor
    Medical Personnel
        Staffing
        Training
Commercial Escorts

Aircraft/Ambulance Section
    Medical Configuration
    Operational Issues
    Aircraft/Ambulance equipment
    Communications

Management and Administration Section
    Management/Policies
    Utilization Review
    Quality Management
    Infection Control

Rotor-Wing Standards
Certificate of the Aircraft Operator
Weather and Weather Minimums
Pilot Staffing and Training
Maintenance
Helipad and Refueling
Community Outreach

Fixed-Wing Standards
Certificate of the Aircraft Operator
Aircraft

Weather and Weather Minimums
Pilot Staffing and Training
Maintenance
Community Outreach

Ground Interfacility Standards
Vehicles
Driver Qualifications
Maintenance and Sanitation
Mechanic
Policies

*Apply to all modes of transport.

---

services needed to be able to have their entire transport program accredited. Although the Commission on Accreditation of Ambulance Services (CAAS) exists for ground emergency services, CAAS does not have standards for critical care transport. Therefore, CAMTS developed the ground standards (critical care standards were already in place) and began to fill this void in 1997 when it offered accreditation for ground critical care services as well as air medical services. In 2000, CAMTS also included basic life support (BLS) and advanced life support (ALS) ground standards to accommodate the transport services that either provided air or critical care ground services and also provided BLS and ALS ground transport.[3,7]

As mentioned previously, most medical professionals understand accreditation because of exposure to the hospital accrediting agency, the Joint Commission. However, in developing an air medical accreditation process, aviation professionals had to be educated on the purpose and goals of accreditation. Although the aviation component was accustomed to regulations, the aviation professionals were not familiar with accreditation and did not understand the need for yet another process when most believed they were already overregulated by the FAA. The fixed-wing community was particularly baffled. Most fixed-wing transport services were owned and managed by private aviation operators who were totally unfamiliar with the term accreditation. CAAMS worked through the National EMS Pilots Association, as one of its member organizations, to try to gain wider acceptance and also developed a formal Aviation Advisory Committee to involve the fixed-wing community, managers from the major EMS Aviation Operators, and the FAA. The purpose of the Aviation Advisory Committee, which meets annually, is to provide updated information and to provide a forum for gathering input from the aviation professionals.

Another challenge facing CAAMS was the volatile healthcare market of the 1990s. Hospitals were closing, merging, or buying up other hospitals, and if transport was part of hospital's system, it suddenly needed to show a positive financial outlook or cease to exist, quite a turnaround from the 1980s when hospitals did not worry about what the helicopter cost as long as it brought patients into the hospital and was available as a visible marketing tool. Therefore, when the focus shifted to the bottom line of the budget, many hospital-based helicopter programs were fighting for survival and had difficulty justifying the cost of accreditation.

Since the year 2000, CAMTS has been meeting the demands of a rapidly changing air medical and ground transport community. A simple one-helicopter program based at one specific hospital is no longer the norm. With private business and aviation companies hiring their own medical teams and outsourcing communication centers, scheduling a site visit has become much more complicated. In many cases, a team of three or more site surveyors is necessary to visit all the satellite bases, maintenance centers, and communication centers that may be a part of a single program.

An increase in the number of applicants for accreditation has also been experienced as state and local EMS agencies move towards requiring CAMTS accreditation. In 2008, nine states (Colorado, Massachusetts, Maryland, Michigan, New Hampshire, New Mexico, Rhode Island, Utah, and Washington) and several county agencies in California and Nevada had regulations that required air medical services to achieve CAMTS accreditation. CAMTS is placed in a potentially litigious position, especially if a medical transport service does not meet the standards and does not receive accreditation. The CAMTS Board of Directors prefers that states provide "deemed status" to CAMTS accredited services for accredited programs that have met or exceeded higher standards than the minimal standards usually required by government agencies. In addition, there are legal challenges to states that require CAMTS accreditation based on the 1978 Airline Deregulation Act (ADA).[8] The primary focus was on the competitive market environment for air carriers. To ensure that states would not undo federal deregulation with regulation of their own, Congress included a preemption provision as follows: "A State, political subdivision of a state, or political authority of at least 2 states, may not enact or enforce a law, regulation, or other provision having the force or effect of law related to *price, route, or service* of an air carrier that may provide air transport." Because some of the CAMTS Accreditation Standards exceed Federal Aviation Regulations (FARs) in terms of pilot training and certain operating criteria, such as higher weather minimums, states that require CAMTS accreditation are being challenged in Federal court.

Many services apply for accreditation and reaccreditation not because they are required to do so by state regulations or by contracts but for the obvious benefits of accreditation such as outside auditing, accreditation as a marketing tool, competitive edge, and reimbursement advantages.[3]

Many medical transport services also find a number of intangible benefits as a result of going through the accreditation process, such as more cohesive working relationships, team building, a revitalized pride, and professionalism among personnel. Along with these benefits, the program receives a listing of the contingencies or areas that do not meet the intent of the accreditation standards or are not in compliance with the accreditation standards. The Commission tracks these areas of contingency and keeps a list of the most cited areas. Box 40-2 lists the most current frequently cited areas of contingency.

Today, 17 member organizations are involved, each sending one representative to serve on the board of directors. Board members make all of the accreditation decisions, create and update policies, and revise the Accreditation Standards. In addition to the founding organizations listed earlier, CAMTS is proud to include the following member organizations:

Aerospace Medical Association (AsMA)
American College of Surgeons (ACS)
Air Medical Physicians Association (AMPA)
Air and Surface Transport Nurses Association (ASTNA)

BOX 40-2	**Frequently Cited Areas of Weakness**

The quality management or performance improvement program lacks follow-up and loop closure.
Medical director is not involved in the interviewing and hiring process for the medical personnel.
Skills maintenance program documentation is weak.
Initial orientation is not well documented.
Continuing clinical experiences are not documented.
No designated Safety Management System exists.
Safety committee does not have representation from communications and maintenance.
No annual drill exists for the postincident/accident plan (PAIP).

American Academy of Pediatrics (AAP)
American Association of Critical Care Nurses (AACN)
American Association of Respiratory Care (AARP)
American College of Emergency Physicians (ACEP)
American College of Surgeons (ACS)
Association of Air Medical Services (AAMS)
Emergency Nurses Association (ENA)
International Association of Flight Paramedics (IAFP)
National Air Transportation Association (NATA)
National Association of Air Medical Communication Specialists (NAACS)
National Association of Neonatal Nurses (NANN)
National Association of State EMS Officials
National EMS Pilots Associations (NEMSPA)

It is the diversity and wealth of experience from the member organization board representatives that provide CAMTS with the strength and integrity to offer accreditation to medical transport services in North American and abroad and to continually improve medical transport services for patients now and in the future.

SUMMARY

Accreditation provides a framework for program evaluation and improvement. It also demonstrates to the public and the patients that a transport program complies with specific standards to ensure safe and competent patient transport.

REFERENCES

1. AIM/FAR: *91,105 Flight crewmembers at stations*, New York, 1998, McGraw-Hill.
2. ASHBEAMS: *Air medical crew national standard curriculum*, Pasadena, CA, 1988, US Department of Transportation.
3. Commission on Accreditation of Air Medical Systems: *Accreditation standards of the commission on accreditation of medical transport systems*, ed 7, Andersonville, SC, 2006, CAAMS.
4. Frazer R: Air medical accidents: 20 year search for information, *AirMed* 5(5):34, 1999.
5. Helicopter Association International: *Helicopters 1948–1998: a contemporary history*, Alexandria, VA, 1998, HAI.

6. Joint Commission on Accreditation: *An introduction to the Joint Commission*, Chicago, 1988, The Commission.

7. Richardson JG: *Health and longevity*, Philadelphia, 1914, Home Health Society.

8. Rhodes M, et al: Field triage for on-scene helicopter transport, *J Trauma* 26(11):963, 1986.

41

STRESS AND STRESS MANAGEMENT

Debra A. Milliner

Transport professionals face a number of situations that challenge both clinical skills and personal reserves. The result of these situations is stress. Left unacknowledged and unprocessed, this stress can be detrimental to transport professionals. To prevent the side effects of stress, transport professionals must understand the causes and strategies that help mitigate the adverse effects of stress and methods that help prevent stress-related diseases. This chapter examines the history of stress and the development of stress research, the pathophysiologic effects of stress, and the methods of stress management in both work and personal environments.

STRESS IN TRANSPORT MEDICINE

The transport environment and the nature of the industry expose transport professionals to frequent stress in both their professional and personal lives. The challenges of transport predispose these individuals to stress not commonly addressed by other professions. Continual changes in healthcare and clinical services provide a tumultuous arena for the provision of care.

Rules and laws govern transport programs and can predispose personnel to stress. Air medical transport programs must deal with rigorous federal regulations to accomplish the daily operations of the aviation programs. Interactions with pilots who are governed by the Federal Aviation Agency can produce conflicts between duty time and the ability to undertake the transport. Ground transport programs face regulations dictated by not only federal agencies but state and local governing bodies. These challenges add stress to the already demanding environment of transport medicine.

Transport professionals are often physically limited by space during the provision of patient care. Transport vehicles, whether ambulance, airplane, or helicopter, are much smaller than any hospital room and require the transport professional to be creative to provide care in such a limited environment. The lack of information about the patient's true diagnosis, especially injury, adds additional stress to the transport team. Research has identified that limitations in the physical working environment add to individual stress.[48] The challenges of providing care during scene transports also can produce stress for the transport professional.[9,10]

Financial considerations can also present stress to the transport team. Changes in insurance coverage, reimbursement, managed care, downsizing, and outsourcing have added challenges to the financial management of transport medicine. Today's programs also are required to frequently examine current service lines and consider the addition of new programs, which require new training and cultural changes within the organization. The fear of restructuring and potential job loss has markedly increased stress in long-term established transport programs. Working conditions have been found to be the greatest predictor of job stress. Regulatory, physical, and financial factors continue to add to the stress of transport healthcare.[35]

THE HISTORY OF STRESS

Stress is a normal component of life. *Stress* is defined by Johnson[27] as the body's reaction to the environment and the changes that occur. Stress occurs not solely because of an event but is dependant on the person's reaction to the event. One must also understand that individuals react differently and what might be considered a stressor for one person does not present stress to another. Stressors in the transport environment vary between individuals, prior training, education, and experience and the resulting effects of the stressor on the person. Stressors in transport also include those produced by patients, referral agencies, bystanders and family members, and management. Stress from weather and the confines of transport vehicles may result in decision making that can prove fatal to all involved. Understanding the nuances of stress in transport is imperative to safe insightful operational decision making.

Stress is not only potentially damaging during transport but can affect individuals on a daily basis. The American Psychological Association (APA) identified that 43% of all adults have some form of adverse health effects from stress. The APA's research also identified that 70% to 90% of all doctor visits are related to stress ailments and symptoms. Stress has been linked to the leading causes of death in adults: heart disease, cancer, accidents, suicide, cirrhosis of the liver, and lung conditions. The Occupational Safety and Health Administration (OSHA) declared stress a work hazard from the associated dangers found in the work environment.[30]

The negative aspects of stress were first postulated by Claude Bernard (1865) with the description of dynamic equilibrium. *Dynamic equilibrium* is the steady state in the internal body where balance is maintained.[21] Bernard noted that external changes in the environment and external factors that affect the internal balance of an organism must be reacted to and compensated for if the organism is to survive. Walter Cannon (1932) coined the phrase *homeostasis* to further define dynamic equilibrium. Cannon recognized that stressors are both physical and emotional and coined the term *fight or flight* to describe the body's physical reaction to those stresses.

Research on the causes and long-term effects of stress began in the past 70 years. Hans Selye identified the correlation of stress with physical symptoms as early as 1936 while doing research as an endocrinologist. He identified the role of the pituitary gland in the stress response. Selye postulated that as the body continues to function under stressful situations, adaptation occurs (general adaptation syndrome) but with exhaustion that can eventually lead to death.[40] Selye introduced the term *stress* and defined it as "mutual actions of forces that take place across any section of the body, physical or psychological."[21]

Selye said, "To be free of stress is to be dead."[28] However, Selye found that stress was both productive and destructive and introduced the concept of *general adaptive syndrome* (GAS). General adaptive syndrome is comprised of three parts: alarm, resistance, and exhaustion.[39] During the *alarm* stage, the body releases adrenaline as a result of a perceived danger. Although the body may not be able to identify or define the threat, preparation is made to respond once the danger is identified.

The next phase, *resistance*, is commonly labeled the fight or flight stage. Marked physiologic events occur from pathophysiologic actions that prepare the body to flee from the perceived danger.[39] The sympathetic nervous system causes:

- Increased respirations increase oxygen levels to supply more oxygen for the body to use.
- Increased blood glucose levels provide energy to help the body react to the stressor.
- Pulse and blood pressure elevate to increase muscular blood flow and improve strength and stamina.
- Muscles tense in preparation to move the body to flee the danger.

- Pupils dilate and allow more light into the eye to aid vision.
- Senses heighten to help identify and avoid the danger.
- Decreased gastric motility and blood shunting to vital organs help the organism survive and send the oxygenated blood where most needed.
- Loosening of bowel and bladder.
- Increased adrenaline levels to increase awareness and accelerate all functions in the body.
- Mobilization of clotting capabilities in preparation for injury to prevent possible hemorrhage.
- Increased perspiration and saliva to help cool the organism.
- Increased hormone production in response to the stimulus and to help the organism's function at peak potential.

The final stage, *exhaustion*, occurs when the stressor has been resisted. If ineffective means of stress reduction are used, the body returns to the alarm stage and becomes further exhausted because all resources have been exhausted. This continual exhaustion can deplete resources until death of the organism occurs.

Holmes and Rahe (1964) developed the Holmes and Rahe *Schedule of Recent Experiences* that awarded numeric rankings to events commonly associated with stress syndrome. These events are common occurrences that affect almost everyone during the life cycle. The most common of these events are death, divorce, loss of a job, moving, and severe illness. The research identified that stressful life events have detrimental effects and have been associated with sudden cardiac death, diabetes, pregnancy and obstetric complications, and increased risk for other diseases.[26] Transport professionals often experience these events while continuing to perform in the high-stress transport environment. Transport professionals are often tasked with the added stress of illness or death of patients and the concurrent personal events of team members.

Categories of Stress

Stress is divided into acute and chronic stress. *Acute stress* is a short-term immediate response to an event. It can be experienced by transport professionals

during a traumatic arrest or during a mass casualty incident. *Chronic stress* occurs with continuous acute stress responses that keep the body continually "on alert" with no relaxation phase.[3] The nature of the transport environment requires a constant state of attention and readiness during all phases of transport in an environment with the potential for conflict, industry hazards, and a constant state of change. Chronic stress can occur when a transport professional does not use adequate stress management tools over an extended period of time.

The two different types of stress are *eustress* and *distress*. Eustress is normal stress that occurs in everyday life or in the work setting. It is beneficial because individuals work and react in a positive productive manner when some stress is involved. Transport professionals work at peak performance when the call is challenging or the patient offers opportunities to perform advanced skills.

Distress is defined by Webster's Dictionary as "great pain, anxiety, or sorrow; acute physical or mental suffering; affliction; trouble." Distress is destructive stress that causes physical and mental conditions to develop in the individual. Distress in the transport arena includes those situations with multiple victims, children, or high-profile transports. Distress causes an individual to be less effective in the provision of care and can predispose the transport team to increased risk for accident and injury. Chronic eustress also predisposes the transport professional to chronic physical and mental health conditions because the team members always remain in a state of alarm.

Burnout can occur when transport professionals experience chronic stress.[2] Burnout can change positive feelings of engagement to negative ones. Transport personnel who were previously engaged and enthusiastic may become apathetic, bitter, impatient, cynical, and exhausted.[2] These psychological and emotional symptoms are often associated with physical manifestations in stress.

HOW STRESS AFFECTS THE BODY

Stress can cause physical and emotional exhaustion as a short-term effect.[27] The severity of the body's response to stress is related to the type of stress, the frequency of stress, and methods of stress management used. Long-term effects include a possible relationship between stress and the development of Alzheimer's disease.[1,4]

The body attempts to create a balance to deal with stress. The initial response to a stressor is stimulation of the sympathetic nervous system. This stimulation produces the fight or flight phenomenon. In response, the parasympathetic nervous system releases hormones to the adrenal glands to help stem the release of cortisol. The cortisol binds with the hormones for transport back to the kidney for excretion. This action helps the body reach homeostasis.

When the stress is resolved, the parasympathetic system responds in an attempt to revert to a state of relaxation. As individuals age, this process becomes more difficult and takes longer to occur. The norepinephrine released during this process helps to improve mood, helps in the creation of new memories, and increases creativity.

EFFECTS OF STRESS ON BODY SYSTEMS

When a stressor occurs, the body's systems initially react to stressful situations during the alarm and resistance phase. However, continued stress produces long-term effects on every system in the body, which leads to exhaustion. Transport professionals should be aware of these symptoms and work to recognize these effects in themselves and in others on the team.

NEUROLOGIC

The nervous system is activated any time a stressor is identified. It signals the release of chemicals and prepares the body for rapid response to the perceived stressor. If stress is continuous, the body does not have time to recover and exhaustion occurs.

All other bodily systems are controlled by the nervous system and thus are affected by this continual stimulation. The affects of stress are not limited to the nervous system; they disrupt the body's homeostasis and leave bodily functions in turmoil.[3]

Continued stress produces initial hyperactivity and excitement that decreases as the stressor is met and mitigated. However, long-term neurologic effects include weakness, sleep pattern disruption, and lethargy. Research has identified that the brain remains hyperactive even after the stress has resolved, but this activity predisposes the individual to depression and anxiety.[49]

ENDOCRINE

Stress affects the immune system. Stress has a direct relationship with blood sugar fluctuations. Long-term effects of stress have been identified in blood sugar fluctuations in diabetes.[37] Individuals with high stress also have higher rates of colds and other infections than individuals with less stress.

CARDIOVASCULAR

The body reacts to stress by increasing heart rate and blood flow. These actions, in conjunction with the production and secretion of stress hormones predispose the individual to hypertension and heart disease. The constant irritation of the circulatory systems leads to inflammation, which is believed to play a role in heart attacks and strokes. Research postulates that cholesterol levels may also be affected by stress.[3,13] Continual stress or the lack of adequate stress mitigation can lead to cardiac disease and myocardial infarction.[29]

RESPIRATORY

During a stressful event, the respiratory drive increases to provide more oxygen during the fight or flight stage of stress. Although tachypnea is harmless in most individuals, those with asthma or chronic respiratory conditions may experience airway compromise. Even short-term stress may cause asthma attacks in those individuals with the disease.[2]

MUSCULOSKELETAL

When an individual perceives stress, the muscles in the body tighten in preparation to flee the event. At the passing of the perceived stressor, the muscles relax. These actions may lead to stress-induced conditions, such as migraine headaches and torticollis, and muscle strain and tension. Chronic muscle tension and fatigue contribute to multiple chronic musculoskeletal conditions.[3]

GASTROINTESTINAL

The gastrointestinal system often responds to stress with nausea or vomiting. Stress can also affect digestion so alteration in nutrient absorption occurs.

Diarrhea and constipation are common symptoms of individuals affected by stress. Changes in appetite or alcohol consumption as an ineffective coping mechanism carry their own consequences.

IMMUNE SYSTEM

Inflammation causes a release of glucocorticoid hormones and cortisol, which trigger the antiinflammatory response. During stressful situations, the body's immune system becomes altered and thus affects the ability of the immune system to response to this event. Psoriasis and eczema are both disorders of the immune system that are affected by long-term stress. Stress not only affects the body's ability to heal, but these conditions cause stress because of the physical appearance and associated pain of the condition, which increases an individual's stress.[14]

REPRODUCTIVE

Stress affects an individual both physically and psychologically. Sexual dysfunction is commonly reported with individuals experiencing stress. These conditions vary from impotence to a lack of sexual desires. Some individuals have sexual addiction patterns associated with continual stress situations.

Individuals can experience issues with reproduction as a result of long-term stress. Stress can cause a disruption in menstruation in both adolescent girls and women. Stress can also cause irregular periods and painful menses.

Males may have decreased production of testosterone with associated reduction in sperm cell production with decreased motility. Males also are susceptible to infections of the reproductive tract, prostate gland, testes, and urinary tract as a result of a depressed immune system associated with extended periods of stress.[3]

PSYCHOLOGIC

Cortisol interferes with the neurotransmitters in the body. Excessive cortisol can cause difficulty in concentration and produce issues with long-term memory retrieval.[45]

Stress also impacts individuals emotionally. Transport team members with high levels of stress may become depressed, anxious, short tempered, argumentative, and disruptive.[37] Individuals exposed to patients who attempt suicide have also been identified at risk for increased stress after the event.[8]

CAUSES OF STRESS

A *stressor* can be defined as "anything that causes stress."[23] Stress can result in job dissatisfaction, reduced work effectiveness, and behavioral and health changes. Stress can also be further differentiated between affective stress and cognitive stress. *Cognitive stress* may result from excessive mental workload. *Affective stress* (emotional stress) occurs when concerns exist about one's personal life.[23] Both types of stress can be detrimental and potentially deadly to individuals in the transport setting.

PERSONAL STRESSORS

Personal stressors come in many forms: family issues, financial worries, home, and management. Although we want to separate home life from career, it is practically impossible to do so.[35]

Personal stressors produce tensions in both home and work settings. Feelings of a loss of control often compound the symptoms of stress in the individual. Recognition of these stressors is often difficult because of the personalization of the issues.[27]

ENVIRONMENTAL STRESSORS

The transport environment provides a variety of *environmental stressors* produced in part by the vehicles used in the movement of patients. Noise, vibration, gravitational forces, and temperature and humidity extremes are the most recognized physical stressors in the transport environment. Limited space availability in most transport vehicles also produces stress for transport team members. Night transports, which produce limited lighting in which to provide patient care, can cause stress in transport crews.

STRESS IN THE WORKPLACE

Stress in the work setting is seldom lacking; rather, an overabundance often exists.[28] Transport medicine produces stress in both clinical care and workplace challenges that occur in the department. Blumen[7] identified the correlation of both self-imposed and externally imposed stressors in relation to helicopter crashes in emergency medical services operations.

Transport team members must realize that the workplace can produce the greatest amount of stress for an employed individual. Once again, the reaction to the stressor is the greatest predictor of detrimental effects rather than the stressor.[23,29,31]

Transport professionals who deal with stress may have difficulty accomplishing tasks. Characteristic problems include poor decision making, lack of concentration, apathy, lack of motivation, and job-related anxiety that can impact patient care.[31]

The perception of job stress has markedly increased over the past decade. The National Institute of Occupational Safety and Health (NIOSH) identified the following statistics:

- 40% of workers report their jobs are extremely stressful.
- 25% view their jobs as the number one stressor in life.
- 75% of all employees believe that on-the-job stress has increased over the past generation.
- 29% of all workers feel extremely stressed at work.
- 26% feel they are burned out.
- Job stress is the greater cause of health symptoms over financial or family problems.[35]

Workplace violence has become commonplace in certain areas of medicine.[24] Emergency healthcare has witnessed an increase in the threats to healthcare providers.[11, 24] Transport professionals are subjected to individuals whose conditions are altered from medical conditions or exposure to drugs and alcohol. These conditions certainly predispose the transport professional to risk of injury during patient care.

Emphasis on punishment in work-related situations must be minimized. Individuals who are punishment sensitive may have a stronger reaction to stressors than employees who are not so predisposed.[47, 41, 44]

Current research lists the major causes of work stress:

- The design of task: Heavy workloads, long work hours and irregular shifts, and hectic tasks.
- Management style: Poor communications, lack of involvement in decision making, and lack of family-oriented policies and procedures.
- Interpersonal relationships: Lack of social support among coworkers and management.
- Work roles: Uncertain job responsibilities, excessive job responsibilities.
- Career concerns: Lack of job security and lack of ability for career growth, advancement, or promotion.
- Environmental conditions: Unsafe or precarious working conditions.[35]

Job performance causes the greatest stress on employees and middle managers. Organizations can reduce employee stress by adjusting organizational culture. The development and initiation of stress management programs in organizations help employees recognize stress in themselves and others.[20,31] An atmosphere that uses nonpunitive quality management allows for reporting of errors without fear, which helps reduce stress. An open work environment that allows employees to seek help through employee assistance programs also encourages transport professionals to share feelings of frustration and stress with trained professionals.[20, 22, 31]

SELF-IMPOSED STRESSORS

Stress is not only produced by external sources but also occurs through *self-imposed stressors*. The inability to manage stress effectively can many times compound stress itself. These self-imposed stressors are often listed using the pneumonic DEATH (drugs, exhaustion, alcohol, tobacco, and hypoglycemia). Drugs, both over-the-counter and prescription, can produce issues with cognition and alertness. Exhaustion from multiple transports, insomnia from stress, and the common practice among transport professionals of multiple jobs also alters cognition and can cause potentially dangerous lack of attentiveness. Alcohol, when not consumed in the work setting, causes dehydration and depressed cognition. Research has shown that after a drinking binge, an individual may need up to 3 days for full return of higher mental and reflex functions to return.[23] Tobacco causes long-term health issues and can predispose the transport professional to hypoxia. An individual with a carboxyhemoglobin (COHb) level of 5% at a cabin altitude of 5000 ft has the equivalent physiologic altitude of 10,000 ft.[23] Hypoglycemia caused by the unpredictable nature of transport and erratic meals causes weakness and decreased alertness or worse. All of these stressors are self imposed and are under the control of the transport individual.[21]

CRITICAL INCIDENT STRESS

Critical incident stress (CIS) can occur with one specific incident or situation. Critical incidents usually involve a perceived threat to a personal physically or the physical health of others. Critical incidents are determined by the effect on a person's sense of safety and security and "competency in the world."[12]

Critical incidents may affect only the individual or may have a global impact. Examples of personal critical incidents include line of duty deaths among emergency medical services (EMS) or law enforcement personnel, assaults, sexual abuse, involvement in unethical acts, suicide or attempted suicide, robbery, or unexpected death of a relative or loved one. Global critical incidents include acts of terrorism, natural disasters, mass casualty homicides, or first response to a mass casualty event (Box 41-1). Critical incident stress can affect anyone associated with the event; however, those incidents represented by greater media attention can increase the risk of critical incident stress.[5,12]

Transport personnel who experience these events, either on a personal or global level, must recognize the potential for the development of long-term physical and psychologic symptoms, especially when the event is of prolonged duration.[12] The most common symptoms that occur among transport professionals include anxiety and fear for personal safety.

POSTTRAUMATIC STRESS DISORDER

Posttraumatic stress disorder (PTSD) occurs when chronic stress symptoms occur and lead to psychiatric illness. PTSD occurs after an individual experiences or witnesses a severe trauma that presents a physical threat to the person or other persons.[19] It differs from critical incident stress by the physical and psychologic responses and the duration of these symptoms.[34]

Posttraumatic stress disorder can also occur as a result of accumulative numerous smaller stress events. These events include death notification by law enforcement officers, verbal or physical abuse from patients or bystanders, and repeated involvement in violent incidents (homicides or motor vehicle crashes).[12,18,32,43]

The initial response to the stressor is fear, helplessness, or horror. After this experience, the individual

---

BOX 41-1 | **What is a Critical Incident?**

A *critical incident* is any event that has an impact stressful enough to overcome the usually effective coping skills of either an individual or a group. Critical incidents are usually sudden powerful events that are outside of the range of ordinary human experience. The following are examples of such events:

1. Line-of-duty death.
2. Serious line-of-duty injury.
3. Coworker suicide.
4. Multicasualty incidents (e.g., Oklahoma City, New York Trade Center, a multivehicle crash on the freeway, airplane crashes).
5. A police-involved shooting (an officer is shot or an officer shoots another individual).
6. Injury or death to a civilian as a result of operational procedures (e.g., fire engine or ambulance versus private vehicle; accidents as the result of high-speed chases).
7. Significant events that involve children, especially injury or death to a child, especially if perpetrated by an adult. Ninety-five percent of the CISDs done in the United States have involved children.
8. Failed mission after extensive effort. Loss of the victim becomes personal for the rescuer.
9. Excessive media interest: Continuous newspaper and television coverage make it impossible to escape the event. Subsequent litigation adds to the memory.
10. Any other powerful event that strikes a chord in the transport provider. One individual's event may not be another's.

experiences "numbness, avoidance or hyperarousal."[19] PTSD most often occurs in natural disasters, mass casualty incidents, war, personal assaults by patients or bystanders, or and diagnosis of a life-threatening medical condition. PTSD has been proven in all age groups, including children, and is most common in women. Symptoms usually occur within 3 months of the incident but may develop months or years later.[19] A diagnosis of PTSD is made through an examination of six criteria (Box 41-2).

Symptoms of PTSD may be either physical or psychologic. Individuals with chronic PTSD frequently have general medical conditions in conjunction with somatic symptoms (Box 41-3). Research has identified that emergency healthcare providers with prior critical incidents are not more vulnerable to PTSD. However, they are more vulnerable to psychologic stress responses when exposed to work-related stress events when they possess previous trauma experiences *and* poor social support.[38] Transport professionals may not identify these symptoms personally but may witness changes among others in the program. The recognition of PTSD symptoms and the physiologic changes associated with the syndrome is imperative for the initiation of coping mechanisms.

BOX 41-2   Criteria for Diagnosis of PTSD

First Criterion

The experiencing of a traumatic event that involves the threat of death or injury
   and
A feeling of helplessness, intense fear, or horror as a result of the experience.

Second Criterion

Persistent reliving of the event through dreams, illusions, hallucinations, flashbacks, and thoughts and intense psychologic distress.

Third Criterion

Avoidance of stimuli related to the event or experience. Three or more of these avoidance strategies must exist:
Avoidance of thoughts, feelings, or conversations associated with the event.
Avoidance of people, places, or events that trigger recollections of the event.
Inability to recall important aspects of the event.
Markedly diminished interest or participation in previously enjoyed events.
Feelings of detachment.
Narrowed range of affect.
Sense of impending doom.

Fourth Criterion

The individual experiences symptoms of hyperarousal. Two or more of these must exist:
Insomnia or difficulty sleeping.
Inability to concentrate.
Hypervigilance.
Emotional outbursts or irritability.
Hypersensitivity and exaggerated startle response.

Fifth Criterion

Duration of the symptoms exceeds a 1-month time period.

Sixth Criterion

The event causes clinically significant distress or functional impairment.

Gore TA, Richards-Reid GM: *Posttraumatic stress disorder, eMedicine*, available at http://www.emedicine.com, accessed June 2008.

BOX 41-3	**Chronic PTSD Symptoms**

A. The traumatic event is persistently experienced in one (or more) of the following ways:

1. Recurrent and intrusive distressing recollections of the event, including images, thoughts, or perceptions.
2. Recurrent distressing dreams of the event.
3. Acting or feeling as if the traumatic event were recurring (includes a sense of reliving the experience, illusions, hallucinations, and dissociative flashback episodes, including those that occur on awakening or when intoxicated).
4. Intense psychologic distress at exposure to internal or external cues that symbolize or resemble an aspect of the traumatic event.
5. Physiologic reactivity on exposure to internal or external cues that symbolize or resemble an aspect of the traumatic event.

B. Persistent avoidance of stimuli associated with the trauma and numbing of general responsiveness (not present before the trauma), as indicated by three (or more) of the following:

1. Efforts to avoid thoughts, feelings, or conversations associated with the trauma.
2. Efforts to avoid activities, places, or people that arouse recollections of the trauma.
3. Inability to recall an important aspect of the trauma.
4. Markedly diminished interest or participation in significant activities.
5. Feeling of detachment or estrangement from others.
6. Restricted range of affect (e.g., unable to have loving feelings).
7. Sense of a foreshortened future (e.g., does not expect to have a career, marriage, children, or a normal life span).

C. Persistent symptoms of increased arousal (not present before the trauma), as indicated by two (or more) of the following:

1. Difficulty falling or staying asleep.
2. Irritability or outbursts of anger.
3. Difficulty concentrating.
4. Hypervigilance.
5. Exaggerated startle response.

D. Duration of the disturbance (symptoms in criteria A, B, and C) is more than 1 month.

E. The disturbance causes clinically significant distress or impairment in social, occupational, or other important areas of functioning.

Reprinted with permission from the *Diagnostic and statistical manual of mental disorders*, ed 4, text revision, Copyright 2000, American Psychiatric Association.

Coping mechanisms for dealing with PTSD are either direct (Box 41-4) or indirect (Box 41-5). Individuals with higher levels of social support are less vulnerable to PTSD and thus may find the coping mechanisms more beneficial.

CRITICAL INCIDENT STRESS MANAGEMENT

Critical incident stress management (CISM) is an interventional protocol designed to help deal with major traumatic events.[12] CISM is highly structured and requires specific standardized training for individuals involved in the processes after a major event. The seven components to CISM are: preincident education, individual crisis or peer support, demobilization, defusing, debriefing, family support, and referral services. Grief and loss sessions are included when deaths are involved.

Grief and loss sessions are used after the death of an individual involved in a critical incident. These sessions help those involved to work through the grief process and deal with the sense of loss involved in the critical incident.[12]

Crisis management briefings are used to keep participants informed "before, during and after crisis to present facts, facilitate a brief, controlled discussion"

BOX 41-4   **Direct Coping Strategies**

Direct coping strategies aim to eliminate or reduce the size of the threat so the person is better able to handle the situation.
1. Enhance health through exercise, adequate rest, and a balanced diet to produce a positive stressor-management effect.
2. Leave the stressful situation.
3. Change problematic aspects of the situation to reduce demand from the environment (e.g., interpersonal working conditions, short staffing, poor lighting, excessive noise).
4. Nurture social support. Social support is an important buffer against stressors. Support can be with selected friends or a self-help group.
5. Learn on one's own with books, tapes, and videos.
6. Increase one's knowledge base with a trained instructor.

From Kivisto J, Couture RT: Stress management for nurses controlling the whirlwind, *Nurs Forum* 32:25-33, 1997.

BOX 41-5   **Indirect Coping Strategies for Stress Management**

Behavioral Interventions

The goal is to act differently so that new and effective coping patterns are acquired.
1. Slow down normal daily activities to enjoy the small pleasures in life.
2. Enjoy more humor in life by reading humorous books, watching humorous films. Allow yourself to laugh.
3. Spend time with positive people.
4. Decrease palliative coping behavior (overeating, abuse of alcohol or nonprescription drugs) and increase positive coping behavior (exercise, proper diet).
5. Take hardiness training (commitment, control, and challenge).
   a. Commitment: Tendency to involve oneself in activities with the environment.
   b. Control: Believing and acting as if one can influence events.
   c. Challenge: Individuals who feel appropriately challenged are more likely to have higher levels of confidence and lower levels of disabling emotions and greater capabilities in using resources than individuals who feel threatened.
6. Reshape behaviors that are characteristic of type A personality traits (e.g., free-floating hostility, sense of time urgency, and insecurity of status associated with a preoccupation with numbers). Like item 1, slow down. It's okay.

Cognitive Interventions

The goal is to develop more realistic, positive, and self-supportive thinking patterns to positively enhance feelings and actions. These strategies are useful when one adds stress to life by exaggerating threat, imagining catastrophes, or putting oneself down.
1. Positive self talk serves to defuse anxiety induced by exaggeration. The individual learns to use fewer self-critical remarks and to be more self encouraging. This enables objective assessment of the real risk in a situation and a focus on personal strengths.
2. Mental imagery involves visualizing relaxing images and has the effect of calming the mind and inducing a more relaxed physiologic state.
3. Thought stopping is a two-step process: recognizing and stopping anxious thoughts, followed by a relaxation technique. The pleasant sensations of relaxation reinforce the thought-stopping process and decrease negative consequences.
4. Stress inoculation: The individual is educated about stress reaction, trained in coping skills, and provided with opportunities to practice these skills.
5. Reframe the stressor. Is the event a threat or is it the individual's perception? For example, does a failing grade make the student a failure? Or can the issue be reframed by saying, "This problem can be fixed if I make some changes." The student must make the changes, but reframing the matter makes it less psychologically devastating.

| BOX 41-5 | **Indirect Coping Strategies for Stress Management—cont'd** |

Physiologic Interventions

The goal is to produce a physical state that is not compatible with the physiologic arousal that is generally associated with stress. This state is referred to as the relaxation response.

1. Learn diaphragmatic breathing. Sit quietly and take slow deep breaths while expanding the abdomen rather than the chest. Relaxed breathing relaxes the person.
2. Practice progressive relaxation. Contract a muscle group for 20 seconds; relax it; progress from one muscle group to another throughout the body.
3. Practice yoga. Many have found it to be beneficial in acquiring a relaxed body and calm state of mind.

and provide information about the critical incident. These briefings may be adjusted as information about the critical incident changes.[12]

Preincident education is formal training for individuals in high-risk professions where critical incidents can occur. This training is offered before an incident occurs through special training sessions taught by professionals trained in CISM.[21]

Individual crisis or *peer support* sessions focus on individuals affected by a critical incident. Interventions are provided by professionals trained in CISM.

Demobilization involves small groups both during and after critical incidents. Demobilization includes individuals that are brought to the incident for rescue and recovery.

Defusing generally lasts 30 to 60 minutes and is a less formal version of debriefing. Defusing is generally conducted within 1 to 4 hours after the traumatic event. It allows individuals to voice concerns in a voluntary nonthreatening way. Defusing is generally not conducted more than 12 hours after the critical incident. Both defusing and debriefing are voluntary and confidential.[21]

Debriefing involves the group involved in the traumatic incident. Debriefing is intended to help the individuals involved recover from the stressful event through open discussion within 24 to 72 hours after the event. Debriefing includes six phases: introduction, fact phase, feeling phase, symptom phase, teaching phase, and reentry.

Family support helps the family members of individuals that are involved in the incident. *Referral services* are used for a recognized need for services outside the CISM realm. These may include but are not limited to mental health services, financial and legal services, clergy, and medical services.[21]

Critical incident stress management must be presented by individuals specifically trained in the process, although defusing is often done routinely by transport professionals after a call. These sessions are informal discussions that allow each team member to voice concerns without fear of retribution or retaliation (Box 41-6).[12,33]

MITIGATING STRESS

Stress can cause deterioration in both body and mind. The body's ability to respond to and mitigate the results of stress depends on the individual's response to the stressor or ability to adapt. When individuals develop healthy methods of managing stress, theses affects can be managed with less detrimental long-term effects. Frequently, transport professionals use alcohol and drugs to help mitigate the effects of stress.[23] These methods actually increase the effects of stress and worsen the physical and emotional manifestations. The key to stress mitigation is balance. Without balance, stressors become overwhelming and the exhaustion phase becomes the norm rather than the anomaly.[28]

Transport team members must also remember that they are part of a team and at times one of the team members may be the one who is suffering from the effects of stress. When this situation is recognized, the transport programs should have resources in place so that members can easily support one another, which may include refusing a transport so that appropriate help can be obtained.

BOX 41-6	**Why is CISM Effective?**

CISM defusing and debriefing interventions are effective because interventions:

1. Occur early—often within hours after the crisis event.
2. Offer the opportunity for catharsis or ventilation that can lower stress levels and help make sense of the trauma.
3. Allow co-workers to verbalize the trauma. Participants verbally reconstruct and express the specific traumas, fears, or regrets they experienced. Using words, they can make concrete the emotions, images, and memories that are keeping them off balance.
4. Provide a behavioral structure with a beginning and end, superimposed on the event that frequently represents chaos, suffering, and unanswerable questions. Research shows that this structured environment within which to "worry" reduces the tendency for worry to interfere with other activities.
5. Provide a psychologic structure for individuals to explore the critical incident from the cognitive or thinking level down through the emotional level and then back again to the everyday world.
6. Provide opportunity for group support. The sense of individual isolation is reduced, useful information is shared, and mutual comfort and help are given. The social network is restored.
7. Offer peer support. People who've been through the same experiences are there to reassure colleagues that life will be OK eventually.
8. Offer education on stress, and teach coping techniques for dealing with the physical and emotional effects of the critical incident on the body and mind.
9. Provide opportunity for follow-up. Additional peer support, mental health assistance, and chaplain involvement are built in for individuals who might like more assistance—even before they ask.
10. Are action oriented. People are not allowed to remain in a state of confusion. Participants in interventions feel their concerns are being taken seriously. They feel group leaders are in control and know what they are talking about.

DIET

A balanced diet is important to help counteract the effects of stress and to help maintain a healthy body.[6] Caffeine appears to be a staple among transport professionals. However, caffeine is a strong stimulant that produces a stress reaction on the body. The avoidance of caffeine helps individuals feel more relaxed and helps sleep patterns.[20] Caffeine is found in coffee, tea, soda, and chocolate. If used, it is best consumed before lunch and with a balanced meal. Alternatives to caffeine, such as green or herbal teas, are acceptable and often healthier.[6]

Alcohol is often used by individuals as a relaxation tool. Alcohol stimulates the secretion of adrenaline and results in nervous tension, irritability, and insomnia, thus increasing stress.[12] Limiting alcohol to a single glass of wine with dinner is a healthier alternative.

Fried foods and high fat foods depress the immune system. Because stress depresses the immune system, transport professionals should restrict intake of fatty fried foods. A supply of healthy alternatives, such as granola or high-protein bars, is helpful in the avoidance of unhealthy fast food options.[6]

Whole grains promote the production of serotonin in the body, which increases a sense of well being. Yellow, green, and leafy vegetables are rich in vitamins and minerals, help boost the production of serotonin, and help boost the immune system, thus helping to counteract the effects of stress on the body.

EXERCISE

Exercise mitigates stress in several ways. Exercising releases endorphins that chemically make an individual feel better. Exercise also stops the production of the chemicals that are produced during the fight or flight phase of stress.[12]

Exercise does not have to be extremely strenuous or take a long period of time. Any movement that engages the cardiovascular and musculoskeletal system produces positive effects.[27] Team sports or activities with another also add to the benefits of exercise (Figure 41-1). Associated weight loss can also prove beneficial as can strength building exercises that improve work performance and reduce the risk of on the job injuries.

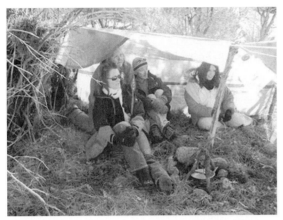

FIGURE 41-1   **Survival training provides an opportunity for team building and stress management.**

LAUGHTER

Laughter has been found to be an effective stress management tool.[1] Laughter allows for the release of endorphins that produce feelings of euphoria and relaxation. Laughter has been proven to benefit both neuroendocrine and cardiac systems and has shown improved clinical courses for chronically and acutely ill individuals.[42] Watching a funny movie, visiting a comedy club, or joking with friends can help relieve stress through humor.

VERBALIZATION OF FEELINGS

Individuals often keep feelings of stress internalized for fear of showing weakness or loss of control.[36] When sharing feelings that involve stress, individuals should not minimize their feelings or the feelings of others. Transport professionals should share their concerns with others but must also be willing to seek professional help when feelings begin to jeopardize their sense of well being.

SLEEP

Although inadequate sleep periods may not solely produce stress among transport professionals, sleep deprivation is associated with increased risk for accident and injury.[15-17,46] Disruption in circadian rhythm and shortened sleep cycles have been found to increase stress and increase the risk for injury and accident in transport professionals.

Transport professionals can minimize the effects of shift work by alleviating secondary jobs, maintaining a consistent sleep pattern when not on duty, and avoiding activities that can disrupt sleep patterns (alcohol, caffeine).

ALTERNATIVE METHODS

Complementary and *alternative therapies* are defined by the National Institutes of Health National Center for Complementary and Alternative Medicine (2002) as:

> "A broad range of healing philosophies, approaches and therapies that mainstream Western medicine does not use, accept, study, understand, or make available. A few of the many CAM (Complementary and Alternative Medicine) practices include the use of acupuncture, herbs, homeopathy, therapeutic massage, and traditional Oriental medicine to promote well-being or treat health conditions."[25]

Alternative methods of stress management vary but include: massage, acupuncture, music therapy, color therapy, meditation, and pet therapy. These methods may be used alone or in conjunction with other stress management tools for a comprehensive program.

SUMMARY

Stress can never be eliminated. Stress and response to stress can be beneficial in a limited scope. Transport individuals must recognize personal stressors and develop methods to mitigate stress both in personal and work settings. Management must also realize their role in stress mitigation among employees.

The secret is learning appropriate stress management. The recognition of stress in oneself and in team members is imperative in the prevention of long-term complications from stress. Through recognition and stress mitigation therapies, the high-stress atmosphere of transport medicine can be managed appropriately.

REFERENCES

1. Alessia K: Stop stressing and start relishing life, *Natural Health Vegetarian Life* 46: Autumn 2008.
2. American College of Emergency Physicians: *Avoid burnout by managing your stress*, available at http://www.acep.org, accessed June 2008.
3. American Psychological Association: *Mind/body health interaction*, APA Help Center from the American Psychological Association, available at http://apahelpcenter.org/articles/article.php?id=141, accessed May 2008.
4. Barry P: Linking stress and senility, *Sci News* 172(1):13, 2007.
5. Battles ED: An exploration of post-traumatic stress disorder in emergency nurses following Hurricane Katrina, *J Emerg Nurs* 33(4):314, 2007.
6. Blackwood A: Food + stress, *body + soul* 24(20):64, 2007.
7. Blumen I: *A safety review and risk assessment in air medical transport*, November 2002.
8. Bohan F, Doyle L: Nurses' experiences of patient suicide and suicide attempts in an acute unit, *Mental Health Pract* 11(5):12, 2008.
9. Boudreaux E, Jones GN, Mandry C, et al: Patient care and daily stress among Emergency Medical Technicians, *Prehosp Disaster Med* 11(3):188, 1996.
10. Boudreaux E, Mandry C: Sources of stress among Emergency Medical Technicians (part 1): what does the research say? *Prehosp Disaster Med* 11(4):296, 1996.
11. Burbeck R, Coomber S, Robinson SM, et al: Occupational stress in consultants in accident and emergency medicine: national survey of levels of stress at work, *Emerg Med J* 19:234, 2002.
12. Cardinal S: *What is a critical stress incident? CISM International*, available at http://www.criticalincidentstress.com/critical_incidents, accessed June 2008.
13. Chandola T, Britton A, Brunner E, et al: Work stress and coronary heart disease: what are the mechanisms? *Eur Heart J* 29(5):640, 2008.
14. Cohen S, Janicki-Deverts D, Miller GE: Psychological stress and disease, *JAMA* 298(14):1685, 2007.
15. Frakes MA, Kelly JG: Off-duty preparation for overnight work in rotor wing air medical programs, *Air Med J* 24(5):215, 2005.
16. Frakes MA, Kelly JG: Shift length and on-duty rest patterns in rotor-wing air medical programs, *Air Med J* 23(6):34, 2004.
17. Frakes MA, Kelly JG: Sleep debt and outside employment patterns in helicopter air medical staff working 24-hour shifts, *Air Med J* 26(1):45, 2007.
18. Goodwin RD: A twin study of post-traumatic stress disorder symptoms and asthma, *Am J Respir Crit Care Med* 176:983, 2007.
19. Gore TA, Richards-Reid GM: *Posttraumatic stress disorder, eMedicine*, available at http://www.emedicine.com, accessed June 2008.
20. Goudreau J, Edmondson G, Conlin M: Dispatches from the war on stress, *Business Week* 4045:74, 2007.
21. Hall Wofford M, Frakes M, Mayberry R: *Transport nurse advanced trauma course*, Denver, CO, 2006, ASTNA.
22. Hanna DR, Romana M: Debriefing after a crisis, *Nurs Manage* 38(8):38, 2007.
23. Hawkins FH: *Human factors in flight*, Burlington, VM, 2002, Ashgate.
24. Holleran RS, editor: Preventing staff injuries from violence, *J Emerg Nurs* 32(6):523, 2006.
25. House of Delegates of the Federation of State Medical Boards of the United States, Inc: *Model guidelines for the use of complementary and alternative therapies in medical practice*, Washington, DC, 2002, NIH.
26. Jacobs GD: The physiology of mind-body interactions: the stress response and the relaxation response, *J Altern Complement Med* 7(1):S-83, 2001.
27. Johnson TD: Address your stress, for a healthier life, *Nations Health* 38(3):24, 2008.
28. Kaye B, Jordan-Evans S: *Love'em or lose'em*, San Francisco, 1999, Berrett-Koehler.
29. Lucini D, Riva S, Pizzinelli P, et al: Stress management at the worksite; reversal of symptoms profile and cardiovascular dysregulation, *Hypertension* 49:291, 2007.
30. Miller LH, Smith AD: *How does stress affect us? APA Help Center from the American Psychological Association*, available at http://apahelpcenter.org/articles/article.php?id=1, accessed May 2008.
31. Milliken TF, Clements PT, Tillman HJ: The impact of stress management on nurse productivity and retention, *Nurs Econ* 25(4):2003, 2007.
32. Milstein JM, Gerstenberger AE, Barton S: Healing the caregiver, *J Altern Complement Med* 8(6):917, 2002.
33. Nachshoni T, Knobler HY, Jaffe E, et al: Psychological guidelines for a medical team debriefing after a stressful event, *Mil Med* 172(6):581, 2007.
34. National Center for Posttraumatic Stress Disorder: *Common reactions after trauma, United States Department of Veterans Affairs*, available at http://www.ncptsd.va.gov/ncmain/ncdocs/fact_shts/fs_commonreactions.html, accessed May 2008.
35. NIOSH working group: *Stress...at work*, National Institute for Occupational Safety and Health for the

CDC, available at http://www.cdc.gov/niosh/stresswk.html, accessed May 2008.

36. North C, Wraa C: *Stress: taming your shadow*, 2000 Critical Care Transport Medicine Conference, April 18, 2000.

37. Pazarino PJ: Stress, MedicineNet.com, available at http://www.medicinenet.com/script/main, accessed May 2008.

38. Regehr C, LeBlanc V, Jelley RB, et al: Previous trauma exposure and PTSD symptoms as predictors of subjective and biological response to stress, *Can J Psychiatr* 52(10):675, 2007.

39. Rosenbluh ES: Stress and its consequences, *J Police Crisis Negotiations* 5(1):79, 2005.

40. Russell JA: Stress milestones. *Int J Biol Stress* 10(1):1, 2007.

41. Sacks SB, Clements PT, Fay-Hillier T: Career perspectives; care after chaos: use of critical incident stress debriefing after traumatic workplace events, *Perspect Psychiatr Care* 37(4):133, 2001.

42. Sahakian A, Frishman WH: Humor and the cardiovascular system, *Altern Ther Health Med* 13(4):56, 2007.

43. Schottenbauer MA, Glass CR, Arnkoff DB, et al: Contributions of psychodynamic approaches to treatment of PTSD and trauma: a review of the empirical treatment and psychopathology literature, *Psychiatry* 71(1):13, 2008.

44. The American Institute of Stress: *Job stress*, available at http://www.stress.org/job.htm, accessed May 2008.

45. The Franklin Institute: *The human brain*, available at http://www.fi.edu/learn/brain/stress.html, accessed May 2008.

46. Thomas F, Hopkins RO, Handrahan DL, et al: Sleep and cognitive performance of flight nurses after 12-hour evening versus 18-hour shifts, *Air Med J* 25(5):216, 2006.

47. Van Der Linden D, Beckers DGJ, Taris TW: Reinforcement sensitivity theory at work: punishment sensitivity as a dispositional source of job-related stress, *Eur J Personality* 21:889, 2007.

48. Vischer JC: The effects of the physical environment on job performance: towards a theoretical model of workspace stress, *Stress Health J Int Soc Invest Stress* 23(3):175, 2007.

49. Wang J, Rao H, Wetmore GS, et al: Perfusion functional MRI reveals cerebral blood flow pattern unders psychological stress, *Proc Natl Acad Sci U S A* 102(49):17804, 2005.

POST-ACCIDENT RESOURCE DOCUMENT

INTRODUCTION

Air medical transport services provide an essential life-saving function in the healthcare and aviation systems. These services are generally high profile in nature and attract positive attention from the media. Although air medical crashes are rare, when they occur, they instantly become an intensely emotional event.

This document describes the various phenomena experienced by members of an air medical program after an aircraft incident. Its intended purposes are to assist air medical program leaders in progressing through the necessary critical functions necessary after a crash and to address the short-term and long-term issues and decisions.

PHASE I: THE FIRST FEW HOURS: INITIAL SHOCK AND REACTION

When an air medical crash occurs, the timeliness and quality of information conveyed may vary depending on the circumstances. Notification of the crash may come to the communications center via scene witnesses (e.g., emergency medical services [EMS], police, fire, and bystanders) or from the media. Rotor-wing crashes, which likely occur during take-off or landing, usually are a witnessed event, whereas a fixed-wing crash may occur in a rural area far from the program's base of operation. With the advent of

scanners, alpha-numeric paging systems, and media access to crash information, flight team members may receive information directly before official notification from a program representative.

POST-ACCIDENT INCIDENT PLAN

The program's post-accident incident plan (PAIP) becomes the road map for the communications center staff to initiate the necessary critical steps that enhance crew survival and limit the program's liability. Priorities are:

- Verification of facts: crash location, other pertinent details.
- Dispatch of rescue crews: civil air patrol, air medical, or ambulance response to the crash site.
- Activation of notification list according to the PAIP.
- Notification of security for crowd control at the base of operation or hospital.

ROLE OF PROGRAM LEADERSHIP

The air medical program administrator's role involves developing organization around the process, ensuring that the PAIP is followed, and ensuring that appropriate roles are assigned. Provision of medical care to the victims of the crash, both air medical crew members and others involved in the crash, should be a high priority. The program leader should also ensure that the appropriate notifications are made to administration, the public relations director, the Part 135 operator (aviation site manager or lead pilot), and regulatory agencies such as the National Transportation Safety Board (NTSB), Federal Aviation Administration (FAA), and state health department. Flight team members must be notified of the event and directed to come to the program site where resources are available and factual information can be shared.

Family Member Notification

As the person in charge, the program leader must ensure that family members of the onboard crew are notified. Ideally, this notification should occur in person. The program leader should send a responsible person to the location of the family members whenever feasible. Often, the media broadcast the information regarding the crash before notification of the family can occur. Minimally, this notification should occur via phone. A private area at the facility, but away from the flight team, should be identified for the family members to gather. An individual should be assigned to provide factual information and to meet the needs of the family members. The program leader should communicate facts only, not speculate.

In the first few hours, a critical incident stress-diffusing session needs to be organized. An agency of choice is identified to conduct this session, and as many crew members as possible should be present.

Dealing with the Media

An appropriate individual must be assigned to deal with the media. The media should have a place to convene away from the crash site or the flight team. A proactive approach to information sharing helps to limit speculation on the part of the media. When possible, one of the program leaders should be designated as a liaison for information sharing with the public relations official.

Decision to Remain in Service

A decision to remain in service may need to be addressed quickly if the program operates multiple aircraft. The program administrator needs to quickly assess whether continued service is appropriate depending on the flight team members' readiness to respond to a request for service. Such a decision should put safety first, keeping in mind that the profound effects on the air medical crew may minimize their effectiveness in providing patient care and in paying attention to safety principles for anywhere from hours to days after a crash. Flight team members need time to seek information and process the events and results of the crash.

During this period, the availability of other air medical transport programs in the area should be considered. If possible, their communications centers are notified of the program's situation and informed that flight requests may be referred to their programs.

The program leader should also identify the scene coordinator, someone from the aviation team (pilot or mechanic) who should be assigned to coordinate activities at the crash site. The role of this individual is to coordinate the efforts of the various investigating agencies and to provide information to these agencies and the program administrator. This individual also is the liaison to the Part 135 operator.

Critical Incident Stress Management

An air medical crash invokes a critical incident stress (CIS) response for many individuals both inside and outside of the program. Therefore, the program leadership must recognize that psychologic assistance in dealing with the stress response and grieving process should be a required step for all members of the air medical team. Details about the assistance (who provides it, how it is provided, and who participates) should be identified in the post-accident incident planning process. Because individuals may not be able to adequately assess their own level of stress response, mandatory participation in the critical incident stress management (CISM) session is beneficial.

The mental health professionals involved in the CIS response can provide crucial assistance in assessment of individual readiness for return to flight. This assessment of all team members, including the program leader, is a crucial component of any PAIP and provides the information needed to determine the right time to return the program to service.

Despite CISM interventions and readiness assessments, air medical team members may experience a wide variety of post-stress phenomenon, such as hypervigilance (e.g., obsession over the sighting of wires in and around the landing zone) or flashbacks (e.g., triggered by a nighttime flight with circumstances similar to the crash). Such phenomena may limit a team member's ability to perform his or her role. Strategies such as doubling up flight team members or adding flight team members on board as staffing and aircraft configurations allow can be helpful as individuals return to perform their role on the aircraft after any critical incident.

Anger is an emotion commonly experienced by flight team members as a normal reaction to catastrophic loss and post-traumatic stress. Although individuals need to work through their anger, if misdirected, this anger may be destructive to the rebuilding process. One-on-one counseling may be necessary to address individual stress reactions to an event.

After a crash, team members are likely to continue in their role as members of the air medical team. This involvement provides an opportunity to experience regular acknowledgment and support from coworkers who can directly relate to their feelings. Commonly, some staff resign 6 to 12 months after a crash. The number of staff resigning is based on numerous factors, such as support both in and outside of work and individual ability to cope with the work-related tragedy.

PHASE II: THE FIRST 24 HOURS: INITIAL DEVELOPMENT OF A PLAN

The decision regarding the continuation of the air medical service is likely to occur in the first 24 hours and is often the ultimate test of the agency's support of the air medical program. If this decision is not addressed in the first few hours, this may become an essential decision to make and communicate to customers. The media can be a good source of distributing this information. Emergency medical services (EMS), public service groups, and communications centers should be notified of the return to service.

MANAGEMENT OF THE MEDIA

Any positive relations developed with the media may pay off as the intense news coverage occurs. Regular news conferences and flight team interviews should be conducted as appropriate. The public needs to know that the flight team can go on and that the program will continue. Providing the human side of this situation to the media may cause a switch in focus from the negative aspects of the event. The local media (television and print) are likely to cover this topic daily for several days to weeks. Flight program staff need to expect this so that they are not overwhelmed by the amount of media coverage.

INTERACTION WITH FAMILY MEMBERS

Interactions with family members of the crash victims should be planned. Program administration needs to contact family members to express concern and to determine whether their needs are being met.

Family members of the air medical team may want to participate in a debriefing. The CISM team may be appropriate for this activity and the staff debriefing. In addition, family members may benefit from meeting with one of the program's pilots and representatives from administration. Their need for information is heightened, especially with regard to program safety. Meeting the needs of team members' families goes a long way in gaining the individual support necessary for return to work in the flight program.

KEEPING LEADERSHIP INFORMED

Daily briefings to the CEO, Board of Directors, and line managers should be provided. The program leadership may have difficulty with use of objective decision-making skills during the crisis. The objectiveness of second-order people can assist with this and validation of decision making.

COMMUNICATION WITH THE AIR MEDICAL TEAM

Updated information from administration, planned CISM interventions, interaction with media, and successes (e.g., positive encounters and support from peers or customers) should be provided. Regular staff meetings and ongoing CISM interventions, such as diffusing, debriefings, one-on-ones, and further individual counseling sessions, may be needed on a daily basis for the first week or two. This time is an opportunity to share information, common feelings, and experiences.

Neighboring air medical programs and the Concern Network should be contacted, if this has not already occurred. The industry recognition and support that results may be beneficial to the staff and program leadership.

LEGAL ISSUES

The legal consequences of a crash quickly become apparent. Attorneys, risk managers, and the insurance carrier should be notified as early as possible. Leadership should be prepared to share the PAIP and steps taken to mitigate the event.

PHASE III: DAYS 2 TO 5: IMPLEMENTATION AND MODIFICATION

During this phase, many of the realities of the crash become evident. The agencies that surround the program need to get back to business, whereas the air medical team members and leadership may continue to experience difficulty in coping with daily encounters and tasks.

CARE OF THE INJURED VICTIMS

In the case of crash survivors, care of the injured crew members may necessitate special attention to confidentiality issues, especially if the care takes place at the program's base hospital or trauma center. Flight team members commonly make regular visits to an injured flight team member. Their preoccupation with the injured team member's medical condition and concern for family members may delay the individual's return to flying.

HUMAN RESOURCES

The human resources department staff is essential in assisting with the processing of forms for injured and deceased employees. The staff may be able to contact the hospital chaplain to coordinate support for the rest of the hospital staff or agency employees.

REPLACEMENT OF THE AIRCRAFT

Plans to replace the aircraft should be underway with a plan for return to service. It is helpful to the flight team to know the plan for going back into service. All equipment on board the aircraft needs to be replaced. Use of the equipment list should ease the process of identification of capital purchases required. When possible, an individual in the purchasing department should be designated to handle the process of timely equipment replacement. Equipment vendors may be able to provide loaner units to facilitate getting the aircraft back into service in a timely manner.

Identification of the tail number for the replacement aircraft may become a sensitive issue for flight team members. Retiring the tail number of the crash vehicle and starting again is often wise. Flight teams may have a useful role in tail number selection. Several tasks appropriate to delegate to the flight team are symbolic of the program moving forward, such as ordering and restocking the replacement aircraft. Opportunities to empower the staff with appropriate decisions may provide a mechanism to move beyond the immediate crisis.

PSYCHOLOGIC SUPPORT FOR STAFF

Ongoing assessment of team readiness to return to work and available ongoing psychologic support are necessary to plan and communicate need. Staff must understand the necessity of ongoing psychologic care, especially if individuals are not coping effectively with the stress. Inappropriate group dynamics may become evident as a coping mechanism, necessitating an intervention for the entire group.

FUNERAL PLANNING

Death in the line of duty often translates to a public funeral, a ritual observed by firefighters, EMS personnel, and police officers. The EMS community is likely to communicate this expectation early. Often, the outpouring of expected involvement cannot be contained and may result in a public funeral. In many cases, the next of kin of the deceased may need to be convinced that a public funeral is in order. A trusted member of the EMS community who has experience in planning a public funeral (e.g., a member of a local fire department) should be identified. This person may be invaluable in planning with the family and program leadership an otherwise overwhelming event. Religious officials need to be involved in the planning along with the family so that the funeral plans are culturally sensitive to meet the needs of the family (e.g., Native American burial practices) and those of the community at large.

In addition, regular meetings with the designated individuals planning the public funeral are necessary to ensure that the air medical program and staff needs are met. Municipal and state police involvement may be necessary to ensure that a processional of rescue vehicles can occur.

The air medical service leadership should consider taking the flight teams out of service to allow attendance at the funerals because participation in this ritual is an essential part of the healing process. Once again, neighboring flight programs can be called to cover air medical transport requests. Several hours of down time after each funeral may be needed before team members can return to service.

MEMORIAL SERVICES

Memorial services may occur in addition to the public funeral. The CISM team and mental health workers can give advice regarding the appropriate timing for the memorial service. The service should provide an opportunity for team members to share personal remarks and eulogies. This service can provide a sense of closure for some team members and an opportunity to move forward in the recovery process.

Participation in the funeral and memorial service is essential for all flight program staff. The aircraft may be taken out of service for this time, and coverage by other air medical services may be requested. A neighboring air medical service can be asked to reposition aircraft to better cover the region, which reduces the chance of air medical team members missing the service and conveys to the community the program's commitment to provide service.

REQUEST FOR MEMORIALS

Individuals or groups in the community may find a need to memorialize the aircraft crash site and deceased crew members. These issues may raise sensitivities with family members and the flight team, especially if suggestions are not consistent with the wishes of the family or flight team. Decisions dealing with these requests can be distracting and time consuming. Keep in mind that these issues do not need to be dealt with right now. An urgent decision is rarely necessary. In many cases, delegating this responsibility to the public relations department may be appropriate.

DELAYED ISSUES

FORMAL INVESTIGATION

As the formal investigation continues, announcements of findings should be shared with key personnel in a timely manner. The program leader may need to adopt a strategy to relay information to air medical teams before media reports. Ongoing regular meetings with the staff may be beneficial.

EVALUATE PROGRAM SAFETY

A plan to evaluate the program's safety program should include a review of:

- Safety and operational policies and procedures.
- Safety education for staff.
- Quality and effectiveness of crew resource management (CRM) training.
- Community outreach safety education.
- Quality of the program's safety culture.

Review of these processes is a necessary step in providing reassurance for all members of the air medical team, administration, and risk management offices, with respect to the program's commitment to safety. A plan to evaluate safety helps to avoid the pitfall of reacting to requests based on stress and emotion rather than methodology. The flight team, operator, and administration should be involved. The effectiveness of the PAIP is evaluated and revised as necessary. An independent safety audit may be the choice to ensure objectivity. A timetable for implementation of recommendations should be developed.

LEGAL ISSUES

We exist in a litigious society, and the number and nature of suits filed may be surprising. The news of such suits may become a significant distraction to the air medical teams as they work to reenter the flight environment. Some issues to keep in mind are:

- Insurance subrogation, the legal doctrine of substituting one creditor for another, can lead to litigation involving customers, which could become an image problem for the program if the insurance provider sues the customer in the name of the operator or aircraft owner. Working closely with the legal department to support and reassure customers may be essential to preserve a positive working relationship.
- Filing deadlines and statutes of limitations should be anticipated so that the flight team and public relations director can be prepared to manage the media. Often, announcements of lawsuit filings appear in the press. Knowledge of lawsuits may generate a negative emotional response by air medical teams. Because safety policy, procedures, and communications logs are likely to be subpoenaed, such documents may be archived as manuals are updated.

Final Outcome of Lawsuits

Several years are often necessary to settle lawsuits that result from an air medical crash. This possibly may be reported in the media. A relationship should be developed with legal counsel regarding their commitment to communication with the program when legal activity is likely to attract the media's interest. Keeping flight teams informed is essential.

EMOTIONAL SUPPORT FOR PROGRAM LEADERSHIP

To perform in the midst of an overwhelmingly emotional event, the leader may deny his or her own feelings of fear, grief, and anger to move the program forward. Although this denial may be necessary initially, if this process goes on for too long, the program may move on and leave the program leadership emotionally destitute and dysfunctional. Program managers must set aside some time to go through a formal grieving process and recognition of the intense impact the event has on them. Professional counseling is needed for all individuals involved. Without this assistance, inappropriate methods of dealing with the stress may eventually impair the long-term effectiveness of the manager. The help of a professional counselor should be sought in a confidential setting, preferably away from the work environment. Time away from work with family and friends needs to be planned.

ANNIVERSARIES

The anniversary of a crash is a time of special recognition for the team and family members. The program leader should be prepared to deal with special requests for time off and recognize that the staff may need to be together. A meeting of the staff with an opportunity to talk about feelings may be beneficial and should be offered to the flight team. Mental health workers should be available if team members need to speak in confidence about their feelings around the anniversary.

Each anniversary is acknowledged in various ways by the staff. If the psychologic needs of the staff and program leadership are regarded as a high priority, it is easier to deal with each anniversary.

BIBLIOGRAPHY

1. Hawkins M: Personal protective equipment in helicopter EMS, *Air Med J* 4(94):123-126, 1994.
2. Dodd R: Factors related to occupant crash survival in emergency medical services helicopters, *Aviation Sci Technol* 1992.
3. Low R, Sousa J, Dufresne D, et al: *IFR capability lowers accident rates of civilian helicopter ambulances: a multifactorial epidemiologic study*, Greenville, NC, 1997, East Carolina University School of Medicine.
4. Schneider C: Dollars and sense, *Air Med* 21(4): 1997.
5. National Transportation Safety Board (NTSB): *Safety study, commercial emergency medical service helicopter operations, report number NTSB/SS-88/01*, Washington, DC, 1988, NTSB.
6. Mitchell J, Everly G: *Critical incident stress debriefing: an operations manual for the prevention of traumatic stress among emergency services and disaster workers*, ed 2, Ellicott City, MD, 1996, Chevron Publishing Corp.
7. Mitchell J, Bray G: *Emergency services stress: guidelines for preserving the health and careers of emergency personnel*, Englewood Cliffs, NJ, 1990, Prentice Hall Publishers.

POST-CRASH ADMINISTRATIVE CHECK LIST

Action Steps	Completion date/time	Comments

I. First 2 Hours

A. Activate PAIP.

   1. Emergency/medical response to crash site.

   2. Complete notification list.

   3. Decide whether to remain in service (multiple aircraft).

   4. Identify and activate:

     a. Scene coordinator.

     b. Base site coordinator.

     c. Accident investigation team.

   5. Identify a coordinator for the media.

   6. Convene flight team members.

     a. Provide updated information.

     b. Plan for initial CISM intervention.

     c. State expectation for ongoing CISM interventions.

B. Notify family members, in person as applicable.

C. Ensure that various coordinators have a checklist.

II. First 24 Hours

A. Liaison with public relations regarding managing the media.

B. Interact with family members.

C. Develop a plan to address flight team family member needs and CISM intervention.

D. Inform leadership of plan.

E. Schedule a meeting with air medical team for information sharing and CISM.

F. Notify attorneys, risk managers, and insurance carrier.

III. First 2 to 5 Days

A. Notify Human Resources, employee benefits, employment status, agency support.

B. Develop and communicate plan for aircraft replacement.

C. Develop and implement a plan for ongoing psychologic support for staff.

D. Designate an individual to plan a public funeral as indicated.

E. Designate individual to plan memorial service.

F. Identify a contact person to deal with requests for memorials.

IV. Delayed Issues: 5 Days to 2 Weeks and Beyond

A. Formal investigation: communicate initial findings.

B. Evaluate program safety.

C. Keep track of legal issues and communicate to staff:

   1. Insurance subrogation.

   2. Filing deadlines/statute of limitations.

   3. Final outcome of lawsuits.

D. Provide emotional support for program leadership. If not already done, it is time to make a plan.

E. Anniversaries: plan meetings with staff and honor requests for time off.

Add items to checklist as necessary.

APPENDIX

B MEDICAL CONDITION LIST AND APPROPRIATE USE OF AIR MEDICAL TRANSPORT

POSITION STATEMENT OF THE AIR MEDICAL PHYSICIAN ASSOCIATION

APPROVED BY THE AMPA BOARD OF TRUSTEES
NOVEMBER 10, 2001

BACKGROUND

The Balanced Budget Act of 1997 initiated a process to convert all Medicare ambulance transport billing (including air) to a fee structure. Previous to this, ambulance reimbursement was done for the private ambulance industry under a fee structure reimbursement (commonly known as part B) and, for hospital-based ambulance service, under cost-based reimbursement (commonly known as Part A).

The new fee structure was developed in a process called Negotiated Rule Making (NRM). The NRM process established relative value units for each type of transport, rural modifiers, cost of living adjusters, and a phase-in schedule. As part of the NRM process, the Medical Conditions Work Group developed the Medical Condition List. This condition list was developed to simplify the issue of medical necessity for each level of transport and to reduce the importance of ICD-9 codes to describe prehospital impressions. The Medical Condition List was developed because ICD-9 codes are not designed to describe prehospital medical conditions. The standardization of medical necessity for different types of conditions created by the Medical Condition List will allow medical necessity to be aligned with appropriate utilization and will improve efficiency and simplify the billing and reimbursement process. The Medical Condition List was under consideration for possible inclusion in the final rule but was not included in the final rule published February 27, 2002. A commitment to develop the medical condition codes over the next 12 months was promised by the Center for Medicare and Medicaid Services (CMS) (formerly HCFA).

AMPA POSITION STATEMENT

AMPA supports the addition and adoption of the Medical Condition List, as submitted by the Medical Conditions Work Group, as a rational method of determining medically appropriate utilization of Medical Transport.

Furthermore, it is AMPA's position, as detailed in the Medical Condition List, that the determination of medical appropriateness for interfacility medical transport is determined by a physician, as documented on a written Certification of Medical Necessity. Medical appropriateness of scene medical transport is determined by the requesting authorized prehospital provider, based on regional policy and their best medical judgment at the time of the request for transport. Further, AMPA supports that the Certificate of Medical Necessity for scene transport can be completed by the EMS control physician, receiving physician, or by the Medical Director of the transport program. AMPA supports that consultation with the transport provider Medical Director is the optimal method of determining the appropriate mode of safe patient transport.

AMPA does not support the use of discharge ICD-9 codes to retrospectively determine medical appropriateness, as this may adversely restrict access to appropriate care and negates the regional, environmental, and situational factors that are also important in determining medical appropriateness.

AMPA does not support a specification of a time needed for land transport as a general Guideline. AMPA feels that when a time specification is made it should be done regionally.

AIR MEDICAL TRANSPORT GUIDELINES, DETAILED AS APPROPRIATE BY THE MEDICAL CONDITION LIST

AMPA supports the NRM workgroup recommendation to replace the list of conditions in section 2120.4 B (Medical Appropriateness) with:

- Acute neurological emergencies requiring emergent/time-sensitive interventions not available at the sending facility.
- Acute vascular emergencies requiring urgent/time sensitive interventions not available at the sending facility.

- Acute surgical emergencies requiring urgent/time sensitive interventions not available at the sending facility.
- Critically ill patients with compromised hemodynamic/respiratory function who require intensive care during transport and whose time of transfer between critical care units must be minimized during transport.
- Critically ill obstetric patients who require intensive care during transport and whose time of transfer between facilities must be minimized to prevent patient/fetal morbidity.
- Acute cardiac emergencies requiring emergent/time-sensitive intervention not available at the sending facility.
- Critically ill neonatal/pediatric patients with potentially compromised hemodynamic/respiratory function, a metabolic acidosis greater than 2 hours post delivery, sepsis, or meningitis.
- Patients with electrolyte disturbances or toxic exposure requiring immediate life-saving intervention.
- Transplantation patients (fixed-wing vs. helicopter).
- Patients requiring care in a specialty center not available at the sending facility.
- Conditions requiring treatment in a Hyperbaric Oxygen Unit.
- Burns requiring treatment in a burn treatment center.
- Potentially life or limb-threatening trauma requiring treatment at a trauma center, including penetrating eye injuries.
- EMTALA physician-certified inter-facility transfer (not a patient request).
- EMS regional or state-approved protocol identifies need for on-scene air transport.

Medical Condition List*

#	On-Scene Condition (general)	On-Scene Condition (specific)	Service Level	Comments and Examples (not all-inclusive)
Emergency Conditions – Non-traumatic				
1	Abdominal pain	With other signs or symptoms	ALS	Nausea, vomiting, fainting, pulsatile mass, distention, rigid, tenderness on exam, guarding
2	Abdominal pain	Without other signs or symptoms	BLS	
3	Abnormal cardiac rhythm/Cardiac dysrhythmia	Potentially life-threatening	ALS	Bradycardia, junctional and ventricular blocks, non-sinus tachycardias, PVC's > 6, bi- and trigeminy, vtach, vfib, atrial flutter, PEA, asystole
4	Abnormal skin signs		ALS	Diaphoresis, cyanosis, delayed cap refill, poor turgor, mottled
5	Abnormal vital signs (includes abnormal pulse oximetry)	With symptoms	ALS	Other emergency conditions
6	Abnormal vital signs (includes abnormal pulse oximetry)	Without symptoms	BLS	
7	Allergic reaction	Potentially life-threatening	ALS	Other emergency conditions, rapid progression of symptoms, prior hx of anaphylaxis, wheezing, difficulty swallowing
8	Allergic reaction	Other	BLS	Hives, itching, rash, slow onset, local swelling, redness, erythema
9	Animal bites/sting/ envenomation	Potentially life or limb-threatening	ALS	Symptoms of specific envenomation, significant face, neck, trunk, and extremity involvement; other emergency conditions
10	Animal bites/sting/ envenomation	Other	BLS	Local pain and swelling, special handling considerations and patient monitoring required
11	Sexual assault	With injuries	ALS	
12	Sexual assault	With no injuries	BLS	
13	Blood glucose	Abnormal – < 80 or > 250, with symptoms	ALS	Altered mental status, vomiting, signs of dehydration, etc.
14	Respiratory arrest		ALS	Apnea, hypoventilation requiring ventilatory assistance and airway management
15	Difficulty breathing		ALS	

(Continued)

Medical Condition List—cont'd

#	On-Scene Condition (general)	On-Scene Condition (specific)	Service Level	Comments and Examples (not all-inclusive)
Emergency Conditions – Non-traumatic—cont'd				
16	Cardiac arrest – Resuscitation in progress		ALS	
17	Chest pain (non-traumatic)		ALS	Dull, severe, crushing, substernal, epigastric, left sided chest pain associated with pain of the jaw, left arm, neck, back, and nausea, vomiting, palpitations, pallor, diaphoresis, decreased LOC
18	Choking episode		ALS	
19	Cold exposure	Potentially life or limb threatening	ALS	Temperature < 95°F, deep frostbite, other emergency conditions
20	Cold exposure	With symptoms	BLS	Shivering, superficial frostbite, and other emergency conditions
21	Altered level of consciousness (non-traumatic)		ALS	Acute condition with Glascow Coma Scale <15
22	Convulsions/Seizures	Seizing, immediate post-seizure, post-ictal, or at risk of seizure & requires medical monitoring/ observation	ALS	
23	Eye symptoms, non-traumatic	Acute vision loss and/or severe pain	BLS	
24	Non-traumatic headache	With neurologic distress conditions	ALS	
25	Non-traumatic headache	Without neurologic symptoms	BLS	
26	Cardiac symptoms other than chest pain	Palpitations, skipped beats	ALS	
27	Cardiac symptoms other than chest pain	Atypical pain or other symptoms	ALS	Persistent nausea and vomiting, weakness, hiccups, pleuritic pain, feeling of impending doom, and other emergency conditions
28	Heat exposure	Potentially life-threatening	ALS	Hot and dry skin, temp > 105°F, neurologic distress, signs of heatstroke or heat exhaustion, orthostatic vitals, other emergency conditions
29	Heat exposure	With symptoms	BLS	Muscle cramps, perfuse sweating, fatigue

Medical Condition List—cont'd

#	On-Scene Condition (general)	On-Scene Condition (specific)	Service Level	Comments and Examples (not all-inclusive)
Emergency Conditions – Non-traumatic—cont'd				
30	Hemorrhage	Severe (quantity)	ALS	Uncontrolled or significant signs of shock, other emergency conditions
31	Hemorrhage	Potentially life-threatening	ALS	Active vaginal, rectal bleeding, hematemesis, hemoptysis, epistaxis, active post-surgical bleeding
32	Infectious diseases requiring isolation procedures/public health risk		BLS	
33	Hazmat exposure		ALS	Toxic fume or liquid exposure via inhalation, absorption, oral, radiation, smoke inhalation
34	Medical device failure	Life or limb-threatening malfunction, failure, or complication	ALS	Malfunction of ventilator, internal pacemaker, internal defibrillator, implanted drug delivery device
35	Medical device failure	Health maintenance device failure	BLS	O2 supply malfunction, orthopedic device failure
36	Neurologic distress	Facial drooping; loss of vision; aphasia; difficulty swallowing; numbness, tingling extremity; stupor, delirium, confusion, hallucinations; paralysis, paresis (focal weakness); abnormal movements; vertigo; unsteady gait/balance; slurred speech, unable to speak	ALS	
37	Pain, acute and severe not otherwise specified in this list	Patient needs specialized handling to be moved: pain exacerbated by movement	BLS	
38	Pain, severe not otherwise specified in this list	Acute onset, unable to ambulate or sit	BLS	Pain is the reason for the transport
39	Pain, severe not otherwise specified in this list		ALS	Use severity scale (7-10 for severe pain), pt. receiving pre-hospital pharmacologic intervention
40	Back pain – non-traumatic (T and/or LS)	Suspect cardiac or vascular etiology	ALS	Other emergency conditions, absence of or decreased leg pulses, pulsatile abdominal mass, severe tearing abdominal pain

(Continued)

	Medical Condition List—cont'd			
#	**On-Scene Condition (general)**	**On-Scene Condition (specific)**	**Service Level**	**Comments and Examples (not all-inclusive)**
Emergency Conditions – Non-traumatic—cont'd				
41	Back pain – non-traumatic (T and/or LS)	New neurologic symptoms	ALS	Neurologic distress list
42	Poisons, ingested, injected, inhaled, absorbed	Adverse drug reaction, poison exposure by inhalation, injection or absorption	ALS	
43	Alcohol intoxication, drug overdose (suspected)	Unable to care for self; unable to ambulate; no risk to airway; no other symptoms	BLS	
44	Alcohol intoxication, drug overdose (suspected)	All others, including airway at risk, pharmacological intervention, cardiac monitoring	ALS	
45	Post–operative procedure complications	Major wound dehiscence, evisceration, or requires special handling for transport	BLS	Orthopedic appliance; prolapse
46	Pregnancy complication/Child-birth/Labor		ALS	
47	Psychiatric/Behavioral	Abnormal mental status; drug withdrawal	ALS	Suicidal, homicidal, hallucinations, violent, disoriented, DT's, withdrawal symptoms, transport required by state law/court order
48	Psychiatric/Behavioral	Threat to self or others, severe anxiety, acute episode or exacerbation of paranoia, or disruptive behavior	BLS	
49	Sick person	Fever with associated symptoms (headache, stiff neck, etc.)	ALS	
50	Sick person	Fever without associated symptoms	BLS	>102 in adults >104 in children
51	Sick person	No other symptoms	BLS	With other emergency conditions
52	Sick person	Nausea and vomiting, diarrhea, severe and incapacitating	ALS	
53	Unconscious, fainting, syncope	Transient unconscious episode or found unconscious	ALS	
54	Near syncope, weakness or dizziness	Acute episode or exacerbation	ALS	
55	Medical/Legal	State or local ordinance requires ambulance transport under certain conditions	BLS	Minor with no guardian; DWI arrest at MVA for evaluation; arrests and medical conditions (psych, drug OD)

Medical Condition List—cont'd

#	On-Scene Condition (general)	On-Scene Condition (specific)	Service Level	Comments and Examples (not all-inclusive)
Emergency Conditions – Trauma				
56	Major trauma	As defined by ACS Field Triage Decision Scheme	ALS	Trauma with one of the following: Glascow <14; systolic BP<90; RR<10 or >29; all penetrating injuries to head, neck, torso, extremities proximal to elbow or knee; flail chest; combination of trauma and burns; pelvic fracture; 2 or more long bone fractures; open or depressed skull fracture; paralysis; severe mechanism of injury including: ejection, death of another passenger in same patient compartment, falls >20′, 20″ deformity in vehicle or 12″ deformity of patient compartment, auto pedestrian/ bike, pedestrian thrown/run over, motorcycle accident at speeds > 20 mph and rider separated from vehicle.
57	Other trauma	Need to monitor or maintain airway	ALS	Decreased LOC, bleeding into airway, trauma to head, face or neck
58	Other trauma	Major bleeding	ALS	Uncontrolled or significant bleeding
59	Other trauma	Suspected fracture/dislocation requiring splinting/ immobilization for transport	BLS	Spinal, long bones, and joints, including shoulder, elbow, wrist, hip, knee, and ankle, deformity of bone or joint
60	Other trauma	Penetrating extremity injuries	BLS	Isolated with bleeding stopped and good CSM
61	Other trauma	Amputation – digits	BLS	
62	Other trauma	Amputation – all other	ALS	
63	Other trauma	Suspected internal, head, chest, or abdominal injuries	ALS	Signs of closed head injury, open head injury, pneumothorax, hemothorax, abdominal bruising, positive abdominal signs on exam, internal bleeding criteria, evisceration
64	Other trauma	Severe pain requiring pharmacologic pain control	ALS	See severity scale

(Continued)

Medical Condition List—cont'd

#	On-Scene Condition (general)	On-Scene Condition (specific)	Service Level	Comments and Examples (not all-inclusive)
Emergency Conditions – Trauma—cont'd				
65	Other trauma	Trauma NOS: it is up to the provider to provide sufficient documentation to support this claim	BLS	Ambulance required because injury is associated with other emergency conditions or other reasons for transport exist, such as special patient handling or patient safety issues
66	Burns	Major – per ABA	ALS	Partial thickness burns > 10% TBSA; involvement of face, hands, feet, genitalia, perineum, or major joints; third degree burns; electrical; chemical; inhalation; burns with preexisting medical disorders; burns and trauma
67	Burns	Minor – per ABA	BLS	Other burns than listed above
68	Lightning		ALS	
69	Electrocution		ALS	
70	Near drowning		ALS	
71	Eye injuries	Acute vision loss or blurring, severe pain or chemical exposure, penetrating, severe lid lacerations	BLS	
Non-Emergency				
72	Bed confined (at the time of transport)	*unable to get up without assistance; and *unable to ambulate; and *unable to sit in a chair or wheelchair	BLS	Patient is going to a medical procedure, treatment, testing, or evaluation that is medically necessary
73	ALS monitoring, required	Cardiac/hemodynamic monitoring en route	ALS	Expectation monitoring is needed before and after transport
74	ALS monitoring, required	Advanced airway management	ALS	Ventilator dependent, apnea monitor, possible intubation needed, deep suctioning
75	ALS monitoring, required	IV meds required en route	ALS	Does not apply to self-administered IV medications
76	ALS monitoring, required	Chemical restraint	ALS	
77	BLS monitoring, required	Suctioning required en route	BLS	Per transfer instructions
78	BLS monitoring, required	Airway control/positioning required en route	BLS	Per transfer instructions

Medical Condition List—cont'd

#	On-Scene Condition (general)	On-Scene Condition (specific)	Service Level	Comments and Examples (not all-inclusive)
Non-Emergency—cont'd				
79	BLS monitoring, required	Third party assistance/attendant required to apply, administer, or regulate or adjust oxygen en route	BLS	Does not apply to patient capable of self-administration of portable or home O_2. Patient must require oxygen therapy and be so frail as to require assistance.
80	Specialty care monitoring	A level of service provided to a critically injured or ill patient beyond the scope of the national paramedic curriculum.	SCT	
81	Medical conditions that contraindicate transport by other means	Patient safety: Danger to self or others. In restraints	BLS	Refer to definition in the CFR – sec. 482. 13(e).
82	Medical conditions that contraindicate transport by other means	Patient safety: Danger to self or others. Monitoring.	BLS	Behavioral or cognitive risk such that patient requires monitoring for safety.
83	Medical conditions that contraindicate transport by other means	Patient safety: Danger to self or others. Seclusion (flight risk)	BLS	Behavioral or cognitive risk such that patient requires attendant to assure patient does not try to exit the ambulance prematurely. CFR sec. 482. 13(f)(2) for definition.
84	Medical conditions that contraindicate transport by other means	Patient safety: Risk of falling off wheelchair or stretcher while in motion	BLS	Patient's physical condition is such that patient risks injury during vehicle movement despite restraints. Indirect indicators include MDS criteria.
85	Medical conditions that contraindicate transport by other means	Special handling en route: Isolation	BLS	Includes patients with communicable diseases or hazardous material exposure who must be isolated from public or whose medical condition must be protected from public exposure; surgical drainage complications
86	Medical conditions that contraindicate transport by other means	Special handling en route: Patient size	BLS	Morbid obesity which requires additional personnel or equipment to transfer

(Continued)

Medical Condition List—cont'd

#	On-Scene Condition (general)	On-Scene Condition (specific)	Service Level	Comments and Examples (not all-inclusive)
Non-Emergency—cont'd				
87	Medical conditions that contraindicate transport by other means	Special handling en route: Orthopedic device	BLS	Backboard, halotraction, use of pins and traction, etc.
88	Medical conditions that contraindicate transport by other means	Special handling en route: >1 person for physical assistance in transfers	BLS	
89	Medical conditions that contraindicate transport by other means	Special handling en route: Severe pain	BLS	Pain must be aggravated by transfers or moving vehicle such that trained expertise of EMT required (pain scale). Pain is present, but is not sole reason for transport.
90	Medical conditions that contraindicate transport by other means	Special handling en route: Positioning requires specialized handling	BLS	Requires special handling to avoid further injury (such as with >grade 2 decubiti on buttocks). Generally does not apply to shorter transfers <1 hour. Positioning in wheelchair or standard car seat inappropriate due to contractures or recent extremity fractures—post-op hip as an example.
Inter-facility				
91	EMTALA-certified inter-facility transfer to a higher level of care	Physician has made the determination that this transfer is needed – Carrier only needs to know the level of care and mode of transport	BLS, ALS, SCT, Air	Excludes patient-requested EMTALA transfer
92	Service not available at originating facility, and must meet one or more emergency or non-emergency conditions		BLS, ALS, SCT, Air	Specify what service is not available
93	Service not covered	Indicates to Carrier that claim should be automatically denied		

*When using this chart, use all codes that apply.

INDEX

Note: Page numbers followed by *b*, *f*, or *t* indicate boxes, figures, or tables, respectively.